THE PERIODONTAL LIGAMENT IN HEALTH AND DISEASE

Second Edition

B K B Berkovitz
BDS MSC PhD LDSRCS
Biomedical Sciences Division
Anatomy and Human Biology Group
King's College London
London

B J Moxham
BSc BDS PhD
Anatomy Unit
School of Molecular and Medical Biosciences
University of Wales, College of Cardiff
Cardiff

H N Newman
BDentSc MDS FRCPath MA PhD ScD
Eastman Dental Institute for Oral Healthcare Sciences
University of London
London

Mosby-Wolfe

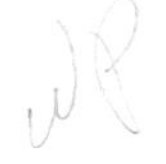

London Baltimore Barcelona Bogotá Boston Buenos Aires Caracas Carlsbad, CA Chicago Madrid Mexico City Milan Naples, FL New York Philadelphia St. Louis Seoul Singapore Sydney Taipei Tokyo Toronto Wiesbaden

Project Managers: Caroline Turner
Roddy Craig

Developmental Editor: Lucy Hamilton

Cover Design: Ian Spick

Illustration: Jenni Miller

Production: Mike Heath

Index: Jill Halliday

Publisher: Geoff Greenwood

Published in 1995 by Mosby-Wolfe, an imprint of Times Mirror International Publishers Limited

Printed by Grafos S.A. sobre papel, Barcelona, Spain

ISBN 0 723 41931 0

For full details of all Times Mirror International Publishers Limited titles, please write to Times Mirror International Publishers Limited, Lynton House, 7–12 Tavistock Square, London WC1H 9LB, England.

A CIP catalogue record for this book is available from the British Library.

Library of Congress Cataloging-in-Publication Data Applied For

Preface

PREFACE - SECOND EDITION

Since the 1980s and early 1990s, there has been a resurgence of interest in the biology and pathobiology of the periodontal ligament. This is most evident from the considerable increase in the number of research papers dealing with this tissue that have been published in the scientific journals, whether concerned specifically with dentistry or oral biology, or more generally with connective tissue biology. In line with these developments, we are pleased to report that the chapters from the original edition of this book have had to be considerably modified to encompass the increased literature. Furthermore, two new chapters reflecting important areas of scientific advancement (cell biology associated with orthodontic tooth movement and reattachment and regeneration of the periodontal ligament) have been added. Consequently, we are tempted to consider this monograph as an entirely new book.

It was our hope, on being invited to produce a new edition, that the increase in research into the periodontal ligament would provide less uncertainty and a firmer base of knowledge than pertained in the early 1980s. It became clear to us, however, that much research still remains to be undertaken, in particular to improve our understanding of the pathobiology of the tissue. For example, although chronic inflammatory periodontal disease remains a common form of tooth loss, our knowledge about the effects of this group of diseases on the periodontal ligament remains poor in comparison with that for the gingival connective tissues.

In the preface to the first edition of this book, we intimated that the scholarship involved in writing books and research monographs is undervalued, especially when performance indicators to assess the quality of research appear to be founded on the notion that there is a "definite" experiment to test any given concept! We continue to believe that reviews are important precisely because of the ever increasing and diverse literature, and that such reviews enable the individual research paper to have a firmer "contextual" basis and provide the multidisciplinary perspective required to close the gaps in our knowledge. Such reviews can still highlight controversy and furnish hypotheses. Where controversy exists, we trust this will not be burdensome to the reader, but will fire the imagination. Again, we dedicate this book to those with this scholarly approach.

PREFACE - FIRST EDITION

This book is built upon the belief that the periodontal ligament is a tissue worthy of study because of its biological interest as a connective tissue adapted to specialized functions, and because clinically it is involved in one of the most common causes of tooth loss in man – chronic inflammatory periodontal disease. Our purpose in writing this book was to gather together knowledge of the periodontal ligament which, having been obtained from diverse disciplines, has been scattered in the literature. As work proceeded, however, we became aware that the book's value lies not only in what information it can supply, but also in revealing the many things which remain to be discovered. It is our fervent hope that this will encourage researchers to greater efforts.

There are two things which this book is not. First, it is not a text dealing with all the tooth-supporting tissues. Although for some topics it has been necessary to widen the field to include tissues other than the periodontal ligament (particularly in those chapters dealing with the periodontal ligament in disease), we have restricted discussion as many texts already cover the periodontium as a whole. However, the periodontium is a complex field of study with an enormous literature and, in our opinion, such texts have not given the periodontal ligament the importance it deserves. Second, we have not concerned ourselves with therapy.

It is clear to us that, if we are to gain a proper understanding of the periodontal ligament, its study must be multi-disciplinary. Furthermore, it is necessary to be aware of how advances in connective tissue biology in general have a bearing upon our study, even if we can only claim a fugitive up-to-dateness.

In choosing authors, we have not only picked colleagues from the various fields of dental sciences and dental surgery who wanted to write specifically about the periodontal ligament but have included some who, because of the lack of information, could only write about the ligament as a connective tissue. We have found both approaches instructive and, perhaps, even those interested primarily in soft connective tissues can also learn from study of the periodontal ligament. We are particularly glad to have been able to bring together colleagues in the fields of periodontal biology and pathology and would be pleased if this resulted in more integrated research.

It is fashionable nowadays for scientists to decry the scholarship involved in writing books, contending that books lend themselves to desultory speculation. Whilst speculation based upon tendentious argument has been discouraged, we believe that reasoned discursiveness is advantageous, furnishing debate and encouraging the development of hypotheses for future research. It is obvious that in any newly emerging area of research there exist uncertainty and extensive gaps of ignorance. Consequently, it is not surprising that, despite our initial intention to present a consistent story, in places different authors maintain different views about some aspects of the biology or pathology of the periodontal ligament. We trust that where controversy exists, this will not be found burdensome to the reader but will fire his imagination. It is to persons such as this that this book is dedicated.

INTRODUCTORY REMARKS

This book has been written primarily for the graduate dentist and dental research worker. Nevertheless, it also contains information which should be of relevance to those engaged in the study of connective tissues in general. For example, even though the periodontal ligament (PDL) is often considered to be specialized, such specializations, being essentially modifications of systems already existing in other connective tissues, provide important insights into how connective tissues are adapted to function. Again, knowledge concerning the biomechanical properties of connective tissues *in vivo* is difficult to obtain without the use of invasive techniques. Because of the nature of the attachment of the tooth, tooth-borne loading allows an examination of such properties with minimum damage. We think it appropriate, therefore, to provide some general and elementary information about the PDL for those without a background in dental science.

The PDL is the fibrous connective tissue that occupies the periodontal space between the root of a tooth and its bony socket (Fig. 1). At the cervical region of the tooth, above the alveolar crest, the PDL merges with the gingival connective tissue. At the root apex, the PDL merges with the dental pulp. Together with cementum, alveolar bone and the lamina propria of the gingiva, the PDL forms the tissue which supports the tooth in the jaw. These supporting tissues are often referred to collectively as the periodontium. This type of attachment is not common to all dentitions, being restricted to mammals and a few groups of reptiles.

Although the term "periodontal ligament" appears to be used most frequently, many other names have been given (e.g. periodontal membrane, alveolo-dental ligament, desmodont, pericementum, dental periosteum and gomphosis). According to many dictionaries (e.g. the Concise Oxford Dictionary, Gould's Medical Dictionary, Black's Medical Dictionary, the Faber Medical Dictionary), a ligament is defined as a band of fibrous tissue binding together skeletal elements. To us, this definition does not seem inappropriate for the PDL.

The average width of the PDL usually is quoted as 0.2 mm. However, the dimensions of the periodontal space vary around the tooth. It has been reported that the periodontal space is often hour-glass shaped, being narrowest in the mid-root region near the fulcrum about which the tooth moves. The PDL usually is widest cervically. Its width also varies according to the functional state of the tissue. Some data show that teeth in heavy function tend to have wider ligaments than non-functioning teeth. Furthermore, the periodontal space appears to narrow slightly with age.

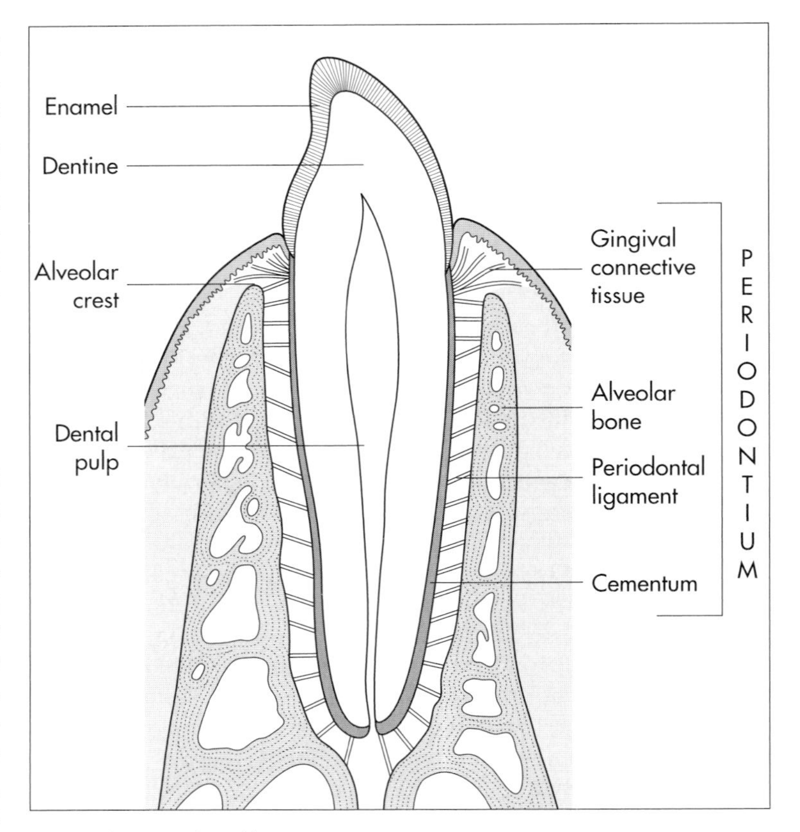

Fig. 1 The periodontal ligament

As other fibrous connective tissues, the PDL consists of a fibrous stroma (mainly collagen) in a gel of ground substance containing cells, blood vessels and nerves. In many respects, the PDL appears to be a specialized fibrous connective tissue. For example, it is comparatively well vascularized and innervated, and it has a relatively high rate of turnover (that of its collagen being many times faster than in skin). It would be wrong, however, to over-emphasize its specializations to the extent of losing sight of the many features it has in common with other fibrous connective tissues. It can be argued that the periodontal ligament has features more in common with fetal than with adult connective tissues. The presence of intercellular contacts between the fibroblasts, the high rate of turnover and the pattern of its collagen fibril diameter distribution are suggestive of it being fetal-like.

Functionally, the PDL is considered primarily to be the tissue responsible for resisting displacing forces impinging upon the tooth. This is usually referred to as the tooth support mechanism. In this capacity the ligament serves to protect the tissues, especially those in the periapical region, against damage. The PDL also is responsible for the processes whereby a tooth attains, and then maintains, its functional position. These processes include the mechanism which generates the forces effecting tooth eruption and the mechanism responsible for drifting of teeth. We should also include the tooth support mechanism, particularly that part which allows recovery following tooth displacement. The cells of the PDL form, maintain and repair not only the ligament itself but also the adjacent alveolar bone and cementum. This ability to rapidly remodel forms the basis of orthodontics. Sensory nerves and receptors within the PDL appear to have an important proprioceptive function and they may play a part in the control of masticatory movements. In addition, sensations of pain from the PDL may have a protective role.

Study of the PDL has attracted the biologist more than the pathologist. Indeed, the term "periodontal disease" is synonymous to most clinicians with chronic inflammatory periodontal disease, because of its association with widespread tooth loss. Curiously, in this condition the PDL ahead of the main lesion remains uninvolved. However, a survey of the literature shows that the PDL is subject to a large number of less frequent disorders. Even if a number of these spread from the surrounding tissues (particularly the overlying gingiva), others originate within the PDL itself (e.g. periodontal cysts). Altogether, it is now clear that the PDL is liable to as wide a range of diseases as other tissues.

ACKNOWLEDGEMENTS

We wish to acknowledge the assistance of many of our colleagues who kindly provided illustrations for this book and who are referred to in the text.

It is with much gratitude that we also acknowledge the following publications and their editors who graciously gave us permission to reproduce the figures listed below:

Figure 2.7: Connective Tissue Research
Figure 3.1, 3.16: Archives of Oral Biology
Figure 3.6, 3.12: Rheumatology
Figure 3.19: Archives of Oral Biology
Figure 6.1: Proceedings of the Finnish Dental Society
Figure 6.2: Journal of Periodontology
Figure 6.3, 6.4: Acta Odontologica Scandinavica
Figure 6.5: Acta Physiologica Scandinavica
Figure 7.4, 7.7: Archives of Oral Biology
Figure 7.8, 7.11: Journal of Anatomy
Figure 7.9, 7.10: Anatomy and Embryology
Figure 7.12, 7.13, 7.14, 7.15, 7.16, 7.17: Journal of Physiology
Figure 8.7–8.21: Journal of Periodontology
Figure 8.24: Journal of Anatomy
Figure 9.2: Journal of Dental Research
Figure 9.4, 9.9: Journal of Oral Pathology
Figure 9.6, 9.11, 9.13, 9.14, 9.15, 9.16: Archives of Oral Biology
Figure 9.7: Journal de Biologie Buccale
Figure 9.8: Scanning Microscopy
Figure 10.1, 10.2, 10.8: Journal of Dental Research
Figure 10.3, 10.9, 10.10, 10.11, 10.12, 10.13, 10.23, 10.25: Archives of Oral Biology
Figure 10.4, 10.15: J Biomech
Figure 10.5: Advances in Oral Biology, Vol 2, Journal of Biomechanics (Edited by PH Staple), Academic Press, London, 1966
Figure 10.6: Oral Science Review
Figure 10.7: Journal of Prosthetic Dentistry
Figure 10.14: Journal of Periodontology
Figure 10.16, 10.17, 10.18: Research in Veterinary Sciences
Figure 10.19: Journal of Periodontal Research
Figure 10.20, 10.21: Current Orthodontic Concepts and Techniques, Vol 1, 2nd edition (edited by TM Grabner and BF Swain), Saunders, Philadelphia, 1975
Figure 10.22: American Journal of Orthodontics
Figure 10.23: European Journal of Orthodontics
Figure 11.4, 11.6, 11.7, 11.8: American Journal of Orthodontics
Figure 14.1, 14.2, 14.3, 14.5, 14.6: Journal of Periodontal Research
Figure 14.4: Parodontologie
Figure 14.15, 14.16, 14.17, 14.18, 14.19: Journal of Endodontics
Figure 15.2: American Journal of Anatomy
Figure 15.3: Archives of Oral Biology
Figure 15.7, 15.12: Journal of Clinical Periodontology
Figure 15.8, 15.9, 15.10, 15.11: International Endodontic Journal
Figure 16.3, 16.4, 16.6, 16.8: Swedish Dental Journal
Figure 16.5: Acta Odontologica Scandinavica
Figure 20.3: Archives of Oral Biology

Chapter 9, table 1: Journal de Biologie Buccale
Chapter 9, table 2: Microvascular Research
Chapter 9, table 3: Archives of Oral Biology
Chapter 10, table 1: Biological Mechanisms of Tooth Eruption, Resorption and Replacement by Implants (edited by Z Davidovitch). EBSCO Media, Alabama, 1988

BKB Berkovitz, BJ Moxham, HN Newman
London 1995

Contents

Chapter 1

Cells of the Periodontal Ligament

BKB Berkovitz, RC Shore

INTRODUCTION

Compared with most connective tissues, the periodontal ligament (PDL) is highly cellular (*Fig. 1.1*). It is estimated that fibroblasts occupy up to 20 per cent of the sheep incisor PDL (Berkovitz, 1988) and between 43 per cent and 55 per cent of the PDL connective tissue of rodents (excluding the vasculature) (Beertsen and Everts, 1977; Shore and Berkovitz, 1979; Shore *et al.*, 1985; Shore *et al.*, 1991). In the mouse, this large percentage is produced by between 10,000 and 20,000 cells per mm^2 (based on a count of nuclear profiles) (McCulloch and Melcher, 1983). However, this cell density may change with age and function (Klingsberg and Butcher, 1960; Cohn, 1965). Undifferentiated mesenchymal cells and epithelial cells may also be present, the latter being found in normal PDL as small clusters – the rests of Malassez, which represent the remnants of the developmental epithelial root sheeth (of Hertwig). Occasional defence cells are found in the normal healthy tissue. The majority of these are macrophages, but eosinophils may also be present. Mast cells may also be found in the vicinity of the neurovascular tissue. In addition to these cells found within the 'body' of the PDL, the cells that maintain and remodel the hard tissues on the borders of the PDL are considered to be part of this tissue – these cells are the cementoblasts, osteoblasts, osteoclasts, and odontoclasts.

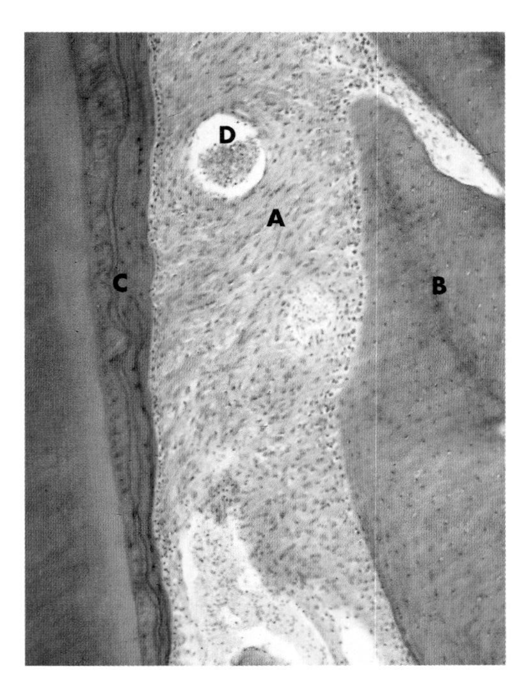

Fig. 1.1 Light micrograph of a longitudinal section of periodontal ligament showing the high cellularity of the tissue. The fibroblasts are arranged perpendicular to the tooth surface in the alveolar crest region, whilst apically they are arranged more obliquely (A). Alveolar bone (B), Cementum (C), Capillary (D). Magnification × 70.

FIBROBLASTS

The fibroblasts lie between the collagen fibres, and although various shapes have been described (Fullmer, 1967; Roberts and Chamberlain, 1978), it is likely that their appearance is governed by the surrounding matrix (Ross, 1968). The determination of the precise shape of PDL fibroblasts is important because of the proposed role for these cells in eruption (see below and Chapter 9). In the zone of the rodent incisor nearest the tooth, the fibroblasts are said to be fusiform, being arranged parallel to the tooth surface (Beertsen *et al.*, 1974). This view was based on examination of the PDL sectioned only in the longitudinal plane. However, if the PDL is sectioned both transversely and longitudinally, it can be deduced that the cells take the form of a flattened irregular disc, approximately 30 μm in diameter (Shore and Berkovitz, 1979; Berkovitz, 1988). This is confirmed by scanning electron microscopy – the spaces between the fibres (in which the cells were located) (Sloan 1978; Picton and Wills, 1981). However, a definitive three-dimensional reconstruction of PDL fibroblasts has yet to be accomplished.

The PDL fibroblast contains a prominent nucleus, which has a single distinct nucleolus and clearly defined nuclear pores (*Fig. 1.2*). When stained with colloidal silver (Crocker and Nar, 1987) it demonstrates either one or two regions of acidic proteins which

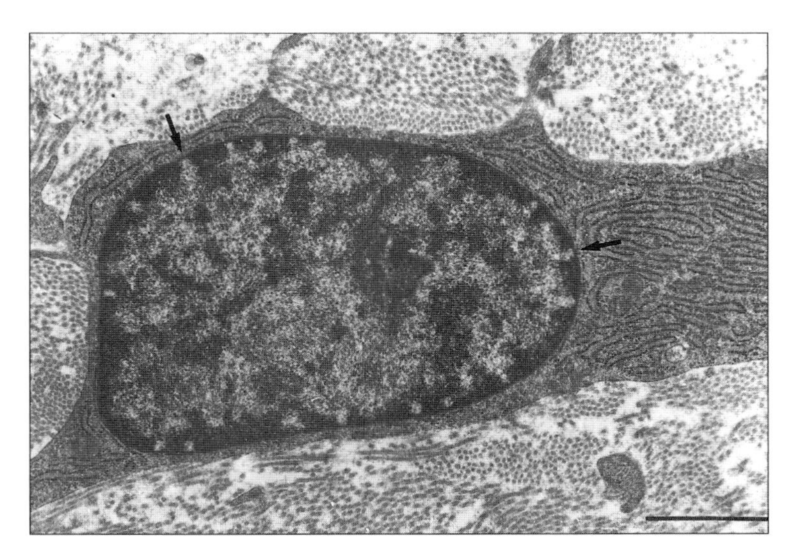

Fig. 1.2 Electron micrograph of a periodontal fibroblast showing a large prominent nucleus with numerous nuclear pores (arrowed). Note the smooth, non-crenulated nature of the nuclear outline. Bar = 2.0μm.

are associated with the nucleolar organizer regions (Shore *et al.*, 1991) (*Fig. 1.3*). An internal dense lamina, characteristic of connective tissue cells, is also found. The nucleus is a flattened disc shape; it has a diameter of approximately 10 µm (Shore and Berkovitz, 1979) and may occupy up to 30 per cent of the cell volume (Beertsen and Everts, 1977; Yamasaki *et al.*, 1987a). Its outline appears relatively smooth, and no published pictures have yet demonstrated any form of crenulation in the *in vivo* state. This may be noteworthy – it has been suggested that periodontal fibroblasts have a role in generating the force of eruption by contraction, in a way similar to myofibroblasts that are responsible for wound contraction (see Chapter 9). However, in certain induced pathological states, such as cyclosporin-induced hypertrophy, crenulated nuclei may be present in a significant number of cells (Yamasaki *et al.*, 1987b). In the aged PDL of both mice and rats, multinucleated fibroblasts may appear, arising either from fusion of mononuclear cells or perhaps by faulty division (Sasaki and Garant, 1993).

As fibroblasts produce the extracellular matrix of the PDL, which demonstrates a very high rate of turnover (Sodek, 1977) (see Chapter 3), the cells contain significant amounts of the organelles involved in protein synthesis and degradation. As one would expect, the synthetic pathway in these cells is the same as that found in other protein-matrix producing cells, such as odontoblasts, ameloblasts, etc. Cho and Garant (1981a) have demonstrated, using tritiated proline in a pulse–chase experiment, that the synthetic pathway is from rough endoplasmic reticulum (RER) to Golgi complex and thence via secretory vesicles to the cell membrane. Their data suggested that a period of approximately 30 minutes was required for the completion of this process. Furthermore, this and a companion study (Cho and Garant, 1981b), in which colchicine was administered, suggested that the passage of the secretory vesicles was microtubule dependent. The RER is found in parallel arrays of cisternae which are coated by ribosome rosettes. The cisternae may or may not be dilated (*Fig. 1.4*). The RER is dispersed throughout the cytoplasm, except for the finest cell processes, and it occupies between 5 per cent and 7 per cent of the cell by volume in the rat incisor (Beertsen and Everts, 1977; Shore *et al.*, 1985; Shore *et al.*, 1991), up to 9 per cent in the rat molar (Shore *et al.*, 1991), and approximately 5 per cent in the human PDL (Yamasaki *et al.*, 1987a). These values do not seem to change when periodontal function changes because of altered occlusal loading (Shore *et al.*, 1982, 1985). The cisternae are generally seen to contain material that is more electron–dense than the surrounding cytoplasm.

The PDL fibroblasts possess a Golgi complex of typical constituents which is found primarily in a juxtanuclear position (Garant and Cho, 1979), although its boundaries are often indistinct and its position not as localized as that of, for example, the osteoblast (c.f. *Figs. 1.5 and 1.8*). The diffuse nature of the Golgi in PDL fibroblasts makes quantitation difficult.

Mitochondria appear to be distributed throughout the cell, except for the finest cell processes. Most published micrographs suggest that their profiles vary from elongated to round. This range of shapes may reflect either an inherent variability of shape or simply the plane of section. The mitochondria possess a characteristically dense intramitochondrial matrix. Quantitative analysis suggests that these organelles occupy approximately

Fig. 1.3 Light micrograph of periodontal fibroblasts stained with colloidal silver. Note the one or two intense areas of staining within the fibroblast nuclei. Magnification, × 800.

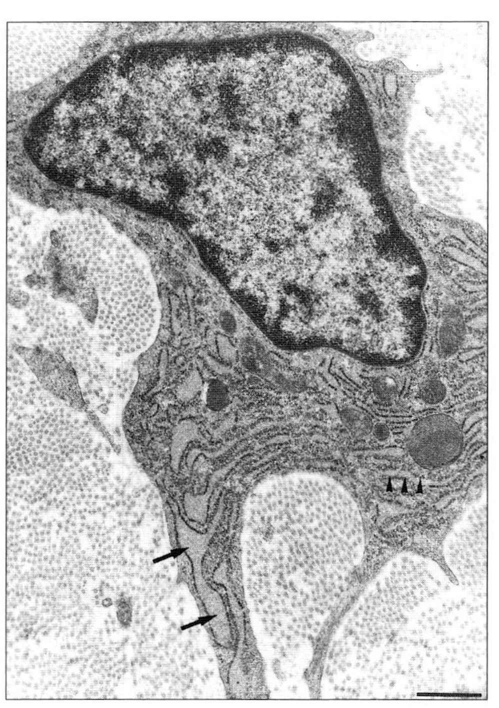

Fig. 1.4 Electron micrograph showing a periodontal fibroblast with numerous cisternae of RER. Note the cisternae may be in the form of parallel arrays (arrow heads) or in a more dilated form (arrows). Bar = 1.0µm.

2–2.5 per cent of the cell by volume in the rat (Shore *et al.*, 1982). This value does not seem to be altered by different occlusal loading levels or eruption rates (Shore *et al.*, 1982, 1985). It also seems remarkably similar between species (Berkovitz, 1988) and between closely related (but functionally different) connective tissues such as PDL and the connective tissue related to the enamel organ of the rodent incisor (Moxham *et al.*, 1991). Slightly higher values (3–3.5 per cent) may be found in human PDL (Yamasaki *et al.*, 1987a).

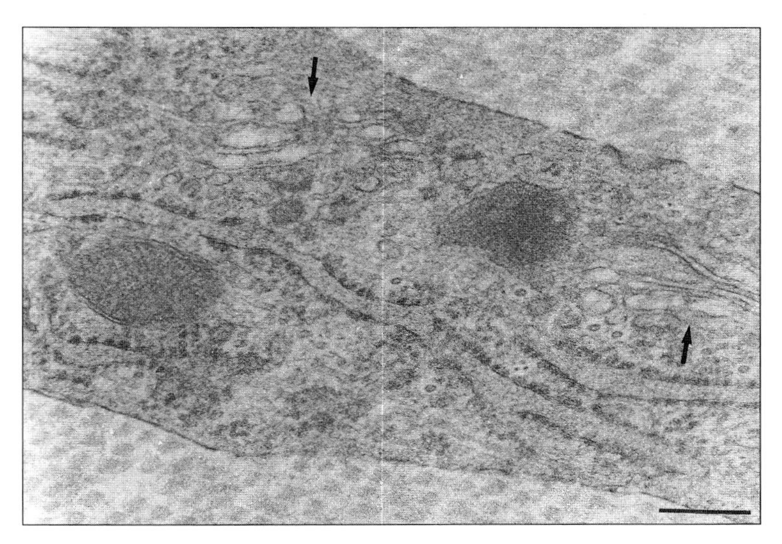

Fig. 1.5 Electron micrograph of two areas of Golgi saccules (arrowed) within a periodontal fibroblast. Bar = 0.25μm.

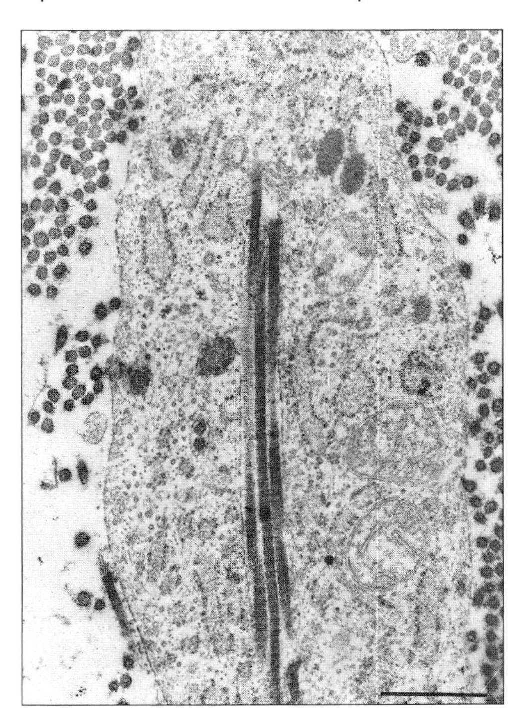

Fig. 1.6 Electron micrograph of a periodontal fibroblast containing three fragments of fibrillar collagen, apparently within a membrane bound vesicle. However, it is possible that they simply lie within a cellular invagination which only appears intracellular because of the plane of section. On the other hand, the orientation of the fibrils compared to that of the extracellular fibrils may suggest a true intracellular location. Bar = 0.4μm.

Lysosomes are present in PDL fibroblasts in the form of large membrane-bound vesicles containing a homogeneous matrix that is more electron-dense than the surrounding cytoplasm. Their numbers are considerably less than in actively phagocytic cells such as macrophages. They occupy approximately 0.5 per cent of the cell in both rat incisor and molar PDL (Shore *et al.*, 1991) and seem to be unaffected by either eruption rate or occlusal loading (Shore *et al.*, 1982, 1985). Even where collagen crosslinking has been disrupted by the administration of a lathyrogen, the volume–density of lysosomes does not significantly increase (Shore *et al.*, 1984).

The structures so far described are typical of those seen in fibroblasts in connective tissues in general. However, PDL fibroblasts also contain significant numbers of other organelles only infrequently seen in adult connective tissues.

There are many reports showing that PDL fibroblasts contain small fragments of collagen fibrils within membrane bound vesicles (Ten Cate, 1972; Listgarten, 1973; Beertsen *et al.*, 1974; Eley and Harrison, 1975; Frank *et al.*, 1976; Shore and Berkovitz, 1979) (*Fig. 1.6*). These are termed 'intracellular collagen profiles'. Three broad types can be observed within the cell:

- a normally banded fibril within an electron-lucent vacuole;
- a normally banded fibril within an electron-dense vacuole (with or without swellings along its length); and
- a fibril where the characteristic banding is lost (*Fig. 1.7*).

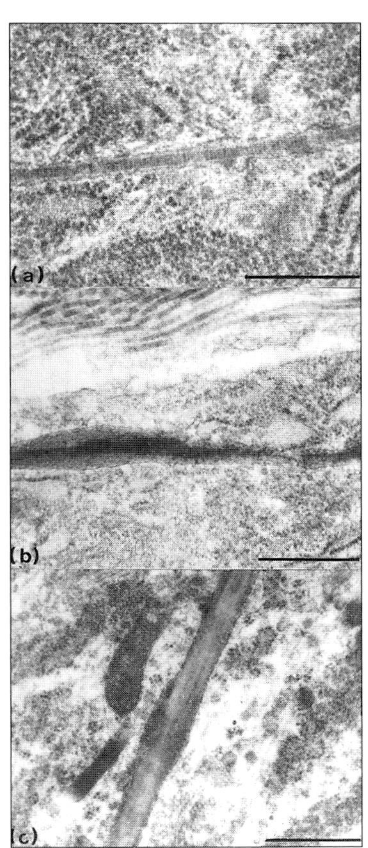

Fig. 1.7 Electron micrograph of three intracellular, collagen-containing vesicles. (a) Banded fibril surrounded by an electron-lucent zone. (b) Banded fibrils surrounded by electron dense material. (c) Fibrils with indistinct banding, surrounded by electron dense material. Bar = 0.75μm.

These three types are thought to constitute the temporal sequence of the intracellular degradation of collagen (Ten Cate *et al.*, 1976). The cell initially phagocytoses a fragment of a collagen fibril (Garant, 1976; Everts and Beertsen, 1988), and the resulting phagosome then fuses with one or more lysosomes to form a phagolysosome. The lysosomal enzymes then degrade the fibril, which consequently loses its characteristic structure.

The degradation of collagen has historically been regarded as an extracellular process. Accordingly, a specific enzyme, collagenase (matrix metalloproteinase-I – MMP-I), is thought to be responsible for cleaving the triple helical portion of the molecules within the fibril into 1/4–3/4 fragments and, together with MMP-IV, it leads to spontaneous denaturation under physiological conditions. The rest of the molecule is then responsive to further proteolysis by gelatinase (MMP-II) and MMP-V. However, before any of this collagenase activity can occur, the glycoproteins such as fibronectin and proteoglycans residing on the fibril surface and masking the collagenase binding site must first be removed by stromelysin (MMP-III) (see also Chapter 4).

If, therefore, degradation of PDL collagen is indeed an intracellular process, the question arises as to why this is so. It may relate to its dense fibrous nature, diffusion of collagenase, collagenase activators, or TIMP (tissue inhibitor of metalloproteinases) being more restricted. Alternatively, the high rate of turnover may require a more controllable degradative system.

However, the PDL may not be unique in possessing this form of degradation. Ten Cate and Deporter (1975) have suggested that collagen degradation is entirely intracellular in all healthy tissues where there is controlled turnover and remodelling. Only in tissues where the changes are pathological or where the degradation is rapid and involves a whole tissue simultaneously does the extracellular pathway have a role. Obviously, where turnover is relatively slow, the restriction on sample area imposed by electron microscopy makes the detection of intracellular collagen profiles a rare event.

A number of problems remain, however, concerning the significance of intracellular collagen profiles. Firstly, it has been suggested that they are not truly intracellular but are merely invaginations of the cell membrane, and that they may, in part, relate to the way the collagen is secreted within a deep cellular invagination so that its orientation can be better controlled (Trelstad and Hayashi, 1979). Secondly, they may result from the internal polymerization of newly synthesized procollagen. Thirdly, it has been suggested that, even if the profiles are intracellular and are involved in degradation of extracellular fibrils, they may not be the major route by which the collagen is catabolized.

Electron-dense markers such as thorium dioxide (Ten Cate *et al.*, 1976), histochemical techniques for the localization of acid and alkaline phosphatases (Deporter and Ten Cate, 1973; Ten Cate and Syrbu, 1974), and serial sectioning of fibroblasts both *in vivo* and *in vitro* (Svoboda *et al.*, 1979; Melcher and Chan, 1981) all provide evidence for the intracellular nature of the collagen fibrils within the profiles and that the collagen had originated in the extracellular compartment.

The possibility of internal polymerization of collagen before secretion has been suggested from the work of Cho and Garant (1981b), in which the number of profiles increased after administration of the antimicrotubule agent, colchicine. The effect of the colchicine was presumed to be inhibition of the normal secretory pathway, leading to an intracellular build-up of procollagen and its subsequent polymerization into banded fibrils.

The possible intracellular polymerization of collagen has also been suggested in other tissues. Michna (1988), using anabolic steroids to enhance synthesis, demonstrated an increase in intracellular collagen profiles in tendon fibroblasts. This increase was linked to the possible increase in need for rapid intracellular degradation of collagen before secretion, as suggested by the work of Bienkowski *et al.* (1978) and Bienkowski and Engels (1981).

However, several points may be made in relation to these findings. Firstly, Everts *et al.* (1985, 1989) and Everts and Beertsen (1987) failed to find an increase in profiles after increased secretion or depolymerization of microtubules, but they did find a complete lack of profiles when phagocytosis was inhibited in an *in vitro* model system. In addition, the morphology of the intracellular collagen in the stimulated tendon, having diameters up to 120 nm (Michna, 1988), suggests that it is unlikely to represent *de novo* polymerization. Fibrils of this size are characteristic of highly stressed extracellular fibrils, a situation unlikely to occur over a very short time period within an intracellular vacuole. Furthermore, it is difficult to see why the cell should attempt to process the procollagen in this way so that a normally banded fibril resulted from a purely intracellular process. Finally, at early time intervals after ^{3}H-proline injection (i.e. 30 minutes), collagen-containing vacuoles were unlabelled – only elongated secretory granules were labelled (Weinstock, 1981).

With regard to the question of whether or not fibrillar phagocytosis is the major route of collagen catabolism in healthy tissues, several reports have indicated a relationship between the number of profiles and the turnover rate of the connective tissue. Stereological analysis of PDL, gingiva, and skin (Svoboda *et al.*, 1981), and of rat incisor and molar PDLs (Shore and Berkovitz, 1979; Shore *et al.*, 1991) have demonstrated some evidence of a positive correlation between the number of profiles and the turnover of the collagen. By relating the total volume of intracellular fibrillar collagen to the turnover rate and volume of extracellular fibrils, it can be calculated that the process of degradation must be completed within about 30–40 minutes if all the collagen is degraded in this way (Shore and Berkovitz, 1979). Some evidence that this may be the case arises from *in vitro* studies using proteinase inhibitors to stop the final degradation of the fibril. Under these conditions, the number of profiles that accumulate inside the cell approaches 100 times as much as that seen normally in a 48-hour period – this also suggests a time of approximately 30 minutes (Everts and Beertsen, 1988).

The microfilaments and microtubules within PDL fibroblasts have been the subject of much controversy about the possible involvement of these organelles in fibroblast traction. The microfilaments are present in the cytoplasm of the cell either as a network that fills the cell processes (Beertsen *et al.*, 1974) or as bundles beneath the cell membrane that resemble stress fibres seen in fibroblasts *in vitro* (Beertsen *et al.*, 1974; Shore and Berkovitz, 1979) (*Fig. 1.8*). Microfilaments of 5–7 nm diameter are found in many cell types, both motile and non-motile. These microfilaments are composed predominantly of polymerized actin (F-actin), although other proteins are present as well (Brinkley, 1982). They are important in membrane ruffling, amoeboid movement, chromosome movement, endocytosis, exocytosis, and cell surface receptor mobility (Allison, 1973; Brinkley, 1982). Their presence within PDL fibroblasts, together with the apparent migration of the cells in an occlusal direction (Beertsen, 1975), has led to the proposal that the fibroblasts generate the eruptive force (Melcher and Beertsen, 1977).

However, data presented by Moxham *et al.* (1991) suggest that the filament bundles within rodent incisor fibroblasts are not polarized. It is possible that the cells undergo continual short-term localized movements that are unrelated to eruptive movements in order to maintain the matrix around them. Indeed, it has been suggested that fibroblasts are responsible for connective tissue morphogenesis, by:

- laying down oriented fibrils in their wake during this type of movement (Garant and Cho, 1979; Trelstad and Hayashi, 1979); or
- laying down fibrils at their leading edge (Garant and Cho, 1989); or
- generating localized areas of tension within the matrix, which subsequently align the randomly secreted collagen (Stopak and Harris, 1982).

As the PDL has an extremely high rate of turnover and therefore a constant need for fibril orientation, this local motility may be of considerable significance in maintaining PDL integrity. That the presence of stress fibres may be linked to fibril orientation rather than to eruption is also suggested by the finding that such stress fibres occur in tenocytes of the achilles tendon of new-born rabbits (Ippolito *et al.*, 1977). These cells are presumably not undergoing highly polarized migratory activity (the subject of fibroblast motility is discussed further in Chapter 9). Stress fibres may be connected to, and colinear with, extracellular filaments via a fibronexus, particularly in inflamed tissue (Singer, 1979; Garant *et al.*, 1982). These sites may be intimately associated with accumulations of the extracellular glycoprotein, fibronectin (Cho *et al.*, 1988). In less inflamed tissue, the fibronectin may be more associated with small attachment plaques around the cell (Cho *et al.*, 1988; Zhang *et al.*, 1993), attached to the membrane via a receptor, integrin-α5 (Steffensen *et al.*, 1992).

Microtubules have also been linked to fibroblast motility, although evidence suggests that their importance may lie in facilitating protein export (Ehrlich and Bornstein, 1972). Indeed, as has already been mentioned, the disruption of micotubules leads to internal accumulation of procollagen (Cho and Garant, 1981b). The microtubules are characterized as non-branching cylinders of approximately 22 nm diameter, which in any one cell may often appear randomly arranged (Shore and Berkovitz, 1979) (*Fig. 1.9*). They are often seen to radiate from centrioles, structures which themselves consist of a hollow tube of microtubules.

A structure frequently associated with the centriole of PDL fibroblasts is a solitary cilium. Beertsen *et al.* (1975) have

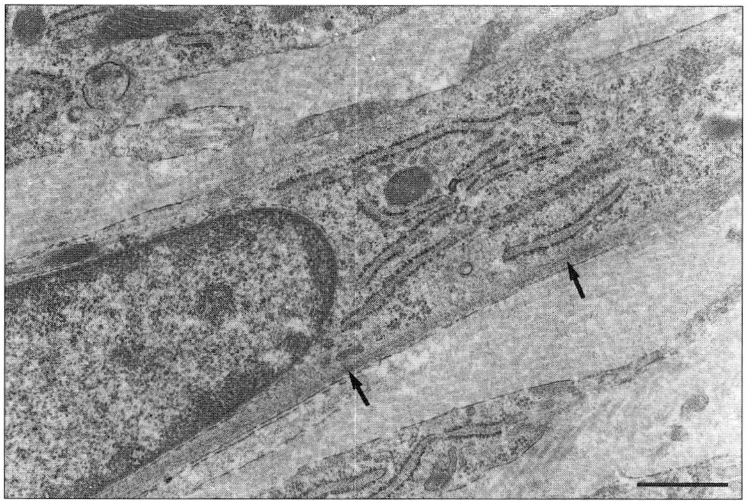

Fig. 1.8 Electron micrograph of a periodontal fibroblast showing a bundle of microfilaments (stress fibre) (arrowed) beneath the cell membrane. Bar = 0.6μm.

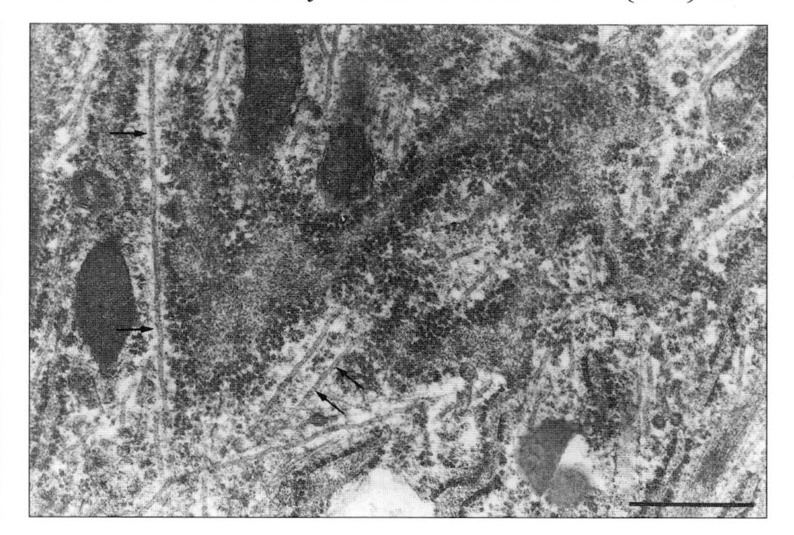

Fig. 1.9 Electron micrograph of a periodontal fibroblast showing numerous microtubules (arrowed). Note their apparent lack of preferential orientation. Bar = 0.5μm.

estimated that solitary cilia are present in more than 70 per cent of rat incisor PDL fibroblasts. These solitary cilia lie within invaginations of the cell membrane with their distal ends protruding into the surrounding matrix (*Fig. 1.10*). The major part of the shaft of the cilium lacks the central doublet of microtubules from the normal 9 + 2 configuration (Beertsen *et al.*, 1975) and appears to lack the dynein side arms associated with the outer doublets (*Fig. 1.11*). Cilia usually occur on motile cells and the free surface of epithelia. Their function in the PDL is unknown, although as they lack the central doublet (and most likely the dynein moeity), Beertsen *et al.* (1975) doubted that they are associated with motility. Their appearance in other non-motile cells is not uncommon (Sorokin, 1962; Fawcett, 1981) – again, in these cells they lack the central tubule doublet. A possible role for these structures may lie in their suggested link with the control mechanism of the cell cycle and inhibition of centriolar activity (Lloyd, 1979). Conversely, however, in neural tissue, the incidence of rudimentary cilia seems to be associated with the most malignant (i.e. the most rapidly proliferating) tissue (Park *et al.*, 1988).

A number of authors have discussed the degree of polarization of PDL fibroblasts and their organelles in relation to collagen secretion and/or motility. Possible polarization can be considered on two levels:

- whether individual cells are polarized in terms of shape and organelle content; and
- whether the population of cells within the tissue as a whole is polarized in a particular orientation.

When considering individual cells, Beertsen *et al.* (1979) and Garant and Cho (1979, 1989) have suggested that both the Golgi complex and the centriolar region of periodontal fibroblasts may be situated between the leading edge of the cell and the posteriorly located nucleus ('periodontal' in this context refers to cells of the transseptal region also). The cell was considered to be secreting matrix from its leading edge. In both mouse and rat PDLs, significant numbers of cells appeared to be polarized in opposing directions, i.e. the population of cells as a whole did not appear to be polarized in a single direction. Some cells may be moving apically while neighbouring cells are moving incisally. This may imply that such polarization may have more to do with organized matrix secretion than eruption. Microtubules have also been considered as indicators of polarity. However, it is difficult to decipher such polarity at the level of the individual cell when considering this organelle.

Some indication of *population* polarity can be gained from counts of microtubules that have been sectioned perpendicular to their long axis in both longitudinal and transverse sections of the PDL. Several investigations have employed this analysis, with conflicting results. Beertsen *et al.* (1979) demonstrated some degree of polarization, but Moxham *et al.* (1991) failed to find any evidence of such an arrangement.

The final element of the cytoskeleton that must be considered are the 'intermediate' filaments (IFs), so called because of their size (approximately 11 nm), which is intermediate between that of the thin (actin) and thick filaments of muscle. There are five classes of IFs, depending on the tissue of origin. Mesenchymal tissues typically express vimentin, a subtype of class III IFs (for review see Steinert *et al.*, 1985; Stewart, 1990). While they generally have a perinuclear distribution, their precise function is unclear (see Geiger, 1987). Their distribution within periodontal fibroblasts appears to depend, to some extent, on species. While published micrographs of rodent and dog PDL, for example, demonstrate a relatively sparse distribution of IFs (e.g. Cho and

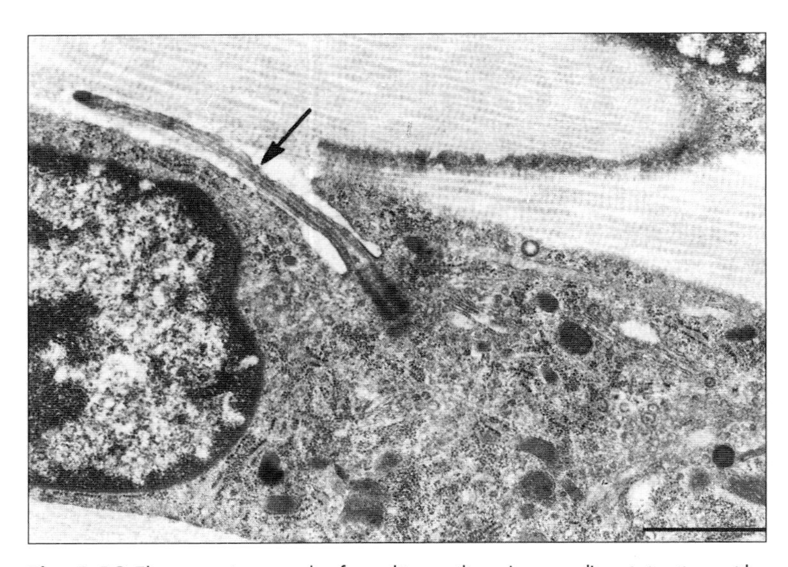

Fig. 1.10 Electron micrograph of a solitary cilium (arrowed), originating within a deep cellular invagination and extending into the extracellular matrix. Bar = 1.0μm.

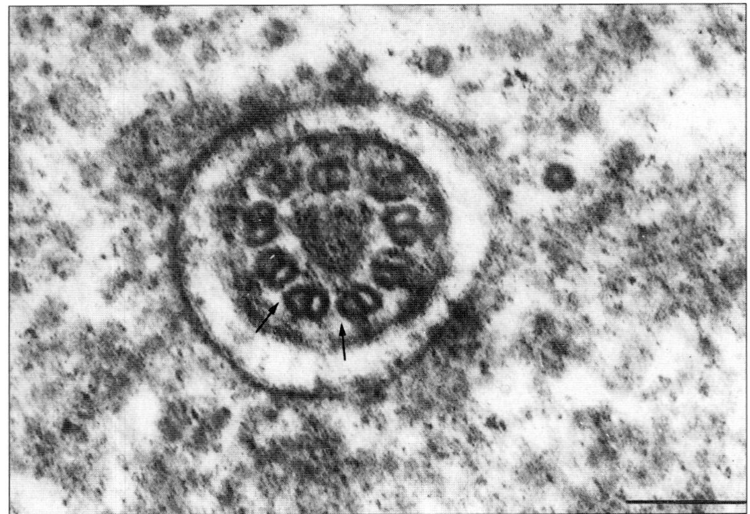

Fig. 1.11 High-power electron micrograph showing a cilium such as that shown in Fig. 1.10 cut transversely to its shaft. Note the absence of the central doublet and the lack of dynein side arms (arrowed). Bar = 100nm.

Garant, 1981; Cho *et al.*, 1988), others, such as human and sheep PDL, may posses significant accumulations of IFs, particularly within cell processes (Yamasaki *et al.*, 1987b; Berkovitz, 1988) (*Fig. 1.12*). In addition, recent work (Webb *et al.*, 1994) suggests that periodontal fibroblasts (but not gingival fibroblasts) and cementoblasts co-express vimentin and *cytokeratin* immediately before and during the active phase of eruption (*Fig. 1.13*). Once eruption has ceased, the expression of cytokeratin ceases also.

One further feature of PDL fibroblasts is the presence of numerous intercellular contacts, contacts not normally being found in significant numbers between fibroblasts of adult connective tissues (Gabbiani, 1979; Moxham *et al.*, 1984). Such structures are normally observed in foetal connective tissues (Ross and Greenlee, 1966; Greenlee and Ross, 1967), between myofibroblasts in healing wounds (Gabbiani, 1979), and between fibroblasts in culture (Gilula, 1972; Pinto da Silva and Gilula, 1972). In the PDL, two major types of contact are seen: gap junctions (*Fig. 1.14*) and simplified desmosomes (macula adhaerens) (*Fig. 1.15*) (Azuma *et al.*, 1975; Beertsen and Everts, 1980; Shore *et al.*, 1981). The gap junctions vary in size between 0.1 μm and 0.5 μm in

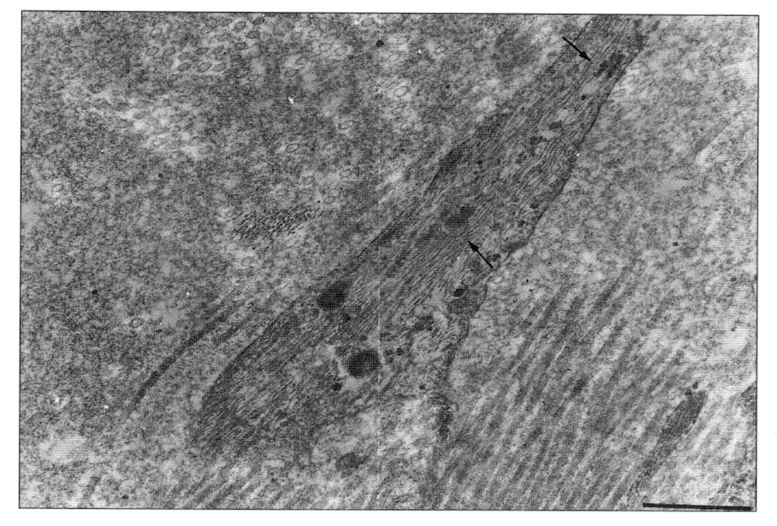

Fig. 1.12 Electron micrograph of fibroblast cell process from the periodontal ligament of the sheep. Note the numerous filaments of the intermediate type (arrowed) which almost fill the cytoplasm. Bar = 1.0μm.

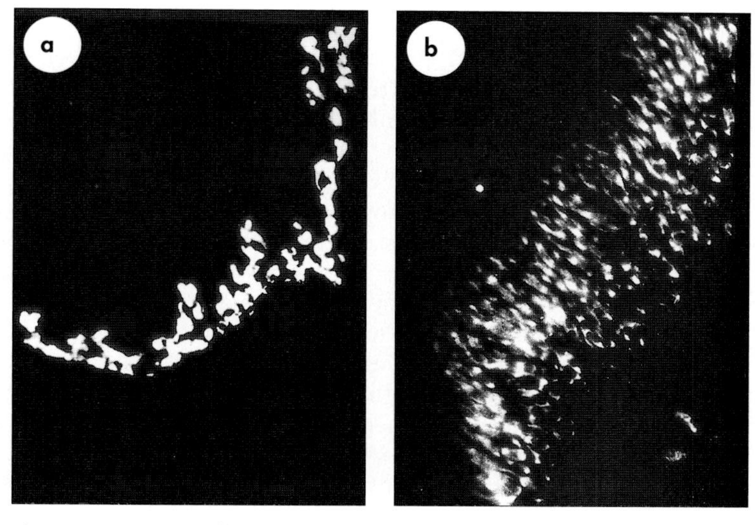

Fig. 1.13 a) Immunofluorescence micrograph of the cementoblasts and follicular fibroblasts adjacent to Hertwig's root sheath of a rat molar, showing labelling with an anti-cytokeratin antibody. b) Immunofluorescence micrograph of the periodontal ligament of an erupting rat molar. Note the labelling of fibroblasts throughout the entire width of the ligament with an anti-cytokeratin antibody. Magnification, × 100. (Courtesy of P. P. Webb.)

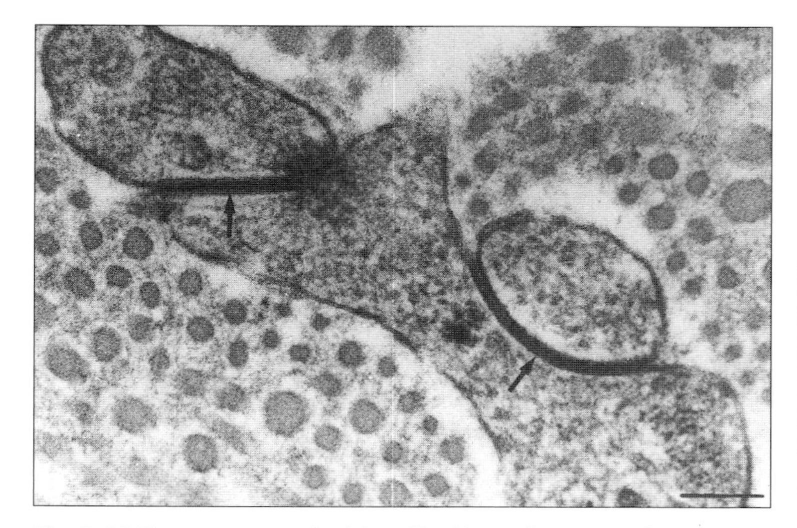

Fig. 1.14 Electron micrograph of three fibroblast cell processes showing intercellular contacts of the gap junction type (arrowed). Bar = 100nm.

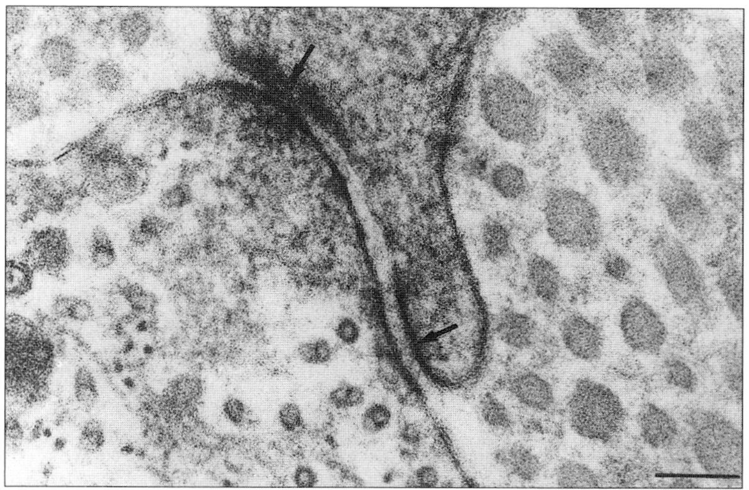

Fig. 1.15 Electron micrograph of two intercellular contacts of the simplified desmosome type (arrowed). Note the filamentous material in the intercellular space. Bar = 100nm.

diameter, with an array of 6–7 nm globular subunits (Beertsen and Everts, 1980). The macula adhaerens are generally smaller, ranging from 0.1–0.4 µm (Beertsen and Everts, 1980; Shore *et al.*, 1981). They lack the intercellular specialization and inserting tonofilaments that are characteristic of the epithelial macula, as seen in the cell rests for example. Frequently, the gap junction and simplified desmosome are found in close association (Shore *et al.*, 1981). An additional (and the most numerous) type of contact reported in the rat PDL is the 'close contact' (Shore *et al.*, 1981) (*Fig. 1.16*), where the cell membranes of opposing cells come to lie in close association without any visible membrane specialization.

It has been suggested that the unusually high number of contacts within the PDL is related to the generation of the eruptive force by the PDL fibroblasts (either by motility or contractility). According to this hypothesis, the intercellular coordination of the process would be achieved via the gap junctions, and the force would be transmitted via the simplified desmosomes. However, it is also possible that these structures are required for the coordination of the constant and high turnover of the matrix. That the numbers of contacts is not directly related to eruption is suggested by the fact that there are a greater number of simplified desmosomes in the connective tissue adjacent to the enamel organ of the rat incisor than in the PDL of this tooth (Shore *et al.*, 1981). The enamel-related connective tissue gains no attachment to the tooth and therefore cannot transmit a force to it. In addition, there are similar numbers in the PDLs of the continously growing rat incisor and the fully erupted rat molar (Shore *et al.*, 1981). However, this data would also indicate no clear-cut relationship with matrix turnover either.

Specific cell surface receptors shown to be present on PDL fibroblasts are those for EGF – epidermal growth factor – (both in dental follicle and fully differentiated PDL) (Thesleff *et al.*, 1987; Topham *et al.*, 1987; Cho *et al.*, 1991) and IL-1β (interleukin-1β) (Saito *et al.*, 1991). In addition, *in vitro* studies suggest the presence of receptors for I-LGF (insulin-like growth factor), PDGF (platelet-derived growth factor), growth hormone (Blom *et al.*, 1992; Matsuda *et al.*, 1992) and parathyroid hormone (Ngan *et al.*, 1988).

The presence of receptors for IL-1β may have considerable significance for the progression of chronic inflammatory periodontal disease. In other connective tissues, an increase in available IL-1β leads to increased collagenase production by fibroblasts *in vitro* (but not intracellular phagocytosis) (Everts *et al.*, 1990). In addition, increase in this cytokine also leads to production of a second cytokine, IL-6, by the fibroblast (Bartold and Haynes, 1991). This response is greater in PDL fibroblasts than in gingival fibroblasts (Shimizu *et al.*, 1992). IL-6 in turn stimulates osteoclastic activity, apparently through an effect on osteoclastogenesis (Löwik *et al.*, 1989). This relationship between the production of IL-1β and IL-6 by periodontal fibroblasts and increased osteoclastic activity may also be important in the tissue response to orthodontic loading (Davidovitch *et al.*, 1988).

It has recently been shown that the cells of the periodontal ligament demonstrate a strong positive staining reaction to cellular retinoic acid-binding protein (CRABP-I) (Berkovitz and Maden, 1993). The presence of receptors for both EGF (Thesleff *et al.*, 1987; Topham *et al.*, 1987; Cho *et al.*, 1991) and CRABP-I may be another example of the foetal-like nature of the PDL. Within the embryonic mouse mandible, the expression of EGF mRNA is controlled by retinoic acid (retinol) (Kronmiller *et al.*, 1993), while the presence of CRABP-I may be important in modulating the action of the retinoic acid by binding any excess within the cell (Mark *et al.*, 1992). Within the fully differentiated PDL, a lack of retinoids (vitamin A deficiency) may lead to necrosis and decreased vascularity (Boyle, 1947; Bryer, 1957).

The role of cytokines and growth factors in the PDL, particularly in relation to orthodontic tooth movement, is discussed in Chapter 00.

CEMENTOBLASTS

Cementoblasts are the cells responsible for secreting the organic (mainly collagenous) matrix of cementum. They therefore have the organelles necessary for protein synthesis and export (*Fig. 1.17*). However, their appearance is dictated by their activity, i.e. the rate at which cementum is being deposited. When active they may appear as a distinct layer of cells on the root surface, somewhat similar to the osteoblastic layer but usually not as regular in arrangement. Apart from their location immediately adjacent to cementum, cementoblasts are often indistinguishable from periodontal fibroblasts. Indeed, as some of the cementoblast cell processes do not approach cementum and their cytoplasmic contents are not polarized, the cells may contribute matrix to the PDL. The synthetic pathway is presumably similar to that of the fibroblast. However, there is little quantitative data relating specifically to cementoblasts, although they appear to have less RER but more mitochondria than PDL fibroblasts (Yamasaki *et al.*, 1987b).

One prominent feature seen in human cementoblasts is the accumulation of numerous glycogen granules, the number decreasing the further the distance from the cementum surface (Yamasaki *et al.*, 1986). They also appear to contain significant quantities of both intermediate and actin filaments. The cell membrane may demonstrate numerous intercellular contacts of both the gap junction and simplified desmosome type (Yamasaki *et al.*, 1987b). The membrane may also possess receptors for growth hormone (Zhang *et al.*, 1993) and (to a limited extent) EGF (Cho *et al.*, 1991). The frequency of EGF receptors appears to be considerably reduced compared to adjacent fibroblasts.

OSTEOBLASTS

Osteoblasts within the PDL are found on the surface of the alveolar bone. Their gross appearance and ultrastructure is similar to that of osteoblasts found elsewhere in the body (for recent reviews see Holtrop, 1990; Schenk *et al.*, 1993). When most active, they form a layer of cuboidal cells, which exhibit a strong basophilic cytoplasm. A prominent nucleus lies towards the basal end of the cell and a pale juxtanuclear area indicates the site of the Golgi complex. Like fibroblasts they are seen to contain a prominent RER and numerous mitochondria and vesicles. The Golgi complex, however, appears more localized and extensive than in the fibroblast (*Fig. 1.18*). Microtubles and microfilaments are present, the latter being particularly prominent beneath the secreting membrane of the cell. The cells do not appear to possess receptors for EGF (Martineau-Doizé *et al.*, 1987). They do contact one another, primarily via gap junctions and also via simplified desmosomes. They also form contacts via gap junctions with osteocytes lying within lacunae in the adjacent bone, thus forming a coordinated system throughout the bone tissue (Holtrop and Weinger, 1972). As bone deposition proceeds, osteoblasts become incorporated in the matrix as osteocytes (in which the organelle content is reduced).

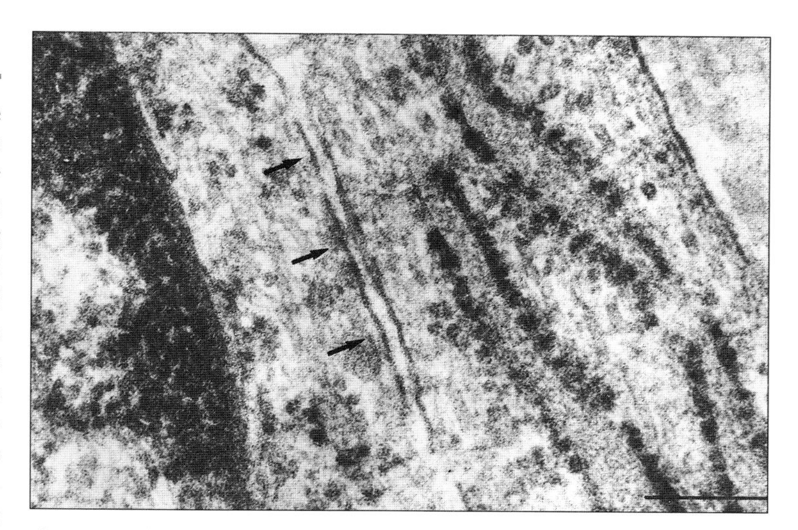

Fig. 1.16 Electron micrograph of two fibroblasts demonstrating an intercellular contact of the 'close contact' type (arrowed). Note the close alignment of the cell membranes but without any apparent specialisation. Bar = 200nm.

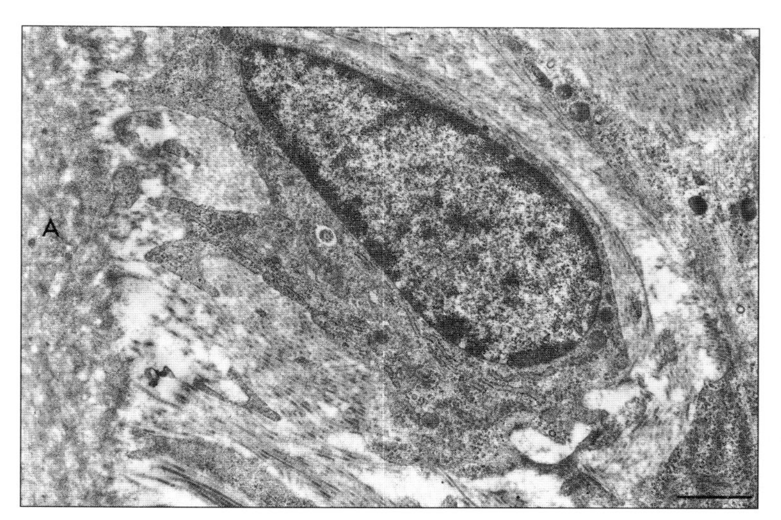

Fig. 1.17 Electron micrograph of a cementoblast lying adjacent to the surface of cementum (A). The cytoplasm contains the organelles involved in protein synthesis, but not in large amounts. Bar = 1.5μm.

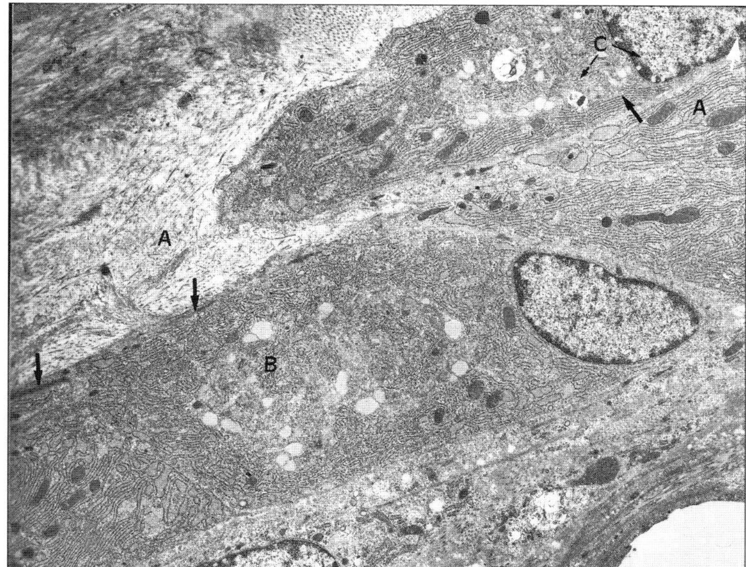

Fig. 1.18 Electron micrograph of osteoblasts lying adjacent to a forming bone surface (A). The cells exhibit extensive arrays of rough endoplasmic reticulum and a prominent Golgi complex (B). Note bundles of microfilaments (arrowed) beneath the cell membrane adjacent to the bone. Inset shows longitudinal section of periodontal ligament with a layer of osteoblasts adjacent to a forming bone surface (A). Note extensive areas of Golgi complex (arrowed) appearing as a pale zone within the cytoplasm. Note also the flattened cells (C) immediately adjacent to the osteoblasts, which may represent osteoblast precursors. Bar = 3.0μm.

Cells that may be osteoblast precursors are often seen beneath the osteoblast layer in the vicinity of adjacent blood capillaries (see *Fig. 1.18*). These cells have a reduced cytoplasm and few organelles. As they proceed through the stages of differentiation from precursor via committed osteoprogenitor to preosteoblast, they first migrate away from the bone surface into the body of the PDL before eventually taking up their functional position (Roberts *et al.*, 1987). Once in the functional state, the cells may remain active for a period of up to 20 days. This compares to a period of approximaely 10 days for periosteal osteoblasts (McCulloch and Heersche, 1988).

When osteogenesis is not occurring, a distinct layer of osteoblasts is absent. Indeed, in other sites in mature animals, osteoblasts (and osteoclasts) are present over only approximately 10–15 per cent of bone surfaces (Jowsey *et al.*, 1965); the remaining 85–90 per cent of the bone surface is covered by flattened cells with scanty cytoplasm, the so-called bone-lining cells.

OSTEOCLASTS

Although it has been claimed that bone resorption may be mediated via osteocytes (Bélanger, 1971), resorption of bone surfaces is accomplished via a distinct cell type, the osteoclast. The osteoclasts found within the PDL on the surface of the alveolar bone are typical of such cells elsewhere in the skeleton, in that:

- they are found within resorption lacunae;
- they are large and multinucleated; and
- they have a 'ruffled border' adjacent to the resorbing surface, enclosed by a smooth 'annular' or 'clear' zone (*Fig. 1.19*)

(For recent reviews of osteoclast structure, see Holtrop, 1990; Schenk *et al.*, 1993).

They do not cover the whole of the resorbing surface at any one time (Owen and Shetlar, 1968); rather they 'service' a much larger area by demonstrating considerable motility (Hancox, 1972; Jones and Boyde, 1977), leaving a trail of continuous resorption pits visible in their wake. On the alveolar periosteal surface of hamsters, the number of osteoclasts per millimetre of linear bone profile has been found to range from 0.1 per millimetre in healthy tissue to 4.5 per millimetre in active periodontal disease (Saffar and Makris, 1986). These figures were subject to large variations between regions and between animals, however. In the sheep incisor PDL, the number of osteoclasts per millimetre also varied, from 0.9 per millimetre in healthy tissue to 1.2 per millimetre in diseased tissue (Shore *et al.*, unpublished data).

The cytoplasm, particularly that part that is adjacent to the ruffled border, is often highly vacuolated or 'foamy', and accumulations of numerous mitochondria may be present throughout the cell, suggesting extreme metabolic activity. Ultrastructurally, the ruffled border itself is composed of many tightly packed infoldings of the cell membrane, which may be coated with fine bristle-like structures (Kallio *et al.*, 1971). In contrast to the cytoplasm adjacent to the ruffled border, that part that is adjacent to the 'annular zone' is denser, as it lacks the large numbers of vacuoles. It has been suggested that this modified area of cell periphery may act to 'seal' the active site of resorption (i.e. the ruffled border) into its own microenvironment, thereby controlling and limiting the lateral spread of acids and enzymes (Malkani *et al.*, 1973). With conventional histological stains, the cytoplasm stains less intensely than adjacent active osteoblasts, suggesting the presence of only small amounts of RER. This characteristic is confirmed by electron microscopy (see *Fig. 1.19*). Numerous free ribosomes may be present, however, suggesting considerable protein production for internal use (Holtrop, 1990). Much of this production will be of enzymes that are destined for the dissolution of the bone matrix. While the bone matrix is, like the PDL, primarily fibrillar collagen, there is no evidence for the presence of intracellular collagen profiles. This may be related to the controlled extracellular environment available to the osteoclast or to the removal of the collagen by subadjacent PDL fibroblasts (Heersche and Deporter, 1979) or by perivascular macrophages (Dorey and Bick, 1977).

The multinucleated cells associated with the resorption of cementum and dentine have sometimes been referred to as cementoclasts and odontoclasts. However, the evidence suggests that all multinucleated resorptive cells involved in the removal of mineralized tissues are morphologically and functionally similar (Yaeger and Kraucunas, 1969; Freilich, 1971; Addison, 1979).

A more detailed discussion of the interactions between osteoblasts and osteoclasts can be found in Chapter 12. The reader is also referred to a recent review by Marks and Popoff (1988).

EPITHELIAL CELLS

Aggregations of epithelial cells are a normal feature of the periodontal ligament. They represent the remains of the developmental epithelial root sheath (of Hertwig), which is involved in mapping out the shape of the root(s) and in the differentiation of root odontoblasts (e.g. Thomas and Kollar, 1988). The epithelial cells also secrete enamel-like proteins onto the root surface (Slavkin *et al.*, 1988; Luo *et al.*, 1991).

The epithelial cell rests (ECR) can be distinguished from the fibroblasts of the PDL in routine histological sections by the close packing of their cuboidal cells and by their tendency to stain more deeply (*Fig. 1.20*). They are unique in being completely surrounded by connective tissue cells (Brunette *et al.*, 1979). Immediately after disruption of the root sheath, the ECR are found in groups of one or two cells, with only a partial basal lamina. Subsequently, the epithelial rests become more cellular and are contained within an almost complete basal lamina with narrowed intercellular spaces. As laminin is chemotactic to epithelial cells, the basal lamina may therefore play a role in the formation, differentiation, and maintenance of the ECR (Hamamoto *et al.*, 1991).

ECR have a high nuclear–cytoplasmic ratio. They exhibit basal cell-like, undifferentiated, and hyperproliferative characteristics, as indicated by expression of cytokeratins 5, 6, 14, 16, and 19 (Salonen *et al.*, 1991). ECR appear most often in cross-section as separate, duct-like clusters of cells (see *Fig. 1.20*). However, when cut tangentially or with serial sectioning, they are seen to form a network of interconnecting strands parallel to the long axis of the root (*Fig. 1.21*) (Simpson, 1965; Valderhaug, 1974). ECR are located closer to the cementum than to the alveolar bone surface, the average distance being 27 µm in the apical region, gradually increasing cervically to 41 µm (Valderhaug and Zander, 1967). The distribution of ECR changes with age: they are less numerous in older individuals and more numerous in children (Reitan, 1961; Simpson, 1965; Wesselink and Beertsen, 1993). Up to the second decade of life, ECR are found most commonly in the apical region of the periodontal ligament, whereas later in life the majority of cell rests are located cervically in the gingiva of the alveolar crest (Reeve and Wentz, 1962). In this cervical region, some of the ECR are presumably derived from the gingival epithelium and the junctional epithelium (Wentz *et al.*, 1950). Grant and Bernick (1969) and Spouge (1984) have drawn attention to possible continuity between the ECR on the one hand and either the reduced enamel epithelium before eruption or the junctional epithelium after eruption on the other hand. Such continuity may be of significance in chronic inflammatory periodontal disease.

As non-functional cells usually disappear, the persistence of ECR suggests that they are not totally inactive and may subserve some, as yet undetermined, function (Spouge, 1980). As previously described, they do change their distribution with age and this is in line with the observation that epithelial rests take up tritiated thymidine, indicating some degree of turnover of these cells (Trowbridge and Shibata, 1967; McCulloch and Melcher, 1983c). Indeed, very intense binding of EGF has been observed in ECR, possibly indicating that such cells could be activated by a local rise in tissue levels of this growth factor (Thesleff, 1987). However, there is no evidence of a direct relationship between the number of EGF receptors and cell proliferation (Thesleff *et al.*, 1987). A possible relationship between epithelial cell rests and periodontal sensory nerve endings has also been described (Lambrichts *et al.*, 1993).

Reitan (1961) observed that on the 'compression' side of teeth that are subjected to orthodontic loading, hyalinization occurred and that, although there was subsequent regeneration of the connective tissue elements of the PDL, there was no regeneration of the ECR. However, Brice *et al.* (1991) have reported the presence of ECR (at the ultrastructural level) in areas of repairing orthodontic root resorption. Indeed, these authors suggest ECR may be involved in mediating repair cementogenesis. After reimplantation studies, Löe and Waerhaug (1961) observed that ankylosis and subsequent root resorption never occurred when a periodontal ligament that contained ECR was retained. These authors suggested that ECR may be the factor in limiting the resorption and may therefore play a role in the maintenance of the periodontal space, a view later supported by Lindskog *et al.* (1983). However, this view was not substantiated by Wesselink and Beertsen (1993). These authors administered the drug 1-hydroxyethylidine-1,1-bisphosphonate, which resulted in a marked reduction in the width of the PDL and produced ankylosis at several sites in the presence of the normal distribution of the ECR.

Ultrastructurally, ECR can be seen to be separated from the surrounding connective tissue by a basal lamina, which may be fragmented (Listgarten, 1975). The nucleus of each cell is prominent, contains condensed heterochromatin, and often shows invaginations (*Fig. 1.22*). The scanty cytoplasm is characterized by the presence of tonofilaments, some of which insert into the desmosomes frequently found between adjacent cells and into the hemidesmosomes between the cells and the basal lamina. Tight junctions are also found between the cells. Abundant mitochondria are distributed throughout the cell, but the scarcity of RER and Golgi complex indicates a lack of significant extracellular protein secretion (Valderhaug and Nylen, 1966; Hamamoto *et al.*, 1989). A primary cilium accompanied by a centriole is often seen in association with root-like structures and the Golgi complex, while the presence of coated pits and vesicles (together with gap junctions) could provide an anatomical basis for cells to exchange 'information' and to respond to changes in the environment (Hamamoto *et al.*, 1989). The ultrastructural appearance of the ECR again indicates that the cells may be more than simply inactive resting cells.

Although ECR show little evidence of cell proliferation *in vivo*, they can be readily cultured *in vitro* from fragments of periodontal ligament, and in such conditions they undergo rapid proliferation (e.g. Brunette *et al.*, 1976; Ragnarsson *et al.*, 1985; Yamasaki and Pinero, 1989). As these cells have been implicated in the aetiology of periodontal cysts, *in vitro* studies have been undertaken primarily to determine what biologically active substances (particularly those related to the degradation of bone and collagen) may be synthesized by the cells and how the cells themselves react to various biologically active molecules.

Following tissue culture of the periodontal ligament, the epithelial component derived from the ECR can be separated from those of the connective tissue elements by differential trypsinization and then identified by specific antibody staining for the presence of keratin and the absence of vimentin (Brunette *et al.*, 1976; Ragnarsson *et al.*, 1985). *In vitro*, the cells proliferate rapidly, with a doubling time of 36 hours and, unlike cells *in vivo*, which appear quiescent, they secrete numerous proteins (Brunette *et al.*, 1979). When cultured, resting cells have an appearance similar to those *in vivo*, although desmosomes are poorly developed and there is no well-defined basal lamina. In

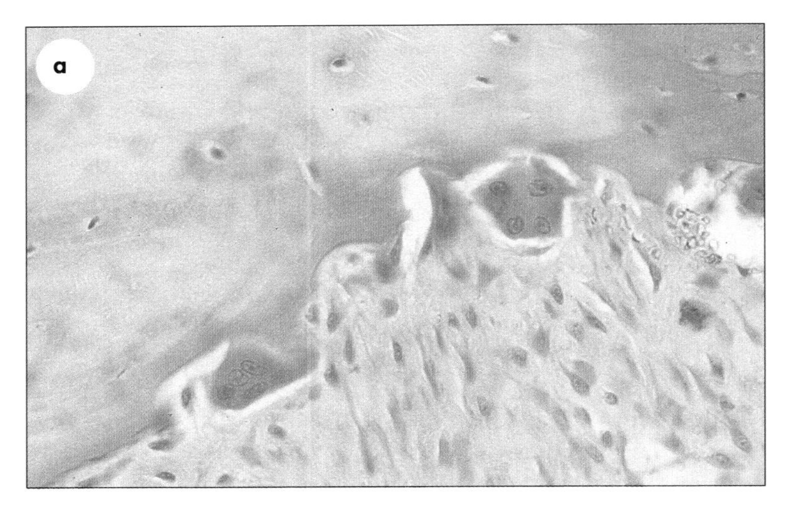

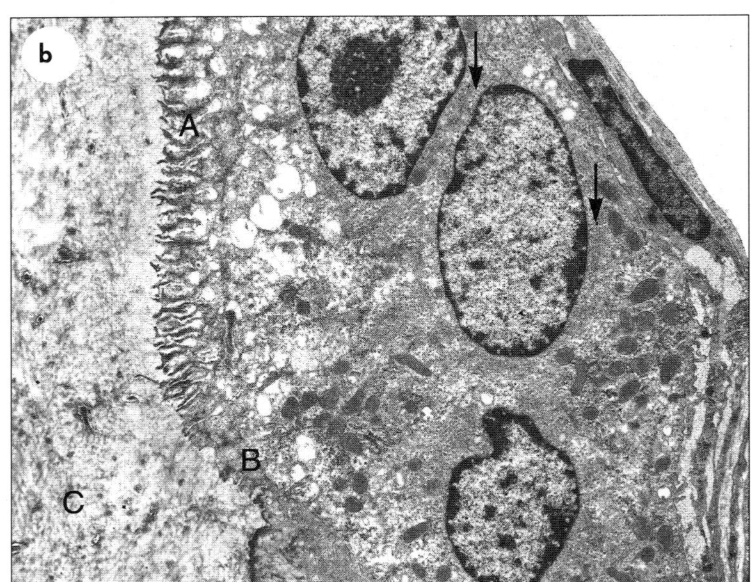

Fig. 1.19 a) Light micrograph of multinucleated osteoclasts within the periodontal ligament. Section stained with haemotoxylin and eosin. b) Electron micrograph of a multinucleated osteoclast showing general distribution of organelles. There is an abundance of vesicles and a lack of mitochondria beneath the brush border (A). Note the lack of microvilli in the 'annular zone' (B). The Golgi complex lies in a juxtanuclear position (arrow) and there is little endoplasmic reticulum. Alveolar bone (C). H & E, × 300.

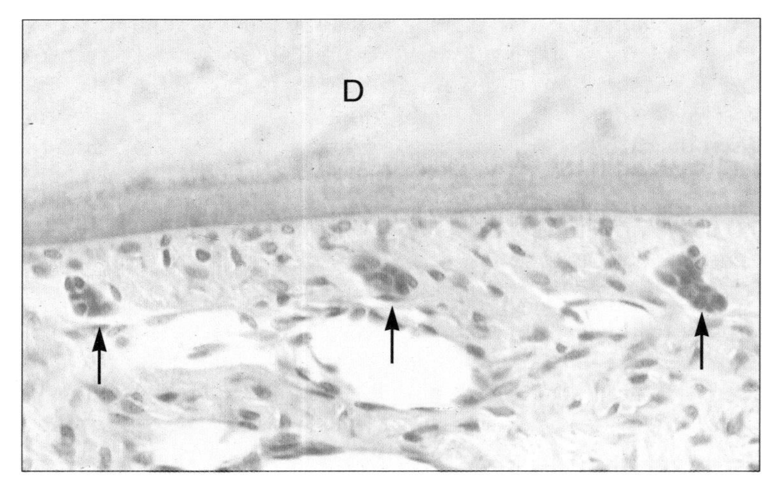

Fig. 1.20 Light micrograph of epithelial cell rests (arrowed) within the periodontal ligament. Dentine (D). H & E, magnification × 200.

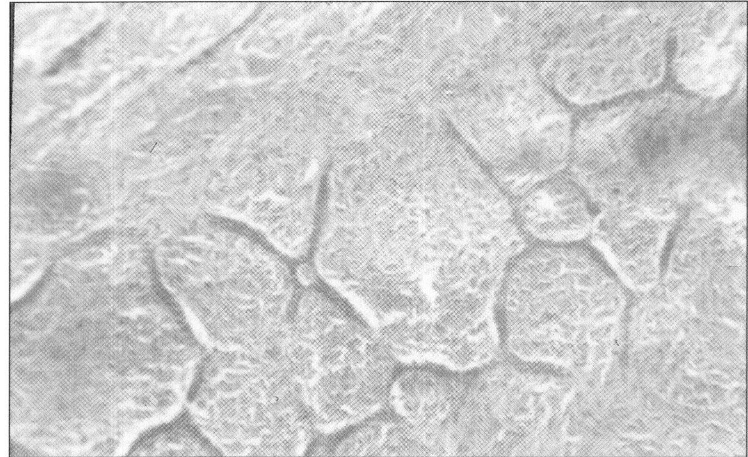

Fig. 1.21 Light micrograph of epithelial cell rests, sectioned tangentially to demonstrate their reticular nature. H & E, magnification, × 160.

proliferating cells *in vitro*, however, there is more cytoplasm, which contains more RER and free ribosomes, and there are newly synthesized actin-containing microfilaments. Furthermore, tonofilaments and desmosomes are less prominent, and there are no gap junctions (Yamasaki and Pinero, 1989). The volume of cells *in vitro* is of the order of 1600 μm^3 (Brunette *et al.*, 1979). Substances known to increase the intracellular concentration of cAMP (e.g. cholera toxin) stimulate the growth of ECR (Brunette, 1984). When cultured in collagen gels, epithelial cell rests have the ability to cause slight gel contraction, as judged by a straightening of the normal wavy alignment of the collagen (Bellows *et al.*, 1981).

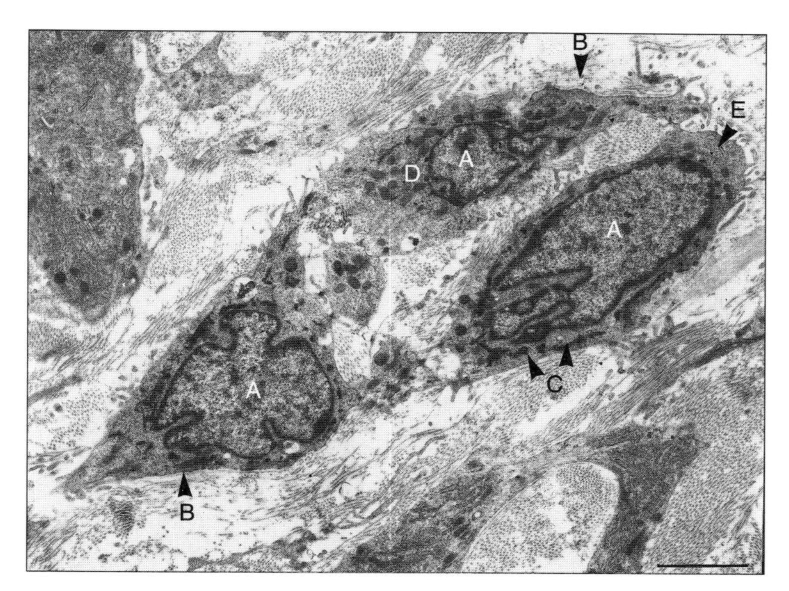

Fig. 1.22 Electron micrograph of an epithelial cell rest. Note the indented nuclei (A), fragmented basal lamina (B), tono-filaments (C), mitochondria (D) and a small amount of rough endoplasmic reticulum (E). Bar = 3.0 µm.

Compared with resting epithelial cells (which contain glycogen, demonstrate succinic dehydrogenase activity, and lack neutral fat droplets), proliferating ECR lack glycogen, exhibit a reduced succinic dehydrogenase activity, and show a significant accumulation of neutral fat droplets. These observations suggest that the endogenous protein synthesis required for cell proliferation is due partly to pentose shunt activity, indicating the ability of these cells to undertake anaerobic glycolysis (Ten Cate, 1965, 1967; Grupe *et al.*, 1967).

As many important cell functions (e.g. growth, motility, attachment, synthetic activity) are largely regulated by the extracellular matrix components, one study has examined the process of attachment of ECR to different extracellular matrix proteins and their expression of fibronectin and integrin receptors. The cells are seen to attach to, and spread rapidly on, fibronectin, vitronectin, and type I collagen. Variability is encountered, as cell lines vary in their attachment to laminin. Some epithelial cells are seen to express the fibronectin gene, while fibronectin can be identified in the tracts left behind by migrating cells. In the early stages of spreading when the cells are separated, the whole cell body stains for integrin, while later staining is limited to cell-to-cell contact areas (Uitto *et al.*, 1992). Between 2 per cent and 7 per cent of total protein secreted *in vitro* by ECR is collagenous and probably related to the basal lamina (Birek *et al.*, 1980). Of the production of glycosaminoglycans, 86 per cent is hyaluronan, 5.6 per cent is heparan sulphate, 5.1 per cent is dermatan sulphate and 3.1 per cent is chondroitin sulphate. These values are not modified when the epithelial cells are co-cultured with periodontal fibroblasts (Merrilees *et al.*, 1983).

ECR have been shown to produce prostaglandin, which *in vitro* can produce bone resorption (Brunette *et al.*, 1979: see page 24). When co-cultured with rat calvaria, the release of calcium into the culture medium indicates that ECR have the capacity to cause resorption. Although prostaglandins and other proteins are produced by the cultured epithelial cells, as bone resorption is not inhibited by the addition of indomethacin (an inhibitor of prostaglandin synthetase), factors other than prostaglandins are thought to be responsible for the resorption (Birek *et al.*, 1980). Various matrix metalloproteinases are released by ECR; these appear to have the ability to degrade collagen fibrils extracellularly (Salonen *et al.*, 1991). Factors that may be involved in the activation of such enzymes are unknown, although the state of differentiation of the cells may be an important consideration (Salonen *et al.*, 1991). Pettigrew *et al.* (1980) also report that ECR can produce a collagenolytic-enzyme inhibitor. ECR have the capacity to degrade collagen intracellularly, as evidenced by the presence of intracellular collagen profiles within the cells when cultured on collagen or demineralized dentine (Birek *et al.*, 1980; Salonen *et al.*, 1991). A lysosomal fraction from the cells has been shown to contain cathepsin D and acid phosphatase (Birek *et al.*, 1980).

CELLULAR CHANGES WITH AGE

A decrease in cellularity of the PDL with age has been reported in the premolars of dogs (Berglundh *et al.*, 1991) and the molars of rats (Klingsberg and Butcher, 1960; Jensen and Toto, 1968; Toto *et al.*, 1975), hamsters (Klingsberg and Butcher, 1960), mice (Toto and Borg, 1968), and monkeys (Klingsberg and Butcher, 1960; Levy *et al.*, 1972). For example, Toto *et al.* (1975) calculated the average cell density to be 93±9 cells per 110 µm^2 at one month, and 69±7 cells per 110 µm^2 at 15 months. Grant and Bernick (1972) and Severson *et al.* (1978) reported a decreased cellularity in the human PDL with age, although no quantitative data was presented. Severson *et al.* (1978) described the presence of fat cells, while Grant and Bernick (1972) and Levy *et al.* (1972) reported evidence of degenerative vascular changes. As atrophic changes within the periodontal ligament have been reported in association with loss of occlusal function (Cohn, 1965, 1966) and cell density and cell kinetics may be responsive to inflammatory change (Tonna and Stahl, 1974), it may be difficult to separate the changes solely related to physiological ageing with those affected by factors such as vascularity and function.

In addition to a reduction in cell density, a decrease in the mitotic index has also been described. (Jenson and Toto, 1968; Toto and Borg, 1968; Toto *et al.,* 1975). Thus, the labelling index of periodontal fibroblasts decreases from 104±3 per 1000 cells at one month to 44±1.5 per 1000 cells at 15 months for rat molars. These authors also suggested that the fibroblasts in ageing tissues had longer 'lives' than those in younger tissues.

Cho and Garant (1984) have described the presence of large, multinucleated fibroblastic cells in aged rats, which account for more than 17 per cent of the cells in the PDL. These differ from osteoclasts at the electron microscope level in that they have considerable amounts of RER, a conspicuous Golgi complex, and intracellular collagen profiles. Sasaski and Garant (1993) expanded on these observations by noting the presence of multiple centrioles, which suggest that the cells arise by cell fusion. The basic fibroblastic nature of the cells is demonstrated by their uptake of tritiated proline and by the presence of acid phosphatase activity associated with phagolysosomes. However, unlike neighbouring mononuclear fibroblasts, alkaline phosphatase is absent from the cell membranes – this may be associated in some way with the formation of the multinuclear state.

CELL KINETICS WITHIN THE PERIODONTAL LIGAMENT

As osteoblasts and cementoblasts of the periodontal ligament become incorporated into alveolar bone and cellular cementum, replacement cells must be provided within the ligament to permit osteogenesis and cementogenesis to continue. PDL fibroblasts are also generated throughout life. The question arises as to whether periodontal fibroblasts, cementoblasts, and osteoblasts all arise from a common precursor or whether each cell type has its own specific precursor cell.

To date, this has not been clarified, mainly owing to the lack of specific markers that help to distinguish precursor cells, such as the preosteoblasts, precementoblasts and prefibroblasts, from each other. However, some information is becoming available. Nuclear size can help distinguish some cell types (e.g. Roberts *et al.*, 1981), while receptors to epidermal growth factor are present during root development on preosteoblasts and periodontal fibroblasts, but not on precementoblasts, cementoblasts, and osteoblasts (Cho *et al.*, 1991).

Studies have shown that approximately 0.5–3 per cent of cells within the PDL are initially labelled (i.e. labelling index) following an injection of tritiated thymidine (e.g. Jensen and Toto, 1968; Toto and Kwan, 1970; Roberts and Jee, 1974; Smith and Roberts, 1980; McCulloch and Melcher, 1983a,b,c; McCulloch *et al.*, (1989). Such variation may be related to diurnal periodicity (with the maximum percent of labelled cells being encountered between 09:00 and 10:00 hours – Roberts, 1975a; Roberts *et al.,* 1979; Singh *et al.*, 1987), or it may be related to location within the ligament or to individual variation (Gould *et al.*, 1982; McCulloch and Melcher, 1983a). With age, there is an overall reduction in the labelling index (Jensen and Toto, 1968; Toto and Borg, 1968; Toto *et al.,* 1975).

Dividing progenitor cells within the periodontal ligament are located predominantly paravascularly (Gould *et al.,* 1982; McCulloch and Melcher, 1983b,c; Roberts *et al.*, 1987) and give rise to cells that can migrate towards the bone and cement surfaces, where they differentiate into osteoblasts and cementoblasts (McCulloch and Melcher, 1983b). McCulloch (1985) identified a population of cells within 10 μm of blood vessels. These cells traversed the cell cycle more slowly than other proliferating cells located further from the blood vessels. This suggested that this population may represent stem cells that are not terminally differentiated but that continue to divide at a slow rate – one daughter cell of each division migrates away from the vessel and undergoes two or three further rapid divisions and differentiates into a fibroblast, osteoblast, or cementoblast; the other daughter cell remains undifferentiated and is capable of unequal mitosis like the original cell.

McCulloch and Melcher (1983c) investigated the relationship between cell density and cell generation within the periodontal ligament. In addition to finding that labelling indices are highest in zones adjacent to blood vessels (which lay mainly next to bone), McCulloch and Melcher (1983c) and McCulloch *et al.* (1989) also reported that labelling indices were significantly higher in the middle of the ligament, where cell density was lower, compared with zones adjacent to bone and cementum, where cell density was higher.

Yee (1979), Gould *et al.* (1980) and Gould (1983) have studied the morphology of progenitor cells in the periodontal ligament. Whilst it may be expected that such cells (identified at their mitotic phase or at their synthetic phase following uptake of tritiated thymidine) would have a relatively undifferentiated appearance (e.g. small size, scarcity of intracellular organelles, and a high nuclear–cytoplasmic ratio), some progenitor cells have been shown to be relatively well-differentiated, containing much RER and even intracellular collagen profiles.

With continuous infusion of thymidine (obtained by using osmotic minipumps), the labelling index rises from about 1 per cent at the beginning to between 30 per cent and 50 per cent by the end of 40–60 days (Gould *et al.*, 1982; McCulloch and Melcher, 1983a). This has been interpreted as indicating that the 50 per cent or more of unlabelled cells have either lost the capacity for mitosis or have cycle times that are longer than 60 days (McCulloch and Melcher, 1983a). The cell cycle time for roughly one half of the cells in the normal periodontal ligament has been calculated to be less than 48 hours, while that of many of the proliferating cells associated with orthodontically stimulated teeth has been calculated to be about 32–36 hours (Roberts, 1975a; Roberts *et al.*, 1981). For PDL fibroblasts, Gould *et al.* (1983) have calculated a turnover time of 45 days, there being a slight increase with age. Although the majority of labelled cells divided within three days after a pulse injection of tritiated thymidine, a measurable population of labelled cells had not divided even after 14 days, being G_2-blocked (McCulloch and Melcher, 1983a).

One of the major problems in studying cell kinetics of the PDL is the heterogeneity of the system (reviewed by McCulloch and Bordin, 1991). Thus, cells incorporating tritiated thymidine may not only be true stem cells, but may also be cells already partially differentiated as preosteoblasts, precementoblasts, and prefibroblasts; however, as previously mentioned, the lack of specific cell markers makes such identification difficult. In a series of investigations, Roberts and co-workers have detailed much information on the cell kinetics of the periodontal osteoblast and have particularly used orthodontically induced osteogenesis as the model system, thereby increasing the number of proliferating osteogenic cells for study within the periodontal ligament. For an account of the origin of bone-forming cells in general, see Marks and Popoff (1988) and Tenenbaum (1991).

Although Roberts and Chase (1981) administered tritiated thymidine after orthodontically induced osteogenesis, they found that the initial layer of osteoblasts was unlabelled. This implies that among the cells of the normal PDL are preosteoblasts that are sufficiently differentiated to become osteoblasts without synthesizing DNA. Indeed, these authors report that approximately half the fibroblast-like cells of periodontal ligament contribute to osteoblast production. Bearing in mind that virtually all cells across the ligament synthesize collagen, as judged by autoradiographic studies using tritiated proline (e.g. Beertsen and Everts, 1977; Rippin, 1978), this might indicate that such preosteoblasts contribute to the formation of periodontal ligament collagen before finally differentiating into osteoblasts (Roberts *et al.*, 1982).

Although there are no specific biochemical markers to distinguish the different connective tissue-type cells in the periodontal ligament, Roberts *et al.* (1981, 1982, 1987) and Roberts and Ferguson (1989) used nuclear size to classify cells in the periodontal ligament after orthodontically induced osteogenesis. In control ligaments, four broad categories of increasing nuclear size could be discerned: A cells (nuclear diameter 40–79 μm^3), B cells (80–119 μm^3), C cells (120–169 μm^3), and D cells (nuclear diameter more than 170 μm^3). The small precursor cells (A cells) are the self-perpetuating source of progenitors, while the committed osteoprogenitor cells (A´ cells) move from their paravascular position and enter an area of relatively low cell density, where they enlarge and differentiate into G_1 preosteoblasts (C cells). This migration suggests that regions of higher cell density may suppress cell proliferation. C cells then synthesize DNA to become G_2 preosteoblasts (D cells), which divide and then migrate towards the bone surface to form osteoblasts. Calculations for cell cycle time during orthodontically induced osteogenesis are: G_1 phase – 21 hours, S phase – 9 hours, G_2 phase – 2.5 hours, M phase – 1.2 hours. Note that population B would represent typical PDL fibroblasts.

The relatively low labelling index seen in the normal physiological state can be significantly increased by various experimental procedures. However, the heterogeneity of the patterns of cell proliferation elicited by orthodontic forces (e.g. Roberts and Chase, 1981), endocrine factors (Roberts, 1975b), trauma (Gould *et al.*, 1979, 1980), and electrical stimulation (Davidovitch *et al.*, 1980) suggests that the progenitor cells are a mixed population with regard to the induction of proliferation (Roberts *et al.*, 1982). For example, in contrast to the primarily paravascular proliferation of traumatized periodontal ligament (Gould *et al.*, 1979, 1980), cells entering the S phase after orthodontic stimulation are widely distributed throughout the tissue and migrate mainly towards alveolar bone to form osteoblasts (Roberts and Chase 1981). Thus, orthodontic pressure and injury may recruit progenitors that are distinctly different cell types (osteogenic versus fibroblastic), or the proliferating progenitors may represent individual components of the same sequence.

As there is no increase in the number of cells within the periodontal ligament with age, the periodontal ligament has been regarded as a slowly renewing tissue (McCulloch and Melcher, 1983b). Homeostatic mechanisms must exist within the tissue whereby cell generation is in equilibrium with cell death or cell migration (McCulloch and Melcher, 1983c). Preliminary studies that mention evidence of some cell death have been presented by Schellens *et al.* (1982) and McCulloch and Melcher (1983a). However, a detailed study has recently been documented by McCulloch *et al.* (1989). These authors quantified the number of cells exhibiting histological evidence associated with 'dying' cells at the ultrastructural level. They calculated that the average number of dying cells is 0.65 per cent, but that this percentage is five times higher within 20 μm of bone and cementum than in the middle of the PDL. As the less cellular regions in this middle zone of the ligament are particularly rich in progenitor cells (McCulloch and Melcher, 1983), McCulloch *et al.* (1989) suggested that progenitor cells born in the midzone of the ligament (and perhaps outside the ligament) migrate to bone and cementum, where they may ultimately die or become incorporated as either osteocytes or cementocytes. These authors also noted that the mechanism of removal of dying cells is obscure but that it is not the result of phagocytosis by macrophages.

In the normal physiological state, few labelled cells appear to be lost from the periodontal ligament by incorporation into bone or cement (McCulloch and Melcher, 1983b). Davidson and McCulloch (1986) tested their data for cell proliferation times against two models. One model assumed that all proliferating cells were homogeneous and proceeded through the cell cycle at a rate described by an exponential distribution. The other model assumed that mitosis produced one proliferating and one differentiated cell, each with a characteristic and distinct lifetime and proliferative capacity. Their data best fitted the latter model.

In modelling the cell kinetics of the periodontal ligament, one could assume that the system is a more or less closed one. However, McCulloch *et al.* (1987) have provided some evidence that raises the possibility that cells may migrate out from the endosteal spaces in the alveolar bone (which are in continuity with the periodontal ligament) and into the ligament, thereby augmenting the populations of fibroblasts, osteoblasts. and cementoblasts. Some support for this is found in the observation that cells derived from bone can synthesize cementum-like and bone-like tissue *in vitro* (Melcher *et al.*, 1986).

In addition to the 'blast' type of cells, the periodontal ligament also contains osteoclasts and odontoclasts. The origin of the osteoclasts has been the subject of a number of recent reviews (e.g. Mundy and Roodman, 1987; Marks and Popoff, 1988; Chambers, 1991; Nijweide and de Grooth, 1991; Burger and Nijweide, 1991). Unlike fibroblasts, osteoblasts, and cementoblasts, which are derived from precursors of connective tissue origin, osteoclasts are derived from haemopoietic stem cells. This extraskeletal origin of osteoclasts implies that osteoclasts are not normal resident cells of the periodontal ligament, but enter the ligament as mononuclear cells from the haemopoetic system as required and then fuse to form the typical large, multinucleated giant cell.

There are three main views concerning the origin of the osteoclast. One is that osteoclasts result from the fusion of monocytes or macrophages, or both. A second view states that osteoclasts share a common progenitor (e.g. promonocyte or monoblast) with cells of the monocyte–macrophage line. A third view suggests that osteoclasts have an origin from a pluripotent haemopoietic stem cell entirely separate from that of the monocyte–macrophage line. As yet, the precise origin of the osteoclast is not known

Within the periodontal ligament, there is evidence that the first cells to form osteoclasts are local preosteoclasts, followed by circulating preosteoclasts (Roberts, 1975b). Little is known about the odontoclast (cementoclast), although it is assumed that its origin is similar to that of the osteoclast.

TISSUE CULTURE STUDIES INVOLVING PERIODONTAL LIGAMENT CELLS

Tissue culture studies have been undertaken on periodontal ligament cells principally to determine:

- cellular properties not readily obtained from *in vivo* investigations, such as cell motility and cell traction;
- what biologically active substances the cells secrete in relation to health and possible disease; and
- how the cells react to certain biologically active molecules.

One of the most difficult aspects of *in vitro* studies is the extrapolation of the results to the *in vivo* situation. Clearly, when cells are removed from their *in vivo* situation and cultured on glass or plastic, their environment totally changes. This is of particular relevance in the case of the periodontal ligament, which can be considered highly specialised in terms of its high metabolic activity and vascularity. Even when cells are cultured in collagen gels, this environment bears little similarity to the dense and specialized extracellular matrix seen *in vivo*. That the environment can readily influence cells *in vitro* is seen from the different appearance of cells when cultured in the presence or absence of collagen gels (e.g. Hay, 1982; Tomasek *et al.*, 1982).

As a case study in the care that must be taken before extrapolating from *in vitro* studies, the example of the effects of prostaglandin on bone can be highlighted. All the *in vitro* studies suggested that this molecule increases bone resorption. However, its effect *in vivo* is to increase bone remodelling with more bone formation, resulting in a net increase in bone mass. Therefore, in situations where osteogenesis is not sustainable, as is the case for most bone organ culture systems, the net effects are catabolic (for discussion of this topic, see Marks and Miller, 1993).

A population of PDL fibroblasts may be obtained by culturing portions of the periodontal ligament as explants, or by immediately releasing the cells from the periodontal ligament with enzymes (reviewed by Sodek, 1983). The whole of the tooth, plus the attachment tissues, has also been grown in organ culture (Melcher and Turnbull, 1976; Duncan *et al.*, 1984). The lack of standardization of culture methods in general does not make it easy to directly compare the results of different authors. Because of the heterogeneous nature of the original cell population of the ligament and because of the difficulties previously referred to concerning the identity of specific cell populations, it is not easy to determine what population of cells is being cultured. Furthermore, the culture technique used may select for a particular subpopulation of cells, while the properties of the cells may change with the number of passages (Murphy and Daniel, 1987).

One of the fundamental questions relating to tissue culture of PDL fibroblasts is how closely the cells resemble those *in vivo*. Although some similarities between the two have been reported (e.g. Rose *et al.,* 1987), Gabbiani (1979) is of the opinion that cultured fibroblasts in general are cytologically very different from fibroblasts *in vivo*, especially with regard to the content and organization of filaments and contractile proteins (i.e. they resemble myofibroblasts more closely); this appears to be supported for PDL fibroblasts by the observations of Bellows *et al.* (1981). In this context, Pender and McCulloch (1991) report that the total actin in PDL fibroblasts *in vitro* is still about three times higher than for gingival fibroblasts. Certainly, the general shape that is seen in tissue culture, which is referred to by most authors as being typical of the fibroblast, is highly elongated and unlike the more rounded cells reported *in vivo* (see page 00). Furthermore, the work of Hou *et al* (1993) seems to indicate that little collagen is secreted extracellularly during culture of PDL fibroblasts (assuming they are not left in confluence for prolonged periods).

Important properties of fibroblasts studied *in vitro* relate to motility and contractility, as these properties may be associated with generating the force of tooth eruption and with orienting the fibres of the periodontal ligament (e.g. Bellows *et al.,* 1981; Garant and Cho, 1989). Fibroblasts have been observed to migrate at rates varying from about 1 μm/minute to 3 μm/minute (Couchman and Rees, 1979; Pouyssegur and Pastan, 1979; Harris *et al.,* 1981;). A rate for periodontal fibroblasts of 12.5 μm/hour can be calculated from data reported by Brunette *et al.* (1976). These rates are of importance if it is believed that the eruptive force is generated by the active migration of periodontal fibroblasts, as eruption rates can reach as high as 1 mm/day (see Chapter 9). However, when considering the rates *in vivo*, one must bear in mind the possible inhibitory effect of the presence of the fibrous extracellular matrix (Bard and Hay, 1975).

Beertsen *et al.* (1974) and Beertsen (1975) suggest that the presence of microfilaments and microtubules within periodontal ligament fibroblasts are consistent with the cells being motile, as such organelles are also evident in fibroblasts migrating *in vitro*. However, there is evidence that well organized stress fibres are not present in actively migrating cells *in vitro* (e.g. Burridge, 1981; Herman *et al.*, 1981; Willingham *et al.,* 1981). Indeed, the presence of stress fibres may reflect the method of tissue culture, as cells moving on planar substrata were found to exhibit stress fibres, which were not evident when cells were moving in collagen gels (Tomasek *et al.,*1982). Wood and Thorogood (1987) also report that migrating mesenchymal cells *in vivo* show an absence of cytoskeletal organization.

Motility of fibroblasts is clearly affected by interactions with components of the extracellular matrix. Knowledge of this process is essential in understanding the regenerative processes associated with periodontal wound healing and guided tissue regeneration (see Chapter 16). In this context, Somerman *et al.* (1992) have observed differences in attachment properties between fibroblasts derived from adult periodontal ligaments compared with those derived from the developing dental follicle.

Melcher and Beertsen (1977) have suggested that the presence of microtubules and microfilaments in cells provides a structural basis for a motile system. Initially, there is extension of cell processes and attachment to collagen fibrils or to other cells; the subsequent withdrawal of these processes could draw the collagen fibrils or cells closer together. Because of the alignment of the fibres, this could then result in movement of the tooth in an occlusal direction. The combination of migration and contraction has been termed 'traction' by Stopak and Harris (1982), and this topic has recently been reviewed by Aubin (1989) and by Aubin and Opas (1989). Some evidence in support of this view has been derived from *in vitro* studies in which monkey PDL fibroblasts were incorporated into three-dimensional collagen gels, resulting in contraction of the gel (i.e. Bellows *et al.*, 1981) – contraction using monkey periodontal fibroblasts has been reported to be greater than with other types of cell, including human gingival fibroblasts.

In this context, Pender and McCulloch (1991) have demonstrated that human PDL fibroblasts have more actin *in vitro* than gingival fibroblasts. Bellows *et al.* (1982) also demonstrated that sufficient tension is developed to bring together fragments of tooth and bone that are initially placed some distance apart within the gel; this contraction is inhibited by colcemid and cytochalasin D, which suggests that microtubules and microfilaments are involved. While confirming that human PDL fibroblasts contract collagen gels, Murphy and Daniel (1987) found that the amount of contraction did not differ significantly between periodontal fibroblasts and fibroblasts derived from human sclera or foreskin, and that human gingival fibroblasts produced the most contraction. Hughes and Issberner (1988) also reported that PDL fibroblasts contract collagen gels less than gingival and oral mucosa fibroblasts. Using strain gauges attached to contracting collagen gels, Kasugi *et al.* (1990) have calculated that the isometric force that can be exerted by a periodontal fibroblast is 5×10^{-8}N (this is 1–2 per cent of the isometric force that can be exerted by a smooth muscle cell). In view of the importance that has been placed on fibroblast motility in generating the force of tooth eruption, it is noteworthy that Harris *et al.* (1981) found that the more motile cells (e.g. macrophages, leucocytes, and transformed fibroblasts) exert the weakest tractional forces.

The most detailed study of the morphology of PDL fibroblasts during gel contraction has been carried out by Bellows *et al.* (1982). The cells appear spindle-shaped. Ultrastructurally, they are similar to myofibroblasts, possessing thick cell coats, considerable amounts of microfilamentous material dispersed throughout the cytoplasm, numerous structures resembling gap junctions, occasional crenulated nuclei, and little RER. In exhibiting these features, however, fibroblasts *in vitro* seem to differ from *in vivo* periodontal fibroblasts, which have an irregular discoid shape, with cytoplasm that contains considerable amounts of RER and microfilamentous material, primarily in the form of stress fibres beneath the cell membrane (Beertsen *et al.*, 1974; Beertsen and Everts, 1977; Shore and Berkovitz, 1979; Berkovitz, 1981). Gap junctions are infrequent *in vivo*, where the more common type of intercellular contact is the simplified desmosome (Shore *et al.*, 1981). Significantly, as contraction of the collagen gel *in vitro* ceases, the morphology of the cultured fibroblasts changes to resemble PDL fibroblasts *in vivo* – the cells assume a more rounded morphology, they exhibit extensive endoplasmic reticulum, and they show few gap junctions but more desmosome-like contacts (Bellows *et al.*, 1982). This change in morphology of fibroblasts during gel contraction is presumably related to a change in function, knowledge of which might enhance our understanding of the role of periodontal fibroblasts *in vivo*.

Whereas the contraction of granulation tissue (containing myofibroblasts) is affected by colchicine, cytochalasin B, 5-hydroxytryptamine, angiotensin, and histamine, no such effect has been demonstrated on strips of uninjured subcutaneous connective tissue (Van den Brenk and Stone, 1974). It would be of obvious interest to know how the PDL reacted *in vivo* to pharmacological agents which affect smooth muscle. Studies on granulation tissue have shown the fibronexus to be the predominant binding site attaching myofibroblasts to each other, gap junctions making up only 4 per cent of such structures (Singer *et al.*, 1984). This led the authors to conclude that the fibronexus may serve to transmit the collective forces generated by the contraction of actin microfilaments within myofibroblasts throughout the granulation tissue, and thereby effect wound contraction. Although the fibronexus has been described as being present in fibroblasts in the transseptal fibre region of the gingiva (Garant *et al.*, 1982), more detailed study reveals that these specialized contact areas are present only in inflamed gingiva (Cho *et al.*, 1988). Larjava *et al.* (1989) compared human granulation tissue fibroblasts in oral chronic inflammatory lesions with gingival fibroblasts with respect to cell surface sialoglycoproteins and the synthesis of extracellular matrix components. Though there were general similarities, the authors concluded that granulation tissue fibroblasts represent a distinct phenotype of fibroblastic cell.

As with the *in vivo* situation, Svoboda *et al.* (1979) have demonstrated the ability of PDL fibroblasts to phagocytose collagen *in vitro*. However, because the number of intracellular collagen profiles increased over time, there is no clear evidence as to whether intracellular degradation occurs in this *in vitro* situation.

Limeback *et al.* (1978) and Limeback and Sodek (1979) have shown that periodontal fibroblasts *in vitro* synthesize both type I and type III collagen in the approximate ratios seen *in vivo*. However, the difference in metabolic rate demonstrated *in vivo* between periodontal ligament, gingival fibroblasts, and skin fibroblasts (Sodek, 1977, 1978) is not reproduced *in vitro* (Limeback *et al.*, 1978; Mariotti and Cochran, 1990). Furthermore, the amount of type III collagen decreases on subculturing (Limeback and Sodek, 1979). Limeback *et al.* (1983) found that primary cultures of periodontal fibroblasts contain a heterogeneous mixture of cells that not only synthesize different levels of collagen but also produce different ratios of type I and type III collagen. Also, 99 per cent of fibroblasts produce both collagen and fibronectin (Connor *et al.*, 1983).

An enzyme that belongs to the neutral-metalloproteinases and that is released in latent form is produced by PDL fibroblasts *in vitro* (Overall and Sodek, 1987; Otsuka *et al.*, 1988), and non-specific and specific gelatinase activities have also been described by Pettigrew *et al.* (1980). Some anticollagenase activity has also been documented (Morris and Harper, 1987; Otsuka *et al.*, 1988). Stopp *et al.* (1989) have reported that the protein content of individual PDL fibroblasts decreases during culture and attainment of cellular confluence; they related this decrease to reduced cell proliferation, reduced *de novo* protein synthesis, and reduced cell volume.

Studies have been undertaken on the nature of the glycosaminoglycans (GAG) synthesized by PDL fibroblasts, chiefly by Merrilees *et al.* (1983), Smalley *et al.* (1984), Mariotti and Cochran (1990), and Larjava *et al.* (1992); these are discussed in Chapter 4.

Like cells *in vivo* (Nojima *et al.*, 1990), periodontal fibroblasts *in vitro* are generally rich in alkaline phosphatase (e.g. Yamashita *et al.*, 1987; Piche *et al.*, 1989; Nojima *et al.*, 1990; Somerman *et al.*, 1990; Arceo *et al.*, 1991; Takeshita *et al.*, 1992). The finding of some cell lines with low levels of this enzyme may reflect the heterogeneity of the cells of the PDL (Piche *et al.*, 1989). PDL fibroblasts can also synthesize the bone-associated proteins, osteonectin and gla-protein (Wasi *et al.*, 1984; Nojima *et al.*, 1990; Arceo *et al.*, 1991). These features show that periodontal fibroblasts have some osteoblast-like properties, which may not be surprising considering that many of the component cells of the ligament are of the osteoblast lineage. In this respect and in some others, periodontal fibroblasts differ from gingival fibroblasts; this may be significant in terms of periodontal wound healing (e.g. Piche *et al.,* 1989; Somerman *et al.,* 1989, 1990, 1992; Mariotti and Cochran, 1990; Matsuda *et al.,* 1992; see also Chapter 16). Indeed, PDL fibroblasts can initiate the formation of mineral-like nodules *in vitro* (Melcher *et al.,* 1986; Arceo *et al.,* 1991). The cells also release a bone resorption inhibition factor (Giniger *et al.,* 1991), as well as prostaglandin (Ngan *et al.,* 1988; Saito *et al.,* 1991). Like true bone cells, Ngan *et al.* (1988) and Saito *et al.* (1990a) report that periodontal fibroblasts respond to parathormone by increased levels of prostaglandins, while Nojima *et al.* (1990) found increased production of cAMP. However, Somerman *et al.* (1990) found that periodontal fibroblasts did not respond to parathormone or calcitonin.

In vitro systems have been designed to subject periodontal fibroblasts to tension or pressure in the hope of obtaining information to aid our understanding of processes such as orthodontic tooth movement. For example, cells respond to mechanical stress by an increase in the amount of type III collagen synthesized (Duncan *et al.,* 1984), and by an elevated synthesis of prostaglandin and cAMP (Ngan *et al.,* 1990). Mechanical stretching reduces F-actin in PDL fibroblasts, unlike the situation for gingival fibroblasts, where the level is rapidly increased (Pender and McCulloch, 1991).

A number of tissue culture studies have been undertaken to determine the effects of various biologically active molecules, especially growth factors and cytokines, on PDL fibroblasts in an attempt to understand and improve periodontal wound healing. Growth factors have been reported as having variable effects, though they are generally mitogenic (Rutherford *et al.,* 1992; Blom *et al.*, 1992; Matsuda *et al.,* 1992; Takeshita *et al.,* 1992). In addition to their possible effects on cell proliferation, growth factors can modulate the rate of protein production by fibroblasts. TGF-β increases the secretion of collagen (Narayanan *et al.,* 1989; Matsuda *et al.,* 1992; Wise *et al.,* 1992). Cytokines (e.g. interleukin 1, tumour necrosis factor, interferon) have also been shown to increase the production of prostaglandin (Davidovitch *et al.,* 1988; Richards and Rutherford, 1988; Ngan *et al.,* 1988; Saito *et al.,* 1990a,b,c; Davidovitch, 1991). They can also increase the production of procollagenase (Richards and Rutherford, 1990) and elevate the level of cAMP (Ngan *et al.,* 1988).

These investigations highlight the importance of interactions between the cytokine-producing cells (such as monocytes and macrophages) and periodontal fibroblasts in both health and disease. These topics are considered further in Chapters 12 and 14.

DEFENCE CELLS

Like other soft fibrous connective tissues, the periodontal ligament contains defence cells, including macrophages, mast cells, and eosinophils. These cells achieve most importance during inflammatory periodontal disease and are considered in Chapters 14.

McCulloch *et al.* (1989) described the detailed distribution of the macrophage in the healthy periodontal ligament using electron microscopy. Among the features which distinguish the macrophage from the fibroblast are numerous microvilli and lysosomes and other membrane-bound vesicles of varying density, and the paucity of RER and Golgi complex (*Fig. 1.23*). These authors found that macrophages comprise just under 4 per cent of the cells of the periodontal ligament and are located close to blood vessels. As the labelling index of perivascular cells is high compared with other regions of the ligament, McCulloch *et al.* (1989) raised the possibility that lymphokines released from macrophages may be involved in cell kinetics. Studies have shown that granules released by mast cells may be phagocytosed by fibroblasts, suggesting that other interactions may occur between mast cells and fibroblasts (Atkins *et al.*, 1985).

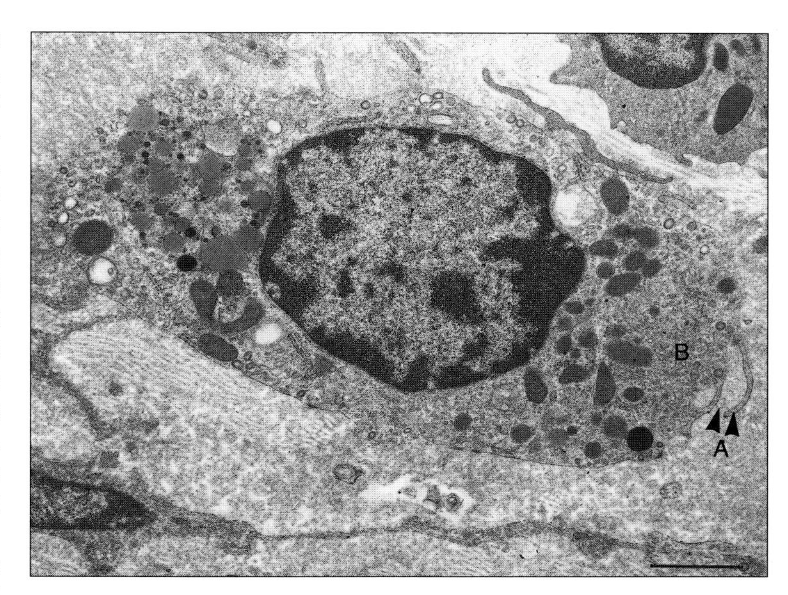

Fig. 1.23 Electron micrograph of a macrophage. There are a larger number of lysosomes and mitochondria. Note the paucity of rough endoplasmic reticulum. A = microvilli, B = Golgi complex. Bar = 1.5 μm.

REFERENCES

Addison WC (1979) The distribution of nuclei in human odontoclasts in whole cell preparations. Arch Oral Biol 23, 1167–1171.

Allison AC (1973) The role of microfilaments and microtubules in cell movement, endocytosis and exocytosis. In: Locomotion of Tissue Cells, pp110–143, Elsevier, Amsterdam.

Arceo N, Sauk JJ, Moehring J, Foster RR, Somerman MJ (1991) Human periodontal cells initiate mineral-like nodules in vitro. J Periodontol 62, 499–503.

Atkins FM, Friedman MM, Subba Rao PV and Metcalfe DD (1985) Interactions between mast cells, fibroblasts and connective tissue components. Int Arch Allergy Appl Immun 77, 96–102.

Aubin JA (1989) The role of the cytoskeleton and cell adhesion in the periodontal ligament during tooth movement. In: The Biology of Tooth Movement (Norton LA and Burstone CJ, eds), pp 201–226, CRC Press, Boca Raton, Florida.

Aubin JA and Opas M (1989) Cell adhesion and contractility. In: Biological Mechanisms of Tooth Eruption and Root Resorption (Davidovitch Z, ed), pp 43–51, EBSCO Media, Birmingham, Alabama.

Azuma M, Enlow DG, Fredrickson RG and Gaston LF (1975) A myofibroblastic basis for the physical forces that produce tooth drift and eruption, skeletal displacement of sutures and periosteal migration. In: Determinants of Mandibular Form and Growth (McNamara JA, ed), pp 179–207, University of Michigan, Michigan.

Bard JBL and Hay ED (1975) The behaviour of fibroblasts from the developing avian cornea. J Cell Biol 67, 400–418.

Bartold PM and Haynes DR (1991) Interleukin-6 production by human gingival fibroblasts. J Periodont Res 26, 339–345.

Beertsen W (1975) Migration of fibroblasts in the periodontal ligament of the mouse incisor as revealed by autoradiography. Arch Oral Biol 20, 659–666.

Beertsen W and Everts V (1977) The site of remodelling of collagen in the periodontal ligament of the mouse incisor. Anat Rec 189, 479–498.

Beertsen W and Everts V (1980) Junctions between fibroblasts in mouse periodontal ligament. J Periodont Res 15, 655–688.

Beertsen W, Everts V and Brekelsman M (1979) Unipolarity of fibroblasts in rodent periodontal ligament. Anat Rec 195, 535–544.

Beertsen W, Everts V and van den Hooff A (1974) Fine structure of fibroblasts in the periodontal ligament of the rat incisor and their possible role in tooth eruption. Arch Oral Biol 19, 1087–1098.

Beertsen W, Everts V and Houtkooper JM (1979) Frequency of occurrence and position of cilia in fibroblasts of the periodontal ligament of the mouse incisor. Cell Tissue Res 163, 415–431.

Bélanger LF (1971) Osteocytic resorption. In: The Biochemistry and Physiology of Bone, Vol. 3 (Bourne GH, ed), pp 240–270, Academic Press, New York.

Bellows CG, Melcher AH and Aubin JE (1981) Contraction and organization of collagen gels by cells cultured from periodontal ligament, gingiva and bone suggest functional differences between cell types. J Cell Sci 50, 299–314.

Bellows CG, Melcher AH and Aubin JE (1982a) Association between tension and orientation of periodontal ligament fibroblasts and exogenous collagen fibres in collagen gels in vitro. J Cell Sci 58, 125–138.

Bellows CG, Melcher AH, Bhargava U and Aubin JE (1982b) Fibroblasts contracting three-dimensional collagen gels exhibit ultrastructure consistent with either contraction or protein secretion. J Ultrastruct Res 78, 178–192.

Berglundh T, Linde J and Sterrett JD (1991) Clinical and structural characteristics of periodontal tissues in young and old dogs. J Clin Periodontol 18, 616–623.

Berkovitz BKB (1981) A critique of the fibroblast migration hypothesis of tooth eruption with a note on the tissue fluid pressure hypothesis. In: Orthodontics: The State of the Art (Barrer HG, ed), pp 239–255, University of Philadelphia Press, Philadelphia.

Berkovitz BKB (1988) Structural observations on the periodontal ligament in relation to the eruptive mechanism. In: Biological Mechanisms of Tooth Eruption and Root Resorption (Davidovitch Z, ed), pp 227–291, EBSCO Media, Birmingham, Alabama.

Berkovitz BKB and Maden M (1993) Cellular retinoic acid binding protein in the periodontal ligament. J Periodontol 64, 392–396.

Bienkowski RS, Cowan MJ, McDonald JA and Crystal RG (1978) Degradation of newly synthesised collagen. J Biol Chem 253, 4356–4363.

Bienkowski RS and Engels CJ (1981) Measurement of intracellular collagen degradation. Analyt Biochem 116, 414–424.

Birek P, Wang H-M, Brunette DM and Melcher AH (1980) Epithelial rests of Malasses in vitro. Lab Invest 43, 61–72.

Blom S, Holmstrup P and Dabelsteen E (1992) The effect of insulin-like growth factor-I and human growth hormone on periodontal ligament fibroblasts morphology, growth pattern, DNA synthesis and receptor binding. J Periodontol 63, 960–968.

Boyle PE (1947) Effects of vitamin A deficiency on the periodontal tissues. Am J Orthod 33, 744–748.

Brice GL, Sampson WJ and Sims MR (1991) An ultrastructural evaluation of the relationship between epithelial rests of Malassez and orthodontic root resorption and repair in man. Aust Orthod J 12, 90–94.

Brinkley BR (1982) The cytoskeleton: a perspective. In: Methods in Cell Biology, volume 24: The Cytoskeleton (Wilson L, ed), pp 1–8, Academic Press, New York.

Brunette DM (1984) Cholera toxin and dibutyl cyclic AMP stimulate the growth of epithelial cells derived from epithelial rests from porcine periodontal ligament. Arch Oral Biol 29, 303–309.

Brunette DM, Heersche JNM, Purdon AD, Sodek J, Moe HK and Assuras JN (1979) In vitro cultural parameters and protein and prostaglandin secretion of epithelial cells derived from porcine rests of Malassez. Arch Oral Biol 24, 199–203.

Brunette DM, Kanoza RJ, Marmary Y, Chan J and Melcher AH (1977) Interactions between epithelial and fibroblast-like cells in cultures derived from monkey periodontal ligament. J Cell Sci 27, 127–140.

Brunette DM, Melcher AH and Moe HK (1976) Culture and origin of epithelial-like and fibroblast-like cells from porcine periodontal ligament explants and cell suspensions. Arch Oral Biol 21, 393–400.

Bryer LW (1957) An experimental evaluation of the physiology of tooth eruption. Int Dent J 7, 432–478.

Burger EH and Nijweide PJ (1991) Cellular origin and theories of osteoclast differentiation. In: Bone, volume 2: The Osteoclast (Hall BK, ed), pp 31–60, CRC Press, Boca Raton, Florida.

Burridge K (1981) Are stress fibres contractile? Nature 294, 691–692.

Chambers TC (1991) Regulation of osteoclast development and function. In: Biology and Physiology of the Osteoclast. (Rifkin BR and Gay CV, eds), pp 337–356, CRC Press, Boca Raton, Florida.

Cho MI and Garant PR (1981a) An electron microscopic radioautographic study of collagen secretion in periodontal ligament fibroblasts of the mouse: I. Normal fibroblasts. Anat Rec 201, 577–586.

Cho MI and Garant PR (1981b) An electron microscopic radioautographic study of collagen secretion in periodontal ligament fibroblasts of the mouse: II. Colchicine-treated fibroblasts. Anat Rec 201, 587–598.

Cho MI and Garant PR (1984) Formation of multinuclear fibroblasts in the periodontal ligaments of old mice. Anat Rec 208, 185–196.

Cho MI, Garant PR and Lee LL (1988) Immunocytochemical in vivo localization of fibronectin-rich contact sites on fibroblasts of normal periodontal ligament and inflamed gingiva. J Periodont Res 23, 230–238.

Cho MI, Lin WL and Garant PR (1991) Occurrence of epidermal growth factor binding sites during differentiation of cementoblasts and periodontal ligament fibroblasts of the young rat: a light and electron microscopic radioautographic study. Anat Rec 231, 14–24.

Cohn SA (1965) Disuse atrophy of the periodontium in mice. Arch Oral Biol 10, 909–920.

Cohn SA (1966) Disuse atrophy of the periodontium in mice following partial loss of function. Arch Oral Biol 11, 95–105.

Connor NS, Aubin JE and Sodek J (1983) Independent expression of type I collagen and fibronectin by normal fibroblast-like cells. J Cell Sci 63, 233–244.

Couchman JR and Rees DA (1979) The behaviour of fibroblasts migrating from chick heart explants: Changes in adhesion, locomotion and growth, and in the distribution of actinomyosin and fibronectin. J Cell Sci 39, 149–165.

Crocker J and Nar P (1987) Nucleolar organizer regions in lymphomas. J Path 151, 111–118.

Davidovitch Z (1991) Tooth movement. Crit Rev Oral Biol Rev 2, 411–450.

Davidovitch Z, Finkelson MD, Steigman S, Shanfeld JL, Montgomery PC, Korostoft E (1980) Electrical currents, bone remodelling, and orthodontic tooth movement. II. Increase in rate of tooth movement and periodontal cyclic nucleotide levels by combined force and electric current. Am J Orthodont 77, 33–47.

Davidovitch Z, Nicolay OF, Ngan PW and Shanfeld JL (1988) Neurotransmitters, cytokines and the control of alveolar bone remodelling in orthodontics. Dent Clin North Am 32, 411–435.

Davidson D and McCulloch CAG (1986) Proliferative behaviour of periodontal ligament cell populations. J Periodont Res 32, 414– 428.

Deporter DA and Ten Cate AR (1973) Fine structural localisation of acid and alkaline phosphatase in collagen containing vesicles of fibroblasts. J Anat 114, 457–461.

Dorey CK and Bick KL (1977) Ultrahistochemical analysis of glycosaminoglycan hydrolysis in the rat periodontal ligament. II: Aryl sulfatose and bone resorption. Calcif Tissue Res 24, 143–149.

Duncan GW, Yen EHK, Pritchard ET and Suge DM (1984) Collagen and prostaglandin synthesis in force-stressed periodontal ligament in vitro. J Dent Res 63, 665–669.

Ehrlich HR and Bornstein P (1972) Microtubules in transcellular movement of procollagen. Nature 238, 257–260.

Eley BM and Harrison JD (1975) Intracellular collagen fibrils in the periodontal ligament of man. J Periodont Res 10, 168–170.

Everts V and Beertsen W (1987) The role of microtubules in the phagocytosis of collagen fibrils by fibroblasts. Collagen Rel Res 7, 1–15.

Everts V and Beertsen W (1988) The cellular basis of tooth eruption: the role of collagen phagocytosis. In: The Biological Mechanisms of Tooth Eruption and Root Resorption (Davidovitch Z, ed), pp 237–242, EBSCO Media, Birmingham, Alabama.

Everts V, Beertsen W and Tigchelaar-Gutter W (1985) The digestion of phagocytosed collagen is inhibited by the proteinase inhibitors leupeptin and E-64. Collagen Rel Res 5, 315–336.

Everts V, Hembry RM, Reynolds JJ and Beertsen W (1989) Metalloproteinases are not involved in the phagocytosis of collagen fibrils by fibroblasts. Matrix 9, 266–276.

Everts V, Wolvius E, Saklatvala J and Beertsen W (1990) Interleukin 1 increases the production of collagenase but does not influence the phagocytosis of collagen fibrils. Matrix 10, 388–393.

Fawcett DW (1981) The Cell, Saunders, Philadelphia.

Frank RM, Fellinger E and Steuer P (1976) Ultrastucture du ligament alvéolo-dentaire du rat. J Biol Buccale 4, 295–313.

Freilich LS (1971) Ultrastructure and acid phosphatase cytochemistry of odontoclasts: Effects of parathyroid extract. J Dent Res 50, 1047–1055.

Fullmer HM (1967) Connective tissue components of the periodontium. In: Structural and Chemical Organisation of Teeth (Miles AEW, ed), pp 349–414, Academic Press, London.

Gabbiani G (1979) The role of contractile proteins in wound healing and fibrocontractive diseases. Methods Achiev Exp Path 9, 187–206.

Garant PR (1976) Collagen resorption by fibroblasts. J Periodontol 47, 380–390.

Garant PR and Cho MI (1979) Cytoplasmic polarisation of periodontal ligament fibroblasts. J Periodont Res 14, 95–106.

Garant PR and Cho MI (1989) Fibroblast migration, cytoplasmic polarity and matrix secretion in the periodontal ligament. In: The Biology of Tooth Movement (Norton LA and Burstone CJ, eds), pp 29–53, CRC Press, Boca Raton, Florida.

Garant PR, Cho MI and Cullen MR (1982) Attachment of periodontal ligament fibroblasts to the extracellular matrix in the squirrel monkey. J Periodont Res 17, 70–79.

Geiger B (1987) Intermediate filaments: looking for a function. Nature 329, 392–393.

Gilula NB, Reeves R and Steinbach A (1972) Metabolic coupling, ionic coupling and cell contacts. Nature 235, 262–265.

Giniger PR, Norton L, Sousa S, Lorenzo JA and Bronner F (1991) A human periodontal ligament fibroblast clone releases a bone resorption inhibition factor in vitro. J Dent Res 70, 99–101.

Gould TRL, Brunette DM and Dorey J (1982) Cell turnover in the periodontal ligament determined by continuous infusion of 3H-thymidine using osmotic minipumps. J Periodont Res 17, 662–668.

Gould TRL, Brunette DM and Dorey J (1983) Cell turnover in the periodontium in health and periodontal disease. J Periodont Res 18, 353–361.

Gould TRL, Melcher AH and Brunette DM (1977) Location of progenitor cells in periodontal ligament of mouse molar stimulated by wounding. Anat Rec 188, 133–141.

Gould TRL, Melcher AH and Brunette DM (1980) Migration and division of progenitor cell populations in periodontal ligament after wounding. J Periodont Res 15, 20–42.

Grant DA and Bernick S (1969) A possible continuity between epithelial rests and epithelial attachment in miniature swine. J Periodontol 43, 87–95.

Grant DA and Bernick S (1972) The periodontium of ageing rats. J Periodontol 43, 660–667.

Greenlee TK and Ross R (1967) The development of the rat flexor digital tendon. A fine structure study. J Ultrastruct Res 18, 354–376.

Grupe HE, Ten Cate AR and Zander HA (1967) A histochemical and radiobiological study of in vitro and in vivo human epithelial cell rest proliferation. Arch Oral Biol 12, 1321–1329.

Hamamoto Y, Nakajima T and Ozawa H (1989) Ultrastructure of epithelial rests of Malassez in human periodontal ligament. Arch Oral Biol 34, 179–185.

Hamamoto Y, Suzuki I, Nakajima T and Ozawa H (1991) Immunohistochemical localisation of lamini in the epithelial rests of Malassez of immature rat molars. Arch Oral Biol 36, 623–626.

Hancox NM (1972) The osteoclast. In: The Biochemistry and Physiology of Bone, Vol. I (Bourne GH, ed), pp 45–69, Academic Press, New York.

Harris AK, Stopak D and Wild P (1981) Fibroblast traction as a mechanism for collagen morphogenesis. Nature 290, 249–251.

Hay ED (1982) Interaction of embryonic cell surface and cytoskeleton with extracellular matrix. Am J Anat 165, 1–12.

Heershe JNM and Deporter DA (1979) The mechanism of osteoclastic bone resorption: a new hypothesis. J Periodont Res 14, 266–267.

Herman IM, Crisona NJ and Pollard TD (1981) Relation between cell activity and the distribution of cytoplasmic actin and myosin. J Cell Biol 90, 84–91.

Holtrop ME (1990a) Light and electron microscopic structure of bone forming cells. In: Bone, volume 1: The Osteoblast and Osteocyte (Eds BK Hall), pp1–39, The Telford Press, New Jersey.

Holtrop ME (1990b) Light and electron microscopic structure of osteoclasts. In: Bone, volume 2: The Osteoclast (Hall BK , ed), pp1–30, CRC Press, Boca Raton, Florida.

Holtrop ME and Weinger JM (1972) Ultrastructural evidence for a transport system in bone. In: Calcium, Parathyroid Hormone and the Calcitonins (Eds RV Talmage and PL Munson), pp365–374, Excerpta Medica, Amsterdam.

Hou L-T, Kollar EJ and Yaeger JA (1993) Modulations of extracellular matrix proteins in cultured oral cells. J Periodont Res 28, 102–114.

Hughes FJ and Issberner JP (1988) Phenotypic variations in contraction of fibroblast derived from the periodontal tissues. J Dent Res 67, 646.

Ippolito E, Natali PG, Postacchini F (1977) Ultrastructural and immunochemical evidence of actin in the tendon cell. Clin Orthop Rel Res 126, 282–284.

Jensen JL and Toto PD (1968) Radioactive labelling index of the periodontal ligament in ageing rats. J Dent Res 47, 149–153.
Jones SJ and Boyd A (1977) Some morphological observations on osteoclasts. Cell Tissue Res 185, 387–397.
Jowsey J, Kelly PJ, Riggs BL, Bianco AJ, Scholz DA and Gershon-Cohen J (1965) Quantitative microradiographic studies of normal and osteoporotic bone. J Bone Joint Surg Am 47A, 785–806.
Kallio DM, Garant PR and Minkin C (1971) Evidence of coated membranes in the ruffled border of osteoclasts. J Ultrastruct Res 37, 169–177.
Kasugi S, Suzuki S, Shibita S, Amano H and Ogura H (1990) Measurements of the isometric contractile forces generated by dog periodontal ligament fibroblasts in vitro. Arch Oral Biol 35, 597–601.
Klingsberg J and Butcher EO (1960) Comparative histology of age changes in oral tissues of rat, hamsters and monkeys. J Dent Res 39, 158–160.
Kronmiller JE, Upholt WB and Kollar EJ (1993) Effects of retinol on the temporal expression of transforming growth factor-α mRNA in the embryonic mouse mandible. Arch Oral Biol 38, 185–188.
Lambrichts I, Creemers J and Van Steenberghe D (1993) Periodontal neural endings intimately related to epithelial rests of Malassez in humans. J Anat 182, 153–162.
Larjava H, Hakkinen L and Rahemtulla F (1992) A biochemical analysis of human periodontal tissue proteoglycans. Biochem J 284, 264–274
Larjava H, Heino J, Kahari VM, Vuorio E (1989) Characterisation of one phenotype of human periodontal granulation-tissue fibroblasts. J Dent Res 68, 20–25.
Levy BM, Dreizen S and Bernick S (1972) Effect of ageing on the marmoset periodontium. J Oral Path 1, 61–65.
Limeback HF and Sodek J (1979) Procollagen synthesis and processing in the periodontal ligament in vivo and in vitro. A comparative study using slab-gel fluorography. Europ J Biochem 100, 541–550.
Limeback HF, Sodek J and Aubin JE (1983) Variations in collagen expression by cloned periodontal ligament cells. J Periodont Res 18, 242–248.
Limeback HF, Sodek J and Brunette DM (1978) Nature of collagens synthesised by monkey periodontal ligament fibroblasts in vitro. Biochem J 170, 63–71.
Lindskog S, Blomlöf L and Hammarstrom L (1983) Repair of periodontal tissues in vivo and in vitro. J Clin Periodontol 10, 188–205.
Lindskog S, Blomlöf L and Hammarstrom L (1988) Evidence for a role of odontogenic epithelium in maintaining the periodontal space. J Clin Periodontol 15, 371–373.
Listgarten MA (1975) Cell rests in the periodontal ligament of mouse molars. J Periodont Res 10, 197–202.
Listgarten MA (1973) Intracellular collagen fibrils in the periodontal ligament of the mouse, rat, hamster, guinea pig and rabbit. J Periodont Res 8, 335–342.
Lloyd C (1979) Primitive model for cell cycle control. Nature 280, 631–632.
Loe H and Waerhaug J (1961) Experimental replantation of teeth on dogs and monkeys. Arch Oral Biol 3, 176–184.
Löwik CWGM, Van der Pluijm GW, Bloys H, Hoekman K, Bijvoet OLM, Aarden LA and Papapoulos SE (1989) Parathyroid hormone (PTH) and PTH-like protein (PLP) stimulate interleukin-6 production by osteogenic cells: a possible role of interleukin-6 in osteoclastogenesis. Biochem Biophys Res Commun 162, 1546–1552.
Luo W, Slavkin HC and Snead MN (1991) Cells from Hertwig's root sheath do not transcribe amelogenin. J Periodont Res 26, 42–47.
Malkani K, Luxembourger MM and Rebel A (1973) Cytoplasmic modifications at the contact zone of osteoclasts and calcified tissue in the diaphyseal growing plate of foetal guinea pig tibia. Calc Tissue Res 11, 258–264.
Mariotti A and Cochran DL (1990) Characterisation of fibroblasts derived from human periodontal ligament and gingiva. J Periodontol 61, 103–111.
Mark MP, Bloch-Zupan A and Ruch JV (1992) Effects of retinoids on tooth morphogenesis and cytodifferentiations, in vitro. Int J Dev Biol 36, 517–526.
Marks SC and Popoff SN (1988) Bone cell biology: the regulation of development, structure, and function in the skeleton. Am J Anat 183, 1–44.
Marks SC and Miller SC (1993) Prostaglandins and the skeleton: The legacy and challenges of two decades of research. Endocrine J 1, 337–334.
Martineau-Doizé B, Lai WH, Warshawsky H and Bergeron JJM (1987) Specific binding sites for epidermal growth factor in bone and incisor enamel organ of the rat. In: Development and Diseases of Cartilage and Bone Matrix (Sen A and Thornhill T, eds), pp 389–399, A.R. Liss, New York.
Matsuda N, Lin WL, Kumar NM, Cho MI and Genco RJ (1992) Mitogenic, chemotactic and synthetic responses of rat periodontal ligament fibroblastic cells to polypeptide growth factors in vitro. J Periodontol 63, 515–525.
McCulloch CAG (1985) Progenitor populations in the periodontal ligament of mice. Anat Rec 211, 258–262.
McCulloch CAG, Barghava U and Melcher AH (1989) Cell death and the regulation of populations of cells in the periodontal ligament. Cell Tissue Res 255, 129–138.
McCulloch CAG and Bordin S (1991) Role of fibroblast subpopulations in periodontal physiology and pathology. J Periodont Res 26, 144–154.
McCulloch CAG and Heersche JNM (1988) Lifetime of the osteoblast in mouse periodontium. Anat Rec 222, 128–135.
McCulloch CAG and Melcher AH (1983a) Continuous labelling of the periodontal ligament of mice. J Periodont Res 18, 231–241.
McCulloch CAG and Melcher AH (1983b) Cell migration in the periodontal ligament of mice. J Periodont Res 18, 339–352.
McCulloch CAG and Melcher AH (1983c) Cell density and cell generation in the periodontal ligament of mice. Am J Anat 167, 43–58.
McCulloch CAG, Nemeth E, Lowenberg B and Melcher AH (1987) Paravascular cells in endosteal spaces of alveolar bone contribute to periodontal ligament cell populations. Anat Rec 219, 233–242.
Melcher AH and Beertsen W (1977) The physiology of tooth eruption. In: The Biology of Occlusal Development (McNamara JA, ed), pp 1–23, University of Michigan, Michigan.
Melcher AH and Chan J (1981) Phagocytosis and digestion of collagen by gingival fibroblasts in vivo: a study of serial sections. J Ultrastruct Res 77, 1–36.
Melcher AH, Cheong J, Cox E, Nemeth E, *et al.* (1986) Synthesis of cementum-like tissue in vitro by cells cultured from bone: A light and electron microscope study. J Periodont Res 21, 592–612.
Melcher AH and Turnbull RS (1976) Organ culture in studies on the periodontium. In: Organ Culture in Biomedical Research. (Balls M and Monnickendam MA, eds), pp149–163, Cambridge University Press, Cambridge.
Merrilees MJ, Sodek J and Aubin JE (1983) Effect of cells of epithelial rests of Malassez and endothelial cells on synthesis of glycosaminoglycans by periodontal ligament fibroblasts in vitro. Dev Biol 97, 146–153.
Michna H (1988) Intracellular collagen fibrils: evidence of an intracellular source from experiments with tendon fibroblasts and fibroblastic tumour cells. J Anat 158, 1–12.
Morris ML and Harper E (1987). The presence of an inhibitor of human skin collagenase in the roots of healthy and periodontally diseased teeth. J Periodont Res 22, 78–80.
Moxham BJ, Berkovitz BKB and Shore RC (1984) Is the periodontal ligament a foetal connective tissue? In: Tooth Morphogenesis and Differentiation (Belcourt AB and Ruch JV, eds), pp 557–566, INSERM, Paris.
Moxham BJ, Shore RC and Berkovitz BKB (1991) A quantitative study of the ultrastructure of fibroblasts within the enamel-related connective tissue of the rat incisor. J Biol Buccale 19, 135–140.
Mundy GR and Roodman GD (1987) Osteoclast ontogeny and function. In: Bone and Mineral Research: 5 (WA Peck WA, ed), pp 209–279, Elsevier, Amsterdam.

Murphy KG and Daniel JC (1987) Human periodontal ligament in vitro: Cell culture passage effect on collagen gel contraction. J Periodont Res 22, 342–347.

Narayanan AS, Page RC and Swanson J (1989). Collagen synthesis by human fibroblasts. Regulation by transforming growth factor-beta in the presence of other inflammatory mediators. Biochem J 260, 463–469.

Ngan P, Saito S, Saito M, Shanfeld J and Davidovitch Z (1990) The interactive effects of mechanical stress and interleukin-1β on prostaglandin E and cyclic AMP production in human periodontal ligament fibroblasts in vitro: Comparison with cloned osteoblastic cells of mouse (MC3T3-E1). Arch Oral Biol 35, 717–725.

Ngan P, Zadeh Y, Shanfeld J and Davidovitch Z (1988) The effect of interleukin-1β and parathyroid hormone on cyclic nucleotide and prostaglandin levels in human periodontal ligament fibroblasts in vitro. In: The Biological Mechanisms of Tooth Eruption and Root Resorption (Davidovitch Z, ed), pp261–267, EBSCO Media, Birmingham, Alabama.

Nijweide PJ and de Grooth R (1991) Ontogeny of the osteoclast. In: Biology and Physiology of the Osteoclast. (Rifkin BR and Gay CV, eds), pp 81–104, CRC Press, Boca Raton, Florida.

Nojima N, Kobayashi M, Shionome M, Suda T and Hasegawa K (1990) Fibroblastic cells derived from bovine periodontal ligaments have phenotypes of osteoblasts. J Periodont Res 25, 179–185.

Otsuka K, Pitaru S, Overall CM and Sodek J (1988) Biochemical comparision of fibroblast populations from different periodontal tissues: characterisation of matrix protein and collagenolytic enzyme synthesis. Biochem Cell Biol 66, 166–176.

Overall CM and Sodek J (1987) Initial characterisation of a neutral metaloproteinase, active on native 3/4 collagen fragments, synthesised by ROS 17/2.8 osteoblastic cells, periodontal fibroblasts, and identified in gingival crevicular fluid. J Dent Res 66, 1271–1282.

Owen M and Shetlar MR (1968) Uptake of 3H-glucosamine by osteoclasts. Nature 220, 1335–1336.

Park P, Manabe S and Ohno T (1988) Incidence and ultrastructure of rudimentary cilia in benign and malignant peripheral nerve tumours. Ultrastruct Path 12, 407–418.

Pender N and McCulloch CAG (1991) Quantitation of actin polymerisation in two human fibroblast sub-types responding to mechanical stretching. J Cell Sci 100, 187–193.

Perera KAS and Tonge CH (1981a) Metabolic turnover of collagen in the mouse molar periodontal ligament during tooth eruption. J Anat 133, 359–370.

Perera KAS and Tonge CH (1981b) Fibroblast cell population kinetics in the mouse molar periodontal ligament and tooth eruption. J Anat 133, 281–300.

Pettigrew DW, Sodek J, Wang H-W and Brunette DM (1980) Inhibitors of collagenolytic enzymes synthesised by fibroblasts and epithelial cells from porcine and macaque periodontal tissues. Arch Oral Biol 25, 269–274.

Piche JE, Carnes DL and Graves DT (1989) Initial characterisation of cells derived from periodontia. J Dent Res 68, 761–767.

Picton DCA and Wills DJ (1978) Viscoelastic properties of the periodontal ligament and mucous membrane. J Prosth Dent 40, 263–272.

Picton DCA and Wills DJ (1981) Visualisation by scanning electron microscopy of the periodontal ligament in vivo in the macaque monkey. Arch Oral Biol 26, 821–825.

Pinto da Silva P and Gilula NB (1972) Gap junctions in normal and transformed fibroblasts in culture. Exp Cell Res 71, 393–401.

Pouyssegur J and Pastan I (1979) The directionality of locomotion of mouse fibroblasts. Exp Cell Res 121, 373–382.

Ragnarsson B, Carr G and Daniel JC (1985) Isolation and growth of human periodontal ligament cells in vitro. J Dent Res 64, 1026–1030.

Reeve CM and Wentz FM (1962) The prevalence, morphology and distribution of epithelial rests in the human periodontal ligament. J Oral Med Oral Surg Oral Path 15, 785–793.

Reitan K (1961) Behaviour of Malassez epithelial rests during orthodontic tooth movement. Acta Odont Scand 19, 443–468.

Richards D and Rutherford RB (1988) The effects of interleukin 1 on collagenolytic activity and prostaglandin-E secretion by human periodontal ligament and gingival fibroblast. Arch Oral Biol 33, 237–343.

Richards D and Rutherford RB (1990) Interleukin-1 regulation of procollagenase mRNA and protein in periodontal fibroblasts in vitro. J Periodont Res 25, 222–229.

Rippin JW (1978) Collagen turnover in the periodontal ligament under normal and altered forces II. Adult rat molars. J Periodont Res 13, 149–154.

Roberts WE (1975a) Cell kinetic nature and diurnal periodicity of the rat periodontal ligament. Arch Oral Biol 20, 465–471.

Roberts WE (1975b) Cell population dynamics of periodontal ligament stimulated with parathyroid extract. Am J Anat 143, 363–370.

Roberts WE, Aubert MM, Sparaga JM and Smith RK (1979) Circadian periodicity of the cell kinetics of rat molar periodontal ligament. Am J Orthodont 76, 316–323.

Roberts WE and Chamberlain JG (1978) Scanning electron microscopy of the cellular elements of rat periodontal ligament. Arch Oral Biol 23, 587–589.

Roberts WE and Chase DC (1981) Kinetics of cell proliferation and migration associated with orthodontically induced osteogenesis. J Dent Res 60, 174–181.

Roberts WE and Ferguson DJ (1989) Cell kinetics of the periodontal ligament. In: The Biology of Tooth Movement. (Norton LA and Burstone CJ, eds), pp 55–69, CRC Press, Boca Raton, Florida.

Roberts WE, Goodwin WCJr and Heiner SR (1981) Cellular responses to orthodontic force. Dent Clin North Amer 25, 3–17.

Roberts WE and Jee WSS (1974) Cell kinetics of orthodontically stimulated periodontal ligament in the rat. Arch Oral Biol 19, 17–21.

Roberts WE, Mozsary PG and Klingler E (1982) Nuclear size as a cell-kinetic marker for osteoblast differentiation. Am J Anat 165, 373–384.

Roberts WE, Wood HB, Chambers DW and Burk DT (1987) Vascularly oriented differentiation gradient of osteoblast precursor cells in rat periodontal ligament: Implications for osteoblast histogenesis and periodontal bone loss. J Periodontol 22, 461–467.

Rose GG, Yamasaki A, Pinero GJ and Mahan CJ (1987) Human periodontal ligament cells in vitro. J Periodont Res 22, 20–28.

Ross R (1968) The connective tissue fiber forming cell. In: Treatise on Collagen, volume 2: Biology of Collagen (Part A) (Gould BS, ed), pp 2–82, Academic Press, London.

Ross R and Greenlee TK (1966) Electron microscopy: attachment sites between connective tissue cells. Science 153, 997–999.

Rutherford RB, Trail-Smith MD, Ryan ME and Charette MF (1992) Synergistic effects on platelet-derived growth factor mitogenesis in vitro. Arch Oral Biol 37, 139–145.

Saffar JL and Makris GP (1986) A morphological and quantitative study of osteoclast changes during the progress of periodontitis in the hamster. J Biol Buccale 14, 255–262.

Saito M, Saito S, Ngan PW, Shanfeld J and Davidovitch Z (1991) Interleukin 1 beta and prostaglandin E are involved in the response of periodontal cells to mechanical stress in vivo and in vitro. Am J Orthodont Dentofac Orthop 99, 226–240.

Saito S, Ngan P, Rosol T, Saito M, Shimuzu H, Shinjo N, Shanfeld J and Davidovitch Z (1991) Involvement of PGE synthesis in the effect of intermittent pressure and interleukin-1 beta on bone resorption. J Dent Res 70, 27–33.

Saito S, Ngan P, Saito M, Kim K, Lanese R, Shanfield and Davidovitch Z (1990b) Effects of cytokines on prostaglandin E and cAMP levels in human periodontal ligament fibroblasts in vitro. Arch Oral Biol 35, 387–395.

Saito S, Ngan P, Saito M, Lanese R, Shanfield J and Davidovitch Z (1990c) Interactive effects between cytokines in PGE production by human periodontal ligament fibroblasts in vitro. J Dent Res 69, 1456–1462.

Saito S, Saito M, Ngan P, Lanese R, Shanfield J and Davidovitch Z (1990a) Effects of parathyroid hormone and cytokines on prostaglandin E synthesis and bone resorption by human periodontal ligament fibroblasts. Arch Oral Biol 35, 845–855.

Salonen J, Uitto V-J, Pan Y-M and Oda D (1991) Proliferating oral epithelial cells in culture are capable of both extracellular and intracellular degradation of interstitial collagen. Matrix 11, 43–55.

Sasaki T and Garant PR (1993) Multinucleated fibroblastic cells in the periodontal ligaments of aged rats. J Periodont Res 28, 65–71.

Schellens JPM, Everts V and Beertsen W (1982) Quantitative analysis of connective tissue resorption in the supra-alveolar region of the mouse incisor ligament. J Periodont Res 17, 407–422 .

Schenk RK, Felix R and Hofstetter W (1993) Morphology of connective tissue: Bone. In: Connective Tissue and Its Heritable Disorders (Royce PM and Steinman B, eds), pp 85–101, Wiley–Liss Inc.

Severson JA, Moffet BC, Kocich V and Selipsky H (1978) A histologic study of age changes in the adult human periodontal joint (ligament). J Periodontol 49, 189–200.

Shimizu N, Ogura N, Yamaguchi M, Goseki T, Shibata Y, Abiko Y, Iwasawa T and Takigichi H (1992) Stimulation by interleukin-1 of interleukin-6 production by human periodontal ligament cells. Arch Oral Biol 37, 743–748.

Shore RC and Berkovitz BKB (1979) An ultrastructural study of periodontal ligament fibroblasts in relation to their possible role in tooth eruption and intra-cellular collagen degradation in the rat. Arch Oral Biol 24, 155–164.

Shore RC, Berkovitz BKB and Moxham BJ (1984) Histological study including ultrastructural quantification, of the periodontal ligament in the lathyritic rat mandibular dentition. Arch Oral Biol 29, 263–273.

Shore RC, Berkovitz BKB and Moxham BJ (1985) The effects of preventing movement of the rat incisor on the structure of its periodontal ligament. Arch Oral Biol 30, 221–228.

Shore RC, Berkovitz BKB and Moxham BJ (1981) Intercellular contacts between fibroblasts in the periodontal connective tissues of the rat. J Anat 133, 67–76.

Shore RC, Berkovitz BKB and Moxham BJ (1982) A quantitative comparison of the ultrastructure of the periodontal ligaments of impeded and unimpeded rat incisors. Arch Oral Biol 27, 423–430.

Shore RC, Kirkham J, Robinson C, Moxham BJ and Berkovitz BKB (1991) An assessment of the control of matrix turnover by a quantitative ultrastructural analysis of fibroblasts of the periodontal ligament in rats. J Biol Buccale 19, 68–73.

Simpson HE (1965) The degeneration of the rests of Malassez with age as observed by the apoxestic technique. J Periodontol 36, 288–291.

Singer II (1979) The fibronexus: a transmembrane association of fibronectin containing fibres and bundles of 5nm microfilaments in hamster and human fibroblasts. Cell 16, 675–685.

Singer II, Kawaka DW, Kazazis DM and Clark RA (1984) *In vivo* co-distribution of fibronectin and actin fibres in granulation tissue: immunofluorescence and electron microscope studies of the fibronexus at the myofibroblast surface. J Cell Biol 98, 2091–2106.

Singh IJ, Sandhu HS and Tonna EA (1987) Autoradiographic evaluation of circadian periodicity in cell proliferation in the periodontal ligament of the young mouse. Arch Oral Biol 32, 377–379.

Slavkin HC, Bringas PJr, Bessem C, Santos V, Nakamura M, Hsu MY, Snead ML, Zeichner-David M and Fincham AG (1988) Hertwig's epithelial root sheath differentiation and initial cementum and bone formation during long-term culture of mouse mandibular first molars using serumless, chemically defined medium. J Periodont Res 23, 249–255.

Sloan P (1978) Scanning electron microscopy of the collagen fibre architecture of the rabbit incisor periodontium. Arch Oral Biol 23, 567–572.

Smalley JW, Shuttleworth CA and Grant ME (1984) Synthesis and secretion of sulphated glycosaminoglycans by bovine periodontal ligament fibroblast cultures. Arch Oral Biol 29, 107–116.

Smith RK and Roberts WE (1980) Cell kinetics of the initial response to orthodontically induced osteogenesis in the rat molar periodontal ligament. Calcif Tissue Int 30, 51–56.

Sodek J (1978) A comparison of collagen and non-collagenous protein metabolism in rat molar and incisor periodontal ligaments. Arch Oral Biol 23, 977–982.

Sodek J (1983) Periodontal ligament: Metabolism. In: Handbook of Experimental Aspects of Oral Biochemistry. (Lazzari EP, ed), pp 183–193, CRC Press, Boca Raton, Florida.

Sodek J (1977) A comparison of the rates of synthesis and turnover of collagen and non-collagenous protein in adult rat periodontal tissues and skin using a microassay. Arch Oral Biol 22, 655–665.

Somerman MJ, Foster RA, Imm GM, Sauk JJ and Archer SY (1989) Periodontal ligament cells and gingival fibroblasts respond differently to attachment factors in vitro. J Periodontol 60, 73–77.

Somerman MJ, Foster RA and Sauk JJ (1992) Biochemical analysis of periodontal cell activities. In: The Biological Mechanisms of Tooth Movement and Craniofacial Adaptation. (Davidovitch Z, ed), pp 291–300, EBSCO Media, Birmingham, Alabama.

Somerman MJ, Young MF, Foster RA, Moehring G, Imm G and Sauk JJ (1990) Characterisation of human periodontal ligament cells in vitro. Arch Oral Biol 35, 241–247.

Sorokin S (1962) Centrioles and the formation of rudimentary cilia by fibroblasts and smooth muscle cells. J Cell Biol 15, 363–377.

Spouge JD (1980) A new look at the rests of Malassez. J Periodontol 51, 437–444.

Spouge JD (1984) The rests of Malassez and chronic marginal periodontitis. J Clin Periodontol 11, 340–347.

Steffensen B, Duong AH, Milam SB, Potempa CL, Wimborn WB, Magnuson VL, Chen D, Zardeneta G and Klebe RJ (1992) Immunohistological localisation of cell adhesion proteins and integrins in the periodontium. J Periodontol 63, 584–592.

Steinert PM, Steven AC and Roop DR (1985) The molecular biology of intermediate filaments. Cell 42, 411–419.

Stewart M (1990) Intermediate filaments: structure, assembly and molecular interactions. Curr Opin Cell Biol 2, 91–100.

Stopak D and Harris AK (1982) Connective tissue morphogenesis by fibroblast traction. Dev Biol 90, 383–398.

Stopp M, Gross J and Lauer HC (1989) Protein content in rabbit periodontal ligament fibroblasts during growth in culture. Cell Biol Int Rep 13, 385–389.

Svobada ELA, Brunette DM and Melcher AH (1979) In vitro phagocytosis of exogenous collagen by fibroblasts from the periodontal ligament: an electron microscope study. J Anat 128, 301–314.

Svoboda ELA, Shiga A and Deporter DA (1981) A stereological analysis of collagen phagocytosis by fibroblasts in three soft connective tissues with differing rates of collagen turnover. Anat Rec 199, 473–480.

Takeshita A, Zhon GN, Hanazawa S, Takara I, Higuchi H, Katayama I and Kitano S (1992) Effect of interleukin-1 beta on gene expressions and functions of fibroblastic cells dervied from human periodontal ligament. J Periodont Res 27, 250–255.

Ten Cate AR (1965) The histochemical demonstration of specific oxidative enzymes and glycogen in the epithelial cell rests of Malassez. Arch Oral Biol 10, 207–213.

Ten Cate AR (1967) The formation and function of the epithelial rests of Malassez. In: The Mechanisms of Tooth Support (Anderson DJ, Eastoe JE, Melcher AH and Picton DCA, eds), pp 80–83, Wrights, Bristol.

Ten Cate AR (1972) Morphological studies of fibrocytes in connective tissue undergoing rapid remodelling. J Anat 112, 401–414.

Ten Cate AR and Deporter DA (1975) The degradative role of the fibroblast in the remodelling and turnover of collagen in soft connective tissue. Anat Rec 182, 1–14.

Ten Cate AR, Deporter DA and Freeman E (1976) The role of fibroblasts in the remodelling of the periodontal ligament during physiologic tooth movement. Am J Orthod 69, 155–168.

Ten Cate AR and Syrbu S (1974) Relationship between alkaline phosphatase activity and the phagocytosis and degradation of collagen by the fibroblasts. J Anat 117, 351–359.

Tenenbaum HC (1991) Cellular origins and theories of differentiation of bone forming cells. In: The Osteoblast. (Hall B, ed), pp 41–69, CRC Press, Boca Raton, Florida.

Thesleff I (1987) Epithelial cell rest of Malassez bind epidermal growth factor intensely. J Periodont Res 22, 419–421.

Thesleff I, Partanen AM and Rihtniemi L (1987) Localization of epidermal growth factor receptors in mouse incisors and human premolars during eruption. Eur J Orthod 9, 24–32.

Thomas FN and Kollar EJ (1988) Tissue interactions in normal murine root development. In: Biological Mechanisms of Tooth Eruption and Root Resorption (Davidovitch Z, ed), pp 145–151, EBSCO Media, Birmingham, Alabama.

Tomasek JT, Hay ED and Fujiwara K (1982) Collagen modulates cell shape and cytoskeleton of embryonic corneal and fibroma fibroblasts: Distribution of actin, alpha-actin, and myosin. Dev Biol 92, 107–122.

Tonna EA and Stahl SS (1974) Comparative assessment of the cell proliferative activities of injured paradontal tissues in ageing mice. J Dent Res 53, 609–622.

Topham RT, Chiego DJ, Gattone VH, Hinton DA and Klein RM (1987) The effect of epidermal growth factor on neonatal incisor differentiation in the mouse. Dev Biol 124, 532–543.

Toto PD and Kwan HW (1970) Doubling time of labelled periodontal cells of rats. J Dent Res 49, 1017–1019.

Toto PD and Borg M (1968) Effect of age changes on the premitotic index in the periodontium of mice. J Dent Res 47, 70–73.

Toto PD, Rubenstein AS, and Gargiulo AW (1975) Labelling index and cell density of ageing rat oral tissues. J Dent Res 54, 553–556.

Trelstad RL and Hayashi K (1979) Tendon fibrillogenesis: Intracellular collagen subassemblies and cell surface changes associated with fibril growth. Dev Biol 71, 228–242.

Trowbridge HO and Shibata F (1967) Mitotic activity in epithelial rests of Malassez. Periodontics 5, 109–112.

Uitto V-J, Larjava H, Peltonen J and Brunette DM (1992) Expression of fibronectin and integrins in cultured periodontal ligament epithelial cells. J Dent Res 71, 1203–1211.

Valderhaugh JP (1974) Epithelial cells in the periodontal membrane of teeth with and without periapical inflammation. Int J Oral Surg 3, 7–16.

Valderhaugh JP and Nylen MV (1966) Function of epithelial rests as suggested by their ultrastructure. J Periodont Res 1, 69–78.

Valderhaugh JP and Zander H (1967) Relationship of epithelial rests of Malassez to other periodontal structures. J Am Soc Periodont 5, 254–258.

Van den Brenk H and Stone MG (1974) Actions and interactions of colchicine and cytochalasin B on contraction of granulation tissue and on mitosis. Nature 251, 327–329.

Wasi S, Otsuka K, Yao KL, Tung PS, Aubin JE, Sodek J and Termine JD (1984) An osteonectin–like protein in porcine periodontal ligament and its synthesis by periodontal ligament fibroblasts. Can J Biochem Cell Biol 62, 470–478.

Webb PP, Benjamin M, Moxham BJ and Ralphs JR (1994) Age related changes in intermediate filament expression in the periodontium of the rat. J Anat (in press).

Weinstock M (1981) Tissue reactions of the periodontal ligament as a factor in ortho–perio treatment. In: Orthodontics – The State of the Art (Barrer HG, ed), pp 79–96, University of Pennsylvania Press, Pennsylvania.

Weinstock M and Leblond CP (1974) Formation of collagen. Fed Proc 33, 1205–1218.

Wentz FM, Weinmann JP and Schour I (1950) The prevalence distribution and morphologic changes of epithelial remnants in the molar region of the rat. J Dent Res 29, 637–646.

Wesselink PR and Beertsen W (1993) The prevalence and distribution of rests of Malassez in the mouse molar and their possible role in repair and maintenance of the periodontal ligament. Arch Oral Biol 38, 399–403.

Willingham MC, Yamada SS, Davies PJA, Rutherford AV, *et al.* (1981) Intracellular localisation of actin in cultured fibroblasts by electron microscopic immunocytochemistry. J Histochem Cytochem 29, 17–37.

Wise GE, Lin F and Fan W (1992) Effects of transforming growth factor-β, on cultured dental follicle cells from rat mandibular molars. Arch Oral Biol 37, 471–478.

Wood A and Thorogood P (1987) An ultrastructural and morphometric analysis of an in vitro contact guidance system. Development. 101, 363–381.

Yaeger JA and Kraucunas E (1969) Fine structure of the resorptive cells in the teeth of frogs. Anat Rec 164, 1–13.

Yamasaki A and Pinero GJ (1989) An ultrastructural study of human epithelial rest of Malassez maintained in a differentiated state *in vitro*. Arch Oral Biol 34, 443–451.

Yamasaki A, Rose GG, Pinero GJ and Mahan CJ (1986) Glycogen in human cementoblasts and PDL fibroblasts. J Periodontol 21, 128–136.

Yamasaki A, Rose GG, Pinero GJ and Mahan CJ (1987a) Ultrastructure of fibroblasts in cyclosporin A induced gingival hyperplasia. J Oral Path 16, 129–134.

Yamasaki A, Rose GG, Pinero GJ and Mahan CJ (1987b) Ultrastructure and morphometric analyses of human cementoblasts and periodontal fibroblasts. J Periodontol 58, 192–201.

Yamashita Y, Sato M and Noguchi T (1987) Alkaline phosphatase in the periodontal ligament of the rabbit and macaque monkey. Arch Oral Biol 32, 677–678.

Yee JA (1979) Response of periodontal ligament cells to orthodontic force: Ultrastructural identification of proliferating fibroblasts. Anat Rec 194, 603–614.

Zhang X, Schuppan D, Becker J, Reichert P and Gelderblom HR (1993) Distribution of undulin, tenascin and fibronectin in the human periodontal ligament and cementum : comparative immunoelectron microscopy with ultra thin cryosections. J Histochem Cytochem 41, 245–251.

Chapter 2
Structural Organization of the Fibres of the Periodontal Ligament

Philip Sloan and D Howard Carter

TYPES OF FIBRES

In common with most other connective tissues, the fibres in the periodontal ligament (PDL.) are mainly collagenous in nature. Although they are structurally associated with other extracellular matrix molecules, including fibronectin and tenascin (*Figs 2.1, 2.2, 2.3, 2.4, 2.5*), it is generally recognized that these molecules are involved in cell–matrix interactions rather than in maintaining the integrity of the tissue (see Chapter 4). However, it has been suggested that tenascin has a structural rǒle in myotendinous insertions (Lukinmaa *et al.*, 1991),

COLLAGEN FIBRES OF THE PERIODONTAL LIGAMENT

At least 18 species of collagen have been isolated from the extracellular matrix of connective tissues (Kielty *et al.*, 1993) and, like most other connective tissues, the collagen of the PDL is largely type I, with lesser amounts of type III, IV, V, VI and XII also present (Butler *et al.,* 1975; Wang *et al.,* 1980; Dublet *et al.,* 1988; Romanos *et al.,* 1991; Romanos *et al.,* 1992; Sloan *et al.,* 1993). Collagen types I, III and V are 'banded' collagen molecules (Burgeson, 1988), which have a characteristic periodicity of 67 nm when stained and examined in the electron microscope, owing to the staggered arrangement of the molecules in the fibril. A satisfactory classification of this family of molecules is yet to be established (Kielty *et al.*, 1993), but they can be divided into two main groups (Olsen, 1989) – fibril collagens and FACIT collagens.

Fibril collagens include collagen types I, III and V. Although collagen type III generally co-distributes with collagen type I (Keene *et al.*, 1987) to form mixed fibrils of infinitely varying proportions (Henkel and Glanville, 1982), a higher proportion of collagen type III is present in foetal tissues (see Berkovitz, 1990), and the molecule has been associated with the argyrophilic reticulin fibre (Melcher and Eastoe, 1969; Eastoe, 1976). Collagen type V also co-distributes with collagen type I, but it can only be demonstrated immunohistochemically by disrupting the fibrils (Bronckers *et al.,* 1986; Burgeson, 1988; Becker *et al.,* 1991). This may indicate that the molecule, which is composed of α_1(V), α_2(V) chains, is present in the cores of the fibrils.

FACIT collagens are 'fibril-associated collagens with interrupted triple helices' (Olsen, 1989). It is suggested that these molecules link the 'fibrillar' collagen fibres and organize the extracellular matrix (Olsen, 1989); collagen type XII and a molecule (undulin), identical to the non-collagenous region of collagen type XIV, have been located in the rat PDL (Dublet *et al.*, 1988; Zhang *et al.,* 1993).

Collagen type VI is a short chain molecule that has only recently been located in the PDL (Romanos *et al.,* 1992; Sloan *et al.,* 1993). It is a microfibril-forming collagen that ramifies the extracellular matrix, but it does not directly associate with the major banded collagen fibrils (von der Mark *et al.,* 1984). The molecule may be central in retaining the integrity and elasticity of the extracellular matrix.

Collagen type IV does not form fibrils and is found in the basement membranes of the neurovascular bundles and epithelial rests of the PDL (Sloan *et al.,* 1993). Although this collagen is specifically associated with basement membranes, it may have a further structural role in maintaining the integrity of the PDL by anchoring the elastic system to the vasculature (see below, pages 47–48).

The fibres of the PDL appear to be similar to those of other supportive connective tissues in that they are composed of an integrated unit of fibrous components (Amenta *et al.*, 1986). Nevertheless, the fibres of the periodontium have the particular structural requirements to withstand intrusive forces from mastication (tooth support) and to accommodate tooth eruption in growing animals (see Chapters 9 and 10). It follows that their disposition is central to our understanding of tooth support and eruption.

In some species and tooth types, the PDL collagen is assembled into fibres at an early stage of the ligament's development (Freeman and Ten Cate, 1971; Berkovitz and Moxham, 1989), while in others (e.g. monkey succedaneous teeth) fibres develop much later (Grant *et al.*, 1972). Even though fibrillogenesis is an extracellular event, the periodontal fibroblast cell processes may play a role in the assembly of the principal fibres (Yamamoto and Wakita, 1992).

The collagen fibril diameters of the mammalian PDL are relatively small, with mean diameters of the order 45–55 nm, with a unimodal distribution (*Figs 2.6, 2.7*) (Berkovitz *et al.*, 1981; Luder *et al.*, 1988). In other connective tissues, e.g. tendon, fibril diameters may reach 250 nm. There is evidence that the diameter of the fibrils increases with maturation in connective tissues (Torp, Bayer and Friedman, 1975; Parry and Craig, 1984) and the small diameter of the fibrils in the PDL could be the result of either the high rate of collagen turnover or the absence of mature collagen fibrils (Berkovitz *et al.*, 1981). Comparative studies have described fibrils measuring up to 250 nm in diameter in the PDL of the crocodile, where collagen turnover is slow (Berkovitz and

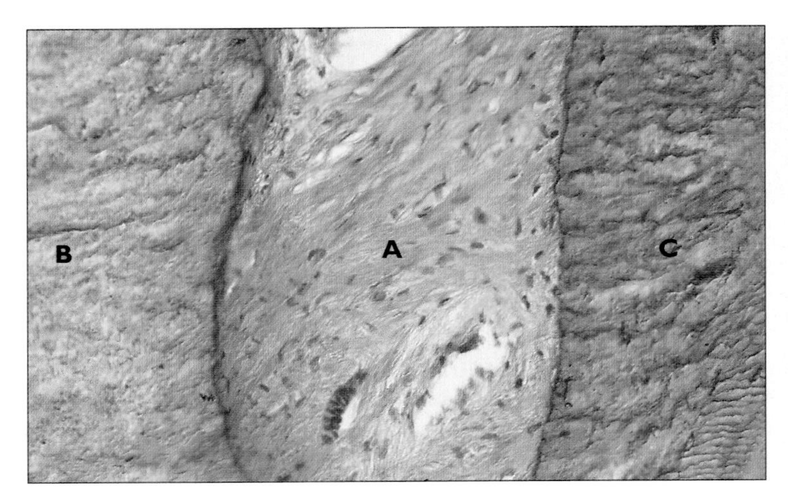

Fig. 2.1 Haematoxylin and eosin (× 140) stained transverse cryosection of human periodontal ligament (A) showing its relation to alveolar bone (B) and cementum (C).

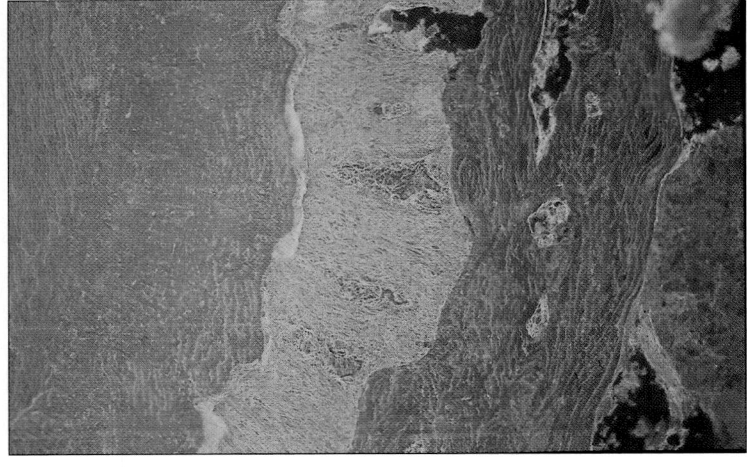

Fig. 2.2 Cryosection of human periodontal ligament. Immunofluorescent stain showing distribution of collagen type I. (× 56)

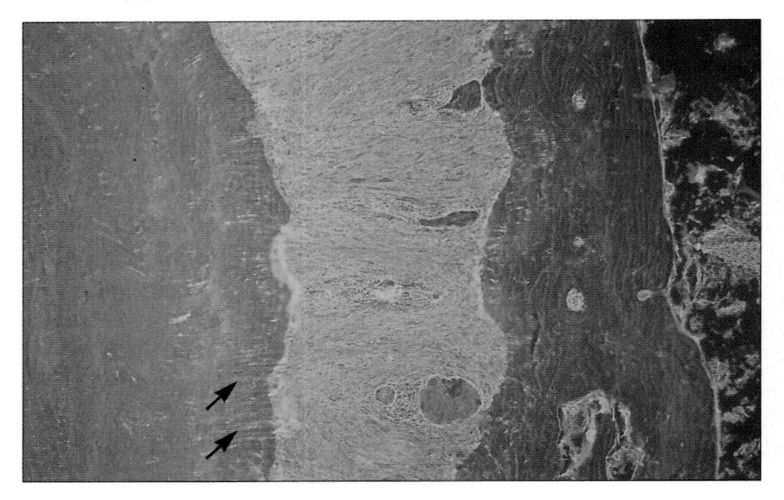

Fig. 2.3 Cryosection of human periodontal ligament stained for collagen type III. Note the staining of the inserting Sharpey fibres (arrows). (× 56)

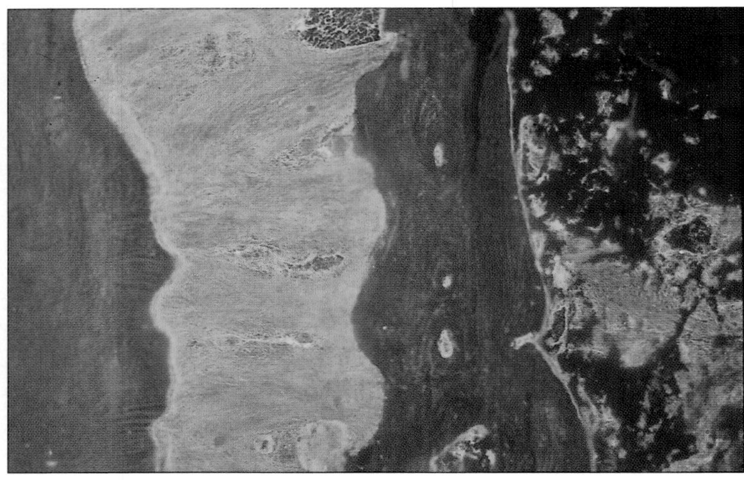

Fig. 2.4 Cryosection of human periodontal ligament stained for fibronectin. (× 56)

Sloan, 1979), but significant differences in fibril diameter are not apparent in the PDL of the continuously growing incisor (higher turnover) and the non-continuously growing molar of the mature rat (lower turnover – Berkovitz and Moxham, 1989). At the same time, there is no increase in fibril diameter in the maturing human PDL (Luder *et al.*, 1988).

It has been suggested that fibril diameter is regulated by the co-polymerization of different collagen molecules (Olsen, 1989). The small diameter of the collagen fibrils in the PDL may then result from a specific fibril composition. There is, however, no comparative evidence to support this because the composition of the fibrils in the PDL appears to be identical to other connective tissues. The determinants of fibril diameter in the PDL therefore await further investigation, and the significance of collagen fibril diameters is discussed further in relation to tooth support in Chapter 10.

'ELASTIC FIBRES' OF THE PERIODONTAL LIGAMENT

In many connective tissues, the collagen fibres are closely associated with an elastic meshwork which may function either as a static elastic element in a pliant composite or as a resilient material (Wainwright *et al.*, 1976; Serafini-Fracassini *et al.*, 1977; Cotta-Pereira *et al.*, 1989). Three fibrous components of the elastic system are generally recognized – oxytalan, elaunin, and elastin.

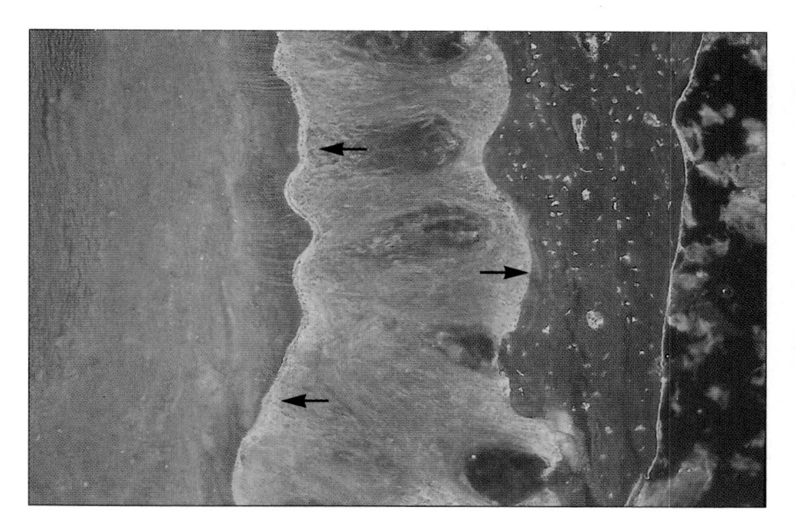

Fig. 2.5 Cryosection of human periodontal ligament, stained for tenascin, showing concentration of staining in the region of the fibrous insertions (arrows). (× 56)

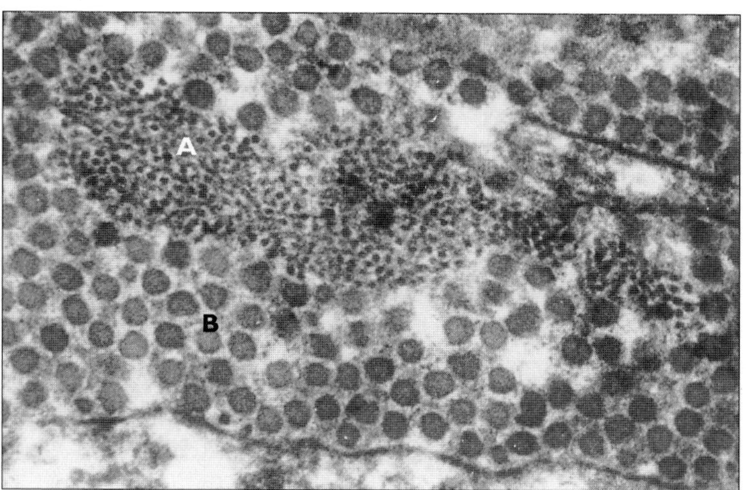

Fig. 2.6 Transmission electron micrograph showing a transversely sectioned oxytalan fibre (A) surrounded by transversely sectioned collagen fibres (B). (Magnification × 95,000.)

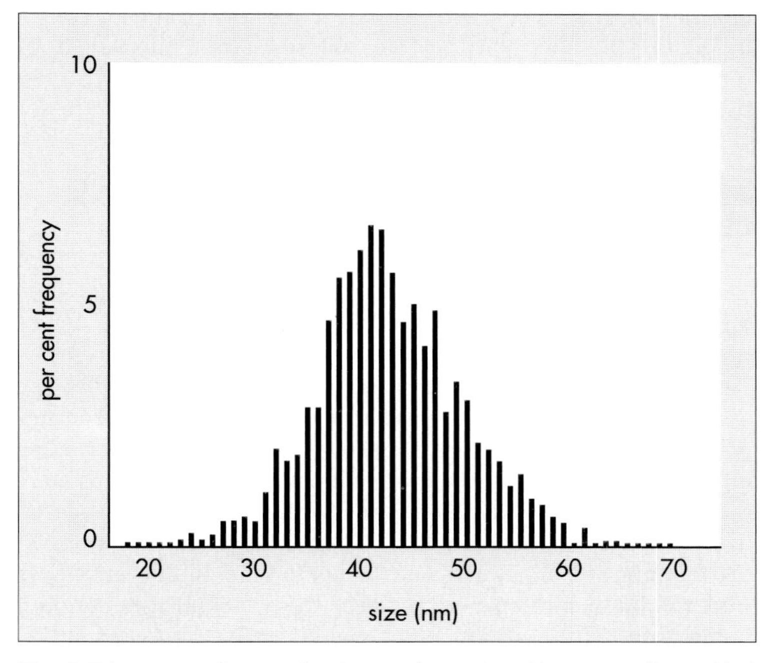

Fig. 2.7 Histogram showing distribution of periodontal ligament collagen fibril diameters (N = 1800). (From Berkovitz *et al.*, 1981.)

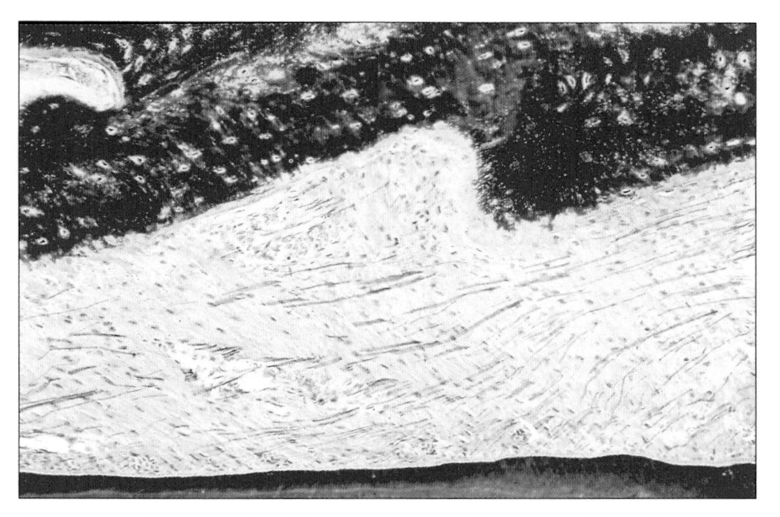

Fig. 2.8 Monkey periodontal ligament showing disposition of oxytalan fibres. (Monopersulphate thionine stain, × 180.)

Oxytalan and elaunin

Oxytalan and elaunin fibres can only be demonstrated with elastin stains after rigorous oxidation procedures at the light microscope level (*Fig. 2.8*) (Fullmer, 1959; Rannie, 1963) and they have frequently been classified as distinct species of elastic fibre. Oxytalan fibres form a three-dimensional meshwork that extends from the cementum to the peripheral periodontal blood vessels (Sims, 1975, 1976). The meshwork itself is largely oriented in the apico-occlusal plane and is interconnected with fine lateral fibrils. Depending on site and species, oxytalan fibres measure between 0.2 and 1.5 μm in diameter in the electron microscope, and it is reported that they occupy 3 per cent of the PDL in humans (Shore,

Moxham, and Berkovitz, 1984). In contrast they measure between 0.5 and 2.5 μm in diameter in the light microscope (Beertsen *et al.*, 1974). In the transmission electron microscope, oxytalan fibres appear similar to developing elastin fibres and are composed of groups of microfilaments embedded within amorphous material (*Fig. 2.9*; see *Fig. 2.6*) (for review, see Fullmer *et al.*, 1974; Shore, Moxham and Berkovitz, 1984). Similarities between the microfibrils of oxytalan fibres and developing elastin fibres have also been described (Sims, 1984) and it is now accepted that oxytalan and elaunin fibres are precursors of the elastin fibre (Franzblau and Faris, 1981; Chavrier *et al.*, 1988).

The similarity between the ultrastructure of oxytalan microfibrils and fibrils of fibronectin has been commented upon (Frank and Nalbandian, 1989). This has been supported by studies in our laboratory (*Fig. 2.10*), which have demonstrated that oxytalan fibres are stained strongly by immunohistochemical stains for fibronectin (Sloan and Carter, 1993). At the same time, these fibrils are stained by the high-iron diamine technique following procedures that oxidize the disulphide linkages to sulphonic acid groups (Sannes *et al.*, 1979; Tagaki *et al.*, 1987; Baba *et al.*, 1988). As it is well established that fibronectin is important for fibroblast adhesion and migration (Yamada, 1989), it is reasonable to suggest that oxytalan fibres play a specific role in fibroblast migration within the periodontal ligament (see also Chapter 9).

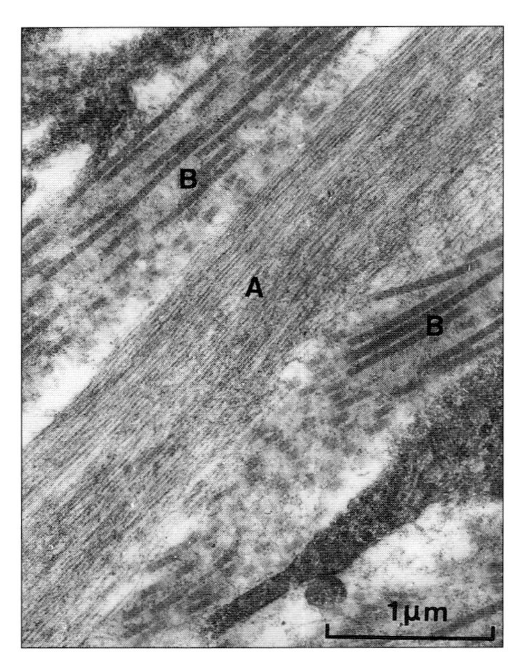

Fig. 2.9 Transmission electron micrograph showing a longitudinally sectioned oxytalan fibre (A) made up of parallel arrays of microfibrils and some collagen fibrils (B). (Magnification × 22,000.)

Elastin

Elastin fibres are only found in the PDL of some species and tooth types. They are composed of a microfibrillar glycoprotein and amorphous elastin, which is a proteinaceous rubber (Ross, 1973; Rosenbloom, 1993). Mature elastin fibres are composed principally of elastin and are contained by arrangements of microfibrils, some of which may remain embedded in the elastin core (Ross, 1973; Kadar, 1974). At the insertion of the elastin fibre, the microfibrils group together to form bundles that are indistinguishable from those that appear in elaunin and oxytalan fibres (Johnson and Pylypas, 1992). The identity of the microfibrillar components of elastin fibres has yet to be fully established, though several microfibril-associated glycoproteins (including fibrillin) have been characterized (Sakai *et al.*, 1986; Gibson *et al.*, 1991; Rosenbloom, 1993).

It has been proposed that the elementary units of elastin are rod-like in shape (Gray *et al.*, 1973), and rod-like structures have been observed using high-resolution ultrastructural techniques in ox elastin (Gotte *et al.*, 1974). The elementary units are probably aggregated into globular protein masses with free solvent in the intervening spaces (Partridge, 1967; Kadar, 1974). Such a model, in which the globular protein masses are compressed or restrained by the hydrophobic tendency, is in accord with the thermodynamic behaviour of elastin (Wainwright *et al.*, 1976).

ARRANGEMENT OF THE PERIODONTAL COLLAGEN FIBRES

FIBRE ARRANGEMENT IN TEETH OF LIMITED GROWTH

Textbook pictures of the fibrous architecture of the PDL are derived from studies published around the turn of the century (Black, 1887, 1899). Groups of principal fibre bundles arranged into gingival, crestal, horizontal, oblique and apical groups were described (*Figs 2.11, 2.12, 2.13*). The fibre bundles were considered to pass directly from cementum to bone, supporting the tooth in the manner of a sling, while at the same time, indifferent fibres were randomly interspersed between the principal fibre bundles. Using both light (Zwarych and Quigley, 1965; Grant *et al.*, 1972) and transmission electron microscopes (Bevelander and Nakahara, 1968; Ten Cate, 1972; Frank *et al.*, 1976), the principal bundles appear to branch into smaller bundles within the ligament to form a continuous plexiform arrangement.

However, persistent technical problems are encountered when preparing the tissues of the periodontium for histological analysis, compounded on the one hand by the difficulties encountered when attempting to deduce three-dimensional arrangements of fibres from two-dimensional sections (Sloan, 1978a), and on the other by the absence of an associated biochemical topography (Carter *et al.*, 1994).

The precise arrangement of the fibres has been the subject of debate, even though the majority of collagen fibrils in the PDL appear to be grouped together to form bundles (Melcher and Eastoe, 1969). Indeed, the apparent disposition of the fibre bundles has varied according to the method of histological preparation (Sloan *et al.*, 1976; Sloan, 1979a,b). For example, the collagen fibres of the PDL appear to be oriented as a random 'indifferent fibre plexus' when ground sections are examined in the scanning electron microscope (Shackleford, 1971, 1973; Svejda and Skach, 1973). This cannot be correlated with either light or transmission electron microscope studies and it is now accepted that the 'indifferent fibre plexus' is an artefact produced by the method of preparation.

Scanning electron microscope studies of the periodontium can be correlated with other histological techniques if the tissues are demineralized and sliced by a razor blade; and using this method the PDL of both the macaque monkey and the human appears to be a continuous band of fibrous tissue (100–150 μm in width) containing prominent neurovascular bundles (Sloan, 1978a,b). The majority of the collagen fibrils appear as bundles in both transverse and longitudinal section and the irregular profiles of the sectioned bundles in the scanning electron microscope suggest that they pursue a complex wavy course (Sloan, 1978b, 1979b). Fibroblasts with extensive flattened cytoplasmic processes are also evident lying between the bundles, and there is an intimate association between the individual fibrils and the cytoplasmic extensions of the fibroblasts, which could facilitate remodelling by intracellular degradation (see also Chapter 1). Close to the cementum, the fibre bundles are 3–10 μm in diameter, while close to the alveolar bone they are 10–20 μm in diameter. The remaining bundles in the PDL are 1–4 μm in diameter. Because of the frequent branching and the wavy course pursued by the anastomosing bundles, it is impossible to trace an intact network of bundles across the periodontal space using bright field microscopy.

The complex relationships between the networks of bundles may be investigated using polarizing microscopy (*Fig. 2.14*). In transverse sections, the birefringence of the collagen suggests that there is a predominance of radiating circumflex fibres that curve around the neurovascular bundles (Sloan, 1978b, 1979a). In longitudinal sections, overlapping networks of anastomosing bundles are evident within the horizontal, oblique, and apical groups. These descend from the alveolar surface and are obliquely orientated to the axis of the tooth.

On the other hand, it has been suggested that the PDL behaves as a thixotropic gel (Kardos and Simpson, 1979). The evidence for this is based primarily on a reinterpretation of the tooth support data of Parfitt (1967). The theory proposes that, until ageing occurs, only the transseptal fibres of the gingiva are polymerized, the remainder persisting as a gel. Application of a force to such a system could cause a change from a gel to a sol, which would result in flow. In order to satisfy the requirements of the theory, the fibres seen in histological preparations must be considered as artefacts, but it is difficult to reconcile this view with the observations of Mashouf and Engel (1975), who found highly organized birefringent collagen fibres in the rat periodontal ligament in fresh undemineralized sections.

FIBRE ARRANGEMENT IN CONTINUOUSLY GROWING TEETH

As the continuously growing incisor of rodents and lagomorphs has been widely used in dental research and in studies of tooth eruption, it will be considered here. Light microscope and scanning electron microscope studies have demonstrated that the PDL of the mature tooth of limited growth is organized into three distinct zones during development and eruption (Eccles, 1959; Kerebel and Balouet, 1967; Levy and Bernick, 1968; Levy *et al.*, 1972; Grant *et al.,* 1972; Beertsen and Everts, 1977; Sloan, 1978b). By the time functional occlusion is reached, however, the collagen fibres are organized as continuous bundles that insert into the alveolar bone and cementum as Sharpey fibres (for further discussion of the development of the PDL see Chapter 8). The collagen fibres of the PDL of continuously growing rodent teeth also appear to be arranged into three zones (*Fig. 2.15*). For many years it was accepted that the collagen fibrils of the outer (alveolar) and inner (cemental) zones in the continuouosly growing incisor were organized into bundles that inserted into the mineralized tissue as Sharpey fibres (Sicher, 1923; Hunt, 1959; Ness and Smale, 1959; Eccles, 1964; Ciancio *et al.*, 1967; Beertsen and Snijder, 1969; Beertsen *et al.,* 1974; Beertsen and Everts, 1977). It was also accepted that the fibres of the middle zone were spliced together to form an intermediate plexus (Sicher 1923, 1942) and that this arrangement facilitated remodelling of the ligament during tooth eruption. The intermediate plexus is now thought to be a histological artefact because the fibres of the middle zone form a continuous branching network of bundles in transverse section rather than an intermediate plexus (Ciancio *et al.*, 1967; Hindle, 1967).

A model has been proposed for the three-dimensional structure of the rabbit PDL which accounts for these observations (Sloan 1978a). It is accepted that the collagen fibrils in the outer and inner zones are organized into round bundles as described in previous studies. The alveolar zone bundles are larger than the cemental zone bundles and the collagen bundles in the alveolar and cemental zones are oriented radially. In the middle zone, however, rather than being organized as an intermediate plexus, the model proposed that the collagen fibrils are arranged into thin sheets that form a series of flattened compartments running along the axis of the tooth (*Fig. 2.16*). This accords with light microscope observations (Sicher, 1923; Hindle, 1967; Ciancio *et al.,* 1967), in that the three fibrous zones are only evident in longitudinal sections. In the same way, the homogeneous appearance of the

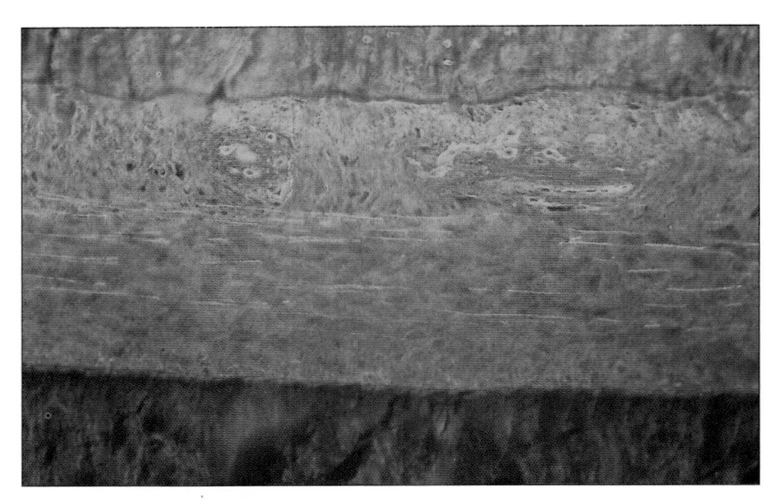

Fig. 2.10 Longitudinal cryosection of rat incisor periodontal ligament. Immunofluorescent stain for fibronectin showing oxytalan fibres. (Magnification × 70.)

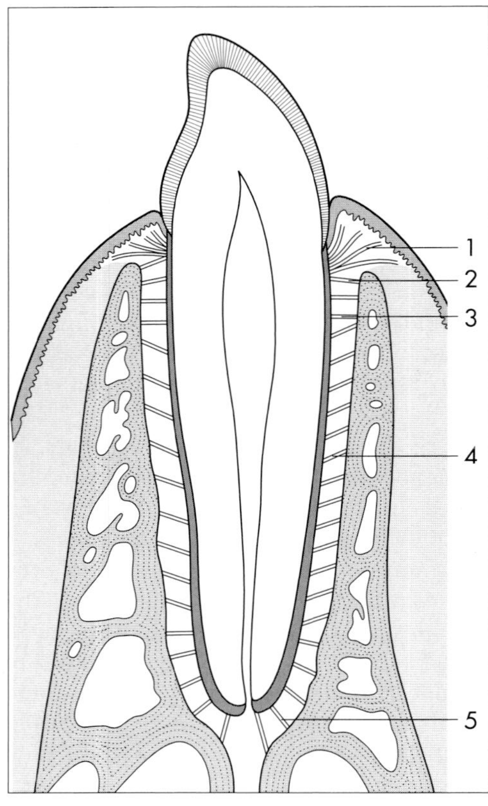

Fig. 2.11 Diagram showing the arrangement of periodontal collagen into groups of principal fibres. 1 – gingival, 2 – crestal, 3 – horizontal, 4 – oblique, 5 – apical.

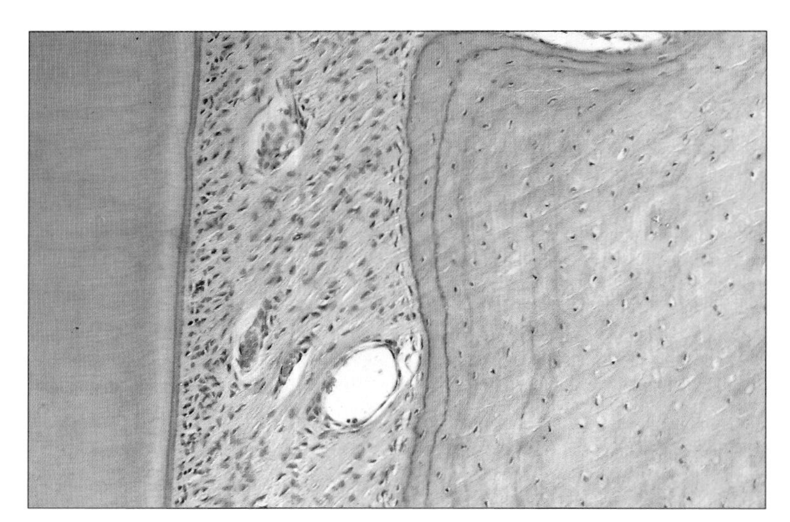

Fig. 2.12 Monkey periodontal ligament showing arrays of oblique fibres and their insertion into the alveolus. (Haematoxylin and eosin stain × 70.)

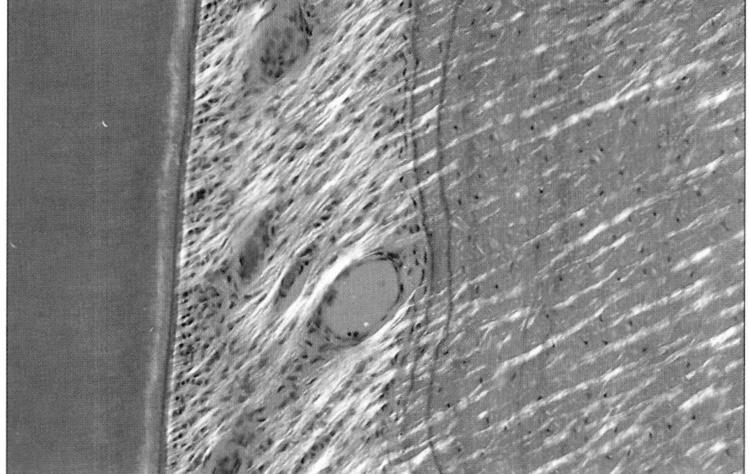

Fig. 2.13 Same field as Fig. 2.12 showing orientation of oblique fibres and their insertion. (Polarized light, magnification × 75.)

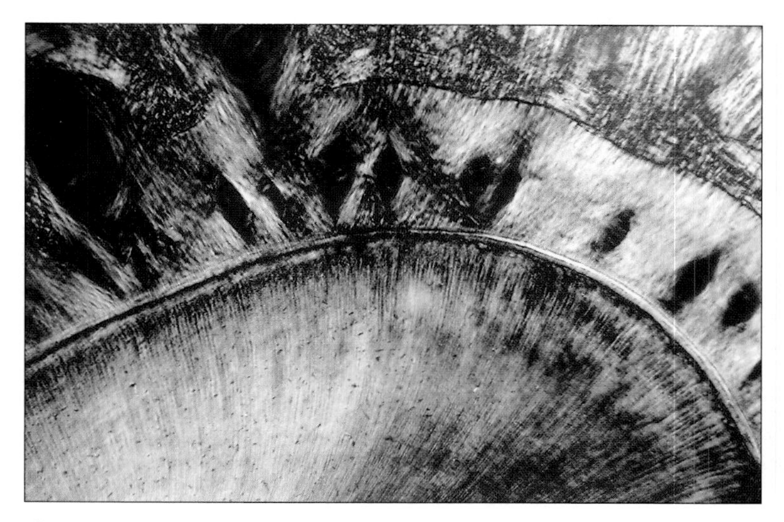

Fig. 2.14 Transverse section of monkey periodontal ligament viewed in polarized light showing the overlapping arrangement of groups of circumflex bundles. (Magnification × 30.)

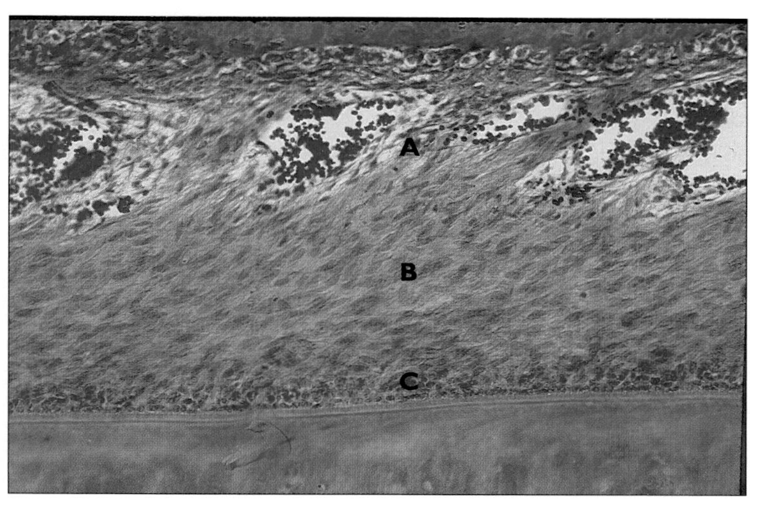

Fig. 2.15 Longitudinal paraffin section showing the three zones of the rabbit incisor periodontal ligament: (A) alveolar, (B) middle, and (C) cemental zones. (Heidenhains azan-trichrome stain × 190.)

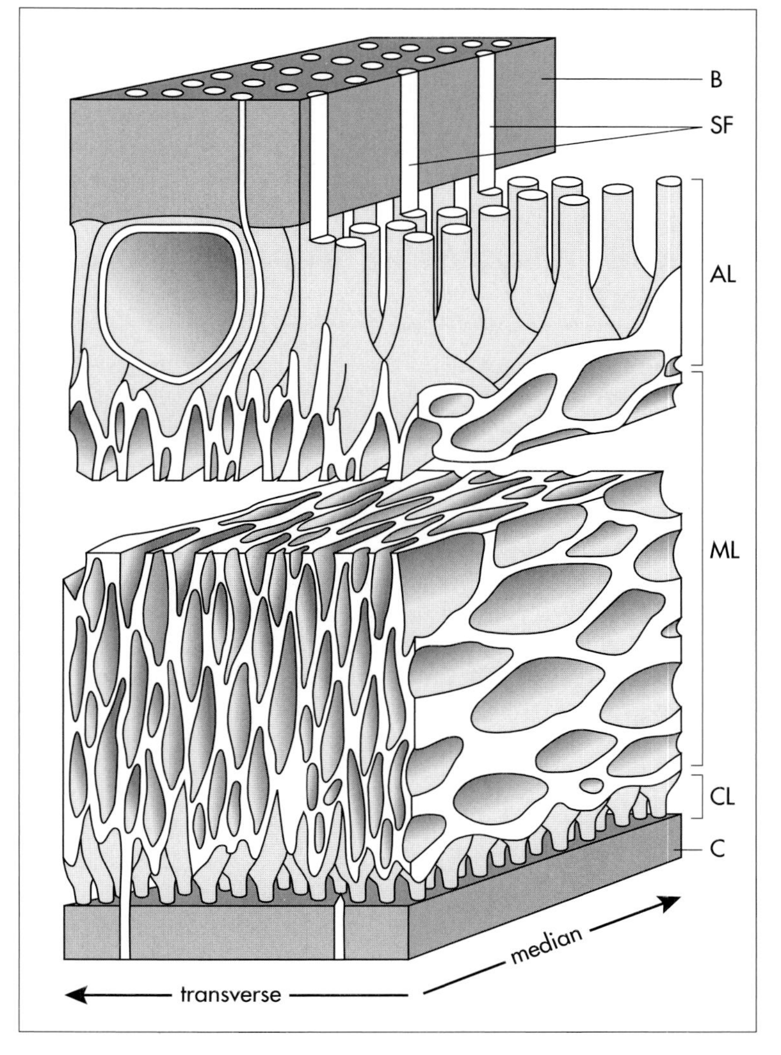

Fig. 2.16 Diagram showing the proposed arrangement of collagen in the periodontal ligament of the continuously growing incisor, showing alveolar bone (B) with inserting Sharpey fibres (SF), which are continuous with ligament bundles in the alveolar layer (AL). The middle layer collagen (ML) is arranged into longitudinally oriented laminates, while the cemental layer (CL) collagen is organized into bundles that insert into cementum (C).

middle zone in the scanning electron microscope in longitudinal section would be due to the sheets of collagen lying in the section plane (whereas in transverse section they would appear to be composed of bundles). Evidence for this arrangement is provided by the flattened morphology of the fibroblast cytoplasmic extensions in the middle zone of the rabbit incisor PDL (Ness and Smale, 1959) and possibly also by biomechanical studies (albeit *in vitro*), which have shown that the strength and resilience of the PDL is greater in the rat molar than in the incisor (Chiba *et al.*, 1990; Komatsu and Chiba, 1993; Chiba and Komatsu, 1993).

Attempts have also been made to determine whether the collagen fibres in the middle zone of the PDL differ from those of the other layers. Using polarizing microscopy, Hindle (1967) concluded that the collagen fibres in the middle zone were less mature than those of the alveolar and cemental zones, on account of their relatively low birefringence. In transverse section, the middle zone collagen appeared as a network of birefringent bundles, whereas in longitudinal section the middle zone collagen showed only patchy birefringence. This can also be explained by the spatial distribution of collagen fibres of the middle zone if they were arranged into sheets (Sloan, 1979a), because the highly oriented collagen fibres would only produce measurable birefringence when the sheet was transversely sectioned. A longitudinal section would include several sheets or parts of sheets of varying orientation, an arrangement which would produce a generally lowered or patchy birefringence (*Fig. 2.17*).

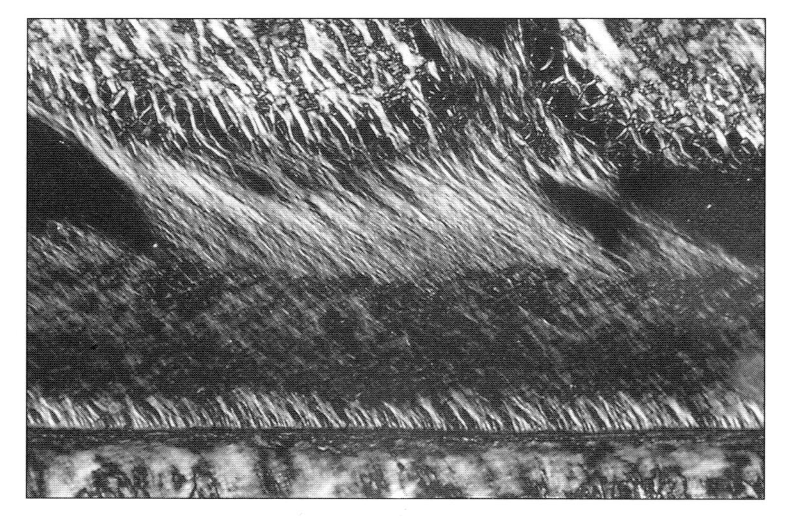

Fig. 2.17 Unstained longitudinal section of rabbit incisor periodontal ligament showing patchy birefringence of the middle zone. (Magnification × 190.)

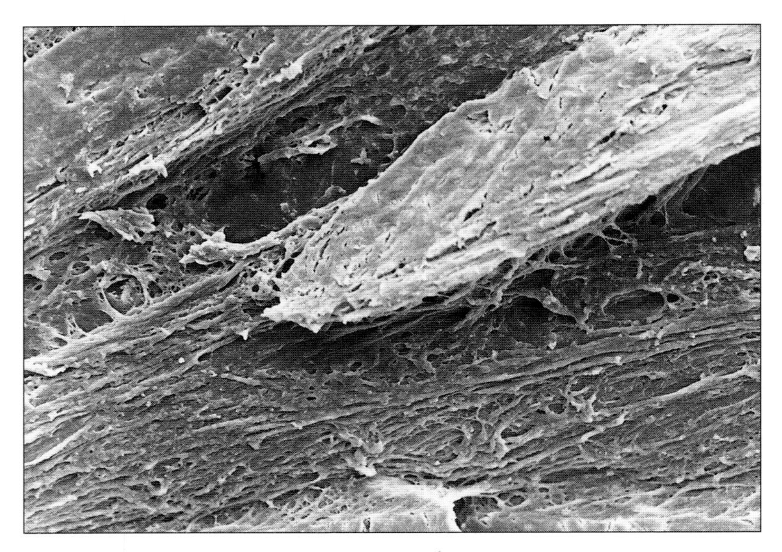

Fig. 2.18 Scanning electron micrographs of longitudinal cryosections of rat incisor periodontal ligament showing inserting alveolar and cemental bundles (arrows). (Magnification × 490.)

More recent scanning electron microscope studies in our laboratory using cryosections of rat incisor (Carter and Sloan, 1994) have confirmed that the middle zone fibrils are arranged as sheets (*Figs 2.18, 2.19, 2.20*).

COLLAGEN TURNOVER IN THE PERIODONTAL LIGAMENT

It is necessary to account for the way in which the differential forces that are generated to effect tooth eruption are transmitted to the tooth. It has been proposed that there is a rapidly remodelling zone of shear within the middle zone of the ligament. The inner cemental zone could then move with the tooth while the outer alveolar zone would remain anchored into the alveolus (Beertsen and Everts, 1977). Much effort has been directed towards identifying the site and the extent of remodelling in the three zones of the erupting periodontal ligament.

Radiolabelling techniques have shown that many apparently stable tissues turn over at the molecular level (e.g. Lapiere, 1967). Measurements of tritiated proline and tritiated glycine uptake in the PDL of erupting teeth have indicated that there is a high turnover of collagen with a half-life varying between 3 and 23 days (Stallard, 1963; Crumley, 1964; Carneiro and Leblond, 1966; Anderson, 1967; Ramos and Hunt, 1967; Thomas, 1967; Magnusson, 1968; Robins, 1972; Skougaard *et al.*, 1970; Carneiro and Fava de Moraes, 1965). In fact, the turnover of collagen in the

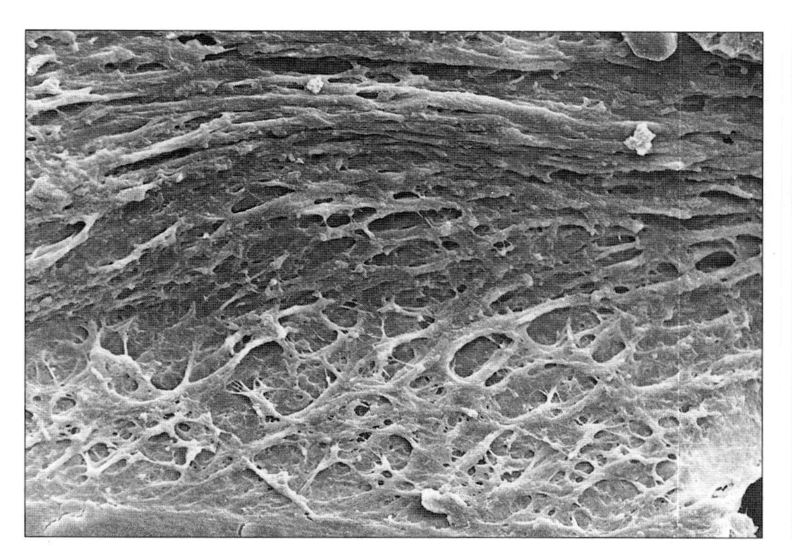

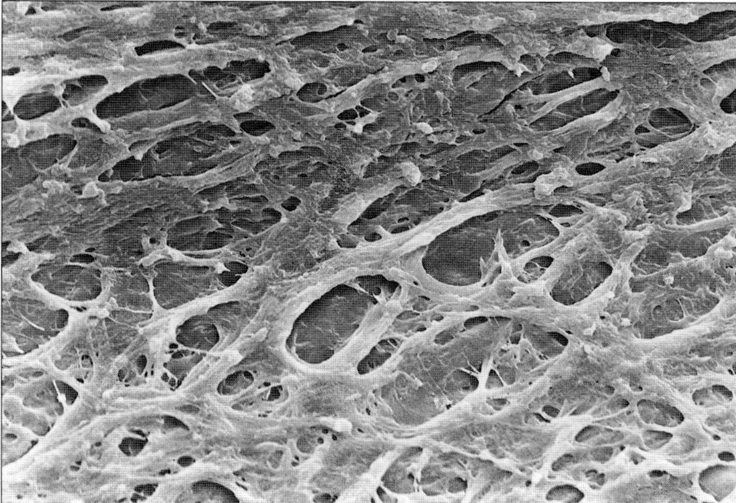

Figs 2.19, 2.20 Scanning electron micrographs showing detail of the middle zone laminates and the bundles of the cemental and alveolar zone. *Fig. 2.20* shows detail of the laminates and their relation to the bundles. (Magnification × 680 – **2.19**; × 1800 – **2.20**.)

PDL is estimated to be several times greater than in skin and oral mucosa (see Sodek, 1989 for review).

These results, however, (which can only be semi-quantitative because uptake of the labelled amino acid precursor alone was measured) failed to demonstrate any layer within the ligament where collagen turnover was localized (though differences in the rate of turnover were noted between apical and crestal regions). Although it has been suggested that the proportion of labelled amino acid precursor taken up specifically into the collagen was not measured by these studies (because proline may also be incorporated into non-collagenous proteins – Laurent, 1987; Sodek and Ferrier, 1988), more refined biochemical microassays have confirmed that hydroxyproline was mainly incorporated into collagen (Sodek, 1977; Sodek *et al.,* 1977).

More precise measurement of collagen turnover can be attained by autoradiographic techniques using tritiated proline administered by intraperitoneal injection (Rippin, 1976a,b). By measuring grain densities in various regions of the PDL and by plotting regression lines of log grain density against time, it was demonstrated that the collagen turnover varied in young rats (i.e. 2.45–6.47 days in the apical and crestal regions respectively). Nevertheless, turnover seemed to occur evenly over the width of the ligament and no distinct layer of rapid remodelling in the middle of the ligament was identified. Rippin (1978) also observed that older rats had a slightly lower turnover rate and that turnover increased in hypofunctional molars. Similar conclusions were also reached by studying the turnover of ground substance using labelled sulphated glycosaminoglycans (Baumhammers and Stallard, 1968). Collagen turnover is also considered in Chapter 3.

Evidence for a 'zone of shear' has been derived from studies that have examined both the pattern of uptake and the subsequent loss of tritiated proline. Grain densities were initially found to be highest in the growing region, but with time there was a shift of the peak of labelling occlusally at a rate comparable with that of tooth eruption (Beertsen and Everts, 1977). This shift was interpreted as evidence for the movement of the inner zone of the PDL. Further support for the presence of a 'zone of shear' has been provided by morphometric analyses of the ligament of the erupting incisor; these analyses have demonstrated that banded fibril-containing phagolysosomes are concentrated in the fibroblasts of the middle zone (Beertsen and Everts, 1977). However, this was not confirmed in another study (Shore and Berkovitz, 1979). Such phagolysosomes are discussed in Chapter 1. Similar phagolysosomes are found in other connective tissues where rapid collagen remodelling events occur, e.g. in the endometrial stroma (Zorn *et al.,* 1989).

It has been shown that the specific degradation and removal of collagen type VI may precede remodelling of the major banded collagen fibrils in the periosteum, periodontium (Everts and Beertsen, 1992) and endometrial stroma (Mulholland *et al.,* 1992).

Despite this, some evidence for a specific zone of remodelling in the rodent incisor has been provided using immunohistochemical studies that enable the preparation of cryosections of the incisor (*Fig. 2.21*) (Carter *et al.*, 1994). The stain for collagen type VI was evident in all zones of the PDL of the fully erupted molars but was absent from the middle zone of the erupting molar and incisor (*Fig. 2.22*) (Sloan *et al.*, 1993). The apparent absence of collagen type VI from the middle zone cannot be explained by the simple lack of collagenous matrix in the region, as stains for collagen type I and III were uniform across the PDL (*Fig. 2.23*), and cross banded collagen fibrils are present (Berkovitz *et al.*, 1981; Berkovitz and Moxham, 1989). This suggests that a specific process of collagen remodelling occurs in this region by intracellular phagocytosis (Sloan *et al.*, 1993). The absence of collagen type VI could either predispose the fibres to further remodelling or it could enable the sheets of collagen to slide past each other. The lack of data supporting these histological observations from tracer studies may simply reflect the poor

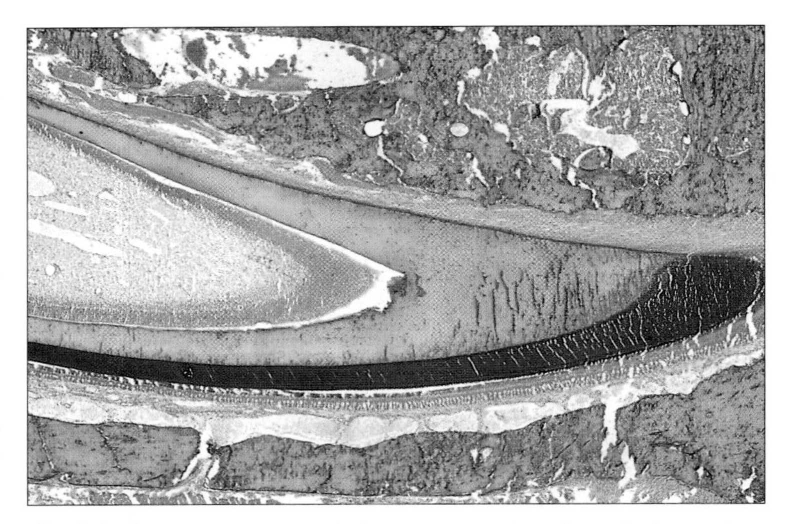

Fig. 2.21 Low-power micrograph showing cryosection of a rat incisor and surrounding tissues. (Haematoxylin and eosin × 20.)

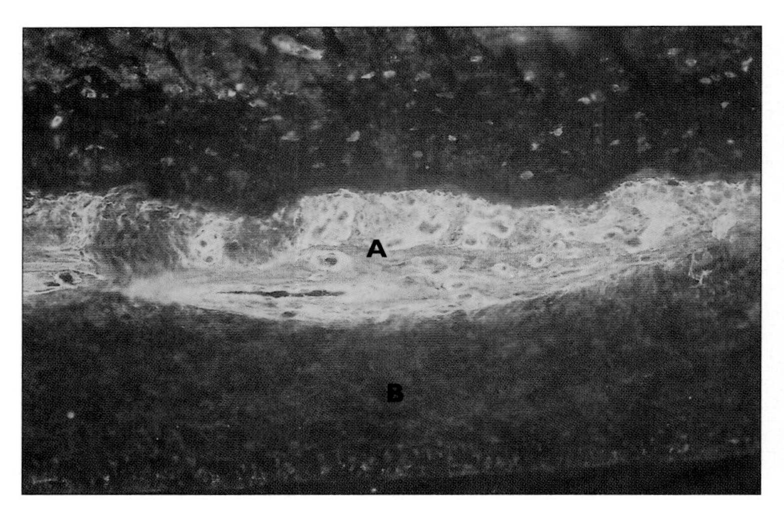

Fig. 2.22 Longitudinal cryosection of rat incisor periodontal ligament showing strong staining of the alveolar zone for type VI collagen (A) and the absence of staining of the middle zone (B). (Magnification × 50.)

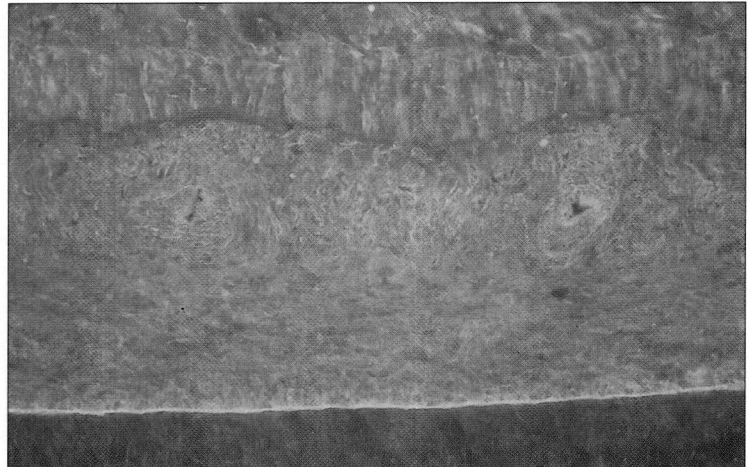

Fig. 2.23 Longitudinal cryosection of rat incisor showing the uniform staining of the periodontal ligament for type III collagen. Note the staining of Sharpey fibres in the alveolar bone. (Magnification × 70.)

resolution of these techniques when assessing turnover in heterogeneous regions of the extracellular matrix or when interpreting results against a background of generally rapid turnover.

The concept of an 'intermediate plexus' or a 'zone of shear' depends not only on histological or radiolabelling studies, but also on functional considerations. In this aspect, there is evidence to suggest that the 'zone of shear' may be restricted to the tissue at the very surface of the root. In a study of the rat incisor ligament following root resection (Berkovitz, Shore and Sloan, 1980), it was found that the PDL persisted for a short distance beneath the erupting tooth fragment lining the vacated socket. Indeed, almost the entire width of the ligament was present and its fibrous architecture was maintained. Examination of the lathyrytic PDL also shows evidence of a cleavage zone adjacent to the tooth (Shore, Berkovitz and Moxham, 1984). Clearly, further more specific immunohistochemical analyses are required to evaluate the nature of the periodontal fibres and remodelling events of the mid– zone.

FUNCTIONAL ADAPTATIONS OF THE COLLAGEN FIBRES OF THE PDL

Current theories of tooth support envisage a multiphasic system involving fibres, ground substance, blood vessels, and fluid, all acting together to resist mechanical forces, and it seems that there is both tension and compression of the tissues (see Chapter 10). Minns *et al.* (1973) showed that the internal orientation of collagen fibres in connective tissues influences the mechanical properties of the tissue and suggested that, in general, collagenous bundles could best resist axially directed forces. The arrangement of the majority of the PDL collagen fibres into horizontal and obliquely directed groups may therefore be adapted to resist such axial forces (which would, at the same time, involve straightening the crimp). The overlapping arrangement of the bundle networks seen in the scanning electron microscope and by polarizing microscopy could also be of importance in resisting rotational forces. Such an arrangement has mechanical advantages over a simple radial arrangement and is often used in engineering (e.g. in arranging the wire spokes of a wheel) (*Figs 2.24, 2.25*; see *Fig. 2.14*).

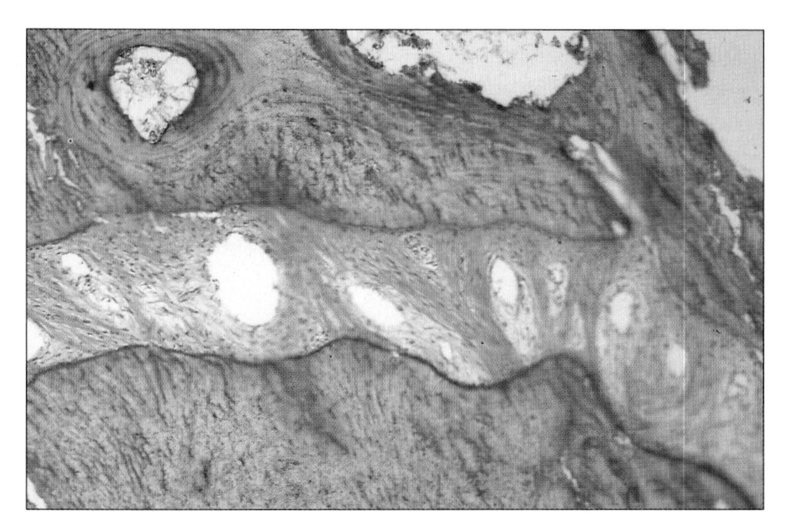

Fig. 2.24 Transverse cryosection of human periodontal ligament showing circumflex and radial arrangements of the principal fibres. (Haematoxylin and eosin × 56.)

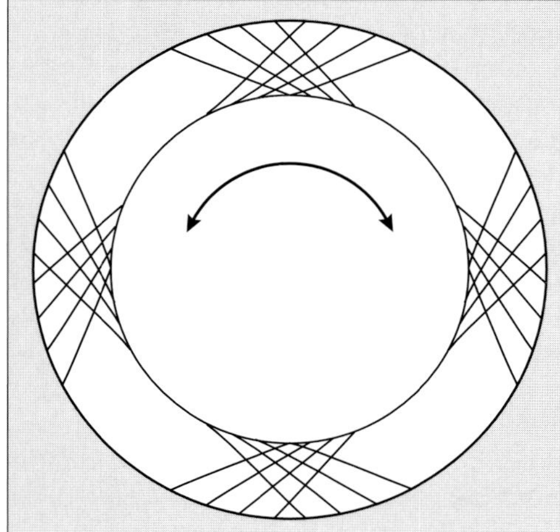

Fig. 2.25 Diagram showing the disposition of the circumflex periodontal fibres in the erupted tooth. When subjected to rotational and intrusive forces, some fibre groups will be in tension.

The overlapping arrangement of the bundles may also be advantageous in resisting intrusive forces, as axial displacement of the tooth would tend to straighten out the fibre bundles and compress the blood vessels. The complex three-dimensional arrangement of the fibres also means that some bundles would always be placed in tension, irrespective of the direction of an applied force. This enables local areas of the PDL to resist compressive forces, a property that might otherwise be impossible on account of the anisotropic properties of the collagenous bundles (Minns *et al.*, 1973).

COLLAGEN CRIMPING

Collagenous tissues exhibit a quantifiable periodicity of structure of variable scale, ranging from submicroscopic to anatomical; the waveform that describes this periodicity has been referred to as a 'crimp' (Diamant *et al.*, 1972; Keller and Gathercole, 1976). In the polarizing microscope, crimping can be recognized by a regular banding of dark lines across a collagenous bundle observed when its axis lies perpendicular to the polarizer directions. It has been suggested that crimping may be due not only to a sharp zig-zag arrangement of collagen fibrils, but also to the microanatomical organization of collagenous sheets and bundles (Gathercole and Keller, 1991). Alternative explanations postulate that the waveform is sinusoidal (reviewed by Viidik, 1980) and that sharp bending is unlikely to exist *in vivo*. However, an accumulating body of evidence from polarizing microscopy, transmission and scanning electron microscopy, biomechanical studies, and x-ray diffraction analysis favours a crimped arrangement (Parry, 1988; Gathercole and Keller, 1991).

Examination of the PDL fibres and other ligaments in polarized light has shown that the collagen fibre bundles have a 'crimped' structure that may itself confer special mechanical properties on the ligament (*Fig. 2.26*). The crimp may be in the form of a well-defined zig-zag in some tissues (e.g. in tendon) with a quantifiable periodicity and angular deflection from the fibre axis (Diamant *et al.*, 1972). A typical stress–strain curve for rat-tail tendon shows that there is an early, easily extensible, non-linear region attributable to straightening out of the crimp (Diamant *et al.*, 1972; Keller and Gathercole, 1976). This may enable the ligament to absorb impact tensile loads without extending the collagen fibrils and without generating heat (Trelstad and Silver, 1981).

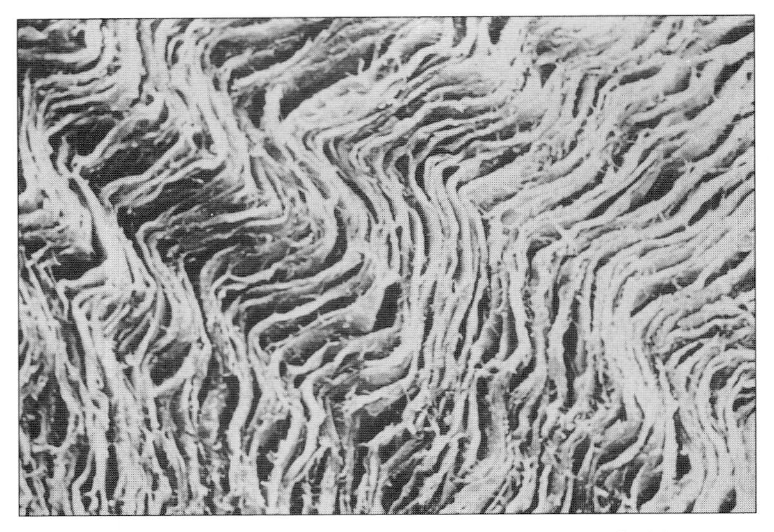

Fig. 2.26 Scanning electron micrograph of transverse section of rabbit periodontal ligament showing crimped arrangement of the fibres (× 1000).

The crimped structure of the collagen fibrils in the PDL is, however, less well defined and, although there is evidence of a biphasic response to tooth loading in the ligament (Moxham and Berkovitz, 1983), further analyses are required to establish whether it has a role in tooth support. It has also been suggested that fibroblast processes in developing collagenous tissues may play a role in fabricating the crimped arrangement (Shah *et al.*, 1982), and consequently that crimping may be an important feature in tooth eruption (Gathercole and Keller, 1991). There is, however, no evidence to suggest that the crimp can generate contractile forces in the collagen molecules.

SHARPEY FIBRES

At their insertions, the collagen bundles of the PDL are embedded into cementum and alveolar bone in a manner similar to a tendon inserting into bone – i.e. in the form of Sharpey fibres. The orientation of the Sharpey fibres in the alveolar bone is similar to that of the adjacent PDL bundles (Melcher and Eastoe, 1969) and they tend to be concentrated in the crestal region. However, a variety of orientations are seen in cementum (Selvig, 1964, 1965;

Yamamoto and Wakita, 1992). Light microscope observations (Quigley, 1970; Cohn, 1972a,b, 1975) have suggested that some Sharpey fibres in mice, hamsters, monkey, and humans pass right through alveolar bone, which implies that there may be continuity between the collagen fibres of the PDL of adjacent teeth. Although the existence of these transalveolar fibres has been disputed (Atkinson, 1978), transalveolar fibres appear to be a major structural feature of the interdental septum in the young mouse (Johnson, 1987).

On the basis of ultrastructural and microradiographic observations, Dreyfuss and Frank (1964) and Selvig (1965) have reported that most of the Sharpey fibres that insert into alveolar bone have unmineralized cores and are separated from each other by lamellar bone fibres which either run parallel to the mineral surface or are randomly arranged. Immunohistochemical studies have shown that Sharpey fibres are enclosed within a sheath of collagen type III (Wang *et al.,* 1980) (*Fig. 2.27*), and it has been suggested that this collagen may not only confer elasticity on the fibres, but also that it maintains the elasticity of the fibres when inserted into bone by preventing their mineralization (Wang *et al.,* 1980; Tung *et al.,* 1985; Huang *et al.*, 1991). Poorly mineralized coarse birefringent fibres, which are recognized by antibodies raised against collagen type III, are also a feature of developing intramembranous bone (Carter *et al.*, 1991) (*Fig. 2.28*), where they appear to form a preliminary framework for the generation of the new trabeculae. Because a proportion of these fibres persist in the mature skeleton, and because they appear to extend from the Sharpey fibres of myotendinous insertions, it was suggested that they were central to the maintenance of skeletal integrity (Carter *et al.,* 1991). If so, the periodontal ligament may be important not only to the maintenance of the dentition, but also to the whole of the periodontal apparatus; this is well illustrated by the atrophy of the alveolar bone that often follows the removal of the teeth and associated PDL (Devlin and Ferguson, 1991).

After the removal of the soft covering connective tissue by enzymatic or chemical means and examination of the surface of alveolar bone and cementum with the scanning electron microscope, it is evident that the peripheral bone surrounding the Sharpey fibres may be mineralized to a level that is slightly above or below the level of the bone surface, depending on their state of development (Boyde 1968, 1972; Boyde and Jones 1968; Jones and Boyde 1972, 1974). Where the fibres insert obliquely, the bone surface exhibits a stepped appearance that indicates that mineralization occurs approximately at right angles to the axis of the fibre (Jones and Boyde, 1972). The mineralized periphery of the fibres may confer some local mechanical advantage for transmitting axially directed forces; while the occurrence of mineralization at approximately right angles to the axis of the fibre suggests that the Sharpey fibres are subjected to tensional forces. The mineral interface also appears concave and this would confer maximum strength to the mineral–collagen interface, which is the weakest part of the fibre bundle (Jones and Boyde, 1972). Distinct clusters of mineralized spheres may be evident within the fibres, but the role of these structures is yet to be established.

THE ARRANGEMENT AND FUNCTIONAL ADAPTATIONS OF THE ELASTIC FIBRES OF THE PDL

Mature elastin fibres have been described in the PDL of deer, pigs, cattle, dogs, and alligators (Fullmer *et al.*, 1974; Soule, 1967; Tagaki *et al.,* 1989) and they are especially prominent in the coronal one-third of the ligament in the herbivores (Fullmer *et al.,* 1974). This suggests that elastin fibres may dampen lateral masticatory stresses and, in this situation, the low modulus and long-range reversible extensibility of elastin would seem to be more important than resilience as a physical property.

In contrast, it has been reported previously that oxytalan alone is present in the PDL of man, monkey, rat, and mouse (Fullmer *et al.,* 1974; Edmunds *et al.,* 1979; Hirayami *et al.*, 1985; Tagaki *et al.,* 1987), and it may be that oxytalan fibres have a specific role in stabilizing the tooth in certain functional situations (even though they appear to be a minor component of the tissue). Consquently, it has been shown that there are few oxytalan fibres in the PDL of unerupted alligator teeth compared with the erupted teeth, where these fibres are numerous and highly interconnected to elastin fibres (Takagi *et al.,* 1989). While it has been reported that orthodontic manipulation of PDL causes lengthening and narrowing of oxytalan fibres in humans (Jonas and Riede, 1980), another study failed to observe any changes in oxytalan fibres in rats (Bowling and Rygh, 1988).

The oxytalan fibres and collagen bundles of the periodontal ligament often appear to interweave at right angles to each other (Simpson, 1967; Edmunds *et al.,* 1979) in a manner similar to elastic ligaments near their insertion (e.g. ligamentum nuchae) (Serafini-Fracassini *et al.,* 1977). It also appears that oxytalan fibres can act in the same way as elastin fibres because they are straightened by forced extrusion and they become wavy with forced intrusion (Sims, 1976). If this is so, an attachment of oxytalan fibres would be necessary, either directly to collagen as proposed by Edmunds *et al.* (1979), or indirectly through the

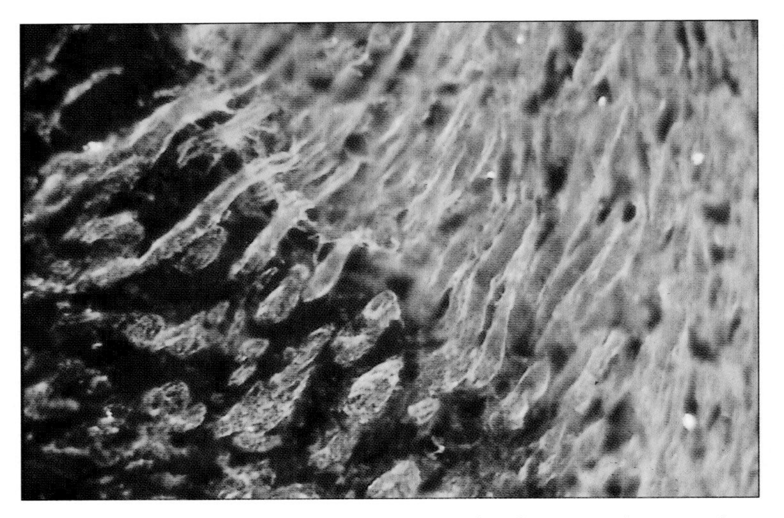

Fig. 2.27 Sharpey fibre insertion showing peripheral staining of inserting bundles with immunofluorescent stain for collagen type III (A – bone). (Magnification × 280.)

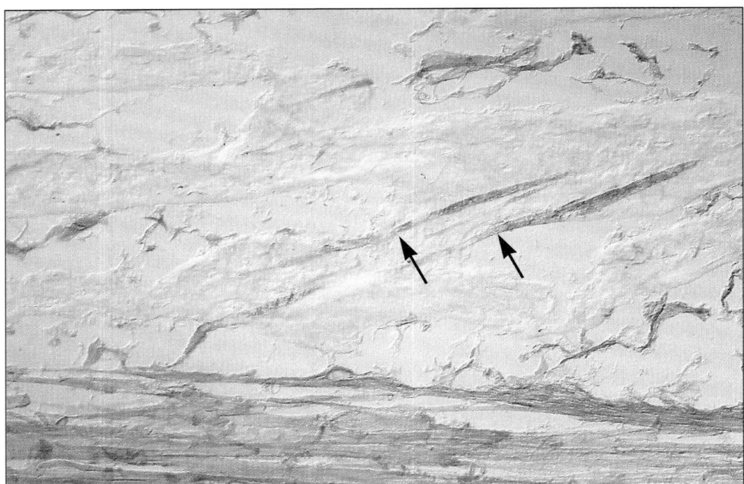

Fig. 2.28 Immunoperoxidase staining for collagen type III showing coarse fibre bundles arising from the periosteum of the femoral anlage and inserting into the primary trabeculae (arrows). (Magnification × 140.)

vasculature. Evidence for such attachments has been presented for the human premolar and mouse molar teeth, in which the largest apical occlusal oxytalan fibres are linked to laterally anastomosing minor fibres that insert into cementum and the connective tissue surrounding neurovascular structures (Fullmer *et al.,* 1974; Sims, 1975, 1976, 1983, 1984). More recently, the association has been confirmed in a study in which the collagenous and cellular elements were removed from the PDL using ultrasonication in sodium hydroxide (Johnson and Pylypas, 1992). It was shown that the elastic system of the mouse was actually composed of irregular, fenestrated sheets of elaunin attached to cementum, alveolar bone, and blood vessels by anchoring filaments of oxytalan. The study indicated that the elastic system of the ligament is not only more extensive than previously appreciated (Freezer and Sims, 1987) but also that the interconnected arrangement of oxytalan and elaunin fibres is similar to that found in other connective tissues (Bock and Stockinger, 1984; Bonnaure-Mallet and Lescoat, 1989).

The close relationship of oxytalan fibres to the periodontal blood vessels and putative nerve endings has lead to the suggestion that the fibres act as part of a mechanoreceptor system which modulates the behaviour of the vessels either directly or indirectly through a more general neural response (Sims, 1983; see also Chapter 5).

It is also possible that the structural integrity of the sliding collagen sheets of the middle zone of the erupting ligament is maintained during eruption by interspersed sheets of elastic elements, anchored on the one hand to the vasculature and on the other to the inserted Sharpey fibres of the cemental and alveolar zones. There is a pressing requirement for a reassessment of the elastic fibre network of the periodontal ligament (including its relationship to the collagen fibres) with regard to both tooth eruption and tooth support.

AGEING OF THE PERIODONTAL FIBRES

Comparatively few studies have been carried out on the effects of ageing on the fibres of the periodontium, and those that have lack any detailed quantification. Qualitative studies of the aged human periodontal ligament have suggested that the main change with age is increased collagen fibrosis and decreased cellularity (Grant and Bernick, 1972). It was also claimed that the fibre bundles were thicker and that the fibre groups seemed to be broader and more highly organized. Areas of hyalinization were present and there was decreased argyrophilia, increased fuchsinophilia, and a reduction in alcian blue-positive areas. Sporadic mineralization of the fibres was also seen. On the other hand, an apparent decrease in the number of periodontal fibres has been reported in aged Galagos primates (Grant *et al.*, 1973) and in human post-mortem tissues (Severson *et al.,* 1978), in which there was also an increase in the size of interstitial spaces. The decrease in collagen fibre content may be the combined result of the decrease in cellularity (Klingsberg and Butcher, 1960; Grant and Bernick, 1972; Severson *et al.,* 1978) and the formation of multinucleated fibroblasts (Sasaki and Garant, 1993). The number of synthesizing connective tissue cells decreases in the ageing PDL of the mouse and rat (Toto and Borg, 1968; Jensen and Toto, 1968) and an age-dependent decrease in the rate of collagen synthesis in the mouse molar periodontal ligament has also been reported (Stahl and Tonna, 1977). Although explanted gingival fibroblasts exhibit reduced collagen synthesis with increasing donor age, this has not been demonstrated in PDL fibroblasts (Johnson *et al.,* 1986).

Severson *et al.* (1978) found that the periodontal alveolar bone surface was smooth and regular in young adults and that the insertions of the PDL fibres were fairly evenly distributed. In older adults, the corresponding surfaces were jagged and uneven and an irregular insertion of fibres was seen. Cementum was thicker in aged tissues and the cemental surface also became irregular with time. This irregularity of the fibre insertions, together with replacement of some of the PDL space by interstitial areas and fat cells, suggests that the structural organization of the ligament degenerates with age.

The recognition of the dividing line between age change and pathological change poses one of the fundamental problems in studying the pathogenesis of chronic inflammatory periodontal disease. Using gnotobiotic rats, Socransky *et al.* (1970) found that age-related changes, including recession of the alveolar crest, occurred within the periodontium in the absence of inflammatory periodontal disease. It has also been shown that in rodents the response of connective tissues to injury is affected by ageing (Holm-Pedersen and Viidik, 1972) and age-related changes to collagen fibres both in structure (Torp *et al.,* 1975) and composition (Bailey and Robins, 1976) have been reported. Furthermore, a gradual recession of alveolar bone in the gnotobiotic rat with increasing age has been reported (Amstad-Jossi and Schroeder, 1978). Whilst the volume density of gingival connective tissue occupied by collagen fibrils was found to remain fairly constant with age, the size and numerical density of the fibroblasts varied greatly. These features may be compared to studies of early inflammatory periodontal disease, in which collagen loss is a prominent feature (Schroeder *et al.*, 1973; Garant, 1976; reviewed by Williams *et al.,* 1992).

The later stages of periodontal disease, however, involve the deeper structure of the ligament, and failure involves the breakdown of the tooth support mechanism. It seems likely that alterations to the collagen fibres of the ligament play a prominent role in the breakdown. At the same time, since in many tissues ageing effects can be attributed to alterations in elastin rather than alterations in collagen (Rosenbloom, 1993), studies are required to determine the effects of ageing on the periodontal elastic network. A greater understanding of the part played by the fibres in normal tooth support would therefore contribute greatly to the understanding of chronic inflammatory periodontal disease.

REFERENCES

Amenta PS, Gay S, Vaheri A and Martinez-Hernandez A (1986) The extracellular matrix is an integrated unit: ultrastructural localization of collagen types I, III, IV, V, VI, fibronectin and laminin in human term placenta. Collagen Res Rel 6, 125–152.

Amstad-Jossi M and Schroeder HE (1978) Age related alterations of periodontal structures around the cemento-enamel junction and of the gingival connective tissue composition in germ-free rats. J Periodont Res 13, 76–90.

Anderson AA (1967) The protein matrixes of the teeth and periodontium in hamsters: a tritiated proline study. J Dent Res 46, 67–78.

Atkinson ME (1978) The development of transalveolar periodontal ligament fibres in the mouse. J Dent Res 57, 151 (abstract).

Baba T, Takagi M, Kagami A, Hishikawa H and Hosokawa, Y (1988) Ultrastructural cytochemical properties of elastin-associated microfibrils and their relation to fibronectin. Histochem J 20, 688–696.

Bailey AJ and Robins SP (1976) Current topics in the biosynthesis, structure and function of collagen. Sci Prog 63, 419–444.

Baumhammers A and Stallard RE (1968) S^{35}-sulfate utilization and turnover by the connective tissues of the periodontium. J Periodont Res 13, 187–193.

Becker J, Schuppan D, Rabanus J, Rauch R, Niechoy U and Gelderblom HR (1991) Immunoelectron microscopic localization of collagens type I, V, VI and of procollagen type III in human periodontal ligament and cementum. J Histochem Cytochem 39, 103–110.

Beersten W and Snijder J (1969) A comparative study on the histological structure of the periodontal membranes of teeth with a continuous and non-continuous eruption. Ned Tijdschr Tandheelk 76, 542–569.

Beersten W, Everts V and van den Hooff A (1974) Fine structure of fibroblasts in the periodontal ligament of the rat incisor and their possible role in tooth eruption. Arch Oral Biol 19, 1087–1098.

Beersten W and Everts V (1977) The site of remodelling of collagen in the periodontal ligament of the mouse incisor. Anat Rec 189, 479–498.

Berkovitz BKB and Sloan P (1979) Attachment tissues of the teeth in *Caiman sclerops* (Crocodilia). J Zool Lond 187, 179–194.

Berkovitz BKB, Shore RC and Sloan P (1980) An histological study of the periodontal ligament of rat mandibular incisor following root resection with special reference to the zone of shear. Arch Oral Biol 25, 235–244.

Berkovitz BKB, Weaver ME, Shore RC and Moxham BJ (1981) Fibril diameters in the extracellular matrix of the periodontal connective tissues of the rat. Conn Tiss Res 8, 127–132.
Berkovitz BKB and Moxham BJ (1989) Tissues changes during tooth eruption. In: Teeth, Vol. 6, Handbook of Microscopic Anatomy (Oksche A and Volbrath L, eds), 2nd edition, pp 21–71, Springer-Verlag, Berlin.
Berkovitz BKB (1990) The structure of the periodontal ligament: an update. Eur J Orthod 12, 51–76.
Bevelander G and Nakahara H (1968) The fine structure of the human peridental ligament. Anat Rec 162, 313–326.
Black GV (1887) Periosteum and peridental membrane. Dent Rev (Wien) 1, 289–302.
Black GV (1899) The fibres and glands of the periodontal membrane. Dental Cosmos Philad XLI, 101–162.
Bock P and Stockinger L (1984) Light and electron microscopic identification of elastic, elaunin and oxytalan fibres in human trachial and bronchial mucosa. Anat Embryol (Berl) 170, 145–153.
Bonnaure-Mallet M and Lescoat D (1989) Development of elastic system fibres in human vocal cords. Acta Anat (Basel) 136, 125–128.
Bowling K and Rygh P (1988) A quantitative study of oxytalan fibres in the transseptal region and tension zones of rat molars following orthodontic movement. Eur J Orthod 10, 13–26.
Boyde A (1968) Scanning electron microscopy of collagen free calcified connective tissue. Beitr Elektronmikroskop Direktabb Obserfl 1, 213–222.
Boyde A (1972) Scanning electron microscope studies of bone. In: The Biochemistry and Physiology of Bone (Bourne GH, ed) 2nd edition, volume 1, pp 259–309, Academic Press, London.
Boyde A and Jones SJ (1968) Scanning electron microscopy of cementum and Sharpey fibre bone. Z Zellforsch 92, 536–548.
Bronckers ALJJ, Gay S, Lyaruu DM, Gay RE and Miller EJ (1986) Localization of type V collagen with monoclonal antibodies in developing dental and peridental tissues of the rat and hamster. Collagen Rel Res 6, 1–13.
Burgeson RE (1988) New collagens, new concepts. Annu Rev Cell Biol 4, 551–577.
Butler WT, Birkedal-Hansen H, Beagle WF, Taylor RE and Chung E (1975) Proteins of the periodontium. Identification of collagen with the $[\alpha1\ (I)]_2$, $\alpha2$ and $[\alpha1\ (III)]_3$ structures in the bovine periodontal ligament. J Biol Chem 250, 8907–8912.
Carneiro J and Fava de Moraes F (1965) Radio-autographic visualization of collagen metabolism in the periodontal tissues of the mouse. Arch Oral Biol 10, 833-848.
Carneiro J and Leblond CP (1966) Suitability of collagenase treatment for the autoradiographic identification of newly synthesised collagen labelled with ^{3}H-glycine or ^{3}H-proline. J Histochem Cytochem 14, 334–344.
Carter DH, Sloan P and Aaron JE (1991) Immunolocalization of collagen types I and III, tenascin and fibronectin in intramembranous bone. J Histochem Cytochem 39, 599–606.
Carter DH, Sloan P and Aaron JE (1994) The cryomicrotomy of the rat dental tissues: A technique for morphological and immunohistochemical analysis. Histochem J 26, 103–109.
Carter DH and Sloan P (1994) The fibrous architecture of the rat periodontal ligament in cryosections examined by scanning electron microscopy. Arch Oral Biol 39, 949–953.
Chavrier C, Hartmann DJ, Couble ML and Herbage C (1988) Distribution and organization of the elastic system fibres in healthy human gingiva: ultrastructural and immunohistochemical study. Histochemistry 89, 47–52.
Chiba M, Yamane A, Ohshima S and Komatsu K (1990) *In vitro* measurement of regional differences in the mechanical properties of the peridontal ligament in the rat mandibular incisor. Arch Oral Biol 35, 153–161.
Chiba M and Komatsu K (1993) Mechanical responses of the periodontal ligament in the transverse section of the rat mandibular incisor at various velocities of loading *in vitro*. J Biomechanics 26, 561–570.
Ciancio SC, Neiders ME and Hazen SP (1967) The principal fibres of the periodontal ligament. Periodontics 5, 76–81.
Cohn SA (1972a) A re-examination of Sharpey's fibres in alveolar bone of the mouse. Arch Oral Biol 17, 255–260.
Cohn SA (1972b) A re-examination of Sharpey's fibres in alveolar bone of the marmoset. Arch Oral Biol 17, 261–269.
Cohn SA (1975) Transalveolar fibres in the human periodontium. Arch Oral Biol 20, 257–259.
Cotta-Pereira G, Guerra-Rodrigo FG and David-Ferrieira JF (1989) Comparative study between the elastic system fibres in human thin and thick skin. Biol Cell 31, 297–302.
Crumley PJ (1964) Collagen formation in the normal and stressed periodontium. Periodontics 2, 53–61.
Devlin H and Ferguson MWJ (1991) Alveolar ridge resorption and mandibular atrophy. A review of the local and systemic factors. Br Dent J 170, 101–102.
Diamant J, Keller A, Baer E, Litt M and Arridge RGC (1972) Collagen ultrastructure and its relation to mechanical properties as a function of ageing. Proc R Soc Lond (Biol) 180, 293–315.
Dreyfuss F and Frank R (1964) Microradiographie et microscopie électronique du cément humain. Bull Group Int Rech Sci Stomat Odontol 7, 167–181.
Dublet B, Dixon E, de Miguel E and van der Rest M (1988) Bovine type XII collagen: amino acid sequence of a 10kDa pepsin fragment from periodontal ligament reveals a high degree of homology with the chicken α_1(XII) sequence. Federation of European Biochemical Societies 223, 177–180.
Eastoe JE (1976) Collagen chemistry and tissue organization. In: The Eruption and Occlusion of Teeth (Poole DFG and Stack MV, eds), pp 247–249. Butterworth, London.
Eccles JD (1959) Studies on the development of the periodontal membrane. The principal fibres of the molar teeth. Dent Prac 10, 31–35.
Eccles JD (1964) The development of the periodontal membrane in the rat incisor. Arch Oral Biol 9, 127–133.
Edmunds RS, Simmons TA, Cox CF and Avery JK (1979) Light and ultrastructural relationship between oxytalan fibres in the periodontal ligament of the guinea-pig. J Oral Path 8, 109–120.
Everts V and Beertsen W (1992) Collagen phagocytosis in periodontal remodelling. In: Biological Mechanisms of Tooth Eruption and Root Resorption (Davidovitch Z, ed), pp 29–36, EBSCO Media, Birmingham, Alabama.
Frank RM, Fellinger E and Steuer P (1976) Ultrastructure du ligament alvéolo-dentaire du rat. J Biol Buccal 4, 295–313.
Frank RM and Nalbandian J (1989) Structure and ultrastructure of the dental pulp. In: Teeth (Berkovitz BKB, Boyde A, Frank RM, *et al.*, eds), pp 249–307, Handbook of Microscopic Anatomy, volume 6, Springer-Verlag, Berlin and Heidelberg.
Franzblau C and Faris B (1981) Elastin. In: Cell Biology of the Extracelllar Matrix (Hay ED, ed), pp 65–93. Plenum Press, New York and London.
Freeman E and Ten Cate AR (1971) Development of the periodontium: an electron microscope study. J Periodontol 42, 387–395.
Freezer SR and Sims MR (1987) A transmission electron microscope stereological study of the mouse molar periodontal ligament. Arch Oral Biol 32, 407–412.
Fullmer HM (1959) Observations on the development of oxytalan fibres in the periodontium of man. J Dent Res. 38, 510–516.
Fullmer HM, Sheetz JH and Narkates AJ (1974) Oxytalan connective tissue fibers: a review. J Oral Path 3, 291–316.
Garant PR (1976) An electron microscopic study of the periodontal tissues of germ free rats and rats mono-infected with *Actinomyces naeslundii*. J Periodont Res (supp) 15, 9-79.

Gathercole LJ and Keller A (1991) Crimp morphology in the fibre-forming collagens. Matrix 11, 214–234.

Gibson MA, Sandberg LB, Grosso LE and Cleay EG (1991) Complementary DNA cloning establishes microfibril associated glycoproteins (MAGP) to be a discrete component of the elastin associated microfibrils. J Biol Chem 266, 7596–7601.

Gotte L, Giro G, Volpin D and Horne RW (1974) The ultrastructural organization of elastin. J Ultrastruct Res 46, 23–34.

Grant D and Bernick S (1972) The periodontium of ageing humans. J Periodontol 43, 660–667.

Grant D, Bernick S, Levy BM and Dreizen S (1972) A comparative study of periodontal ligament development in teeth with and without predecessors in marmosets. J Periodontol 43, 162–169.

Grant D, Chase J and Bernick S (1973) Biology of the periodontium in primates of the Galago species. I. The normal periodontium in young animals. II. Inflammatory periodontal disease. III. Lability of cementum. IV. Changes in ageing: ankylosis. J Periodontol 44, 540–550.

Gray WR, Sandberg LB and Foster JA (1973) Molecular model for elastin structure and function. Nature 246, 461–466.

Henkel W and Glanville RW (1982) Covalent crosslinking between molecules of type I and type III collagen. The involvement of the N-terminal, nonhelical regions of the alpha 1(I) and alpha 1(III) chains in the formation of intermolecular crosslinks. Eur J Biochem 122, 205–213.

Hindle MO (1967) The intermediate plexus of the periodontal membrane. In: The Mechanisms of Tooth Support (Anderson DJ, Eastoe JE, Melcher AH and Picton DCA, eds), pp 66–67, Wright, Bristol.

Hirayami H, Takagi M and Toda Y (1985) Histochemical studies of oxytalan fibres in monkeys Jpn J Oral Biol 27, 933–941.

Holm-Pedersen P and Viidik A (1972) Tensile properties and morphology of healing wounds in old and young rats. Scand J Plast Reconstr Surg 6, 24–35.

Huang YH, Ohsaki Y and Kurisu K (1991) Distribution of type I and type III collagen in the developing periodontal ligament of mice. Matrix 11, 25–35.

Hunt AM (1959) A description of the molar teeth and investing tissues of normal guinea pigs. J Dent Res 38, 216–243.

Jensen JL and Toto PD (1968) Radioactive labelling index of the periodontal ligament in ageing rats. J Dent Res 47, 149.

Johnson BD, Paye NC, Narayanan AS and Pieters HP (1986) Effect of donor age on protein and collagen synthesis *in vitro* by human diploid fibroblasts. Lab Invest 55, 490–496.

Johnson RB (1987) A classification of Sharpey's fibers within the alveolar bone of the mouse: a high voltage electron microscope study. Anat Rec 217, 339–347.

Johnson RB and Pylypas SP (1992) A re-evaluation of the distribution of the elastic meshwork within the periodontal ligament of the mouse. J Periodont Res 27, 239–249.

Jonas IE and Riede UN (1980) Reaction of oxytalan fibers in human periodontium to mechanical stress. J Histochem Cytochem 28, 211–216.

Jones SJ and Boyde A (1972) A study of human root cemental surfaces as prepared for and examined in the SEM. Z Zellforsch 130, 318–337.

Jones SJ and Boyde A (1974) The organization and gross mineralization patterns of the collagen fibres in Sharpey fibre bone. Cell Tissue Res 148, 83–96.

Kadar A (1974) The ultrastructure of elastic tissue. Path Europ 9, 133–146.

Kardos TB and Simpson LO (1979) A theoretical consideration of the periodontal membrane as a collagenous thixotropic system and its relationship to tooth eruption. J Periodont Res 14, 445–451.

Keene DR, Sakai LY, Bachinger HP and Burgeson RE (1987) Type III collagen can be present on banded collagen fibrils regardless of fibril diameter. J Cell Biol 104, 2393–2402.

Keller A and Gathercole LJ (1976) Biophysical and mechanical properties of collagen in relation to function. In: The Eruption and Occlusion of Teeth (Poole DFG and Stack MV, eds), pp 262–266, Butterworth, London.

Kerebel B and Balouet G (1967) Observations sur le plexus intermédiaire du ligament paradontal. Actualités Odontostomat 80, 395–409.

Kielty CM, Hopkinson I and Grant ME (1993) Collagen: the collagen family: structure, assembly and organization in the extracellular matrix. In: Connective Tissue and its Heritable Disorders (Royce PM and Steinmann B, eds), pp 103–147. Wiley–Liss, New York.

Klingsberg J and Butcher EO (1960) Comparative histology of age change in oral tissues of rat, hamster and monkey. J Dent Res 39, 158.

Komatsu K and Chiba M (1993) The effect of velocity of loading on the biomechanical responses of the periodontal ligament in transverse sections of the rat molar *in vitro*. Arch Oral Biol 38, 369–375.

Lapiere CM (1967) Mechanisms of collagen fibre remodelling. In: The Mechanisms of Tooth Support (Anderson DJ, Eastoe JE, Melcher AH and Picton DCA, eds), pp 20–24, Wright, Bristol.

Laurent GJ (1987) Dynamic state of collagen: pathways of collagen degradation *in vivo* and their possible role in the regulation of collagen mass. Am J Physiol 252, C1–C9.

Levy BM and Bernick S (1968) Development and organisation of the periodontal ligament of deciduous teeth in marmosets. J Dent Res 47, 27–33.

Levy BM, Dreizen S and Bernick S (1972) The Marmoset Periodontium in Health and Disease. Karger, Basel.

Luder HU, Zimmerli I and Schroeder HE (1988) Do collagen fibrils of the periodontal ligament shrink with age? J Periodont Res 23, 46–52.

Lukinmaa PL, Mackie EJ and Thesleff I (1991) Immunohistochemical localization of the matrix glycoproteins tenascin and the ED-sequence-containing form of cellular fibronectin in human permanent teeth and periodontal ligament. J Dent Res 70, 19–26.

Magnusson B (1968) Tissue changes during molar tooth eruption. Trans R Schools Dent Stockh Umea 13, 1–122.

Mashouf K and Engel MB (1975) Maturation of periodontal connective tissue in the newborn rat incisor. Arch Oral Biol 20, 161–166.

Melcher AH and Eastoe JE (1969) The connective tissues of the periodontium. In: Biology of the Periodontium, (Melcher AH and Bowen WH, eds), pp 167–343, Academic Press, London.

Minns RJ, Soden PD and Jackson DS (1973) The role of the fibrous components and ground substance in the mechanical properties of biological tissues: a preliminary investigation. J Biomech 6, 153–165.

Moxham BJ and Berkovitz BKB (1983) Continuous monitoring of the position of the ferret mandibular canine tooth to enable comparisons with the continuously growing rabbit incisor. Arch Oral Biol 28, 477–481.

Mulholland J, Aplin JD, Ayad S, Hong L and Glasser SR (1992) Loss of collagen type VI from rat endometrial stroma during decidualization. Biol Reprod 46, 1136–1143.

Ness AR and Smale DE (1959) The distribution of mitoses and cells in the tissues bounded by the socket wall of the rabbit mandibular incisor. Proc R Soc Biol 151, 106–128.

Olsen BR (1989) The next frontier: Molecular biology of extracellular matrix. Connect Tissue Res 23, 115–121.

Parfitt GJ (1967) The physical analysis of the tooth supporting structures. In: The Mechanisms of Tooth Support (Anderson DJ, Eastoe JE, Melcher AH and Picton DCA, eds), pp 154–156, Wright, Bristol.

Parry DAD and Craig AS (1984) Growth and development of collagen fibrils in connective tissue. In: Ultrastructure of the connective tissue matrix (Ruggeri A and Motta PM, eds), pp 34–64, Martinus Nijhoff Publishers, Boston.

Parry DAD (1988) The molecular and fibrillar structure of collagen and its relationship to the mechanical properties of connective tissue. Biophys Chem 29, 195–209

Partridge SM (1967) Diffusion of solutes in elastin. Biochim Biophys Acta 140, 132–141.
Quigley MB (1970) Perforating (Sharpey's) fibres of the periodontal ligament and bone. Ala J Med Sci 7, 336–342.
Ramos AM and Hunt AM (1967) Remodelling of the periodontal ligament of guinea pig molars. In: The Mechanisms of Tooth Support (Anderson DJ, Eastoe JE, Melcher AH and Picton DCA, eds), pp 107–112, Wright, Bristol.
Rannie I (1963) Observations on the oxytalan fibres of the periodontal membrane. Trans Eur Orthodont Soc 39, 127–136.
Rippin JW (1976a) Collagen turnover in the periodontal ligament under normal and altered functional forces. I. Young rat molars. J Periodont Res 11, 101–107.
Rippin JW (1976b) Collagen turnover in rat molar periodontal ligament. In: The Eruption and Occlusion of Teeth (Poole DFG and Stack MV, eds), pp 304–305, Butterworth, London
Rippin JW (1978) Collagen turnover in the periodontal ligament under normal and altered functional forces. II Adult rat molars. J Periodont Res 13, 149–154.
Robins MW (1972) Collagen metabolism in the periodontal ligament of the rat incisor. J Dent Res 51, 1246.
Romanos GE, Schröter-Kermani C, Hinz N, Wachtel HC and Bernimoulin JP (1991) Immunohistochemical localization of collagenous components in healthy periodontal tissues of the rat and marmoset (*Callithrix jacchus*). II. Distribution of collagen types IV, V and VI. J Periodont Res 26, 323–332.
Romanos GE, Schröter-Kermani C, Hinz N, Wachtel HC and Bernimoulin JP (1992) Immunohistochemical localization of collagenous components in healthy periodontal tissues of the rat and marmoset (*Callithrix jacchus*). I. Distribution of collagen types I and III. J Periodont Res 27, 101–110.
Rosenbloom J (1993) Elastin. In: Connective Tissue and its Heritable Disorders (Royce PM and Steinmann B, eds), pp 167–188, Wiley–Liss, New York.
Ross R (1973) The elastic fibre, a review. J Histochem Cytochem 21, 199–208.
Sakai LY, Keene DR and Engvall E (1986) Fibrillin, a new 350-kD glycoprotein, is a component of extracellular microfibrils. J Cell Biol 103, 2499-2509.
Sasakai T and Garant PR (1993) Multinucleated fibroblastic cells in the periodontal ligaments of aged rats. J Periodont Res 28, 65–71.
Sannes PL, Spicer SS and Katsuyama T (1979) Ultrastructural localisation of sulfated complex carbohydrates with a modified iron diamine procedure. J Histochem Cytochem 27, 1108–1111.
Schroeder HE, Munzel-Pedrazzoli S and Page RC (1973) Correlated morphometric and biochemical analysis of gingival tissue in early chronic gingivitis in man. Arch Oral Biol 18, 899–923.
Scott JE and Burton SM (1984) Selective demineralization of hard tissues in organic solvents: retention or extraction of proteoglycan? J Microsc 134, 291.
Selvig KA (1964) An ultrastructural study of cementum formation. Acta Odont Scand 22, 105–120.
Selvig KA (1965) The fine structure of human cementum. Acta Odont Scand 23, 423–441.
Serafini-Fracassini A, Field JM, Smith JW and Stephens WGS (1977) The ultrastructure and mechanics of elastic ligaments. J Ultrastruc Res 58, 244–251.
Severson JA, Moffett BC, Kokich V and Seplipsky H (1978) A histologic study of age changes in the adult human periodontal joint (ligament). J Periodontol 49, 189–200.
Shackleford JM (1971) Scanning electron microscopy of the dog periodontium. J Periodont Res 6, 45–54.
Shackleford JM (1973) The indifferent fibre plexus and its relationship to principal fibers of the periodontium. Am J Anat 131, 427–442.
Shah JS, Palacios E and Palacios L (1982) Development of crimp morphology and cellular changes in chick tendons. Dev Biol 94, 299–504
Shore RC and Berkovitz BKB (1979) An ultrastructural study of periodontal ligament fibroblasts in relation to their possible role in tooth eruption and intracellular collagen degradation in the rat. Arch Oral Biol 24, 155–164.
Shore RC, Berkovitz BKB and Moxham BJ (1984) Histological study, including ultrastructural quantification, of the periodontal ligament in the lathyritic rat mandibular dentition. Arch Oral Biol 29, 263–273.
Shore RC, Moxham BJ and Berkovitz BKB (1984) Oxytalan fibres in the periodontal ligament. In: Tooth Morphogenesis and Differentiation (Ruch J and Belcourt AB, eds), Colloquium of the Institut de la Santé et de la Recherche Médicale, 125, 565–572.
Sicher H (1923) Über die Fixation und das Wachstum dauernd wachsender Zähne. Korresp Bl Zahnärzte 49, 332–343.
Sicher H (1942) Tooth eruption: the axial movement of continuously growing teeth. J Dent Res 21, 201–210.
Simpson HE (1967) A three-dimensional approach to the microscopy of the peridontal membrane. Proc R Soc Med 60, 537–542.
Sims MR (1975) Oxytalan-vascular relationships observed in histologic examination of the periodontal ligaments of man and mouse. Arch Oral Biol 20, 713–717.
Sims MR (1976) Reconstitution of the human oxytalan system during orthodontic tooth movement. Am J Orthod 70, 38–58.
Sims MR (1983) Electron-microscopic affiliations of oxytalan fibres, nerves and the microvascular bed in the mouse periodontal ligament. Arch Oral Biol 28, 1017–1024.
Sims MR (1984) Ultrastructural analysis of the microfibrillar component of mouse and human periodontal oxytalan fibers. Connect Tissue Res 13, 59-67.
Skougaard MR, Levy BM and Simpson J (1970) Collagen metabolism in skin and periodontal membrane of the marmoset. Scand J Dent 78, 256–262.
Sloan P (1978a) Scanning electron microscopy of the collagen fibre architecture of the rabbit incisor periodontium. Arch Oral Biol 23, 567–572.
Sloan P (1978b) Microanatomy of the periodontal ligament in some animals possessing teeth of continuous and limited growth. PhD thesis, University of Bristol.
Sloan P (1979a) Polarising microscopy of the rodent periodontal ligament. J Dent Res 53, 118.
Sloan P (1979b) Collagen fibre architecture in the periodontal ligament. J R Soc Med 72, 188–191.
Sloan P, Shellis RP and Berkovitz BKB (1976) Effect of specimen preparation on the appearance of the rat periodontal ligament in the scanning electron microscope. Arch Oral Biol 21, 633–635.
Sloan P, Carter DH, Kielty C and Shuttleworth CM (1993) An immunohistochemical study examining the role of collagen type VI in the rat periodontal ligament. Histochem J 25, 523–530.
Sloan P and Carter DH (1993) Fibronectin is associated with oxytalan fibres in the rat periodontal ligament. J Dent Res (in press).
Socransky SS, Hubersak C and Propas D (1970) Induction of periodontal destruction in gnotobiotic rats by a human oral strain of *Actinomyces naeslundii*. Arch Oral Biol 15, 993–995.
Sodek J (1977) A comparison of the rates of synthesis and turnover of collagen and non-collagen proteins in adult rat periodontal tissues and skin using a microassay. Arch Oral Biol 22, 655–665.
Sodek J, Brunette DM, Feng J, *et al.* (1977) Collagen synthesis is a major component of protein synthesis in the periodontal ligament of various species. Arch Oral Biol 22, 647–653.
Sodek J and Ferrier JM (1988) Collagen remodelling in rat periodontal tissues: compensation for precursor reutilization confirms rapid turnover of collagen. Collagen Rel Res 8, 11–21.

Sodek J (1989) Collagen turnover in periodontal ligament. In: The Biology of Tooth Movement (Norton LA and Berstone CJ, eds), pp 157–181, CRC Press, Boca Raton, Fl.

Soule JD (1967) Oxytalan fibres in the periodontal ligament of the caiman and the alligator (*crocodilia, reptilia*). J Morphol 122, 169–174.

Stahl SS and Tonna EA (1977) H^3-proline study of ageing periodontal ligament matrix formation. Comparison between matrices adjacent to either cemental or bone surfaces. J Periodont Res 12, 318–322.

Stallard RE (1963) The utilization of ^{3}H-proline by the connective tissue elements of the periodontium. Periodontics 1, 185–188.

Svejda J and Skach M (1973) The periodontium of the human tooth in the scanning electron microscope. J Periodontol 44, 478–484.

Tagaki M, Baba T, Baba H and Toda Y (1987) Ultrastructural cytochemistry of oxytalan fibres in monkey periodontal ligaments with the high iron diamine method. Histochem J 19, 75–84.

Takagi M, Kazama T, Shimada K, Hosokawa Y and Hishikawa, H (1989) Differentiation distribution and ultrastructural staining of oxytalan and elastic fibers in the periodontal ligament of *Al.ligator mississippiensis*. Anat Rec 225, 279–287.

Ten Cate AR (1972) Morphological studies of fibrocytes in connective tissue undergoing rapid remodelling. J Anat 112, 401–414.

Thomas NR (1967) The properties of collagen in the periodontium of an erupting tooth. In: The Mechanisms of Tooth Support (Anderson DJ, Eastoe JE, Melcher AH and Picton DCA, eds), pp 102–106. Wright, Bristol.

Torp S, Bayer E and Friedman B (1975) Effects of age and mechanical deformation on the ultrastructure of tendon. In: Structure of Fibrous Biopolymers (Atkins EDT and Keller A, eds), pp 223–250, Butterworth, London.

Toto PD and Borg M (1968) Effects of age changes of the premitotic index in the periodontium of mice. J Dent Res 47, 70.

Trelstad RL and Silver FH (1981) Matrix assembly. In: Cell Biology of Extracellular Matrix (Hay ED, ed), pp 179–215, Plenum Press, New York and London.

Tung PS, Domenicucci C, Wasi S and Sodek J (1985) Specific immunohistochemical localization of osteonectin and collagen types I and III in fetal and adult porcine dental tissues. J Histochem Cytochem 33, 531–540.

Viidik A (1980) Interdependence between structure and function in collagenous tissues. In: Biology of Collagen (Viidik A and Vuust J, eds), pp 257–280, Academic Press, London.

Von der Mark H, Aumailley M, Wick G, Fleischmajer R and Timpler R (1984) Immunochemistry, genuine size and tissue localization of collagen VI. Eur J Biochem 142, 493–502.

Wainwright SA, Biggs WD, Currey JD and Gosline JM (1976) Mechanical Design in Organisms, pp 116-119, Edward Arnold, London.

Wang HM, Nanda V, Rao LG, Melcher AH, Heersche HNM and Sodek J (1980) Specific immunohistochemical localization of type III collagen in porcine periodontal tissues using peroxidase-antiperoxidase method. J Histochem Cytochem 28, 1215–1223.

Williams DM, Hughes FJ, Odell EW and Farthing PM (eds) (1992) The normal periodontium. In: Pathology of Periodontal Disease, Chapter 2, pp 17–31, Oxford University Press, Oxford.

Yamada KM (1989) Fibronectin domains and receptors. In: Fibronectin. Biology of Extracellular Matrix: A Series (Mosher DF, ed), pp 88–90, Academic Press, London.

Yamamoto T and Wakita M (1992) Bundle formation of principal fibers in rat molars. J Periodont Res 27, 20–27.

Zhang X, Schuppan D, Becker J, Reichart P and Gelderblom HR (1993) Distribution of undulin, tenascin and fibronectin in the human periodontal ligament and cementum: comparative immunoelectron microscopy with ultra-thin cryosections. J Histochem Cytochem 41, 245–251.

Zorn TMT, Bijovsky AT, Bevilacqua EMAF and Abrahamsohn PA (1989) Phagocytosis of collagen by mouse decidual cells. Anat Rec 225, 96–100.

Zwarych PD and Quigley MB (1965) The intermediate plexus of the periodontal ligament: history and further observations. J Dent Res 44, 383–391.

Chapter 3
The Biochemistry of the Fibres of the Periodontal Ligament
J Kirkham, C Robinson

INTRODUCTION

The extracellular matrix of the periodontal ligament (PDL) comprises two major compartments – the fibres and ground substance. These components, seen in the electron microscope as an insoluble fibrillar network surrounded by an apparently less ordered, thixotropic gel, have evolved to meet the functional requirements of tooth support and, arguably, tooth eruption (see Chapters 9 and 10). The fibrous elements are able to provide the tissue with tensile strength, while the ground substance is capable of dissipating compressional forces (see Chapter 4).

The apparently loosely organized, reticular structure of the extracellular matrix disguises the fact that this compartment is subject to a high degree of order and control. This results in a matrix that not only provides both tensile and compressional strength but also determines the movement of other components (such as ions and small molecules) throughout the tissue. In addition, the matrix provides positional information for the cellular elements.

Collagen and the elastin family (i.e. elastin, elauin and oxytalin; see Chapter 2) together make up the fibrous elements of the PDL. Collagen is the most abundant of these and it is often presumed to be the most important in terms of tooth support. A great deal of work has been carried out on connective tissue collagen, including that of the PDL, providing a wealth of data in recent years. Much less is known about the minor fibrous components.

COLLAGEN FIBRE BIOCHEMISTRY

GENERALIZED CONNECTIVE TISSUE COLLAGEN FIBRE BIOCHEMISTRY

Collagen, which is the most abundant protein in the animal kingdom, is now understood to comprise a large family of related but genetically distinct proteins (Kuhn, 1986; Miller and Gay, 1987; Kielty *et al.*, 1993). Collagens are secreted primarily but not exclusively by fibroblasts, though many other cell types have also been shown to produce collagen (including some epithelial cells – Trelstad and Slavkin, 1974).

Although some 18 different collagen types (not all of which form fibres) have now been described, all share to a greater or lesser degree common features of basic molecular structure and homology of conserved amino acid sequence. This is the collagen triple helix or 'superhelix', which arises because of the primary sequence of the component polypeptide chains (known as 'α-chains'). Fibrous collagens in particular demonstrate this feature. The fibrous collagens are defined by their ability to undergo spontaneous (though not necessarily self-regulated) fibrillogenesis, which results in the formation of insoluble fibres with highly ordered macromolecular superstructures.

GENETIC ORGANIZATION

The unusual primary sequence of amino acids in the fibrous collagens is related directly to their genetic organization (reviewed by Chu and Prockop, 1993). The α1(I) chains of type I collagen are encoded by 41 small exons, most of which comprise of 54 bp and code for 6 [GLY-X-Y] repeats (Boedtker *et al.*, 1983). The remainder either code for two or three $[GLY\text{-}X\text{-}Y]_6$ repeats or contain a 9 bp deletion, corresponding to one [GLY-X-Y] (*Table 3.1*). The evidence provided by the genetic organization suggests, therefore, that fibrillar collagens are evolved from an ancestral molecule based upon the repetition of a [GLY-X-Y] sixfold repeat and that modern collagens are the result of gene duplication.

Table 3.1
Exon arrangement for type I collagen α1(I) chain. (Based on data from Boedtker *et al.*, 1983).

Exon Length	Number of $[GLY\text{–}X\text{–}Y]_6$	Number of Exons
54	1	21
108	2	9
162	3	1
45	$1\ [GLY\text{–}X\text{–}Y]_5$	5
99	$1 + 1\ [GLY\text{–}X\text{–}Y]_5$	5

CLASSIFICATION OF COLLAGEN TYPES

At least 25 different gene sequences have been described encoding for collagenous polypeptides (reviewed by Kielty *et al.*, 1993). Together these give rise to 13 distinct collagen types, which are designated I to XIII. A further type XIV collagen has also recently been reported based upon cDNA data.

All of the collagen types consist of three polypeptides (the α-chains) and, although homologous in part, these vary widely in the amount of their structure which is in the form of the classic triple helix. Many contain relatively small segments of triple helix with non-helical interruptions.

The collagens can be divided into three groups. The first and most abundant group is the fibrous collagens. These collagens are all in the form of uninterrupted helices that are highly conserved. These collagens are types I, II, III, V, and XI .

The second group is the high molecular weight collagens, which contain numerous intervening non-helical sequences, resulting in many stretches of interrupted helices. These collagens are those found in association with basement membranes (e.g. types IV and VII). They do not form fibres but can nevertheless form superaggregates of reticular-type networks via end-to-end association and parallel arrays. These structures are characteristically cross-linked by disulphide bridges, in addition to the LYS derived cross-links described on pages 62–65.

The third group is the short-chain collagens and consists of types VI, VIII, IX, X, XII and XIII. All contain numerous intervening non-helical domains but relatively little is known regarding their supermolecular organization. The large globular domains characteristic of some of these collagen types (e.g. type X) place them far away from the fibre-forming collagens that conform to the classical stereotype for collagen structure. Indeed, type IX collagen may be classified as a proteoglycan, with chondroitin or dermatan sulphate side chains, or both.

A summary of the various collagen types is shown in *Table 3.2*.

COLLAGEN TYPES WITHIN THE PERIODONTAL LIGAMENT

The PDL contains mostly fibrils of type I collagen as well as a significantly high proportion of type III fibrils (Butler *et al.*, 1975; Sodek and Limeback, 1979; Shuttleworth and Smalley, 1983). This amount of type III collagen is unusually high for a mature connective tissue (approximately 20 per cent of the total collagen) and is more characteristic of a foetal connective tissue (Epstein, 1974). Immunolocalization of types I and III collagen in the PDL has revealed that the two types follow similar wide distribution patterns associated with the major fibrils throughout the tissue (Becker *et al.*, 1990). Similar studies have also shown that the minor collagens, types V and VI, are also present (Becker *et al.*, 1990; Romanos *et al.*, 1991; Lukinmaa and Waltimo, 1992). Type V cross-reactivity was seen with aggregated unbanded 12 nm filaments localized in the tissue spaces between major fibres, whereas antibodies to type VI collagen cross-reacted with microfilaments interconnecting single fibrils. Further information on the distribution and organization of PDL collagen is given in Chapter 2.

Following pepsin digests of bovine PDL, Yamauchi *et al.* (1986) reported the presence of a low molecular weight collagenous component containing unusually high proportions of cysteine. This was later found to share over 90 per cent sequence homology with type XII collagen derived from chick, based on cDNA-deduced data (Dublet *et al.*, 1988). This component is probably in the form of a homotrimer. Type XII collagen is of the FACIT (Fibril-Associated Collagens with Interrupted Helices) class (Dublet *et al.*, 1987), suggesting a role for this molecule in the three-dimensional organization of the major collagen fibrils in the PDL.

A role for type XII collagen in fibrillogenesis was supported by the work of Karimbux *et al.* (1992), who demonstrated (using Northern blot analysis coupled with *in situ* hybridization) that type XII expression was both spatially and temporally restricted in the rat molar. These authors showed that, while expression of type I collagen was widespread throughout the PDL and tended to decrease with age, expression of type XII collagen was greatest in the PDL adjacent to alveolar bone and increased with maturity.

It is possible that the different sub-populations of cells within the PDL each express collagen differently in terms of both type and amount. Limeback *et al.* (1983) showed that different primary cell lines cultured from porcine PDL produced different amounts and different types of collagen *in vitro*. This is further supported by data showing that collagen distribution throughout the sheep PDL follows consistent site-specific patterns that are not simply a mirror image of total protein content (Kirkham *et al.*, 1989, 1991) (*Fig. 3.1*).

Western blotting using polyclonal antibodies raised to types I, III, IV, V and VI collagens revealed the presence of all of these in neutral salt-soluble extracts of sheep PDL (*Fig. 3.2*). The sizes of these fragments suggests that all of these collagens are undergoing remodelling in the tissue (see below).

GENERAL STRUCTURE OF FIBROUS COLLAGENS

All collagens are made up of three polypeptide chains (i.e. they are trimeric). These chains (α-chains) may be identical (homotrimers) or different (heterotrimers). However, the three polypeptide chains are organized into a three-stranded helical structure known as the collagen triple helix (Ramachandran and Kartha, 1954; Ramachandran, 1967; Miller and Gay, 1982). This is readily illustrated using type I collagen (which is the most abundant of the fibrous collagens) as the classical example.

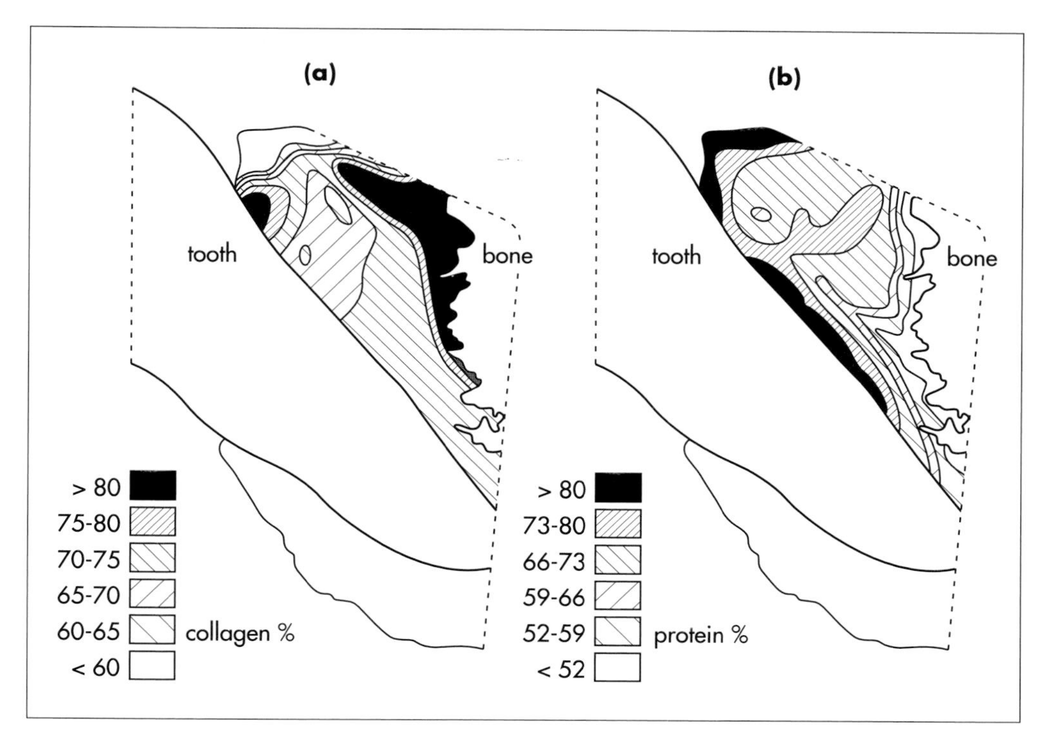

Fig. 3.1 (a) Typical distribution pattern of collagen in the sheep periodontium. Collagen percentage of total tissue protein was calculated from hydroxyproline content following amino acid analysis. Highest concentrations of collagen can be seen adjacent to alveolar bone and immediately beneath the gingival sulcus region. (b) Typical distribution pattern of protein concentration in the sheep periodontium. Protein percentage of tissue dry weight was calculated from total amino acids recovered following amino acid analysis. In contrast to collagen, highest concentrations of protein can be seen adjacent to cementum and in the epithelial region of the tissue. (From Kirkham *et al.*, 1989. Reproduced by permission of the publishers.)

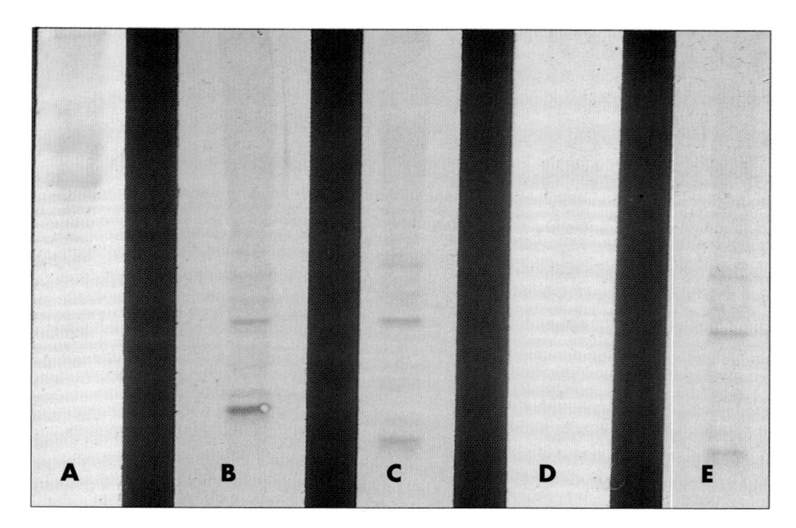

Fig. 3.2 Western blot showing cross-reactivity of specific components in neutral salt extracts of sheep PDL with antibodies raised to (A) type I collagen; (B) type III collagen; (C) type IV collagen; (D) type V collagen and (E) type VI collagen. Cross-reactivity with components of low molecular weight indicates the presence of degraded fragements of all of these collagen types in the tissue. (Antibodies kindly supplied by Dr S Ayad, University of Manchester.)

Table 3.2 The collagen super family. (Based on data from Kuhn, 1986; Kielty et al., 1993; Chu and Prockop, 1993.)

Collagen type	Gene size (kB)	Number of exons (sequenced total)	Chains	Mr of a chains	Aggregation and macromolecular structure	Special characteristics	Tissue location	Reported in PDL?
I	18 (Pro-a1) 38 (Pro-a1)	44/51 15/52	$[a1(I)]\ [a2(I)]_2$ $[a1(I)]_3$	95 K	Tropocollagen arrayed in 67 nm quarter stagger, forming large-diameter, banded fibrils	97% uninterrupted helix	Skin, bone, tendon, ligament. Widespread in connective tissues	Yes (approx. 80%)
II	30 (Pro-a1)	53/53	$[a1(II)]_3$	95 K	67 nm staggered array forming small-diameter banded fibrils	High in HYL and HYL+CHO compared with I and III; > 90% uninterrupted helix	Cartilage, vitreous, nucleus pulporus	No
III	44 (Pro-a1)	36/52	$[a1(III)]_3$	110 K	67 nm staggered array forming small-diameter fibrils	> 90% uninterrupted helix; co-expressed with I (may form part of same fibril); high HYP; CYS; sulphated TYR	Foetal skin, tendon, aorta, reticulin fibres	Yes (approx 20%)
V		6/– (a2)	Variable heter- or homotrimer plus splice products $[a1(V)]_2\ [a2(V)]$ $[a1(V)]\ [a2(V)]$ $[a3(V)]_3$ etc	115–125 K	Possible staggered array; forms fine banded fibrils *in vitro*	Extensively processed; often co-expressed with I and II; large globular domains at N- and C-termini; uninterrupted helix	Widespread, especially fetal connective tissue; also ligament, tendon, bone, pericellular	Yes (minor)
XI		6/– (a2)	[a1(XI)] [a2(XI)] [a3(XI)]		Forms fine fibrils; may copolymerize with Type II	Closely related to V; high HYL+CHO; [a3(XI)] similar to [a1(II)]	Cartilage	No
IV	100 (a1)	52/52	$[a1(IV)]_2\ [a2(IV)]$, also [a3(IV)] [a4(IV)] [a5(IV)]	185 K, 170 K	End-to-end association forming reticular network	Interrupted helix; large globular domain; disulphide bonds; high degree of flexibility	Basement membranes network	Yes
VII			$[a1(VII)]_3$	~ 300 K	Centrosymmetrical aggregate of anti-parallel dimers in parallel arrays, forming 'fibrils'	Extended helical domain containing non-helical interruptions; triantennary globular domains at C-terminal	Anchoring filaments, skin, oral mucosa, cervix	

VI		6/– (α2)	[α1(VI)] [α2(VI)] [α3(VI)]	150 K 150 K 270 K	Microfibrils forming extensive network in soft connective tissues; intracellular aggregation to dimers and tetramers, then end-to-end association in extracellular matrix	Short helical domain; very large globular N- and C-terminal domains; high CYS content	Widespread, skin, cornea, tendon, ligament	Yes (minor)
VIII			[α1(VIII)]$_3$, also [α2(VIII)]	61 K	Little known; may form hexagonal lattice network	Similar to X; synthesis possibly by endothelial cells; short chain helix with interruptions.	Descemet's membrane, fetal heart	
X	5 (α1)	3/3	[α1(X)]$_3$	59 K	Little known; forms fine filaments and possibly a hexagonal lattice	Similar to VIII; short interrupted helical domain; large globular C-terminal; high denaturation temperature (47°C); collagenase-susceptible; high MET; high hydrophobicity	Hypertrophic and mineralizing cartilage, pericellular matrix	No
IX	100 (α1) 10 (α2)	19/– 32/–	[α1(IX)] [α2(IX)] [α3(IX)]		Not fibrous but associated with other collagen fibrils via helical domain covalent x-link to type II	Some homology with XII; short chain helix with interruptions; S–S bonded; PG: CS/DS on α2	Cartilage, vitreous	No
XII		7/– (α1)	[α1(XII)]$_3$	220 K		Some homology with IX; large non-helical N domain; two short helical domains	Tendon, ligaments	Yes (minor)
XIV			[α1(XIV)]$_3$			Some homology with XII	Fetal skin and tendon	
XIII		10/– (α1)	[α1(XIII)]$_3$	Possibly tissue specific, < 70 K		Unique gene organization; not yet isolated from tissue	Fetal epidermis, intestinal mucosa	

Primary structure

Each polypeptide chain in type I collagen contains 1056 amino acid residues, over 90 per cent of which are in the form of the repeating tri-residue motif [GLY-X-Y], where X is often proline and Y is often hydroxyproline. Together, these two imino acids account for over 20 per cent of all residues. It is this high proportion of imino acids, coupled with the presence of glycine at every third residue, which confers the characteristic conformation to collagen molecules (Ramachandran and Ramakrishnan, 1976).

Secondary, tertiary and quaternary structure

The α-chains each form an extended polyproline helix with left handed symmetry and an average of 3.3 amino acid residues per turn (pitch is approximately 3 nm) (Ramachandran, 1967; Traub and Piez, 1971). The structure of the individual α-chain is shown in *Fig. 3.3*. The three polypeptide chains are then wound around each other to form the collagen triple helix in what is often described as a 'rope-like' fashion, producing a semi-rigid structure that is long and thin (300 nm × 1.5 nm), as shown in *Fig. 3.4*. The triple helix has right handed symmetry with a pitch of approximately 10 nm. The entire helical structure is stabilized

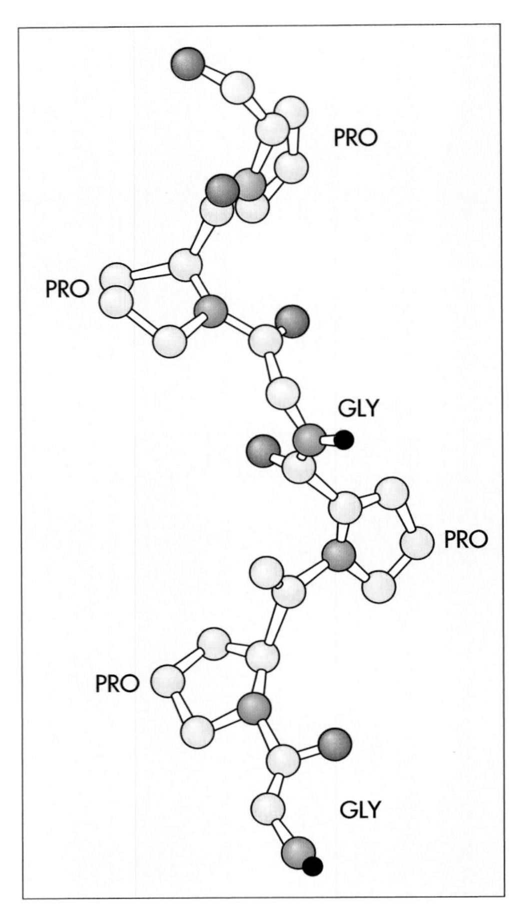

Fig. 3.3 Model showing structure of a short sequence of a single collagen α-chain in the triple helical domain. Two tripeptide [GLY–PRO–PRO] repeats are also shown.

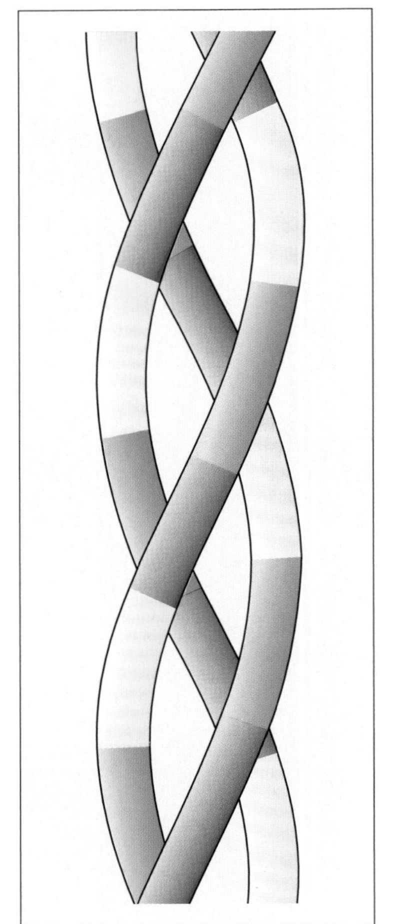

Fig. 3.4 Diagrammatic representation of collagen triple helical structure.

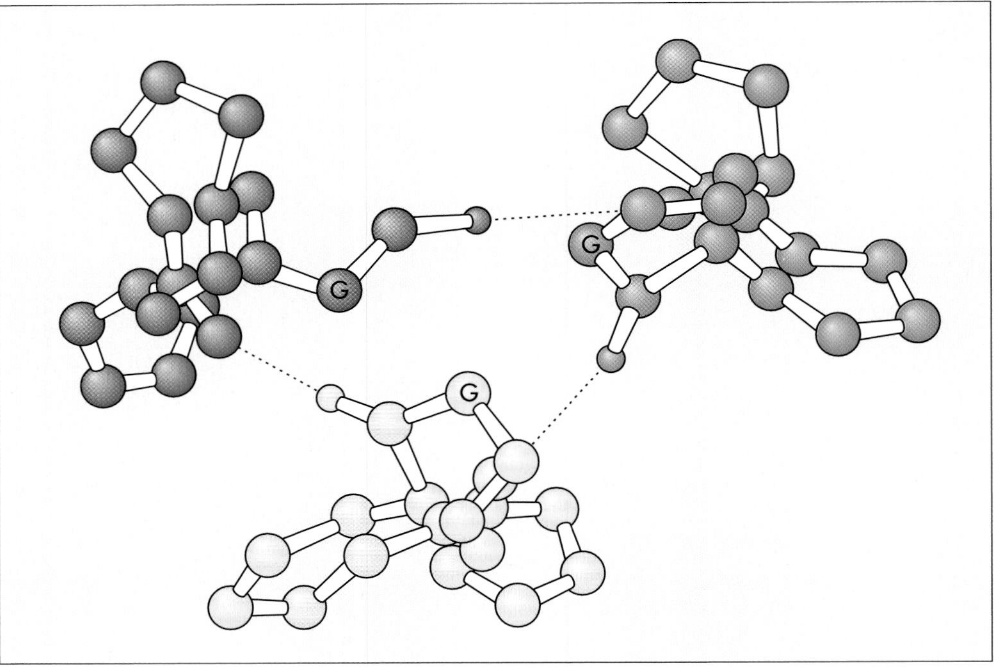

Fig. 3.5 Model showing relationship between α-chains in a cross-section of the collagen triple helix. The three individual α-chains are shown in different colours. Hydrogen bonds are shown as dotted lines. Glycine residues (G) are centrally positioned within the helix while the large pyrrolidine rings are on the outside.

by interchain H bonding with the rigid five-membered pyrrolidine rings of the proline and hydroxyproline lying on the outside of the helix (*Fig. 3.5*). These have a stabilizing effect on the helical structure by limiting rotation of the peptide bond.

Glycine, with its small side chain (-H), is essential for the adoption of the triple helical conformation, as it is the only amino acid capable of fitting into the tightly packed centre of the helix. Genetic mutations resulting in substitution of glycine inevitably result in malformation of the helix, e.g. in some forms of osteogenesis imperfecta (Cohn *et al.*, 1988; Pruchno *et al.*, 1991; Deak *et al.*, 1991).

The proportion of hydroxyproline residues is also an important determinant in helix stability due to their extra capability for H-bonding. Non-hydroxylated triple helices have been shown to be denatured *in vitro* at temperatures below 37°C (Berg and Prockop, 1973; Rosenbloom *et al.*, 1973).

Type I collagen has 338 [GLY-X-Y] repeats per α-chain, accounting for some 95 per cent of the total structure in the form of uninterrupted triple helix. However, the N- and C- termini of the α-chains do not contain the [GLY-X-Y] motif, which results in a non-helical conformation at the ends of the molecule (Kuhn, 1986). These regions are referred to as the teleopeptides and, unlike the triple-helical central domain, are particularly susceptible to proteolytic attack (Starkey *et al.*, 1977; Burleigh, 1977; Nakano and Scott, 1987; Maciewicz *et al.*, 1987).

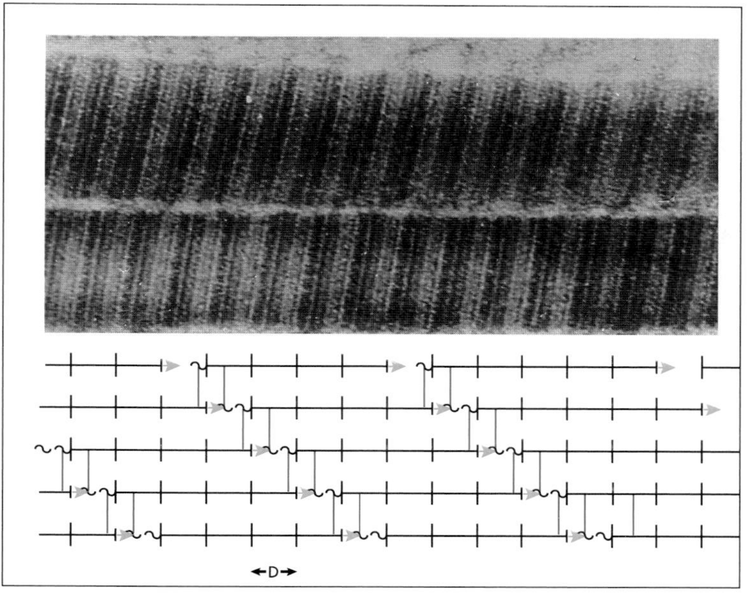

Fig. 3.6 (top) Appearance of collagen fibrils in the transmission electron microscope. Selective staining of specific regions of the triple helix gives rise to the characteristic cross-banded appearance. This distance (approximately 67 nm) is the 'D' period, arising from the alignment of stained tropocollagen molecules as shown (bottom) Alignment of tropocollagen molecules in a quarter stagger array forming cross-banded fibrils as shown (top). C-termini of individual tropocollagen molecules are shown as blue arrowheads. Fibrils are stabilized by covalent bonds (shown in red) forming between modified LYS and HYL residues in the non-helical teleopeptides and other LYS–HYL residues in the helical domain in adjacent tropocollagen molecules. (Based on data from Kuhn, 1986.)

THE HIERARCHY OF COLLAGEN STRUCTURE – FIBRILLOGENESIS

The basic structure described above results in long, rope-like, collagen molecules, which can be thought of as the basic unit of fibrillar structure. Nomenclature becomes a problem at this point because different authors use a variety of terms to describe the same structures. The basic trimeric structure described above will be referred to in this review as 'tropocollagen'. The relationship between tropocollagen and the fibrillar structures seen in the transmission light and electron microscopes is explained by the ability of the tropocollagen molecules to form stable supermolecular aggregates (Veis and Payne, 1988). This tendency is determined by a number of contributing factors but the relative distribution of polar and non-polar amino acid residues along the triple-helical domain appears to be the most important.

However, it is also important to bear in mind the role played by other matrix molecules, notably the proteoglycans decorin (PG-S2) and fibromodulin (in cartilage) in the assembly of tropocollagen into fibrils (Scott, 1984; Heinegard and Oldberg, 1993); this is discussed in Chapter 4.

The ordered arrangement of millions of tropocollagen molecules results in the formation of the classical cross-banded collagen fibrils seen in the transmission electron microscope. This arrangement has been described as a quarter stagger parallel array. It is brought about by aggregation of the tropocollagen in an end-to-end manner with corresponding rows of similarly arranged molecules aligned in parallel but displaced from each other by one quarter of their length (*Fig. 3.6*). The characteristic cross-banded appearance is conferred by the resulting alignment of specific regions of the individual tropocollagen molecules, known as the 'D' period. This corresponds to the even spacing of five charged regions within the triple-helical domains; these charged regions take up heavy metal stains (such as those used in electron microscopy) in a characteristic way. Each charged region is separated by a distance of approximately 67 nm (depending upon the tissue) from the next, so that when the staggered array of tropocollagen molecules described above occurs, a cross-banded fibril results.

COLLAGEN STRUCTURE IN THE PERIODONTAL LIGAMENT

Using x-ray diffraction, Gathercole *et al.* (1987) showed that the D period for the major fibrils of human PDL was 65 nm, i.e. slightly less than the 67 nm described above. The 65 nm periodicity is also characteristic of dermal collagens (Brodsky *et al.*, 1980), and the two tissues share a number of other common features. This smaller axial arrangement is possibly due to the presence of specific non-collagenous components implicated in the process of fibrillogenesis, notably the small proteoglycans, which are more rich in glucuronate in PDL and dermis compared to tendon, which has classical 67 nm periodicity (Brodsky *et al.*, 1980). Measuring directly from electron micrographs, Moxham (1985) quoted an average of 57 nm for the axial periodicity of PDL collagen, which may be related to functional considerations (e.g. whether the tissue is subjected to predominantly tensional versus compressional forces).

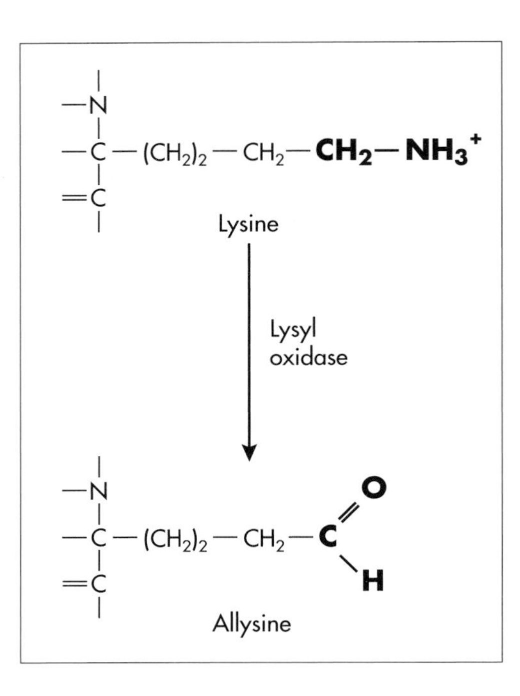

Fig. 3.7 Oxidative deamination of lysine to produce the aldehyde derivitive, allysine.

COLLAGEN CROSS-LINKING

GENERAL STRUCTURE AND FORMATION OF COLLAGEN CROSS-LINKS

Collagen fibrils are stabilized by intermolecular and intramolecular cross-links, which form immediately upon correct alignment of the tropocollagen monomers. Without the formation of these cross-links, the fibrils formed are dysfunctional (Bailey *et al.*, 1974). Most cross-links arise by formation of strong covalent bonds that arise between enzymatically modified lysine (LYS) and hydroxylysine (HYL) residues at the non-helical terminal domains of the teleopeptides, and other LYS/HYL residues positioned within the helical domain (Light and Bailey, 1980).

Both LYS and HYL can be oxidatively deaminated by the copper-dependent enzyme lysyl oxidase (Pinnell and Martin, 1968; Harris, 1976; Tanzer, 1976) to produce their corresponding aldehydes (often known as 'Allysine' and 'Hydroxyallysine' respectively) (*Fig.* 3.7). This step appears to occur in the very earliest stages of fibrillogenesis since the enzyme binds to the fibrillar surface (Cronlund *et al.*, 1985) and this would be precluded as fibrillogenesis progresses.

Following this initial oxidative controlling step, covalent cross-links are spontaneously formed via two possible routes (Eyre, 1987; Last *et al.*, 1990). The first of these, based upon allysine, is characteristic of skin, cornea and sclera. The second, based upon hydroxyallysine, is characteristic of bone, ligament, tendon and foetal skin. The ratio of the two forms appears to be tissue specific.

ALLYSINE-BASED CROSS-LINKS

There are two major types of cross-links arising from the condensation of allysine residues. The first of these (*Fig. 3.8*) results in the formation of an aldol condensation product and is the basis of most intramolecular cross-linkages that give rise to β-chains (dimeric α-chains). It has been suggested that these intramolecular cross-links may take part in further intermolecular cross-linking via reaction with either histidine or other hydroxylysine residues to form aldol histidine (Tanzer *et al.*, 1973) and hydroxymerodesmosine (Masuda *et al.*, 1976) (*Fig. 3.9*). However, other workers have suggested that these structures represent preparation artefacts (Light and Bailey, 1982).

The second allysine-based cross-link forms between adjacent tropocollagen molecules, between allysine in the teleopeptide domain of one tropocollagen molecule and LYS or HYL in the helical domain of another (Bailey and Peach, 1968). An aldimine (or Schiff's base) results, which then condenses further to form the covalent cross-link, dehydrohydroxylysinonorleucine (see *Fig. 3.8*), which in turn yields hydroxylysinonorleucine (HLNL) on borohydride reduction. Cross-links that can be obtained following borohydride reduction in this way are referred to as reducible cross-links.

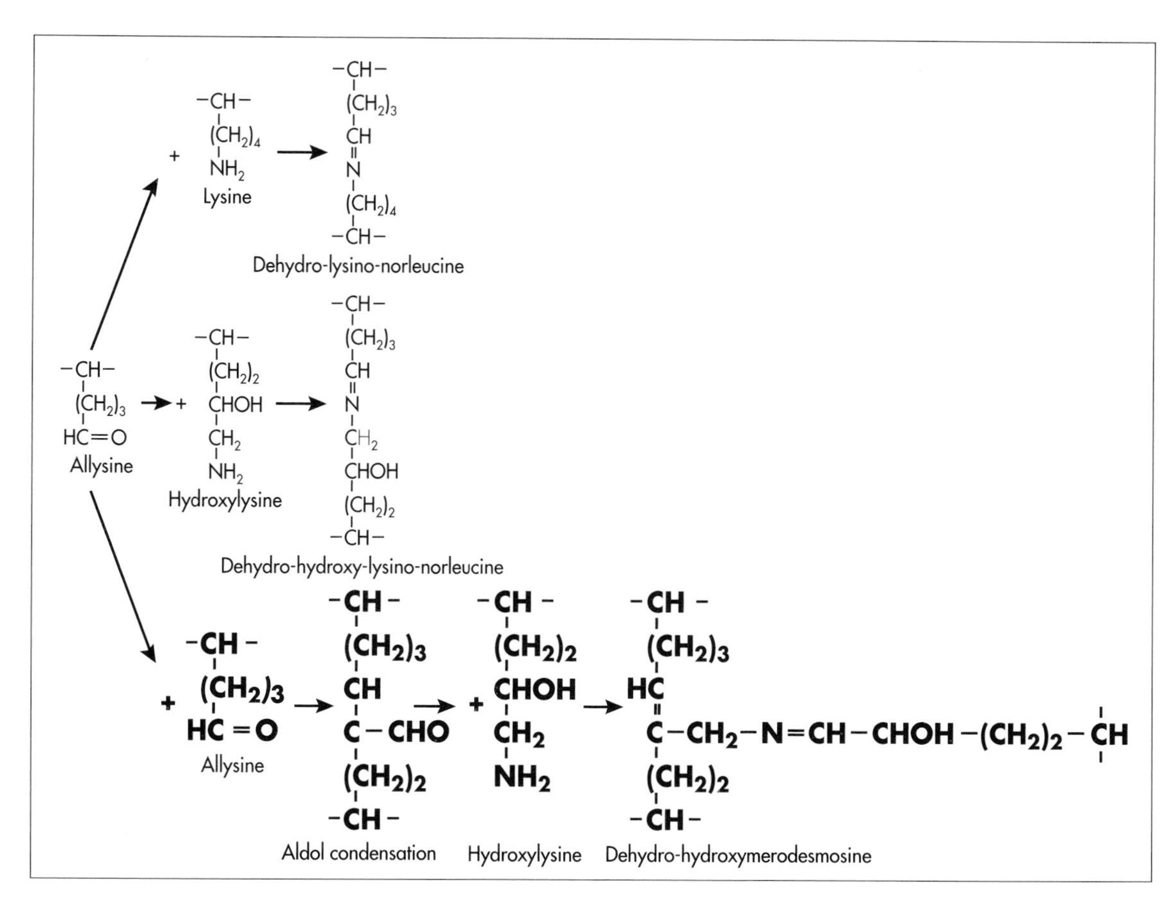

Fig. 3.8 Allysine-based reducible cross-links found in collagen. The aldol condensation product pathway is the basis of most intra-chain cross-links and gives rise to β-chains.

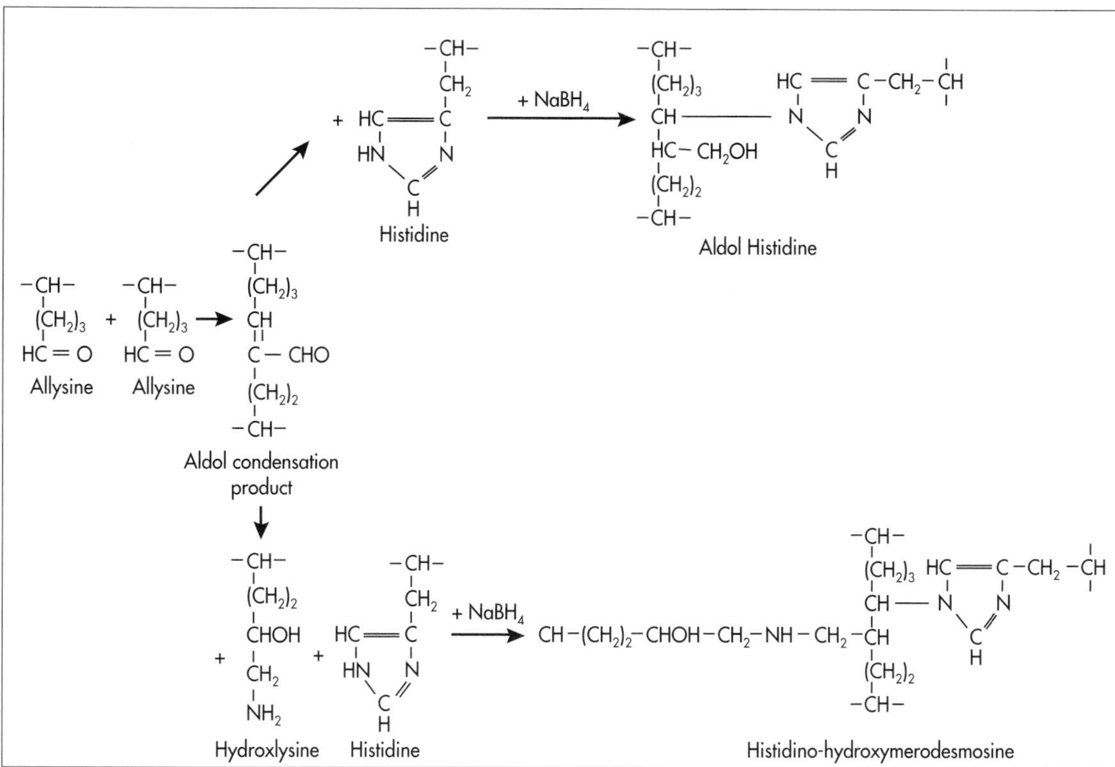

Fig. 3.9 Allysine-based cross-links forming histidino-based linkages identified following borohydride reduction.

HYDROXYALLYSINE-BASED CROSS-LINKS

Intermolecular reducible cross-links also arise via condensation of hydroxyallysine residues with HYL (Mechanic and Tanzer, 1970). This forms dehydrodihydroxylysinonorleucine, which yields dihydroxylysinonorleucine (DHLNL) after borohydride reduction. Dehydro-dihydroxy-lysinonorleucine can then undergo an Amadori rearrangement, which results in the formation of the ketoimine, hydroxylysino-5-oxo-norleucine (*Fig. 3.10*), which is more stable.

AGE-RELATED CHANGES IN CROSS-LINKS

With increasing age, the number of reducible cross-links as described above decreases, being replaced by more stable, less well-defined non-reducible cross-links (Robins *et al.*, 1973; Mechanic *et al.*, 1974; Moriguchi and Fujimoto, 1978; Eyre *et al.*, 1988). These confer greater stability but less elasticity to the fibrils, which become accordingly less soluble. Two examples of this type of cross-link include hydroxylysyl-pyridinoline (arising from three HYL residues) and lysyl-pyridinoline (arising from two HYL and one LYS residues) (Kielty *et al.*, 1993). Pyridinoline-based cross-links of this type were first isolated and partially characterized by Fujimoto *et al.* (1978). The structures of these non-reducible cross-links, which show characteristic fluorescence, are shown in *Fig. 3.11*.

SUGAR-BASED CROSS-LINKS

There is some evidence to suggest that collagen fibrils (particularly in tissues with low turnover rates) can also be stabilized by sugar-derived cross-links. These arise following the non-enzymatic glycosylation of tropocollagen (usually via the aldehyde group of glucose and a free amino group on LYS or HYL) to form a Schiff's base. They can then go on to form condensation products such as those described above, including non-reducible cross-links following modification and reaction with other free amino groups (Kielty *et al.*, 1993).

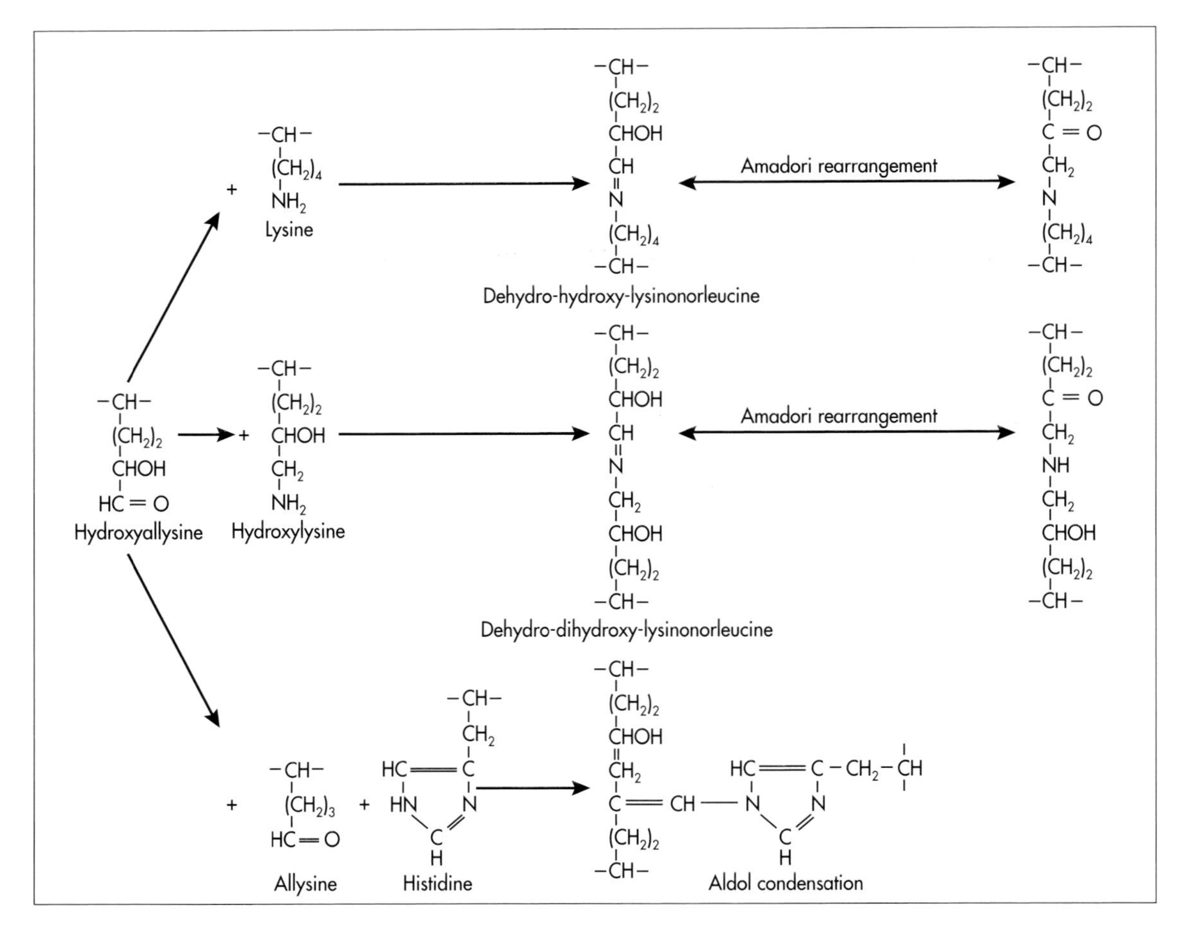

Fig. 3.10 Hydroxyallysine-based cross-links found in collagen.

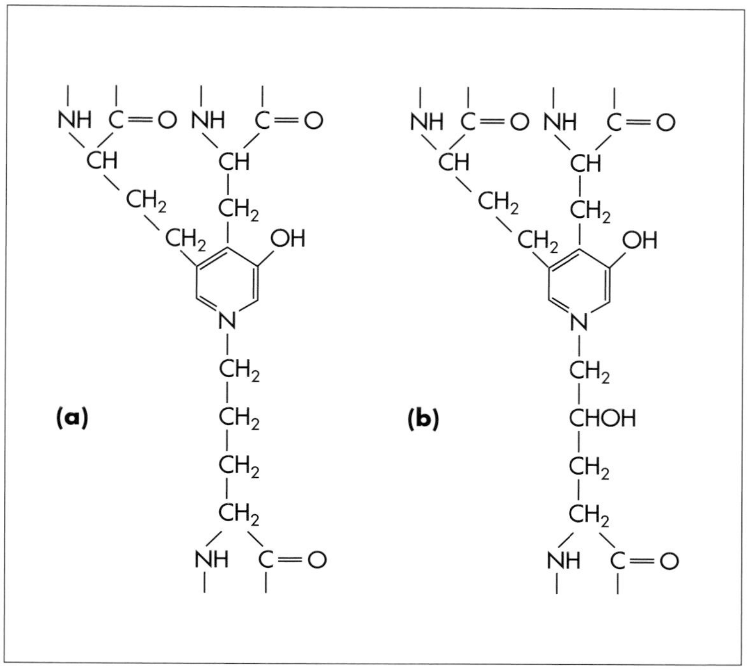

Fig. 3.11 Structures of two non-reducible cross-links in collagen: (a) hydroxylysylpyridinoline (arising from three HYL residues) and (b) lysyl-pyridinoline (arising from two HYL residues and one LYS residue).

COLLAGEN CROSS-LINKS IN THE PERIODONTAL LIGAMENT

Early reports suggested that the major collagenous cross-linkage in bovine PDL was DHLNL, with HLNL contributing only a minor proportion of the total reducible cross-links that were isolated (Pearson *et al.*, 1975). Later work (Kuboki *et al.*, 1981) calculated the ratio of DHLNL: HLNL in bovine PDL collagen to be approximately 0.3 (compared with 0.5 for pulp and 0.18 for gingival collagen). This placed the PDL in a category similar to skin (Bailey and Shimokomaki, 1971) rather than bone and dentine, where the dihydroxy form predominates (Mechanic *et al.*, 1971). In contrast, Ranta (1978) calculated the ratio of DHLNL: HLNL to be between 1.1 and 1.9. This ratio did not change with either age or tissue location.

In a more recent and comprehensive investigation, Yamauchi and co-workers (1986) carried out a complete characterization of the cross-linkages in bovine PDL type I collagen, including sequence analysis. These authors reported the ratio of DHLNL:HLNL to be 1.3, which was apparently unique to this tissue. Cross-links comparable in structure to those of a range of other tissues were found between α1-chain teleopeptides and helical loci. However, cross-linkage of the α2-chain that involves HYL at residue 87 in the helical domain, which was isolated from the PDL in this study, had not been previously reported.

Non-reducible cross-links were also investigated by these authors and found to make up only a very small proportion of the total. In addition, the reducible cross-links were found to be associated with O-linked carbohydrate on specific hydroxylysine residues, suggesting that glycosylation might provide a means of maintaining the fibrils in an 'immature state', perhaps permitting a higher rate of collagen turnover in this tissue (see below). This concept of a foetal state for the PDL is discussed further in Chapter 8.

GENERAL BIOSYNTHESIS OF FIBROUS COLLAGENS

PROCOLLAGEN

The spontaneous fibrillogenesis displayed by certain tropocollagen molecules presents an apparent paradox – how are these molecules exported into the extracellular matrix in an unaggregated form? The presence of a soluble precursor form of collagen was predicted many years before its ultimate isolation and characterization (Schmitt, 1960). Studies using fibroblasts and chondrocytes *in vitro* and tissue explants demonstrated that the fibre-forming collagens (in common with many other exported proteins) were synthesized as a larger precursor (Fessler and Smith, 1970; Bellamy and Bornstein, 1971; Goldberg *et al.*, 1972; Burgeson *et al.*, 1972). This precursor molecule was eventually called procollagen. Procollagen is now synonymous with the soluble precursor of the fibrous collagens. Only type I procollagen will be discussed here.

Procollagens have a molecular weight which is up to 50 per cent greater than that of the final tropocollagen molecule (Martin *et al.*, 1975). This is due to peptide extensions at both the N- and the C-termini (Schofield and Prockop, 1973; Kuhn, 1986). These extensions are known as propeptides and are essentially non-helical. The propeptides are not identical, with the C-terminal propeptide being much larger (approximately 246 amino acids) than the N-terminal propeptide (139 amino acids for the pro α1(I) chain and 57 amino acids for the shorter pro α2(I) chain) (Bernard *et al.*, 1983). The appearance of the procollagen molecule as revealed by electron microscopy consists of the long triple-helical central portion with a large globular domain at the C-terminal and a smaller, hook-like extension at the N-terminal (Kielty *et al.*, 1993). This flexible hook-like region is due to the sequence of amino acids of the N-terminal propeptide (Kuhn, 1986). Cysteine residues at the terminus of the molecule participate in disulphide intrachain bonding. Adjacent to this is a brief stretch of triple helix, which is responsible for the hook. This is followed by the non-helical teleopeptide (Fietzek and Kuhn, 1976) (*Fig. 3.12*).

The C-terminal propeptide, which forms a large, globular domain, is glycosylated at an ASN-X-SER/THR locus (Sandell *et al.*, 1984) and contains stabilizing interchain disulphide bonds in addition to intrachain bonds (Forster and Freedman, 1984). The C-terminal propeptide has been shown to be essential for triple-helix assembly (Prockop *et al.*, 1976).

Both propeptides are susceptible to proteolytic cleavage (Martin *et al.*, 1975). Indeed, cleavage of the propeptides is a necessary prerequisite for fibrillogenesis in the extracellular matrix. Failure to remove the N-terminal propeptide results in the inherited condition of dermatosparaxis in cattle and sheep, in which accumulations of partially processed procollagen molecules arise with concomitant failure to form fibres (Schofield and Prockop, 1973). The ultimate fate of the cleaved propeptides remains a matter of some conjecture, however, and there is some evidence to suggest that they may have a role in the control of collagen biosynthesis at the pre-translational level (Wiestner *et al.*, 1979; Wu *et al.*, 1986).

SYNTHESIS OF PROCOLLAGEN

Procollagen biosynthesis begins at the ribosomes on the rough endoplasmic reticulum (RER) and involves extensive co-translational and post-translational modifications, which are controlled by some nine or ten different enzymes (Kivirikko and Myllyla, 1985). Pre-pro α-chains are initially synthesized containing a signal peptide sequence at the N-terminal. This appears to be a typical signal peptide – approximately 25 amino acids in length, hydrophobic, and highly conserved (Yamada *et al.*, 1983). The role of the signal peptide is in translocation of the pro α-chains into the lumen of the RER, after which it is cleaved at a GLY-GLN sequence in pre-pro α1-chains and at a SER-GLN/GLY sequence in pre-pro α2 chains. This cleavage is catalysed by non-specific signal peptidase activity in the RER (Kivirikko and Myllyla, 1982a).

HYDROXYLATION OF PROLINE AND LYSINE

Hydroxylation of PRO and LYS residues is apparently initiated as a co-translational event that occurs on the nascent α-chains during chain elongation at the ribosome (Kivirikko and Myllyla, 1980). Hydroxylation is catalysed by three hydroxylase enzymes with specific target sequences, as shown in *Table 3.3*.

All of the hydroxylases require Fe^{2+}, α-ketoglutarate, O_2, and ascorbic acid. The reaction produces CO_2 and succinate (Kivirikko and Myllyla, 1985) (*Fig. 3.13*). The role of ascorbic acid is indirect; it probably plays a part in the regeneration of Fe^{2+} following uncoupling of the α-ketoglutarate decarboxylation reaction (Myllyla *et al.*, 1984). The role of hydroxyproline and hydroxylysine in helix stability and intermolecular cross-linkage (see page 64) is an important one and failure of this mechanism (e.g. in vitamin C deficiency) results in a range of pathologies (Bailey *et al.*, 1974), including scurvy, hydroxylysine-deficient disease, lathyrism, and Menkes' kinky hair syndrome.

Hydroxylation also continues as a post-translational modification in the lumen of the RER, but ceases after triple-helix formation (Kivirikko and Myllyla, 1985).

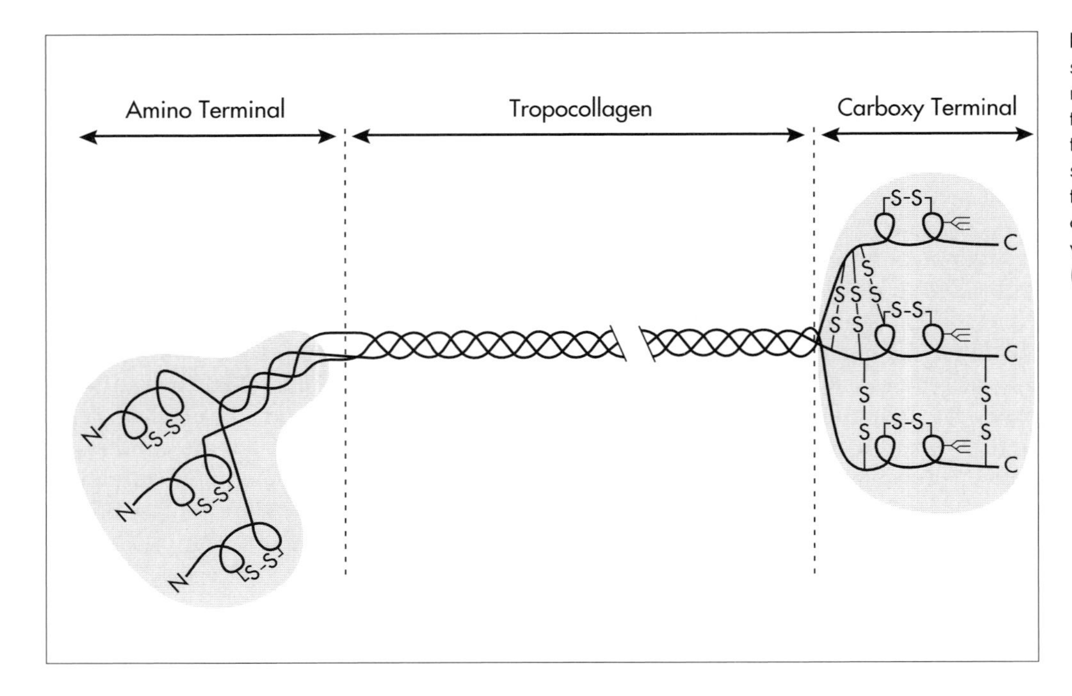

Fig. 3.12 Diagrammatic representation of the structure of type I procollagen. Both N- and C-termini contain stabilizing intrachain disulphide bonds in the propeptide regions. The N-terminal also contains a short stretch of triple helix, which is responsible for the characteristic appearance in the electron microscope. Disulphide bonds between pro α-chains are a feature of the C-terminal propeptide, which is also glycosylated via N-linked sugars. (Based on data from Kuhn, 1986.)

Table 3.3
Target sequence and product for hydroxylase enzymes. (Based on data from Kivirikko and Myllyla, 1980).

Enzyme	Target	Product
Prolyl-4-hydroxylase	–X–PRO–GLY–	4-Hydroxyproline
Prolyl-3-hydroxylase	–PRO–4HYP–GLY–	3-Hydroxyproline
Lysyl-hydroxylase	–X–LYS–GLY–	5-Hydroxylysine

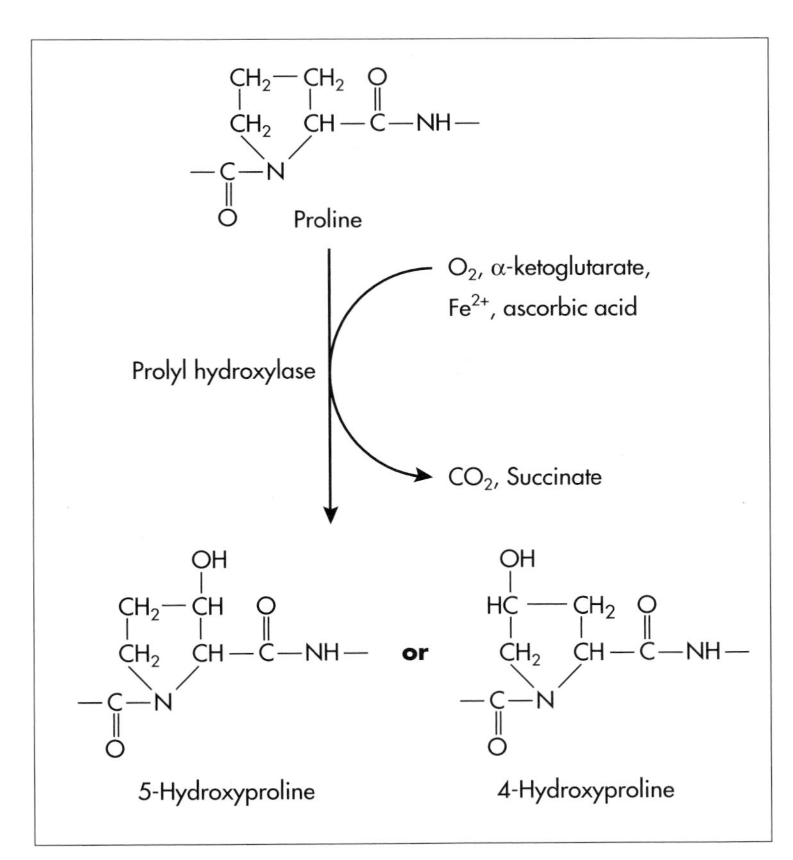

Fig. 3.13 Hydroxylation of proline via the prolyl hydroxylase catalysed reaction (see also *Table 3.3*).

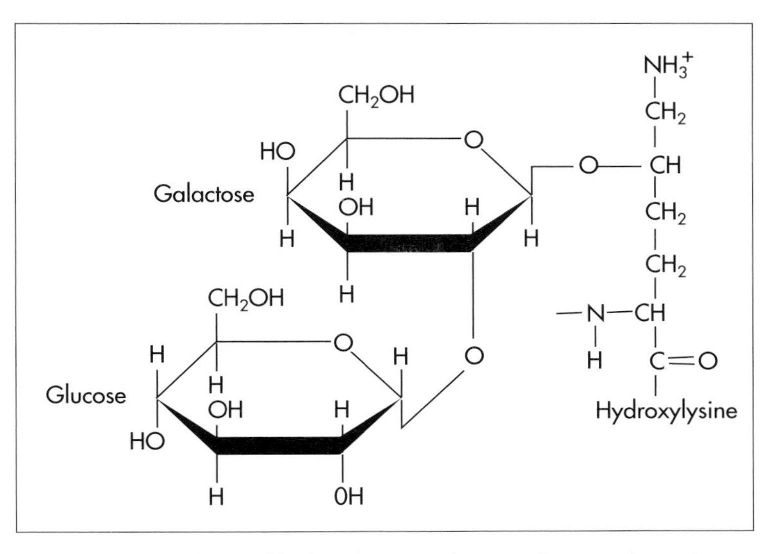

Fig. 3.14 Glycosylation of hydroxylysine residues in collagen. Either galactose or glucosyl-galactose (illustrated) are O-linked in a reaction catalysed by transferase enzymes utilizing UDP-activated precursor sugars.

GLYCOSYLATION OF HYDROXYLYSINE AND ASPARAGINE

Collagen is a glycoprotein, and the addition of -O-linked carbohydrate to some hydroxylysine residues in the triple-helical domain also occurs at the co-translational and post-translational levels (Kivirikko and Myllyla, 1980). The amount of glycosylation varies with tissue and age, but essentially two carbohydrate residues are involved. These are the monosaccharide galactose and the disaccharide glucosyl-galactose, formed by the addition of glucose to *in situ* galactose residues (Kivirikko and Myllyla, 1979, 1982b) (*Fig. 3.14*). The reactions are catalysed by hydroxylysyl galactosyl transferase and galactosyl hydroxylysyl glucosyl transferase respectively, utilizing the activated (UDP) sugars in the presence of bivalent cations (preferably Mn^{2+}) (Kivirikko and Myllyla, 1979, 1982b). The significance of these sugars is not yet fully understood, though a role in fibril organization has been suggested.

The propeptide extensions are also subject to glycosylation at the C-terminal via N-linkages (*Fig. 3.15*) to asparagine residues in a ASN-X-SER/THR sequence (Sandell *et al.*, 1984). These are synthesized on carrier lipids and transferred via carrier proteins on to the nascent chains (Kivirikko and Myllyla, 1985). The significance of these N-linked oligosaccharides is unknown.

HELIX FORMATION

Triple-helix formation is initiated via the association of the three C-terminal propeptides. A role for the signal peptide in the assembly of two α1 chains and one α2 chain at a common site at the rough endoplasmic reticulum membrane has been suggested (Kirk *et al.*, 1987). Chain alignment begins by non-covalent (particularly hydrophobic) interactions at the C-terminal propeptide (Fessler *et al.*, 1981). The C-terminal end of the triple helical domain consists of a highly conserved stretch of 3–10 repeating GLY-PRO-HYP motifs which stabilize the propagating helix. This alignment is further stabilized by interchain disulphide bond formation in the propeptide domain (Forster and Freedman, 1984). The enzyme, protein, disulphide isomerase, which has wide substrate specificity (Freedman and Hillson, 1980), is required for correct cis/trans conformational alignment and rearrangement of (incorrect) disulphide bridges.

Subsequent further folding of the collagen triple helix proceeds rapidly after the initial stabilization of the C-terminal propeptides, which is the rate-determining step for helix formation (Fessler *et al.*, 1981).

The fully associated trimeric procollagen molecule is then exported from the cell via the Golgi apparatus in the classical secretory pathway. Once outside the cell, in the extracellular matrix, further processing occurs by endopeptidase activity (Kivirikko and Myllyla, 1985), which cleaves the N- and C-propeptides, leaving the tropocollagen molecule, which can then aggregate and form fibres as described above. Removal of the propeptides is achieved via at least two specific endopeptidases, procollagen-C-proteinase and procollagen-N-proteinase, which cleave at the C- and N- termini respectively (Kivirikko and Myllyla, 1985). These are both enzymes of the matrix metalloproteinase class as described below.

There is some evidence to suggest that, at least in the case of type I procollagen, degradation may proceed via an intracellular route. Bienowski *et al.* (1978) suggested that fibroblasts may produce collagen in excess of their normal requirements, a fraction of which is broken down intracellularly before becoming incorporated into fibrils. A role for this route in rapidly meeting inreased demand for collagen has been suggested (Berkovitz, 1990).

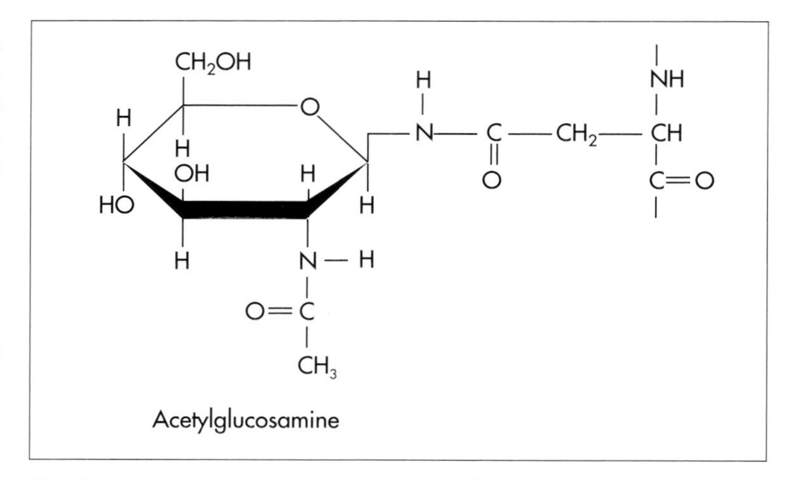

Fig. 3.15 Example of N-linked glycosylation of asparagine residues.

METABOLISM OF THE FIBROUS COLLAGENS

GENERAL FEATURES OF COLLAGEN DEGRADATION

Breakdown of the collagenous matrix is a normal event in tissues undergoing morphogenesis, morphostasis and growth. However, it is vital that this process is subject to rigid control, as failure to maintain an appropriate balance between degradation and synthesis can lead to net destruction or net gain, resulting, for example, in pathological conditions such as chronic inflammatory periodontal disease or hypertrophic scar tissue formation.

The fibrillar collagens are subject to fragmentation, owing to physical wear and tear on the tissue and to the action of highly reactive free radicals (Murphy and Reynolds, 1993). However, collagen breakdown is also under stringent cellular control mediated via a group of proteolytic enzymes – the matrix metalloproteinases (reviewed by Murphy and Reynolds, 1993). This is a group of endopeptidases, which share some degree of sequence homology and which are characterized by their metal binding properties and neutral pH optima. Matrix metalloproteinases (or MMPs) all contain Zn^{2+} at their active site and require Ca^{2+} as stabilizer. All are secreted as inactive precursors, which are often self-activated and are inhibited by tissue inhibitor of metalloproteinases (TIMP). MMPs are secreted by connective tissue cells (predominantly fibroblasts) but are also produced by some leucocytes (polymorphonuclear neutrophil leucocytes and macrophages).

Fibrillar collagen is very resistant to proteolytic degradation in its triple-helical domain (Kuhn, 1986). Two matrix metalloproteinases (collagenases) are capable of cleaving the helix at a single locus, resulting in two fragments of 3/4 and 1/4 molecular lengths from the N-terminus (Highberger *et al.*, 1979). The triple-helical conformation is rapidly lost after cleavage, and the resulting denatured molecule is then exposed to the action of less specific proteases which degrade the collagen further (Burleigh, 1977).

The non-helical teleopeptides are far more susceptible to proteolysis (Starkey *et al.*, 1977; Burleigh, 1977; Nakano and Scott, 1987; Maciewicz *et al.*, 1987). Their degradation effectively weakens the cross-links in the collagen fibrils, which in turn improves the efficacy of collagenases, presumably by facilitating access to the collagenase locus.

The six major matrix metalloproteases effective in collagen degradation are shown in *Table 3.4*.

The control of these enzymes is clearly important in maintaining tissue morphostasis. Primary control is exerted by the production of the inhibitor molecule, TIMP, which forms irreversible complexes with the MMPs via non-covalent interactions (Welgus *et al.*, 1985) . TIMP itself is a highly conserved glycoprotein (M_r is approximately 30 K). It is secreted by fibroblasts and macrophages (Murphy and Docherty, 1988). Co-ordinated production of both matrix metalloproteinases and TIMP is presumably under both temporal and spatial control.

Profiles of collagen fibrils are also seen in fibroblasts, probably as a result of phagocytosis (Ten Cate and Deporter, 1975; Garant, 1976; Shore and Berkovitz, 1979). These can be further degraded by lysosomal enzymes (notably cysteine proteases), which operate at acidic pHs. In contrast to the extracellular degradation of collagen, this intracellular pathway of collagen phagocytosis and subsequent breakdown does not appear to involve matrix metalloproteinases (Everts and Beertsen, 1992).

Matrix metalloproteinases are also known to be inducible enzymes, and the cytokines, particularly interleukin-1, seem to play an important role in the control of their expression (Gowen *et al.*, 1984). Certain growth factors and hormones have also been shown to affect the expression of these enzymes. Interleukin-1, tumour necrosis factor (TNF) (Dayer *et al.*, 1985), platelet-derived growth factor (PDGF) (Bauer *et al.*, 1985), transforming growth factor-β (TGFβ) (Edwards *et al.*, 1987) and fibroblast growth factor (FGF) (Phadke, 1987) have all been shown to increase production of matrix metalloproteinases. TGFβ also increases TIMP production. These molecules are discussed further in Chapter 12. In contrast, glucocorticoids and retinoids have been shown to inhibit MMP production (Clark *et al.*, 1987) and both of these also increase the production of TIMP.

Table 3.4 Connective tissue matrix metalloproteinases. Based upon data from Murphy and Reynolds (1993).

Matrix metalloproteinase	Mr	Source	Substrate	Comments
Interstitial collagenases (2)	55 K 75 K	Fibroblasts, macrophages Polymorphonucleocytes	Single locus on native collagens types I, II, III, and X generating 3/4 and 1/4 fragments Some activity against denatured collagen	Plasmin activation? Stromelysin activation?
Gelatinases (2)	72 K 95 K	Fibroblasts Macrophages, polymorphonucleocytes Tumours	Type IV collagen Denatured collagen Non-helical teleopeptides of fibrillar collagens types V, VII, XI	Some activity against denatured collagen Denatured collagen
Stromelysins (2)	57 K (both)	Fibroblasts, macrophages	Type IV cross-links Type IX collagen Propeptides of I, II, III	Plasmin activation? Various proteases

METABOLISM OF COLLAGEN IN THE PERIODONTAL LIGAMENT

The earliest manifestations of vitamin C deficiency (scurvy) were seen as intraoral lesions and tooth loosening (Hunt and Paynter, 1959), which indicated that the periodontal tissues were subject to rapid turnover of collagen. Use of radiolabelled proline and its subsequent incorporation into hydroxyproline has enabled a great deal of work to be carried out, which has since confirmed this. Interpretation of radiolabelling data is often difficult, however, owing to the effects of recycling and reutilization of tracer and to the fact that most connective tissues contain pools of collagen that may be turning over at different rates (e.g. intracellular and extracellular degradation of procollagen; breakdown of salt-soluble – non-fibrillar non-cross-linked – collagen, and ultimate degradation of insoluble collagen fibrils). These criteria are reviewed by Sodek (1989).

The earliest attempts to determine collagen turnover in the PDL used autoradiographic techniques (Stallard, 1963; Crumley, 1964; Carneiro and Fava de Moraes, 1965; Carneiro and Leblond, 1966; Skougaard *et al.*, 1970; Skougaard and Levy, 1971). These studies (mostly using ^{3}H-labelled proline) suggested that turnover of collagen in the periodontal tissues was rapid. However, the technique fails to discriminate between specific radiolabelling of collagen and incorporation of the tracer into other proteins, many of which (particularly intracellular proteins) turn over at a much higher rate than extracellular proteins.

Orlowski (1976, 1978), overcame these difficulties in part by measuring the specific activity of hydroxyproline 24 hours after injection with ^{3}H-proline. Turnover in the PDL was found to be higher than that of the gingiva, with a half life of around 9.5 days and a turnover time of 13.5 days for the rat incisor PDL.

In an attempt to address the problem of recycling of radio tracer and the influence of different collagen pools turning over at different rates, Sodek (1976, 1977) utilized a novel short-term approach to measure incorporation of ^{3}H-labelled proline into newly synthesized (and therefore salt-extractable) and mature collagen in the rat molar PDL, gingiva, alveolar bone and skin. Hydroxyproline-specific activities for these tissues revealed that the rate of collagen synthesis in the PDL was twice that in gingiva, four times that in skin, and six times that in alveolar bone. This study also showed that the conversion of newly synthesized collagen into mature insoluble collagen was highly efficient in the PDL compared with the other tissues (which showed up to 50 per cent degradation of newly synthesized collagen). This supported the suggestion of Guis and Slootweg (1973) based upon collagen extractability, that newly synthesized tropocollagen matured rapidly in bovine PDL. The half life of mature collagen in rat molar PDL was calculated by Sodek to be 1 day, compared with 5 days in gingiva, 6 days in alveolar bone and 15 days in skin. Subsequent studies (Sodek, 1978) comparing molar and incisor PDLs calculated a longer half life of 3 days for mature collagen in the incisor ligament.

Imberman *et al.* (1986) applied the so-called 'pool expansion' technique in order to determine the half life of collagen in the rat incisor and molar PDLs; they then compared these with those of the skin, gingiva, and palatal mucosa. This approach involves the injection of ^{3}H-proline in the presence of excess amounts of unlabelled tracer in an attempt to eliminate the problem of tracer reutilization. These authors calculated the half lives of collagen to be: 7.8 days for incisor PDL, 8.8 days for molar PDL, 150 days for incisor gingival tissue, 8.8 days for molar gingiva, 50 days for skin and 21 days for palatal mucosa.

Finally, using Poole's approach (1971), Sodek and Ferrier (1988) attempted to validate the apparently rapid rate of collagen turnover in the periodontal tissues of the rat. This involved compensation for the reutilization of radiolabel by use of decay curves based upon the decay of the radioactive precursor. This study yielded half life values for mature, insoluble collagen as 3 days for molar PDL, 6 days for incisor PDL, and 10 days for gingiva.

The discrepancies between values reported by different workers using a variety of techniques clearly indicate the difficulties involved in obtaining definitive data for collagen turnover rates in the PDL and other connective tissues in general. However, the general consensus is that the turnover of collagen in PDL is unusually high. This may have important implications in the aetiology of chronic inflammatory periodontal disease (see Chapter 14), such that an imbalance in the synthesis and degradation process may result in net collagen loss (Page and Ammons, 1974).

The rate of turnover of specific collagen types has received less attention. However, Sodek and Limeback (1979) showed that types I and III collagen are metabolized at similar rates in the PDL and gingiva of the rat molar and incisor both *in vivo* and *in vitro*. These results, together with the reported co-expression of types I and III collagens (Gay *et al.*, 1976) have prompted the suggestion that these collagens may be controlled coordinately (Sodek, 1989).

Turnover of collagen in the periodontal tissues may be related, at least in part, to their functional loading. Early autoradiographical work by Crumley (1964) suggested an increase in protein metabolism in the stressed periodontium (see Chapter 15). However, later work by Rippin (1976, 1978), also using autoradiography, indicated increased protein metabolism in the crestal region of the hypofunctional PDL of the rat molar. Kanoza *et al.* (1980) determined the effects of PDL hypofunction biochemically by removing rat molars from occlusion. These workers demonstrated an increase in collagen remodelling in the hypofunctional ligament involving both collagen type I and type III. Seemingly conflicting reports may be due to the possibility of site-specific differences in collagen metabolism within the PDL (Beertsen and Everts, 1977; Sodek, 1989; Kirkham *et al.*, 1991). Sodek (1989) suggested that the differences in turnover rate with tooth type might be due to the direction of the functional loading on the tissue, i.e. tensional as opposed to compressional. This could be an important consideration when tooth attachment is lost during chronic periodontitis (Kirkham *et al.*, 1992).

Finally, perhaps related to the constraints described above, turnover of collagen in the PDL also appears to be in some way linked with rate of eruption, though opinions vary as to the extent and consistency of this relationship (Berkovitz, 1990). Rippin (1976, 1978) reported an increase in collagen turnover with reactivated eruption following extraction of opposing teeth, but no such increase was observed when eruption was accelerated in the rat incisor (Van den Bos and Tonino, 1984). The precise relationship between rate of eruption and PDL collagen turnover remains obscure.

COLLAGEN METABOLISM AND PERIODONTAL DISEASE

Chronic inflammatory periodontal disease (CIPD) clearly involves the net destruction of collagen in the extracellular matrix (*Fig. 3.16*). The precise aetiology of CIPD remains obscure, however, and the unusually rapid rate of collagen turnover in this tissue raises the possibility that the pathology is related to a disturbance in the host synthesis/degradation pathway (Page and Ammons, 1974). Low-level, persistent bacterial infection could conceivably result in chronic inflammation leading to cytokine production and induction of matrix metalloproteinases by host cells (Meikle *et al.*, 1986, 1989; Murphy and Reynolds, 1993).

In support of this, collagenase activity has been shown to be greater in the presence of inflammatory periodontal disease. Christner (1980) reported collagenase activity in human periodontal tissue only in PDLs from teeth that had suffered loss of attachment. In addition, collagenase levels were found to vary with degree of inflammation in biopsy tissue from gingivitis patients (Overall *et al.*, 1987).

Levels of tissue-derived collagenase were also found to be higher in gingival crevicular fluid from patients suffering from CIPD compared with healthy controls (Larivee *et al.*, 1986; Villela *et al.*, 1987) and these levels were reduced by periodontal treatment.

Other proteolytic enzymes have also been implicated in the pathological destruction of the periodontal extracellular matrix. Heath and co-workers (1982) reported the production of all three types of matrix metalloproteinases by inflamed gingival tissue explants *in vitro*. Matrix metalloproteinase activity of the gelatinase type was also seen to increase with disease at specific sites in the periodontium of the sheep (Smith, 1992) (*Fig.* 3.17).

Phagocytosis and intracellular lysosomal digestion of collagen is known to play an important role during normal collagen turnover (Garant, 1976; Birek *et al.*, 1980; Wang, 1982) and it is

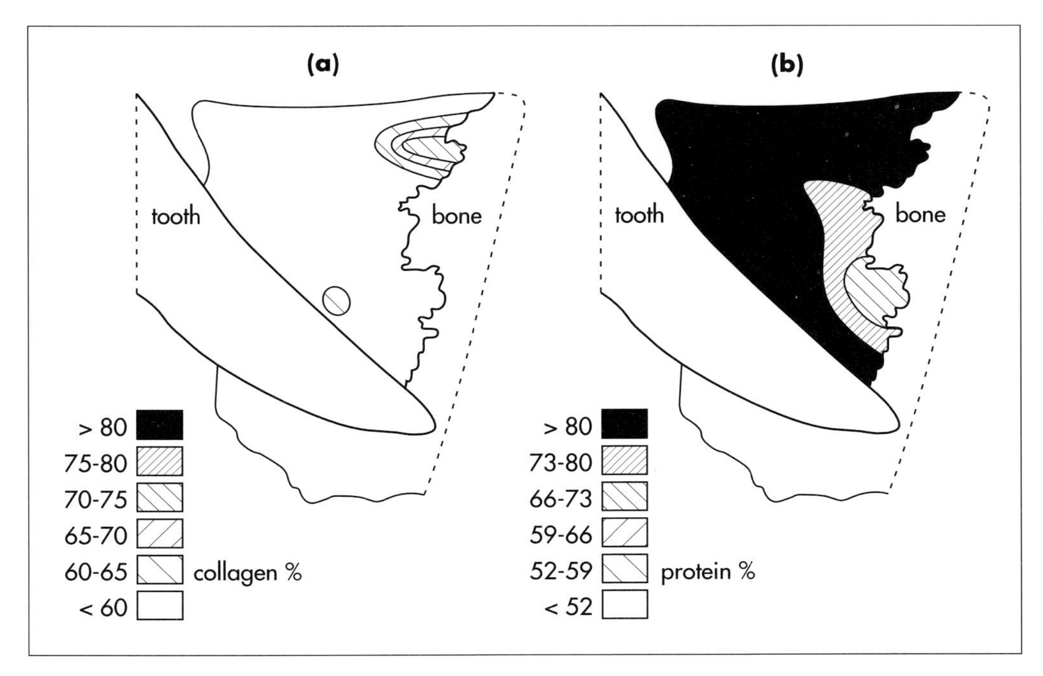

Fig. 3.16 (a) Effect of chronic inflammatory periodontal disease on collagen distribution in the sheep periodontium. Concentrations of collagen can be seen to be drammatically reduced when compared with healthy tissue (see *Fig. 3.1a*). Collagen percentage of total tissue protein was calculated from hydroxyproline content following amino acid analysis. (b) Effect of periodontal disease on protein distribution in the sheep periodontium. Protein concentrations can be seen to be increased when compared with healthy tissue (see *Fig. 3.1b*). Protein percentage of tissue dry weight was calculated from total amino acids recovered following amino acid analysis. (From Kirkham *et al.*, 1989. Reproduced by permission of the publishers.)

possible that this pathway may also be abnormal during CIPD. It is also possible that inhibitor production could be affected by the disease process, which would in turn affect the activity of the enzymes. Sandholm (1986) suggested that susceptibility to CIPD may be related to inhibitor availability. This was supported by the findings of Morris and Harper (1987), who reported decreased amounts of TIMP in chronically inflamed periodontal tissue.

MINERALIZATION OF COLLAGEN

One important aspect of collagen biochemistry which has received relatively little attention in the PDL is that of mineralization. In calcified dental tissues, such as alveolar bone, dentine, and cementum (but not enamel), collagen fibres are mineralized along their length and cores with hydroxyapatite crystals (Weiner and Traub, 1986; Glimcher, 1989). The nucleation and control of crystal growth in these tissues has been extensively investigated and is reviewed elsewhere (see Glimcher, 1989; Weiner and Traub, 1992). However, some collagen fibres in the PDL insert into bone and cementum and are effectively mineralized in these areas. These insertions are known as Sharpey's fibres because of their resemblance to similar insertions described in tendon (Quigley, 1970; Shackleford, 1971) (see also Chapter 2).

Previous work has suggested that Sharpey's fibres represent an embedding of the PDL fibres by entrapment in the advancing mineral front (Selvig, 1965). This well-defined interface between mineralized and non-mineralized collagen in the PDL implies some form of strict control mechanism which retains the width (approximately 200 μm in the case of human PDL) of unmineralized fibres.

It is possible that the failure of PDL fibres proper to mineralize *in vivo* may be due to a number of interrelated causes. Cross-linkage of fibrils in PDL is known to be different from bone (see page 65) and this could lead to restriction of access of mineral ions to nucleation sites in the hole zones, where collagen mineralization is generally thought to be initiated (Glimcher, 1989). This may in turn be related to degrees of collagen glycosylation, collagen assembly and the presence or absence of specific fibre-associated proteins and proteoglycans.

Alternatively, control of collagen mineralization could be mediated via expression of specific spatially restricted enzymes, such as alkaline phosphatase. Beertsen and van den Bos (1992) used an *in vitro* system to demonstrate the role of alkaline phosphatase in the mineralization of different collagenous substrates. These authors suggested that alkaline phosphatase activity could play a key role in collagen calcification *in vivo*.

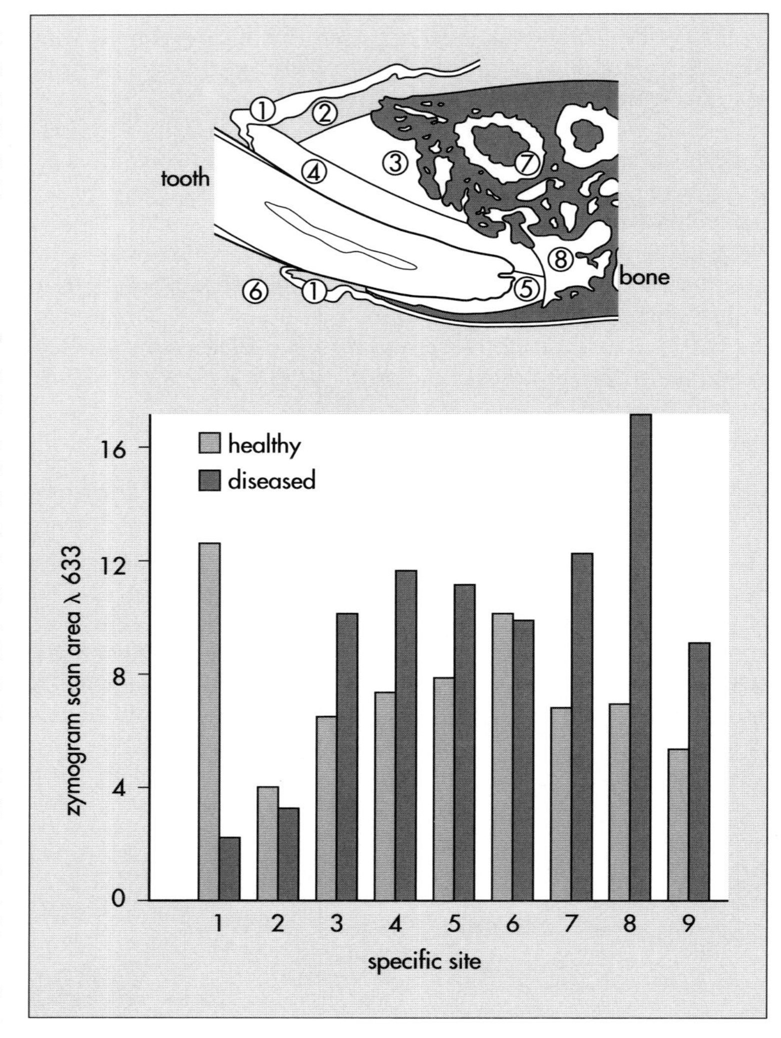

Fig. 3.17 Site-specific gelatinase activity in healthy and diseased sheep periodontal tissue. Gelatinase activity measured using a zymographic technique followed by densitometry. Increased activity can be seen associated with chronic inflammatory periodontal disease compared with healthy tissue.

Yamashita and co-workers (1987) showed the presence of alkaline phosphatase in rabbit and monkey PDL, which was similar to that of bone. Further studies using the larger PDL from the sheep revealed that most of this activity was located in tissue adjacent to alveolar bone but not in the bulk of the unmineralized PDL (Smith, 1992).

The presence and/or absence of inhibitors or nucleating sites could also be responsible for the control of mineralization. Glycosylaminoglycans have been implicated in this respect, with chondroitin sulphate (which predominates in mineralized tissues) being replaced mainly by dermatan sulphate in soft unmineralized tissues. This mechanism finds some support in experiments that have shown that PDL collagen will mineralize *in vitro* if incubated in solutions metastable with respect to hydroxyapatite at pH 7.4 but only if the glycosylaminoglycans are first removed (Kirkham *et al.*, 1993). The resulting hydroxyapatite crystals are small, thin plates that can be seen to align in parallel with the collagen fibrils (*Fig. 3.18*). The role of the ground substance in mineralization is discussed in more detail in Chapter 4.

This aspect of PDL physiology is clearly an important area, which could provide an ideal opportunity for studies on the control of crystal growth in mineralized tissues.

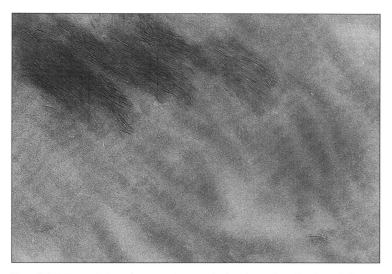

Fig. 3.18 Transmission electron micrograph showing mineralization of sheep PDL collagen fibrils *in vitro*. Freeze-dried PDL was treated with glycosylaminoglycan (GAG) degrading enzymes prior to incubation in solutions saturated with respect to hydroxyapatite at pH 7.0. Small plate-like crystals can be seen aligned in parrallel with the collagen. No crystals were seen in control specimens which were not pre-treated to remove GAGs.

BIOCHEMISTRY OF THE MINOR FIBRES

MINOR FIBRES IN GENERAL CONNECTIVE TISSUE

Collagen, as described above, is by far the most abundant of the fibrous proteins found in connective tissues and is largely responsible for its tensile strength. However, in addition to these major fibres, there is a second network of minor fibres, often intimately associated with the collagen, which confers a different set of properties. These are the elastic fibres. There are three types of elastic fibre, which are histochemically and ultrastructurally distinct: mature elastic fibres (sometimes referred to as elastin fibres), elauin and oxytalan (Cotta-Pereira *et al.*, 1977). These three fibre types are closely related and together appear to represent a developmental continuum. Mature elastic fibres consist of a microfibrillar component surrounding an amorphous core of elastin protein; elauin is seen as bundles of microfibrils embedded in a relatively small amount of amorphous elastin; and oxytalan appears to consist of the microfibrillar component only (Cotta-Pereira *et al.*, 1976; Bock and Stockinger, 1984). Thus, elauin and oxytalan have been described as 'immature' elastic fibres, which can be distinguished histochemically by the need for oxidation of tissue sections prior to staining with elastin stains.

Mature elastic fibres are now recognized as consisting of two ultrastructurally distinct, though intimately associated, components. The first of these is an amorphous core of a polymeric protein which has an affinity for anionic stains – this is elastin protein itself, contributing more than 90 per cent of the mature elastic fibres (for a review, see Rosenbloom, 1993). The amorphous elastin is surrounded by a microfibrillar component, which forms bead-like microfibrils of 10–15 nm diameter and has an affinity for cationic stains.

Progress in the biochemical analysis of these two components was initially slow, owing to their great insolubility and the difficulties in obtaining purified extracts, as elastic fibres are often closely interwoven with collagen (Partridge, 1962). However, based upon techniques originally described by Ross and Bornstein (1969), mature elastic fibres that were ultrastructurally homogeneous were extracted. Further characterization by electrophoresis of these isolated fibres revealed a mixture of proteins and glycoproteins (Ross and Bornstein, 1969; Cleary and Gibson, 1983).

ELASTIN

Elastin is a single gene product that yields a highly insoluble, amorphous, hydrophobic protein with the ability to form aggregates based upon stable covalent cross-linkages (Rosenbloom, 1993). The amino acid composition reveals that approximately one-third of all residues are glycine (Starcher and Galione, 1976) but, unlike collagen, these residues are not evenly distributed throughout the length of the elastin molecule; most workers agree that the conformation of elastin is that of a random coil (Torchia and Piez, 1973). In addition to glycine, elastin contains approximately 10–15 per cent proline and some 40 per cent hydrophobic residues (*Fig. 3.19*). A small amount of hydroxyproline is also present but, in contrast to collagen, hydroxylation is not a necessary prerequisite for fibre formation (Uitto *et al.*, 1976), and the function of this imino acid in elastin is unknown.

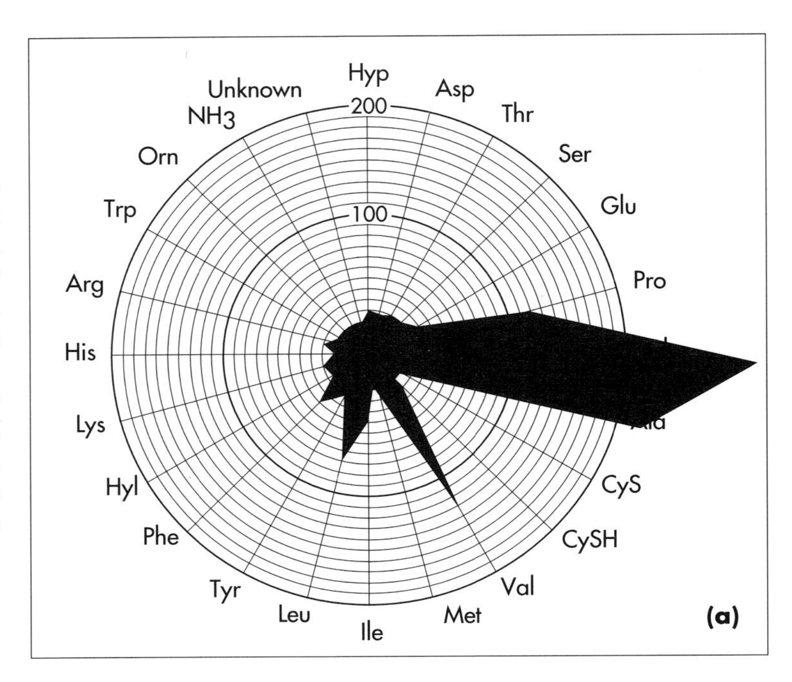

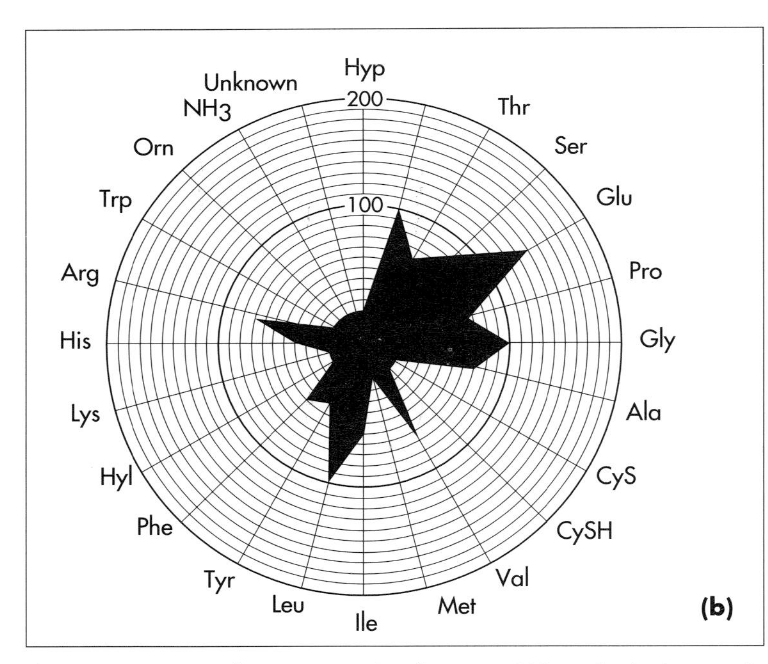

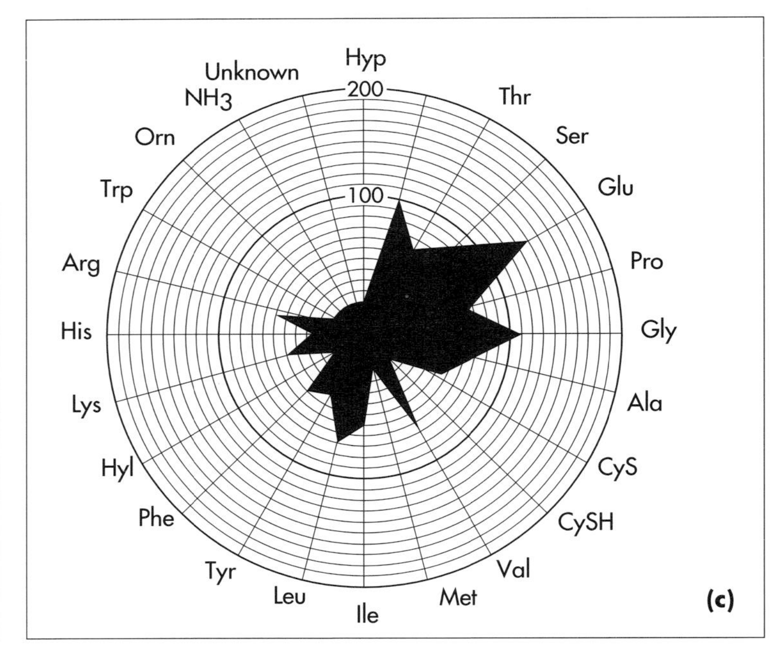

Fig. 3.19 Amino acid compositions (residues per 1000 residues), shown as Rose diagrams, comparing the compositions of (a) elastin, (b) oxytalan, and (c) microfibrillar proteins. (Based on compositions published by Sodek, 1978.)

The amino acid composition of elastin is similar between species, but there is some variability, which indicates a progressive increase in hydrophobicity with evolution (Sage and Gray, 1979). The presence of some degree of repeating structure and the similarities to collagen have led to suggestions that these fibrillar proteins may be distantly related (Smith *et al.*, 1981). Like collagen, elastin is secreted as a soluble precursor, tropoelastin (M_r 73 K), which contains no cross-links and appears to be the monomeric unit of elastin (Sandberg *et al.*, 1969, 1971).

The high degree of insolubility of elastin is due to the extensive covalent cross-links between tropoelastin molecules, which seem to occur at approximately every 70 residues on the polypeptide chain (Paz *et al.*, 1982; Eyre *et al.*, 1984). These arise from lysine residues in a similar manner to the cross-links in collagen. The same enzyme – lysyl oxidase – is utilized in both cases; this enzyme seems to operate on the insoluble form of elastin in a way similar to that seen for collagen fibrils. The enzyme converts the amino group of lysine to the aldehyde derivative, after which spontaneously formed covalent cross-links occur. There is no hydroxylysine (and effectively no histidine) in elastin (Starcher and Gallione, 1976), so the cross-links formed are between lysine and allysine residues only.

Dehydrolysinonorleucine (forming between allysine and lysine residues) and aldol condensation products (forming between allysine residues) are the two most important bifunctional cross-links (Paz *et al.*, 1982; Eyre *et al.*, 1984). Dehydromerodesmosine (*Fig. 3.20*) has also been implicated as a possible trimeric cross-link, and tetrafunctional cross-links may occur in elastin. These are the desmosine cross-links, which appear to arise from three allysine residues and one lysine residue, forming a pyridinium ring that is alkylated in four positions (*Fig. 3.21*). Differences in the position of alkylation give rise to the structural isomer isodesmosine (see *Fig. 3.21*). Although these cross-linkages have the potential capability of uniting up to four different polypeptide chains, it is thought that they actually form between two molecules only, with two LYS residues on each (Eyre *et al.*, 1984). The precise route (and indeed there may be more than one) to these cross-links remains equivocal, but an oxidation step is required, prompting the suggestion by Rosenbloom (1993) that this could be coordinated with the reduction of dehydrolysinonorleucine cross-links.

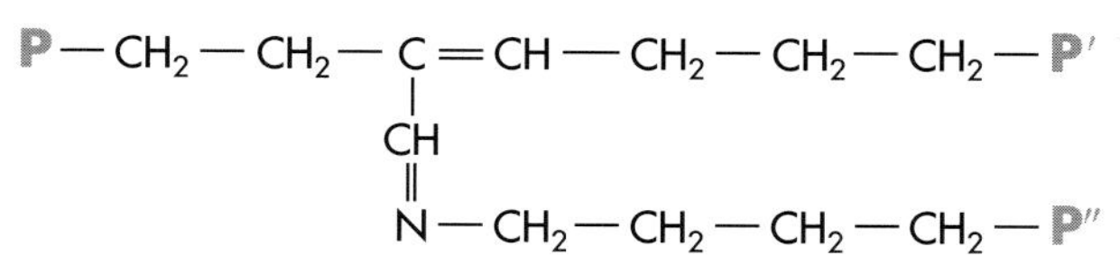

Dehydromerodesmosine

Fig. 3.20 Structure of dehydromerodesmosine, a potential trimeric cross-link in elastin.

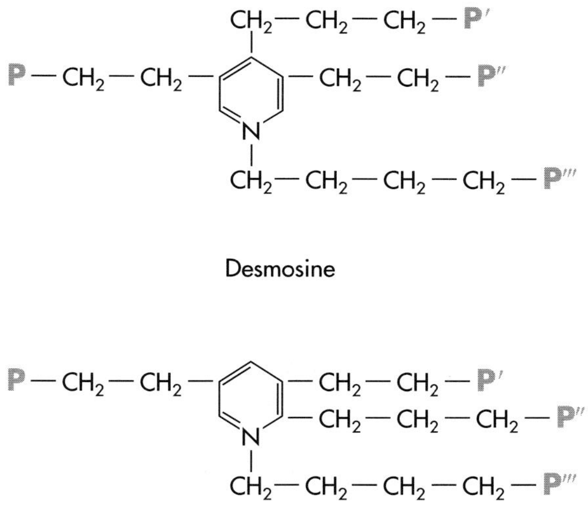

Desmosine

Isodesmosine

Fig. 3.21 Structures of desmosine and isodesmosine, possible tetrameric cross-links in elastin.

MICROFIBRILLAR PROTEINS

The microfibrillar component of elastic fibres is known to precede the deposition of elastin itself (Fahrenbach *et al.*, 1966; Shcwartz and Fleischmajer, 1986) and is presumed to be responsible for the alignment of soluble tropoelastin monomers prior to their incorporation into insoluble aggregates. Early work suggested that the microfibrillar component consisted of more than one protein type (Sear *et al.*, 1978) and subsequent studies have supported this (Cleary and Gibson, 1983; Cleary, 1987). The microfibrils formed by these proteins can occur independently from elastin in some tissues (e.g. PDL) and in this case they have been classified separately as oxytalan fibres (see below) (Fullmer and Lillie, 1958). Where bundles of microfibrils are found surrounded by an elastin matrix, they are classified as elauin fibres (Cotta-Pereira *et al.*, 1976).

Microfibrillar proteins are also extremely difficult to isolate and purify. They are highly insoluble, containing numerous disulphide cross-links, leading to difficulties in distinguishing between 'true' microfibrillar proteins and microfibril-associated proteins (Cleary and Gibson, 1983). In contrast to elastin, evidence points to the involvement of a number of different proteins and glycoproteins. Early studies by Sear *et al.* (1978) isolated a 150 KDa glycoprotein that was associated with elastic-microfibrils in bovine nuchal ligament and human skin (see below). However, this was later shown to be the α-chain of type VI collagen by Gibson *et al.*, (1986).

A 31 KDa microfibril-associated glycoprotein, rich in glutamic acid, proline and cysteine, was isolated by Gibson *et al.* (1986) from bovine nuchal ligament. Antibodies raised to this glycoprotein were used to immunolocalize the antigen to both the microfibrillar component of mature elastic fibres and to non-elastin-associated microfibrils in a range of tissues (Gibson and Cleary, 1987). Antibodies to this 31 K component also recognized at least two other microfibrillar proteins with molecular weights of 78 KDa and 340 KDa respectively. It was suggested that this larger, 340 KDa component might represent the major subunit of the microfibril, probably equivalent to the 350 KDa glycoprotein fibrillin described in human tissue (Sakai *et al.*, 1986).

MINOR FIBRES OF THE PERIODONTAL LIGAMENT

The elastic elements of the periodontium have been less well characterized than the collagen fibres. Most workers agree that the PDL appears to contain oxytalan fibres (Fullmer, 1959; Simpson, 1967; Sims, 1973; 1975). Early reports describing the presence of 'elastin' in PDL from some species probably relate to differences in nomenclature and to the presence of mature elastic fibres in gingival tissue and some vasculature. In a recent study re-evaluating the elastic fibre network in the PDL of the murine molar, Johnson and Pylypas (1992) confirmed the presence of oxytalan fibres but, in addition, showed that elauin also contributed significantly towards the elastic elements of the tissue.

Most of the studies carried out on elastic fibres of the PDL have used a histological approach (Fullmer, 1960; Sheetz *et al.*, 1973; Fullmer *et al.*, 1974; Edmunds *et al.*, 1979). However, much less is known about their biochemical characteristics and it has become clear that the range of fibres observed histologically represent variations on the two component theme described above.

Oxytalan fibres in the periodontal ligament

The most abundant elastic fibre described in the PDL is the oxytalan fibre (see Chapter 2). For many years it was known that these fibres, which tend to run axially (in contrast to the more obliquely oriented collagen fibres), stained with characteristic elastic stains only after oxidization of the tissue section. These fibres were first described by Fullmer and Lillie (1958) and were later proposed as immature or modified elastin fibres by Fullmer (1960). The staining properties described above, together with the size of these fibres (in the 10–16 nm range), suggested that the oxytalan fibre was analogous, perhaps identical, to the microfibrillar component of elastin (Sodek, 1978).

Sodek (1978) suggested that oxytalan fibres in the rat PDL were chemically related to the microfibrillar component of mature elastic fibres containing elastin (based on amino acid compositional data). The similarity in the compositions is shown in *Fig. 3.19*.

Shuttleworth and Smalley (1983) isolated a 140 K glycoprotein from bovine PDL which was also apparently produced by PDL fibroblasts *in vitro* (Smalley *et al.*, 1981). This 140 KDa component showed cross-reactivity with antisera raised to microfibrillar proteins (Kewley *et al.*, 1977). Immunohistochemistry revealed that the antisera recognized epitopes that are associated with major collagen fibrils and are found in proximity to elastic fibres. Other authors also described a glycoprotein of similar size found in extracts of human skin and bovine nuchal ligament (Sear *et al.*, 1981). Later work showed that this glycoprotein was in fact α-chains of type VI collagen (Gibson *et al.*, 1986). Type VI collagen is also a glycoprotein which forms microfibrils in an extensive network throughout the extracellular matrix of most soft connective tissues (Timpl and Engel, 1987) and the distribution pattern for this macromolecule would account for the confusion in earlier reports. Elastic fibres are considered further in Chapter 2.

SUMMARY

The major fibrous protein of the PDL is type I collagen, with type III collagen present in unusually high quantities (about 20 per cent of collagen present). Types IV, V, VI and XII have also been detected, albeit in much smaller amounts.

Periodontal ligament collagen is also unusual in its supermolecular arrangement, rapid assimilation into fibrils, absence of non-reducible cross-links with age and ratio of DHLNL:HLNL reducible cross-links compared with other soft connective tissues. These factors may all be related to the extremely rapid rate of collagen turnover in the ligament.

Collagen degradation is mediated by interstitial collagenases. Increased collagenase activity appears to be associated with chronic inflammatory periodontal disease and could be cytokine mediated.

The minor fibres of the PDL seem to comprise predominantly oxytalan, with some elauin but no mature elastic fibres, indicating an 'immature' or foetal-like connective tissue. Oxytalan fibres appear to be derived from microfibrillar proteins, which are as yet poorly characterized and probably arise from more than one gene product.

The biochemistry of the fibres of the collagen of the PDL suggests that this is an unusual connective tissue, with many foetal-like characteristics. This may be related to tissue function and may represent an important factor in the aetiology of chronic inflammatory periodontal disease.

ACKNOWLEDGEMENTS

The authors wish to thank the Agricultural and Food Research Council of Great Britain for their support of the work carried out at Leeds, and Mr Simon Strafford for his help with the illustrations.

REFERENCES

Bailey AJ and Peach CM (1968) Isolation and structural identification of a labile intermolecular crosslink in collagen. Biochem Biophys Res Comm 33, 812–819.

Bailey AJ, Robins SP and Balian G (1974) Biological significance of the intermolecular crosslinks of collagen. Nature 251, 105–109.

Bailey AJ and Shimokomaki MS (1971) Age-related changes in the reducible cross-links of collagen. FEBS Lett 16, 86–88.

Bauer EA, Cooper TW, Huang JS, Altman J and Deuel TF (1985) Stimulation of in vitro human skin collagenase expression by platelet-derived growth factor. Proc Natl Acad Sci USA 82, 4132–4136.

Becker J, Schuppan D, Rabanus JP, Reuch R, Niechoy U and Gelderblom HR (1990) Immunoelectron microscopic localisation of collagen type I, V, VI and of procollagen type III in human periodontal ligament and cementum. J Histochem Cytochem 39, 103–110.

Beertsen W and Everts V (1977) The site of remodelling of collagen in the periodontal ligament of the mouse incisor. Anat Rec 189, 479–498.

Beertsen W and van den Bos T (1992) The role of alkaline phosphatase in the mineralization of collagenous substrates. In: The Mechanisms of Tooth Movement and Craniofacial Adaptation (Ed Z Davidovitch), pp 181–185, Ohio State University, Columbia, Ohio.

Bellamy G and Bornstein P (1971) Evidence for procollagen, a biosynthetic precursor of collagen. Proc Natl Acad Sci USA 68, 1138–1142.

Berg RA and Prockop DJ (1973) The thermal transition of a non-hydroxylated form of collagen: Evidence for a role for hydroxyproline in stabilizing the triple helix of collagen. Biochem Biophys Res Comm 52, 115–120.

Berkovitz BKB (1990) Structure of the periodontal ligament. Eur J Orthod 12, 51–76.

Bernard MP, Chu ML, Myers JC, Ramirez F, Eikenberry EF and Prockop DJ (1983) Nucleotide sequences of complementary deoxyribonucleic acids for the pro-alpha I-chain of human type-I procollagen. Statistical evaluation of structures that are conserved during evaluation. Biochem 22, 5213–5223.

Bienowski RS, Cowan MJ, McDonald JA and Crystal RG (1978) Degradation of newly synthesised collagen. J Biol Chem 253, 4356–4363.

Birek P, Wang HM, Brunette DM and Melcher AH (1980) Epithelial rests of Malassez in vitro. Phagocytosis of collagen and the possible role of their lysosomal enzymes in collagen degradation. Lab Invest 43, 61–72.

Bock P and Stockinger L (1984) Light and electron microscopic identification of elastic, elaunin and oxytalan fibres in human tracheal and bronchial mucosa. Anat Embryol 170, 145–153.

Boedtker H, Fuller F and Tate V (1983) The structure of collagen genes. Int Rev Connect Tissue Res 10, 1–63.

Boyde A and Jones SJ (1968) Scanning electron microscopy of cementation and Sharpey fibre bone. Zeit Zellfersch Mikroscop Anat 92, 536–548.

Brodsky B, Eikenberry EF and Cassidy K (1980) An unusual collagen periodicity in skin. Biochim Biophys Acta 621, 162–166.

Burgeson RE, Wyke AW and Fessler JH (1972) Collagen synthesis by cells II: Secretion of a disulphide linked material. Biochem Biophys Res Comm 48, 892–897.

Burleigh MC (1977) Degradation of collagen by non-specific proteinases. In: Proteinases in Mammalian Cells and Tissues. (Barrett AJ, ed), pp 285–309, Elsevier, Amsterdam.

Butler WT, Birkedal-Hansen H, Beagle WF, Taylor RE and Chung E (1975) Proteins of the periodontium. Identification of collagen with the (1 (I)) 2 and (1 (III)) structures in the bovine periodontal ligament. J Biol Chem 250, 8907–8912.

Carneiro J and Fava de Moraes F (1965) Radiographic visualisation of collagen metabolism in the periodontal tissues of the mouse. Arch Oral Biol 10, 833–848.

Carneiro J and Leblond CP (1966) Suitability of collagenase treatment for the autoradiographic identification of newly synthesised collagen labelled with 3H-glycine or 3H-proline. J Histochem Cytochem 14, 334–344.

Christner P (1980) Collagenase in the human periodontal ligament. J Periodontol 51, 455–461.

Chu M and Prockop DJ (1993) Collagen: Gene structure. In: Connective Tissue and its Heritable Disorders (Royce PM and Steinmann B Eds), pp 149–165, Wiley–Liss, New York.

Clark SD, Kobayashi DK and Welgus HG (1987) Regulation of the expression of tissue inhibitor of metalloproteinases and collagenase by retinoids and glucocorticoids in human fibroblasts. J Clin Invest 80, 1280–1288.

Cleary EG (1987) The microfibrillar component of the elastic fibres. Morphology and biochemistry. In: Connective Tissue Disease. Molecular Pathology of the Extracellular Matrix (Uitto J and Perejda AJ, eds), pp 55–81, Marcel Dekker, New York.

Cleary EG and Gibson MA (1983) Elastin-associated microfibrils and microfibrillar proteins. Int Rev Connect Tissue Res 10, 97–207.

Cohn DH, Apone S, Eyre DR, *et al.* (1988) Substitution of cysteine for glycine within the carboxyl-terminal telopeptide of the 1 chain of type I collagen produces mild osteogenesis imperfecta. J Biol Chem 263, 14605–14607.

Cotta-Pereira G, Guerra Rodrigo F and Bittencourt-Sampaio S (1976) Oxytalan, elaunin and elastic fibres in the human skin. J Invest Derm 66, 143–148.

Cotta-Pereira G, Guerra Rodrigo F and David-Ferreira JF (1977) The elastic system fibres. In: Elastin and Elastic Tissue (Sandberg LB, Gray WR and Franzblau C Eds), pp 19–30, Plenum Press, New York.

Cronlund AL, Smith BD and Kagan HM (1985) Binding of lysyl oxidase to fibrils of type I collagen. Connect Tissue Res 14, 109–119.

Crumley PJ (1964) Collagen formation in the normal and stressed periodontium. Periodontics 2, 53–61.

Dayer JM, Beutler B and Cerami A (1985) Cachectin/tumor necrosis factor stimulates collagenase and prostaglandin E2 production by human synovial cells and dermal fibroblasts. J Exp Med 162, 2163–2168.

Deak SB, Scholz PM, Amenta PS, *et al.* (1991) The substitution of arginine for glycine 85 of the 1(I) procollagen chain results in mild osteogenesis imperfecta. J Biol Chem 266, 21827–21832.

Dublet B, de Miguel E and van der Rest M (1987) Type IX and type XII collagens: A new class of extracellular matrix components. In: Protides of the Biological Fluids (Peeters H, ed), pp 411–414, Pergamon Press, Oxford.

Dublet B, Dixon E, de Miguel E and van der Rest M (1988) Bovine type XII collagen: Amino acid sequence of a 10 kDa pepsin fragment from periodontal ligament reveals a high degree of homology with the chicken I(XII) sequence. FEBS Lett 233, 177–180.

Edmunds RS, Simmons TA, Cox CF and Avery JK (1979) Light and ultrastructural relationship between oxytalan fibres in the periodontal ligament of the guinea pig. J Oral Path 8, 109–120.

Edwards DR, Murphy G, Reynolds JJ, *et al.* (1987) Transforming growth factor beta modulates the expression of collagenase and metalloproteinase inhibitor. EMBO J 6, 1899–1904.

Epstein EHJR (1974) Human skin collagen. Release by pepsin digestion and preponderance in foetal life. J Biol Chem 249, 3225–3231.

Everts V and Beertsen W (1992) Collagen phagocytosis in periodontal remodelling. In: The Biological Mechanisms of Tooth Movement (Davidovitch Z, ed), pp 29–36, Ohio State University, Colombus, Ohio.

Eyre DR (1987) Collagen cross-linking amino acids. Methods Enzymol 144, 115–139.

Eyre DR, Dickson IR and van Ness K (1988) Collagen cross-linking in human bone and articular cartilage. Age-related changes in the content of mature hydroxypyridinium residues. Biochem J 252, 495–500.

Eyre DR, Paz MA and Gallop PM (1984) Cross-linking in collagen and elastin. Annu Rev Biochem 53, 717–748.

Fahrenbach WH, Sandberg LB and Cleary EG (1966) Ultrastructural studies on early elastogenesis. Anat Rec 155, 563–575.

Fessler I, Timpl R and Fessler JH (1981) Assembly and processing of procollagen type III in chick embryo blood vessels. J Biol Chem 256, 2531–2537.

Fessler JH and Smith LA (1970) Collagen synthesis by cells in culture. In: Chemistry and Molecular Biology of the Intercellular Matrix (Balarzis EA, ed), p 411, Academic Press, New York.

Fietzek PP and Kuhn K (1976) The primary structure of collagen. Int Rev Connect Tissue Res 7, 1–60.

Forster SJ and Freedman RB (1984) Catalysis by protein disulphide-isomerase of the assembly of trimeric procollagen from procollagen polypeptide chains. Biosci Rep 4, 223–229.

Freedman RB and Hillson DA (1980) Formation of disulphide bonds. In: The Enzymology and Post-translational Modification of Proteins (Freedman RB and Hawkins HC, eds), pp 157–212, Academic Press, London.

Fujimoto D, Moriguchi T, Ishida T and Hayashi H (1978) The structure of pyridinoline, a collagen crosslink. Biochem Biophys Res Comm 84, 52–57.

Fullmer HM (1959) Observations on the development of oxytalan fibres in the periodontium of man. J Dent Res 38, 510–516.

Fullmer HM (1960) A comparitive histochemical study of elastic, pre-elastic and oxytalan connective tissue fibres. J Histochem Cytochem 8, 290–295.

Fullmer HM and Lillie RD (1958) The oxytalain fiber: a previously undescribed connective tissue fiber. J Histochem Cytochem 6, 425–430.

Fullmer HM, Sheetz JH and Narkates AJ (1974) Oxytalan connective tissue fibres: A review. J Oral Path 3, 291–316.

Garant PR (1976) Collagen resorption by fibroblasts. J Periodontol 47, 380–390.

Gathercole LJ, Porter S and Scully C (1987) Axial periodicity in periodontal collagens. Human periodontal ligament and gingival connective tissue collagen fibres possess a dermis-like D-period. J Periodont Res 22, 408–411.

Gay S, Martin GR, Muller PK, Timpl R and Kuhn K (1976) Simultaneous synthesis of types I and III collagen by fibroblasts in culture. Proc Natl Acad Sci USA 73, 4037–4040.

Gibson MA and Cleary EG (1987) The immunohistological localisation of microfibril-associated glycoprotein (MAGP) in elastic and non-elastic tissues. Immun Cell Biol 65, 345–356.

Gibson MA, Hughes JL, Fanning JC and Cleary EG (1986) The major antigen of elastin-associated microfibrils is a 31-KDa glycoprotein. J Biol Chem 261, 11429–11436.

Glimcher MJ (1989) Mechanism of collagen calcification: Role of collagen fibrils and collagen-phosphoprotein complexes in vitro and in vivo. Anat Rec 224, 139–153.

Goldberg B, Epstein EH and Sherr CJ (1972) Precursors of collagen secreted by cultured human fibroblasts. Proc Natl Acad Sci USA 69, 3655–3659.

Gowen M, Wood DD, Ihrie EJ, Meats JE and Russell RGG (1984) Stimulation by human interleukin 1 of cartilage breakdown and production of collagenase and proteoglycanase by human chondrocytes but not by human osteoblasts in vitro. Biochim Biophys Acta 797, 186–193.

Guis MB and Slootweg RN (1973) A biochemical study of collagen in the periodontal ligament from erupting and non-erupting bovine incisors. Arch Oral Biol 18, 253–263.

Harris ED (1976) Copper-induced activation of aortic lysyl oxidase in vivo. Proc Natl Acad Sci USA 73, 371–374.

Heath JK, Gowen M, Meikle MC and Reynolds JJ (1982) Human gingival tissues in culture synthesise three metalloproteinases and a metalloproteinase inhibitor. J Periodont Res 17, 183–190.

Heinegard D and Oldberg A (1993) Glycosylated Matrix Proteins. In: Connective Tissue and its Heritable Disorders (Royce PM and Steinmann B, eds), pp 189–209, Wiley–Liss inc., New York.

Highberger JH, Corbett C and Gross J (1979) Isolation and characterisation of a peptide containing the site of cleavage of the chick skin collagen 1(I) chain by animal collagenases. Biochem Biophys Res Comm 89, 202–208.

Hunt AM and Paynter KJ (1959) The effects of ascorbic acid deficiency in the teeth and periodontal tissues of guinea pigs. J Dent Res 38, 232–243.

Imberman M, Ramamurthy N, Golub L and Schneir M (1986) A reassessment of collagen half-life in rat periodontal tissues: Application of the pool-expansion approach. J Periodont Res 21, 396–402.

Johnson RB and Pylypas SP (1992) A re-evaluation of the distribution of the elastic meshwork within the periodontal ligament of the mouse. J Periodont Res 27, 239–249.

Kanoza RJJ, Kelleher L, Sodek J and Melcher AH (1980) A biochemical analysis of the effect of hypofunction on collagen metabolism in the rat molar periodontal ligament. Arch Oral Biol 25, 663–668.

Karimbux NY, Rosenblum ND and Nishimura I (1992) Site-specific expression of collagen I and XII mRNAs in the rat periodontal ligament at two developmental stages. J Dent Res 71, 1355–1362.

Kewley MA, Steven FS and Williams G (1977) Preparation of specific antiserum towards the microfibrillar protein of elastic tissues. Immunology 32, 483–489.

Kielty CM, Hopkinson I and Grant M (1993) The collagen family: structure, assembly and organization in the extracellular matrix. In: Connective Tissue and its Heritable Disorders (Royce PM and Steinmann B, eds), pp 103–147, Wiley–Liss inc., New York.

Kirk TZ, Evans JS and Veis A (1987) Biosynthesis of type I procollagen. Characterisation of the distribution of chain sizes and extent of hydroxylation of polysome-associated pro-alpha-chains. J Biol Chem 262, 5540–5545.

Kirkham J, Robinson C and Shore RC (1991b) Rates of protein turnover at specific sites of the rat incisor periodontal ligament. J Biol Buccale 19, 61–67.

Kirkham J, Robinson C and Spence J (1989) Site-specific variations in the composition of healthy sheep periodontia. Arch Oral Biol 34, 405–411.

Kirkham J, Robinson C and Spence J (1991a) Effect of periodontal disease ('broken mouth') on the distribution of matrix macromolecules in the sheep periodontium. Arch Oral Biol 36, 257–263.

Kirkham J, Robinson C and Spence J (1992) The effect of periodontal disease on GAG distribution in the sheep periodontium. Arch Oral Biol 37, 1031–1037.

Kirkham J, Shore RC and Robinson C (1993) Effect of glycosylaminoglycan removal on mineralisation of periodontal ligament in vitro. J Dent Res 72, 713 (Abstract 209).

Kivirikko KI and Myllyla R (1979) Collagen glycosyltransferases. Int Rev Connect Tissue Res 8, 23–72.

Kivirikko KI and Myllyla R (1980) Hydroxylation of prolyl and lysyl residues. In: The Enzymology of Post-translational Modification of Proteins (Freedman RB and Hawkins HC, eds), pp 53–104, Academic Press, London.

Kivirikko KI and Myllyla R (1982a) Post-translational modifications. In: Collagen in Health and Disease (Weiss JB and Jayson MJV, eds), pp 101–120, Churchill Livingstone, Edinburgh.

Kivirikko KI and Myllyla R (1982b) Post-translational enzymes in the biosynthesis of collagen. Intracellular enzymes. Methods Enzymol 82, 245–304.

Kivirikko KI and Myllyla R (1985) Post-translational processing of procollagens. Ann NY Acad Sci 460, 187–201.

Kuboki Y, Takagi T, Sasaki S, Saito S and Mechanic GL (1981) Comparative collagen biochemistry of bovine periodontium, gingiva and dental pulp. J Dent Res 60, 159–163.

Kuhn K (1986) The collagen family – variations in the molecular and supramolecular structure. Rheumatology 10, 29–69.

Larivee J, Sodek J and Ferrier JM (1986) Collagenase and collagenase inhibitor activities in crevicular fluid of patients receiving treatment for localised juvenile periodontitis. J Periodont Res 21, 702–715.

Last JA, Armstrong LG and Reiser KM (1990) Biosynthesis of collagen crosslinks. Int J Biochem 22, 559–564.

Light ND and Bailey AJ (1980) The chemistry of collagen cross-links. Purification and characterisation of crosslinked polymeric peptide material from mature collagen containing unknown amino acids. Biochem J 185, 323–381.

Light ND and Bailey AJ (1982) Covalent cross-links in collagen. In: Methods in Enzymology (Cunningham LW and Frederiksen DW, eds), pp 360–372, Academic Press, London.

Limeback HF and Sodek J (1979) Procollagen synthesis and processing in periodontal ligament in vivo and in vitro. Eur J Biochem 100, 541–550.

Limeback HF, Sodek J and Aubin JE (1983) Variation in collagen expression by cloned periodontal ligament cells. J Periodont Res 18, 242–248.

Limeback HF, Sodek J and Brunette DM (1978) Nature of collagens synthesised by monkey periodontal ligament fibroblasts in vitro. Biochem J 170, 63–71.

Lukinmaa PL and Waltimo J (1992) Immunohistochemical localisation of types I, V, and VI collagen in human permanent teeth and periodontal ligament. J Dent Res 71, 391–397.

Maciewicz RA, Etherington DJ, Kos J and Turk V (1987) Collagenolytic cathepsins of rabbit spleen: A kinetic analysis of collagen degradation and inhibition by chicken cystatin. Coll Rel Res 7, 295–304.

Martin GR, Byers PH and Piez KA (1975) Procollagen. Adv Enzymol 42, 167–191.

Masuda M, Karube S, Hayashi Y, Shindo H and Igarashi M (1976) Direct measurement of collagen crosslinks with automatic amino acid analyser – identification of peaks due to crosslinks. FEBS Lett 63, 245–249.

Mechanic G and Tanzer ML (1970) Biochemistry of collagen crosslinking: isolation of a new crosslink, hydroxylysinohydroxynorleucine, and its reduced precursor, dihydroxynorleucine, fron bovine tendon. Biochem Biophys Res Comm 41, 1597–1604.

Mechanic GL, Kuboki Y, Shimokawa H, Nakamoto K, Sasaki S and Kawanishi Y (1974) Collagen cross-links: direct quantitative determination of stable structural cross-links in bone and dentine collagens. Biophys Res Comm 60, 756–763.

Mechanic GL, Tanzer ML and Gallop PM (1971) The nature of cross-links in collagen from mineralised tissues. Biophys Res Comm 45, 644–653.

Meikle MC, Atkinson SJ, Ward RV, Murphy G and Reynolds JJ (1989) Gingival fibroblasts degrade type I collagen films when stimulated with tumour necrosis factor and interleukin 1: Evidence that breakdown is mediated by metalloproteinases. J Periodont Res 24, 207–213.

Meikle MC, Heath JK and Reynolds JJ (1986) Advances in understanding cell interactions in tissue resorption. Relevance of the pathogenesis of periodontal diseases and a new hypothesis. J Oral Path 15, 239–250.

Miller EJ and Gay S (1982) Collagen: An overview. Methods Enzymol 82, 3–32.

Miller EJ and Gay S (1987) The collagens: An overview and update. Methods Enzymol 144, 3–41.

Moriguchi T and Fujimoto D (1978) Age-related changes in the content of the collagen cross-link. J Biochem 84, 933–935.

Morris ML and Harper E (1987) The presence of an inhibitor of human skin collagenase in the roots of healthy and periodontally diseased teeth. J Periodont Res 22, 78–80.

Moxham BJ (1985) Studies on the mechanical properties of the periodontal ligament. In: Current Topics in Oral Biology (Lisney SJW and Mathews B, eds), pp 73–82, University of Bristol Press, Bristol.

Murphy G and Docherty AJP (1988) Molecular studies on the connective tissue metalloproteinases and their inhibitor TIMP. In: The Control of Tissue Damage (Glauert AM, ed), pp 223–241, Elsevier, Amsterdam.

Murphy G and Reynolds JJ (1993) Extracellular matrix degradation.In: Connective Tissue and its Heritable Disorders (Royce PM and Steinmann B, eds), pp 287–316, Wiley–Liss inc., New York.

Myllyla R, Majamaa K, Gunzler V, Hanauske-Abel HM and Kivirikko KI (1984) Ascorbate is consumed stoichiometrically in the uncoupled reactions catalysed by prolyl 4-hydroxylase and lysyl hydroxylase. J Biol Chem 259, 5403–5405.

Nakano T and Scott PG (1987) Postpartum changes and certain properties of the proteolytic activity from involuting rat uterus that degrades the C-telopeptide of type I collagen. Biomed Res 8, 359–367.

Orlowski WA (1976) The incorporation of H3-proline into the collagen of the periodontium of a rat. J Periodont Res 11, 96–100.

Orlowski WA (1978) Biochemical study of collagen turnover in rat incisor periodontal ligament. Arch Oral Biol 23, 1163–1165.

Overall CM, Wiebken OW and Thonard JC (1987) Demonstration of tissue collagenase activity in vivo and its relationship to inflammation severity in human gingiva. J Periodont Res 22, 81–88.

Page RC and Ammons WF (1974) Collagen turnover in the gingiva and other mature connective tissues of the marmoset *Saguinus oedipus*. Arch Oral Biol 19, 651–658.

Partridge SM (1962) Elastin. Adv Protein Chem 17, 227–302.

Paz MA, Keith DA and Gallop PM (1982) Elastin isolation and cross-linking. Methods Enzymol 82, 571–578.

Pearson CH, Wohllebe M, Carmichael DJ and Chovelon A (1975) Bovine periodontal ligament. An investigation of the collagen, glycosylaminoglycan and insoluble glycoprotein components at different stages of tissue development. Connect Tissue Res 3, 195–206.

Phadke K (1987) Fibroblast growth factor enhances the interleukin-1-mediated chondrocytic protease release. Biochem Biophys Res Comm 142, 448–453.

Pinnell SR and Martin GR (1968) The cross-linking of collagen and elastin: enzymic conversion of lysine in peptide linkage to α-aminoadipic-δ-semialdehyde (allysine) by an extract from bone. Proc Natl Acad Sci U S A 61, 708–716.

Poole B (1971) The kinetics of the disappearance of labelled leucine from the free leucine pool of rat liver and its effects on the apparent turnover of catalase and other hepatic proteins. J Biol Chem 246, 6587–6591.

Prockop DJ, Berg RA, Kivirikko KI and Uitto J (1976) Intracellular steps in the biosynthesis of collagen. In: Biochemistry of Collagen (Ramachandran GN and Reddi AH, eds), pp 163–273, Plenum Press, New York.

Pruchno CJ, Cohn DH, Wallis GA, Willing MC, Starman BJ, Zhang X and Byers PH (1991) Osteogenesis imperfecta due to recurrent point mutations at CpG dinucleotides in the COLIAI gene of type I collagen. Hum Genet 87, 33–40.

Quigley MB (1970) Perforating (Sharpey's) fibres of the periodontal ligament and bone. Ala J Med Sci 7, 336–342.

Ramachandran GN (1967) Structure of collagen at the molecular level. In: Treatise on Collagen (Ramachandran GN, ed), pp 103–183, Academic Press, New York.

Ramachandran GN and Kartha G (1954) Structure of Collagen. Nature 174, 269–270.

Ramachandran GN and Ramakrishnan C (1976) Molecular Structure. In: Biochemistry of Collagen (Ramachandran GN and Ramakrishnan C, eds), pp 45–84.

Ranta H (1978) Age-related changes in collagen cross-linking. Changes in bovine dentine and periodontal ligament and description of a new type of non-reducible cross-link. Proc Finn Dent Soc 74, 3–64.

Rippin JW (1976) Collagen turnover in the periodontal ligament under normal and altered functional forces. I. Young rat molars. J Periodont Res 11, 101–107.

Rippin JW (1978) Collagen turnover in the periodontal ligament under normal and altered functional forces. II. Adult rat molars. J Periodont Res 13, 149–154.

Robins SP, Shimokomaki M and Bailey AJ (1973) The chemistry of collagen cross-links. Age-related changes in the reducible components of intact collagen fibres. Biochem J 131, 771–780.

Romanos GE, Schroter-Kermani C, Hinz N, Wachtel HC and Bernimoulin J-P (1991) Immunohistochemical localisation of collagenous components in healthy periodontal tissues of the rat and marmoset (Callithrix jacchus). II. Distribution of collagen types IV, V and VI. J Periodont Res 26, 323–332.

Rosenbloom J (1993) Elastin. In: Connective Tissue and its Heritable Disorders (Royce PM and Steinmann B, eds), pp 167–188, Wiley–Liss, Inc., New York.

Rosenbloom J, Harsch M and Jiminez S (1973) Hydroxyproline content determines the denaturation temperature of chick tendon cartilage. Arch Biochem Biophys 158, 478–484.

Ross R and Bornstein P (1969) The elastic fibre. I. The separation and partial characterisation of its macromolecular components. J Cell Biol 40, 366–381.

Sage H and Gray WR (1979) Studies on the evolution of elastin. I. Phylogenetic distribution. Compend Biochem Phys 64, 313–327.

Sakai LY, Keene DR and Engvall E (1986) Fibrillin, a new 350-kD glycoprotein, is a component of extracellular microfibrils. J Cell Biol 103, 2499–2509.

Sandberg LB, Weissman N and Gray WR (1971) Structural features of tropoelastin related to the sites of cross-links in aortic elastin. Biochem 10, 52–56.

Sandberg LB, Weissman N and Smith DW (1969) The purification and partial characterisation of a soluble elastin-like protein from copper-deficient porcine aorta. Biochem 8, 2940–2945.

Sandell LJ, Prentice HL, Kravis D and Upholt WB (1984) Structure and sequence of the chicken type II procollagen gene. Characterisation of the region encoding the carboxyl-terminal teleopeptide and propeptide. J Biol Chem 259, 7826–7834.

Sandholm L (1986) Proteases and their inhibitors in chronic inflammatory periodontal disease. J Clin Invest 13, 19–26.

Schmitt FO (1960) Contributions of molecular biology to medicine. pp 725–749, Academic Medicine, New York.

Schofield JD and Prockop DJ (1973) Procollagen – a precursor form of collagen. Clin Orthops 97, 175–195.

Schwartz E and Fleischmajer R (1986) Association of elastin with oxytalan fibres of the dermis and with extracellular microfibrils of cultured skin fibroblasts. J Histochem Cytochem 34, 1063–1068.

Scott JE (1984) The periphery of the developing collagen fibril. Biochem J 218, 229–233.

Sear CHJ, Grant ME and Jackson DS (1981) The nature of the microfibrillar glycoproteins of elastin fibres. Biochem J 194, 587–598.

Sear CHJ, Kewley MA, Jones CJP, Grant ME and Jackson DS (1978) The identification of glycoproteins associated with elastic-tissue microfibrils. Biochem J 170, 715–718.

Selvig K (1965) The fine structure of human cementum. Acta Odont Scand 23, 423–441.

Shackleford JM (1971) Scanning electron microscopy of the dog periodontium. J Periodont Res 6, 45–54.

Sheetz JH, Fullmer HM and Narkates AJ (1973) Oxytalan fibres: Identification of the same fibre by light and electron microscopy. J Oral Path 2, 254–263.

Shore RC and Berkovitz BKB (1979) An ultrastructural study of periodontal ligament fibroblasts in relation to their possible role in tooth eruption and intracellular collagen degradation in the rat. Arch Oral Biol 24, 155–164.

Shuttleworth CA and Smalley JW (1983) Periodontal Ligament. Int Rev Connect Tissue Res 10, 211–247.

Simpson HE (1967) A three dimensional approach to the microscopy of the periodontal membrane. Proc R Soc Med 60, 537–542.

Sims MR (1973) Oxytalan fibres of molars in the mouse mandible. J Dent Res 52, 797–803.

Sims MR (1975) Oxytalan-vascular relationships observed in histological examination of the periodontal ligaments of man and mouse. Arch Oral Biol 20, 713–717.

Skougaard MR, Frandsen A and Baker DG (1970) Collagen metabolism of skin and periodontal membrane in the squirrel monkey. Scand J Dent Res 78, 374–377.

Skougaard MR and Levy BM (1971) Collagen metabolism in periodontal membrane of the marmoset, influence of periodontal disease. Scand J Dent Res 79, 518–522.

Smalley JW, Grant ME, Wilson NHF and Shuttleworth CA (1981) Non-collagenous proteins of periodontal ligament. J Dent Res 60, Abs. 179.

Smith AJ (1992) A Biochemical Investigation of the Sheep Periodontium PhD thesis, University of Leeds.

Smith DW, Sandberg LB, Leslie BH, Wolt TB, Minton ST, Myers B and Rucker RB (1981) Primary structure of a chick tropoelastin peptide: Evidence for a collagen-like amino acid sequence. Biochem Biophys Res Commun 103, 880–885.

Sodek J (1976) A new approach to assessing collagen turnover by using a micro-assay. A highly efficient and rapid turnover of collagen in the rat periodontal tissues. Biochem J 160, 243–246.

Sodek J (1977) A comparison of the rates of synthesis and turnover of collagen and non-collagen proteins in the adult rat periodontal tissues and skin using a microassay. Arch Oral Biol 22, 655–665.

Sodek J (1978) A comparison of collagen and non-collagenous protein metabolism in rat molar and incisor periodontal ligaments. Arch Oral Biol 23, 977–982.

Sodek J (1989) Collagen turnover in periodontal ligament. In: The Biology of Tooth Movement (Norton LA and Burstone CJ, eds), pp 157–181, CRC Press, Boca Raton.

Sodek J and Ferrier JM (1988) Collagen remodelling in rat periodontal tissues: Compensation for precursor reutilization confirms rapid turnover of collagen. Coll Rel Res 1, 11–21.

Sodek J and Limeback HF (1979) Comparison of rates of synthesis, conversion and maturation of type I and type III collagens in rat periodontal tissues. J Biol Chem 254, 10496–10502.

Stallard R (1963) The utilisation of 3H-proline by the connective tissue elements of the periodontium. Periodontics 1, 185–188.

Starcher BC and Galione MJ (1976) Purification and comparision of elastins from different animal species. Anal Biochem 74, 441–447.

Starkey PM, Barrett AJ and Burleigh MC (1977) The degradation of articular collagen by neutrophil proteinases. Biochim Biophys Acta 483, 386–397.

Tanzer ML (1976) Crosslinking. In: Biochemistry of Collagen. (Ramachandran GA and Reddi AH, eds), pp 137–162, Plenum Press, New York.

Tanzer ML, Housley T, Berube L, Fairweather R, Franzblau C and Gallop PM (1973) Structure of two histidine-containing cross-links from collagen. J Biol Chem 248, 393–402.

Ten Cate AR and Deporter DA (1975) The degradative role of the fibroblast in the remodelling and turnover of collagen in soft connective tissue. Anat Rec 182, 1–14.

Timpl R and Engel J (1987) Type VI collagen. In: Structure and Function of Collagen Types (Mayne R and Burgeson RE, eds), pp 105–143, Academic Press, Orlando.

Torchia DA and Piez KA (1973) Mobility of elastin chains as determined by 13C nuclear-magnetic resonance. J Mol Biol 76, 419–424.

Traub W and Piez KA (1971) The chemistry and structure of collagen. Adv Protein Chem 25, 243–352.

Trelstad RL and Slavkin HG (1974) Collagen synthesis by the epithelial enamel organ of the embryonic rabbit tooth. Biochem Biophys Res Comm 59, 443–449.

Uitto J, Hoffman HP and Prockop DJ (1976) Synthesis of elastin and procollagen by cells from the embryonic aorta. Differences in the role of hydroxyproline and the effects of proline analogs on the secretion of the two proteins. Arch Biochem Biophys 173, 187–200.

Van den Bos T and Tonino GJM (1984) Composition and metabolism of the extracellular matrix in the periodontal ligament of impeded rat incisors. Arch Oral Biol 29, 893–897.

Veis A and Payne K (1988) Collagen fibrillogenesis. In: Collagen: Biochemistry (Nimni ME, ed), pp 113–137, CRC Press, Boca Raton, Fl.

Villella B, Cogen RB, Bartolucci AA and Birkedal-Hansen H (1987) Collagenolytic activity in crevicular fluid from patients with chronic adult periodontitis, localised juvenile periodontitis and gingivitis, and from healthy control subjects. J Periodont Res 22, 381–389.

Wang HM (1982) Detection of lysosomal enzymes derived from pig periodontal fibroblasts and their ability to digest collagen fibrils and proteoglycan. Arch Oral Biol 27, 715–720.

Weiner S and Traub W (1986) Organization of hydroxyapatite crystals within collagen fibrils. FEBS Lett 206, 262–266.

Weiner S and Traub W (1992) Bone structure: from angstroms to microns. FASEB J 6, 879–885.

Welgus HG, Jeffery JJ, Eisen AZ, Roswitt WT and Stricklin GP (1985) Human skin fibroblast collagnase: interaction with substrate and inhibitor. Coll Rel Res 5, 167–169.

Wiestner M, Krieg T, Horlein D, Glanville RW, Fietzek P and Muller PK (1979) Inhibiting effect of procollagen peptides on collagen biosynthesis in fibroblast cultures. J Biol Chem 254, 7016–7023.

Wu CH, Donovan CB and Wu GY (1986) Evidence for pre-translational regulation of collagen synthesis by procollagen propeptides. J Biol Chem 261, 10482–10484.

Yamada Y, Mudryj M and de Crombrugghe B (1983) A uniquely conserved regulatory signal is found around the translation initiation site in three different collagen genes. J Biol Chem 258, 14914–14919.

Yamashita Y, Sato M and Noguchi T (1987) Alkaline phosphatase in the periodontal ligament of the rabbit and macaque monkey. Arch Oral Biol 32, 677–678.

Yamauchi M, Katz EP and Mechanic GL (1986) Intermolecular cross-linking and stereospecific molecular packing in type I collagen fibrils of the periodontal ligament. Biochem 25, 4907–4913.

Chapter 4
The Ground Substance of the Periodontal Ligament

G Embery, RJ Waddington, RC Hall

INTRODUCTION

The ground substance, along with the other extracellular matrix components of connective tissues, is synthesized by cells of the fibroblast family. In oral tissues, this includes periodontal ligament and gingival fibroblasts, osteoblasts, cementoblasts, and odontoblasts. Much of our knowledge of the biology of the periodontal ligament (PDL) derives from the studies of the extracellular matrices of more accessible tissues such as cartilage, skin, and bone. Although studies on the PDL have not received the same attention, data emerging from the relatively few workers in this area are now beginning to unravel the chemical–structural aspects of the PDL that help to explain its unique anatomical position and physiological function.

In common with all connective tissues, the ground substance of PDL can be described as a gel-like matrix in which are embedded the cellular and fibrous components, such as collagen. Broadly speaking, two types of glycoconjugates, namely glycoproteins and proteoglycans, together with hyaluronan, form the major constituents of the ground substance. This classification encompasses a wide range of compounds, each of which appear specific in its distribution and occurrence. Likewise, glycoconjugates within the ground substance exhibit very varied biological functions, which are of importance in maintaining the structural integrity of the tissue.

PROTEOGLYCANS

Without doubt, the bulk of investigations of the chemistry of the ground substance has centred on the proteoglycans. The combination of more sensitive extraction and analytical techniques and the application of molecular biology has led to a vast increase in knowledge of these macrosubstances.

CORE PROTEINS

In essence, proteoglycans (PG) are composed of specific core proteins to which one or more glycosaminoglycan (GAG) chains are covalently attached via a specific sequence, usually the trisaccharide galactose–galactose–xylose. Perhaps the main PG studied is aggrecan, which is a member of the class of secretory aggregating PG and is found in cartilage (Wight *et al.*, 1991).

Advances in molecular biology have permitted the defining of amino acid sequence for at least six PG core proteins. They range widely in molecular size. The smallest is 20 kDa – this is known as serglycin owing to its complement of 24 consecutive serine–glycine repeats (Bourdon *et al.*, 1985). It is located in storage granules of mast cells.

Another PG is decorin, with a core protein size of 36 kDa and so named because it 'decorates' collagen fibrils (Krusius and Ruoslahti, 1986). It is present in a wide range of tissues and is characterized by leucine-rich sequences that interact with the fibrillar collagens of many connective tissues.

The syndecan family of PG are named from the Greek *syndein*, 'to bind together', and have core proteins in the order of 32kDa; these core proteins contain a COOH-terminal cytoplasmic domain, a hydrophobic domain that connects the plasma membrane, and an extracellular domain that bears the GAG chains (Gallagher and Lyon, 1989).

Versican, another aggregating PG that, like aggrecan, interacts with hyaluronic acid, is present in human fibroblasts and has a core protein of 260 kDa. It shows sequence homology with aggrecan in its -NH_2 terminal G1 and -COOH terminal G3 domains, but it is clearly a different gene product since versican lacks a G2 domain and thus differs in the region where chondroitin sulphate chains attach.

An up-to-date list of the classification of the range of PG obtained from a wide range of connective tissues is given in *Table 4.1*. It is now apparent that there is no model structure for PG other than an association between GAG and core proteins. With the exception of heparin and hyaluronic acid, the linkage is at the GAG-reducing end via a seryl O-glycosidic linkage (chondroitin sulphate, dermatan sulphate, or heparan sulphate) or via an N-linkage to asparagine (typified by keratan sulphate). A list of the diagrammatic structures of selected PG is shown in *Fig. 4.1*.

In addition to GAG chains, oligosaccharides are associated with the core protein, which has made protein sequencing difficult unless detailed purification techniques are applied. In the large aggregating PG, the oligosaccharides feature as link glycoproteins and are involved in aggregation and disaggregation phenomena.

GLYCOSAMINOGLYCANS

Although the primary characteristics of PG reside in the core protein sequences, the GAG still remain the main structural determinants and an accessible means by which identification and classification may be achieved. GAG are linear polymers of disaccharide repeat sequences, which contain a hexosamine (usually D-N-acetylglucosamine or D-N-acetylgalactosamine) and

Table 4.1 Classification and structural–biological properties of proteoglycans

Name	Number of glycosaminoglycans	Type	Core protein Mr (kDa)	Tissue
Large aggregating proteoglycans				
Aggrecan	100	CS	208–221	Cartilage
	20–30	KS	265	Fibroblasts
Versican	12–15	CS		
Non-aggregating proteoglycans				
Biglycan	2	CS/DS	38–45	Connective tissue cells
Decorin	1	CS/DS	36–45	Connective tissue cells
Fibromodulin	1	KS	42	Connective tissue cells
Cell surface proteoglycans				
Syndecan	1–3	CS	31	Epithelia
	1–2	HS	82–88	Fibroblasts
Fibroglycan	2–4	HS	49–90	Fibroblasts
Glypican	3–4	HS	62	Epithelia
CD 44	?	CS or HS	?	Lymphocytes
Basement membrane proteoglycan				
Perlecan	2–15	HS	400	Basement membrane
Intracellular proteoglycan				
Serglycin	10–15	CS/DS/HS/ heparin	10–19	Myeloid cells

D-N-sulphoamidoglucosamine in heparin or heparan sulphate, and a hexuronic acid, either D-glucuronic acid or D-iduronic acid. With the exception of hyaluronic acid, the GAG are sulphated and covalently attached to the core protein at the reducing terminus.

Chondroitin sulphates are composed of D-glucuronic acid and D-N-acetylgalactosamine linked by alternating 1–3 and 1–4 glycosidic bonds. Ester sulphate is present on either the C4 or C6 of the N-acetylgalactosamine residues. Both undersulphated and oversulphated isomers have been identified. Such compounds are strictly galactosaminoglycuronoglycans, and they share structural properties with dermatan sulphate, which is a galactosaminoiduronoglycan since a large proportion of uronic residues are represented by the C5 epimer L-iduronic acid. Dermatan sulphate has much in common with chondroitin-4-sulphate, as it bears a 4-sulphated moiety on the D-N-acetylgalactosamine residue. Sulphate groups have also been identified on the C6 of the galactosamine and on the uronic acid residues (Fransson *et al.*, 1974).

Heparan sulphate and heparin contain disaccharide sequences consisting of N-acetylglucosamine and a hexuronic acid, which may be D-glucuronic acid or L-iduronic acid. The most important characteristic of these compounds is, however, the variable presence of N-sulphated glucosamine residues. D-glucuronic acid predominates in heparan sulphate, whereas L-iduronic features more so in heparin. Variable degrees of 0-sulphation are also found, including C-2 on iduronic acid, and C-6 and C-3 on glucosamine; there is a high degree of α-glycosidic linkage.

Hyaluronic acid, currently termed hyaluronan, is a non-sulphated GAG. It has the highest Mr value of all GAG (106 kDa), and it is composed of N-acetylglucosamine and D-glucuronic acid. It is not strictly a PG since its synthetic assembly is independent of a core protein, although its association with protein in a large molecular-size secretory PG, such as aggrecan, place it in the PG series.

Although not detected in periodontal tissues (with the exception of the bone of various species – Waddington, Embery

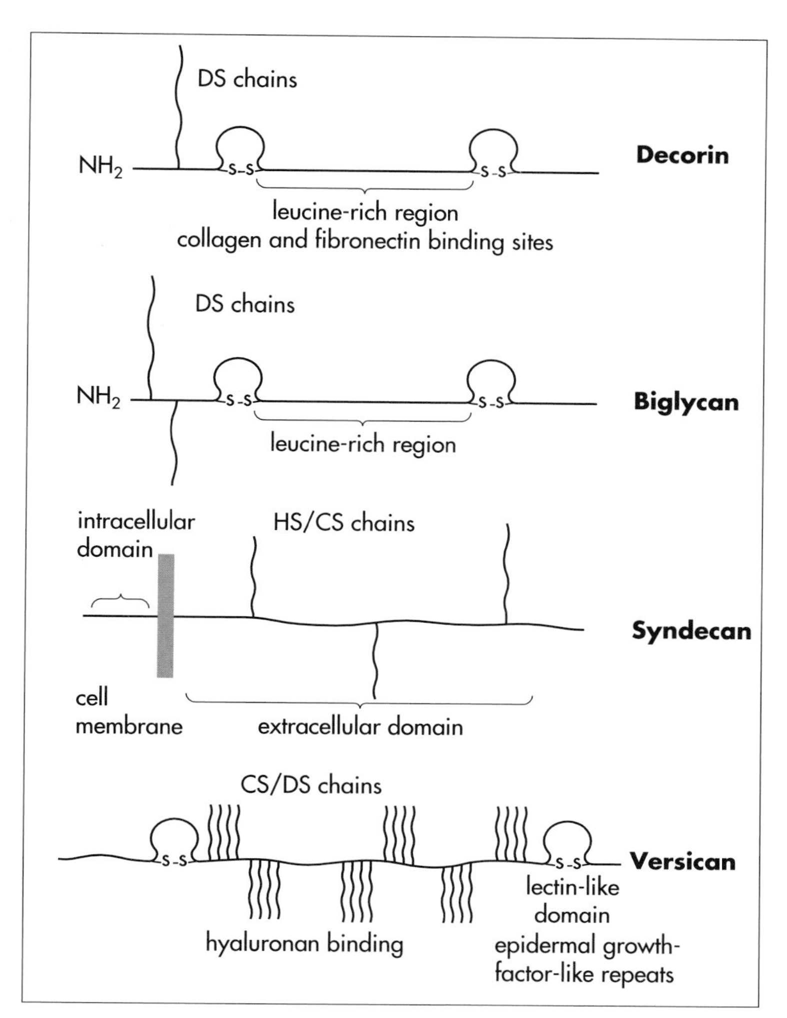

Fig. 4.1 Diagrammatic representation of proteoglycan structures, showing the main features of decorin, biglycan, syndecan, and versican. Further details on these proteoglycans are also given in this table.

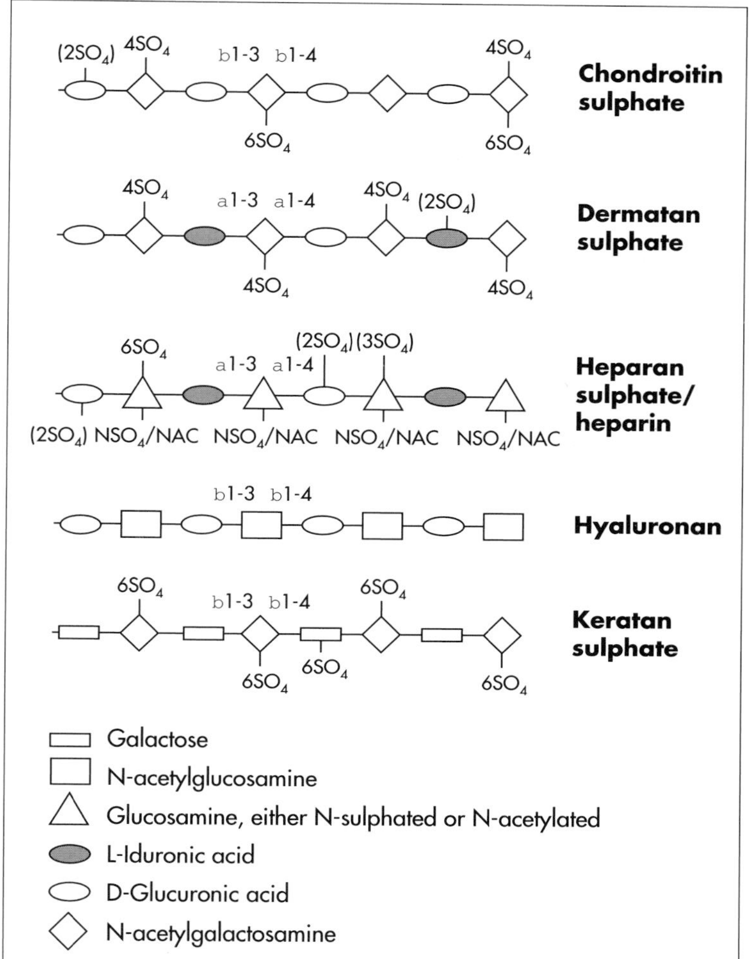

Fig. 4.2 Comparative structures of the repeating units of selected glycosaminoglycans. The structures are diagrammatic and depict the types of glycosidic linkages, sulphation patterns, hexosamine, and hexuronic acid residues present in the major glycosaminoglycans.

and Last, 1988), keratan sulphate is unique among GAG in not possessing hexuronic acid. Rather, it is composed of disaccharide sequences of N-acetylglucosamine and D-galactose, and possesses O- and N-linked sequences to the core protein.

A schematic representation of the repeating disaccharide structure of GAG is given in *Fig. 4.2.*

BIOSYNTHESIS OF GLYCOSAMINOGLYCANS AND PROTEOGLYCANS

In view of the rapid turnover of the collagenous and non-collagenous components of the extracellular matrix of the PDL, some detail of the biosynthetic events is necessary for a complete picture of ground substance biology. No detailed studies have been carried out on the PDL *per se*, but it is unlikely that the synthetic events and control mechanisms differ from those of the fibroblast family of other tissues that have been studied more.

As in most fibroblasts, PG metabolism in the PDL is a highly regulated, dynamic process. In healthy tissue this process is in a steady state, where synthesis and catabolism are closely matched so that the tissue content of the PG remains the same over a given time (Hascall *et al.*, 1991).

Biosynthesis of core proteins

The core proteins of the PG are synthesized in the rough endoplasmic reticulum (RER), like other proteins. All those PG whose sequence is known have N-terminal, hydrophobic signal sequences, which are removed co-translationally. Some, such as the core proteins of aggrecan and decorin, are released into the lumen while others, such as syndecan, remain embedded in membrane. With the exception of serglycin, all core proteins have

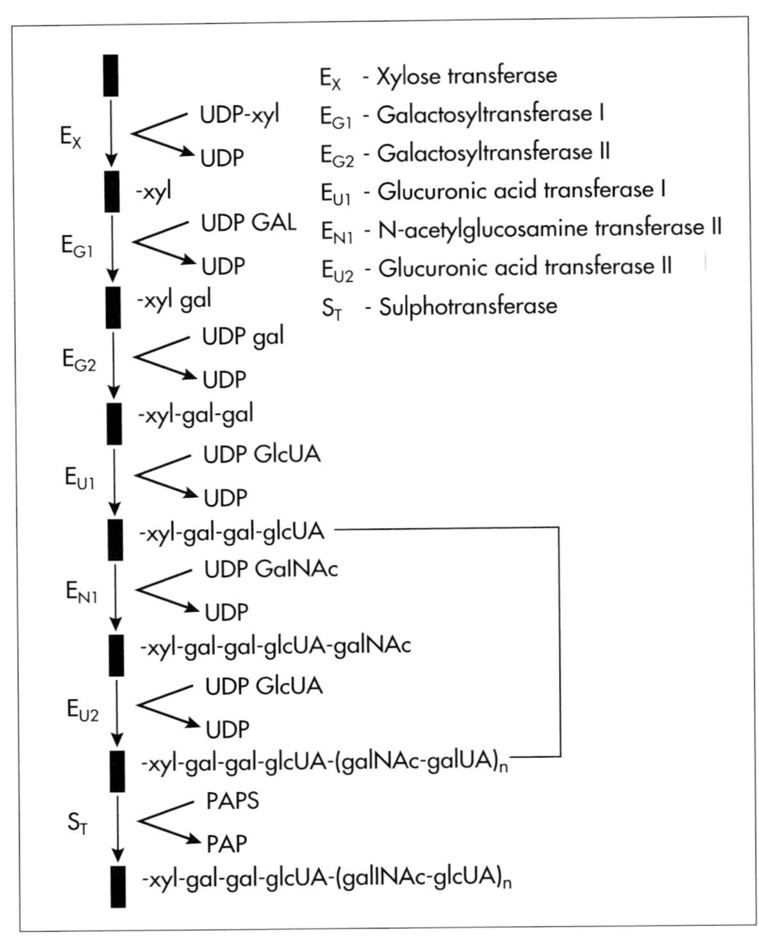

Fig. 4.3 Schematic diagram representing the synthesis of CS chains. Chondroitin sulphate chains are added to the core protein in the Golgi. With the exception of xylose transferase, which adds xyloses to hydroxyls on appropriate serines (Ex), to initiate the GAG chains, all enzymes required to synthesize a particular GAG appear to be organized into multienzyme complexes in the trans-Golgi. After xylose addition, each of the enzymes required for the completion of the linkage region – i.e. galactosyltransferase 1 (EG1), galactosyltransferase 2 (EG2) and glucuronic transferase 1 (EU1) – and then to elongate the backbone – Ga1NAc transferase 2 (EN1), and the distinct glucuronic acid transferase 2 (EU2) – adds an appropriate sugar from a UDP-sugar donor. Some evidence suggests that a second GalNAc transferase is actually required for chain elongation, and this is shown in the model. The sugars are transferred sequentially to the non-reducing end of the growing chain to form glycosidic bonds of the correct anomeric configurations (α or β), and in the correct linkages with the release of UDP. The UDP sugars are synthesized in the cytosol of the lumen and transported by an antiport mechanism into the Golgi lumen. This mechanism effectively recycles the UMP and supplies sufficient amounts of the activated sugars in the Golgi to meet the biosynthetic demands. Phosphadenosinephosphosulphate (PAPS) is the metabolically active form of sulphate required by sulphotransferases (St) to add sulphate esters to the elongating chains; it is also synthesized in the cytosol and transported into the Golgi by an antiport mechanism that exchanges one PAPS for one AMP. Two sulphate transferases, one to form 4-0-sulphate and the other 6-0-sulphate on the Ga1NAc, are the predominant ones for the synthesis of CS on most CS-PGs.

one or more asparagine-X-serine (threonine) sites, the consensus sequence required to initiate synthesis of N-linked oligosaccharides.

N-asparagine-linked oligosaccharide synthesis utilizes a lipid-linked oligosaccharide precursor. This contains nine mannose moieties and three glucose moieties linked to two N-acetylglucosamine residues which are assembled on dolichol pyrophosphate (for review, see Kornfield and Kornfield, 1985; Schachter, 1986). The dolichol moiety is embedded in the membrane of the RER with the oligosaccharide projecting into the lumen. A specific enzyme transfers the entire oligosaccharide onto the carboxyamido side chain of an asparagine in a nascent core protein, provided the recognition amino acid sequence – asparagine-X-serine (threonine) – is accessible. An N-glycosylamine bond is formed, with the release of the dolichol pyrophosphate. Once the polypeptide synthesis is complete, the resulting molecule moves through the RER to the different Golgi compartments, where it can be further processed with the addition of sialic acid.

In the trans-Golgi compartment, 0-linked oligosaccharides are synthesized (Lohmander *et al.*, 1986; Hanover *et al.*, 1982). These oligosaccharides are abundant in mucins and are found in many PGs. They are initiated by a glycosyl transferase that transfers Ga1NAc from UDP-Ga1NAc onto the hydroxyl of either the serine or the threonine in the protein core to form an a-glycosidic bond. Specific sugars are then added sequentially to appropriate hydroxyl groups on non-reducing terminals. The pathway for the schematic biosynthesis of chondroitin sulphate is shown in *Fig. 4.3.*

Biosynthesis of glycosaminoglycans

Sulphated GAGs

The biosynthesis of GAG chains, with the exception of keratan sulphate, is initiated by the transfer of xylose from UDP-xylose to the hydroxyl group of the protein core residue, this reaction being catalysed by xylosyl transferase. With the exception of this enzyme, all remaining enzymes required for the synthesis of the GAG chain appear to be organized into multi-enzyme complexes in the trans-Golgi. Using a radio-labelled precursor of xylose, Lohmander *et al.* (1986) have shown that, in the CS chains in aggrecan, xylose may be added 10 minutes before the remainder of the chain is synthesized. This indicates that xylose transferase may be active in either an early Golgi or a late RER compartment.

Following xylose addition, the linkage region is extended by the transfer of galactose from UDP-galactose by galactosyltransferase I, and then coupled by the addition of a second galactose residue, catalysed by galactosyltransferase II. The type of GAG chain synthesized appears to be determined by the glycosylated protein (Stevens *et al.*, 1982; Bourdon *et al.*, 1986). The carbohydrate backbone is formed by the alternate transfer of N-acetylhexosamine and glucuronic acid units from the corresponding UDP sugars. The sugars are transferred sequentially to the non-reducing end of the chain, where they grow to form either α- or β-

glycosidic bonds with the release of UDP. Sulphate esters from phosphoadenosine-phosphosulphate (PAPS) are added to the carbohydrate polymer by sulphotransferases, and can subsequently be subjected to further modification. These include 5-epimerase, for conversion of some of the D-glucuronic acid to L-iduronic acid and for 2-0-sulphation of some of the iduronic acids in both classes of GAGs. In heparin and heparan sulphate, N-deacetylation coupled with N-sulphation occurs. Further, specific enzymatic 3-0-sulphation of GlcNAc and 2-0-sulphation on glucuronic in heparin and heparan sulphate, while rare, appears to have important biological consequences, namely potential anticoagulant and antimitotic activities respectively.

Once GAG chain elongation is initiated, the completion of the PG structure is rapid, e.g. within a minute for aggrecan. The mature PG are then packaged into vesicles and translocated from the trans-Golgi to their final location. Hyaluronic acid synthesis differs from that of PG as it is not localized in the Golgi, but is associated with the cytoplasmic side of the plasma membrane. Studies show that hyaluronic acid is elongated at its reducing end by adding UDP-N-acetylglucosamine (or UDP-glucuronic acid) with displacement of UDP from the UDP-glucuronosyl (or UDP-N-acetylglucosaminyl) residue, which occupies the reducing end. This reaction is catalysed by hyaluronic acid synthetase (Prehm, 1989). The elongating hyaluronic acid molecule appears to be extruded directly into the extracellular space. This is consistent with the inability of most studies to provide convincing evidence for a covalently bound protein core (Mason *et al.*, 1982).

PROTEOGLYCANS AND GLYCOSAMINOGLYCANS IN PERIODONTAL LIGAMENT

Early studies on the GAG present in the PDL were investigated by autoradiography (Baumhammers and Stallard, 1968), by histochemical procedures (Mashouf and Engel, 1975) and by electron microscopy (Plecash, 1974). Even now there have been few attempts to extract and identify them from tissue extracts, the first major attempt being credited to Munemoto *et al.* (1970), who used papain treatment of bovine PDL from erupted molar teeth. These workers detected hyaluronic acid, chondroitin-4-sulphate, chondroitin-6-sulphate, dermatan sulphate, heparan sulphate and an undersulphated chondroitin sulphate. The presence of the chondroitin-6-sulphate is disputed by other workers, who could not detect this isomer in bovine, canine, or human gingival tissues (Sakamoto *et al.*, 1978; Embery, *et al.*, 1979). The observations were, however, corroborated by Pearson *et al.* (1975) and Gibson (1979). In these studies, dermatan sulphate was shown to be the principal GAG present in the PDL, in the form of two distinct PG types characterized as proteodermatan sulphate and a mixed hybrid PG containing dermatan sulphate and chondroitin-4-sulphate. The GAG chains had Mr values of 18–20 kDa and numbered two or three chains per PG unit. The low levels of serine and threonine were of significance as were the higher amounts of leucine, isoleucine, lysine, and histidine. The core protein Mr estimates were 60–70 kDa, with an overall Mr of 130 kDa for the proteodermatan sulphate molecule. This compares with 90 kDa for skin.

The mixed DS–CS hybrid PG was more heterogenous than proteodermatan sulphate and of larger average molecular size. L-iduronate corresponds to about 7 per cent of dermatan sulphate periods, and two galactosaminoglycan chains with Mr values of 32k Da and 20k Da were identified. The mixed hybrid PG and the proteodermatan sulphate undergo self-aggregation to form aggregates in the order of 600 kDa, although not in the form of the aggregates induced by hyaluronic acid similar to those of aggrecan and versican. Further work by Pearson and Pringle (1986) confirmed the presence of dermatan sulphate PG in bovine PDL and demonstrated that both versican and decorin were present. The study also demonstrated that the decorin molecule isolated from bovine PDL shares immunological properties with decorin obtained from bovine gingiva, dental pulpl, and skin.

Studies by Embery *et al.* (1987) on intrusive loading of monkey PDL detected hyaluronic acid, dermatan sulphate, chondroitin-4-sulphate and heparan sulphate. The latter might originate from other tissue sources, since it had not been previously reported in the PDL.

A topographical distribution of the extracellular matrix of the sheep periodontium in the healthy and diseased states has been made by Kirkham *et al.* (1989) and Kirkham *et al.* (1992). The GAG concentrations were highest adjacent to alveolar bone. Increasing disease severity was accompanied by a decrease in dermatan sulphate and a concomitant increase in chondroitin-4-sulphate. In a further study related to the rate of tooth eruption, the sulphated GAG content of PDL under accelerated, normal, and impeded eruption regimes was measured in view of the possible importance of the contribution by ground substance to the degree of hydration (Kirkham *et al.*, 1993). The sulphated GAG content increased fourfold during accelerated eruption but decreased to a corresponding extent in the absence of eruption.

In a further series of unpublished findings, Walker, Moxham and Embery (1994) have identified changes in the GAG and PG composition of sheep PDL with age using a panel of monoclonal antibodies towards selected compounds, including chondroitin-4-sulphate, dermatan sulphate, keratan sulphate, and oversulphated chondroitin.

With the exception of the above studies, the major data on PDL PG has stemmed from the use of culture systems using ligament and gingival fibroblasts. The field has recently been well reviewed by Rahemtulla (1992) in a treatise on oral PG.

Various studies have reported that PDL fibroblasts synthesize hyaluronic acid, heparan sulphate, dermatan sulphate, and a copolymeric chondroitin sulphate–dermatan sulphate GAG of bovine (Shuttleworth and Smalley, 1983; Smalley *et al.*, 1984), human (Mariotti and Cochran, 1990), and porcine (Merrilees *et al.*, 1983) origin. The most comprehensive study has been made by Larjava *et al.* (1992) using human PDL fibroblast cultures. The PG in these cultures were labelled with radiosulphate, and the products were analysed by SDS-PAGE and agarose gel electrophoresis. Newly synthesized PG were extracted from the medium, cell membrane, and extracellular matrix fractions in the presence of protease inhibitors. Using combinations of chondroitinase and heparatinase digestions and immunochemical procedures, seven major PG were detected. These were versican; a high molecular weight chondroitin sulphate PG, decorin; a dermatan sulphate PG; a membrane-associated sulphate PG; two medium or matrix-associated heparan sulphate PG, and a 91 kDa membrane-associated chondroitin sulphate PG. Overall, versican and decorin were found in the matrix and medium fractions. Two heparan sulphate PG of large molecular size were associated with the cell membrane fraction and two further heparan sulphate PG, distinct from those of the cell membrane, were detected in the medium and extracellular matrix fraction.

Larjava *et al.* (1992) claim that the 91 kDa chondroitin sulphate PG is related to the newly designated PG family member, CD 44, which is called the hermes antigen or ECM receptor III. In unpublished studies, Larjava *et al.* have noted the production of CD 44 by periodontal fibroblasts; this can be identified by immunoprecipitation using specific antibodies. Although such work yields vital information on the genetic potential of these cells to express the matrix proteins stated, discrepancies are noted between the structure and content of cell culture techniques by comparison with *in vivo* tissue analysis.

PROTEOGLYCANS AND GLYCOSAMINOGLCYANS IN GINGIVAL TISSUES

Most studies on the PG and GAG of the periodontium have been performed on gingival tissues. It is likely that some degree of contamination of PDL samples by gingival epithelial and connective tissue occurs. In view of the close anatomical proximity of the gingiva, some comment on its ground substance components is warranted.

Early histochemical studies demonstrated the presence of GAG (then called acid mucopolysaccharides) in gingival tissues (Quintarelli, 1960; Thonard and Scherp, 1962). The localization of the GAG led to the biochemical identification of these compounds using selective isolation and characterization techniques.

The work of Ciancio and Mather (1971) on healthy gingiva showed the presence of chondroitin-4-sulphate and chondroitin-6-sulphate isomers. In contrast Hiramatsu *et al.* (1978) detected only chondroitin-4-sulphate and dermatan sulphate in porcine gingival extracts. Hyaluronic acid and heparan sulphate have been detected in minor amounts (Sakamoto *et al.*, 1978) in bovine gingiva, a finding confirmed by Embery *et al.* (1979), who also showed the presence of chondroitin-4-sulphate and dermatan sulphate in human gingival tissue. This in turn was corroborated by Bartold *et al.* (1981), confirming that there were trace amounts of keratan sulphate in human gingival tissues.

Of significance is the finding that hyaluronic acid accounts for 20–30 per cent of the total GAG content of human gingiva. This is one of the highest concentrations of this GAG in any tissue in the body and is of importance in later sections of this review with reference to markers of tissue activity. The only detailed study on gingival epithelium has been carried out by Bartold *et al.* (1981), who showed that heparan sulphate accounted for 60 per cent of the epithelial GAG, with hyaluronic acid, chondroitin-4-sulphate and dermatan sulphate making up the remainder. The molecular size of the hyaluronic acid was double that of the underlying connective tissue, and there was evidence of aggregation of these molecules.

Using a specific probe raised towards the hyaluronic acid-binding region of aggrecan from cartilage, Tammi *et al.* (1990) demonstrated the presence of hyaluronic acid in gingival epithelium and buccal epithelium. This was localized at the surfaces and intercellular spaces of the basal and spinous cells.

Fewer studies have been carried out on the PG of gingival tissue. The first reported observation arose from the work of Dziewiatkowski *et al.* (1977) on bovine gingiva. By using caesium chloride density centrifugation and gel chromatography, these workers isolated a PG which contained 8 per cent protein, 30 per cent hexuronic acid, 32 per cent hexosamine, and 15 per cent ester sulphate, and which was rich in glycine, serine, and threonine. The PG promoted fibrillogenesis of salt-soluble collagen *in vitro* and also inhibited fibrillogenesis of acid-soluble collagen. Embery *et al.* (1979) isolated a PG from human gingiva that contained chondroitin-4-sulphate and dermatan sulphate. This PG was rich in aspartic acid, glutamic acid, serine, and threonine, and it resembled a PG from the skin. Three distinct PG fractions were isolated by Bartold *et al.* (1983), data later confirmed by Purvis *et al.* (1984) using $CaCl_2$-soluble extracts of human gingival tissue. The association of heparan sulphate (Mr 12 K) with the highest molecular size PG fraction (Mr 200 kDa), which also contained chondroitin-4-sulphate and hyaluronic acid, was of interest in picturing the molecular association of the molecules *in vivo*. Dermatan sulphate was notably absent from the highest molecular weight fraction and was present with hyaluronic acid and chondroitin-4-sulphate in the lower size PG fractions.

A proteodermatan sulphate has been identified in bovine gingiva. It contained 30 per cent protein, 20 per cent uronic acid, 25 per cent hexosamine, and a core protein of 55 kDa (Tomioka, 1981). Two distinct PG were reported in gingival tissue by Pearson and Pringle (1986) using 4 M guanidinium extraction, anion exchange, and Sepharose CL-4B chromatography. The smaller of the PG had a core protein of 55 kDa; the GAG was only represented by dermatan sulphate characterized as decorin.

The ease of maintenance of gingival fibroblasts in culture has been helpful in investigating the synthesis of PG using labelled sulphate, glucosamine, and selected amino acids such as leucine. The ability of gingival fibroblasts to incorporate ^{35}sulphate into covalently bound macromolecules has been demonstrated by Hassell and Stanek (1983) and by Hassell *et al.* (1986). In more detailed investigations, Bartold and Page (1985) showed that gingival fibroblasts were able to synthesize and secrete hyaluronic acid, heparan sulphate, and dermatan sulphate. Whereas dermatan sulphate was the predominant GAG secreted into the medium, heparan sulphate was correspondingly associated with cell membrane extracts. Further studies revealed that gingival fibroblasts secreted both chondroitin sulphate and dermatan sulphate into the medium, and that chondroitin sulphate and heparan sulphate PG were retained in the cell membrane fractions (Bartold and Page, 1987).

The ability of cultured fibroblasts derived from normal and inflamed gingiva to synthesize PG was also demonstrated by Bartold and Page (1986). These workers studied the *in vitro* proliferation rates and PG derived from age-matched and sex-matched donors. Fibroblasts from inflamed gingiva demonstrated a slower growth rate than cells from healthy tissue. The rate of ^{35}sulphate incorporation into cell-associated PG and the subsequent release of these PG into the culture medium showed no significant differences between the healthy and inflamed groups. However, heparan sulphate and chondroitin sulphate were depleted in the medium of the inflamed fibroblasts, whereas dermatan sulphate levels were elevated. Overall, the intracellular pool of PG was found to be greatly diminished in the inflamed tissue fibroblast layers.

Bartold and Page had also noted previously (1986b) that gingival fibroblast cells from donors of different ages synthesized and secreted PG to different degrees – the proportion of high molecular weight PG decreased with increasing age of the donor, and the proportion of heparan sulphate increased with a parallel loss of chondroitin sulphate and dermatan sulphate.

GLYCOPROTEINS AND OTHER NON-COLLAGENOUS PROTEINS IN PERIODONTAL LIGAMENT

There have been comparatively few attempts to study in detail the non-collagenous glycoproteins in the PDL. This is partly because the amounts present will be less than the PG present. In addition, such molecules are less well defined than the PG, in that they contain a greater array of neutral sugars such as mannose, galactose, and fucose, and because they lack hexuronic acid in a repeat disaccharide unit.

However, with the advent of specific antibodies, a clearer picture of molecules such as fibronectin and tenascin is beginning to emerge at the histochemical level.

Few detailed reports on the biochemistry of the glycoproteins of the PDL have been cited since the review by Pearson (1982) in the previous edition of this book. The main published source still remains that of Pearson *et al.* (1975), an investigation into the glycoprotein components of bovine PDL at different stages of tissue development. For comparison, these workers compared their data with that of other dermal or tendon material. Non-collagen glycopeptides were released after papain digestion of the NaCl-

Table 4.2 Neutral sugar compositions of non-collagen glycopeptides and glycoproteins.*

	% of total neutral sugar				g per 14 g Hyp
	Gal	Man	Glc	Fuc	Total
Bovine periodontal ligament					
Unerupted	46	37	10	7	0.77
Erupted	45	35	12	8	0.57
Occluded	45	30	20	5	1.0
CR occluded	25	28	44	3	—
Bovine dental pulp	43	33	15	9	0.77
CR dental pulp	33	34	27	6	—
Cementum	45	29	18	8	0.9
Predentine	38	27	23	12	2.2
Bovine dermis	53	25	13	9	0.1
Rabbit skin SGP	46	31	10	13	—
Pig aorta SGP	39	52	9	—	—
Bovine tendon GP	54	29	5	12	—

*Results shown for the soft dental tissue and bovine dermis refer to non-collagen glycopeptides isolated after papain digestion of the NaCl-insoluble matrices or the bacterial collagenase-insoluble residues (CR) of the latter. The glycopeptides of cementum and predentine were derived from decalcified matrices. In all these analyses, neutral sugars were determined by ion-exchange chromatography of acid hydrolysates.

insoluble matrices or the bacterial collagenase-insoluble residues of the latter. The neutral sugar components are shown in *Table 4.2*. In all instances, galactose predominated over mannose, whereas fucose occurred as a minor constituent. Glucose was present in all tissue extracts. Since this sugar is relatively low in concentration in glycoproteins, the authors suggested it arose from the contaminating lipids of the cell membranes.

The results demonstrated a remarkable similarity between the glycopeptides of the PDL and those of other tissues. However, the neutral sugar composition of the PDL collagenase-insoluble fractions showed some differences (see *Table 4.2*), since mannose was approximately equal to galactose and glucose was significantly increased. The mannose–galactose ratio was closer to that of the aortic structural protein.

The collagenase-insoluble residues contain a large part of the NaCl-insoluble glycoproteins of bovine ligament. The presence of structural protein was deduced from the dissolutions of the residue in 6 M urea – 0.M 2-mercaptoethanol followed by aggregation and precipitation if the urea is removed by dialysis in the presence of reducing agents.

The neutral sugar contents of pure glycoproteins of soft dental tissues are not known, but it is unlikely that they exceed those of skin and tendon glycoproteins, especially as the bacterial collagenase-insoluble residues contain only 2–4 per cent hexose. The neutral sugar values in *Table 4.2* show that the insoluble matrices of the dental tissues contain relatively large amounts of non-collagenous glycoproteins, in the order of 10–20 g per 100 g of collagen. Even higher amounts of hexose were detected in the whole PDL and gingiva (Michalites and Orlowski, 1977) and in dental pulp (Orlowski, 1974), presumably owing to the presence of serum glycoproteins in addition to readily soluble connective tissue glycoproteins (Anderson, 1976).

This background implies that non-collagenous glycoproteins of the ground substance of soft dental tissue may be quantitatively as important as the PG content. It is difficult to equate these findings to histochemical observations, since the bulk of the histochemical studies have involved staining procedures such as the PAS reaction. This method visualizes only small portions of the glyco residues, some of which may be masked or obscured histochemically owing to associated interaction with other connective tissue components such as protein and lipid. PAS granules have been detected in nearly all cells of the PDL of the developing rat incisor (Mashouf and Engel, 1975).

The PDL shares with other soft dental tissues a high cellular content and makes it difficult to ascribe locations to glycoproteins. Biochemical procedures often leave uncertainties as to whether the glycoproteins are related to the cell surface or whether they are structural components of the connective tissue ground substance. Interpretation is also hindered by the knowledge that the extrahelical regions of the procollagen contain oligosaccharides, which bear some resemblance to the non-collagen glycopeptides that contain mannose and glucosamine (Clark and Kefilades, 1978). Sear *et al.* (1977) also showed that elastin fibres contain an apparently specific type of microfibrillar glycoprotein which has characteristics similar to fibronectin and other structural glycoproteins.

With the availability of specific antibodies to certain glycoproteins, a clearer picture of their distribution in various tissues has emerged. Zhang *et al.* (1993) have studied the ultrastructural localization of three distantly related glycoproteins of the extracellular matrix – undulin, tenascin, and fibronectin – in decalcified sections of human PDL and cementum. Undulin was found to be associated with tightly packed major collagen fibrils but not with microfibrils, indicating that this protein may be involved in the supramolecular and functional organization of collagen fibrils into flexible bundles. Tenascin was found on globular masses between less densely packed collagen fibrils, thus displaying a pattern quite distinct from that of undulin. Fibronectin was noted in bulky material between the cross-striated fibrils, often surrounding individual fibrils like garlands, and in the microfibrillar meshwork extending from cross-striated fibrils. The three glycoproteins displayed a distinct and unique pattern of distribution in the PDL, which can be correlated with their molecular structure and potential functions.

The glycoproteins mentioned in the study by Zhang *et al.* (1993) belong to the now well-characterized group of substances that includes fibronectin, laminin, and other cell interactive glycoproteins. The field, which has been reviewed by Yamada (1991), indicates the presence of such molecules in many tissue sources, although it has not been extensively studied in the PDL. An association between fibronectin and oxytalan fibres is described in Chapter 2.

FIBRONECTIN

Perhaps the most widely studied structural glycoprotein is fibronectin. Although it is encoded by a single gene, 20 different forms of human fibronectin sub-units exist. However, all fibronectin molecules conform to the same model pattern (*Fig. 4.4a*), which consists of two polypeptide chains, each of 250 kDa.

The molecule is generally present in loose connective tissue and in embryonic (but not always adult) basement membranes. Fibronectin appears to be lost upon full maturation of most connective tissues (Linder *et al.*, 1975; Hassall *et al.*, 1978). However, there is a continued presence within the PDL, which may reflect the foetal-like role of fibronectin and the failure of the PDL to mature. Immunofluorescent localization of fibronectin has shown its uniform distribution throughout the PDL (Connor *et al.*, 1984; Takita *et al.*, 1987) in association with collagen fibres and at specific sites at the cell–collagen interface (Pitaru *et al.*, 1987). Each fibronectin molecule studied is characterized by a series of structural and functional domains. These include a centrally located cell-binding region with a crucial Arg-Gly-Asp-Ser (RGD) amino acid sequence, to which a variety of cells, including fibroblasts, can attach. The molecules also possess binding

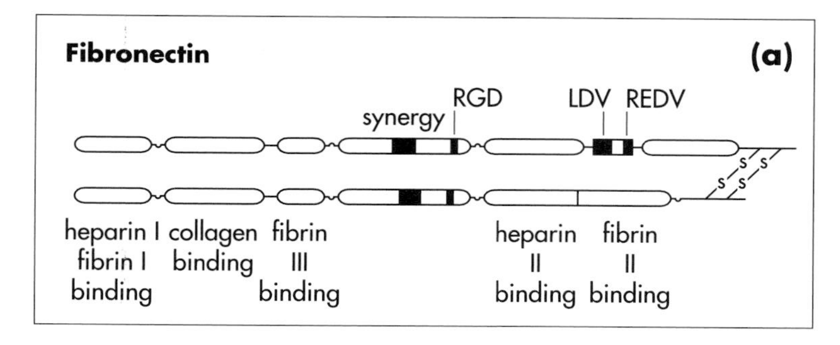

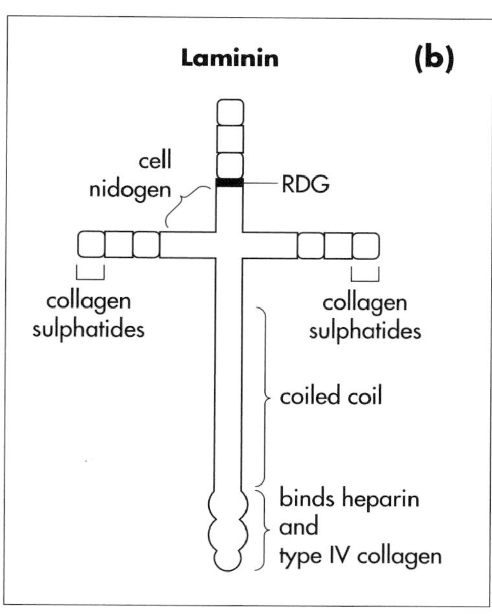

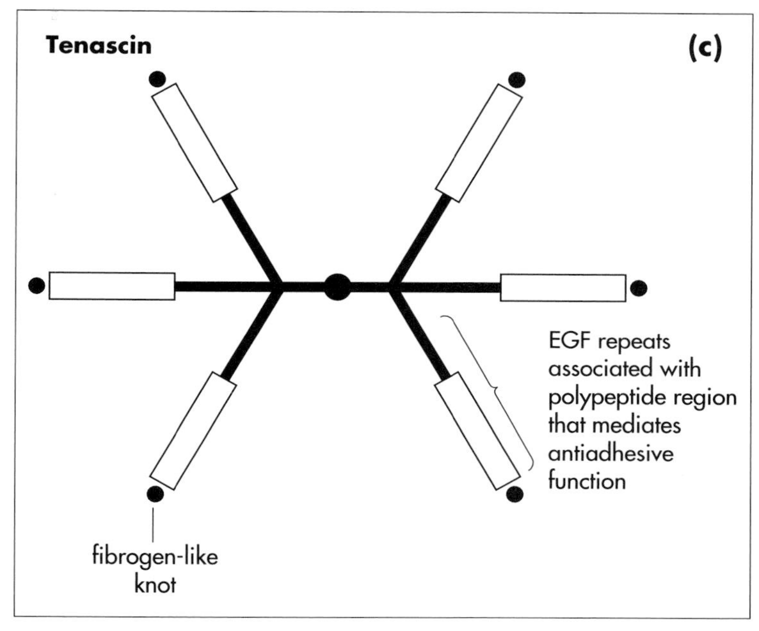

Fig. 4.4 Schematic structures of representative structural glycoproteins found in ground substance – (a) fibronectin (b) laminin (c) tenascin.

domains for collagen, heparin, and fibrin, in addition to matrix-assembly regions, which, although poorly defined, are nevertheless considered of major importance in the maintenance of the integrity of the connective tissue structure.

LAMININ

Laminin is a major glycoprotein component of basement membranes (Kleinman *et al.*, 1993). It is implicated in a variety of functions, including cell adhesion, migration, and differentiation. Laminin is a cross-shaped molecule with a large multiglobulated globular domain consisting of three sub-units linked by disulphide bonds. The molecule possesses a neurite-binding region and terminal amino acid domains for heparin, nitrogen, and collagen. It also has a central cell interactive region. Its molecular size can be up to 1,000,000 kDa (*Fig.* 4.4b). It is associated with the epithelial cell rests of the PDL (see Chapter 1).

VITRONECTIN AND THROMBOSPONDIN

A further multifunctional glycoprotein is vitronectin, which was first identified as a cell-attachment factor with a high affinity for glass surfaces. It is a 75 kDa molecule that has a cell-attachment domain mediated through receptors of the integrin family, including $\alpha v\beta 3$, $\alpha 111G\beta 3$, and $\alpha v\beta 5$. It possesses a cryptic heparin-binding domain that is exposed after surface adsorption. A larger glycoprotein composed of a trimer of identical sub-units is thrombospondin. Each sub-unit is 140 kDa and the sub-units are linked by disulphide bonds. The molecule possesses cell-, heparin-, calcium-, and fibronectin-binding domains. The glycoprotein appears to be involved in cell regulation and cell attachment – particularly in the enhancement or inhibition of attachment.

TENASCIN AND ENTACTIN

Tenascin, also known as cytotactin, is a star-shaped six-membered sub-unit structure, again linked by disulphide bridges. The characteristic feature of the molecule is a central knot (Erickson and Bourdon, 1989). Tenascin is unusual in that it mediates both adhesive and repulsive interactions, in addition to binding fibronectin and certain PG. Expression of the protein is closely associated with the morphogenetic aspects of connective tissue function, including cell migration, wound healing, and tumourgenesis. Tenascin binds in particular to chondroitin sulphide PG via divalent cations.

Lukinmaa *et al.* (1991) have detected tenascin by immunochemical localization in the attachment zone of periodontal ligament, at the interface between mineralized and non-mineralized tissues. This observation has led to the suggestion that tenascin possesses functional roles in cell differentiation during the formation of mineralized matrix and in mediating mechanical stress.

Entactin (nidogen) is a dumbbell-shaped glycoprotein consisting of two globular domains. One of these domains binds to laminin and type IV collagen; the other is a self-aggregation site that leads to clusters of variable-sized self-aggregated units. The molecule has particular roles to play in the organization of the basement membrane (*Fig. 4.4c*).

CATABOLISM OF PROTEOGLYCANS AND GLYCOPROTEINS OF THE GROUND SUBSTANCE

There has been an extensive increase in our understanding of the degradation of the components of the extracellular matrix of many tissues. Although the bulk of the studies have been carried out on non-dental tissues, it is almost certain that the same mechanisms apply to the PDL. In view of the degradative role of tissue factors in the health of the PDL and the high metabolic turnover of this tissue in the normal state, an update on the catabolic events involved is worthy of mention. For example, the work of Sodek (1977) has indicated that PDL is one of the most metabolically active tissues in the body. The turnover rate for mature collagen in the PDL was found to be five times faster than that of gingiva, six times faster than that of bone, and 15 times faster than that of skin. Furthermore, the half lives of insoluble collagen and sulphated GAG have been shown to be extremely short, at 9.7 and 1.7 days respectively (Van den Bos and Tonino, 1984).

Most of our knowledge in this area relates to the catabolism of PG, where in most (if not all) connective tissues it occurs as a result of the activity of the resident connective tissue cells and infiltrating cells. It is tightly regulated by a complex interplay of cell–cell and cell–matrix interactions, involving the production of enzymes, activators, and inhibitors, and regulatory molecules such as growth factors.

The endopeptidases (proteinases) are the key enzymes in the degradative processes, since the protein components of most matrix macromolecules are the predominant determinants of tissue structure and function. Exopeptidases and glycosidases play a secondary role in the degradative processes (Murphy and Reynolds, 1993). In *in vitro* experiments, matrix macromolecules can be degraded by endopeptidases from the four major classes (metallo-, serine, cysteine and aspartic active site residues) (Murphy and Reynolds, 1993).

The current view is that degradation of the extracellular matrix (ECM) takes place in two steps – in the initial step, the degradation of the matrix is an extracellular process; this degradation ranges from fine modification of the glycoproteins associated with the cell to clipping of the cross-linked insoluble collagen and elastin that form the basis of the matrix (Murphy and Reynolds, 1993). This process may be supplemented by a second step – physical disruption (e.g. by free radicals) in inflammatory situations, (Freeman and Crapo, 1982; Bartold *et al.*, 1984), injury, and infection.

Except in special circumstances, such as bone resorption or other situations where the cell is in close apposition to its matrix, extracellular degradation is thought to occur at neutral pH values. Consequently, proteinases of the metallo- and serine families will be optimally functional and could be responsible for the initial phase of the degradative process. The connective tissue cells synthesize and secrete an important group of matrix metalloproteinases (MMP), which can synergistically digest all the components of the ECM. After the initial proteolytic attacks on the matrix, the fragments generated may be phagocytosed by local cells for additional intracellular degradation by lysosomal proteinases, such as the cathepsins B, L and D.

The MMP constitute an important family of structurally and functionally homologous metal-dependent proteinases. Their substrate specificity varies greatly, from the broadly reactive to the highly specific (*Table 4.3*). They generally exhibit poor peptidase activity and are specifically involved in cleavage at Gly-X- bonds, where X is usually a hydrophobic amino acid (e.g. leucine or isoleucine) present in large proteins, such as those located in the ECM (Davies *et al.*, 1992). In mammalian cells, this gene family includes both fibroblast and polymorphonucleocytes (PMN), types of interstitial collagenase, two types of gelatinase (or type IV collagenase) referred to as PMN gelatinase, 92 kDa gelatinase, fibroblast gelatinase, or 72 kDa type gelatinase, at least three stromelysins, and a truncated metalloproteinase, (PUMP-1), which lacks the C-terminal domain present in other MMP. The MMP are also discussed in relation to degradation of collagen in Chapter 3.

The chief characteristics of the MMP are:

1. The catalytic mechanism is dependent on zinc at the active centre. All MMP contain the zinc-chelating motif (VAAHEXGH), which follows the pattern of proteins that contain zinc, with the fourth site of the zinc tetrahedron available for catalysis (Van Wart and Birkedal-Hansen, 1990). Ca^{2+} is also required for the stabilization of the proteins, although the molecular mechanism for this requirement is unknown.
2. The proteinases are secreted in an inactive proform (zymogens) (Sellers *et al.*, 1978) and are activated in the extracellular milieu, although the precise mechanism of activation is unknown. Plasmin has been strongly implicated in collagenase and stromelysin activation *in vitro* and in cell model systems (Werb *et al.*, 1977; Gavriolovic *et al.*, 1985; Gavriolovic and Murphy, 1989).
3. The inactive precursors are activated by a variety of proteinases or organo-mercurials (Stetler-Stevenson *et al.*, 1989). Examples of activators include plasmin, trypsin, tryptase, kallikreinin, and cathepsin B (Werb *et al.*, 1977).
4. Metal-chelating agents such as EDTA and 1,10-phenanthroline block their activity and can be reversed by the action of exogenous zinc (Davies *et al.*, 1992).
5. Activation is accompanied by a loss of Mr of 10 kDa (Woessner, 1991).
6. They are optimally active at neutral pH (Davies *et al.*, 1992).

Table 4.3 Matrix metalloproteinases and their various substrates*	
MMP	**Principle matrix substrates**
Interstitial collagenase (52 kDa)	Collagen I, II, III, VII, X
PMN collagenase 75 kDa)	Collagen I, II, III Gelatin
PMN gelatinase (92 kDa)	Collagen IV, V Gelatin
72 kDa gelatinase (matrilysin)	Collagen IV, V, VII, X Gelatin Fibronectin Elastin
92 kDa gelatinase (Invadolysin)	Collagen IV, V, VII Gelatin Proteoglycan Fibronectin Elastin
Stromelysin-1 (53 kDa)	Collagen II, IV, V, IX Procollagen peptides Proteoglycan link protein Fibronectin Laminin
Stomelysin-2 (53 kDa)	Collagen III, IV, V Gelatin Proteoglycan core protein Fibronectin Laminin
PUMP-1 (28 kDa)	Collagen III, IV Gelatin Proteoglycan Fibronectin Elastin

*The Mr of the enzymes may vary, depending on the source and species from which they are extracted. (From Murphy and Reynolds, 1993; Woessner, 1991; Davies et al., 1992.)

7. The cDNA sequences show highly conserved regions across both enzyme types (55 per cent homology between interstitial collagenase and stromelysin-1) as well as across specific species (75 per cent between human, rabbit and rat stromelysin). The extent of sequence conservation is different for the various domains (Murphy and Docherty, 1988; Goldberg *et al.*, 1986; Whitham *et al.*, 1986.

8. The enzymes cleave one or more components of the ECM (Woessner, 1991).

9. Their activity is regulated by a secreted specific inhibitor, tissue inhibitor of metalloproteinases (TIMP) (Sellers *et al.*, 1979; Cawston, 1986).

MMP play a major role in the remodelling events that occur in normal morphogenesis, wound healing, bone and growth plate remodelling, and uterine resorption. In addition, they play a role in pathological processes that occur in joint destruction, rheumatoid arthritis, osteoarthritis, tumour invasion in neoplasia, periodontitis, and osteoporosis.

A number of control mechanisms regulate the activities of MMP; these include inhibition by the stoichiometric complexing of the activated enzyme with natural inhibitors such as TIMP. One of the striking features of the MMP is that they are inducible, i.e. their synthesis and secretion seem to be controlled by factors that alter gene expression.

There is now much evidence for the central role of several cytokines, polypeptide growth factors (eg basic fibroblast growth factor (Edwards *et al.*, 1987), platelet-derived growth factor (Bauer *et al.*, 1985) and hormones in this process). IL-1 (Gowen *et al.*, 1984), and tumour necrosis factor (Dayer *et al.*, 1985; Brenner *et al.*, 1989) are among the most potent inhibitors.

It is clear that the initiation of tissue breakdown must result from an imbalance of active MMP over TIMP. Human plasma contains a super-family of serine proteinase inhibitors, the serpins, which are synthesized in the liver (reviewed by Carrell and Barwell, 1986). They are generally glycoproteins with a single polypeptide chain that acts by presentation of a potential cleavage site for the target enzyme, e.g. α1-proteinase inhibitor complex, which is an important regulator of PMN elastase (Travis and Salvesen, 1989; Heidtmann and Travis, 1986). The plasminogen activators are some of the potentially most important regulators of connective tissue degradation because of their control over the rate of plasmin generation in local extracellular locations.

DEGRADATION OF PROTEOGLYCANS

The protein cores of PG types seem to be generally susceptible to the action of many proteinases. The variation in cleavage patterns between types has not been determined, but most of the work carried out on chondroitin sulphate aggregates seems to be applicable to the general situation. All proteinases appear to cleave at similar loci, with an initial cleavage adjacent to the hyaluronate binding region, releasing almost intact monomers, and with a second cleavage within the chondroitin sulphate-rich region (Roughley, 1977; Campbell *et al.*, 1986). Further cleavages between clusters of GAG side chains associated with extended regions of the core can occur, but these vary more widely. These cleavages generate small peptides with attached carbohydrate chains that are no longer trapped in the collagen network. Stromelysin has been shown to degrade the protein core at multiple sites and to be active over a broad pH range (Galloway *et al.*, 1983). The serine protease, cathepsin G, and lysosomal proteinases have been shown to cleave the protein core at multiple cleavage sites in vitro (Roughley and Barrett, 1977).

There is no evidence for the cleavage of GAG at extracellular sites (Tyler, 1985), except in the case of heparan sulphate. Since heparan sulphate is involved in cell–cell and cell–matrix interactions, as well as binding to fibronectin and types I, II and V collagens, its degradation may represent a significant part of the signalling mechanism of cells.

The intracellular digestion of GAG chains occurs through the initial action of lysosomal endoglycosidases and sulphatases, working from the non-reducing terminus (reviewed by Poole, 1986).

The majority of extracellular matrix glycoproteins, such as fibronectin and laminin, are sensitive to proteinases and are susceptible to the action of many serine proteinases, such as plasminogen activator (Quigley *et al.*, 1987), PMN elastase, cathepsin G (Heck *et al.*, 1990), and MMP stromelysin (Galloway *et al.*, 1983; Okada *et al.*, 1986).

It is now clear that no one proteinase can be considered of overriding importance in matrix turnover, and that a complex cascade of events best explains how matrix destruction occurs.

PERIODONTAL LIGAMENT DESTRUCTION

The connective tissue destruction that occurs in chronic inflammatory periodontal disease is mediated by proteolytic enzymes that are assumed to be released by invading PMN, macrophages, and bacterial enzymes (see Chapter 14). Recent evidence suggests that invasion of the gingival tissues by intact bacteria may occur in severe and advanced forms of inflammatory periodontal disease, but most observations support the view that bacterial invasion is not a feature of periodontitis. It has been hypothesized that the local tissue response to bacterial products may be of greater significance in the pathogenesis of the disease (Meikle *et al.*, 1986), and that the induction of MMP may be an important process. A critical step may be the interaction of bacterial antigens with inflammatory cells (Heath *et al.*, 1987), resulting in the production of MMP. Thus, cytokines may induce the connective tissues of the periodontium to 'self destruct' through the stimulation of MMP production (Meikle *et al.*, 1989), much in the manner suggested for cartilage.

Clinical evidence corroborates this hypothesis with the finding of increased collagenase activity in the crevicular fluid of patients who have periodontitis compared to the activity observed in control patients (Larivee *et al.*, 1986; Villela *et al.*, 1987). This collagenase appears to be tissue derived, rather than being derived from PMNs (Villela *et al.*, 1987). TIMP levels could be assayed only in the control patients (Larivee *et al.*, 1986). In addition, collagenase levels were significantly lower in patients following periodontal treatment. Increased collagenase activity has been demonstrated from explants of inflamed gingiva (Overall *et al.*, 1987), and MMP activities from all three groups of MMP have been demonstrated when inflamed gingiva was cultured (Heath *et al.*, 1982).

FUNCTIONAL ROLE OF PROTEOGLYCANS IN GROUND SUBSTANCE

PG form a diverse family of macromolecules and have been ascribed a diverse number of functions. Many of these functions are determined by the nature, distribution, and concentration of the extracellular components derived from studies on a range of connective tissues other than the PDL, but they may be equally applicable within the PDL (*Fig. 4.5*).

The biomechanical functions of PG and GAG are mainly attributable to their highly polyanionic nature carried largely on the polysaccharide chains. Firstly, PG within a collagenous fibre network have been described as molecular springs (Muir, 1982) capable of generating a Donnan osmotic pressure (reviewed by Comper and Laurent, 1978; Carney and Muir, 1988). PG extracted from cartilage adopt an extended configuration, capable of occupying a volume of 50 ml/g dry weight (Wight *et al.*, 1991), whereas within a connective tissue matrix they occupy volumes of 10 ml/g or less.

The PG exert a swelling pressure entrapped within the collagen matrix. External pressure applied to a tissue will result in a loss of fluid, increasing the effective swelling pressure as PG concentration increases. Fluid loss is restored once the external load is removed, and the fluid flow and the maintenance of a hydrated state is controlled by PG present. Thus, connective tissues such as PDL or cartilage may easily withstand compressive loads. This Donnan osmotic pressure is unaffected by the extent of aggregation of the PG (Myers, Armstrong and Mow, 1984). Small concentrations of hyaluronan or PG will exert a significant effect, and mixed systems (e.g. ones containing PG and serum components) exert a Donnan osmotic pressure greater than the sum of the swelling pressures of the individual solutes at an equivalent concentration (Ogston, 1970; Wiederhielm *et al.*, 1976).

A chondroitin-sulphate PG (probably versican) has been identified using electron microscopy techniques in blood vessels (Salisbury and Wagner, 1981; Kapoor *et al.*, 1986; Morgelin *et al.*, 1989) and arterial smooth muscle cells (Wight and Hascall, 1983; Chang *et al.*, 1983). Versican-rich areas are interweaved with filamentous hyaluronic acid and it has been suggested that they provide resistance to compressive forces, such as those generated by the cardiovascular system. The highly vascular nature of the

PDL suggests that versican may perform a similar function in resisting compressive forces.

PG solutions also exhibit viscoelastic properties, a resistance to flow in response to a shear pressure (Mow *et al.*, 1984). The shear properties of PG in solution are proportional to the extent of aggregation of these macromolecules. Thus, non-aggregated PG are able to diffuse through a connective tissue with relative ease, whereas aggregated PG are fixed within the collagen network (Mow *et al.*, 1984).

The dermatan sulphate PG, DS-PG1 (or biglycan), is widely distributed in the extracellular matrix of soft connective tissues such as skin (Pearson *et al.*, 1983; Pearson and Gibson, 1982), sclera (Coster and Fransson, 1981; Coster *et al.*, 1981), and PDL (Pearson and Gibson, 1982). This PG, which differs from DS-PG II (or decorin) in its core protein primary structure, is capable of self-association (Rosenberg *et al.*, 1986). Although the dermatan sulphate chains themselves are capable of self-association (Fransson *et al.*, 1982), the process is likely to involve the core protein.

Hydrophobic interactions are probably important, since self-association is temperature dependent (it is most effective at temperatures of 37°C or less), and disrupted by chaotropic agents such as 6 M urea. The ineffectual nature of 2 M sodium chloride confirms self-association and is not stabilized via electrostatic interactions alone (Pearson and Gibson, 1982). Aggregates of apparent molecular weights of up to 600 000 have been observed in periodontal tissues. However, super-aggregates of apparent molecular weights of 3×10^6 (Obrink, 1972) and 39×10^6 (Coster, 1979) have been reported in cartilage. PG, therefore, are likely to contribute little to the viscoelastic properties of stress-bearing connective tissues; rather, they maintain the collagen network in a favourable conformation to resist shear forces (Carney and Muir, 1988).

The entrapped PG and other glycoproteins, together with the collagen matrix, are all capable of sterically excluding other macromolecules from their molecular environment (Ogston, 1970; Comper and Laurent, 1978). This steric hindrance gives rise to the filtration and exclusion properties in defining the passage of certain macromolecules within connective tissues. The diffusion of some large molecules, such as antibodies, is therefore likely to be hindered, while the retention of biologically active molecules, such as enzymes, would result in raised concentrations and activity within a localized environment.

The nature and distribution of the PG within the tissue is likely to be of great importance, capable of imposing a directional bias in the movement of certain molecules such as procollagen through the ground substance (Laurent, 1977). The steric exclusion effects have also been described as an influential factor on collagen fibril formation (Carney and Muir, 1988). Comper and Laurent (1978) have demonstrated that the exclusion effects from connective tissues are dependent on the tissue's polysaccharide content. In view of the low GAG content of PG in PDL compared to PG in cartilage, the steric exclusion effects are probably derived mainly from the collagen fibres, with similar conclusions drawn for other fibrous connective tissues such as skin (Comper and Laurent, 1978).

In exhibiting the physicochemical properties described so far, PG are heavily involved in maintaining the structural integrity of connective tissues. PG, alongside other glycoconjugates, have also been implicated in a host of biological functions. These include specific functions relating to the development, remodelling, and repair of a connective tissue known to maintain a high metabolic activity; collagen turnover in the PDL is much faster than that of skin (Sodek, 1977) and is considered further in Chapter 3.

Most, if not all, of the PG in the extracellular matrix can bind to other matrix macromolecules. This interaction is generally mediated via the GAG chains with a particular binding site on the matrix protein. Such binding domains for heparin have previously been identified on the glycoproteins fibronectin (Hynes *et al.*, 1984) and laminin (Martin *et al.*, 1984). Decorin has also been

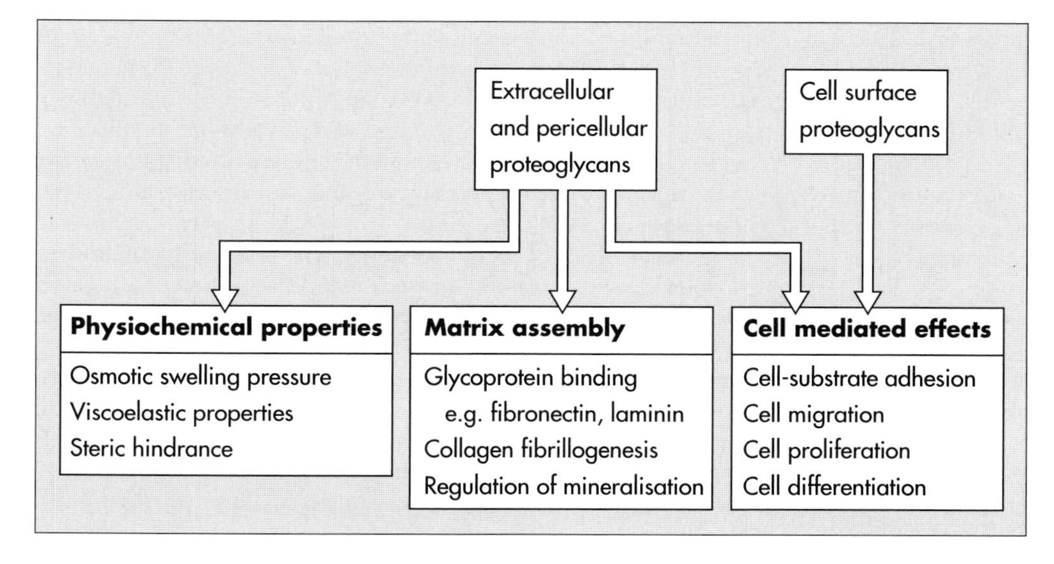

Fig. 4.5 Functional roles of proteoglycans showing the proposed properties of extracellular, pericellular and cell surface types.

shown to bind collagen and glycoproteins such as fibronectin through its core protein (Obrink, 1973a; Vogel *et al.*, 1986; Lewandowska *et al.*, 1987; Schmidt *et al.*, 1987). The binding of decorin to collagen has proved to be quite specific and, along with other PG, may be of importance in the regulation of collagen fibril formation.

PG have been implicated in the promotion of interactions between a variety of extracellular matrix components, helping in their assembly and in their holding together. Such a role for PG has been proposed by Ruoslahti and Pierschbacher (1987), who suggest that PG might enhance the interaction between other matrix components, type I collagen, and fibronectin. Similarly, extracellular heparan sulphate PG can precipitate with laminin and type IV collagen to form a tertiary complex that resembles extracellular matrix (Oldberg and Ruoslahti, 1982; Martin *et al.*, 1984; Kleinman *et al.*, 1986).

Various studies have provided indirect evidence of the involvement of PG in the control of mineralization. In the PDL, PG are thought to function in the inhibition of mineralization. Early studies by Howell and co-workers (1969) led to suggestions that hyaluronate and PG aggregates (but not PG sub-units) are able to shield embryonic mineral clusters, with calcification proceeding only upon dispersion of the aggregates. Indeed, in cartilage there is an apparent loss in the large aggregating PG immediately prior to mineralization, owing to modification of the PG rather than loss of the entire molecule (Howell and Pita, 1976; Buckwalter *et al.*, 1987).

PG have been demonstrated to bind to the mineral face of growing hydroxyapatite crystals (Fujisawa and Kuboki, 1991). Hall *et al.* (1993) showed that hyaluronan, dermatan sulphate, and chondroitin sulphate all inhibit hydroxyapatite crystal growth with an increasing potency, although calcium-binding studies, using equilibrium dialysis to the GAG could not account for this inhibitory effect, as only chondroitin-4-sulphate showed any significant binding.

The presence of decorin bound to collagen fibres has implicated this PG in the inhibition of mineralization. Decorin binds to collagen fibres at specific sites at the gap zone along the collagen fibre (Scott and Haigh, 1985), which electron distribution studies have indicated as the sites of mineral deposition within calcified tissues (White *et al.*, 1977). This has led to suggestions that decorin acts by blocking the sites for initiation of mineralization, a proposal strengthened by the demonstration of the inability of dermatan sulphate to bind free calcium (Hall *et al.*, 1993).

The PG present on the cell surface appear to contribute in a number of other biological functions. These include regulation of extracellular matrix formation; cell-substrate adhesion, leading to cell migration; regulation of cell proliferation; and binding and internalization of extracellular components. Several modes of interaction of PG with the cell surface have been proposed. This may be via direct insertion of the core protein into the plasma membrane, such as occurs with the heparan sulphate–chondroitin sulphate PG of syndecan or CD 44 (Saunders *et al.*, 1989). Insertion into the plasma membrane may occur via a phosphatidylinositol moiety covalently attached to the core protein (Ishihara *et al.*, 1987).

Syndecan and CD 44 possess conserved cytoplasmic domains containing potential phosphorylation sites (Jalkanen *et al.*, 1991), and this has led to the view that these molecules are important in signal transduction during cell adhesion. Considering the well-established role of phosphatidylinositol in cell signalling, PG attached to the cell surface via this molecule may perform similar signal transduction roles.

PG are also capable of binding directly, via non-covalent interactions, with cell-surface receptor sites for either the GAG chains or the core protein, or via indirect means that involve a second extracellular macromolecule, such as the glycoproteins fibronectin or vitronectin, acting as a bridge between the PG and a cell-surface receptor such as integrin (Toole, 1991). In general, attachment of the PG to the cell surface via non-covalent interactions does not involve a specific ARG–GLY–ASP sequence as utilized by other matrix glycoproteins such as fibronectin and integrins.

Just as cell adhesive responses are promoted by cell surface PG, PG within the extracellular matrix are also capable of interfering with cell adhesion. Small interstitial dermatan sulphate PG readily inhibit the capacity of fibroblasts to adhere to a fibronectin substratum (Rosenberg *et al.*, 1986). The PG in the extracellular matrix competitively interact with other extracellular matrix glycoprotein ligands, such as fibronectin, thereby blocking the interaction of the ligand with the cell-surface receptor (Winnemoller *et al.*, 1991; Lewandowska *et al.*, 1991). Steric exclusion effects of large interstitial PG (such as versican) at the cell surface may also play a role in preventing the interaction of cell receptors with a specific ligand in the extracellular matrix (Yamagata *et al.*, 1989).

Extracellular matrix deposition is mediated via interaction of matrix components and cell-surface receptors (McKeown-Longo and Mosher, 1985) for the involvement of cell-surface PG in matrix deposition. Evidence is derived from studies on malignantly transformed cells containing undersulphated heparan sulphate. These cells bind matrix proteins with reduced affinity, indicating a lack of matrix deposition (David and van den Berghe, 1983; Robinson *et al.*, 1984).

The migration of cells through the extracellular matrix proceeds via the continual formation and disruption of adhesion sites between the cell-surface receptors and the matrix ligands as the cell changes shape. The process also involves a corresponding change in the pericellular environment, replacing the dense fibrous matrix, which withholds the cell, with a more open network. A variety of studies have shown PG to influence cell migration, with a number of mechanisms proposed. This is clearly relevant when considering the possible role of fibroblast motility in tooth eruption (see Chapter 9), cell homoeostasisand collagen fibre orientation (see Chapter 2).

Chondroitin sulphate PG have been strongly implicated in promoting cell migration. Malignant cells express increased amounts of chondroitin sulphate, which leads to reduced adhesiveness of these cells (Iozzo, 1985). In addition, the removal of a chondroitin sulphate PG, immunologically similar to CD 44 and present on the surface of mouse melanoma cells, prevents their migration and invasion into a collagen type I substratum, although the cells still remained attached to the matrix (Faassen *et al.*, 1992). In each of these studies, chondroitin sulphate PG were proposed to act via destabilization of the adhesion sites with extracellular matrix ligands, thereby promoting cell migration. Not all cells possess this chondroitin sulphate PG on their cell surface, and other cell-surface PG have been implicated in cell migration. An increase in syndecan has been demonstrated in migrating and proliferating vascular epithelial and endothelial cells in response to wound healing (Elenius *et al.*, 1991), although the precise role of the PG is unclear.

Heparan sulphate membrane-intercalated PG may link intracellular cytoskeletal and extracellular matrix components in facilitating the spread of cells such as fibroblasts on a substratum (Woods *et al.*, 1985). During the formation of cell–cell matrix adhesion sites, these cell-surface PG concentrate in ruffled areas, and later, after interaction with an immobilized extracellular ligand, cause organization of actin into stress fibres (Woods *et al.*, 1986; Izzard *et al.*, 1986).

The presence of certain PG within the extracellular matrix also appears to be critical for cell migration. For example, Kinsella and Wight (1986) demonstrated that stationary vascular endothelial cells produce an extracellular matrix rich in heparan sulphate PG. Upon induction to migrate, an extracellular matrix rich in chondroitin sulphate and dermatan sulphate was produced, presumably conveying a destabilizing effect upon the adhesion sites. In a separate example, heparan sulphate and chondroitin sulphate have been shown to significantly increase the activation of plasminogen, which in turn activates metalloproteinases (such as collagenase) to produce the proteolytic events associated with cell migration. Circumstantial evidence also suggests that hyaluronan plays a role in cell migration, with a significant but transient rise in the GAG associated with increased cell motility that is seen during inflammation, wound healing, tumour invasion, and morphogenesis (Toole, 1991). The process appears to involve either a specific cell-surface hyaluronan receptor (Boudreau *et al.*, 1991) or CD-44 (Lesley *et al.*, 1990).

Recent studies have suggested that chondroitin sulphate PG inhibit cell migration via steric exclusion mechanisms. Areas enriched with chondroitin sulphate PG have been implicated in the prevention of axonal outgrowth of retinal cones (Brittis *et al.*, 1992) and neural crest migration in chick embryos (Perris *et al.*, 1991). In both these studies removal of the chondroitin sulphate resulted in new cell outgrowth.

A number of investigations have implicated different PG in the regulation of cell differentiation and proliferation, with a number of mechanisms proposed. Evidence to suggest that PG play a role in cell differentiation is mainly derived from studies on cartilage development. Chondrocyte differentiation from fibroblast-like mesenchymal cells is associated with an initiation in the synthesis of aggrecan (Goetinck, 1982), thereby possibly destabilizing cell adhesion, which is a prerequisite for maintaining cell differentiation (West *et al.*, 1979). Heparin has also been suggested as a regulatory factor in chondrocyte differentiation (San Antonio *et al.*, 1987) but mechanisms for its actions are not clear.

Cell-surface PG have been identified as receptors for a number of growth factors, thus influencing cell proliferation or metabolism (see Chapters 1 and 12). Heparan sulphate cell-surface PG present on fibroblasts have been described as receptors for platelet-derived growth factor and epidermal growth factor (Rapraeger *et al.*, 1991). A cell-surface chondroitin sulphate PG or heparan sulphate PG that binds TGF-β with high affinity and specificity has been characterized from Chinese hamster ovary cells (Cheifetz and Massague, 1989) and fibroblasts (Segarini and Seyedin, 1987). The binding of the growth factor is via the core protein rather than the GAG chains. Studies indicate, however, that this cell-surface receptor does not directly mediate the effect of the growth factor (Boyd and Massague, 1989); rather it may act as a storage site or regulator for TGF-β action.

Extracellular matrix PG, such as the small interstitial dermatan sulphate PG, also possess a binding affinity for growth factors such as TGF-β (Yamaguchi *et al.*, 1990), thereby neutralizing its effect and inhibiting cell proliferation. Suggestions have been made that these PG function as protectors of these growth factors from proteolysis (Vlodavsky *et al.*, 1991; Damon *et al.*, 1989) and as regulators for their release and activity. Moreover, TGF-β is also capable of increasing the expression of a number of extracellular matrix components in various cell systems, with the induction of PG as high as twenty-fold (Bassols and Massague, 1988). Extracellular matrix PG, such as decorin, may act as a feedback regulator for the activity of growth factors.

There is evidence to suggest that heparin and heparan sulphate also display an anti-proliferative effect on various cells. This inhibitory effect is exerted by heparan sulphate PG produced by confluent, but not sub-confluent, cultures of smooth muscle cells (Fritze *et al.*, 1985) and vascular endothelial cells (Castellot *et al.*, 1981). Further, the heparan sulphate PG produced by lung endothelial cells proved to be a more potent inhibitor of cell proliferation than commercial heparin (Benitz *et al.*, 1990). The inhibition by heparin and heparan sulphate PG appears to suppress entry of the cells into the S phase of cell growth (Castellot *et al.*, 1987; Pukac *et al.*, 1990).

The mechanism by which these PG inhibit cell growth is still far from clear. Castellot *et al.* (1985) have demonstrated that heparin is bound directly by smooth muscle cell followed by internalization. These observations, together with the identification of heparan sulphate as a constituent of the nuclear fraction in liver cells (Fedarko and Conrad, 1986) and its inhibitory effect on DNA polymerase *in vitro* (Winterbourne and Salisbury, 1981; Furukawa and Bhavanadan, 1983), have led to suggestions that this is the mechanism by which heparin and heparan sulphate influence cell proliferation.

PROTEOGLYCAN–COLLAGEN INTERACTION

The interaction of PG with collagen is now recognized as being of great functional importance, particularly with regard to the architecture and geometry of the PDL. The precipitation, growth, and calcification of collagen fibres are all likely to be controlled by the collagen–proteoglycan interaction.

Numerous studies have investigated the interaction of GAG and PG with collagen. The interaction depends mainly on electrostatic forces, which are readily disrupted by raising the salt concentration (Obrink, 1973a; Toole and Lowther, 1968), and which are probably significant at physiological pH and ionic strength. *In vitro* studies of the GAG–collagen interaction have shown that, in general, GAG interact more strongly with collagen with increasing charge density and chain length, and, that the reaction is dependent upon the secondary structure of the polysaccharide chain.

Those GAG rich in iduronic acid, dermatan sulphate, heparin, and heparan sulphate interacted strongly with collagen gels (Obrink, 1973a; Obrink and Sundelof, 1973). The interaction of heparan sulphate with collagen gels was also dependent upon the core protein and was abolished upon its removal, although involvement of the GAG chains was confirmed by the competitive inhibitory effect of heparin (Obrink and Wasteson, 1971). High molecular weight chondroitin sulphate chains bound to collagen gels (Mathews, 1970), but chondroitin sulphate and heparan sulphate did not interact with collagen fibrils that had been reconstituted under physiological conditions. (Koda and Bernfield, 1984). Heparin was shown to interact with both collagen gels and fibres (Obrink and Wasteson, 1971; Koda and Bernfield, 1984). The interaction of hyaluronan or keratan sulphate with collagen was negligible (Obrink, 1973a).

In vitro studies have shown that GAG and PG also affect fibrillogenesis of collagen. Collagen fibril formation occurs spontaneously and rapidly at physiological pH and ionic strength, at 37°C. Dermatan sulphate, heparan sulphate, and heparin, which all strongly interact with collagen, accelerated nucleation and fibril growth at 4°C (Obrink, 1973a; Obrink and Sundelof, 1973c). Chondroitin sulphate and keratan sulphate displayed little effect (Gross and Kirk, 1958; Wood and Keech, 1960). Hyaluronan, however, enhanced fibrillogenesis, possibly by the exhibition of steric exclusion effects (Obrink, 1973a).

The data available for the effect of PG on fibrillogenesis is occasionally contradictory. Aggregated chondroitin sulphate cartilage PG were shown either to inhibit fibril growth (Oegema *et al.*, 1975; Obrink, 1973b) or to have little effect (Chandrasekhar *et al.*, 1984). These PG bound strongly with type I collagen molecules, via strong electrostatic interaction of the GAG chains, although the core protein was also able to interact with type I collagen following removal of the chondroitin sulphate chains (Oegema *et al.*, 1975; Toole, 1976).

Similarly, the small dermatan sulphate PG inhibited fibrillogenesis in vitro, and interacted with type I collagen via both its GAG and protein moieties (Vogel *et al.*, 1984). Both the large chondroitin sulphate PG and the small dermatan sulphate PG were incorporated into the collagen fibrils (Scott *et al.*, 1986; Obrink, 1973a,b). However, the presence of the GAG chains, chondroitin sulphate or dermatan sulphate, during fibril formation did not lead to their subsequent incorporation (Oegema *et al.*, 1975; Obrink, 1973b). These results suggested that the complexes formed between the GAG or PG and collagen are broken during aggregation with other collagen molecules (Scott, 1988). Indeed, chondroitin sulphate PG entrapped in collagen fibrils were not in equilibrium with the surrounding solution and were lost with time (Oegema *et al.*, 1975).

Recent studies by Scott and co-workers have visualized the interaction of dermatan sulphate PG with collagen fibrils by electron microscopy using the cationic reagent, cupromeronic blue. This electron-dense dye (at a particular critical electrolyte concentration) specifically stains for the GAG chains associated with PG, which are maintained in an extended configuration that closely resembles their condition in the native tissue. The tissue electron density was 'intensified' using uranyl acetate to visualize the collagen fibres. Using this technique, a number of tissues rich in type I collagen have been studied. PG filaments were visualized on the outside of tendon collagen fibrils from rat tail in a regular orthogonal array spaced at a distance equivalent to the repeat 'D' distance (approximately 62 nm) (Scott and Orford, 1981). The PG filaments were localized mainly at the 'd' band, with a few at the 'c' band, both in the gap zone. In addition, other PG were seen parallel to the fibril surface spanning the gap between the adjacent D-spaced PG filaments (Scott, 1980), while PG filaments of varying length and thickness, but no definite orientation, were seen between the collagen fibrils (Scott and Orford, 1981). Biochemical analysis and resistance to hyaluronidase digestion suggested that the PG arranged orthogonal to the collagen fibril was rich in dermatan sulphate (Scott and Orford,1981). Similar arrangements of PG in relation to collagen fibrils have been demonstrated in skin and sclera (Scott and Haigh, 1985). No orthogonally arranged gap-zone-associated PG were identified in bone organic matrix (Scott and Haigh, 1985). This finding has led to the interpretation of an inhibitory role for these dermatan sulphate PG during calcification.

These studies also suggested a role for PG in collagen fibril radial growth. In foetal tendon, such growth occurs within a hyaluronan- and PG-rich environment (Scott *et al.*, 1981). The fibrils, which are very thin, showed D-periodic PG attachment (Scott, 1980) and the presence of dermatan sulphate (Scott *et al.*, 1981). Interestingly, during expansion of the collagen fibrils associated with muscle loading, there was a striking loss of hyaluronan and chondroitin sulphate from the extracellular matrix, which then became rich in dermatan sulphate (Scott *et al.*, 1981; Scott and Hughes, 1986). These observations have led to the suggestion that high concentrations of hyaluronan and PG may control the radial expansion and cross-linking of collagen fibrils (Scott *et al.*, 1981). *In vivo*, collagen fibrils grow radially, despite the presence of PG at the fibril surface, which are probably displaced during fusion of the collagen monomers. The PG therefore may perform some regulatory role in controlling the rate of growth and fusion of collagen fibrils (Scott, 1988). The possible functional significance of collagen fibril diameters and the nature of the ground substance in terms of tooth support is discussed in Chapter 10.

GROUND SUBSTANCE AND CHRONIC INFLAMMATORY PERIODONTAL DISEASE

The accumulation of dental plaque in the subgingival and supragingival regions of periodontal tissues inevitably leads to chronic gingivitis and ultimately to chronic periodontitis. The presence of bacterial enzymes and various other products such as lipopolysaccharide initiates a degradative response of the periodontal tissues, leading to loss of structural integrity. Whether the bacterial products act directly or as initiators of host response, or both, is not clear, but the range of experimental evidence designed to examine changes in the ground substance of the periodontium is beginning to shed light on the process.

Histochemical findings by Dewar (1955) indicated a loss of GAG from inflammatory sites in gingiva, a finding supported by the biochemical analysis of GAG in diseased and healthy gingival tissues by Ciancio and Mather (1971). In contrast, Embery *et al.* (1979) showed that the types and quantities of GAG in non-inflamed and severely inflamed human gingival tissue did not differ, a finding corroborated by Bartold and Page (1986b).

Embery *et al.* (1979) also showed that the protein core of PG undergoes structural modification in severe inflammation, causing release of free GAG such as chondroitin-4-sulphate and dermatan sulphate, which then remain apparently unchanged. The reason for this lack of change is unknown, but it may be due to lack of specific hydrolytic enzymes or the inhibition of hydrolytic enzymes by serum factors such as macroglobulins. This concept is important, since it counters standard thinking, which links the presence of hydrolytic enzymes in oral fluids with inflammatory periodontal disease state and degradation of connective tissue. This alteration in overall PG structure rather than the liberated constituent GAG during CIPD is also supported by the work of Bartold and Page (1986a).

These workers also showed that gingival fibroblasts, from patients with normal and inflamed gingiva, studied *in vitro* to assess the influence of inflammation on PG and hyaluronan synthesis, demonstrated an increase in high molecular weight hyaluronic acid in inflamed tissue. There was also an increase in dermatan sulphate PG, a decrease in chondroitin sulphate PG, and an overall reduction in the pool of PG.

Purvis *et al.* (1987), investigating the molecular weight profiles of PG from normal, inflamed, and severely inflamed gingival tissues, showed parallel changes in the GAG profiles of these tissues. Changes were evident in the molecular size of the PG, with a higher proportion of low molecular weight proteoglycans featuring in the more inflamed tissues. The relative amounts of chondroitin sulphate and dermatan sulphate also varied within the three types of tissue, with the DS–C4S ratio being highest in the severely inflamed tissue, indicating selective degradation of the PG present.

The proteinases capable of degrading periodontal tissue have been discussed already, and enzymes capable of depolymerizing GAG via hydrolytic routes include hyaluronidases, chondroitinases and glucuronidases (Kennedy, 1979).

Bacterial enzymes capable of depolymerizing the GAG constituents of ground substance are also present in dental plaque and general oral flora. Several species of oral bacteria in plaque have hyaluronidase activity (Tam and Chan, 1985; Tipler and Embery, 1985). In human gingival crevicular fluid, the bacterial hyaluronidase activity is higher at inflamed areas than at normal sites (van Palenstein-Helderman and Hoogeveen, 1976), and correlates with an increase in the number of Gram-positive bacteria. Bacterial hyaluronidases are distinguishable from those of mammalian origin by their different pH optima (Hopps and Prout, 1972) and by the nature of the enzymatic mechanism. Bacterial hyaluronidase operates via an elimination reaction resulting in the production of Δ-4, 5 unsaturated oligo- and disaccharides, whereas the mammalian enzyme functions via a hydrolytic cleavage process (Tipler and Embery, 1985). Hyaluronidase and chondroitinase are produced by oral streptococci (Schultz-Haudt and Sherp, 1955) and have been isolated from peptostreptococci (Tam and Chan, 1985) and certain staphylococci (Burnett and Sherp, 1968). Strains of *P. gingivalis* and *B. melaninogenicus*, both of which are implicated in CIPD, are also sources of these enzymes (Steffen and Hentges, 1981; Tipler and Embery, 1985). Recently Smith *et al.*, (1991) described a wide range of proteolytic enzymes present in the membranous vesicles of *P. gingivalis* that may act as virulence factors in ground substance breakdown.

CLINICAL AND PHYSIOLOGICAL ASPECTS OF GROUND SUBSTANCE

Changes in the ground substance of the developing PDL are evident during tooth eruption. Gibson (1979) reported data on three groups of bovine developing incisors, where Group 1 consisted of dental follicle, Group 2 had developed a PDL ,and Group 3 had discernible Sharpey's fibres.

The marked decrease in hyaluronate from Group 1 to Group 2 is similar to that which occurs during embryonic development of other connective tissues, e.g. skin (Kawamoto and Nagai, 1976). This may be responsible for the decrease in water content and cell-free spaces during differentiation (Fisher and Solursh, 1977). The fall in hyaluronate (probably due to hyaluronidase activity) coincides with the onset of cytodifferentiation (Toole, 1979). Exogenous hyaluronate inhibited the synthesis of sulphated GAG by chondrocytes (Solursh *et al.*, 1980) but not by skin fibroblasts (Wiebkin and Muir, 1973). In bovine PDL, both types of sulphated GAG chains increased slightly (on a dry basis) between Groups 1 and 2 and more markedly between Groups 2 and 3. Subsequently, dermatan sulphate (and presumably proteodermatan sulphate) showed little change on a dry weight basis and decreased to some extent relative to collagen content. On the other hand, the sulphated galactosaminoglycans associated with PG1 continued to increase over the whole period of eruption, only falling in the final stages. This increase was most noticeable when expressed relative to the collagen content.

These results raise questions about the role of PG in tooth eruption. If PG are involved, it seems more likely to be PG1 than proteodermatan sulphate, not only because of the quantitative changes, but also on account of the probable locations of the PG in the tissues. An interfibrillar location of PG1 would allow a fuller expression of its ability to influence osmotic pressure and swelling of the tissue compared with proteodermatan sulphate, which is more intimately associated with collagen fibrils. The latter association might partly 'tie up' the dermatan sulphate chains and reduce their effect on tissue swelling, a similar action to that observed when GAG in umbilical cord or cornea were allowed to interact with polycations (Gelman and Silberberg, 1976; Comper and Laurent, 1978). Hyaluronate, like PG1, will be less affected by interactions with collagen. However, the content of this glycosaminoglycan was almost constant during eruption.

Thus, PG1 may have a controlling influence on the internal osmotic pressure of bovine PDL during tooth eruption. Because of the non-ideal behaviour of GAG and PG, the effects of small changes in concentration on osmotic pressure are amplified (Comper and Laurent, 1978; Urban *et al.*, 1979). An increase in osmotic pressure arising from an increasing concentration of PG1 may be opposed by an osmotic pull on the interstitial water by the plasma proteins over the capillary wall, and the physical swelling of the tissue will be opposed by the 'elastic contribution' of the collagen fibres (Comper and Laurent, 1978).

There is some evidence of a relationship between ground substance and tooth mobility (see Chapter 10). Picton (1984) studied axial mobility and changes in rest position over 3-hour periods. No loads were applied to 10 teeth but all were displaced into their sockets to a sustained level by a screw for 3 hours. Mobility decreased for those teeth that were intruded a distance equivalent to less than 800 mN force, but it increased after greater intrusion. Vascular changes were considered to play no part and it is more likely that aggregation of PG occurred in the periodontal ground substance where there was little or no displacement of the tooth. Displacement would have generated tension in the collagen fibres of the PDL, leading to smaller PG proteoglycan molecules being formed and a consequent increase in mobility.

In a further study, Embery *et al.* (1987) investigated changes in the PDL ground substance associated with short-term intrusive loadings in macaque monkeys. PG-like fractions were isolated from the ligaments of teeth undergoing various degrees of intrusive loadings. The PG were characterized by their molecular-size profiles on Sepharose 4B, by the presence of uronic acid in the separated fractions, and by the electrophoretic detection of constituent GAG, including heparan sulphate, hyaluronic acid, dermatan sulphate, and chondroitin-4-sulphate. The high molecular weight fraction, peak I (estimated minimum size, $2{\times}10^6$ Da) of the normal functioning (stressed) ligament was reduced by 70 per cent, compared with ligament left undisturbed for 3 hours. There was a decrease in peak I size between 0.25 N and 1 N loadings of approximately 72 per cent. The 4 N loadings produced a further decrease followed by an increase during a 3-hour undisturbed recovery phase. From this it was suggested that changes in the structure of ground substance components of the PDL, particularly in the aggregated forms of the PG present, could explain apparent changes in tooth mobility.

One further aspect relating to the study of ground substance components is the evidence for age-related changes. Weinstein *et al.* (1992) investigated the incorporation of ^{3}H-glucosamine and ^{35}sulphate into gingival segments isolated from rats in the age range 4–18 weeks. Two distinct PG fractions differing in degree of sulphation were obtained by ion-exchange chromatography. Incorporation of both labels in the undersulphated fraction increased with age; there was a pronounced decrease with age in the sulphated PG fraction. The undersulphated PG showed an age-dependent decrease in hyaluronic acid, and increases in dermatan and chondroitin-4-sulphate and chondroitin-6-sulphate. Gel filtration of the sulphated PG fraction yielded high and low molecular weight PG, the GAG of which were particularly rich (61–76 per cent) in dermatan sulphate. Smaller quantities of chondroitin 4-sulphate, chondroitin-6-sulphate, and heparan sulphate were also present. All GAG showed a decrease in content with age.

One concluding aspect is the recognition that ground substance components may feature as biomarkers of PDL destruction. An extensive series of studies recently reviewed by Embery *et al.*

(1991) have pointed to a chondroitin-4-sulphate PG in gingival crevicular fluid tentatively identified as decorin. This putative marker is evident in clinical situations where relatively rapid alveolar bone resorption is occurring, e.g. orthodontic movement and acute periodontitis. It possesses a protein core in the range 56–71 kDa, which shows a close similarity to the parent PG present in alveolar bone. Such a biochemical approach is in principle more sensitive than the usual clinical indices. With further details of the ground substance components of PDL constantly emerging, the possibility arises of their use as biomarkers for the study of PDL in health or disease.

REFERENCES

Anderson JC (1976) Glycoproteins of the connective tissue matrix. Int Rev Connect Tissue Res 7, 251–322.

Bartold PM, Wiebkin OW and Thonard JC (1981) Glycosaminoglycans of human gingival epithelium and connective tissues. Connect Tissue Res 9, 99–106.

Bartold PM and Page RC (1985) Isolation, identification and quantification of glycosaminoglycans synthesized by human gingival fibroblasts in vitro. J Periodont Res 20, 284–292.

Bartold PM and Page RC (1986a) The effect of chronic inflammation on gingiva; connective tissue proteoglycans and hyaluronic acid. J Oral Path 15, 367–374.

Bartold PM and Page RC (1986b) Proteoglycans synthesised by cultured fibroblasts derived from normal and inflamed human gingiva in vitro. Cell Dev Biol 22, 407–417.

Bartold PM and Page RC (1987) Isolation and characterization of proteoglycans synthesized by human gingival fibroblasts in vitro. Arch Biochem Biophys. 253, 399–412.

Bartold PM, Wiebkin OW and Thonard JC (1983) Proteoglycans of human gingival epithelium and connective tissue. Biochem J 211, 119–127.

Bartold PM, Wiebkin OW and Thonard JC. (1984) The effect of oxygen derived free radicals on gingival proteoglycans and hyaluronic acid. J Periodont Res 19, 390–400.

Bassols A and Massague J (1988) Transforming growth factor-β regulates the expression and structure of extracellular matrix chondroitin/dermatan sulphate proteoglycans. J Biol Chem 263, 3039–3045.

Baumhammers A and Stallard RE (1968) ^{35}sulphate utilisation and turnover by the connective tissues of the periodontium. J Periodont Res 3, 187–193.

Beaven LA, Davies M, Couchman JR, Williams, MA and Mason RM (1989) *In vivo* turnover of the basement membrane and other heparan sulphate proteoglycans of rat glomerulus. Arch Biochem Biophys. 269, 579–585.

Benitz WE, Kelley RT, Anderson CM, Lorant DE and Bernfield M (1990) Endothelial heparan sulphate proteoglycan. I. Inhibitory effects on smooth muscle cell proliferation. Am J Respir Cell Mol Biol 2, 13–24.

Boudreau N, Turley E and Rabinovitch M (1991) Fibronectin, hyaluronan and a hyaluronan binding protein contribute to increased ductus arteriosus smooth muscle cell migration. Dev Biol 143, 235–247.

Bourdon MA, Oldberg A, Pierschbacher M and Ruoslahati E (1985) Molecular cloning and sequence analysis of a chondroitin sulphate proteoglycan cDNA. Proc Natl Acad Sci USA 82, 3121–3125.

Bourdon MA, Shiga M and Ruoslahati E (1986) Identification from cDNA of the precursor form of a chondroitin sulphate proteoglycan core protein. J Biol Chem 261, 12534–12537.

Boyd FT and Massague J (1989) Transforming growth factor-β inhibition of epithelial cell proliferation linked to the expression of a 53-kDa membrane receptor. J Biol Chem 264, 2272–2278.

Brenner DA, O'Hara M, Angel P, Chojkier M and Karin M (1989) Prolonged activation of Jun and collagenase genes by tumour necrosis factor-α . Nature 337, 661–663.

Brittis PA, Canning DR and Silver J (1992) Chondroitin sulphate as a regulator of neuronal patterning in the retina. Science 255, 733–736.

Buckwalter JA, Rosenberg LC and Ungar R. (1987) Changes in proteoglycan aggregates during cartilage mineralisation. Calcif Tissue Int 41, 228–236.

Burnett GW and Sherp HW (1968) Oral Microbiology and Infectious Diseases, 3rd edition, p 442, Williams and Wilkins, Baltimore.

Campbell IK, Roughley PJ and Mort JS. (1986) The action of human articular cartilage metalloproteinases on proteoglycans and link protein. Similarity between products of degradation in situ and in vitro. Biochem J 237, 117–122.

Carney SL and Muir H (1988) The structure and function of cartilage proteoglycans. Physiol Rev 68, 858–910.

Carrell RW and Barwell DR (1986) Serpins: The superfamily of plasma serine proteinase inhibitors. In: Proteinase Inhibitors (Barrett AJ and Salvesen G, eds) pp 403–420, Elsevier, Amsterdam.

Castellot JJ, Addonizio ML, Rosenberg R and Karnovsky MJ (1981) Cultured endothelial cells produce a heparin-like inhibitor of smooth muscle cell growth. J Cell Biol 90, 372–379.

Castellot JJ, Wong K, Herman B, et al. (1985) Binding and internalization of heparin by vascular smooth muscle cells. J Cell Physiol 124, 13–20.

Castellot, JJ, Wright, TC and Karnovsky MJ (1987) Regulation of vascular smooth muscle cell growth by heparin and heparin sulphates. Semin Thromb Hemost 13, 489–503.

Cawston TE (1986) Protein inhibitors of metallo-proteinase. In: Proteinase Inhibitors (Barrett AJ and Salvesen G, eds) pp 589–610, Elsevier, Amsterdam.

Chandrasekhar S, Kleinman HK, Hassell JR, Martin G, Termine J and Trelstad RL (1984) Regulation of type I collagen fibril assembly by link proteins and proteoglycans. Collagen Rel Res 4, 323–328.

Chang Y, Yanagishita M, Hascall VC and Wight TN (1983) Proteoglycans synthesized by smooth muscle cells derived from monkey (Macaca nemistrina) aorta. J Biol Chem 258, 5679–5688.

Cheifetz S and Massague J (1989) Transforming growth factor-β (TGF- β) receptor proteoglycan. Cell surface expression and ligand binding in the absence of glycosaminoglycan chains. J Biol Chem 264, 12025–12028.

Ciancio SG and Mather ML (1971) Acid mucopolysaccharides in gingivitis and periodontitis. J Period Res 6, 188–193.

Clark CC and Kefalides NA (1978) Localisation and partial composition of the oligosaccharide units on the propeptide extension of type I procollagen. J Biol Chem 253, 47–51.

Comper CD and Laurent TC (1978) Physiological function of connective tissue polysaccharides. Physiol Rev 58, 255–315.

Connor NS, Aubin JE and Melcher AH (1984) The distribution of fibronectin in rat tooth and periodontal tissues. An immunogluorescence study using monoclonal antibody. J Histochem Cytochem 32, 565–572.

Coster L and Fransson LA (1981) Isolation and characterisation of dermatan sulphate proteoglycans from bovine sclera. Biochem J 193, 143–153.

Coster L (1979) Dermatan sulphate proteoglycans. Thesis, University of Lund.

Coster L, Fransson LA, Sheehan J, Nieduszynski IA and Phelps CF (1981) Self-association of dermatan sulphate proteoglycans from bovine sclera. Biochem J 197, 483–490.

Damon DH, Lobb RR, D'Amore PA and Wagner JA (1989) Heparin potentiates the action of acidic fibroblast growth factor by prolonging its biological half-life. J Cell Physiol 138, 221–226.

David G and van den Berghe H (1983) Transformed mouse mammary epithelial cells synthesize under sulphated basement membrane proteoglycan. J Biol Chem 258, 7338–7344.

Davies M, Martin J, Thomas GJ and Lovett DH (1992) Proteinases and glomerular matrix turnover. Kidney Int. 41, 671–678.

Dayer J-M, Beutler B and Cerami A (1985) Cachectin/tumour necrosis factor stimulates collagenase and prostaglandin E_2 production by human synovial cells and dermal fibroblasts. J Exp Med 162, 2163–2168.

De Clerk YA, Yean TD, Ratskin BJ, Lu HS and Langley KE (1989) Purification and characterisation of two related metalloproteinase inhibitors secreted by bovine aortic epithelial cells. J Biol Chem 264, 7445–7453.

Dewar MR (1955) Observations on the composition and the metabolism of normal and inflamed gingivae. J Periodontol 26, 29–39.

Dziewiatkowski DD, La Valley SJ and La Valley JA (1977) Characterisation of a proteoglycan from bovine gingiva. J Dent Res 56, 327 (abstract).

Edwards DR, Murphy G, Reynolds JJ, *et al.* (1987) Transforming growth factor modulated the expression of collagenase and metalloproteinase inhibitor. EMBO J 6, 1899–1904.

Elenius K, Vainio S, Laata M, Salmivirta M and Thesleff I (1991) Induced expression of syndecan in healing wounds. J Cell Biol 144, 585–595.

Embery G, Oliver WM and Stanbury JB (1979) The metabolism of proteoglycans and glycosaminoglycans in inflamed human gingiva. J Periodont Res 14, 512–519.

Embery G, Picton DC and Stanbury JB (1987) Biochemical changes in periodontal ligament ground substance associated with short-term intrusive loading in adult monkeys (*Macaca fasicularis*) Arch Oral Biol 32, 545–549.

Embery G, Waddington RJ and Last KS (1991) The connective tissues of the periodontium and their breakdown products in gingival crevicular fluid as markers of periodontal disease susceptibility and activity. In: Risk Markers for Oral Diseases Vol. 3: Periodontal Diseases (Johnson NW, ed), Cambridge University Press, Cambridge.

Erikson HP and Bourdon MA (1989) Ann Rev Cell Biol 5, 71–92.

Faassen AE, Schrager JA, Klein DJ, Oegema TR, Couchman JR and McCarthy JB. (1992) A cell surface chondroitin sulphate proteoglycan immunologically related to CD44 is involved in type I collagen mediated melanoma cell motility and invasion. J Cell Biol 116, 521–531.

Fedarko NS and Conrad HE (1986) A unique heparan sulphate in the nuclei of heptatocytes: Structural changes with the growth state of the cells. J Cell Biol 102, 587–599.

Fisher M and Solursh M (1977) Glycosaminoglycan localization and role in maintenance of tissue spaces in the early chick embryo. J Embryol Exp Morph 42, 195–207.

Flenniken AM and Williams BRG (1990) Developmental expression of endogenous TIMP gene and a TIMP-lacZ fusion gene in transgenic mice. Genes Dev 4, 1094–1106.

Fransson LA, Coster L, Malmstrom A and Sjoberg I (1974) The copolymer structure of pig skin dermatan sulphate. Characterisation of D-glucuronic acid-containing oligosaccharide isolated after controlled degradation of oxydermatan sulphate. Biochem J 143, 369–378.

FranssonLA, Coster L, MalmstromA and Sheehan J (1982) Self-association of sclera proteodermatan sulphate. Evidence for interaction via the dermatan sulphate side-chains. J Biol Chem 257, 6333–6338.

Freeman BA and Crapo JD (1982) Biology of disease. Free radicals and tissue injury. Lab Invest 47, 412–426.

Frisch SM and Werb Z (1989) Molecular biology of collagen degradation. In: Collagen: Molecular Biology (Olsen BR and Nimni ME, eds), pp 85–108, CRC Press, Boca Raton, Fl.

Fritze LMS, Reilley CF and Rosenberg RD (1985) An antiproliferative heparan sulphate species produced by post-confluent smooth muscle cells. J Cell Biol 100, 1041–1049.

Fujisawa R and Kuboki Y (1991) Preferential adsorption of dentin and bone acidic proteins on the (100) face of hydroxyapatite crystals. Biochem Biophys Acta 1075, 56–60.

Furukawa K and Bhavanadan VP (1993) Influences of anionic polysaccharides on DNA synthesis in isolated nuclei and by DNA polymerase alpha: correlation of observed effects with properties of the polysaccharides. Biochim Biophys Acta 740, 466–475.

Gallagher JT and Lyon M (1989) Molecular organization and functions of heparan sulphate. In: Heparin (Lane D and Lindahl U, eds), pp 135–158, Edward Arnold, London.

Galloway WA, Murphy G, Sandy JD, Gavrilovic J, Cawston TE and Reynolds JJ (1983) Purification and characterisation of a rabbit bone metalloproteinase that degrades proteoglycan and other connective tissue components. Biochem J 209, 741–752.

Gavrilovic J and Murphy G (1989) The role of plasminogen in cell-mediated collagen degradation. Cell Biol Int Rep 13, 367–375.

Gavrilovic J, Reynolds, JJ and Murphy G (1985) Inhibition of type I collagen film degradation by tumour cells using a specific antibody to collagenase and their specific tissue inhibitor of metalloproteinase (TIMP) Cell Biol Int Rep 9, 1097–1107.

Gelman RA and Silberberg A (1976) The effect of a strongly interacting macromolecular probe on the swelling and exclusion properties of loose connective tissues. Connect Tissue Res 4, 79–90.

Gibson GJ (1979) Proteoglycans of the periodontal ligament. Thesis, University of Alberta.

Goetinck PF (1982) Proteoglycans in developing embryonic cartilage. In: Glycoconjugates, Vol. 3 (Horowitz MI, ed), pp 197–229, Academic Press, New York.

Goldberg GI, Whilhelm SM, Kronberger A, Bauer EA, Grant GA and Eisen AZ (1986) Human fibroblast collagenase. Complete primary structure and homology to an oncogene transformation-induced rat protein. J Biol Chem 261, 6600–6605.

Gowen M, Wood DD, Ihrie EJ, Meats JE and Russell RGG (1984) Stimulation by human interleukin-1 of cartilage breakdown and production of collagenase and proteoglycans by human chondrocytes, but not by human osteoblasts in vitro. Biochem Biophys Acta 797, 186–193.

Gross J and Kirk D (1958) The heat precipitation of collagen from neutral salt solutions, some rate-regulating factors. J Biol Chem 233, 355–360.

Hall RC, Shellis RP, Rose RK and Embery G (1993) Influence of glycosaminoglycans and fluoride on hydroxyapatite formation *in vitro*. J Dent Res 72, 699.

Hanover JA, Elting J, Mintz GR and Lennarz WJ (1982) Temporal aspects of the N- and O-glycosylation of human chorionic gonadotropin. J Biol Chem 257, 10172-10177.

Hascall VC (1988) Proteoglycans: the chondroitin sulphate/keratan sulphate proteoglycans of cartilage. ISI Atlas Sci Biochem 1, 189–198.

Hascall VC, Heinegard DK and Wight TN (1991) Proteoglycans. Metabolism and pathology. In: Cell Biology of the Extracellular Matrix (Hay ED, ed), 2nd Edition, pp 149–175, Plenum Press, New York.

Hascall VC, Luyten FP, Plaas AHK and Sandy JD (1990) Steady state metabolism of proteoglycans in bovine articular cartilage explants. In: Methods in Cartilage Research (Maroudas A and Keuttner K, ed), pp 108–112, Academic Press, New York.

Hascall VC, Morales TI, Hascall GK, Handley CJ and McQuillan DJ (1983) Biosynthesis and turnover of proteoglycans in organ culture of bovine articular cartilage. J Rheumatol Suppl 10, 45–52.

Hassall JR, Pennypacker JP, Yamada KM and Pratt PM (1978) Changes in cell surface proteins during normal and vitamin A-inhibited chondrogenesis in vitro. Ann NY Acad Sci 312, 406–409.

Hassel TM and Stanek EJ (1983) Evidence that healthy human gingiva contains functionally heterogeneous fibroblast subpopulation. Arch Oral Biol 28, 617–625.

Hassell JR, Kimura JH and Hascall VC (1986) Proteoglycan core protein families. Ann Rev Biochem 55, 539–567.

Heath JK, Atkinson SJ, Hembery RM, Reynolds JJ and Meikle MC (1987) Bacterial antigens induce collagenase and prostaglandin E_2 synthesis in human gingival fibroblasts through a primary effect on circulating mononuclear cells. Infect Immun 55, 2148–2154.

Heath JK, Gowen M, Meikle MC and Reynolds JJ (1982) Human gingival tissues in culture synthesize three metalloproteinases and a metalloproteinase inhibitor. J Periodont Res 17, 183–190.

Heck LW, Blackthorn WD, Irwin MH and Abrahamson,DR (1990) Degradation of basement membrane laminin by human neutrophil elastase and cathepsin. G Am J Path. 136, 1267–1274.

Heidtmann H and Travis J (1986) Human 1 proteinase inhibitor. In: Proteinase Inhibitors (Barrett AJ and Salversen G, eds), pp 457–476, Elsevier, Amsterdam.

Hiramatsu M, Abe I and Minami N (1978) Acid mucopolysaccharides in porcine gingiva. J Periodont Res 13, 224–231.

Hopps RM and Prout RES (1972) Identification of tissue and bacterial hyaluronidase in human saliva. J Periodont Res 7, 236–241.

Howell DS and Pita JC (1976) Calcification of growth plate cartilage with special reference to studies on micropuncture fluids. Clin Orthop 118, 208–229.

Howell DS, Pita JC, Marquez JF and Gatter RA (1969) Demonstration of macromolecular inhibitors of calcification and nucleational factors in fluid from calcifying sites in cartilage. J Clin Invest 48, 630–641.

Hynes RO, Schwarzbauer JE and Tamkun JW (1984) Fibronectin: a versatile gene for a versatile protein. In: Basement Membranes and Cell Movement. Ciba Foundation Symposium 108 (Porter R and Whelan J, eds), pp 75–85, Pitman Press, London.

Iozzo RV (1985) Neoplastic modulation of extracellular matrix. J Biol Chem 260, 7464–7473.

Ishihara M, Fedarko NS and Conrad HD (1987) Involvement of phosphatidylinositol and insulin in the co-ordinate regulation of proteoheparan sulphate metabolism and hepatocyte growth. J Biol Chem 262, 4708–4716.

Izzard CS, Radinsky R and Culp LA (1986) Substratum contacts and cytoskeletal reorganisation of BALB/c 3T3 cells on a cell-binding fragment and heparin-binding fragments of plasma fibronectin. Exp Cell Res 165, 320–336.

Jalkanen M, Jalkanen S and Bernfield M (1991) Binding of extracellular molecules by cell surface proteoglycans. In: Biology of Extracellular Matrix: Receptors for Extracellular Matrix (Ed Hay ED), pp 1–37, Academic Press, Orlando.

Kapoor R, Phelps CF and Wight TN (1986) Physical properties of chondroitin sulphate/dermatan sulphate proteoglycans from bovine aorta. Biochem J 240, 575–583.

Kawamoto T and Nagai Y (1976) Developmental changes in glycosaminoglycans, collagen and collagenase activity in embryonic chick skin. Biochem Biophys Acta 437, 190–199.

Kennedy JF (1979) Proteoglycans – biological and chemical aspects in human life, pp 206–220, Elsevier, Amsterdam

Kinsella MG and Wight TN (1986) Modulation of sulphated proteoglycan synthesis by bovine aortic endothelial cells during migration. J Cell Biol 102, 679–687.

Kirkham J, Robinson C and Spence J (1989) Site specific variations in the biochemical composition of healthy sheep periodontium. Arch Oral Biol 34, 405–411.

Kirkham J, Robinson C, Smith AJ and Spence JA (1992) The effect of periodontal disease on sulphated glycosaminoglycan distribution in the sheep periodontium. Arch Oral Biol 37, 1031–1037.

Kirkham J, Robinson C, Phull JK, Shore RC, Moxham BJ and Berkovitz BKB (1993) The effect of rate of eruption on periodontal ligament glycosaminoglycan content and enamel formation in the rat incisor. Cell Tissue Res 274, 413–419.

Kleinman HK, McGarvey ML, Hassell JR, et al. (1986) Basement membrane complexes with biological activity. Biochemistry 25, 312–318.

Kleinman HK, Weeks BS, Schnaper HW, Kibbey MC, Yamamura K and Grant DS (1993) The laminins: a family of basement membrane glycoproteins important in cell differentiation and tumour metastases. Vitam Horm 47, 161–186.

Koda JE and Bernfield M (1984) Heparan sulphate proteoglycans from mouse mammary epithelial cells: basal extracellular proteoglycan binds specifically to native type I collagen fibrils. J Biol Chem 259, 11763–11770.

Kornfeld R and Kornfeld S (1985) Assembly of asparagine-linked oligosaccharides. Annu Rev Biochem 54, 631–664.

Krusius T and Ruoslahti E (1986) Primary structure of an extracellular matrix proteoglycan core protein deduced from cloned cDNA. Proc Natl Acad Sci USA 83, 7683–7687.

Lajava H, Hakkinen L and Rahmetulla F (1992) A biochemical analysis of human periodontal tissue proteoglycans. Biochem J 284, 267–274.

Larivee J, Sodek J and Ferrier JM (1986) Collagenase and collagenase inhibitor activities in crevicular fluid of patients receiving treatment for localised juvenile periodontitis. J Periodont Res 21, 702–715.

Laurent TC (1977) Interaction between proteins and glycosamino-glcyans. Fed Proc 36, 24–27.

Lesley J, Schult R and Hyman R (1990) Binding of hyaluronic acid to lymphoid cell line is inhibited by monoclonal antibodies against Pgp-1. Exp Cell Res 187, 224–233.

Lewandoska K, Choi HU, Rosenberg LC, Zardi L and Culp LA (1987) Fibronectin-mediated adhesion of fibroblasts: inhibition by dermatan sulphate proteoglycan and evidence for a cryptic glycosaminoglycan-binding domain. J Cell Biol 105, 1443–1454.

Lewandowska K, Choi HU, Rosenberg LC, Sasse J, Neame PJ and Culp LA (1991) Extracellular matrix adhesion-promoting activities of a dermatan sulphate proteoglycan-associated protein (22K) from bovine fetal skin. J Cell Sci 99, 657–668.

Lindner E, Vahari A, Ruoslahti E and Wartiovaara J (1975) Distribution of fibroblast surface antigen in the developing chick embryo. J Exp. Medicine 142, 41–49.

Lohmander LS, Hascall VC, Yanagishita M, Kuettner KE and Kimura JH (1986) Post-translational events in proteoglycan synthesis: Kinetics of synthesis of chondroitin sulfate and oligosaccharides on the core protein. Arch Biochem Biophys 250, 211–227.

Lukinmaa PL, Mackie EJ and Thesleff I (1991) Immunohistochemical localization of the matrix glycoproteins – tenascin and the ED-sequence-containing form of cellular fibronectin in human teeth and periodontal ligament. J Dent Res 70, 19–26.

Mariotti A and Cochran DL (1990) Characterisation of fibroblasts derived from human periodontal ligament and gingiva. J Periodontol 61, 103–111.

Martin GR, Kleinman HK, Terranova VP, Ledbetter S and Hassell JR (1984) The regulation of basement membrane formation and cell-matrix interaction by defined supramolecular components. In: Basement Membranes and Cell Movement. Ciba Foundation Symposium, 108 (Porter R and Whelan J, eds), pp 197–209, Pitman Press, London.

Mashouf K and Engel MB (1975) Maturation of periodontal ligament connective tissue in newborn rat incisor. Arch Oral Biol 20, 161–166.

Mason RM, Kimura JH and Hascall VC (1982) Biosynthesis of hyaluronic acid in cultures of chondrocytes from the Swann rat chondrosarcoma. J Biol Chem 257, 2236–2245.

Mathews MB (1970) The interactions of proteoglycans and collagen-model systems. In: Chemistry and Molecular Biology of the Intercellular Matrix (Balazs EA, ed), Vol. 2, pp 1155–1169, Academic Press, London and New York.

McKeown-Longo PJ and Mosher DF (1985) Interaction of the 70,000-mol-wt amino terminal fragment of fibronectin with the matrix-assembly receptor of fibroblasts. J Cell Biol 100, 364–374.

Meikle MC, Atkinson SJ, Ward RV, Murphy G and Reynolds JJ (1989) Gingival fibroblasts degrade type I collagen films when stimulated with tumour necrosis factor and interleukin 1: Evidence that breakdown is mediated by metalloproteinases. J Periodont Res 24, 207–213.

Meikle MC, Heath JK and Reynolds JJ (1986) Advances in understanding cell interactions in tissue resorption. Relevance to the pathogenesis of periodontal diseases and a new hypothesis. J Oral Pathol 15, 239–250.

Merrilees MJ, Sodek J and Aubin JE (1983) Effect of cells of epithelial rests of Malassez and endothelial cells on synthesis of glycosaminoglycans by periodontal ligament fibroblasts in vitro. Dev Biol 92, 146–153.

Mickalite C and Orlowski WA (1977) Study of the non-collagenous components of the periodontium. J Dent Res 56, 1023–1026.

Morgelin M, Paulsson M, Malmstrom A and Heinegard D (1989) Shared and distinct structural features of interstitial proteoglycans from different bovine tissues revealed by electron microscopy. J Biol Chem 264, 12080–12090.

Mow VC, Mak AF, Lai WM, Rosenberg LC and Tang LH (1984) Viscoelastic properties of proteoglycan subunits and aggregates in varying solution concentrations. J Biomech 17, 325–338.

Muir H (1982) Proteoglycans as organisers of the intercellular matrix. Biochem Soc Trans 11, 613–622.

Munemoto K, Iwayawa Y, Yoshida M, Sera M, Aona M and Yokomiza I (1970) Isolation and characterisation of acid mucopolysaccharides of bovine periodontal membrane. Arch Oral Biol 15, 369–382.

Murphy G and Docherty AJP (1988) Molecular studies on the connective tissue metalloproteinases and their inhbitor TIMP. In: The Control of Tissue Damage (Glavert AM, ed), pp 223–241, Elsevier, Amsterdam.

Murphy G and Reynolds JJ (1993) Extracellular matrix degradation. In: Connective Tissues and Inheritable Disorders (Eds Royce PM and Steinmann B), pp 287–316, Wiley–Liss, New York.

Myers ER, Armstrong CG and Mow VC (1984) Swelling pressure and collagen tension. In: Connective Tissue Matrix (Hukins DWL, ed), pp 161–168, Macmillan, London.

Obrink B and Sundelof LO (1973c) Light scattering in the study of associating macromolecules. The binding of glycosaminoglycans to collagen. Eur J Biochem 37, 226–232.

Obrink B and Wasteson A (1971) Nature of the interaction of chondroitin 4-sulphate and chondroitin sulphate-proteoglycan with collagen. Biochem J 121, 227–233.

Obrink B (1972) Isolation and partial characterisation of a dermatan sulphate proteoglycan from pig skin. Biochem Biophys Acta 264, 354–361.

Obrink B (1973a) A study of the interactions between monomeric tropocollagen and glycosaminoglycans. Eur J Biochem 33, 387–400.

Obrink B (1973b) The influence of glycosaminoglycans on the formation of fibres from monomeric tropocollagen in vitro. Eur J Biochem 34, 129–137.

Oegema TR, Laidlow J, Hascall VC and Dziewiatknowski DD (1975) The effect of proteoglycans on the formation of fibrils from collagen solutions. Arch Biochem Biophys 170, 698–709.

Ogston AG (1970) The biological functions of the glycosaminoglycans. In: Chemistry and Mollecular Biology of the Intercellular Matrix (Balazs EA, ed), pp 1231–1240, Academic Press, London.

Okada Y, Nagese H and Harris ED (1986) A metalloproteinase from human rheumatoid synovial fibroblasts that digests connective tissue matrix components. Purification and characterisation. J Biol Chem 261, 14245–14255.

Oldberg A and Ruoslahti E (1982) Interactions between chondroitin sulphate proteoglycan, fibronectin and collagen. J Biol Chem 257, 4859–4863.

Orlowski WA (1974) Analysis of collagen, glycoproteins and acid mucopolysaccharides in bovine and porcine dental pulp. Arch Oral Biol 19, 255–258.

Overall CM, Wiebkin OW and Thonard JC (1987) Demonstration of tissue collagenase activity in vivo and its relationship to inflammation severity in human gingiva. J Periodont Res 22, 81–88.

Pearson CH (1982) The ground substance of the periodontal ligament. In: The Periodontal Ligament in Health and Disease. (Berkovitch BKB, Moxham BJ and Newman HN, eds), pp 119–149, Peramon Press, Oxford.

Pearson CH and Gibson GJ (1982) Proteoglycans of bovine periodontal ligament and skin. Biochem J 201, 27–37.

Pearson CH and Pringle GA (1986) Chemical and immunochemical characterisation of proteoglycans in bovine and gingiva and dental pulp. Arch Oral Biol 31, 541–548.

Pearson CH, Wohllebe M, Carmichael DJ and Chovelon A (1975) Bovine periodontal ligament. An investigation of the collagen, glycosaminoglycan and insoluble glycoprotein components at different stages of development. Connect Tissue Res 3, 195–206.

Pearson CH, Winterbottom N, Fackre DS, Scott PG and Carpenter MR (1983) The NH_2-terminal amino acid sequence of bovine skin proteodermatan sulphate. J Biol Chem 258, 15101–15104.

Perris R, Krotoski D, Lallier T, Domingo C, Sorrell M and Bronner–Fraser M. (1991) Spatial and temporal changes in the distribution of proteoglycans during avian neural crest development. Development 111, 583–599.

Picton DC (1984) Changes in axial mobility of undisturbed teeth and following sustained intrusive forces in adult monkeys (Macaca fasicularis) Arch Oral Biol 29, 959–964.

Pitaru S, Aubin JE, Bhargava U and Melcher AH (1987) Immunoelectron microscopic studies on the distributions of fibronectin and actin in a cellular dense connective tissue: the periodontal ligament of the rat. J Periodont Res 22, 64–74.

Plecash JM (1974) Proteoglycans of the rate periodontium. PhD Thesis, University of Alberta, Edmonton, Canada.

Poole AR (1986) Proteoglycans in health and disease: structures and functions. Biochem J 236, 1–14.

Prehm P (1989) Identification and regulation of the eukaryotic hyaluronate synthase. Ciba Found Symp 143, 21–40.

Pukac, LA, Castellot JJ, Wright TC, Caleb BL and Karnovsky MJ (1990) Heparin inhibits c-fos and c-myc mRNA expression in smooth muscle cells. Cell Regul 1, 435–443.

Purvis JA, Embery G and Oliver WM (1984) Molecular size distribution of proteoglycans in human inflamed gingival tissue. Arch Oral Biol 29, 573–579.

Quigley JP, Gould LI, Schwimmer R and Sullivan LM (1987) Limited cleavage of cellular fibronectin by plasminogen activator purified from transformed cells. Proc Natl Acad Sci USA, 2776–2780.

Quintarelli G (1960) Histochemistry of gingiva. IV. Preliminary investigation of the mucopolysaccharides in connective tissues. Arch Oral Biol 2, 227–284.

Rahmetulla F (1992) Proteoglycans of oral tissues. Crit Rev Oral Biol Med 3, 135–162.

Rapraeger AC, Krufka A and Olwinb B. (1991) Requirement of heparan sulphate for bFGF-mediated fibroblast growth and myoblast differentiation. Science 252, 1705–1798.

Roberts AB, Heine UI, Flanders KC and Sporn MB (1990) Co-localisation of TGF-β 1 and collagen I and collagen III, fibronectin and glycosaminoglycans during lung branching morphogenesis. Development 109, 29–36.

Robinson J, Viti M and Hook M (1984) Structure and properties of an under-sulphated heparan sulphate proteoglycan synthesised by a rat hepatoma cell line. J Cell Biol 98, 946–953.

Rosenberg LC, Choi HU, Poole AR, Lewandowska K and Culp LA (1986) Biological roles of dermatan sulphate proteoglycans. In: Functions of the Proteoglycans. Ciba Foundation Symposium 124 (Evered E and Whelan J, eds), pp 47–60, John Wiley and Son, Chichester.

Roughley PJ (1977) The degradation of cartilage proteoglycans by the tissue proteinases. Proteoglycan heterogeneity and the pathway of proteolytic degradation. Biochem J 167, 639–646.

Roughley PJ and Barrett AJ (1977) The degradation of cartilage proteoglycans by tissue proteinases. Proteoglycan structure and its susceptibility to proteolysis. Biochem J 167, 629–637.
Ruoslahti E and Pierschbacher MD (1987) New perspectives in cell adhesion: RGD and integrins. Science 238, 491–497.
Sakamoto N, Okamoto H and Okuda K (1978) Glycosaminoglycans and quantitative analyses of bovine gingival glycosaminoglycans. Arch Oral Biol 23, 983–987.
Salisbury B and Wagner W (1981) Isolation and preliminary characterization of proteoglycans dissociatively extracted from human aorta. J Biol Chem 256, 8050–8057.
San Antonio JD, Winston BM and Tuan RS (1987) Regulation of chondrogenesis by heparan sulphate and structurally related glycosaminoglycans. Dev Biol 123, 17–24.
Saunders S, Jalkanen M, O'Farrell S and Bernfield M (1989) Molecular cloning of syndecan, a membrane proteoglycan. J Cell Biol 108, 1547–1556.
Schachter H (1986) Biosynthetic controls that determine the branching and microheterogeneity of protein-bound oligosaccharides. Biochem Cell Biol 64, 163–181.
Schmidt G, Robenek H, Harrach B, *et al.* (1987) Interaction of small dermatan sulphate proteoglycan from fibroblasts with fibronectin. J Cell Biol 104, 1683–1691.
Schultz-Haudt SD and Sherp HW (1955) Production of chondrosulphatase by microorganisms isolated from human gingival crevices. J Dent Res 34, 725 (abstract).
Scott JE and Haigh M (1985) Proteoglycan-type I collagen fibril interactions in bone and non-calcifying connective tissues. Biosci Rep 5, 71–81.
Scott JE and Hughes EW (1986) Proteoglycan–collagen relationships in developing chick and bovine tendons. Influence of the physiological environment. Connect Tissue Res 14, 267–278.
Scott JE and Orford CR (1981) Dermatan sulphate-rich proteoglycans associates with rat tail-tendon collagen at the d band in the gap region. Biochem J 197, 213–216.
Scott JE (1980) Collagen-proteoglycan interactions. Localisation of proteoglycan in tendon by electron microscopy. Biochem J 187, 887–891.
Scott JE (1988) Proteoglycan-fibrillar collagen interactions. Biochem J 252, 313–323.
Scott JE, Orford CR and Hughes EW (1981) Proteoglycan–collagen arrangements in developing rat tail tendon. An electron-microscopical and biochemical investigation. Biochem J 195, 573–581.
Scott PG, Winterbottom N, Dodd CM, Edwards E and Pearson CH (1986) A role for disulphide bridges in the protein core in the interaction of proteodermatan sulphate and collagen. Biochem Biophys Res Commun 138, 1348–1354.
Sear CHJ, Grant ME and Jackson DA (1977) Biosynthesis and release of glycoproteins by human skin fibroblasts in culture. Biochem J 168, 91–103.
Segarini PR and Seyedin SM (1987) The high molecular weight receptor to transforming growth factor-β contains glycosaminoglycan chains. J Biol Chem 263, 8366–8370.
Sellers A, Murphy G, Meikle MC and Reynolds JJ (1979) Rabbit bone collagenase inhibitor blocks the activity of other neutral metalloproteinases. Biochem Biophys Res Commun 87, 581–587.
Sellers A, Reynolds JJ and Meikle MC (1978) Neutral metalloproteinases of rabbit bone. Separation in latent forms of distinct enzymes that when activated degrade collagen, gelatin and proteoglycans. Biochem J 171, 492–496.
Shore RC, Berkovitz BK and Moxham BJ (1985) The effect of preventing the movement of the rat incisor on the structure of its periodontal ligament. Arch Oral Biol 30, 221–228.
Shuttleworth CA and Smalley JW (1983) Periodontal ligament. Int Rev Connect Tissue Res 10, 211–247.
Smalley JW, Shuttleworth CA and Grant ME (1984) Synthesis and secretion of sulphated glycosaminoglycans by bovine periodontal ligament fibroblasts cultures. Arch Oral Biol 29, 107–116.
Smith AJ, Greenman J and Embery G (1991) Detection and possible biological role of chondroitinase and heparinase enzymes produced by Porphyromonas gingivalis WSO. J Dent Res 70, 705.
Sodek J (1977) A comparison of the rates of synthesis and turnover of collagen and non-collagenous proteins in adult rat periodontal tissues and skin using a microassay. Arch Oral Biol 22, 655–665.
Solursh M, Hardingham TE, Hascall VC and Kimura JH. (1980) Separate effects of exogenous hyaluronic acid on proteoglycan synthesis an deposition in pericellular matrix by cultured chick embryo limb chondrocytes. Dev Biol 75, 121–129.
Steffen EK and Hentges DJ (1981) Hydrolytic enzymes of anaerobic bacteria isolated from human infections. J Clin Microbiol 14, 153–156.
Stetler-Stevenson WG, Krutzsch HC, Wacher MP, Marguiles IMK and Liotta LA (1989) The activation of human type IV collagenase proenzyme sequence identification of the major conversion product following organo-mercurial activation. J Biol Chem 264, 1353–1356.
Stetler-Stevenson WG, Kutzsch HC and Liotta LA (1989) Tissue inhibitor of metalloproteinase (TMP-2): A new member of the metalloproteinase inhibitor family. J Biol Chem 264, 17374–17378.
Stevens RL, Schwartz LB, Austen LF, Lohmander LS, Kimura JH (1982) Effects of tunicamycin on insulin binding and on proteoglycan synthesis and distribution in Swarm rat chondrosarcoma cell cultures. J Biol Chem 257, 5745–5750.
Takita K, Ohsaki Y, Nakata M and Kurisu K (1987) Immunofluorescence localization of type I and type III collagen and fibronectin in mouse dental tissues in late development and during molar eruption. Arch Oral Biol 32, 273–279.
Tam TC and Chan ECS (1985) Purification and characterisation of hyaluronidase from oral Peptostreptococcus species. Infect Imm 47, 508–513.
Tammi R, Tammi M, Hakkinen L and Larjava H (1991) Histochemical localisation of hyaluronate in human oral epithelium using a specific hyaluronate-binding probe. Arch Oral Biol 35, 219–224.
Thonard JC and Scherp HW (1962) Histochemical demonstration of acid mucopolysaccharides in human gingival epithelial intracellular spaces. Arch Oral Biol 7, 125–136.
Tipler LS and Embery G (1985) Glycosaminoglycan depolymerising enzymes produced by anaerobic bacteria isolated from the human mouth. Arch Oral Biol 30, 391–396.
Tomioka S (1981) Extraction and purification of proteodermatan sulphate from bovine gingiva. J Osaka Odont Soc 44, 587–592.
Toole BP (1979) Morphogenic role of glycosaminoglycans (acid mucopolysaccharides) in brain and other tissues. In: Neuronal Recognition (Barondes S, ed) pp 275–329, Plenum Press, New York.
Toole B (1991) Proteoglycans and hyaluronan in morphogenesis and differentiation. In: Cell Biology of Extracellular Matrix, (Hay ED, ed) 2nd edition, pp 305–341, Plenum Press, New York.
Toole BP and Lowther DA (1968) Dermatan sulphate-protein: isolation from and interaction with collagen. Arch Biochem Biophys 128, 567–578.
Toole BP (1976) Binding and precipitation of soluble collagens by chick embryo cartilage proteoglycan. J Biol Chem 251, 895–897.
Travis J and Salvesen G (1989) Human plasma proteinase inhibitors. Annu Rev Biochem 52, 655–709.
Tyler JA (1985) Chondrocyte mediated depletion of articular cartilage PG in vitro. Biochem J 225, 493–507.
Urban JPG, Maroudas A, Bayliss MT and Dillon J (1979) Swelling pressures of proteglycans at the concentrations found in cartilagenous tissues. Biorheol 16, 447–464.
van den Bos T and Tonino GJM (1984) Composition and metabolism of the extracellular matrix in the periodontal ligament of impeded and unimpeded rat incisors. Arch Oral Biol 29, 893–897.

van Palenstein-Helderman WH and Hoogeveen CJCM (1976) Bacterial enzymes and viable counts in crevices of non-inflamed gingiva. J Periodont Res 11, 25–34.

Van Wart HE and Birkedal-Hansen H (1990) The cystein switch: a principle of regulation of metalloproteinase activity with potential applicability to the entire matrix metalloproteinase gene family. Proc Natl Acad Sci USA 87, 5578–5582.

Villela B, Cogen RB, Bartolucci AA and Birkedal-Hansen (1987) Collagenolytic activity in crevicular fluid from patients with chronic adult periodontitis, localised juvenile periodontitis and gingivitis, and from health control subjects. J Periodont Res 22, 381–389.

Vlodavsky I, Bar-Shavit R, Ishai-Michaeli R, Bashkin P and Fuks Z (1991) Extracellular sequestration and release of fibroblast growth factor: A regulatory mechanism. Trends Biochem Sci 16, 268–271.

Vogel KG, Keller EJ, Lenhoff RJ, Campbell K and Koob TJ (1986) Proteoglycan synthesis by fibroblast cultures initiated from regions of adult bovine tendon subjected to different mechanical forces. Eur J Cell Biol 41, 102–112.

Vogel KK, Paulsson M and Heinegard D (1984) Specific inhibition of type I and type II collagen fibrillogenesis by the small proteoglycan of tendon. Biochem J 223, 587–597.

Waddington RJ, Embery G and Last KS (1988) The glycosaminoglycan constituents of alveolar basal bone of the rabbit. Connect Tissue Res 17, 171–180.

Weinstein M, Liau YH, Slomiany A and Slomiany BL (1992) Glycosaminoglycan pattern in gingival proteoglycans of rat with age. Arch Oral Biol 37, 323–330.

Werb Z, Mainardi CL, Vater CA and Harris ED (1977) Endogenous activation of latent proteinases by rheumatoid synovial cells. Evidence of a role of plasminogen activator. N Engl J Med 296, 1017–1023.

West CM, Lanza R, Rosenbloom J, Lowe M and Holtzer H (1979) Fibronectin alters the phenotypic properties of cultured chick embryo chondroblasts. Cell 17, 491–501.

White SM, Hulmes DJS, Miller A and Timmins PA (1977) Collagen–mineral axial relationship in calcified turkey leg tendon by x-ray and neutron diffraction. Nature 266, 421–425.

White TN, Heinegard DK and Hascall VC (1991) Proteoglycans: structure and function. In: Cell Biology of Extracellular Matrix (Hay ED, ed), pp 45–78, Plenum Press, New York.

Whitham SE, Murphy G, Angel P, Rahmsdorf HJ, Smith BJ, Lyons A, Harris TJR, Reynolds JJ, Herlich P and Docherty AJP (1986) Comparison of human stromelysin and collagenase by cloning and sequence analysis. Biochem J 240, 913–916.

Wiebkin OE and Muir H (1973) The inhibition of sulphate incorporation on isolated adult chondrocytes by hyaluronic acids. FEBS Lett 37, 42–46.

Wiederhielm CA, Fox JR and Lee DR (1976) Ground substance mucopolysaccharides and plasma proteins: their role in capillary water balance. Am J Physiol 230, 1121–1125.

Wight TN, Heinegard DK and Hascall VC (1991) Proteoglycans, structure and function. In: Cell Biology of the Extracellular Matrix (Hay ED, ed) 2nd edition, Plenum Press, New York.

Wight TN and Hascall VC (1983) Proteoglycans in primate arteries. III. Characterization of the proteoglycans synthesized by arterial smooth muscle cells in culture. J Cell Biol 96, 167–176.

Winnemoller M, Schmidt G and Kresse H (1991) Influence of decorin on fibroblast adhesion. Eur J Cell Biol 54, 10–17.

Winterbourne DJ and Salisbury JG (1981) Heparan sulphate is a potent inhibitor of DNA synthesis in vitro. Biochem Biophys Res Commun 101, 30–37.

Woessner JF (1991) Matrix metalloproteinases and their inhibitors in connective tissue remodelling. FASEB J 5, 2145–2154.

Wood GC and Keech MK (1960) The formation of fibrils from collagen solutions. 1. The effect of experimental conditions: kinetic and electron microscope studies. Biochem J 75, 588–598.

Woods A, Couchman JR, Johansson S and Hook M (1986) Adhesion and cytoskeletal organization of fibroblasts in response to fibronectin fragments. EMBO J 5, 665–670.

Woods A, Couchman JR and Hook M (1985) Heparan sulphate proteoglycans of rat embryo fibroblasts. J Biol Chem 260, 10872–10879.

Yamada KM (1991) Fibronectin and other cell interactive glycoproteins. In: Cell Biology of the Extracellular Matrix (Hay ED, ed), 2nd edition, pp 111–146, Plenum Press, New York.

Yamagata M, Suzuki S, Akyama S, Yamada KM and Kimata K (1989) Regulation of cell-substrate adhesion by proteoglycans immobilised on extracellular substrates. J Biol Chem 264, 8012–8018.

Yamaguchi Y, Mann DM and Rouslahti E (1990) Negative regulation of transforming growth factor- by the proteoglycan decorin. Nature 346, 281–284.

Yanagishita M and Hascall VC (1987) Proteoglycan metabolism by rat ovarian granulosa cells in vitro. In: Biology of Proteoglycans (Wight T and Mecham R, eds), pp 105–128, Academic Press, New York.

Zhang X, Schuppan D, Becker J, Reichart P and Gelderblom HR (1993) Distribution of undulin, tenascin and fibronectin in the human periodontal ligament and cementum: comparative immunoelectron

Chapter 5
The Morphology of the Vasculature of the Periodontal Ligament

Milton R Sims

INTRODUCTION

The periodontal ligament (PDL) microvascular bed (MVB) is considered to play a major role in tooth support and physiological function (Wills *et al.*, 1976; Walker, 1980; Moxham and Berkovitz, 1982a; Aars, 1983), erupton (Moxham and Berkovitz, 1982b) and tooth pulsation (Parfitt, 1960; Ng *et al.*, 1981). Moreover, it is now established that a functional interrelationship exists between the vascular and extravascular fluid systems in the PDL (Cooper *et al.*, 1990; Tang and Sims, 1992). Nevertheless, knowledge of the MVB geometry and structure remains limited, although there have been three major reviews of the histology of this peripheral blood system (Saunders and de Röckert, 1967; Edwall, 1982; Schroeder, 1986).

Only recently have ultrastructural details of the MVB anatomy and distribution been published for teeth of limited growth (Berkovitz *et al.*, 1984; Freezer and Sims, 1987; Lew *et al.*, 1989; Clark *et al.*, 1991; Parlange and Sims, 1993). The vasculature of continuously growing teeth has also been described with light microscopy (Kindlova and Matena, 1959; Carranza *et al.*, 1966; Matena, 1973; Moe, 1981), and electron microscopy (Wong and Sims, 1983; Berkovitz *et al.*, 1984), but little data resulted (Moxham *et al.*, 1985, 1987; Blaushild *et al.*, 1992). Furthermore, comparisons of MVB ultrastructure across species remains limited (Freezer and Sims, 1987; Wong and Sims, 1987; Lee *et al.*, 1991; Parlange and Sims, 1993) and require further investigation.

MICROSCOPIC TECHNIQUES

LIGHT MICROSCOPY

Diverse methods have been applied to study this specialized MVB, including histological staining and perfusion with radiopaque substances, chemical precipitates, india ink and plastic microspheres (Schroeder, 1986). Furthermore, the consequences of tooth movement upon MVB morphology have received considerable attention (Castelli and Dempster, 1965; Reitan, 1985; Rygh *et al.*, 1986; Rygh, 1989). While valuable morphological information has been elicited from these investigations, all the findings are based on visual interpretations, without quantification of the experimental changes from the marked vascular variability that affects animals (Sims, 1987a).

The advent of latex perfusion techniques (Kindlova and Matena, 1959, 1962) stimulated PDL research by providing vascular corrosion casts for evaluation. Nevertheless, these casts are difficult to interpret accurately because of their flexibility, and the limitations of focal depth with light microscopy. Subsequently, the long standing morphological concept of a paired PDL arterial and venous system (Kindlova and Matena, 1962) has proved to be untenable (Weekes and Sims, 1986b).

SCANNING ELECTRON MICROSCOPY

During the past 15 years, scanning electron microscopy (SEM) of rigid, synthetic resin, vascular corrosion casts (Murakami, 1971; Murakami *et al.*, 1973; Gannon, 1981; Lametschwandtner *et al.*, 1990) has afforded graphic evidence of the complexity of the MVB architecture (Kishi and Takahashi, 1977; Kawato *et al.*, 1988). When combined with three-dimensional imaging (Nowell and Lohse, 1974; Hodde, 1981; Weekes and Sims, 1986a, 1986b; Wong and Sims, 1987; Lee *et al.*, 1990, 1991) this technique reveals the complex patterns of vascular anastomoses present within the PDL and their comprehensive links with the adjacent bone and gingival tissues.

Corrosion casting has the disadvantage that the relationship to other structures can be lost (Edwall, 1982) unless enzyme digestion is employed (Kawato *et al.*, 1988) or histological studies are used as a supplement (Gannon, 1985). Plastic shrinkage of 10–15 per cent may affect vessel size and introduce distortion (Lametschwandtner *et al.*, 1990). Comparisons of luminal and external diameters with different techniques may also heighten the impression of shrinkage. Even so, existing studies provide good correlation of vessel size between the various techniques in mouse (Sims, 1983b; Wong and Sims, 1987; Freezer and Sims, 1987), rat (Weekes and Sims, 1986a, 1986b; Tang and Sims, 1992), and marmoset (Douvartzidis, 1984; Parlange and Sims, 1993) as well as with immersion fixation for transmission electron microscopy (TEM) of the PDL of man (Foong, 1993).

TRANSMISSION ELECTRON MICROSCOPY

TEM is required to establish the microstructural anatomy of the vessel wall and the related tissues. This technique also enables examination and analysis of the passage of small tracer molecules across the endothelial wall (Cooper *et al.*, 1990). Importantly, stereological studies can be applied to derive some parameters, including physiological function (Gundersen *et al.*, 1988; Nyengaard *et al.*, 1988).

Early studies (Bevelander and Nakahara, 1968; Frank *et al.*, 1976) described human PDL vessels as thin-walled with a variable lumen calibre and a basement membrane. Corpron *et al.* (1976) reported mouse molar capillary endothelium as having luminal microvilli, tight junctions, pores and openings, a basement membrane and an incomplete pericyte layer. Fenestrated capillaries approximated the osteoblasts. Small arterioles with myoendothelial junctions and incomplete muscular coatings were occasionally observed.

These initial TEM observations have been greatly extended (Sims, 1983a; Freezer and Sims, 1987; Lew *et al.*, 1989; Cooper *et al.*, 1990; Clark *et al.*, 1991; Parlange and Sims, 1993; Tang and Sims, 1992; Tang *et al.*, 1993; Chintakanon and Sims, 1994). Nevertheless, many microanatomical features of the endothelial wall remain to be defined at the qualitative and quantitative levels.

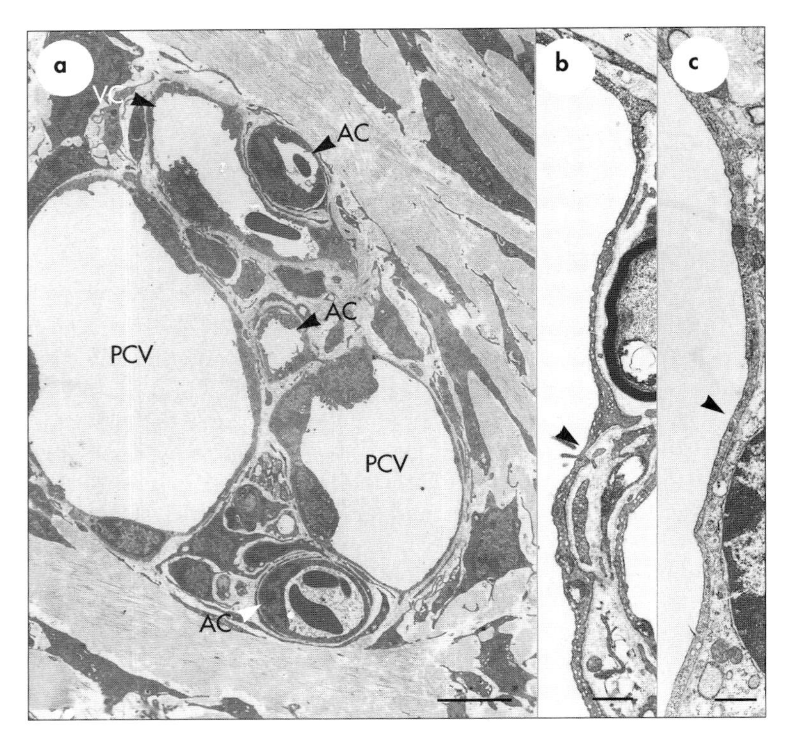

Fig. 5.1 (a) Vessels and neural complex in the mouse molar cervical PDL region adjacent to the alveolar bone. Bar = 5 μm; AC – arterial capillary; PCV – postcapillary sized venule; VC – venous capillary. (b) Thin endothelial wall (arrowhead) of a cervical region postcapillary-sized venule. Bar = 1 μm. (c) Thin endothelial wall (arrowhead) of a large apical collecting venule. Bar = 1 μm.

ANATOMY AND DISTRIBUTION

Morphologically and volumetrically, the rat (Weekes and Sims, 1986b), mouse (Wong and Sims, 1987), and marmoset MVB (Lee *et al.*, 1991) principally consist of a venous system made up of axially aligned, postcapillary sized venules (PCV) and collecting venules (CV). The PCV have a mean diameter of 20 μm, but range from 10 μm to 25 μm (Weekes and Sims, 1986b; Wong and Sims, 1987; Lee *et al.*, 1991), whereas CV have diameters of more than 30 μm. Arterial capillaries (AC) and venous capillaries (VC) contribute a small but significant component to the MVB. The MVB is also fed directly by terminal arterioles (TA) and arteriovenous anastomoses (AVA) with no interposing VC bed (Weekes and Sims, 1986b; Wong and Sims, 1987). Characteristic of VC, PCV, and CV are their very thin endothelial walls and large lumen volume to wall ratios (*Fig. 5.1*).

The PDL and gingival vascular beds communicate by way of an extensive system of anastomoses (Hayashi, 1932; Cohen, 1960; Bernick, 1962; Castelli and Dempster, 1965; Egelberg, 1966; Kindlova, 1967; Saunders and de Röckert, 1967; Levy *et al.*, 1972; Weekes and Sims, 1986a, 1986b; Wong and Sims, 1987; Lee *et al.*, 1991). Generally the PDL vessels arise from the alveolar bone or gingival vessels (Schroeder, 1986).

SEM studies (Kishi and Takahashi, 1977) and light microscopy (Egelberg, 1966; Kindlova, 1968; Hock and Nuki, 1971; Hock, 1975; Kindlova and Trnkova, 1972) show that a circular venous system, located just below the epithelial attachment, defines the coronal limit of the MVB. This circulus consists of a single 10–15 μm diameter vessel in rat and mouse molars (Weekes and Sims, 1986a; Wong and Sims, 1987) and as many as four vessels in marmoset premolars (Lee *et al.*, 1991). The circulus in the mouse (Wong and Sims, 1987) is similar to that in the rat (Kindlova and Matena, 1962; Kindlova, 1965; Carranza *et al.*, 1966; Weekes and Sims, 1986a) and the dog (Egelberg, 1966; Ichikawa *et al.*, 1977). Glomerular formations arise from the circulus and extend into the crevicular region (Weekes and Sims, 1986a, 1986b; Wong and Sims, 1987), but they are not present in the PDL as claimed by Kindlova and Matena (1962).

Vessels in the mouse PDL form a network with some tracts (Wong and Sims, 1987), a network in the macaque (Kindlova, 1965), but a palisade in the rat (Kindlova and Matena, 1962; Weekes and Sims, 1986b). In most regions of the marmoset premolar, the vessels form a network (Lee *et al.*, 1991) but, where larger vessels exist, a palisade arrangement occurs (*Fig. 5.2*).

Differing MVB patterns have been defined for the coronal, middle, and apical thirds of mouse molars (Wong and Sims, 1987). Vascular configuration in the middle third corresponds with descriptions of Bernick (1962) and Castelli and Dempster (1965). Relatively few arterioles have been observed, possibly because of the presence of short arteriovenous shunts, as in the rat (Weekes and Sims, 1986b).

Three specific MVB patterns have been identified in rat molar PDL (Weekes and Sims, 1986b). These occur alongside the buccal and lingual walls, the interdental septum, and the interradicular septum. In the buccal and lingual PDL the principal vessels course occluso-apically in tracts of three to six vessels. Each tract comprises intertwining capillaries of 6–10 μm diameter and 20 μm PCV. Capillary intertwining also occurs in the mouse (Wong and Sims, 1987). A horizontal intercommunicating plexus of fine lateral branches was not seen, although it was reported in other studies (Kindlova and Matena, 1962; Kindlova, 1965; Castelli and Dempster, 1965; Carranza *et al.*, 1966; Garfunkel and Sciaky, 1971; Kishi and Takahashi, 1977); neither was a dual network observed as noted in some species (Castelli and Dempster, 1965; Garfunkel and Sciaky, 1971; Kishi and Takahashi, 1977).

The interdental region is similar to the buccal and lingual zones but the vessels are more closely packed and drain into the alveolar bone (Weekes and Sims, 1986b). Over the interradicular septum a random, anastomosing system of repeating venule segments run a sinuous occluso-apical course for 100–400 μm before re-entering the bone to drain into PCV or small diameter CV. A few 60 μm diameter CV are present in the PDL. A venous ampulla straddles the mouse molar mandibular septum (Sims, 1987b), but in the maxillary molars the ampulla is replaced by smaller vessels of 30 μm diameter.

Around the interradicular septum of rats (Weekes and Sims, 1986b) the arteriolar supply from the alveolus to the PDL opposite the vertical walls is greater than at the crest. One or two arterioles join the middle of a venular segment or enlarge into PCV of 15–30 μm in diameter. However, arterioles are not plentiful and do not course through the PDL for any distance. Arterioles are not reported to be abundant in the mid-PDL region of mice or marmosets (Wong and Sims, 1987; Lee *et al.*, 1991). By contrast, Takahashi and Matsuo (1991) illustrate an even arterial distribution via the alveolar wall of dog premolars.

Apically, the MVB changes to an enveloping venous plexus of anastomosing PCV and CV supplied by arterioles and arteriovenous shunts (Wong and Sims, 1987). Vascular shunts, not unlike the arteriovenular bridges of Forsslund (1959), are present throughout the PDL (Sims, 1983b, 1987b; Weekes and Sims, 1986b; Lee *et al.*, 1991). A dense apical plexus occurs in other species (Kindlova and Matena, 1962; Garfunkel and Sciaky, 1971).

Vascular loops extending at right angles to the axial vessels are present in the cervical and apical regions of rats (Weekes and Sims, 1986b) and mice (Wong and Sims, 1987). Lee *et al.* (1991) describe the marmoset loops as being capillaries 50-100 μm in length. Bernick (1962) relates similar loops to cellular cementum formation. An alternative view is that such loops provide the capillary supply to the neural groups (Griffin, 1972; Griffin and Harris, 1974; Sims, 1984; Freezer and Sims, 1989).

Although the MVB of the PDL, gingiva, and palate have distinct, but interconnected, regional patterns, their venous drainage is directed into the PDL as well as the deeper gingival vessels (Wong and Sims, 1987; Weekes and Sims, 1986a, 1986b). Generally the PDL vascular bed has a rich anastomosis with the bone medulla (Edwall, 1982). Coronal third PDL drainage of mouse (Wong and Sims, 1987) and rat (Kindlova and Matena, 1962; Castelli and Dempster, 1965) is similar. A short drainage route extends to the cervical, interradicular, and medullary vessels, and a long route goes via the PCV and CV vessels to exit through the apex to medullary vessels as in man (Castelli, 1963). In mice, some regions of the ligament MVB drain via the medullary vessels into 50 μm diameter venules located interdentally deep to the molar apices. The medullary pattern is similar to humans (Castelli, 1963).

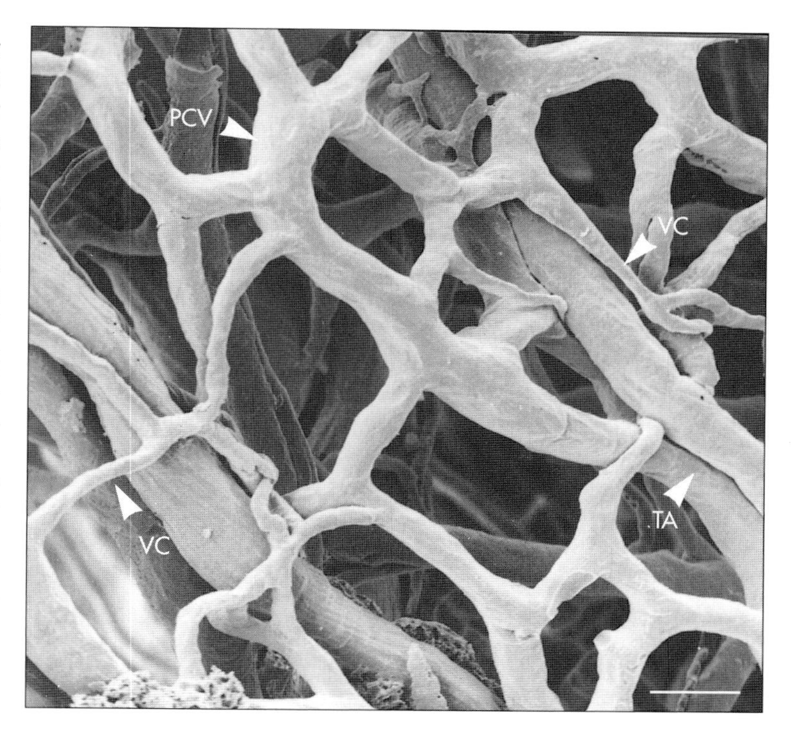

Fig. 5.2 Corrosion cast of the PDL microvasculature in the cervical region of a marmoset mandibular premolar. Bar = 30 μm; PCV – postcapillary-sized venule; VC – venous capillary; TA – terminal arteriole. (Reproduced by courtesy of D Lee.)

Except for the interradicular septum, blood flow in the rat molar is from the gingival to apical region (Weekes and Sims, 1986b). However, the interradicular arrangement indicates a potential for vascular tidal flow to occur in either direction and provide for counter-current exchange (Weekes and Sims, 1986a, 1986b) as in other microvascular beds (Hock and Nuki, 1971). The numerous anastomoses (Forsslund, 1959) also suggest that vascular tidal flow can occur in different directions throughout the PDL.

In continuously growing mouse incisors, the inner layer of the enamel-related zone MVB forms a dense complex of anastomosing vessels 10–15 μm in luminal diameter (Wong and Sims, 1983). The system has a ladder-like appearance. Laterally, a longitudinal venous vessel (70–100 μm in luminal diameter) extends from the gingival to the apical region and demarcates the cementum zone boundary. At the mesial and distal limits, the enamel-related zone vessels coalesce to form an irregular, longitudinal vessel some 30 μm in diameter. Between the anastomosing system and the alveolar wall is a plexus of large venous vessels. The cementum-related zone has a loose vessel network 10–15 μm in luminal diameter arranged at right angles to the boundary vessel. In the occlusal third, the network forms a dual layer; it consolidates to a single layer in the middle third. The vessels adjacent to the cementum are large and interconnect freely in the coronal region, whereas those adjacent to the alveolus are finer and have fewer anastomoses. Both maxillary and mandibular incisors are said to be similar.

VESSEL CATEGORIES

Precise vessel classification requires electron microscopy. Bevelander and Nakahara (1968) identified PDL vessels that resemble capillaries. Avery *et al.* (1975) and Corpron *et al.* (1976) specified mouse vessels as capillaries, fenestrated capillaries, and small arterioles. Frank *et al.* (1976) were less specific, noting that the rat molar MVB consisted mainly of continuous capillaries and a few fenestrated vessels. None of the authors provided the basis for their nomenclature.

The non-dental microcirculation has been defined as a collection of the smallest components of the cardiovascular channels, comprising the arterioles, the blood capillaries and venules. Applying the categorization criteria of other MVB (Wiedeman, 1963; Rhodin, 1967, 1968; Simionescu and Simionescu, 1984, 1988) to perfused PDL, Freezer and Sims (1987) differentiated size-specific capillary and venular vessels. Subsequent studies of mouse molars (Sims *et al.*, 1994), rat molars (Lew *et al.*, 1989; Cooper *et al.*, 1990; Clark *et al.*, 1991), marmoset incisors (Parlange and Sims, 1993; Chintavalakorn, 1993), and the premolars of man (Foong, 1993) have identified eight categories of vessel profile applicable to these species. There are venous capillaries and postcapillary-sized venules, which are pericytic or apericytic. The other vessels are collecting-sized venules, arterial capillaries, terminal arterioles, and arteriovenous anastomoses.

The TA and AVA are separately identifiable histologically and with corrosion casts from their luminal size, nuclei imprints, wall configuration, pathways and vascular connections (Weekes and Sims, 1986b; Wong and Sims, 1987; Lee *et al.*, 1991). For PCV and CV classification, luminal diameter is given preference over the thin-walled morphology, since their marked reduction in investing cells is atypical of other microvascular beds (Rhodin, 1967, 1968) – hence the use of the terms postcapillary-sized venules and collecting-sized venules for the PDL vessels.

The categorization of vessel profiles according to the presence (p-VC, p-PCV) or absence (a-VC, a-PCV) of pericytes does not imply that these pericytic and apericytic entities form separate vascular trees (Sims, 1986). On the contrary, this anatomical difference represents morphological variations along the VC and PCV that are attributable to the irregular investment of pericytes.

Continuously growing mouse incisors (Wong and Sims, 1983) and rat incisors (Blaushild *et al.*, 1992) also have a predominantly venous MVB. On the cementum- and enamel-related aspects, their luminal morphology and distribution correspond with arterioles, capillaries, sinusoidal vessels, PCV, and CV. The upper incisor MVB is also reported to be similar. Kindlova and Matena (1959) Garfunkel and Sciaky (1971), Wong and Sims (1983) and others have provided observations on the rat incisor MVB. However, Blaushild *et al.* (1992) have published the only detailed classification of rat incisor cementum-associated components, and they describe them as small arterioles, terminal arterioles, capillaries, postcapillary venules, and sinusoids.

VESSEL SIZES

In the non-dental MVB, vessel sizes have been defined by Wiedeman (1963), Movat and Fernando (1964), Rhodin (1967, 1968) and Simionescu and Simionescu (1984). According to Wiedeman (1963), diameter alone is not sufficient to classify vessels, owing to autoregulatory mechanisms, and classification should be based on position and function. However, Movat and Fernando (1964) maintained that venules could only be distinguished from capillaries by size. Wiedeman (1963) expressed the opinion that vessel diameters may vary from species to species.

On present evidence, the values for PDL vessel lumina are comparable between species and with the microvascular beds of other tissues. Dental vessel luminal sizes have been designated as follows (Freezer and Sims, 1987; Lew *et al.*, 1989; Clark *et al.*, 1991; Tang and Sims, 1992; Parlange and Sims, 1993; Chintavalakorn, 1993; Foong, 1993):

- p-VC and a-VC – 1.5–10.0 μm;
- p-PCV and a-PCV – 10.0–30.0 μm;
- AC – 1.5–7.0 μm;
- CV – 30–160 μm; and
- AVA-TA 11-60 μm.

The largest ranges exist for the PCV and CV. Of note is the finding that mouse luminal vessel sizes in corrosion casts (Wong and Sims, 1987), immersion fixed specimens (Sims, 1987a), and glutaraldehyde-perfused PDL (Sims *et al.*, 1994) do not reveal significant differences in luminal diameters.

Perfusion of mouse incisors reveals great variation in MVB luminal sizes (Wong and Sims, 1983). A long 70–100 μm diameter vessel demarcates the cementum-related MVB from the enamel PDL zone. The latter has a 10–15 μm anastomosing system with an underlying venular plexus. Diameters of the principal cementum-related venous vessels range from 10–15 μm. For the rat incisor, Blaushild *et al.* (1992) categorize the MVB vessels on the cementum-related PDL as small arterioles with an inner diameter of 20–80 μm, terminal arterioles with a 5–15 μm diameter, capillaries up to 10 μm, postcapillary venules of 10–40 μm, and sinusoids exceeding 40 μm.

VESSEL VOLUME

The PDL is unusual in being a connective tissue with a vascular volume three to seven times that of a routine ligament. Blood volume estimates in teeth of limited growth vary from 1–20 per cent according to species, site, tissue techniques, width and depth effects, method of analysis, extent of function, and age (*Fig. 5.3*). It is also relevant whether a resting or operant vascular bed is defined.

For humans, the incisor and premolar values are quoted as 2–4 per cent (Götze, 1976, 1980), 11 per cent (Sims, 1980), and 9.5 per cent (Foong, 1993). Non-human primates have recorded values of 0.5–1 per cent (Wills *et al.*, 1976), 8.3 ± 0.4 per cent (Douvartzidis, 1984), 11.26 ± 2.72 per cent (Parlange and Sims, 1993) and 10.3 per cent (Chintavalakorn, 1993). Marmoset apical volumes are estimated at 11 per cent (Crowe, 1989), and 10.7 per cent (Weir *et al.*, unpublished data).

Mouse molar MVB volume estimates include 7.7 ± 0.6 per cent (Gould *et al.*, 1977), 17 per cent (Sims, 1980), 7.46–9.24 ± 1.19 per cent (Freezer and Sims, 1987), 10.9 per cent (Sims, 1987a), 8.5 ± 1.37 per cent in young PDL and 9.7 ± 2.14 per cent in one-year-old PDL (Sims *et al.*, 1994). Rat molar data include 22.1 per cent (Moxham *et al.*, 1985), 20 per cent (Lew *et al.*, 1989), and 23.1 per cent (Clark *et al.*, 1991). The only volumetric data for continuously growing rat teeth is provided by Moxham *et al.* (1985), who recorded 50 per cent near the growing base, and by Blaushild *et al.* (1992), who calculated that blood vessels occupy 47 ± 2 per cent in the apical half and 4 ± 2 per cent at the incisal end.

Most studies have not distinguished between luminal volume and the inclusion of the vessel wall. Wall thickness adds 24 per cent to the marmoset lumen, which increases the MVB volume from 11.3 per cent to 14.9 per cent of the PDL (Parlange and Sims, 1993). For humans, the wall adds 3 per cent (Foong, 1993); in young mouse it adds 2 per cent compared with 4 per cent in one-year-old mice (Freezer and Sims, 1987; Sims *et al.*, 1994).

Garfunkel and Sciaky (1971) have noted MVB depth effects in the rat molar PDL. Progressive blood volume increases with depth have been recorded in the PDL of human (Götze, 1976) and marmoset molars (Douvartzidis, 1984). Depth has a quadratic effect on total MVB volume in mouse molars (*Fig. 5.4*) with larger

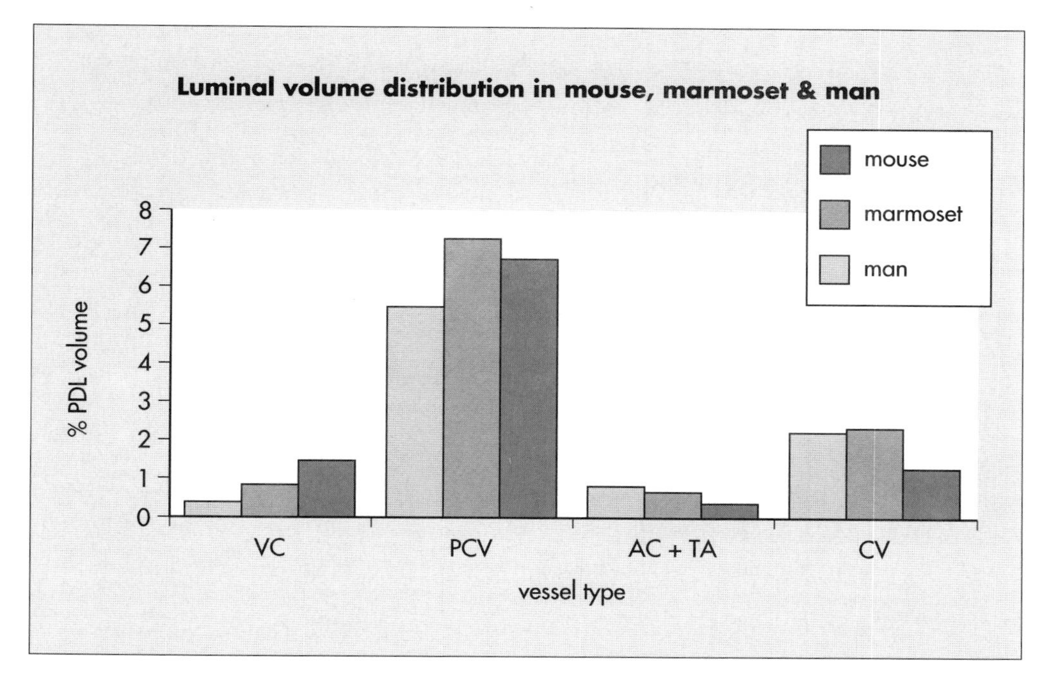

Fig. 5.3 Blood volume of vessel groups as a percentage of the PDL for the mouse molar, marmoset incisor, and human premolar. VC – venous capillaries; PCV – postcapillary-sized venules; AC + TA – arterial capillaries plus terminal arterioles; CV – collecting venules.

volumes in the cervical and apical regions (Sims, 1987a; Sims *et al.*, 1994). This pattern corresponds with the marmoset incisor (Parlange and Sims, 1993), but not with humans (Foong, 1993).

VESSEL DISTRIBUTION

Blood vessel disposition may vary according to species, tooth type, and depth (Götze, 1976; Sims, 1987a). Left and right jaw side differences are not significant in the mouse (Sims *et al.*, 1994) or humans (Foong, 1993). The mesial root of the mouse mandibular molar also shows characteristic differences on each aspect (Sims, 1987a). Vascular apportionment alters according to PDL circumferential thirds (Freezer and Sims, 1987; Parlange and Sims, 1993; Chintavalakorn, 1993; Foong, 1993; Sims *et al.*, 1994), and age (see *Fig. 5.3*).

Fig. 5.5 illustrates the MVB luminal distribution in the mouse molar (Sims *et al.*, 1994), marmoset incisor (Chintavalakorn, 1993) and human premolar (Foong, 1993) across PDL circumferential thirds. *Tables 5.1* and *5.2* highlight the variation according to vessel category. The dominance of a-PCV is evident. Further information on pericytic and a-pericytic vessel profiles has been

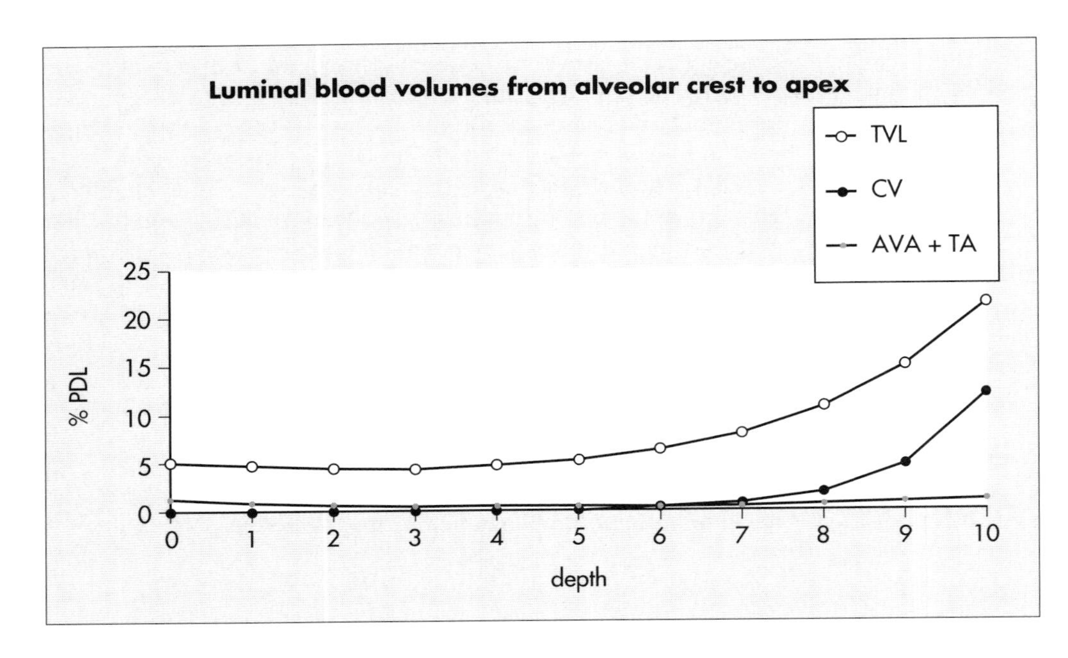

Fig. 5.4 Total blood volume distribution (TVL) for mouse molar between the cervical (depth 0) and apical (depth 10) regions. Arterial (arteriovenous anastomoses plus terminal arterioles) and collecting venule (CV) contributions are shown for comparison.

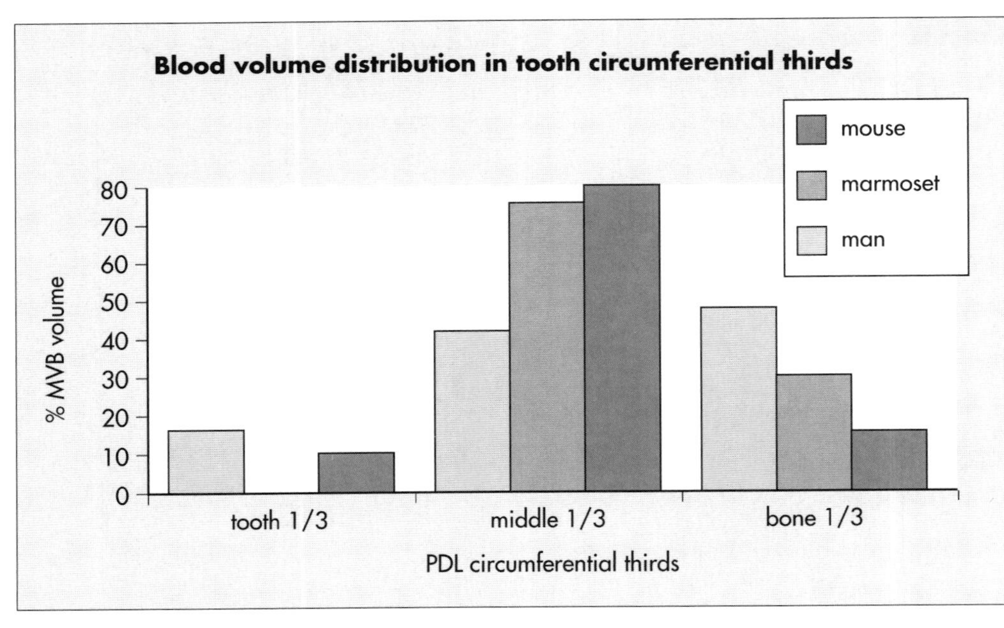

Fig. 5.5 Luminal volume across the PDL circumferential thirds for mouse molar, marmoset incisor, and human premolar.

Table 5.1 Model of vessel lumen volume distribution in young mouse molar across PDL circumferential thirds as a percentage of the total ligament.

	Tooth third	Middle third	Bone third	PDL mean
Pericytic venous capillaries	0.2	0.3	0.0	0.2
Apericytic venous capillaries	0.0	0.6	0.1	0.2
Pericytic postcapillary-sized venules	0.0	0.6	2.9	1.2
Apericytic postcapillary-sized venules	1.4	2.9	8.4	4.2
Arterial capillaries	0.0	0.2	0.5	0.2
Collecting venules	1.3	2.7	1.2	1.7

Table 5.2 Model of the percentage distribution of vessel luminal categories across the circumferential thirds of young mouse molar PDL.

	Tooth Third	Middle Third	Bone Third
Pericytic venous capillaries	40	60	0
Non-pericytic venous capillaries	0	86	14
Pericytic postcapillary-sized venules	0	17	83
Non-pericytic postcapillary-sized venules	11	23	66
Arterial capillaries	0	29	71
Collecting venules	25	52	23
Arteriovenous anastomoses plus terminal arterioles	0	60	40
Pericytic venous capillaries plus non-pericytic venous capillaries	17	75	8
Pericytic postcapillary-sized venules plus non-pericytic postcapillary-sized venules	9	21	70

provided for mice (Freezer and Sims, 1987), rats (Cooper *et al.*, 1990; Tang and Sims, 1992), marmosets (Parlange and Sims, 1993), and humans (Foong, 1993).

Freezer and Sims (1987) found that only 30 per cent of the mouse PCV are pericytic. Pericytic vessels have not been found in the PDL tooth third. Crowe (1989) differentiated apical a-VC and a-PCV as making up 67 per cent and 59 per cent of the VC and PCV, respectively, in the marmoset maxillary incisor apex. Thus, the greatest proportion of the most active vessels consisted of an endothelial tube in profile. Chintavalakorn (1993) surveyed the marmoset incisor PDL and determined that 64 per cent of the MVB volume is contained within a-PCV. The middle PDL circumferential third holds 86 per cent of the blood in a-PCV.

Pericytic vessels in young and one-year-old mouse PDL total 1.1 per cent and 0.8 per cent of PDL volume and 13.2 per cent and 26.7 per cent of MVB volume, respectively (Sims *et al.*, 1994). The apericytic vessels comprise 4.6 per cent and 3.8 per cent of total PDL volume, and 53.7 per cent and 38.4 per cent of total microvascular volume, respectively. Thus, there is a particular reduction of the PCV with age, implying a loss in physiological efficiency. The a-PCV, which are considered to have a major exchange role (Tang and Sims, 1992; Tang *et al.*, 1993), are particularly affected. In other tissues, the arrangement of pericytes along capillaries, and their similarities to smooth muscle cells, has led to the proposal that they are involved in local control of capillary blood flow (Buchanan and Wagner, 1990).

ENDOTHELIAL AND PERIVASCULAR CELLS

The microstructure of the PDL vessel wall is imprecisely documented (Rhodin, 1984). Corpron *et al.* (1976) reported an endothelial cell lining enclosed by basement membrane with or without surrounding perivascular cells. Microvilli and nuclei protruded into the lumen. Cytoplasmic features included numerous microvesicles, scattered ribosomes, small oval mitochondria, fenestrae, pores, and junctional complexes. Small peripheral arterioles had an incomplete muscular coating. For some of these structures, quantitative data are still lacking.

Freezer (1984) described pericytes in mouse molar PDL as elongated cells with little cytoplasmic branching and a basement lamina that was continuous with that of the endothelium. These cells were more commonly associated with vessels with a luminal diameter of 4µm to 8 µm. Where the luminal diameter was greater than 20 µm, the pericyte investment usually appeared to be absent or incomplete. There are no extant studies of the muscle cells.

Rhodin (1967, 1968) defined the ultrastructure of five types of vascular wall elements: endothelial cells, veil cells, pericytes, primitive smooth muscle cells, and smooth muscle cells. Pericytes were stated to be the precursor cells of smooth muscle cells, while the primitive smooth muscle cell represented an intermediate type between pericytes and 'true' smooth muscle cells. The structure of the pericyte was said to be similar to the fibroblast. These and many other aspects of the PDL vessel walls require investigation.

Endothelial and perivascular cells demonstrate close affiliations with oxytalan fibres (Sims, 1983a, 1983b). A study of statistical correlations between these structures (Freezer and Sims, 1988) in mouse molar PDL showed that significant associations exist for oxytalan fibres in the vessel walls of a-PCVs ($p < 0.05$) and p-VC ($p < 0.01$). These attributes may be indicative of functional relationships.

FENESTRAE

Endothelial fenestrae occur in the PDL microvascular bed of mouse molars (Corpron *et al.*, 1976; Sims, 1983b), rat incisors and molars (Frank *et al.*, 1976; Rygh, 1976; Shore *et al.*, 1984; Moxham *et al.*, 1985; Moxham *et al.*, 1987; Lew *et al.*, 1989; Clark *et al.*, 1991), and humans (Gilchrist, 1978). Fenestrae are found in VC, AC, and PCV (Lew *et al.*, 1989; Clark *et al.*, 1991). As in the non-dental MVB (Majno, 1965; Casley-Smith, 1971, 1983; Renkin, 1979; Simionescu and Simionescu, 1984; Milici *et al.*, 1985), fenestrae are confined to attenuated portions of the PDL endothelium.

Fenestrae are labile, circular, transcellular, vascular windows. They are present in groups of two to six units, and almost all possess diaphragms 5–6 nm thick (Clark *et al.*, 1991), though these diaphragms are absent in 10 per cent of AC (Lew *et al.*, 1989). Central knob-like structures (Rhodin, 1962; Friederici, 1969) from 15 nm to 20 nm in diameter are reported in PDL diaphragms (Lew *et al.*, 1989). Fenestral diameters range from 30 nm to 59 nm in mouse molars (Corpron *et al.*, 1976), with mean values of 52 nm for rat incisors and molars (Moxham *et al.*, 1985). Lew *et al.* (1989) and Clark *et al.* (1991) record mean diameters of 54.2 nm and 51.5 nm in the rat molar apical region. Across different tissues, the calculated frequency values of PDL fenestrae show great variation (Clementi and Palade, 1969; Simionescu *et al.*, 1974).

Lew *et al.* (1989) and Clark *et al.* (1991) find no fenestral size differences between vessels; this accords with other MVB (Casley-Smith, 1971). The claim (Corpron *et al.*, 1976) of obvious fenestral polarity (Clementi and Palade, 1969) owing to preferential vessel location is not supported by studies of the PDL apical region in rats (Lew *et al.*, 1989). In the study by Lew *et al.* (1989), fenestrae were 7.5 times more prevalent per mm^2 on the venous side than the arterial side. Clark *et al.* (1991) recorded a 12-fold increase in prevalence, similar to patterns in other microvascular beds (Casley-Smith, 1971). It is not known whether there are differences between species in the structure, frequency, or distribution of PDL fenestrae.

A quantitative study (Moxham *et al.*, 1985) of the number and distribution of fenestrated capillaries in rat incisor and molar PDL shows a greater density of fenestrae for the molar than the continuously erupting incisor. Furthermore, more fenestrae were present in erupting molars than in fully erupted molars (Moxham *et al.*, 1987). These authors suggest that the irregular pattern of fenestral distribution noted along the length of the incisor PDL might be associated with pressure differentials necessary for tooth eruption.

Simionescu *et al.* (1974) and Milici *et al.* (1985) noted that differences in the density and distribution of fenestrae are tissue specific. Fenestrae are dispersed in clusters, which may be large and irregular or small and more clearly outlined. In other tissues, fenestrae are considered adaptations to the need for greater than normal permeability (Casley-Smith *et al.*, 1975, Milici *et al.*, 1985) and it is thought that they play a more important role than junctions and vesicles (Casley-Smith *et al.*, 1975). If the fenestrated vessels of the PDL reflect the functional capacity reported in other MVB (Levick and Smaje, 1987), further investigation is indeed warranted.

ENDOTHELIAL CELL JUNCTIONS

Apart from the abstract by Corpron *et al.* (1976) and the paper by Tang *et al.* (1993), endothelial junctions are ignored in the PDL dental literature. Chintakanon and Sims (1994) have used goniometer tilting to examine ultrastructurally and to classify 200 apparent 'tight' junctions in both normal and extrusively tensioned rat molar PDL. These 'tight' regions have proved to be one of close, tight, or open junctions. No gap junctions were observed.

Close junctions formed 80 per cent of all the junctions. The width of the close junctional region was approximately 5nm to 6 nm. In the non-junctional close region, the width increased by 9.4 per cent with tension ($p < 0.01$). The width variation could imply that there was an increase in fluid and substrate exchange through the close regions.

Tight junctions, where the opposing membranes are fused, were confirmed in 16 per cent of the junction population, and were found to be common in the luminal third (87.5 per cent). The tight regions in the middle third or abluminal third were found only in the apical levels. The proportion of tight junctions was not significantly different among various vascular segments and there was no difference in the tight region location between the experimental and control samples. Tension caused no detectable change in tight junction width. Ultrastructurally, the tight junctions were similar to those reported in the dental pulp (Tabata and Semba, 1987).

Open junctions had an incidence of 4 per cent and were only detected in the thin-walled VC and PCV. These types of vessels are considered to be more leaky and more sensitive to stimulation than other types of vessels (Casley-Smith, 1979, 1983; Tang and Sims, 1992). The pore sizes ranged from 136 nm to 1231 nm. Junction depth was found to have a positive correlation with the endothelial wall thickness across the middle of the junction ($p < 0.001$)

The type of junction and its orientation are known to be important in cell permeability. The close junction incidence in this PDL study was high compared with the 5 per cent found in dog muscular capillaries (Casley-Smith *et al.*, 1975) and the 7 per cent in mouse diaphragm capillaries (Casley-Smith, 1983). This difference implies that the MVB of the PDL is highly permeable via the close junction route, and that different regions of the junction complex provide selective permeability to different sizes of molecules. Close junctions are claimed to be more common in PCV (Simionescu *et al.*, 1978), although this association is denied by others (Bundit and Wissig, 1978; Casley-Smith, 1983).

Three-dimensional junction organization may be simple or complex (Casley-Smith, 1983; Bundgaard, 1984) and may vary between the vascular bed segments. Junction properties can be altered by physiological requirements and by experimental manipulation (Schneeberger and Lynch, 1984) as well as by injury (Cotran, 1967; Casley-Smith and Window, 1976). Current data suggests that when the PDL is placed in tension, the close junctions of both VC and PCV provide major pathways for fluid and molecular transport (Cooper *et al.*, 1990; Tang *et al.*, 1993; Chintakanon and Sims, 1994).

NEURAL ASSOCIATIONS

The PDL blood vessels are closely associated with myelinated and unmyelinated nerves (Griffin, 1972; Griffin and Harris, 1974; Sims, 1983a, 1983b; Byers, 1985; Byers *et al.*, 1986). Sims (1983a, 1983b) demonstrated PDL vessels were related to autonomic and myelinated nerves, which suggested that they might have vasoconstriction and vasodilation roles.

Ultrastructurally, the PDL contains a variety of anatomically discrete structures in juxtaposition to periodontal blood vessels (Freezer and Sims, 1989). These structures include nerve endings contiguous with K-cells, partially exposed terminal axons, preterminal and terminal axons protruding into the vessel wall (Sims, 1984), and lamellated receptors (Berkovitz, 1990).

Freezer and Sims (1988) provide statistically significant data on mouse molar associations between PDL cells, blood vessels, oxytalan fibres, and nerves by constructing a mathematical model for normal PDL. From this study it is hypothesized that, morphologically and functionally, PCV may function as tube or tunnel capillaries in the control of vessel permeability (Intaglietta and de Plomb, 1973). Moreover, K-cells (Beertsen *et al.*, 1974) have a statistically significant correlation with perivascular oxytalan fibres ($p < 0.05$), myelinated and unmyelinated axons ($p < 0.05$ and $p < 0.01$, respectively), and PCV ($p < 0.01$), which contain most of the blood volume. A positive relation also exists between K-cells and a-PCVs ($p < 0.01$).

A further statistical association occurs between myelinated and unmyelinated nerves related to blood vessel walls ($p < 0.01$). These previously unreported relationships of complex structures may delineate operant mechanisms that could influence functional tooth support and tooth movement.

VASCULAR AGEING

It is claimed that arteriosclerotic changes and a reduction in luminal volume characterize the aged human and marmoset MVB (Bernick *et al.*, 1969; Grant and Bernick, 1970, 1972; Bradley, 1972; Levy *et al.*, 1972). These histological findings are disputed by Seversen *et al.* (1978) from their evaluation of human PDL.

Using mouse molar PDL as a model (Sims *et al.*, 1994), the MVB luminal volume density is found to increase from 8.5 per cent ± 1.37 SE in young PDL to 9.7 per cent ± 2.14 SE in one-year-old PDL (*Table 5.3*). There is no significant difference in luminal diameters between young and aged PDL. The mean width of the aged PDL halved from 119.9±16.9 μm to 60.0±10.6 μm. Narrowing of human PDL with age has also been reported by Coolidge (1937).

Significant regional shifts in aged PDL altered the MVB distribution of a-VC, p-PCV, a-PCV, CV, and AVA-TA ($p < 0.01$). A two-fold increase in aged AVA-TA input ($p < 0.01$) bypassed the capillary bed to be shunted directly into the increased volume of CV.

From these stereological data, functional consequences can be derived; these show that the mean PDL cross-sectional area for which one capillary is responsible dropped with age from 2117 μm^2 to 1451 μm^2. Similarly, the average thickness of the PDL sheet served by a capillary was reduced from 52.5 μm to 27.5 μm. Both sets of numbers mean the average diffusion distance was greatly reduced in aged animals, with the possibility of functional impairment. Quantitative data for MVB ageing in humans are not available. Whether any accompanying aged changes occur in associated structures, such as the neural system and oxytalan fibre meshwork, remains to be determined.

LYMPHATIC VESSELS

Despite the traditional lymphatic illustrations in textbooks, evidence for a lymphatic system in the PDL (Edwall, 1982) is a controversial subject. Schweitzer (1907) described a rich lymphatic capillary bed in the foetal PDL. Box (1949) concluded that substantial evidence existed for the presence of PDL lymphatics.

In 1968, Levy and Bernick histologically described lymphatic vessels in marmoset PDL. It is likely that Levy and Bernick misinterpreted PCV as lymphatics (Parlange and Sims, 1993). Ruben *et al.* (1971) reported the demonstration of PDL lymphatics by back perfusion of cervical lymph nodes in the dog. However, the anatomical validity of such a technique is questionable.

Table 5.3 Model of the MVB lumen volume distribution in young and old mouse molar PDL as a percentage of periodontal ligament thirds

		Tooth third	Middle third	Bone third
As percentage of total PDL	Young Old	1.4 1.6	3.4 4.8	3.9 3.4
As percentage of total MVB	Young Old	15.6 16.7	39.7 48.5	44.7 34.8
As percentage of each PDL third	Young Old	4.1 5.2	9.8 12.9	11.9 11.0

Lindhe (1988) concludes that lymphatic capillary walls are histologically difficult to identify. Nevertheless, Schroeder (1986) re-affirmed that the histological evidence favoured the presence of PDL lymphatics. At the ultrastructural level, Casley-Smith (1977) listed the significant features of lymphatic capillaries. Using this classification Gilchrist (1978) claimed to confirm the existence of lymph-like vessels in the human PDL. Barker (1982), using TEM examination, also reported the presence of lymphatics in the alveolar bone of humans, adjacent to the PDL.

Currently, there is no conclusive ultrastructural evidence of PDL lymphatic capillaries. Nevertheless, a tantalizing clinical fact is that a PDL abscess is associated with swollen cervical lymph nodes. Clearly, lymph drainage exists, but the system and its pathways have yet to be convincingly demonstrated.

SUMMARY AND FUTURE RESEARCH

At the ultrastructural level, our knowledge of the MVB is limited. Neither individual tooth MVB differences within a dentition nor variations between species have been definitively assessed. Apart from the blood volume, there is the additional fluid micro-environment provided by the water-rich sol phase of tissue channels and lymph flow in the interstitial compartment. Clearly, a combination of techniques is needed to elucidate the relationships existing between structure and function (Sobin and Tremer, 1977) in the MVB of the PDL.

A definition of the operant and total vascular beds is required. As yet, we lack an understanding of the basis for the control of tidal and vascular flow. Perfusion techniques indicate that both collateral flow mechanisms and functional shut-off systems reside within the microvascular bed.

The paradox of the lymphatic system remains unanswered. This also applies to the anatomical basis for fluid and macromolecular transfer across the MVB wall. Furthermore, uncertainty also exists about extrapolation from animal experiments to the situation in humans.

Care must, however, be taken in interpreting results of quantitative histological and ultrastructural investigations on the microvasculature. Not only is it conceivable that studies involving intravascular perfusions (at different pressures and with fluids having different osmotic pressures) alter the diameters of vessels, it is also well established from physiological studies that, unless the animal under study dies instantly, there will be reactive, compensatory mechanisms in a vascular bed, which differ from tissue to tissue and which will significantly modify measurements of blood volume.

REFERENCES

Aars H (1983) Effects of sympathetic nerve activity on changes in the position and mobility of the rabbit incisor tooth. Acta Physiol Scand 116, 423–428.

Avery JK, Corpron RE, Lee SD and Morawa AP (1975) Ultrastructure of terminal blood vessels in mouse periodontium. J Dent Res 54, 108 (abstract).

Barker JH (1982) Lymphatic vessels in human alveolar bone. Lymphology 15, 1–13.

Beertsen W, Everts V and van den Hoof A (1974) Fine structure and possible function of cells containing leptomeric organelles in the periodontal ligament of the rat incisor. Arch Oral Biol 19, 1099–1100.

Berkovitz BKB (1990) The structure of the periodontal ligament: an update. Eur J Orthod 12, 51–76.

Berkovitz BKB, Shore RC and Moxham BJ (1984) Ultrastructural studies on the developing periodontal ligament. In: Tooth Morphogenesis and Differentiation (Ruch JV and Belcourt AB, eds), volume 125, pp 545–556, Colloquium of the Institut National de la Santé et de la Recherche Médicale.

Bernick S (1962) Age changes in the blood supply to molar teeth of rats. Anat Rec 144, 265–274.

Bernick SE, Levy BM and Patek P (1969) Studies on the biology of the periodontium of marmosets VI. Arteriosclerotic changes in the blood vessels of the periodontium. J Periodont 40, 355–358.

Bevelander G and Nakahara H (1968) The fine structure of the human periodontal ligament. Anat Rec 162, 313–326.

Blaushild N, Michaeli Y and Steigman S (1992) Histomorphometric study of the periodontal vasculature of the rat incisor. J Dent Res 71, 1908–1912.

Box KF (1949) Evidence of lymphatics in the periodontium. J Can Dent Assoc 15, 8–19.

Bradley JC (1972) Age changes in the vascular supply of the mandible. Br Dent J 132, 142–144.

Buchanan RA and Wagner RC (1990) Associations between pericytes and capillary endothelium in the eel rete mirabile. Microvasc Res 39, 60–76.

Bundgaard M (1984) The three-dimensional organization of tight junctions in a capillary endothelium revealed by serial section electron microscopy. J Ultrastruc Res 88,1–17.

Bundit V and Wissig SL (1978) Comparison of the permeability of capillaries, venous capillaries and small venules to protein tracers. J Cell Biol 79, 384a (abstract).

Byers MR (1985) Sensory innervation of periodontal ligament of rat molars consists of unencapsulated Ruffini-like mechanoreceptors and free nerve endings. J Comp Neurol 231, 500–518.

Byers MR, O'Connor TA, Martin RF and Dong WK (1986) Mesencephalic trigeminal sensory neurones of cat. Axon pathways and structure of mechanoreceptive endings in periodontal ligament. J Comp Neurol 250, 181–191.

Carranza FA Jr, Itoiz ME, Cabrini RL and Dotto CA (1966) A study of periodontal vascularization in different laboratory animals. J Periodont Res 1, 120–128.

Casley-Smith JR (1971) Endothelial fenestrae in intestinal villi: differences between the arterial and venous ends of the capillaries. Microvasc Res 3, 49–68.

Casley-Smith JR (1977) Lymph and lymphatics. In: Microcirculation (Kaley G and Altura B , eds), volume 1, pp 421–502, University Park Press, Baltimore and London.

Casley-Smith JR (1979) The fine structure of the microvasculature in inflammation. Bibl Anat 17, 36–53.

Casley-Smith JR (1983) The structure and functioning of the blood vessels, intersititial tissues and lymphatics. In: Lymphology (Foldi M and Casley-Smith JR, eds), pp 27–164, Schattauer, Stuttgart.

Casley-Smith JR, O'Donoghue PJ and Crocker KWJ (1975) The quantitative relationships between fenestrae in jejunal capillaries and connective tissue channels: proof of 'tunnel capillaries'. Microvasc Res 3, 49–68.

Casley-Smith JR and Window J (1976) Quantitative morphological correlations of alterations in capillary permeability, following histamine and moderate burning in the mouse diaphragm; and the effects of benzopyrones. Microvasc Res 11, 279–305.

Castelli WA (1963) Vascular architecture of the human adult mandible. J Dent Res 42, 786–792.

Castelli WA and Dempster WT (1965) The periodontal vasculature and its responses to experimental pressures. J Am Dent Assoc 70, 890–905.

Chintakanon K and Sims MR (1994) Ultrastructural morphology of vascular endothelial junctions in periodontal ligament. Aust Dent J 39, 105–110.

Chintavalakorn S (1993) TEM stereology of blood vessels and nerves in marmoset periodontal ligament following incisor crown fracture, endodontic therapy, orthodontic extrusion and long term retention. MDS thesis, University of Adelaide, South Australia.

Clark AB, Sims MR and Leppard PI (1991) An analysis of the effect of tooth intrusion on the microvascular bed and fenestrae in the apical periodontal ligament of the rat molar. Am J Orthod and Dentofacial Orthop 99, 21–29.

Clementi F and Palade GE (1969) Intestinal capillaries. I. Permeability to peroxidase and ferritin. J Cell Biol 41, 33–58.

Cohen L (1960) Further studies into the vascular architecture of the mandible. J Dent Res 39, 936–946.

Coolidge ED (1937) The thickness of the human periodontal membrane. J Am Dent Assoc 24, 1260–1270.

Cooper SM, Sims MR, Sampson WR and Dreyer CW (1990) A morphometric, electron microscopic analysis of tissue channels shown by ionic tracer in normal and tensioned rat molar apical periodontal ligament. Arch Oral Biol 35, 499–507.

Corpron RE, Avery JK, Morawa AP and Lee SD (1976) Ultrastructure of capillaries in mouse periodontium. J Dent Res 55, 551.

Cotran RS (1967) The fine structure of the microvasculature in relation to normal and altered permeability. In: Physical Basis of Circulatory Transport (Reeve EB and Guyton AC, eds), p 249, WB Saunders, Philadelphia.

Crowe PR (1989) A TEM investigation of extrusion and root canal therapy on the marmoset periodontal ligament. MDS thesis, University of Adelaide, South Australia.

Douvartzidis I (1984) A morphometric examination of the periodontal ligament vasculature of the marmoset molar. MDS thesis, University of Adelaide, South Australia.

Edwall LGA (1982) The vasculature of the periodontal ligament. In: The Periodontal Ligament in health and Disease (Berkovitz BKB, Moxham BJ and Newman HN, eds), pp 151–171, Pergamon Press, Oxford.

Egelberg J (1966) The blood vessels of the dento-gingival junction. J Periodont Res 1, 163–179.

Foong KWC (1993) A TEM stereological investigation of the blood vessels in human mandibular premolar periodontal ligament. MDS thesis, University of Adelaide, South Australia.

Forsslund G (1959) The structure and function of the capillary system in the gingiva in man. Acta Odont Scand 17, suppl 26 (thesis).

Frank RM, Felinger E and Stever P (1976) Ultrastructure du ligament alveolo-dentaire du rat. J Biol Buccale 4, 295–313.

Freezer SR (1984) A study of periodontal ligament mesial to the mouse mandibular first molar. MDS thesis, University of Adelaide, South Australia.

Freezer SR and Sims MR (1987) A transmission electron-microscope stereological study of the blood vessels, oxytalan fibres and nerves of mouse-molar periodontal ligament. Arch Oral Biol 32, 407–412.

Freezer SR and Sims MR (1988) Statistical correlations between cells, blood vessels, oxytalan fibres and nerves in mouse periodontal ligament. Aust Orthod J 14, 227–230.

Freezer SR and Sims MR (1989) Morphometry of the neural structure of the mouse periodontal ligament mesial to the mandibular first molar. Aust Orthod J 11, 30–37.

Friederici HHR (1969) On the diaphragm across fenestrae of capillary endothelium. J Ultrastruct Res 27, 373–375.

Gannon BJ (1981) Preparation of microvascular corrosion casting media: procedure for partial polymerization of methyl methacrylate using ultraviolet light. Biomed Res 2, 233.

Gannon BJ (1985) Vascular Casting Workshop. 10th Congress of New Zealand Electron Microscope Society.

Garfunkel A and Sciaky I (1971) Vascularization of the periodontal tissues in the adult laboratory rat. J Dent Res 50, 880–887.

Gilchrist DR (1978) Ultrastructure of periodontal blood vessels. MDS thesis, University of Adelaide, South Australia.

Götze W (1976) Quantitative Untersuchungen zur Verteilung der Blutgefässe im Desmodont. Dtsch Zahnärztl Z 31, 428–430.

Götze W (1980) Über den Volumenanteil von Faserbündelabschnitten und Blutgefässen in Desmodont menschlicher Frontzähne. Dtsch Zahnärztl Z 35, 1103–1104.

Gould TR, Melcher AH and Brunette DM (1977) Location of progenitor cells in periodontal ligament of mouse molar stimulated by wounding. Anat Rec 188, 133–141.

Grant D and Bernick S (1970) Arteriosclerosis in periodontal vessels of ageing humans. J Periodont 41, 170–173.

Grant D and Bernick S (1972) The periodontium of ageing humans. J Periodont 43, 660–667.

Griffin CJ (1972) The fine structure of end-rings in human periodontal ligament. Arch Oral Biol 17, 785–797.

Griffin CJ and Harris R (1974) Innervation of human periodontium. I. Classification of periodontal receptors. Aust Dent J 19, 51–56.

Gundersen HJG, Bendtsen TF, Korbo L, *et al.*; (1988) Some new, simple and efficient stereological methods and their use in pathological research and diagnosis. APMIS 96, 379–394.

Hayashi S (1932) Untersuchungen über die arterielle Blutversorgung des Periodontiums. Dtsch Mschr Zahnheilk 50, 145–179.

Hock J and Nuki K (1971) A vital microscopy study of the morphology of normal and inflamed gingiva. J Periodont Res 6, 81–88.

Hock J (1975) Gingival vasculature around erupting deciduous teeth of dogs and cats. J Clin Periodontol 2, 44–50.

Hodde KC (1981) Cephalic vascular patterns in the rat. A scanning electron microscopic (SEM) study of casts. Doctoral dissetation, University of Amsterdam, Amsterdam.

Ichikawa T, Watanabe O and Yamamura T (1977) Vascular architecture in oral tissues by vascular casts method for scanning electron microscopy. E Bibl Anat 15, 544–546.

Intaglietta AM and de Plomb EP (1973) Fluid exchange in tunnel and tube capillaries. Microvasc Res 6, 153–168.

Kawato F, Matsuo M, Kishi Y and Takahashi K (1988) Microcirculation and bone remodeling. SEM observation of the vascular changes in periodontal ligament applied to extrusive tooth movement. Microcirculation Annual, pp 67–68, Japanese Society for Microcirculation.

Kindlova M (1965) The blood supply of the marginal periodontium in the *Macacus rhesus*. Arch Oral Biol 10, 869–874.

Kindlova M (1967) Glomerular vascular structures in the periodontium. In: The Mechanisms of Tooth Support. A Symposium (Anderson DJ, Eastoe JE, Melcher AH and Picton DCA, eds), pp 76–79, Wright, Bristol.

Kindlova M (1968) Development of vessels in the marginal periodontium in rats. J Dent Res 47, 507.

Kindlova M and Matena V (1959) Blood circulation in the rodent teeth of the rat. Acta Anat 37, 163–192.
Kindlova M and Matena V (1962) Blood vessels of the rat molar. J Dent Res 41, 650–660.
Kindlova M and Trnkova H (1972) The vascular arrangement beneath the sulcular and junctional epithelium in different degrees of cellular infiltration of dog gingiva. J Periodont Res 7, 323–327.
Kishi Y and Takahashi K (1977) A scanning electron microscope study of the vascular architecture of the periodontal membrane. Jpn J Oral Biol 19, 192–207.
Lametschwandtner A, Lametschwandtner V and Weiger T (1990) Scanning electron microscopy of vascular corrosion casts – technique and applications: updated review. Scanning Electron Microsc IV, 889–941.
Lee D, Sims MR, Sampson WJ and Dreyer CW (1990) Stereo-pair three-dimensional imaging of microvascular architecture in primate dental tissues. Aust Orthod J 11, 251–255.
Lee D, Sims MR, Dreyer CW and Sampson WJ (1991) A scanning electron microscope study of microcorrosion casts of the microvasculature of the marmoset palate, gingiva and periodontal ligament. Arch Oral Biol 36, 211–220.
Levick JR and Smaje LH (1987) An analysis of the permeability of a fenestra. Microvasc Res 33, 233–256.
Levy BM and Bernick S (1968) Studies on the biology of the periodontium of marmosets. V. Lymphatic vessels of the periodontal ligament. J Dent Res 47, 1166–1170.
Levy BM, Dreizen S and Bernick S (1972) Effect of aging on the marmoset periodontium. J Oral Path 1, 61–65.
Lew K, Sims MR and Leppard PI (1989) Tooth extrusion effects on microvessel volumes, endothelial areas and fenestrae in molar apical periodontal ligament. Am J Orthod and Dentofacial Orthop 96, 221–231.
Lindhe J (1988) Textbook of Clinical Periodontology. Munksgaard, Copenhagen.
Majno G (1965) The ultrastructure of the vascular membrane. In: Handbook of Physiology (Hamilton WF and Dow P, eds), pp 293–375, Waverley Press, Baltimore.
Matena V (1973) Periodontal ligament of a rat incisor tooth. J Periodont 44, 629–635.
Milici AJ, L'Hernault N and Palade GE (1985) Surface densities of diaphragmed fenestrae and transendothelial channels in different murine capillary beds. Circ Res 56, 709–717.
Moe H (1981) Adaptation of arterioles to moving capillaries. Acta Anat 109, 369–377.
Movat HV and Fernando NVP (1964) The fine structure of the terminal vascular bed. IV. The venules and their perivascular cells (pericytes, adventitial cells). Exp Mol Pathol 3, 98–114.
Moxham BJ and Berkovkitz BKB (1982a) The periodontal ligament and physiological tooth movements. In: The Periodontal Ligament in Health and Disease (Berkovitz BKB, Moxham BJ and Newman HN, eds), pp 213–245, Pergamon Press, Oxford.
Moxham BJ and Berkovitz BKB (1982b) The effect of external forces on the periodontal ligament – the response to axial loads. In: The Periodontal Ligament in Health and Disease (Berkovitz BKB, Moxham BJ and Newman HN, eds), pp 247–266, Pergamon Press, Oxford.
Moxham BJ, Shore RC and Berkovitz BKB (1985) Fenestrated capillaries in the connective tissues of the periodontal ligament. Microvasc Res 30, 116–124.
Moxham BJ, Shore RC and Berkovitz BKB (1987) Fenestrated capillaries in the periodontal ligaments of the erupting and erupted molar. Arch Oral Biol 32, 477–481.
Murakami T (1971) Application of the scanning electron microscope to the study of the fine distribution of the blood vessels. Arch Histol Jpn 32, 445–454.
Murakami T, Unehira M, Kawakami H and Kubotsu A (1973) Osmium impregnation of methyl methacrylate vascular casts for scanning electron microscopy. Arch Histol Jpn 36, 119.
Ng GC, Walker TW, Zingg W and Burke PS (1981) Effects of tooth loading on the periodontal vasculature of the mandibular fourth premolar in dogs. Arch Oral Biol 26, 189–195.
Nowell JA and Lohse CL (1974) Injection replication of the microvasculature for SEM. Scanning Electron Microsc I, 267–274.Nyengaard JR, Bendtsen TF and Gundersen HJG (1988) Stereological estimation of the number of capillaries, exemplified by renal glomeruli. APMIS 4, 92–99.
Parfitt GJ (1960) Measurement of the physiological mobility of individual teeth in an axial direction. J Dent Res 39, 608–618.
Parlange LM and Sims MR (1993) A TEM stereological analysis of blood vessels and nerves in marmoset periodontal ligament following endodontics and magnetic incisor extrusion. Eur J Orthod 15, 33–44.
Reitan K (1985) Biomechanical principles and reactions. In: Orthodontics. Current Principles and Techniques (Graber TM and Swain BF, eds), pp 101–192, WB Saunders, Philadelphia.
Renkin EM (1979) Regulation of capillary morphology to transport of fluid and large molecules: a review. Acta Physiol Scand Suppl 463, 81–91.
Rhodin JAG (1962) The diaphragm of capillary endothelial fenestrations. J Ultrastruct Res 6, 171–185.
Rhodin JAG (1967) The ultrastructure of mammalian arterioles and precapillary sphincters. J Ultrastruct Res 18, 181–223.
Rhodin JAG (1968) Ultrastructure of mammalian venous capillaries, venules, and small collecting veins. J Ultrastruct Res 25, 452–500.
Rhodin JAG (1984) Architecture of the vessel wall. In: Handbook of Physiology (Renkin EM and Michel CC, eds), volume IV, pp 1–31, American Physiological Society, Baltimore.
Ruben MP, Prieto-Hernandez JR, Gott FK, Kramer GM and Bloom AA (1971) Visualization of lymphatic microcirculation of oral tissues. II. Vital retrograde lymphography. J Periodont 42, 265–272.
Rygh P (1976) Ultrastructural changes in tension zones of rat molar periodontium incident to orthodontic tooth movement. Am J Orthod 70, 269–281.
Rygh P (1989) The periodontal ligament under stress. In: The Biology of Tooth Movement (Norton LA and Burstone CJ, eds), pp 10–27, CRC Press, Florida.
Rygh P, Bowling K, Hovlandsdal L and Williams S (1986) Activation of the vascular system: A main mediator of periodontal fibre remodeling in orthodontic tooth movement. Am J Orthod 89, 453–468.
Saunders RL and de Röckert CH (1967) Vascular supply of dental tissue including lympatics. In: Structural and Chemical Organization of Teeth (Miles AEW, ed), volume 1, pp 199–245, Academic Press, London.
Schneeberger EE and Lynch RD (1984) Tight junctions: their structure, composition and function. Circ Res 55, 723–733.
Schroeder HE (1986) The Periodontium. Springer-Verlag, Berlin.
Schweitzer G (1907) Über die Lymphgefasse des Zahnfleisches und der Zähne beim Menschen und Zähne. Arch Mikrosk Anat 69, 807–908.
Seversen JA, Moffett BC, Kokich V and Selipsky H (1978) A histological study of age changes in the adult human periodontal joint (ligament). J Periodont 49, 189–200.
Shore RC, Moxham BJ and Berkovitz BKB (1984) Fenestrated capillaries in the periodontal ligament. J Dent Res 63, 513.
Simionescu M and Simionescu N (1984) Ultrastructure of the microvascular wall: functional correlations. In: Handbook of Physiology (Renkin EM and Michel CC, eds), pp 41–101, American Physiological Society, Baltimore.
Simionescu N and Simionescu M (1988) The cardiovascular system. In: Cell and Tissue Biology (Weiss L, ed), 6th edtion, pp 354–400, Urban and Schwarzenberg, Baltimore.
Simionescu N, Simionescu M and Palade GE (1974) Morphometric data on the endothelium of blood capillaries. J Cell Biol 60, 128–152.
Simionescu N, Simionescu M and Palade GE (1978) Structural basis of permeability in sequential segments of the microvasculature. 1. Bipolar microvascular fields in the diaphragm. Microvasc Res 15, 1–16.
Sims DE (1986) The pericyte – a review. Tissue Cell 18, 153–174.

Sims MR (1980) Angular changes in collagen cemental attachment during tooth movement. J Periodont Res 15, 638–645.
Sims MR (1983a) Electron-microscopic affiliations of oxytalan fibres, nerves and the microvascular bed in the mouse periodontal ligament. Arch Oral Biol 28, 1017–1024.
Sims MR (1983b) The microvascular venous pool and its ultrastructural associations in mouse molar periodontal ligament. Aust Orthod J 8, 21–27.
Sims MR (1984) Ultrastructural evidence of nerve and oxytalan fibre associations in human periodontal ligament. Arch Oral Biol 29, 565–567.
Sims MR (1987a) A model of the anisotropic distribution of microvascular volume in the periodontal ligament of the mouse mandibular molar. Aust Orthod J 10, 21–24.
Sims MR (1987b) Ultrastructure of the venous ampulla in the interradicular microvascular bed of the mandibular molars of *mus musculus*. J Morphol 191, 217–224.
Sims MR, Leppard PI, Sampson WJ and Dreyer CW (1994) Microvascular luminal changes in aged mouse periodontal ligament. Unpublished data.
Sobin SS and Tremer HM (1977) Three-dimensional organization of microvascular beds as related to function. In: Microcirculation (Kaley G and Altura BM), pp 43–68, University Park Press, Baltimore.
Tabata S and Semba T (1987) Examination of blood capillaries in rat incisor pulp by TEM of thin sections and freeze fracture replicas. J Electron Microsc 36, 283–293.
Takahashi K and Matsuo M (1991) Scanning electron microscopic observation of periodontal ligament. Quintessence 10, 13–23.
Tang MFP and Sims MR (1992) A TEM analysis of tissue channels in normal and orthodontically tensioned rat molar periodontal ligament. Eur J Orthod 14, 433–444.
Tang MFP, Sims MR, Sampson WJ and Dreyer CW (1993) Evidence for endothelial junctions acting as a fluid flux pathway in tensioned periodontal ligament. Arch Oral Biol 38, 273–276.
Walker TW (1980) A model of the periodontal vasculature in tooth support. J Biomech 13, 149–157.
Weekes WT and Sims MR (1986a) The vasculature of the rat molar gingival crevice. J Periodont Res 21, 177–185.
Weekes WT and Sims MR (1986b) The vasculature of the rat molar periodontal ligament. J Periodont Res 21, 186–194.
Wiedeman MP (1963) Dimensions of blood vessels from distributing artery to collecting vein. Circ Res 12, 375–378.
Wills DJ, Picton DCA and Davis WIR (1976) A study of the fluid systems of the periodontium in macaque monkeys. Arch Oral Biol 21, 175–185.
Wong RST and Sims MR (1983) Morphology of the enamel–cementum microvascular junction of the mouse incisor. Aust Orthod J 8, 49–50.
Wong RST and Sims MR (1987) A scanning electron-microscopic, stereo-pair study of methacrylate corrosion casts of the mouse palatal and molar periodontal microvasculatures. Arch Oral Biol 32, 557–566.

Chapter 6

The Physiology of the Vasculature of the Periodontal Ligament

LGA Edwall and H Aars

INTRODUCTION

The periodontal ligament (PDL) undoubtedly has unique functions among the connective tissue in the mammalian body. Its ability to tolerate high intermittent pressures during mastication, as well as more continuous pressure – for instance during orthodontic treatment – combined with its ability to detect small tactile stimuli is impressive. The vasculature in the PDL is adapted to these conditions, and it plays a central role in the functions of the ligament.

The primary role for the blood circulation in the PDL is to provide exchanges of substrate and metabolites between blood and the periodontal tissues, including the dentine. This circulation may also play a part in tooth support and eruption, as well as in the sensory functions of the ligament.

This review is concerned primarily with the basic physiology of the blood circulation that supplies the PDL in health, but some remarks will also apply to pathophysiological conditions. For information concerning the role of the vasculature in the eruptive mechanism and tooth support, see Chapters 9 and 10.

BLOOD FLOW

Blood flow as studied directly by vital microscopy

One of the major difficulties encountered in studies of the microcirculation of the PDL relates to the fact that the major blood supply of the ligament is derived from the surrounding alveolar bone as well as from periapical vessels. Consequently, a window cut in the bone for intravital observation of blood flow is likely to disturb detrimentally the blood supply to the ligament. However, Gängler and Merte (1979a) have described a technique using the rat mandibular incisor, which they claim minimizes this disturbance. The mandible is divided at the symphysis to allow alveolar bone, dentine, and pulp to be removed from the lateral side until only a thin layer of dentine remains, through which the PDL blood flow can be observed under transmitted light. Using this technique, Gängler and Merte (1983) studied the effects of force application on the periodontal blood circulation, having previously (Gängler and Merte, 1979b) compared the resting blood flow in the PDL and gingival microcirculations. In the latter work, the linear flow velocity was measured in various types of vessels in both tissues and was found to be about the same for each type, i.e. a capillary flow rate of 0.02–0.04 mm per second and a venular flow rate of 0.1 μm per second. These values are 2–10 times smaller than those found in alveolar bone marrow (Brånemark, 1961). It is difficult to work out whether such differences are real, whether they are due to experimental difficulties (e.g. maintaining blood flows at normal rates), or whether they represent species differences. Since the capillaries of the bone marrow have diameters of 8 μm (Brånemark, 1961) compared with diameters of 5–7 μm for PDL capillaries (Gängler and Merte, 1979b), it is possible that a slower blood flow in the PDL is to be expected.

Blood flow as studied by indirect techniques

Whenever a new technique is developed, it is first used on oral tissues that are more accessible than the PDL. Thus, using radiolabelled microspheres of diameter 15±5 μm, Meyer (1970) and Path and Meyer (1977) reported flow in alveolar bone in the range of 0.1–0.5 ml/min per gram. Kaplan *et al.* (1978b) found slightly lower values, of about 0.1 ml/min per gram. Comparisons between blood flow in mandibular alveolar bone and in gingiva were made by Kaplan *et al.* (1978a) from studies using radiolabelled microspheres and a diffusible tracer (^{86}Rb). They reported significantly higher flow values in the gingiva (0.5 ml/min per gram in gingiva and 0.1 ml/min per gram in alveolar bone). Only recently has the technique been applied to the study of blood flow in the PDL. Kvinnsland *et al.* (1989, 1992) calculated flow relative to tissue volume. In rat molars, flow in the PDL on average measured 1.7 ml/min per cm^3, about four times as much as the rate observed simultaneously in the pulp.

Another indirect method to study local blood flow involves the measurement of the local clearance of a diffusible tracer, inert, radioactive tracer injected directly into the tissue. This technique was devised by Kety (1949). Kety used radioactive sodium, but nowadays the inert lipid soluble gas ^{133}Xe or ^{125}I as iodide is more commonly used. These tracers (especially Xe) pass so rapidly from the tissue to the blood that in most instances the rate of washout from the injection site is limited only by blood flow. If the tissue in which the injected depot is located is perfused uniformly and constantly with blood, the rate at which the tracer washout has a mono-exponential function. Thus, when tracer concentration is plotted against time on semilog paper, the washout curve forms a straight line. The slope of this curve is related to the rate of blood flow. For example, the curve becomes horizontal if blood flow is arrested suddenly.

It must be emphasized that, since this technique reflects the rate of exchange of solutes between tissue and blood, the nutritive function of the blood flow is accentuated. Consequently, blood shunted away from capillaries via arteriovenous anastomoses will not be discerned by this technique.

Edwall and Kindlová (1971) used tracer disappearance techniques to obtain some measure of blood flow in various oral tissues, including the PDL. Although the method did not allow quantitative calculations of blood flow, their results suggested that there were no significant differences between the rates of disappearance of tracers in PDL, gingiva, dental pulp, and alveolar submucosa. This contrasts with the difference between periodontal and pulp blood flow as estimated with the microsphere technique (Kvinnsland *et al.*, 1989, 1992). It is possible that the difference is caused by a higher degree of arteriovenous shunting in the pulp. Furthermore, the discrepancy might be related to the complexity of the periodontal vascular bed: the injection of 10–20 μl of tracer fluid into the periodontal space in the bifurcation area of a mandibular molar might have resulted in spread of the depot fluid into the adjacent alveolar bone. Therefore, the data of Edwall and Kindlová (1971) for the PDL probably reflected a combined effect in both the ligament and the adjacent bone. A more specific measure of ligament blood flow was obtained by Edwall (1988), in studies in which the PDL was approached from the pulp chamber and the tracer reached the ligament by diffusing through a thin layer of root cementum.

Laser Doppler flowmetry (LDF) is the most recent development in recording of tissue blood flow. This technique is based on the principle that light hitting a moving particle is reflected with a slightly altered wavelength, while reflections from a static surface retain the original wavelength. Light is transmitted to and returned from the tissue by means of fibreoptics. The difference in emitted and reflected wavelength is used to calculate the average linear velocity of flow and the relative amount of moving blood cells. The product of the two – the flux – is a measure of blood flow in the tissue. The technique is non-invasive, and it does not disturb the tissues. One drawback is that the penetration depth of the light is often uncertain, and consequently the relative contribution from small superficial and deeper, larger vessels may vary.

The LDF has been extensively used in studies of circulation, including experimental and clinical studies of blood circulation in oral tissues. The validity of the technique has been tested in the tooth pulp by comparing evoked changes in flow with this and other methods. Edwall *et al.* (1987a) simultaneously measured blod flow in the dental pulp with LDF and local ^{125}I-clearance, and found a good correlation between the two during sympathetic stimulation of the cervical sympathetic trunk and infusion of Substance P (SP). However, upon stimulation of the inferior alveolar nerve, the LDF signal showed an increase while the local clearance rate was unaffected or even decreased. This indicates that the two methods reflect flow changes in different parts of the pulpal vascular bed, and that the flow is unevenly distributed to these parts during antidromic stimulation of the inferior alveolar nerve. Significant correlations between the LDF signal and pulpal blood flow measured with H_2-clearance (Okabe *et al.*, 1989) or ^{133}Xe-washout (Kim *et al.*, 1990) have since been reported in dogs. In the latter study, flow was changed by intra-arterial injection of noradrenaline.

LDF has been used to study the effects of orthodontic forces on periodontal blood flow in humans, by introducing a 0.45 mm (outer diameter) probe into the gingival pocket (Hertrich and Raab, 1990). In cats, Sasano *et al.* (1992) investigated the changes occurring in cervical and apical PDL blood flow during application of external forces (*Fig. 6.1*). Access to the ligament was provided by paring away mandibular bone from the labial side until the periodontal vascular network was visible through a thin layer of bone. The same approach was used to study the effects on ligament blood flow of stimulating the sympathetic and sensory nerves to the maxillary canine in cats (Karita *et al.*, 1989). It is worth remembering, however, that such removal of alveolar bone

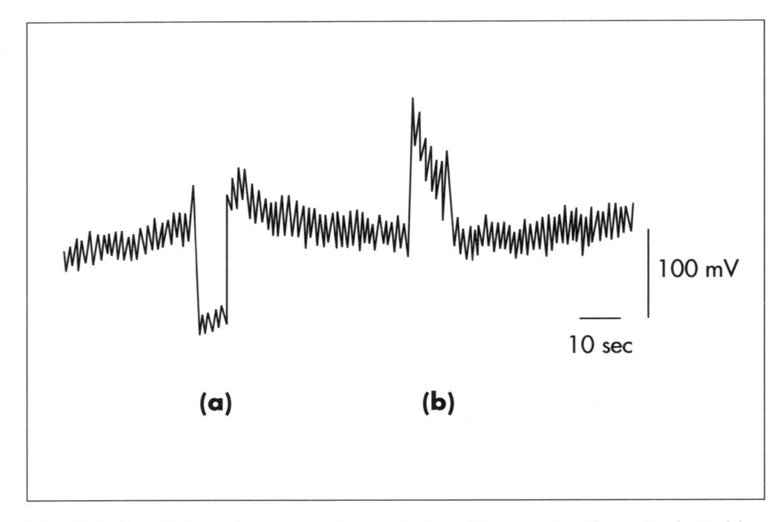

Fig. 6.1 Blood flow changes in the periodontal ligament in the cat, elicited by mechanical stimulation of the canine tooth in (a) labiolingual and (b) linguo-labial direction. Laser Doppler flowmetry. (From Karita *et al.*, 1989.)

is apt to interfere with the circulation of blood in the ligament. Also, as will be discussed below, the circulation will be affected by the accompanying activation of afferent nerves in the area.

Linden (1975) assessed the effects of stimulating the cervical sympathetic trunk on the PDL by monitoring temperature changes within the tissue. This technique offers another possibility for indirectly assessing changes in PDL blood flow, though precise data cannot be provided.

BLOOD VOLUME CHANGES MONITORED BY PLETHYSMOGRAPHIC TECHNIQUES

Plethysmography involves the measurement of volume changes in the tissue under study. If the venous outflow can be obstructed intermittently, the technique can measure total blood flow. Unfortunately, it is not possible to measure precisely volume changes in the PDL or to control venous outflow. Thus, plethysmography can only hint at changes in blood flow within the PDL.

Packman *et al.* (1977) used photoelectric plethysmography to monitor changes in the microcirculation of the human PDL. Light was conducted to and from the periodontal tissues either via miniature fibreoptics placed within the roots of endodontically treated teeth or by transilluminating the ligament from the gingiva. Rapid variations of light absorption were thought to represent vascular changes. At rest, pulsatile changes that were synchronous with the heart beat were recorded. However, their results may reflect not only circulatory changes in the PDL but also relate to changes in the alveolar bone and, in the case of transillumination, in the gingiva.

Another way to use the principle of plethysmography in investigations of the periodontal vasculature involves monitoring changes in tooth position. A number of studies have reported that the ligament allows minute movements of the tooth that are synchronous with pulsatile changes in blood pressure (e.g. Hofmann and Diemer, 1963; Körber, 1963, 1970; Körber and Körber, 1965). The amplitude of movement is usually less than 0.5 μm (e.g. Hofmann and Diemer, 1963; Körber and Körber, 1965), the pulsatile movements axially being less than those labially (*Fig. 6.2*). These tooth movements can be interpreted only in terms of pulsatile changes in local tissue and blood pressures. Using displacement transducers that are sensitive enough to allow continuous monitoring of tooth position, it has been possible to study tooth position in rabbit and rat incisors and ferret and cat canines (Matthews and Berkovitz, 1972; Moxham, 1979a,b; Burn-Murdoch and Picton, 1978; Myhre *et al.*, 1979; Aars, 1982a,b, 1983a,b; Aars and Linden, 1982; Moxham and Berkovitz, 1983). Many of these studies report clear-cut changes following experimental interference with the vascular system, and it seems that the resting position of the tooth is influenced by the arterial blood pressure via the periodontal vessels. This influence was studied indirectly by Edwall *et al.* (1987b), who recorded simultaneously the intra-alveolar tooth position and the local clearance of ^{125}I from the PDL. They demonstrated parallel changes in these parameters during both vasoconstriction and vasodilatation (*Fig. 6.3*). However, venous stasis will increase the interstitial fluid pressure (Kristiansen and Heyeraas, 1989) and extrude the tooth, but reduce the flow. Thus, while circulatory evoked changes in tissue pressure within the PDL will always elicit changes in tooth position, in the absence of venous stasis the position may also

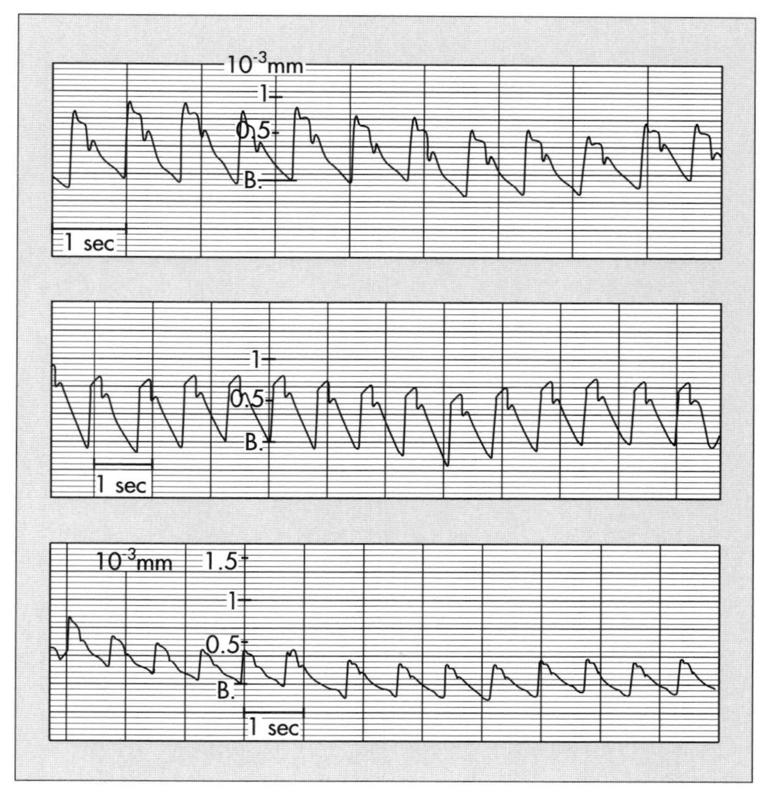

Fig. 6.2 Periodontal pulse in three different subjects. (From Körber, 1970)

offer an indirect estimate of changes in ligament blood flow without interfering with the tissue itself. Such techniques have also been used to investigate the vasomotor control of the periodontal vasculature and to study the mechanisms of tooth support and eruption.

THE MEASUREMENT OF INTERSTITIAL PRESSURES IN THE PERIODONTAL LIGAMENT

Schärer and Hayashi (1969) were the first to report on PDL tissue pressure, recording changes in pressure following force application. Subsequently, Lamb and Van Hassel (1972) and Palcanis (1973) studied the pressures during resting conditions and following traumatic occlusion, tissue damage, and infiltration of Lidocaine with adrenaline. The resting tissue pressure in the canine tooth of the dog was seen to average 9–10 mmHg above atmospheric pressure. Trauma was found to double the pressure. Infiltration of the vasoconstrictor agent reduced the PDL tissue pressure. Others have found a negative pressure in the PDL (Walker *et al.*, 1978). It is known from studies of pulpal interstitial pressure (e.g. Nähri, 1978; Tønder and Kvinnsland, 1983) that marked pressure gradients occur over a distance of only a few millimetres within the tissue. It is possible, therefore, that the tissue pressures recorded in the PDL reflect very localized pressures at the sites of measurement. Kristiansen and Heyeraas (1989) studied the interstitial fluid pressure in rat PDL. They approached the PDL from the pulp chamber, puncturing the thinned cementum with glass pipettes that had a tip diameter of 2–4 μm. With an average mean arterial pressure of 125 mmHg, mean interstitial pressure averaged 15 mmHg. This tissue pressure showed heart synchronous oscillations, but mean pressure remained stable up to 90 minutes after pipette insertion. Mean pressure was increased by venous stasis and reduced after cardiac arrest. There was no indication that the measurement caused inflammatory reactions, which would have distorted the pressure. This technique therefore appears eminently suitable as a research tool for monitoring tissue pressure in the PDL.

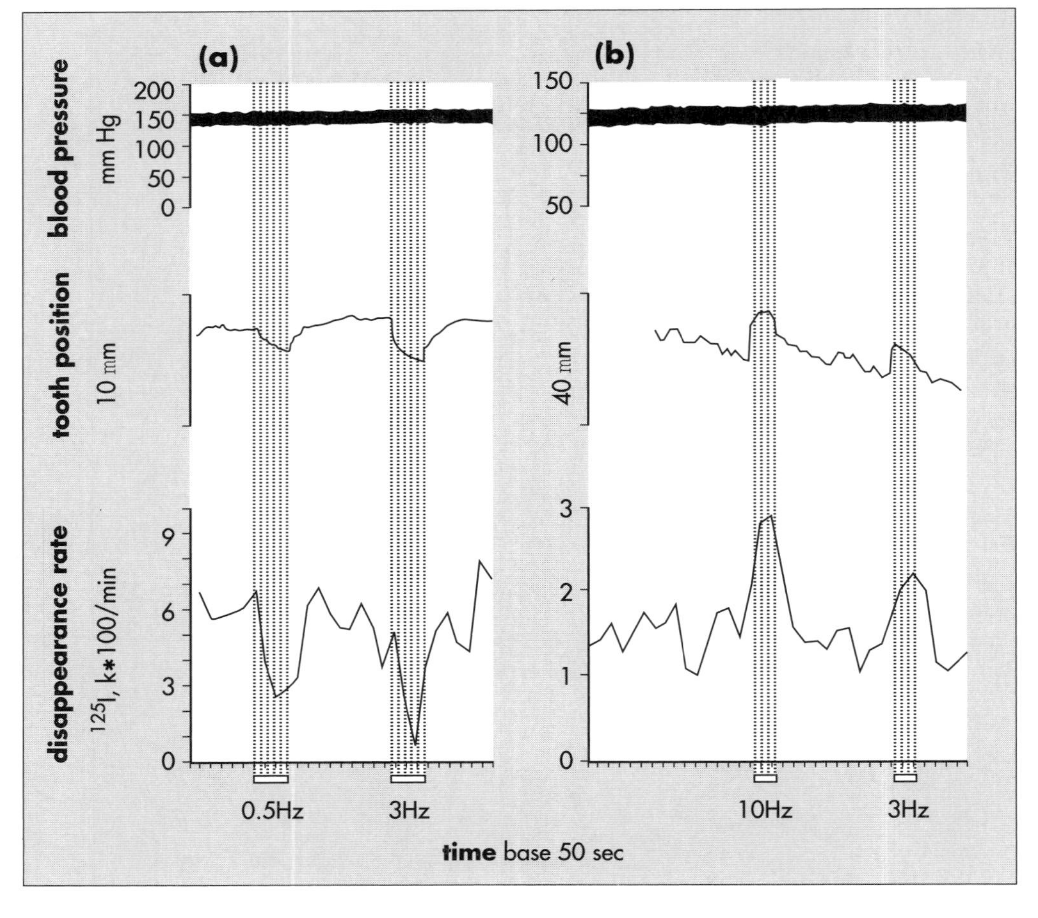

Fig. 6.3 Effects of electrical stimulation of efferent and afferent nerves on tooth position and periodontal ligament blood flow in a cat. Blood flow measured as the disappearance rate of radioactive tracer. (A) Sympathetic nerve stimulation. (B) Stimulation of inferior alveolar nerve, after pretreatment with phentolamine. (Modified from Edwall *et al.*,1987b.)

CONTROL OF THE PDL BLOOD FLOW

Efferent nerves

The vascular control in the PDL has recently attracted much attention. Using tracer disappearance techniques, Edwall and Kindlová (1971) studied the effects of sympathetic nerve activation on blood flow in the PDL and other oral structures in the dog. They reported that the washout rates were reduced after sympathetic activation and that there was a clear frequency–response relationship between the stimulation frequency and the reduction of nutritive blood flow. Sympathetic nerve stimulation induced reduction of up to 70 per cent in the tracer washout rate in all the oral tissues investigated with the exception of the PDL, where the response was higher (about 90 per cent reduction).

Monitoring the tooth position, Moxham (1979b) and Myhre *et al.* (1979) found the rabbit incisor to be intruded by intravascular injection of noradrenaline (*Fig. 6.4*). Moxham (1981) reported that the eruption rate of the rabbit mandibular incisor showed a transient increase after section of the ipsilateral cervical sympathetic trunk, and that stimulation of the peripheral end of the nerve produced intrusive movements of the incisor, although without a clear dose–response relationship. Aars (1982a) observed an extrusion of about 7 μm of the maxillary incisor after bilateral section of the cervical sympathetic trunk in rabbits. Subsequent electrical stimulation of the sectioned nerves made the tooth move back into its socket, and the position held prior to nerve section was obtained with stimuli of about 0.5 Hz. The rapid intrusive movements in response to sympathetic nerve stimulation increased with a rise in stimulation frequency – the maximum (of about 12 μm) was reached with 20 Hz, and 70 per cent of maximum intrusion occurred at 2 Hz (*Fig. 6.5*). The response sometimes varied between stimulation of low- and high-

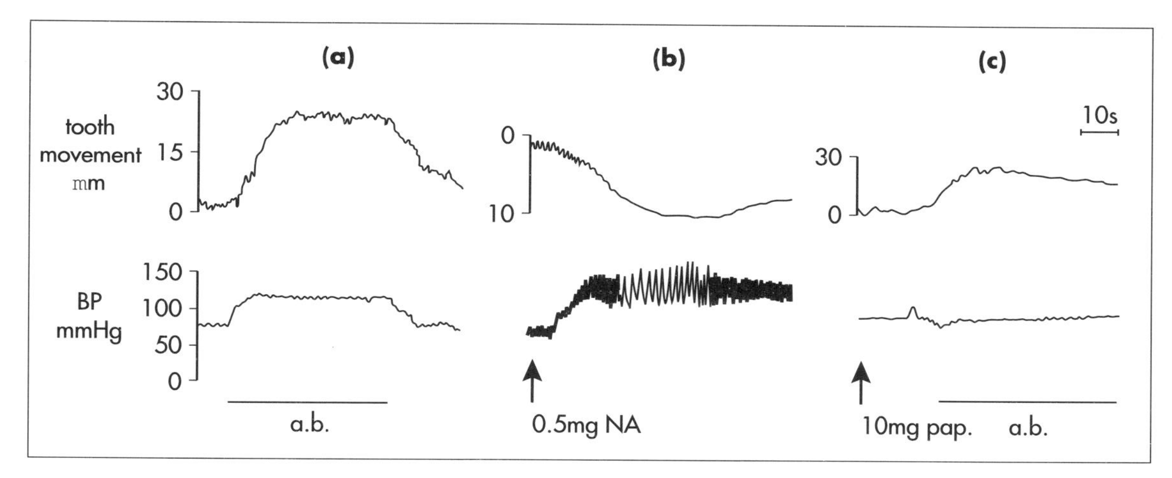

Fig. 6.4 Changes in position of rabbit incisor resulting from (a) alteration of arterial blood pressure, (b) intravenous injection of noradrenaline, and (c) intravenous injection of papaverine. Arterial blood pressure was changed or maintained by inflation of a balloon positioned in the descending aorta. (Modified from Myhre et al.,1979.)

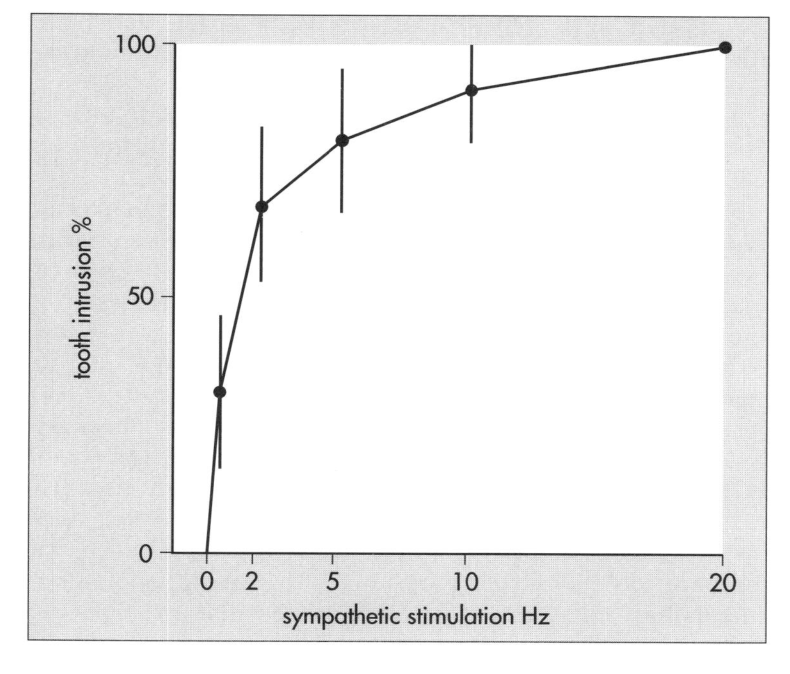

Fig. 6.5 Intrusive movement of the maxillary incisor in response to bilateral sympathetic nerve stimulation in rabbits. Stimulation periods of 20–30 seconds; the changes in position are related to individual responses to 20 Hz stimulation. Mean ± standard deviation. (From Aars 1982a.)

threshold fibres, suggesting the existence of different populations of nerve fibres projecting to periodontal vessels. Variations between evoked responses in different oral tissues might also have contributed: stealing of perfusion pressure, caused by vasodilatation in larger neighbouring tissues, is likely to be as relevant to the periodontal circulation as it is to the tooth pulp (Tønder, 1976; Liu *et al.*, 1990).

Maximum intrusive response to sympathetic nerve stimulation was slightly less for the cat maxillary canine (Aars and Linden, 1982) than for the rabbit incisor, but the relative sensitivity to stimulation was about the same. More recently, sympathetic nerve stimulation has been shown to produce a frequency-dependent reduction in the ligament blood flow in cats, as recorded with a clearance technique (Edwall *et al.*, 1987b; Edwall, 1988) (see *Fig. 6.3*) or laser Doppler flowmetry (Karita *et al.*, 1989).

It is important to note that the circulation of blood in the PDL responds not only to electrical stimulation of sympathetic nerves, but also to more physiological, reflex changes in sympathetic activity. Thus, the position of the tooth has been found to be sensitive to changes in sympathetic nerve activity evoked by haemorrhagic hypotension or electrical stimulation of the aortic baroreceptor nerve (Aars, 1983a). Furthermore, the response to an abrupt rise in arterial pressure, causing extrusion, was more pronounced after sympathectomy (Aars, 1983a). The overall conclusion is that the sympathetic nervous system exerts a powerful influence on circulation in the PDL, and that this control is operative at physiological, low levels of activity.

Administration of the α-adrenoceptor antagonist phentolamine markedly reduced the intrusive response to sympathetic stimulation in rabbits (Aars, 1982a), as it did in cats (Aars and Linden, 1982). Similarly, the sympathetically evoked reduction in ligament blood flow was significantly reduced by phentolamine (Edwall and Gazelius, 1988; Karita *et al.*, 1989). It is thus well established that the reduction of blood flow in the PDL during stimulation of sympathetic nerves is mainly mediated by α-adrenoceptors.

Edwall and Gazelius (1988) studied the reduction in ligament blood flow caused by local arterial infusion of adrenaline or noradrenaline, as well as by electrical sympathetic nerve stimulation in cats. They noted that while each of three different α-adrenoceptor blocking agents almost abolished the effects of the catecholamines, a component of the response to electrical sympathetic stimulation was resistant to α-blockade. This component disappeared after administration of guanethidine, which is known to inhibit the release of noradrenaline and neuropeptide Y (NPY). The two transmitters probably co-exist in the same nerve fibres. Based on these findings, they concluded that the sympathetic regulation of blood flow in the PDL was mediated by postjunctional α_1- and α_2-adrenoceptors, and possibly by non-adrenergic vasoconstriction. The role of NPY in this non-adrenergic vasosconstriction is strengthened by the demonstration of NPY-immunoreactivity in the superior cervical ganglion, the dental pulp, and the oral mucosa in cats (Edwall *et al.*, 1985). In this study, guanethidine abolished the phentolamine-resistant vasoconstriction, without interfering with the response to infused NPY.

Storage vesicles typical of adrenergic nerve fibres have recently been found along periapical arterioles in extracted human teeth (Nakamura *et al.*, 1992). Heyeraas *et al.* (1993) observed NPY-immunoreactive fibres in periapical vessels of the ligament in cats, but noted that they were much more numerous in large blood vessels in the mandibular canal. One may conclude that a fall in ligament blood flow during sympathetic nerve stimulation is caused by vasoconstriction in vessels both outside and inside the PDL.

Aars (1982a,b) reported that β-adrenoceptor blockade produced by infusion of propranolol or more specific β-antagonists extruded the tooth, whereas infusion of isoprenaline reversed or prevented this movement. In line with this observation, the intrusion of the tooth caused by phentolamine (Aars, 1982a) was quite likely due to dominance of β-agonist action of circulating catecholamines after α-blockade. Also, β-receptor antagonists reduced the intrusive response to stimulation of the cervical sympathetic trunk (Aars, 1982b). These results indicate a double adrenergic control of the blood vessels serving the PDL:

(i) sympathetically innervated α-adrenoceptors mediating constriction of precapillary vessels; and

(ii) humoral factors mediating dilatation of post capillary resistance vessels through activation of β_2-adrenoreceptors.

Pre-junctional β_1- and β_2-receptors, enhancing the intrusive response to sympathetic nerve stimulation, may also be present, although functional evidence of their presence was not found in other experiments (Aars, 1982a; Aars and Linden, 1982).

The results reported by Aars (1982a,b) also suggest that both the pre- and postcapillary resistance vessels were under the influence of a sympathetic tone (nervous and humoral) during the experiment; nerve transection and propranolol both induced extrusion. Since the experiments were performed under general anaesthesia, however, it cannot be stated to what extent such sympathetic tone is present in the conscious animal.

Cholinergic pathways have not so far been found to play an important part in the regulation of the periodontal circulation, even if the fibres are there. Thus, Nakamura *et al.* (1992) observed small clear vesicles in human periodontal nerve fibres, typical of cholinergic fibres, and Kato *et al.* (1990) found nerve fibres containing vasointestinal peptide (VIP) in the apical and furcal regions of the PDL in mice, most of them associated with blood vessels. However, the functional correlates of these fibres are mostly unknown, although injection of acetylcholine (Moxham, 1979b) and VIP (Edwall, 1988) has been shown to elicit vasodilatation and increased flow in the PDL. However, Aars (1982a) found no effects of atropine on the resting position of the tooth or on its intrusive response to sympathetic nerve stimulation, and Karita *et al.* (1989) noted that atropine was without effect on the often biphasic responses to electrical stimulation of the superior alveolar nerve in cats. Consequently, although present evidence suggests the existence of efferent vasodilator pathways to the vasculature of the PDL, we still do not know how to stimulate or trigger activity in these nerves. In the tooth pulp, atropine-sensitive active nervous vasodilatation has recently been shown to be evoked by isometric hand grip or dynamic exercise in humans (Aars *et al.*, 1992, 1993), while non-adrenergic, non-cholinergic vasodilatation has been found to occur in the gingiva (Aars *et al.*, 1993).

Linden (1975) investigated the effects of nerve stimulations and transections on PDL temperature. Stimulation of the cervical sympathetic trunk was associated with a fall in ligament temperature, which was prevented by transection of the inferior alveolar nerve and hence the sympathetic fibres to the area.

Afferent nerves

When Linden (1975) stimulated the distal end of the transected inferior nerve, the full effect of sympathetic stimulation on PDL temperature could not be reproduced. Presumably this was due to the fact that the inferior alveolar nerve, apart from containing sympathetic nerve fibres, possesses fibres that have a vasodilator function. Gazelius and Olgart (1980) subsequently reported that antidromic stimulation of the transected inferior alveolar nerve induced a biphasic vascular response in the pulp, which was converted to a clear-cut increase in pulp blood flow after α-adrenoceptor blockade. Their findings suggested that the dilator effect was mediated by Substance P (SP). Since then, nerve fibres that contain SP-related peptide and calcitonin gene-related peptide (CGRP) have been found in the PDL in cats, mice, and rats (Wakisaka *et al.*, 1985; Silverman and Kruger, 1987; Kato *et al.*, 1990, 1992; Kvinnsland and Kvinnsland, 1990; Kvinnsland *et al.*, 1991; Saito *et al.*, 1991; Kvinnsland and Heyeraas, 1992; Heyeraas *et al.*, 1993). Double immunostaining has indicated that the two peptides co-exist in the same nerve fibres in the tooth pulp (Wakisaka *et al.*, 1987). The two have a very similar distribution in the PDL (Kato *et al.*, 1992), where they are mostly confined to the blood vessels in the apical and middle part of the ligament.

The CGRP- and SP-containing nerve fibres are known to be thin sensory fibres, involved in the transmission of pain. Release of the peptides, as in the classical axon reflex, causes vasodilatation and increased vascular permeability, leading to protein extravasation and oedema formation – all indices of neurogenic inflammation. Thus, as in the pulp (Gazelius and Olgart, 1980), Edwall *et al.* (1987b) found that antidromic stimulation of the inferior alveolar nerve in cats treated with phentolamine led to increases in PDL blood flow and concomitant extrusive movement of the tooth, effects which could be mimicked by local intra-arterial injections of SP (see *Fig. 6.3*). Similarly, Karita *et al.* (1989) investigated the effects on PDL blood flow by stimulating the distal end of the cut superior alveolar nerve in cats. They found three different responses: an increased blood flow, a decreased blood flow, and a biphasic change in blood flow. The decreasing component was almost abolished by phentolamine, and the increase in flow disappeared after pretreatment with capsaicin, indicating that the former was due to activation of sympathetic vasoconstrictor fibres in the superior alveolar nerve, the latter to antidromic stimulation of sensory fibres.

Activation of sensory nerves might also explain the results obtained by Sasano *et al.* (1993). They observed that, while application of histamine to the pulp evoked a rise in blood flow in the pulp as well as in the PDL, only the pulpal response disappeared after washing out the histamine. Unless histamine had reached the ligament by diffusion, the persistence of vasodilatation in the ligament suggests that histamine had activated pulpal branches of sensory nerves serving both tissues.

Other regulatory influences

Little is known of pressure autoregulation of the periodontal circulation. The rather small circulatory response to bilateral carotid artery occlusion, as evidenced by minor or no intrusive effect in rabbits and cats, in spite of a reduction in lingual or ear arterial pressure of roughly 50–80 per cent (Aars and Linden, 1982; Aars, 1982a), might be interpreted as evidence of autoregulation. The more so, since sympathetic nerve activity would be expected to rise, owing to a fall in carotid sinus baroreceptor activity. The fact that the tooth moved much more in response to electrical stimulation of the sympathetic nerves than it did in response to carotid occlusion implies that the nervously mediated vasoconstriction produced a more severe reduction in local vascular and tissue pressures. The lack of tooth movements in response to arterial hypotension caused by aortic nerve stimulation (Aars, 1983a) might also suggest autoregulation. However, the hypotension caused marked intrusion after the sympathetic nerves had been cut, suggesting that, with intact nerves, the effect of arterial hypotension on the periodontal circulation had been compensated for by the neurologically mediated fall in vascular resistance. The tooth moved into its socket during haemorrhagic hypotension (Aars, 1983a), illustrating that autoregulation (if present) in this case was unable to override the effects of an increase in sympathetic nerve activity. Furthermore, the tooth will be extruded by a rise in arterial or venous pressure (Myhre *et al.*, 1979, Aars, 1983a,b), and periodontal interstitial pressure follows alterations in arterial and venous pressures (Kristiansen and Heyeraas, 1989).

On the whole, existing evidence therefore indicates that periodontal tissue pressure and the position of the tooth will change in response to sudden alterations in arterial pressure. Direct recordings of periodontal blood flow during changes in arterial pressure have, to our knowledge, not been made. However, as periodontal blood flow has been shown to change in parallel with the position of the tooth, at least during stimulation of efferent and afferent nerves (Edwall *et al.*, 1987b), present knowledge suggests that autoregulation has little if any influence on PDL blood flow.

As studied by vital microscopy, venular diameter and flow velocity increased in the ligament when temperature of the superfused saline was changed from 37°C to 27°C or 42°C (Gängler and Merte, 1980). The physiological significance of this observation is uncertain, however, since the technique involves considerable tissue injury.

THE NUTRITIVE ROLE OF THE PDL VASCULATURE

Wasserman *et al.* (1941) demonstrated that pulpless teeth continue to take up phosphorus via the cementum of the root and that about 10 per cent of the amount of phosphorus taken up by normal teeth during 24 hours enters via the PDL. Gilda *et al.* (1943) performed similar experiments and reported that 25 per cent of the phosphorus uptake during 36 hours had entered via the ligament vasculature. Stüben and Spreter von Kreudenstein (1960) reported similar results for penicillin. Thus there is good evidence that substances pass from the vessels of the PDL into the hard tissues of the root.

FUNCTIONAL ASPECTS OF THE PERIODONTAL CIRCULATION

The vascularization and circulation of blood in the PDL contributes importantly to the mechanical and possibly to the sensory functions of the ligament. Thus, the immediate position of the tooth is influenced not only by external forces, but by the vascular and, therefore, the insterstitial pressure in the PDL (Myhre *et al.*, 1979; Moxham, 1981; Aars, 1982a,b, 1983a; Aars and Linden, 1982; Kristiansen and Heyeraas, 1989). Similarly, the acute mobility of the tooth, as evidenced by its movement in response to acute loading with external forces, depends to a certain degree upon vascularly mediated changes in resting position of the tooth (Aars and Linden, 1982; Aars, 1983a,b). Most importantly, the ability of the tooth to undergo abrupt displacement requires an immediate shift in vascular volumes within the PDL (see *Fig. 6.1*). Blood is immediately moved from compression zones to tension zones or out of the alveolus (Packman *et al.*, 1977; Ng *et al.*, 1981; Gängler and Merte, 1983; Sasano *et al.*, 1992). In humans, Hertrich and Raab (1990) studied the effects of intrusive forces of 0.1–0.5 N on periodontal blood flow in a central maxillary incisor, as measured with laser Doppler technique. They observed a graded reduction within 1–2 seconds, but blood flow returned towards control level if the force was maintained. There are numerous reports on morphometric changes in the periodontal vasculature secondary to application of external forces (Rygh *et al.*, 1986, Nakamura *et al.*, 1986a,b; Lew *et al.*, 1989; Göz *et al.*, 1992). In studies of rat molars with fluorescent microspheres, periodontal blood flow was found to be slightly increased by orthodontic forces acting over several days (Kvinnsland *et al.*, 1989, 1992), but these authors did not distinguish between flow in various zones of the ligament.

Since the sensory function of the PDL depends on the mobility of the tooth, which again may change with the resting position, the sympathetic nervous system through its vascular actions may serve to alter the response of periodontal mechanoreceptors to loading of the tooth. This line of reasoning is suggested by the marked sympathetic inhibitory effects on periodontal mechanoreceptor discharge in response to loads applied to the cat's canine tooth (Cash and Linden, 1982), and on the tooth-tap-evoked digastric muscle reflex in rabbits (Aars *et al.*, 1988; Aars and Brodin, 1989). It is still uncertain, however, if this effect of sympathetic nerve activity is caused by a direct effect on the receptors or whether it is mediated by the alteration in position and mobility of the tooth.

SUMMARY AND CONCLUDING REMARKS

1. Vital microscopic studies suggest that blood flow may be slower in the PDL than in alveolar bone (perhaps owing to a rich network of anastomosing vessels in the ligament). Blood flow in the ligament has been reported to be about equal to or somewhat higher than flow in the dental pulp, the difference in part depending on the applied methods of measurement.

2. Other techniques for estimation of changes in ligament blood flow include microspheres, tracer washout, laser Doppler flowmetry, and interstitial tissue pressure. The recording of changes in tooth position offers the only known way of obtaining estimates of changes in vascular and tissue pressure in the ligament without disturbing the tissue.

3. Changes in vascular volume or tissue pressure in the periodontal ligament influence the resting position and, therefore, the mobility of the tooth.

4. The resting tissue pressure in the PDL of the dog and rat is 10–15 mmHg above atmospheric pressure; the pressure is increased by tissue damage and reduced by infiltration of a vasoconstrictor agent.

5. Activation of sympathetic nerves to the jaws in a dose-dependent manner reduces blood flow in the PDL. The vasoconstriction is mediated by post-junctional α_1- and α_2-adrenoceptors and possibly by peptidergic (NPY) receptors.

6. A double adrenergic vasomotor control of the PDL has been proposed: α-adrenoceptors inducing constriction of precapillary resistance vessels; and β-adrenoceptors mediating dilatation of post-capillary resistance vessels.

7. The ligament circulation is probably influenced by efferent vasodilator nerves, but when and how these nerves are activated remains unknown.

8. The vasodilator axon reflex is operative in the ligament, inducing neurogenic inflammation.

9. The validity of conclusions based on animal studies is probably limited to gross circulatory changes, since the microcirculation is apt to be disturbed by the tissue trauma induced in most studies of PDL blood flow.

10. Among the basic information still lacking is knowledge of:

- the trophic and circulatory functions of the many peptides found in the ligament, and of the interaction between adrenergic, peptidergic and other agents involved in tissue damage;
- the interaction between nutritional blood flow through exchange vessels and shunted blood flow through arteriovenous shunts;
- the lymphatic drainage and its function in the ligament; and
- the role of circulatory parameters in clinical conditions such as bruxism, traumatic occlusion, pulpal or periodontal inflammation and orthodontic treatment.

REFERENCES

Aars H (1982a) The influence of sympathetic nerve activity on axial position of the rabbit incisor tooth. Acta Physiol Scand 116, 417–421.

Aars H (1982b) The influence of vascular β-adrenoceptors on the position and mobility of the rabbit incisor tooth. Acta Physiol Scand 116, 423–428.

Aars H (1983a) Effects of sympathetic nerve activity on changes in the position of the rabbit incisor tooth evoked by acute alterations in arterial blood pressure. Arch Oral Biol 28, 497–500.

Aars H (1983b) Effects of sympathetic nerve activity on acute mobility of the rabbit incisor tooth. Acta Odont Scand 41, 287–292.

Aars H and Brodin P (1989) Reflex changes in sympathetic activity affect the tooth tap-digastric reflex in rabbits. Proc Finn Dent Soc 85, 379–382.

Aars H, Brodin P and Bjørnland T (1988) Sympathetic modulation of the jaw-opening reflex in anaesthetized rabbits. Acta Physiol Scand 134, 319–325.

Aars H, Brodin P and Andersen E (1993) A study of cholinergic and β-adrenergic components in the regulation of blood flow in the tooth pulp and gingiva in man. Acta Physiol Scand 148, 441–447.

Aars H, Gazelius B, Edwall L and Olgart L (1992) Effects of autonomic reflexes on tooth pulp blood flow in man. Acta Physiol Scand 146, 423–429.

Aars H and Linden RWA (1982) The effects of sympathetic trunk stimulation on the position and mobility of the canine tooth of the cat. Arch Oral Biol 27, 399–404.

Brånemark PI (1961) Experimental investigation of microcirculation in bone marrow. Angiology 12, 293–305.

Burn-Murdoch RA and Picton DCA (1978) A technique for measuring eruption rates in rats of maxillary incisors under intrusive loads. Arch Oral Biol 23, 563–566.

Cash RM and Linden RWA (1982) Effects of sympathetic nerve stimulation on intra-oral mechanoreceptor activity in the cat. J Physiol 329, 451–463.

Edwall B (1988) An application of iodide clearance technique to monitor local changes in periodontal ligament blood flow. Acta Odont Scand 46, 119–126.

Edwall L and Gazelius B (1988) Effects of the alpha-adrenoceptor antagonists phentolamine, phenoxybenzamine and idazoxan on sympathetic blood flow control in the periodontal ligament of the cat. Acta Odont Scand 46, 127–133.

Edwall B, Gazelius B, Fazekas A, Theodorsson-Norheim E and Lundberg J M (1985) Neuropeptide Y (NPY) and sympathetic control of blood flow in oral mucosa and dental pulp in the cat. Acta Physiol Scand 125, 253–264.

Edwall B, Gazelius B, Berg JO, Edwall L, Hellander K and Olgart L (1987a) Blood flow changes in the dental pulp of the cat and rat measured simultaneously by laser Doppler flowmetry and local ^{125}I clearance. Acta Physiol Scand 131, 81–91.

Edwall B, Berg JO, Aars H, Gazelius B and Edwall L (1987b) Acute changes in intra-alveolar tooth position and local clearance of ^{125}I from the periodontal ligament. Acta Odont Scand 45, 415–421.

Edwall L and Kindlová M (1971) The effect of sympathetic nerve stimulation on the rate of disappearance of tracers from various oral tissues. Acta Odont Scand 29, 387–400.

Gazelius B and Olgart L (1980) Vasodilatation in dental pulp produced by electrical stimulation of the inferior alveolar nerve in the cat. Acta Physiol Scand 108, 181–186.

Gängler P and Merte K (1979a) Die vitalmikroskopische Untersuchung der periodontalen Blutzirkulation an Ratteninzisivus. Zahn Mund Kieferheilkd 67, 129–136.

Gängler P and Merte K (1979b) Die System- und Mikrozirkulation des Periodontiums – vitalmikroskopische und histologische Untersuchungen an Ratteninzisivi. Zahn Mund Kieferheilkd 67, 459–466.

Gängler P and Merte K (1980) Die Reaktivität der periodontalen Blutzirkulation auf thermische Reize. Zahn Mund Kieferheilkd 68, 762–768.

Gängler P and Merte K (1983) Effects of force application on periodontal blood circulation. J Period Res 18, 86–92.

Gilda JE, McCauley MC and Johansson EG (1943) Effect of pulp extirpation on the metabolism of phosphorus in the teeth of a dog as indicated by radioactive phosphorus. J Dent Res 22, 200.

Göz GR, Rahn BA and Schulte-Mönting J (1992) The effects of horizontal tooth loading on the circulation and width of the periodontal ligament – an experimental study on beagle dogs. Eur J Orthod 14, 21–25.

Hertrich K and Raab WHM (1990) Reaktive Änderung der parodontalen Mikrozirkulation bei kieferorthopädischen Kräften. Fortschr Kieferorthop 51, 253–258.

Heyeraas KJ, Kvinnsland I, Byers MR and Jacobsen EB (1993) Nerve fibers immunoreactive to protein gene product 9.5, calcitonin gene-related peptide, substance P, and neuropeptide Y in the dental pulp, periodontal ligament, and gingiva in cats. Acta Odont Scand 51, 207-221.

Hofmann M and Diemer R (1963) Die Pulsation des Zahnes. Dtsch Zahnärztl Zschr 18, 1268–1274.

Kaplan ML, Davis MA and Goldhaber P (1978a) Blood flow measurements in selected oral tissues in dog using radiolabelled microspheres and rubidium^{86}. Arch Oral Biol 23, 281–284.

Kaplan ML, Jeffcoat MK and Goldhaber P (1978b) Radiolabeled microsphere measurements of alveolar bone blood flow in dogs. J Periodont Res 13, 304–308.

Karita K, Izumi H, Tabata T, Kuriwada S, Sasano T and Sanjo D (1989) The blood flow in the periodontal ligament regulated by the sympathetic and sensory nerves in the cat. Proc Finn Dent Soc 85, 289–294.

Kato J, Ichikawa H, Wakisaka S, Matsuo S, Sakuda M and Akai M (1990) The distribution of vasoactive intestinal polypeptides and calcitonin gene-related peptide in the periodontal ligament of mouse molar teeth. Arch Oral Biol 35, 63–66.

Kato J, Tanne K, Ichikawa H, *et al.* (1992) Distribution of calcitonin gene-related peptide and substance P-immunoreactive nerve fibers and their correlation in the periodontal ligament of the mouse incisor. Acta Anat 145, 101–105.

Kety SS (1949) Measurement of regional circulation by the local clearance of radioactive sodium. Am Heart J 38, 321–328.

Kim S, Liu M, Markowitz K, Bilotto G and Dörscher-Kim J (1990) Comparison of pulpal blood flow in dog canine teeth determined by the laser Doppler and the ^{133}Xenon washout methods. Arch Oral Biol 35, 411–413.

Kristiansen AB and Heyeraas KJ (1989) Micropuncture measurements of interstitial fluid pressure in the rat periodontal ligament. Proc Finn Dent Soc 85, 295–300.

Kvinnsland I, Heyeraas KJ and Byers MR (1991) Regeneration of calcitonin gene-related peptide immunoreactive nerves in replanted rat molars and their supporting tissues. Arch Oral Biol 36, 815–826.

Kvinnsland I and Kvinnsland S (1990) Changes in CGRP-immunoreactive nerve fibres during experimental tooth movement in rats. Eur J Orthod 12, 320–329.

Kvinnsland I and Heyeraas KJ (1992) Effect of traumatic occlusion on CGRP and SP immunoreactive nerve fibre morphology in rat molar pulp and periodontium. Histochemistry 97, 111–120.

Kvinnsland S, Heyeraas K and Øfjord ES (1989) Effects of experimental tooth movement on periodontal and pulpal blood flow. Eur J Orthod 11, 200–205.

Kvinnsland S, Kristiansen AB, Kvinnsland I and Heyeraas KJ (1992) Effect of experimental traumatic occlusion on periodontal and pulpal blood flow. Acta Odont Scand 50, 211–219.

Körber K (1963) Oszillographie der Parodontaldurchblutung. Dtsch Zahnärztebl Z 17, 271–277.

Körber K (1970) Periodontal pulsation. J Periodontol 41, 382–390.

Körber KH and Körber E (1965) Patterns of physiological movement in tooth support. In: Mechanisms of tooth support (Anderson DJ, Eastoe JE, Melcher AH and Picton CA, eds), pp148–153, Wright, Bristol.

Lamb RE and van Hassel HJ (1972) Tissue pressure in the periodontal ligament. J Dent Res 51, (special issue), 240.

Lew K, Sims MR and Leppard PI (1989) Tooth extrusion effects on microvessel volumes, endothelial areas, and fenestrae in molar apical periodontal ligament. Am J Orthod Dentofacial Orthop 96, 221–231.

Linden RWA (1975) Intraoral mechanoreceptors: a study in man and animals. PhD thesis, Bristol University.

Liu M, Kim S, Park DS, Markowitz K, Bilotto G and Dörscher-Kim J (1990) Comparison of the effects of intra-arterial and locally applied vasoactive agents on pulpal blood flow in dog canine teeth determined by laser Doppler velocimetry. Arch Oral Biol 35, 405–410.

Matthews B and Berkovitz BKB (1972) Continuous recording of tooth eruption in the rabbit. Arch Oral Biol 17, 817–820.

Meyer MW (1970) Distribution of cardiac output to oral tissues in dogs. J Dent Res 49, 787–794.

Moxham BJ (1979a) Recording the eruption of the rabbit mandibular incisor using a device for continuously monitoring tooth movements. Arch Oral Biol 24, 889–899.

Moxham BJ (1979b) The effects of some vaso-active drugs on the eruption of the rabbit mandibular incisor. Arch Oral Biol 24, 681–688.

Moxham BJ (1981) The effects of section and stimulation of the cervical sympathetic trunk on eruption of the rabbit mandibular incisor. Arch Oral Biol 26, 887–891.

Moxham BJ and Berkovitz BKB (1983) Continuous monitoring of the position of the ferret mandibular canine tooth to enable comparisons with the continuously growing rabbit incisor. Arch Oral Biol 28, 477–481.

Myhre L, Preus HR and Aars H (1979) Influences of axial load and blood pressure on the position of the rabbit's tooth. Acta Odont Scand 37, 153–159.

Nakamura TK, Nakahara H, Nakamura M, Kiyomura H and Tokioka T (1992) Fine structure of adrenergic nerve fibers in human periodontal ligament. J Periodont Res 27, 569–574.

Nakamura M, Nakamura TK, Yoshikawa M and Kiyomura H (1986a) Vascular changes in pressure zones of rat molar periodontium following orthodontic tooth movement. J Jpn Orthod Soc 45, 126–134.

Nakamura M, Nakamura TK, Yoshikawa M, *et al.* (1986b) Scanning electron microscopic study of vascular changes of periodontal ligaments following experimental tooth movement in rats. J Jpn Orthod Soc 45, 568–573.

Ng GC, Walker TW, Zingg W and Burke PS (1981) Effects of tooth loading on the periodontal vasculature of the mandibular fourth premolar in dogs. Arch Oral Biol 26, 189–195.

Nähri M (1978) Activation of dental pulp nerves of the cat and the dog with hydrostatic pressure. Proc Finn Dent Soc 74, suppl V, 1–64 (thesis).

Okabe E, Todoki K and Ito H (1989) Direct pharmacological action of vasoactive substances on pulpal blood flow: an analysis and critique. J Endod 15, 473–477.

Packman H, Shoher I and Stein RS (1977) Vascular responses in the human periodontal ligament and alveolar bone detected by photoelectric plethysmography. J Periodontol 48, 194–200.

Palcanis KG (1973) Effect of the occlusal trauma on interstitial pressure in the periodontal ligament. J Dent Res 52, 903–910.

Path MG and Meyer MW (1977) Quantification of pulpal blood flow in developing teeth in dogs. J Dent Res 56, 1245–1254.

Rygh P, Bowling K, Hovlandsdal L and Williams S (1986) Activation of the vascular system: a main mediator of periodontal fibre remodeling in orthodontic tooth movement. Am J Orthod 89, 453–468.

Saito I, Ishii K, Hanada K, Sato O and Maeda T (1991) Responses of calcitonin gene-related peptide-immunopositive nerve fibres in the periodontal ligament of rat molars to experimental tooth movement. Arch Oral Biol 36, 689–692.

Sasano T, Kuriwada S, Sanjo D, Izumi H, Tabata T and Karita K (1992) Acute response of periodontal ligament blood flow to external force application. J Periodont Res 27, 301–304.

Sasano T, Shoji N, Kuriwada S and Sanjo D (1993) Acute response of periodontal ligament blood flow to an application of histamine solution to the dental pulp and the gingival sulcus. Jpn J Conserv Dent 36, 557–561.

Schärer P and Hayashi Y (1969) A qualitative study on intraperiodontal pressure. Parodontologie 23, 3–10.

Silverman JD and Kruger l (1987) An interpretation of dental innervation based upon the patttern of calcitonin gene-related peptide (CGRP)–immunoreactive thin sensory axons. Somatosens Res 5, 157–175.

Stüben J and Spreter von Kreudenstein T (1960) Experimentelle Untersuchungen über die Beteiligung des Zahnmarks am Stoffaustausch zwischen Blut und Dentinliquor. Dtsch Zahnärztl Z 15, 967–971.

Tønder KJH (1976) Effect of vasodilating drugs on external carotid and pulpal blood flow in dogs: 'stealing' of dental perfusion pressure. Acta Physiol Scand 97, 75–87.

Tønder KJH and Kvinnsland I (1983) Micropuncture measurements of interstitial fluid pressure in normal and inflamed dental pulp in cats. J Endod 9, 105–109.

Wakisaka S, Ichikawa H, Nishikawa S, Matsuo S, Takano Y and Akai M (1987) The distribution and origin of calcitonin gene-related peptide-containing nerve fibers in feline dental pulp. Histochemistry 86, 585–589.

Wakisaka S, Nishikawa S, Ichikawa H, Matsuo S, Takano Y and Akai M (1985) The distribution and origin of substance P-like immunoreactivity in the rat molar pulp and periodontal tissues. Arch Oral Biol 30, 813–818.

Walker TW, Ng GC and Burke PS (1978) Fluid pressures in the periodontal ligament of the mandibular canine tooth in dogs. Arch Oral Biol 23, 753–765.

Wasserman F, Blayney JR, Groetzinger G and De Witt TG (1941) Studies on the different pathways of exchange of minerals in teeth with the aid of radioactive phosphorus. J Dent Res 30, 389–398.

Chapter 7

The Innervation of the Periodontal Ligament

RWA Linden, BJ Millar, BJJ Scott

INTRODUCTION

Stimulation of teeth can evoke the sensations of touch and pain. The detection of forces applied to the teeth is attributed to mechanoreceptors in the periodontium, particularly those in the periodontal ligament (PDL). The periodontium is defined as the tissues that invest and support the teeth, i.e. the gingivae, cementum, PDL, and alveolus. The electrophysiological response properties of the receptors that respond to a force applied to a tooth were first studied by Pfaffmann (1939a,b). However, by then histologists had described a variety of nerve endings within the PDL (Dependorf, 1913; Kadanoff, 1929; Lewinsky and Stewart, 1936, 1937a,b; van der Sprenkel, 1936; Brashear, 1936; Bradlaw, 1939). The receptors were subsequently described as periodontal mechanoreceptors by Ness (1954), and recently the term 'periodontal ligament mechanoreceptor' has been used to identify specifically those receptors with mechanosensitive properties which are known to be within the PDL (Linden and Millar, 1988a).

The PDL receives an innervation from both myelinated and unmyelinated neurones. Most research work on the physiology of the neurones that innervate the PDL has been carried out on the larger diameter fibres (Aβ). These are known to respond to forces applied to the teeth and supporting structures. Less is known about the smaller fibres in the PDL, particularly the Aδ and the C fibres. Pain can be evoked by direct stimulation of the PDL or by heavy pressure applied to a normal tooth, or sometimes by light pressure applied to a tooth with a periodontal abscess. It is assumed that the Aδ and C fibres are involved with the reception of noxious stimuli.

Activity of receptors that respond to forces applied to the teeth and their supporting structures has been reported by many workers in a variety of species, and recordings have been made from a number of sites:

- peripheral nerves: Pfaffmann, 1939b; Ness, 1954; Wagers and Smith, 1960; Yamada *et al.*, 1961; Matthews, 1965; Yamada, 1967; Kizior *et al.*, 1968; Hannam, 1968, 1969a,b, 1970; Sakada and Kamio, 1970, 1971; Sakada and Onodera, 1974a,b; Hannam and Farnsworth, 1977; Linden 1984; Cash and Linden, 1982b; Johansson and Olsson, 1976; Fujita, 1987; Karita and Tabata, 1985; Tabata and Karita, 1986, 1993; Loescher and Robinson, 1989a; Millar *et al.*, 1989; Mengel *et al.*, 1992, 1993;
- trigeminal ganglion: Kerr and Lysak, 1964; Beaudreau and Jerge, 1968; Mei *et al.*, 1970, 1975, 1977; Appenteng *et al.*, 1982; Cash and Linden, 1982a; Linden and Scott, 1988, 1989a; Dong *et al.*, 1985,1993; Linden *et al.*, 1994;
- mesencephalic nucleus of the fifth nerve: Corbin and Harrison, 1940; Jerge, 1963a; Smith *et al.*, 1967; Smith and Marcarian, 1968; Cody *et al.*, 1972; Goodwin and Luschei, 1975; Linden, 1978; Amano and Iwasaki, 1982; Cash and Linden, 1982a; Passatore and Filippi, 1983; Passatore *et al.*, 1983; Linden and Scott, 1988, 1989a,b; Linden *et al.*, 1994;
- trigeminal nuclei: Kruger and Michel, 1962; Eisenman *et al.*, 1963; Jerge, 1963b; Kawamura and Nishiyama, 1966; Kirkpatrick and Kruger, 1975; Woda *et al.*, 1983, Olsson *et al.*, 1986, 1988; Tabata and Karita, 1991 a,c;
- thalamus: Yokota *et al.*, 1988; Karita and Tabata, 1991; Tabata and Karita, 1991b;
- cerebral cortex: Darian-Smith, 1986; Dubner and Sessle, 1971; Lund and Sessle, 1974; Mei *et al.*, 1977; Tabata *et al.*, 1986.

This activity has been attributed in the past to receptors situated in the periodontium. Most previous electrophysiological studies did not investigate the exact site of the receptor terminals that were stimulated when a force was applied to the tooth crown. These receptors could have been situated in any part of the periodontium and stimulated when the tooth moved within the alveolus. Receptors some distance away from the tooth and its surrounding structures (such as in the sutural tissues – Linden, 1978) may also have been stimulated.

There have been numerous histological studies that have reported on the observed neural structures, which have been described as nerve terminals. Histologists have attempted to attribute these putative nerve terminals with the response characteristics reported in physiological studies. Only recently have there been combined studies in which PDL mechanoreceptors were studied physiologically, located, marked, and then subjected to histological investigation (Millar *et al.*, 1989; Linden *et al.*, 1994). Histological studies on the periodontal innervation have been carried out in various species:

- human: Dependorf, 1913; Kadanoff, 1929; Lewinsky and Stewart, 1936, 1937b; Yamazaki, 1948; Held and Baud, 1955; Bernick, 1957; Rapp *et al.*, 1957; Falin, 1958; Bernick, 1959; Simpson, 1966; Kadanoff, 1967; Griffin and Harris, 1968, 1974a,b; Griffin, 1972; Griffin and Spain, 1972; Harris and Griffin, 1974a,b; Stella, 1975; Maeda *et al.*, 1990a; Lambrichts *et al.*, 1992, 1993;
- cat: Brashear, 1936; Lewinsky and Stewart, 1937a,b; Kizior *et al.*, 1968; Sakada, 1974; Byers and Dong, 1989; Miyake, 1990; Millar *et al.*, 1989, 1994; Linden *et al.*, 1994;
- monkey: Bradlaw, 1939; Bernick, 1952, 1957; Itoh *et al.*, 1981; Maeda, 1987; Byers and Dong, 1989;
- mouse: van der Sprenkel, 1936; Lewinsky and Stewart, 1937b; Corporon *et al.*, 1974; Everts *et al.*, 1977; Freezer and Sims,1987, 1989; Sato *et al.*, 1989; Kato *et al.*, 1992;
- rat: Bernick, 1956; Hattyasy, 1959; Beertsen *et al.*, 1974; Byers and Holland, 1977; Pimenidis and Hinds, 1977; Berkovitz and Shore, 1978; Berkovitz *et al.*, 1983; Marfurt and Turner, 1983; Byers 1985; Maeda *et al.*, 1987; Sato *et al.*, 1988; Byers and Dong, 1989; Maeda *et al.*, 1990b, 1991; Byers, 1990;
- mole: Lewinsky and Stewart, 1937b; Kubota and Osanai, 1977;
- guinea pig: Bernick, 1966; Sato *et al.*, 1989;
- hamster: Kannari *et al.*, 1991; Sato *et al.*, 1989;
- dog: Okabe, 1940; Tokumitsu, 1956; Sato *et al.*, 1992;
- marmoset: Bernick and Levy, 1968;
- crocodile: Kolmer, 1925; Berkovitz and Sloan, 1979;
- ferret: Lewinsky and Stewart, 1937b; Holland, 1988, 1991;
- hedgehog: Lewinsky and Stewart, 1937b;
- rabbit: Lewinsky and Stewart, 1937b.

These studies provide an overall understanding of the anatomy of the innervation of the PDL, although species differences exist. It may be that many of the early studies, particularly those using light microscopy, were not actually observing nerve endings but a variety of neural structures. Furthermore, there has been a tendency for authors to introduce a variety of descriptions, which may have masked similarities. Hannam (1982), in the first edition of this book, suggested 'that differences in technique and standards of preparation, as well as the natural enthusiasm for describing detail, undoubtedly contributed to this impressive array of descriptive terms, making comparison ever difficult'.

In this chapter the physiology and histology of the innervation of the PDL will be described. From a number of recent studies, there is compelling evidence that there is only a single type of PDL mechanoreceptor – a Ruffini ending. There are a number of putative roles for these receptors, which will be discussed. The structure and function of receptors innervated by Aδ and C fibres is considered.

GENERAL ANATOMY OF NERVES SUPPLYING THE PERIODONTAL LIGAMENT

The trigeminal nerve innervates the PDL from either its maxillary nerve or inferior alveolar nerve branches. The majority of nerve fibres supplying the PDL pass through foraminae in the alveolar bone to enter the PDL space close to the tooth apex, while others enter via the lateral aspect of the alveolar wall (Dependorf, 1913; Lewinsky and Stewart, 1936; Okabe, 1940; Held and Baud, 1955; Bernick, 1957; Rapp *et al.*, 1957; Kadanoff, 1967; Kizior *et al.*, 1968; Itoh *et al.*, 1981; Byers, 1985; Maeda *et al.*, 1987; Miyake, 1990). The nerve fibres run coronally from the apical region in bundles parallel to the cementum surface. Those fibres that enter the PDL through the lateral aspect of the alveolar wall divide into ascending and descending branches to form a plexus with the nerve fibres that run coronally from the apical area.

In some species, it appears that the innervation is most dense in the apical region, with only a few fibres reaching the PDL at the cervical margin (Kubota and Osanai, 1977; Freezer and Sims, 1987; Holland, 1991; Loescher and Holland, 1991; Linden *et al.*, 1994). Byers (1985) showed, in rat molar PDL, that the diameter of myelinated axons decreased as the axon travelled towards the cervical margin from the apex. Furthermore, Loescher and Holland (1991) found in the cat that more axons were present in the mesial and distal aspects. Many authors have described bundles of myelinated and non-myelinated nerve fibres lying adjacent to blood vessels and running parallel to the long axis of the tooth in various species (cat: Kizior *et al.*, 1968; mouse: Freezer and Sims, 1987; rat: Byers, 1985; monkey: Itoh *et al.*, 1981). However, Okabe (1940) has been the only worker to describe a dense innervation midway between the apex and cervical margin in the dog.

The PDL can be conveniently divided, for descriptive purposes, into an inner (cementum-related or avascular) part, which occupies about one-third of the PDL space, and an outer (alveolar or vascular) part, which occupies the remaining two-thirds. In the majority of studies, the blood vessels and nerve bundles have been described as running in the outer part of the PDL close to the alveolar bone. *Fig. 7.1* illustrates a large bundle of nerves and blood vessels in the outer third with a smaller bundle of nerves and blood vessels in the middle third. Single myelinated and unmyelinated fibres have been observed in the avascular inner third of the PDL (Griffin and Spain 1972, Byers 1985; Millar *et al.*, 1989). An electron micrograph (*Fig. 7.2*) shows an axon, which supplies a PDL mechanoreceptor, sectioned through the final node of Ranvier. The main bundles of nerve fibres give off branches that run towards the cementum, reaching the inner third of the PDL (Itoh *et al.*, 1981; Millar *et al.*, 1989). *Fig. 7.3* shows a myelinated nerve running in the inner third of the PDL to supply a mechanoreceptor. Sympathetic neurones are present in the PDL, but there is no evidence for a parasympathetic innervation of the PDL.

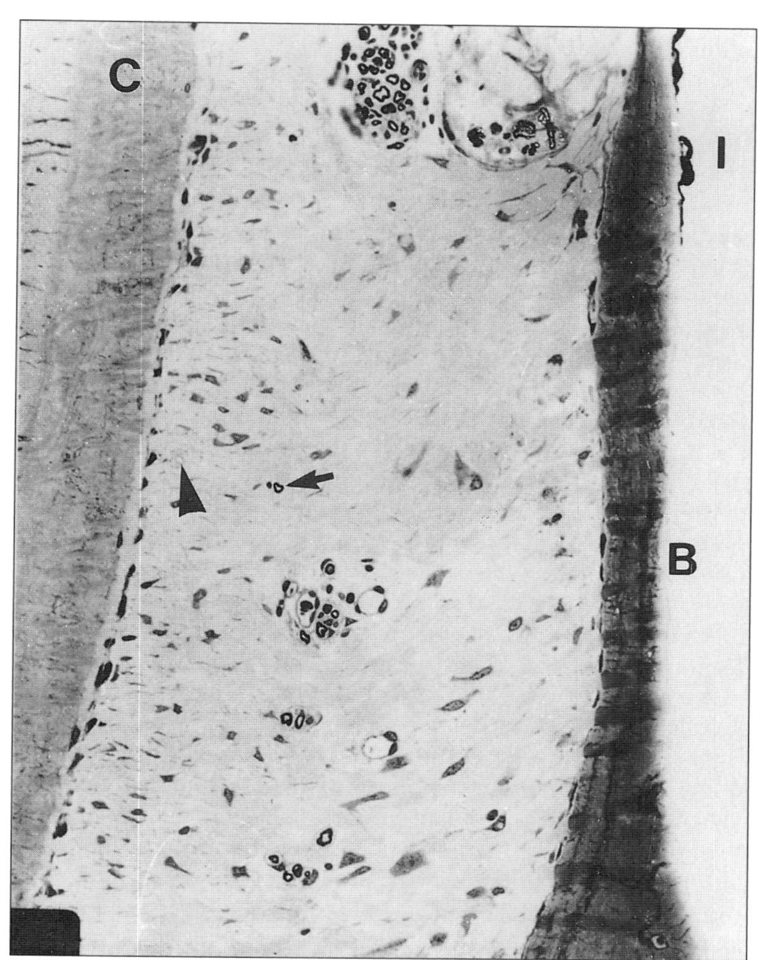

Fig. 7.1 Low-power light microscopy view of the PDL of the lower left canine of the cat showing a large bundle of nerves and blood vessels in the outer third and a smaller bundle of nerves in the middle third. Also seen is an ink-mark (I), pared away alveolar bone (B), and cementum (C). A Ruffini nerve terminal (arrowhead) is shown with an associated myelinated nerve (arrow). The collagen bundles are seen to run from lower left to upper right and the Ruffini nerve terminal is in that part of the PDL that is in line with the ink mark. The ink mark was placed over a physiologically located PDL mechanoreceptor which had its cell body in the trigeminal ganglion. Magnification × 150. (From Linden *et al.*, 1994.)

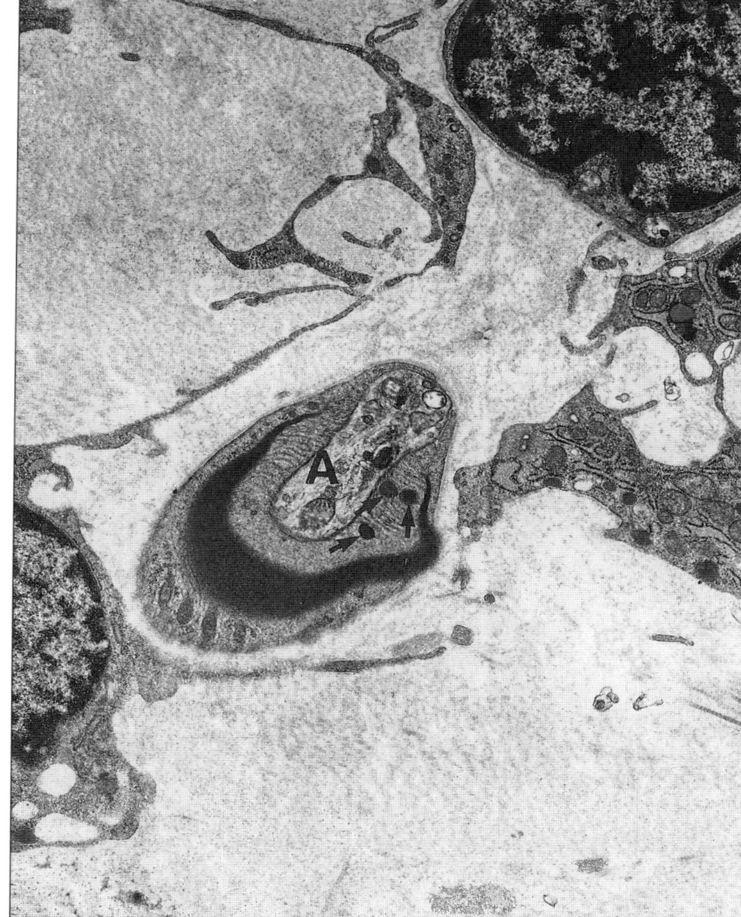

Fig. 7.2 The axon supplying a cat canine PDL mechanoreceptor, which is myelinated with a diameter of 3.5 μm. In the cytoplasmic lamellae of the Schwann cell of the first node of Ranvier there are dense core granules visible (arrows). In the axon (A) an accumulation of mitochondria, clear vesicles, and lamellated bodies are present. Magnification × 10 000. (From Millar *et al.*, 1994.)

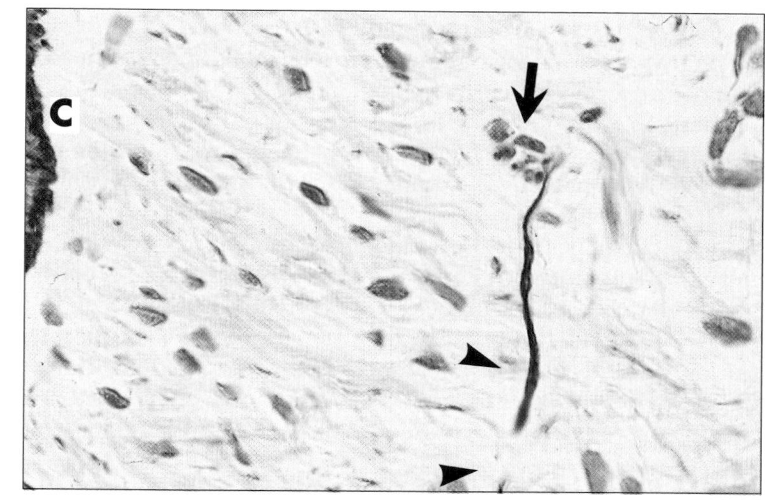

Fig. 7.3 A silver-stained section of a cat canine PDL Ruffini terminal (arrow) with its afferent myelinated axon (arrowheads) observed under an ink-spot after physiological recordings were made. The cementum of the adjacent root surface is indicated (C). Magnification × 670. (From Millar *et al.*, 1989.)

PHYSIOLOGY OF PERIODONTAL MECHANORECEPTORS

In most of the studies in which recordings have been made from neurones that respond when a force is applied to teeth, there has been no way of knowing where in the periodontium, if at all, the receptor was situated. Nevertheless, there are many similarities in the response characteristics between all of the receptors studied, and in this section these properties will be reviewed.

RATE SENSITIVITY, FORCE THRESHOLDS, AND ADAPTATION PROPERTIES

Some of the earliest studies on periodontal mechanoreceptors indicate that the frequency of discharge of the neurones is affected by the rate at which the forces are applied to the teeth (Pfaffmann, 1939a; Hannam, 1969a). Forces as low as 10-60 mN applied to the tooth have been shown to stimulate neurones in the periodontium (Pfaffmann, 1939a; Jerge, 1963a; Beaudreau and Jerge, 1968). In the cat, however, thresholds as high as 800 mN have also been reported (Linden and Millar, 1988a). The threshold is dependent on the rate at which the force is applied (Linden and Millar, 1988b). The force threshold and the sensitivity of the receptors depend on the temperature at the receptor site (Linden and Millar, 1994) with a maximum sensitivity at approximate body temperature. The response of mechanical stimuli to the tooth is temporarily increased following a period of sinusoidal vibration (Linden and Millar, 1989).

In the past, the periodontal mechanoreceptors have been classified into three types according to their adaptation rates: slowly adapting, rapidly adapting, and spontaneously discharging. However, there is a wide range of adaptation properties ranging from very rapidly adapting to very slowly adapting and spontaneously discharging, with no clear distinction between these so-called sub-groups (for review see Linden, 1990).

Cash and Linden (1982b) devised a technique to locate receptors in the PDL of the mandibular canine tooth of the cat by removing the gingival tissues over the labial aspect of the PDL and paring away the overlying bone (see *Fig. 7.1*). Indeed, it was possible to pare down the bone such that only a 'tissue-paper-thin' layer was left overlying the PDL. Receptors could then be located by mechanical stimulation with tungsten wire and electrical stimulation. In these experiments, recordings were made from functionally single fibres dissected from the inferior alveolar nerve. It was noted that the more slowly adapting receptors appeared to be situated in the apical third of the PDL and the rarer, more rapidly adapting, receptors appeared to be situated just below the 'fulcrum' of the tooth. Cash and Linden (1982b) suggested that there may be only one type of PDL mechanoreceptor and that the rate of adaptation (and possibly other response properties) was dependent on the position of the receptor within the PDL.

In a subsequent study (Linden and Millar, 1988a), the view that there may be only one type of mechanoreceptor was investigated in more detail. A relation between the position of the receptor relative to the fulcrum of the tooth and the adaptation properties was observed. There was also a relation between the position of the receptor and the threshold of the receptor to a lateral force applied to the crown of the tooth. It was found that the receptors situated close to the fulcrum of the tooth had the highest thresholds to a force applied to the crown, whereas those at the apex had the lowest threshold. There was a grading of force threshold for receptors situated between these two sites (*Fig. 7.4A*). There was also a grading of adaptation time such that the most rapidly adapting receptors were positioned near the fulcrum of the tooth and the most slowly adapting receptors were positioned near the apex of the tooth (*Fig. 7.4B*). An example of three mechanoreceptors located in the PDL of a mandibular canine tooth and their response to the same force applied to the tooth crown is shown in *Fig. 7.5*. It was shown that the receptors responded maximally when the area of the PDL in which they were present was stretched. If the tooth is considered to rotate about its fulcrum when a force is applied to the crown of the tooth at right angles to its long axis, then varying degrees of displacement of the tooth root about the fulcrum relative to the surrounding alveolar bone will occur. This graded displacement is greatest at the apex of the tooth and reduces at the fulcrum for any given force. Therefore, the receptors situated at the apex will receive the greatest displacement and, consequently, the greatest stimulus when a lateral force is applied to the crown of the tooth. These receptors appear to have a low force threshold and would adapt out slowly, if at all. In contrast, the receptors situated near the fulcrum would receive less stimulus (i.e. less displacement) for the same applied force. This might explain why they have the higher thresholds and adapt rapidly.

Furthermore, Linden and Millar (1988b) showed that the threshold of PDL mechanoreceptors also depended on the rate of force application at the crown tip, and all of the receptors studied had rate-sensitive thresholds. The degree of rate sensitivity appeared to be graded across the adaptation properties. It was shown that the rate sensitivity of a particular receptor was related both to the adaptation properties and to the force threshold at a constant ramp rise time.

These observations, taken together, provide strong support for the view that the response characteristics of a receptor depend on the position of the receptor and the rate, magnitude, and direction of the force applied to the crown of the tooth. However, Loescher and Robinson (1989a) could not establish a similar relationship between the position of the receptor and threshold or adaptation rates. This might be due to differences in experimental methodology. Further support for the hypothesis

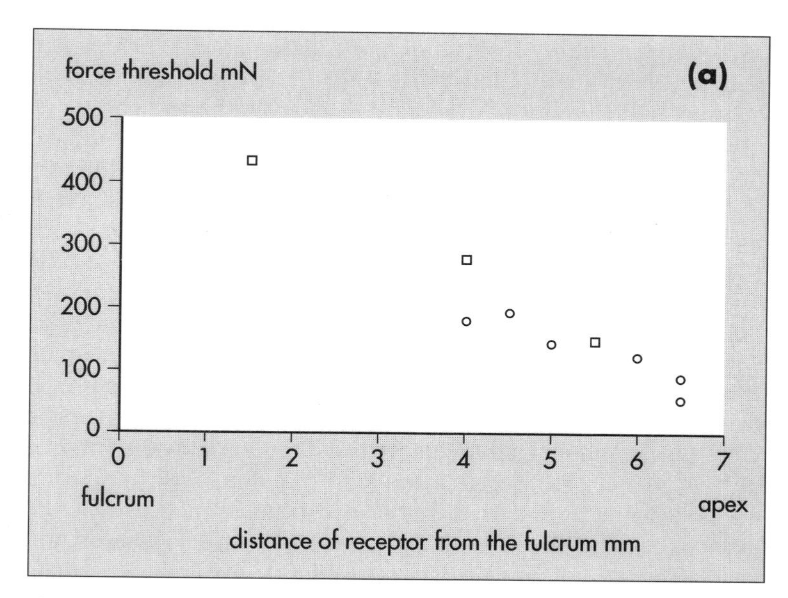

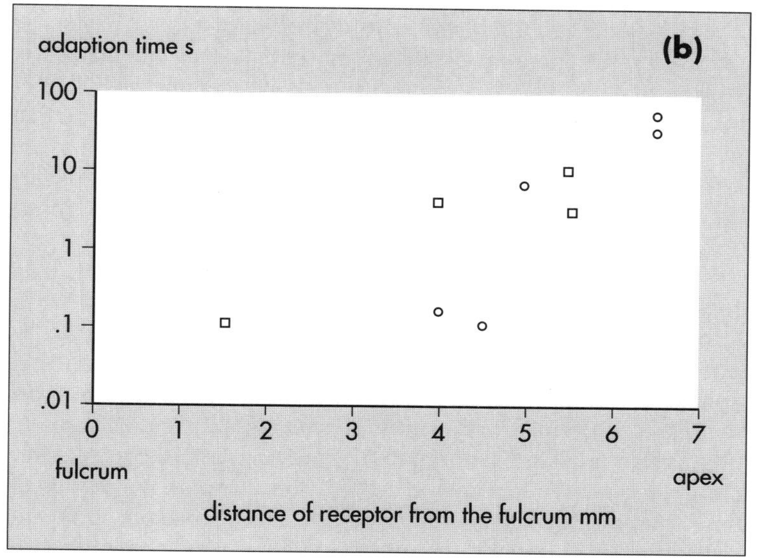

Fig. 7.4 (a) Graph of the relation between the force threshold of nine located PDL mechanoreceptors to a ramp-plateau force (rise time 50 ms) plotted against the position of the receptor relative to the fulcrum. Data from two cats (□ & O) and the relation is significant ($P < 0.001$). (b) Graph of the relation between adaptation time of nine located PDL mechanoreceptors to a force of 1 N shown on a logarithmic scale, against the position of the receptor relative to the fulcrum. Data from two cats (□ & O) AUQ and the relation is significant ($p < 0.02$). (From Linden and Millar, 1988a.)

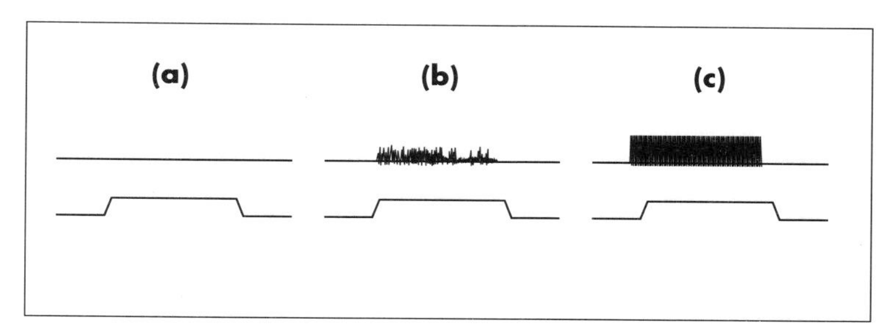

Fig. 7.5 The response from three PDL mechanoreceptors to suprathreshold ramp-plateau stimuli (1 N, 50 ms rise time). The receptors were located within the same cat canine PDL: (a) – 1.5 mm, (b) – 3.0mm; (c) – 5.5 mm from the fulcrum.

that the response properties of PDL mechanoreceptors are related to their position in the PDL has been shown in a recent study in which the peripheral nerve was sectioned and the neurones allowed to reinnervate the PDL (Linden and Millar, 1992). The relationship between the threshold of the reinnervated receptors and their positions in the PDL, and the relationship between the adaptation properties and position was investigated. It was found that these relations were broadly similar to normal PDL mechanoreceptor neurones. It was concluded that these observations gave further support to the view that the response properties depended on the position of the receptor in the PDL. Again, Loescher and Robinson (1989b), in a similar study on reinnervated neurones, could not establish any such relationships.

Some studies have identified neurones that spontaneously discharge in the absence of a mechanical stimulus (e.g. Wagers and Smith, 1960; Hannam, 1969b). These have always been found in peripheral nerve recording studies in which a peripheral nerve has been cut. Cash and Linden (1982a) showed that this spontaneous discharge could be related to cutting sympathetic nerves, which they demonstrated could exert an inhibitory influence upon the discharge of PDL mechanoreceptors.

RECEPTOR FIELDS

The majority of neurones respond to mechanical stimulation of a single tooth (Beaudreau and Jerge, 1968; Hannam, 1970; Linden, 1978; Tabata and Karita, 1986; Linden and Scott, 1989a). Studies in which action potentials have been recorded from neurones in peripheral nerves have revealed periodontal mechanoreceptors that respond when mechanical stimuli are applied to more than one tooth (Hannam, 1970; Sakada and Kamio, 1971; Sakada and Onodera, 1974a; Johansson and Olsson, 1976; Tabata and Karita, 1986; Trulsson, 1993). This has also been reported for periodontal mechanoreceptors in studies recording in the trigeminal ganglion (Kerr and Lysak, 1964; Beaudreau and Jerge, 1968) and the trigeminal mesencephalic nucleus (Jerge, 1963a; Linden, 1978). The explanation of the multiple tooth stimulation could be because the neurones are branched or because the application of force to one tooth causes movement of an adjacent tooth, owing to mechanical coupling.

Branched fibres, giving pulpal and gingival branches, have been reported in the inferior alveolar nerve in cats (Lisney and Matthews, 1978; Robinson, 1979). However, there is no convincing evidence for the branching of single neurones to supply more than one PDL mechanoreceptor. The alternative explanation to branched axons is that, when a force is applied to one tooth, adjacent teeth that are mechanically coupled by direct contact or through transseptal fibres, are stimulated, and PDL mechanoreceptors associated with this adjacent tooth respond (Hannam, 1970; Tabata and Karita, 1986; Johansson and Olsson, 1976; Trulsson, 1993). Tabata and Karita (1986) and Tabata *et al.* (1994) suggested that pressure applied to one tooth influences an adjacent tooth mechanically, and they considered that multiple-tooth units were very few in number compared with single-tooth units. This concept is supported by the finding that most of the multiple-tooth units involve adjacent teeth (Jerge, 1963a; Beaudreau and Jerge, 1968; Hannam, 1970; Sakada and Onodera, 1974a; Tabata and Karita, 1986; Trulsson, 1993) and show a gradual decline in sensitivity when moving to the first, second, and third adjacent tooth away from the most sensitive tooth (Trulsson, 1993).

A recent study by Millar *et al.* (1994) has shown that a direct relationship, without intervening bone, existed between the mandibular canine and first premolar tooth roots in the cat. An area, representing a window in the alveolar septal bone, extended 2–3 mm from the apex towards the tooth crown. Nerve terminals were observed amongst the collagen bundles in the PDL between the roots of the two teeth using light and electron microscopy. This suggests that a PDL mechanoreceptor can respond to forces applied to adjacent teeth; movement of both teeth need not occur. In conclusion, the evidence suggests that any multiple-tooth response is likely to be due to mechanical coupling between teeth.

None of the early studies indicated the exact stimulus needed to initiate an impulse in the neurones. Furthermore, it was not possible to locate the exact site of the receptors within the PDL. Early attempts to locate PDL mechanoreceptors in physiological studies were made using destructive techniques (Ness, 1954; Mei *et al.*, 1975). Actual location has been carried out by dissecting away the overlying tissues and thinning the alveolar bone, followed by punctate and electrical location of the receptors (Cash and Linden, 1982b; Linden and Millar, 1988a,b, 1989, 1994; Linden and Scott, 1988, 1989a; Loescher and Robinson, 1989a,b; Linden *et al.*, 1994). Receptors marked in this way have been studied morphologically by light and electron microscopy (Millar *et al.*, 1989, Linden *et al.*, 1994) (see *Fig. 7.1*).

CONDUCTION VELOCITIES AND FIBRE DIAMETERS

The conduction velocities of the afferent fibres from periodontal mechanoreceptors have been determined in several studies and have a range of 26–87 m/s^{-1} with a mean of 54 m/s^{-1} (Hannam, 1968; De Lange *et al.*, 1969; Linden, 1978; Takagi, 1982; Linden and Millar, 1988a; Linden and Scott, 1989a). These correspond to conduction velocities of the larger Aβ group of fibres.

Myelinated nerves in the PDL have a diameter of 1–16 μm and unmyelinated nerves have a diameter of 0.3–1 μm (Griffin and Harris, 1968; Sakada and Kamio, 1970; Kubota and Osanai, 1977; Millar *et al.*, 1989).

In any discussion of the conduction velocities of periodontal mechanoreceptor fibres, it should be stated that the velocities are dependent on the conditions in which the stimuli are applied. This can be illustrated by findings from a group of neurones in which microelectrode recordings were made in the trigeminal mesencephalic nucleus (Linden and Scott, 1989a). The neurones were initially identified by electrical stimulation of the inferior alveolar nerve, and it was possible to calculate their peripheral conduction velocities from this site of stimulation. However, the authors located the sites of the receptors in the PDL itself and were also able to stimulate electrically at this site and to calculate conduction velocities. It was found that the conduction velocities of the neurones were significantly lower when the neurones were stimulated at the receptor site (mean 33±7 m/s^{-1}) compared with more proximal stimulation in the inferior alveolar nerve (mean 47±9 m/s^{-1}). This could not be explained by the extra conduction distance or by the effects of a lower surface temperature in the more exposed part of the PDL. It was thought that the change in conduction velocity was likely to be due to narrowing of the axon and myelin sheath in the terminal part of the neurone. This has been shown to occur in cutaneous mechanoreceptors (Halata and Munger, 1985). Furthermore, in studies in which electron microscopy was performed on a small number of mechanoreceptors located in the PDL (Millar *et al.*, 1989), it was found that the axons were of a narrower diameter in the area close to the receptor terminals than those running in bundles in the PDL. It is noteworthy that similar observations were made on C fibres in the PDL, in which recordings were made from fine filaments dissected from the inferior alveolar nerve. The conduction velocity determined from electrical stimulation of the PDL was 1.1±0.5 m/s^{-1} and from stimulation of the inferior alveolar nerve it was 1.7±0.8 m/s^{-1} (Mengel *et al.*, 1992). It is also likely that conduction velocities may alter when the fibre size of the neurones changes in the central nervous system, and therefore conduction velocities probably give information of limited use.

DIRECTIONAL SENSITIVITY

Many workers have identified directional sensitivity of the neurones that respond when forces are applied to the teeth (Pfaffmann, 1939a; Wagers and Smith, 1960; Jerge, 1963a; Kerr and Lysak, 1964; Beaudreau and Jerge, 1968; Hannam, 1969a, 1970; Mei *et al.*, 1975; Johansson and Olsson, 1976; Linden, 1978; Cash and

Linden, 1982b; Tabata and Karita, 1986; Linden and Scott, 1989a; Loescher and Robinson, 1989a). Forces applied in the direction of maximum sensitivity result in a greater frequency and duration of discharge of the neurone than forces applied to other surfaces of the tooth. Furthermore, the threshold force is lowest if applied in this direction (Ness, 1954; Karita and Tabata, 1985). Trulsson *et al.* (1992) demonstrated that individual periodontal mechanoreceptive afferents provided ambiguous information regarding the direction of a force applied to the teeth. However, they still suggested that such information may have an important role in the control of mastication.

PHYSIOLOGY OF PERIODONTAL Aδ AND C FIBRES

AFFERENT NEURONES

The PDL receives an innervation from small myelinated and unmyelinated fibres (Byers, 1984, 1985). Mengel *et al.* (1993) have studied the Aδ group of fibres by making recordings from fine nerve filaments from the inferior alveolar nerve. The neurones were identified as Aδ by their conduction velocities as determined from electrical stimulation of the PDL. The mean conduction velocity was 11 ± 7.7 m/s^{-1}. The thresholds of the electrical stimuli required were inversely related to the conduction velocities (i.e. the higher the threshold of a single fibre, the lower the conduction velocity). It was suggested that this was in accordance with findings that show a correlation between conduction velocity and diameter and an inverse correlation between electrical threshold and fibre diameter (hence an inverse correlation between threshold and conduction velocity). Although the forces were not quantified, much higher intensities were required for activation of the Aδ fibres compared to the weak forces necessary to activate Aβ mechanoreceptive neurones. The latter were also observed but not studied in detail. The Aδ fibres responded most strongly when stimulated from one direction, but they also responded to pressure from other directions with a lower frequency. There was practically no adaptation in the 10 second activation time. Some neurones responded to cold stimulation but the response latency was quite variable. Some also responded to heat or the application of potassium chloride. However, the experiments provided no quantitative description of the response characteristics of the recorded Aδ fibres to non-electrical stimuli because the accurate location of the receptive areas of the fibres could not be determined.

Similar observations have been made on C fibres in the PDL (Mengel *et al.*, 1992). A large proportion of the fibres tested responded either to heat (60 per cent) or to cold (74 per cent) applied to the PDL. Half of the fibres tested were activated by potassium chloride, which typically showed an irregular discharge that started after a long latency. The duration of this discharge could be up to 3 minutes. However, the authors were forced to conclude that the results provided little information on the response characteristics of the neurones. Clearly, this is an area which requires further study.

EFFERENT NEURONES

Unmyelinated fibres have also been reported in the PDL and they may have a vasomotor function (Kerebel 1965; Griffin and Harris 1968; Schroeder 1986; Karita *et al.*, 1989). Sympathetic fibres in the PDL are mostly unmyelinated. The most profound physiological effect of sympathetic autonomic activity in the PDL is upon regional blood flow (see Chapter 6). This sympathetic innervation can modulate vascular pressure (see Edwall and Kindlova, 1971; Aars, 1978; Moxham, 1979,1981; Aars and Linden, 1982; Cash and Linden, 1982a). There is no evidence for a parasympathetic innervation of the PDL.

There is evidence that sensory nerve endings in the PDL release their contents under loading. These substances or signal molecules include vasoactive neuropeptides and may act upon capillary endothelial cells or be introduced to specific receptors on various cell types in the PDL, thus contributing to the regulation of their activities. These and other aspects are discussed in more detail in Chapter 12.

MORPHOLOGY OF THE NERVE ENDINGS IN THE PDL

The PDL nerve endings have been studied in several species using various histological techniques: decalcified sections, dissection of the PDL from the roots of extracted teeth, labelling with axonally transported markers, and immunohistochemical techniques. The density of the nerve endings, similar to the distribution of nerves, is greatest in the apical part of the PDL.

Kubota and Osanai (1977) showed, in the shrew, a higher density of free nerve endings and their nerve fibres in the apical part of the PDL, particularly in the maxilla. In an immunohistochemical study of five species of rodent, Sato *et al.* (1989) showed more nerve endings on the lingual aspect compared with the labial aspect of the PDL. The nerve endings in the PDL are usually described as being situated in the inner third, although Kannari *et al.* (1991) found endings in the outer third of the PDL in hamster incisors. A variety of nerve terminals have been described using light and electron microscopy, some in conjunction with labelling with axonally transported markers.

LIGHT MICROSCOPY

Some of the problems for early investigators were the difficulty of obtaining specimens of human PDL, the complexity of preparation, and the need to examine many sections (Simpson, 1966). Dependorf (1913) described nerve bundles forming coarse and fine networks and ending in fine, pointed processes in the cementoblast region. Human specimens obtained after judicial hanging (Kadanoff, 1929) and from victims of accidental death (Falin, 1958) have been used. Kadanoff (1929) described loops of nerves passing into and out of the cementum to end in the PDL itself. His specimens appeared to be less damaged than those of Dependorf (1913). Van der Sprenkel (1936) observed terminal rings close to the bony alveolus, and Lewinsky and Stewart (1936), also studying extracted teeth, found fine arborizations with terminal knob-like bodies. Bernick (1952) could not find organized endings in monkey PDL *in situ* while describing spindle-like structures in extracted human teeth. This could be due to tissue destruction when obtaining PDL from extracted teeth.

In a review of the early work on the innervation of the PDL (Lewinsky and Stewart, 1937b), Black (1887) is cited as having described the innervation in detail, including the presence of a few Pacinian corpuscles near the gingival margin.

Organized endings in the PDL have been described as:

- spindle or knob like (Bernick, 1952; Simpson, 1966; Stella, 1975);
- twisted or coiled endings (Lewinsky and Stewart, 1936; Rapp *et al.*, 1957; Griffin and Harris, 1968; Kizior *et al.*, 1968; Griffin and Spain, 1972);
- unencapsulated Ruffini-like (Rapp *et al.*, 1957);
- elongated spindle-like (Bernick, 1959);
- knob-like (Simpson, 1966).

A recent paper by Sato *et al.* (1992) using immunohistochemistry, light and electron microscopy of the PDL of the dog showed that light microscopy revealed tree-like nerve endings that differed from the Ruffini endings commonly seen in rodents. Using the electron microscope, however, the endings appeared similar to the Ruffini endings of rodents as described by others. This may, in part, help explain the difficulties in describing the nerve endings using light microscopy alone.

ELECTRON MICROSCOPY

PDL mechanoreceptors have been described by numerous authors as organized endings (Everts *et al.*, 1977; Berkovitz and Shore, 1978; Nakamura *et al.*, 1982; Berkovitz *et al.*, 1983; Schulze *et al.*, 1993b), by others as Ruffini-like (Byers, 1985; Nakamura *et al.*, 1986; Maeda *et al.*, 1989; Kato *et al.*, 1992; Lambrichts *et al.*, 1992), and by others as Ruffini endings (Millar *et al.*, 1989; Kannari 1990; Kannari *et al.*, 1991; Sato *et al.*, 1992; Maeda *et al.*, 1991; Linden *et al.*, 1994).

Organized endings

Everts *et al.* (1977) found organized endings in mouse PDL; this was confirmed by Berkovitz and Shore (1978). Nakamura *et al.* (1982) studied PDL from human premolar teeth and described elliptical, encapsulated corpuscles adjacent to blood vessels close to cementum, midway between apex and gingival surface. At the centre was a dilated unmyelinated nerve fibre of 1–5 µm diameter, surrounded, sometimes incompletely, by a Schwann cell as well as basal lamina. They considered these structures to be similar to Pacinian corpuscles. This may suggest a species difference as such receptors have not been reported in many species. Lamellated corpuscles (*Fig. 7.6*) have been observed in *Monodelphis domestica* (Schulze *et al.*, 1993b). Berkovitz *et al.* (1983) described a lamellated nerve corpuscle in the PDL of the rat incisor (*Fig. 7.7*) and numerous others in the Caiman (Berkovitz and Sloan, 1979).

Following the physiological classification of periodontal mechanoreceptors into rapidly adapting, slowly adapting, and spontaneously discharging receptors, there has been a tendency for histologists to describe a number of different morphological types of receptor. An extreme example of this is seen in a series of papers published by Griffin and co-workers in the 1970s, in which they describe, in human PDL, free nerve endings and simple, complex, and compound mechanoreceptors; they then speculate as to their physiological functions (Griffin and Harris, 1968, 1974a,b; Griffin and Malor, 1974; Griffin and Spain, 1972; Griffin, 1972; Harris and Griffin, 1974a,b). Nakamura *et al.* (1986) described round and oval endings of 10–25 µm diameter, mainly in the apical region of human PDL. They found the terminal axons had similar cytoplasmic components to the Golgi tendon organ of the cat and the Ruffini-like mechanoreceptor in the rat PDL. They considered that there may be two types of PDL mechanoreceptor, corresponding to two physiological types.

Ruffini and Ruffini-like endings

A Ruffini corpuscle consists of a myelinated axon with its endings and terminal glial cells (Halata, 1988). The Ruffini nerve ending is incompletely surrounded by terminal Schwann cells with finger-like protrusions anchored in adjacent collagen bundles. The terminal Schwann cells cover the nerve terminals and also send processes into the connective tissue. The presence of a capsule depends on the structure of the surrounding tissue (Halata, 1988). Ruffini corpuscles have been identified physiologically and studied morphologically in the hairy skin of the cat (Chambers *et al.*, 1972) and monkey (Biemesderfer *et al.*, 1978). In ultrastructural studies, Ruffini corpuscles have been described in skin (Munger,

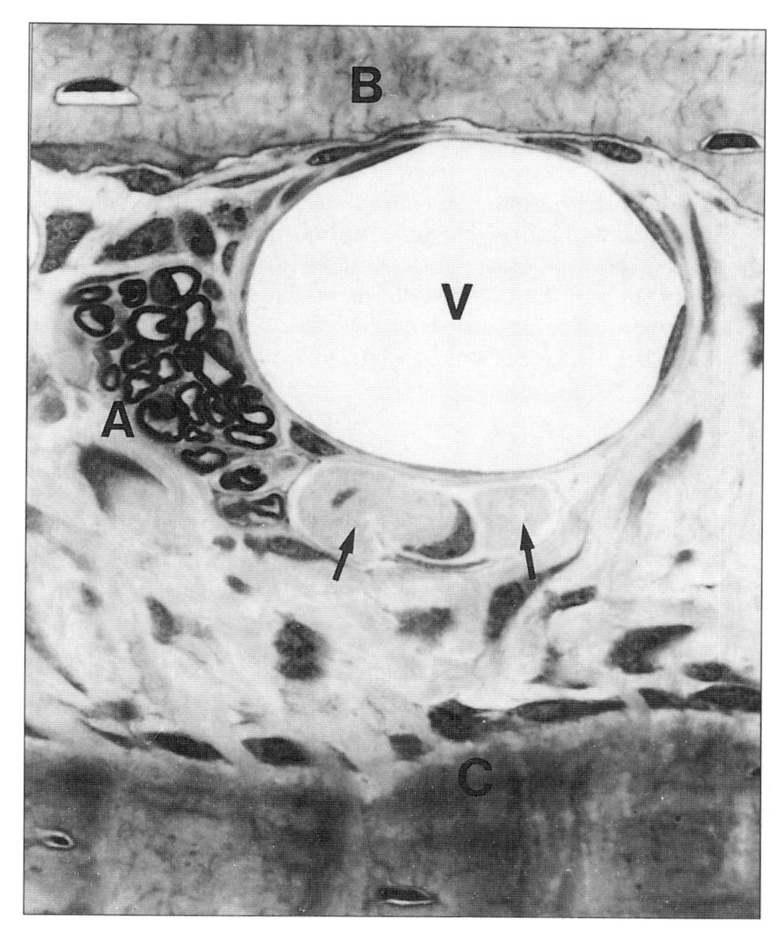

Fig. 7.6 Lamellated corpuscles (arrows) in the periodontal ligament of *Monodelphis domestica* also showing a blood vessel (V), myelinated axons (A), mandibular bone (B), and cementum (C). Magnification × 2180. (Courtesy of Professor Z Halata.)

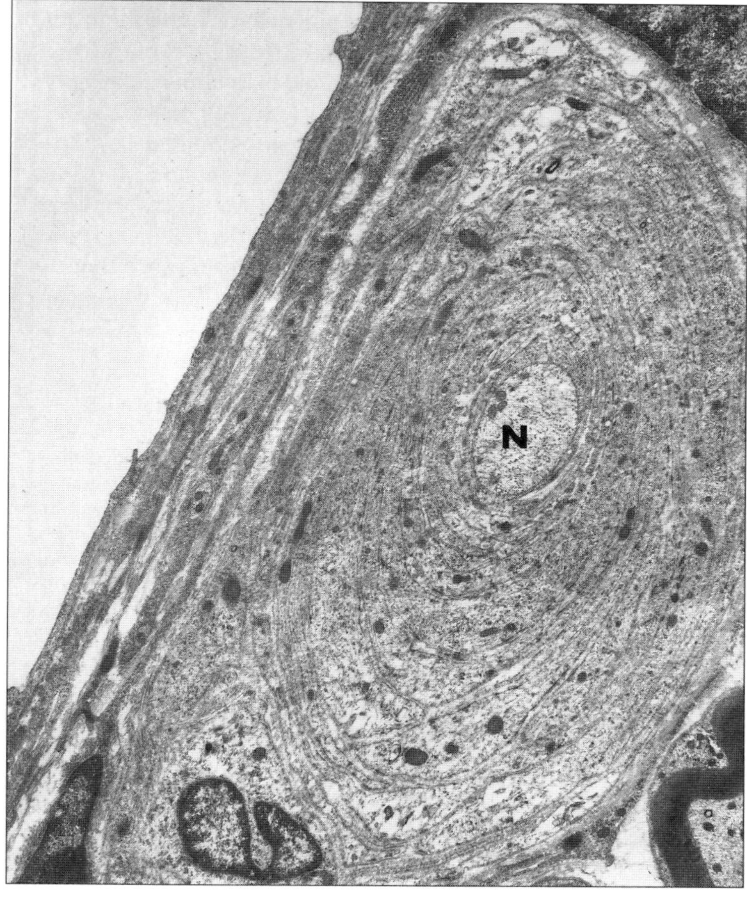

Fig. 7.7 Electron micrograph of a lamellated nerve terminal from the PDL of the rat incisor. A central neurite (N) is seen to be surrounded by circularly arranged cell processes. Magnification × 7500. (From Berkovitz *et al.*, 1983.)

1971; Chambers *et al.*, 1972; Biemesderfer *et al.*, 1978; Halata, 1977, 1988; Halata *et al.*, 1985). Ruffini terminals have also been described ultrastructurally in association with hairs, the pilo-Ruffini complex (Biemesderfer *et al.*, 1978; Munger and Halata, 1984), knee joints (Halata, 1977), and in the primate eyelid (Halata and Munger, 1980). The typical Ruffini corpuscles in the dermis of the skin and in the lamina fibrosa of joint capsules have a cylindrical form and an incomplete perineurial capsule. These structures are similar to the structure of Golgi tendon organs (Schoultz and Swett, 1972); both Golgi tendon organs and Ruffini corpuscles are stretch receptors.

Ruffini and Ruffini-like endings have been reported in the PDL of several species:

- mouse: Everts *et al.*, 1977;
- rat: Byers, 1985; Maeda *et al.*, 1991;
- cat: Linden, 1984; Byers *et al.*, 1986; Millar *et al.*, 1989; Byers and Dong, 1989;
- human: Lambrichts *et al.*, 1992;
- hamster: Kannari, 1990; Kannari *et al.*, 1991;
- dog: Sato *et al.*, 1992;
- *Monodelphis domestica*: Schulze *et al.*, 1993b.

The above papers, taken together, suggest that the PDL Ruffini terminal is unencapsulated and that the nerve endings are incompletely surrounded by the terminal Schwann cells. *Figs 7.8, 7.9, 7.10* illustrate the morphological features of located PDL Ruffini nerve endings. Finger-like protrusions appear to contact and anchor in the collagen bundles. The terminal Schwann cells partially cover the nerve terminals and also send processes into the connective tissue. Kannari (1990) described axon terminals covered by thick Schwann sheaths derived from more than two terminal Schwann cells.

Byers (1985) described four types of nerve ending. The endings were unencapsulated and had a varied structure of Ruffini-like endings. The majority of studies describe the organized terminals as unencapsulated, although Miyake (1990) described both free nerve endings and encapsulated endings in the cat PDL.

Until recently there has been no positive correlation between physiological and morphological studies, and Schroeder (1986) concluded that one of the areas concerning the sensory nerve supply to the PDL that lacked clarity was the lack of agreement between morphological and physiological aspects of the PDL. This follows half a century of observation and speculation.

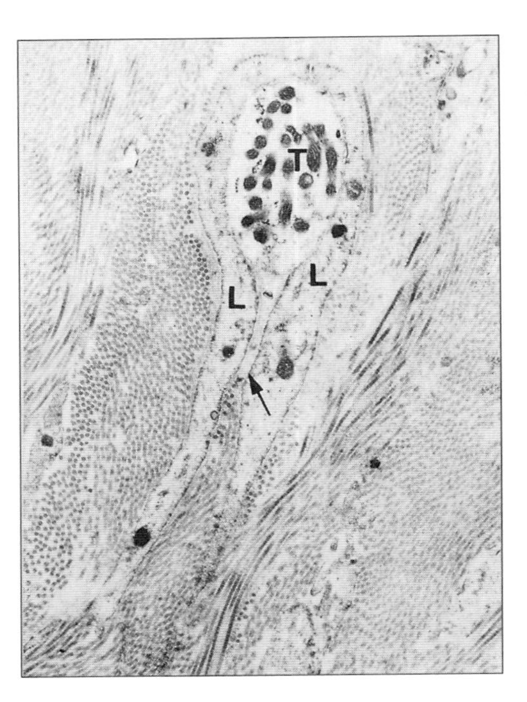

Fig. 7.8 Electron micrograph of a Ruffini terminal (T) located under an ink-mark with Schwann cell lamellae (L). A finger-like protrusion from the terminal is arrowed. Magnification × 9500. (From Millar *et al.*, 1989.)

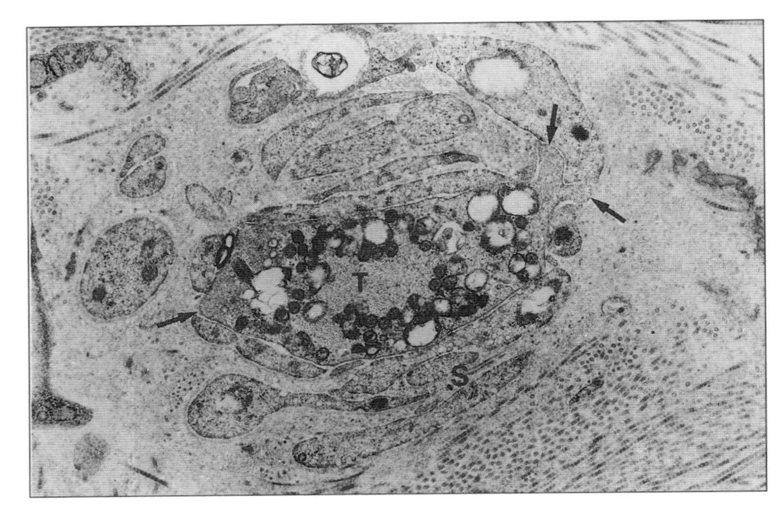

Fig. 7.9 A high-power view of a PDL mechanoreceptor that has its cell body in the trigeminal ganglion. The nerve terminal (T) is surrounded by up to five cytoplasmic lamellae of the terminal Schwann cell (S). There are typical pinocytotic vesicles in the cytoplasmic lamellae of the terminal Schwann cell. From uncovered sides of the nerve terminal, finger-like protrusions (arrows) with clear vesicles pierce into the surrounding tissue. Magnification × 10, 290. (From Linden *et al.*, 1994.)

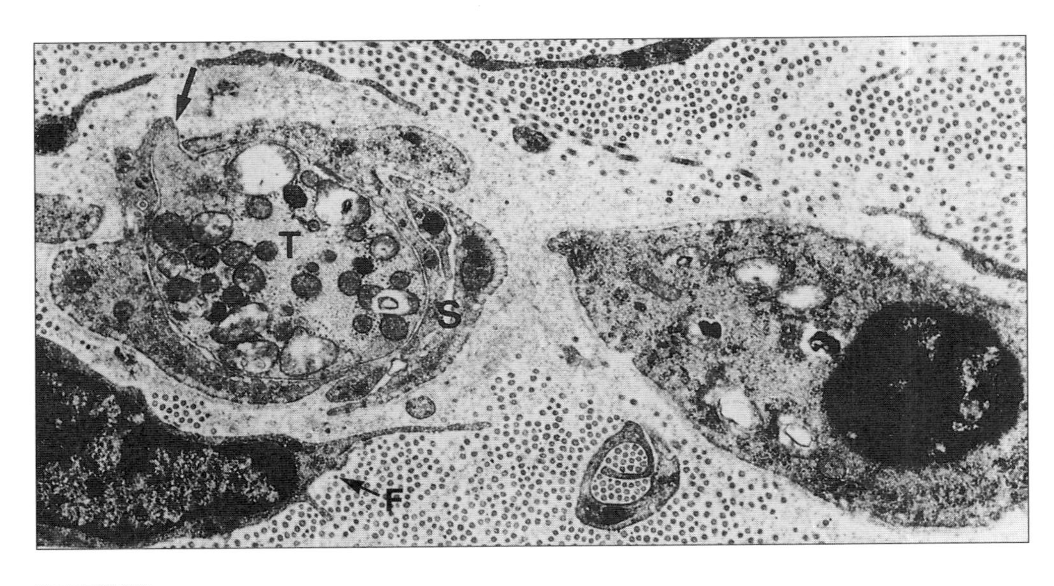

Fig. 7.10 The Ruffini nerve terminal (T) of a PDL mechanoreceptor that had its cell body in the mesencephalic nucleus. A finger-like protrusion (arrow) is seen. In the protrusion of the nerve terminal there are clear vesicles. The terminal Schwann cell (S) makes onion-like oriented cytoplasmic lamellae around the nerve terminal. F– fibroblast. Magnification × 13, 096. (From Linden *et al.*, 1994.)

Correlation of histological descriptions with physiological response properties of putative mechanoreceptors has been attempted in many past studies. However, only in the last five years has there been any attempt to correlate the physiological and morphological characteristics of PDL mechanoreceptors in single studies. Physiological studies over the past decade led to the view that there is only a single type of PDL mechanoreceptor (Cash and Linden, 1982a; Linden and Millar, 1988a,b, 1989, 1992, 1994). A comparison of the response characteristics of the proposed single type of PDL mechanoreceptor with the known properties of other mechanoreceptors suggested that they may well be type SAII (Ruffini) receptors, as described by Chambers *et al.* (1972).

A correlative study (Millar *et al.*, 1989) was carried out on electrophysiologically identified and located PDL mechanoreceptors in anaesthetized cats to test the hypothesis that PDL mechanoreceptors are Ruffini terminals. PDL mechanoreceptors were electrophysiologically identified from functionally single fibres and were located by electrical and punctate stimuli in the PDL of the mandibular canine. The response characteristics were typical of those recorded in earlier studies. The receptor loci were marked and these regions were studied histologically using light and electron microscopy. Under each ink-marked region, Ruffini terminals and smaller terminals resembling free nerve endings were observed. The Ruffini terminals were unencapsulated and the majority had diameters of 2–3 μm. PDL mechanoreceptors with intermediate adaptation properties were shown to have emanated from Ruffini terminals. since the conduction velocities observed eliminated the free nerve endings.

Kannari *et al.* (1991) used immunohistochemistry for neurofilament protein (NFP) and electron microscopy to study PDL Ruffini endings in the hamster. This study revealed a linkage between the axon terminals of the Ruffini endings and the surrounding collagen filaments. The axon terminals were enveloped by multiple layers of the basal lamina, which were penetrated by collagen filaments. The irregularly arranged collagen filaments were sandwiched between electron-dense laminae of the multilayered basal lamina.

Lambrichts *et al.* (1992) described various terminals in PDL from extracted human teeth ranging from simple, small, Ruffini-like structures (without a capsule and ensheathed with Schwann cells) to single and clustered lamellated endings. In addition, they found compound small Ruffini corpuscles (some with incomplete capsules) with ensheathing cells, and free nerve endings.

It is now clear that the Ruffini endings described in the PDL are similar to those previously described in other tissues. The differences between the Ruffini corpuscles in other tissues and those in the PDL are to be found only in the whole corpuscle and not in the nerve terminal itself. It has been suggested that the structure of the terminals depends on the structure of the connective tissue (Byers, 1985; Halata, 1988). The finger-like processes of the nerve terminals and the thin cytoplasmic lamellae of the Schwann cells are anchored in the connective tissue and probably increase the receptive field of the nerve terminals. Finger-like processes have also been described in Pacinian corpuscles (Loewenstein, 1971), and Spencer and Schaumberg (1973) consider that these may be the sites of mechanical transduction.

The presence or absence of a capsule appears to depend on the structure of the surrounding tissue (Halata *et al.*, 1985; Halata, 1988). Ruffini terminals in the PDL do not appear to have a capsule; perhaps there is sufficient suitably aligned collagen present to transmit the tissue displacement (or stretch) to the nerve terminal.

Ruffini end organs, described in cat knee joints, have been shown to be slowly adapting mechanoreceptors and sensitive to capsular stretching (Grigg and Hoffmann, 1984). Zimny *et al.* (1986) considered it likely that the Ruffini endings they described in the anterior cruciate ligament have similar characteristics. Likewise, the PDL mechanoreceptor may respond to stretch in the tissue. The similarity between mechanoreceptors in the cat knee and the PDL was highlighted by Ness (1954) following the work of Boyd (1954).

It is hypothesized (Chambers *et al.*, 1972; Halata, 1977) that tension in collagen fibres deforms the nerve processes and results in nerve activation. Therefore, as proposed by Halata (1977), the Ruffini terminals are able to monitor the tension of several bundles of collagen, explaining the observed directional sensitivity as shown in the knee joint capsule (Grigg and Hoffmann, 1984). This explanation could equally apply to the mechanoreceptors in the PDL. Various studies have confirmed that receptors respond when the part of the ligament in which they are situated is subjected to stretch. It is considered that mechanical deformation of the collagen bundles causes channels to open under membrane loading (transduction). Ions pass across the membrane and cause depolarization to produce the generator potential (see Grigg, 1986; Sachs, 1988a,b; Kruger, 1988; Kannari *et al.*, 1991).

Sims (1981, 1983a,b) described a relation between oxytalan fibres, blood vessels and nerves (see Chapter 5). He went on to postulate that these oxytalan fibres played a role in mechanoreception in the PDL. He extended the hypothesis to include the existence of a stretch-sensitive proprioceptor system consisting of oxytalan fibres, nerves, and blood vessels with similarities between PDL mechanoreceptors and baroreceptors. Oxytalan fibres are pre-elastin fibres (see Freezer and Sims, 1987; Berkovitz, 1990); they consist of bundles of microfibrils and are found close to Schwann cells. Freezer and Sims (1989) described a variety of anatomically discrete neural structures in juxtaposition to blood vessels in mouse molar PDL, which they felt was part of an associated oxytalan fibre meshwork. In the recent study by Millar *et al.* (1989), thin fibrils (possibly oxytalan fibres) were seen in some places to be close to the myelinated axons and close to the nerve terminals. These fibres were seen only around small parts of nerve terminals. There was no close relation observed between the blood vessels and the Ruffini nerve terminals. A direct functional relationship between putative PDL mechanoreceptors and oxytalan fibres has not been demonstrated experimentally.

TRACER STUDIES OF NERVE PATHWAYS IN THE PDL

A variety of axonally transported substances have been used to identify the pathways between cell bodies and nerve terminals. Capra *et al.* (1984) showed that the pulp and PDL receive discrete innervations. Marfurt and Turner (1983) used horseradish peroxidase in the trigeminal ganglion and reported its transport to molar PDL, but terminals were not described. Pimenidis and Hinds (1977) used tritiated proline and described free and organized nerve endings in the rat PDL following injection into the trigeminal ganglion. The technique of immunohistochemistry has also been applied to identify nerve terminals in the PDL using neurofilament protein and glia-specific S-100 protein (Maeda 1987; Maeda *et al.*, 1989; Sato *et al.*, 1988, 1992). Wakisaka *et al.* (1985) investigated the presence of the neurotransmitter Substance P in rat molar PDL and found immunoreactivity localized along the blood vessels in the middle and apical parts of the PDL. Maeda (1987) showed in the monkey that thick nerve bundles entered the PDL through slits in the alveolar wall, with thinner bundles entering higher up the wall. Sato *et al.* (1988) showed that nerves entered the lingual aspect of rat incisor PDL through slits in the alveolar wall in the mid-part of the socket and then immediately formed Ruffini-like corpuscles. The enamel-related connective tissue contained free nerve endings only, and it is considered that only the PDL proper is subjected to sufficient tension during mastication to stimulate the Ruffini endings that respond to stretch. Unlike the Ruffini terminals in the cat (Millar *et al.*, 1989) the endings were restricted to the alveolar wall aspect of the PDL. This may reflect the continuous growth of the rat incisor. Immunostaining for S-100 protein suggested that the PDL nerves were mostly covered by a Schwann cell sheath.

Everts *et al.* (1977), Berkovitz and Shore (1978), and Maeda *et al.* (1989) have described the ultrastructure of Ruffini terminals and ensheathed Schwann-like cells associated with rat incisors. The Ruffini terminals were close to the alveolar wall in the PDL and had axoplasmic processes similar to those in the cat (Millar *et al.*, 1989), which extend to contact nearby collagen bundles. Everts *et al.* (1977) and Maeda *et al.* (1989) reported that the nucleus associated with the Schwann cells was often indented, having a kidney-shaped outline that partly surrounds the nerve terminals and their finger-like processes. Maeda *et al.* (1990b) showed that non-specific cholinesterase is a useful marker to distinguish terminal Schwann cells from ordinary Schwann cells, and they discussed the possible involvement of these specialized Schwann cells in a mechanoreceptive capacity. Maeda *et al.* (1991) used immunostaining for laminin and described a special type of terminal Schwann cell in the rat incisor with well developed rough endoplasmic reticulum and a multilayered structure.

Kannari *et al.* (1991) used a combination of immunohistochemistry for neurofilament protein and electron microscopy to give a detailed account of the relation between PDL Ruffini endings in the hamster and the surrounding collagen filaments. Sato *et al.* (1992) showed in the dog a dense distribution in the apical region and a sparse distribution in the coronal two thirds. Axon terminals were slightly thicker than the preterminal portions and were similar to endings previously described as free nerve endings. Under electron microscopy the terminals resembled Ruffini endings, but using the light microscope the endings were tree-like and differed from the Ruffini endings that are commonly seen in rodents. These authors stated that knobbed endings, corpuscular (lamellated and glomerular) endings, and free nerve endings were rarely encountered in the PDL of incisors and canines of the dog.

FREE NERVE ENDINGS

Free nerve endings have been described in the PDL (Dependorf, 1913; Kadanoff, 1929; Lewinsky and Stewart, 1936; Simpson, 1966; Kubota and Osanai, 1977; Byers, 1985; Millar *et al.*, 1989; Lambrichts *et al.*, 1992). The free nerve endings contain neurotubules, neurofilaments, and vesicles. A typical PDL free nerve ending is seen in *Fig. 7.11*.

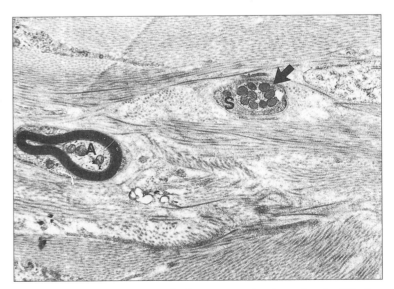

Fig. 7.11 Electron micrograph of a free nerve ending (arrow) in the PDL of the cat mandibular canine tooth with its terminal Schwann cell (S). A = myelinated axon. Magnification × 10,000. (From Millar *et al.*, 1989.)

Although terminals supplied by Aδ and C fibres can give rise to mechanosensitive responses (reviewed by Wall and McMahon 1985) and have been reported in the PDL, the conduction velocities would be considerably less than those reported for PDL mechanoreceptors supplied by Aβ fibres. Terminals supplied by Aδ or C fibres could be the 'type II periodontal mechanoreceptors' described by Mei *et al.* (1977). Mei and his co-workers could only stimulate these receptors with extraction type forces, heating to 50–55°C or injecting bradykinin directly into the PDL. It is unlikely that their so-called type II mechanoreceptors are true mechanoreceptors; it seems more probable that they are nociceptors.

The small nerve terminals observed in the PDL have the same morphology as the free nerve endings in cat hairy skin, as described by Kruger *et al.* (1981). They considered the function of these free nerve endings to be nociceptive, and there is no reason to suggest otherwise for their role in the PDL.

MORPHOLOGY OF NERVE ENDINGS IN OTHER RELATED TISSUES

Although the PDL is the primary subject of this review, brief reference will now be made to adjacent tissues because of their possible functional involvement when a tooth is loaded.

CEMENTUM

Nerve endings in cementum have been studied in many investigations on the innervation of the periodontium. Early studies described free nerve endings in cementum (Dependorf, 1913; van der Sprenkel, 1936; Bernick, 1957). Some studies have reported nerve fibres that appear to loop into and out of the cementum (Kadanoff, 1929; Lewinsky and Stewart, 1936; Rapp *et al.*, 1957; Byers and Holland, 1977), while others describe free nerve endings in the cementoblast layers (Dependorf, 1913; van der Sprenkel, 1936; Bernick, 1957; Weill *et al.*, 1975). Itoh *et al.* (1981) showed nerve fibres terminating in the subcementoblastic and cementoblastic layer, some running parallel to the cementum surface.

Large terminals have been reported close to the cementum, but no terminals have actually been observed in the cementum in studies by Byers and Holland (1977), Byers (1985), and Millar *et al.* (1989). However, Weill *et al.* (1975) have described endings in cementum in an autoradiographic study.

PERIOSTEUM

The periosteum contains free nerve endings, complex unencapsulated corpuscles, and encapsulated corpuscles (for review see Sakada 1983). Free and organized endings with diameters of 3–10 μm have been described in cat periosteum by Sakada and Aida (1971).

The alveolar periosteum has some complex unencapsulated and free nerve endings and Golgi-Mazzoni type mechanoreceptors (Sakada, 1971). The response properties of the free nerve endings and Ruffini-type endings in the cat mandibular molar periosteum have been evaluated (Hada, 1990). Slowly adapting Ruffini-type endings and free nerve endings were found as well as fast adapting free nerve endings and unencapsulated endings.

GINGIVA AND MUCOSA

The innervation of the human gingiva has been described by Jurjiewa, 1913; Kadanoff, 1929; Lewinsky and Stewart, 1938; Gairns and Aitchinson, 1950; Rapp *et al.*, 1957; Dixon, 1961; Balogh and Csiba, 1967; Plenk and Raab, 1970; Stella, 1975. Free nerve endings are found in the basal layers of the epithelium (Byers and Holland, 1977). Free gingival fibres form loops and end in knob-like swellings. Encapsulated Krause-like and Meissner-like endings have also been described in the lamina propria of the gingiva as well as compact and loose unencapsulated whorls. The innervation of the gingiva has been described in several species as rich. Yamamoto and Sakada (1986) described free nerve endings, bush-like nerve endings, Merkel cell-neurite complexes, and encapsulated corpuscles in the gingiva and alveolar mucosa of the shrew. Schulze *et al.* (1993a) have described free nerve endings (innervated by Aδ and C fibres), Merkel nerve endings, and lamellated corpuscles in the gingiva and mucosa of *Monodelphis domestica*.

Sakada (1983) described Merkel cell-neurite, encapsulated, unencapsulated, and free nerve endings in the mucosa. He considered that there is no real difference between the mechanoreceptors in the mucosa from those in the periosteum. Yamamoto and Sakada (1983) reported free nerve endings, encapsulated and bush-like endings in mouse labial mucosa.

CENTRAL REPRESENTATION OF NEURONES THAT INNERVATE THE PDL

Physiological studies on the central representation of neurones that innervate the PDL have been carried out using microelectrodes placed into the trigeminal ganglion or central nervous system in several species. Recordings have been made from neurones that respond to small forces applied to the teeth. However, no central representation studies have been carried out on neurones that respond to noxious stimulation to the PDL.

RECORDINGS FROM FIRST-ORDER NEURONES

The cell bodies of the primary afferent neurones that respond to forces applied to the crown of the tooth are situated in two anatomically distinct sites – the trigeminal ganglion (Gasserian ganglion) and the trigeminal mesencephalic nucleus. Many studies have shown the presence of neurones in the trigeminal ganglion which respond to forces applied to ipsilateral teeth (e.g. Kerr and Lysak, 1964; Beaudreau and Jerge, 1968; Mei *et al.*, 1970, 1975; Appenteng *et al.*, 1982; Cash and Linden, 1982a; Linden and Scott, 1989a).

Neurones in the trigeminal mesencephalic nucleus also respond when forces are applied to the ipsilateral teeth (e.g. Corbin and Harrison, 1940; Jerge, 1963a; Cody *et al.*, 1972; Linden, 1978; Amano and Iwasaki, 1982; Cash and Linden, 1982a; Passatore and Filippi, 1983; Passatore *et al.*, 1983; Dessem *et al.*, 1988; Linden and Scott, 1989a). Linden (1978) confirmed, using electrophysiological techniques of orthograde and retrograde electrical stimulation, that these were primary afferent neurones. Most neurones in the mesencephalic nucleus respond to forces applied to single teeth. However, Linden (1978) also found a group of neurones in the nucleus that responded to forces applied to all of the maxillary teeth, both contralateral and ipsilateral, as well as to forces applied to the nose and hard palate. These were called type P neurones, and one suggested site for these receptors was in the palatomaxillary suture. In all of these studies, either when recording in the trigeminal ganglion or in the mesencephalic nucleus, the precise sites of the mechanoreceptors were not known.

Linden and Scott (1989a) located the positions of the receptors in the labial aspect of the PDL of the mandibular canine tooth while recording in the trigeminal ganglion. They found that the mechanoreceptors were situated in the whole area of the PDL between the fulcrum and apex of the tooth (*Fig. 7.12*). They also looked at the directional sensitivity of the 104 recorded neurones. These data, together with the knowledge that the neurones responded maximally when the area of the PDL in which they were present was placed into tension, suggested that the mechanoreceptors were distributed equally around the whole circumference of the tooth root (*Fig. 7.13*). There appear to be some differences in observations from anatomical studies in which autoradiography was performed following the injection of the trigeminal ganglion with tritiated amino acids (Byers and Matthews, 1981; Byers and Dong, 1989). Labelled neurones were found over a wide area of the PDL, although it appeared unclear whether these were in fact labelled mechanoreceptors.

Linden and Scott (1989a) located the sites of the mechanoreceptors in the labial aspect of the PDL of the mandibular canine tooth when recordings were made in the mesencephalic nucleus (*Fig. 7.14*). In contrast to the situation when recordings were made in the trigeminal ganglion, the located receptors were situated in a discrete area of the PDL intermediate in position between the

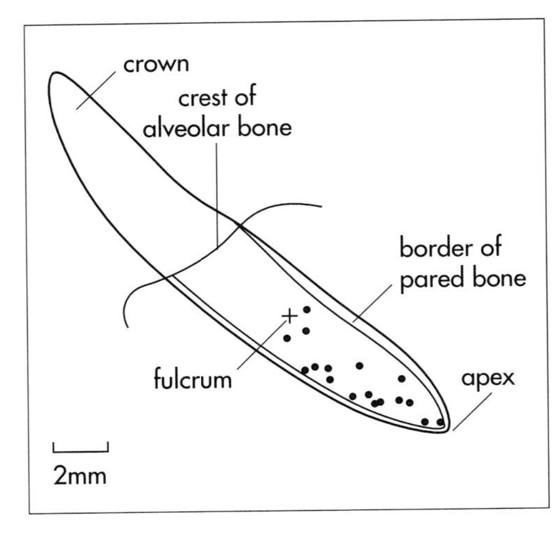

Fig. 7.12 A diagram showing the position of the located receptors when recordings were made in the trigeminal ganglion. (From Linden and Scott, 1989a.)

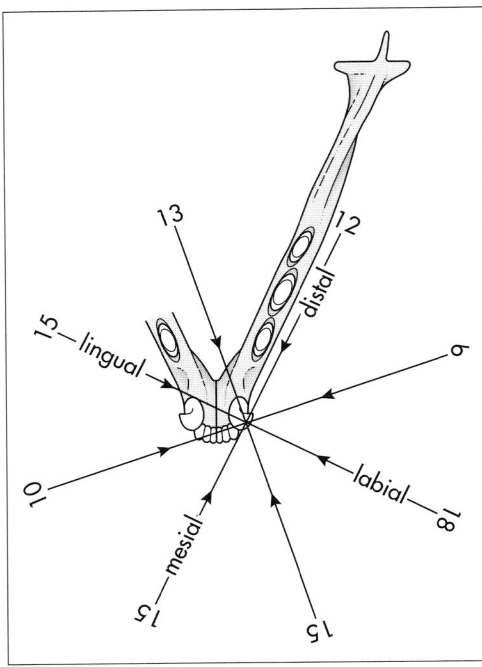

Fig. 7.13 Plan view of the left mandible illustrating the direction of maximum sensitivity of mechanoreceptors represented in the trigeminal ganglion. The numbers denote the number of mechanoreceptors with maximum sensitivity in each direction. (From Linden and Scott 1989a.)

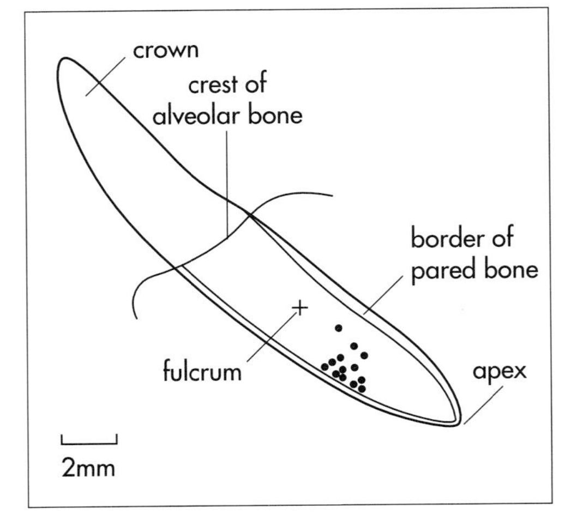

Fig. 7.14 A diagram to show the position of the located receptors when recordings were made in the mesencephalic nucleus. (From Linden and Scott, 1989a.)

fulcrum and apex of the tooth. The variance in the position of the mechanoreceptors whose cell bodies lie in the trigeminal ganglion was significantly greater than the variance in position of the mechanoreceptors whose cell bodies lie in the mesencephalic nucleus. Byers *et al.* (1986) found, through an autoradiographic study, that there was a heavy concentration of putative nerve endings in the apical part of the PDL when the mesencephalic nucleus was injected with tritiated proline. The differences of suggested location of the receptor terminals between the anatomical and physiological studies are difficult to resolve.

In the electrophysiological location study of Linden and Scott (1989a), in which recordings were made in the mesencephalic nucleus, the directional sensitivities of all of the mechanoreceptors recorded in the mesencephalic nucleus were also studied (*Fig. 7.15*). It was found that there was an uneven distribution of mechanoreceptors around the tooth root; the majority (approximately 70 per cent) were situated in an area extending from the labial to the mesial aspect of the PDL.

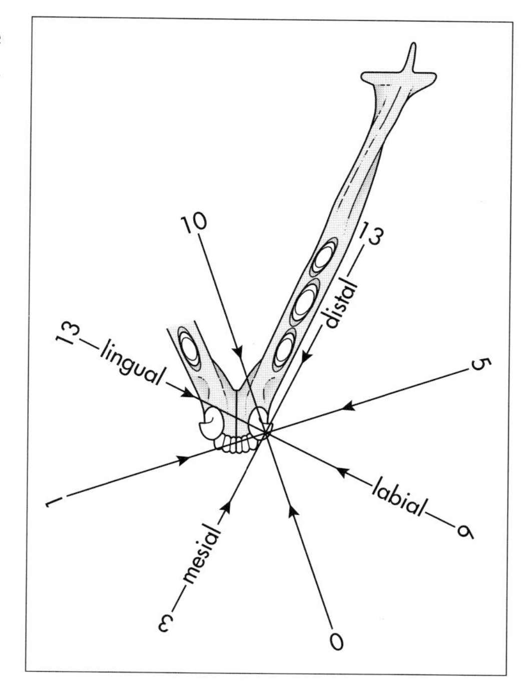

Fig. 7.15 Plan view of the left mandible illustrating the direction of maximum sensitivity of mechanoreceptors represented in the mesencephalic nucleus. The numbers denote the number of mechanoreceptors with maximum sensitivity in each direction. (From Linden and Scott, 1989a.)

These observations were further reinforced by a retrospective examination of data collected in the study by Linden (1978). Recording in the mesencephalic nucleus, the directional sensitivity of 157 mechanoreceptors which responded to a force applied to the mandibular canine tooth had been observed, but a comparison of them had not been made. It was found on re-examination of these data that most of the receptors responded maximally when a force was applied to the same area of the crown of the tooth, as in the more recent study (*Fig. 7.16*).

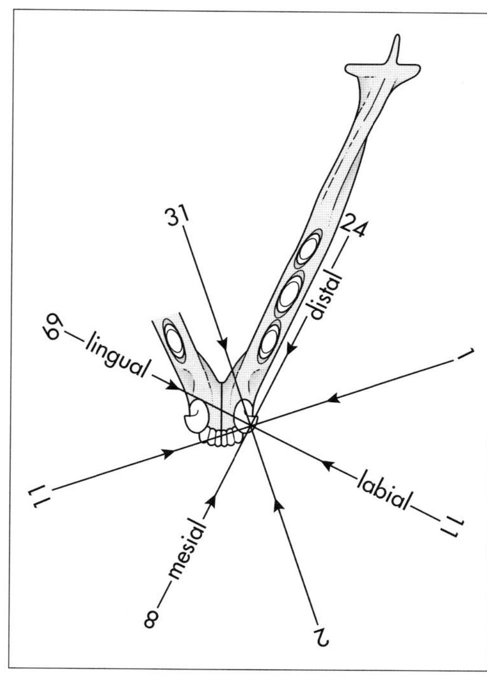

Fig. 7.16 Plan view of the left mandible illustrating the direction of maximum sensitivity of mechanoreceptors represented in the mesencephalic nucleus from an earlier study by Linden (1978). The numbers denote the number of mechanoreceptors with maximum sensitivity in each direction. (From Linden and Scott 1989a.)

It appears, therefore, that the receptors of neurones with their cell bodies in the trigeminal ganglion have a much more even distribution in the PDL (at least in the PDL of the cat mandibular canine tooth) than those with their cell bodies in the mesencephalic nucleus. The reasons for these differences in the distributions are not yet clear. It may be due to the result of the development of the tooth and PDL, or it may reflect different functional roles of the two groups of neurones.

Neurones with their cell bodies in the trigeminal ganglion have a range of adaptation properties, ranging from very rapidly adapting to very slowly adapting, when forces are applied to the teeth (Kerr and Lysak 1964; Beaudreau and Jerge 1968). Linden and Scott (1989a) found that a large number of the mechanoreceptive neurones with cell bodies in the trigeminal ganglion were slowly adapting in that they did not adapt out to a prolonged force applied to the crown of the tooth. Mechanoreceptors that adapted out in a few seconds were found, as also were a few that were very rapidly adapting and gave only a few impulses during a sustained application of a force to the tooth. When recordings have been made in the mesencephalic nucleus, no canine PDL mechanoreceptor neurones with very slowly adapting properties have been found (Jerge 1963a; Linden 1978; Linden and Scott 1989a). These observations, together with observations made on the location of the mechanoreceptors in the PDL (Linden and Scott 1989a), appear to correlate well with those described earlier in that the response characteristics of PDL mechanoreceptors depend on their position in the ligament.

A recent correlative morphological study (Linden *et al.*, 1994) was carried out to compare the morphology of a PDL mechanoreceptor with its cell body in the trigeminal ganglion with one with its cell body in the mesencephalic nucleus. The receptors were electrophysiologically identified and located in the PDL using punctate and electrical stimuli. They were then studied using light and electron microscopy. One receptor was studied by recording from its cell body in the mesencephalic nucleus and the other by recording from its cell body in the trigeminal ganglion. Ruffini nerve endings were observed under the areas marked. The results indicate that PDL mechanoreceptors with cell bodies in the mesencephalic nucleus and those with cell bodies in the trigeminal ganglion can both be Ruffini endings. Furthermore, there were no apparent morphological differences between the two PDL mechanoreceptors studied.

CENTRAL PROJECTIONS TO THE TRIGEMINAL NUCLEI

Recordings from neurones that respond to forces applied to the teeth have been made from the main sensory nucleus, the spinal trigeminal nucleus (oralis, interpolaris, and caudalis), and the supratrigeminal nuclei (Kruger and Michel, 1962; Eisenman *et al.*, 1963; Jerge, 1963b; Kawamura and Nishiyama, 1966; Kirkpatrick and Kruger, 1975; Woda *et al.*, 1983; Olsson *et al.*, 1988). Kawamura and Nishiyama (1966) found that in the cat, the canine tooth had the most prominent representation. In the majority of the studies, the neurones responded to mechanical stimulation of more than one tooth but there is general agreement that mechanical stimulation of only ipsilateral teeth stimulates the neurones. These neurones also display directional sensitivity in that their response is dependent upon the direction in which the force is applied to the tooth (Kirkpatrick and Kruger, 1975; Woda *et al.*, 1983). Recordings have also been made during mastication (Olsson *et al.*, 1986, 1988). Some of the neurones that responded to mechanical stimulation of the teeth were modulated during chewing; they were less excitable during jaw closure than the occlusal phase of mastication.

Tabata and Karita (1991c) recorded activity from periodontal mechanosensitive units in the trigeminal main sensory nucleus of the cat. They found that the majority of recorded units were single tooth units which responded maximally to the canine tooth. They studied the directional sensitivity of the units and found that 73 per cent had single tooth responses and 27 per cent had multiple tooth responses. They found that the majority of the single tooth neurones were of the slowly adapting type and showed directional sensitivity to mechanical stimulation. Multiple-tooth units had receptive fields that most frequently included both the canine and incisor teeth together. Some units responded to teeth and to stimulation of intraoral mucosa or the facial area of skin. The threshold force required for the neurones to respond to mechanical force applied to the canine tooth was less than 0.05 N in most of the units. There was evidence for a somatotopic distribution of neurones, with the mandibular neurones located dorsally and the maxillary units located ventrally. However, many units tended to be distributed in the border region between the two divisions. This was a similar result to that already reported in the main sensory nucleus by Kruger and Michel (1962) and Eisenman *et al.* (1963). Tabata and Karita (1991c) concluded from their studies that the response properties of the units in the main sensory nucleus resembled fairly closely those of the primary afferent neurones. It should be stated, however, that the finding of multiple receptive fields does appear to be different from that of primary afferent neurones.

In the trigeminal spinal nuclei, Tabata and Karita (1991a) have also looked at the responses of periodontal mechanosensitive neurones. They found that the majority of the units in the nucleur oralis were single tooth. In the nucleus interpolaris more than half were multiple-tooth units and in the nucleus caudalis all were multiple-tooth units. The neurones were predominantly sensitive to forces applied to the canine tooth. In this nucleus also, there was evidence for directional sensitivity of the neurones and slowly adapting responses to pressure applied to the teeth. In a later study, Tabata and Karita (1992) looked specifically at the response fields of periodontal mechanosensitive neurones in the trigeminal sensory complex while applying mechanical stimulation to the canine tooth in many different directions. It was found that almost all of the slowly adapting periodontal mechanosensitive neurones were directionally selective to stimulation and that they responded over a broad range of directions.

It is not clear whether the directional sensitivity response of the neurones is a result of a transmission of similar information from the primary afferent neurones. This could be true, but it is also known from anatomical studies using horseradish peroxidase that there is much branching of primary afferent neurones with collaterals given off into different regions of the trigeminal nuclei (Shigenaga *et al.*, 1988; Bae *et al.*, 1993). This also may be true of the receptive fields of the neurones and the response properties.

PROJECTIONS TO THALAMUS AND SOMATOSENSORY CORTEX

Neurones in the nucleus ventralis posteromedialis of the thalamus respond to forces applied to contralateral and ipsilateral teeth (Yokota *et al.*, 1988). Karita and Tabata (1991) studied the response characteristics of periodontal mechanosensitive neurones in the thalamus. They found that a large number of neurones were responsive to a light mechanical stimulus to the teeth. A larger proportion of these neurones were rapidly adapting than the proportion that were slowly adapting. Many of the units responded to stimulation of contralateral teeth and fewer responded to the ipsilateral side; 21 per cent of the neurones responded to bilateral stimulation of the teeth. Therefore, it appears that the receptive fields of the thalamus neurones are very much larger than those observed either at the primary afferent neurones or at the level of the trigeminal nuclear complex. However, the thresholds of the units to mechanical stimulation were similar to that in primary afferent neurones. The authors concluded that the high incidence of multiquadrant units shows the existence of vigorous convergence of input fibres to the thalamus. Directionally sensitive units were much less frequent in the thalamus than in the primary afferents or the trigeminal nuclear complex. It therefore appears that directional sensitivity information becomes less important as the higher centres are reached.

Tabata and Karita (1991b) have also examined the response properties of the periodontal mechanosensitive neurones of the thalamus in the cat and found slowly and rapidly adapting neurones. Their observations suggested to them that the slowly adapting units received periodontal inputs from the trigeminal nuclear complex, whereas the rapidly adapting units received their inputs polysynaptically from other pathways. Woda *et al.* (1983) found that neurones in the trigeminal main sensory nucleus which respond to mechanical stimulation of the teeth do project to the thalamus. In contrast, none of the periodontal units recorded in the nucleus oralis of the spinal trigeminal nucleus were antidromically activated by stimulation of the contralateral or ipsilateral ventrobasal thalamus (Olsson *et al.*, 1988). Taken together, these observations do not appear to provide a complete understanding of the neural pathways involved.

Recordings have been made in the somatosensory cortex (S1) from neurones that respond to forces applied to the teeth (Lund and Sessle, 1974; Tabata *et al.*, 1986; Taira, 1987a,b). Lund and Sessle (1974) suggested that the pathway from periodontal mechanoreceptors to S1 includes two relays; one in the trigeminal brain stem nuclei and the other in the thalamic nuclei. Tabata *et al.* (1986) studied a number of cortical neurones that were sensitive to mechanical stimulation of the teeth and these were found in the caudal part of the coronal gyrus. They responded to transient mechanical stimulation of the tooth. With sustained forces applied to the tooth, the cortical neurones fired strongly at the outset and also after removal of the force, but the responses for the duration of the stimulus were indistinguishable from the spontaneous activity seen when there was no overt stimulus applied. These responses appeared to be modulated by transient mouth opening.

In a later study, Watanabe *et al.* (1991) observed the discharge patterns of these neurones in more detail. It appeared that jaw opening did not influence any phases of the responses of the neurones to suprathreshold stimulation, nor did it influence spontaneous activity or the sizes of the receptive fields. However, jaw opening did affect the initial burst phase of the response to threshold stimulation. The reason for this is unknown.

CEREBELLUM

There is some evidence to suggest a direct and relayed projection of periodontal mechanoreceptors to the cerebellum (Taylor and Elias 1984; Nomura and Mizuno 1985; Elias *et al.*, 1987). However, the functional significance of this is unclear.

DISCUSSION OF CENTRAL CONNECTIONS OF PDL MECHANORECEPTORS

There have been many studies carried out in which recordings have been made in the trigeminal nuclei, and these have been discussed above. However, no study has yet been able to correlate conclusively how activity in a single primary afferent neurone affects the neurones in the trigeminal nuclei. Researchers have no idea of how information on direction of force application, amplitude, duration, rate of force application, etc, is processed at this level.

In our laboratory, we have attempted to study this problem by looking at actions of impulses from primary afferent PDL mechanoreceptive neurones on neurones in the trigeminal nuclei. Primary afferent neurones in the trigeminal ganglion which responded to forces applied to the mandibular canine tooth were recorded intracellularly with a glass microelectrode. Simultaneously we recorded extracellularly from a single neurone in the main sensory nucleus which also responded to forces applied to the mandibular canine tooth. When a pair of neurones had been identified, experiments were performed to determine if there was any evidence for linkage between the two. This was carried out by applying small currents (nanoamps) which were known to be sufficient to cause an action potential in the primary afferent neurones, while monitoring the response from the electrode in the main sensory nucleus. Single pulses and trains of stimuli were applied, depending on how long it was possible to record from the pair of neurones. Despite the technical difficulties, we were able to record simultaneously from a small number of pairs of neurones. However, we could find no evidence of linkage between them. It is possible that, for a neurone in the trigeminal nucleus to respond, there has to be sufficient excitatory activity in the neurones that connect synaptically with it to allow discharge of the neurone. It is likely that spatial and temporal summation of impulses from primary afferent neurones would be required and, of course, there may be inhibitory neurones that also synapse with the neurone. In the intracellular stimulation experiments that we carried out, the failure to demonstrate a linkage may have been because intracellular stimulation of one primary afferent neurone, even with a train of impulses, may simply have been insufficient to cause enough excitatory synaptic transmitter to be released. An alternative, and equally possible, explanation is that there was no linkage between the small number of pairs of primary afferent and trigeminal nuclei neurones studied.

Processing of information from primary afferent PDL mechanosensitive neurones is a complex process. Anatomical studies, although useful to show the connections of neurones, cannot show how impulses in the primary afferent neurones interact with those of other neurones. Electrophysiological studies on trigeminal nuclei neurones have provided only the most basic information on how action potentials are generated. Clearly, much more work is required to understand exactly how information from forces applied to the teeth is processed at the level of the brain stem. This, of course, is also true at the level of the thalamus and the somatosensory cortex, an even more challenging problem.

THE FUNCTIONS OF PDL MECHANORECEPTORS

TOUCH THRESHOLDS

Stewart (1927) was the first to record touch thresholds of human teeth, and in his experiments he stated that some pulpless teeth were also examined. There appeared to be very little difference in touch thresholds between the pulpless teeth and normal teeth. Pfaffmann (1939a) recorded from cat peripheral nerves in response to forces applied to the teeth and noted that the response was not affected by removal of the pulp and cautery of the apical canal. These observations suggested that receptors that respond to forces applied to the teeth are not in the pulp but are located within the PDL or supporting structures. In contrast, Loewenstein and Rathkamp (1955), in humans, found the thresholds of pulpless teeth were higher. Linden (1975) looked at the touch thresholds of the normal central maxillary incisor and the contralateral non-vital central incisor in humans by applying force along the longitudinal aspect of the tooth using an electromechanical force generator. No differences in the touch thresholds were found.

It is now accepted that it is the mechanoreceptors situated in the periodontium which mediate sensation when forces are applied to the teeth. However, Dong *et al.* (1985) claim to have found intradental (pulpal) mechanoreceptors that respond to forces applied to the teeth, but their results were not confirmed in later experiments by Matthews (1986). It has been suggested that, in the experiments of Dong *et al.* (1985), the stimulating electrodes that were placed into the tooth could well have inadvertently stimulated nerves outside the tooth. Recently, in a study by Dong *et al.* (1993), the response properties of periodontal mechanoreceptors and so-called 'intradental mechanoreceptors' have been investigated by making recordings from cells in the trigeminal ganglion. The authors state that there was a response profile observed for all intradental mechanoreceptors. The units responded only to a rapid mechanical transient force (a tap), only rapidly adapting discharges were observed, and there was no directional sensitivity. Unfortunately, no records of the single intradental mechanoreceptor units in response to mechanical stimulation of the teeth were shown in this paper. It seems unlikely that the authors could be certain that, when a rapid tap was applied to the tooth, they were not stimulating neurones in the PDL despite the way the force was applied. Therefore, the evidence for intradental mechanoreceptors remains far from conclusive at the present time.

MASTICATORY SALIVARY REFLEX

There is convincing evidence that periodontal mechanoreceptors play a role in the reflex of salivation which occurs on chewing food. Lashley (1916) recorded bilateral parotid flow and showed that chewing on a piece of rubber between the molar teeth resulted in an increased flow on both sides, with a greater response on the ipsilateral side than on the contralateral side. Kerr (1961) confirmed these findings and concluded that receptors in the PDL were responsible for this secretion. Anderson *et al.* (1985) confirmed, in the rabbit, that the greatest parotid salivary secretion was on the side on which the animal was chewing. Furthermore, there was a relationship between masticatory force and the salivary flow. Hector and Linden (1987) attempted in humans to focus more precisely on the role of periodontal mechanoreceptors in the reflex of salivation. They restricted the area of the mechanical stimulation to the teeth and their supporting structures by using specifically constructed bite platforms, and they controlled the magnitude of the stimulus by monitoring the rectified and integrated electromyographic activity from the masseter muscle. Certain areas around the mouth were anaesthetized. It was found that anaesthesia of two to three inputs produced significant reductions in ipsilateral flow, but anaesthesia of a single input was not always effective. The data from these experiments provided substantial evidence in support of the hypothesis that intraoral mechanoreceptors and particularly periodontal mechanoreceptors contribute to the masticatory—salivary reflex. These, of course, are not the only receptors that contribute to salivary flow during mastication, since gustatory inputs from the facial and the glossopharyngeal nerve provide a substantial contribution to the afferent input to the reflex (Watanabe and Dawes 1988).

Lee and Linden (1992b) carried out experiments on human subjects to determine if there was synergism between an olfactory stimulus and a strong salivary stimulus such as mastication. In some experiments the masticatory stimulus was provided by subjects chewing on base gum (i.e. no sweetener and no flavour). Constant biting force was achieved by supplying visual feedback to the subject from electromyographic activity recorded from the masseter muscle. During this chewing, salivary flow was recorded from the parotid duct using a modified Lashley cup and cannula. Odorous stimuli from peppermint or orange were introduced by placing the test odour in a nebulizer and bubbling air through it so that the resulting odour was administered to the subject by a face mask. No evidence was found, however, that smell had any effect on the stimulated parotid salivary flow. Smell has been shown to increase submandibular salivary flow above resting levels (Lee and Linden 1992a). No studies have been carried out to determine if there is synergism between olfactory stimuli and masticatory stimuli in the submandibular gland.

REFLEXES OF MASTICATORY MUSCLES

Human and animal studies have shown that tapping or fast transient forces applied to the teeth will cause a reflex jaw opening (Hannam and Matthews, 1969; Aars *et al.*, 1988; van Steenberghe *et al.*, 1989; Lund, 1990). It is generally accepted that PDL mechanoreceptors are involved in this reflex. Dessem *et al.* (1988) found that stimulation of low threshold periodontal mechanoreceptors caused an inhibition of jaw closing muscles but not an excitation of the digastric muscle. In humans, stimulation of periodontal mechanoreceptors does not cause an increase in the digastric muscle activity (Matthews, 1975). However, inhibition of the masseter muscle has been observed following either a tooth tap (Goldberg, 1971; Sessle and Schmitt, 1972; van der Glas *et al.*, 1985) or tooth contact (Hannam *et al.*, 1969). Local anaesthesia applied around the tooth abolished the inhibition in one study (Sessle and Schmitt 1972) but this was not found in another similar investigation (Hannam *et al.*, 1970). Yamamura and Shimada (1992) looked at the mechanism that controlled such reflexes in lightly anaesthetized rats. They recorded motor unit activity in the masseter and temporal muscles in response to pressure applied to either a maxillary incisor or maxillary molar tooth. It was found that if the background activity in the motor units was low, incisal or molar stimulation elicited excitatory reflexes. However, if the background activity was high, there were inhibitory reflexes in response to forces applied to the teeth. Their results suggested that different patterns of jaw reflexes could be elicited depending on the background activities in the motor units themselves.

The so called 'silent period' observed in the masseter muscle in response to forces applied to the teeth has been demonstrated in many studies (for a description of the jaw reflexes, see Matthews 1975). The problem is that the silent period is very variable in its presence, number of periods, and duration. Brodin *et al.* (1993) studied the reflex responses evoked in the human masseter muscle by controlled mechanical stimulation applied to the incisor tooth. They applied slow pushes and brisk taps varying between 0.5 N and 3 N. They found that slow pushes evoked long latency, primarily excitatory responses in the muscle. This was in contrast to most previous studies, although Lavigne *et al.* (1987) had found evidence in the rabbit that periodontal mechanoreceptors provide positive feedback to the jaw closing muscles during mastication. In the experiments of Brodin *et al.* (1993), the force probe was held in contact with the tooth. Presumably the purpose of this was to prevent unwanted acoustic or vibratory responses occurring when a force was applied to the tooth by the probe. The force probe was held in contact with the tooth between ramps and taps with a force of 0.5–1 N, and the ramp forces and fast transient forces (taps) were superimposed on the background force. It should be stated, however, that a force of this magnitude, applied horizontally to the labial aspect of the tooth, would definitely be able to stimulate the majority of receptors in the PDL, some even at maximal frequency. Other receptors (e.g. the rapidly adapting neurones) would be likely to have adapted out because of the constant force being applied to the tooth. Therefore, one must question whether a force of the nature applied in the experiments of Brodin *et al.* (1993), together with the preloading of the tooth that occurred between each force application, is in fact responsible for the excitatory response observed in this study. Brodin *et al.* (1993) concluded that the most likely explanation for the different responses evoked by the pushes and taps is that the patterns of different afferent activity elicited by the slow and fast tooth displacements activated different interneuronal pathways to the motor neurones. However, as discussed, it could be the particular experimental procedure that accounts for the observations.

One of the main problems in almost all of the studies investigating reflex effects in masticatory muscles in which mechanical stimuli have been used, either as a tap or as a fast transient, is that the stimulus is likely to excite neurones with receptors that are some distance from the periodontium as well as the PDL mechanoreceptors themselves. Therefore, it is possible that neurones with receptors distant to the periodontium could also be contributing to the reflexes and, because of this, it has been difficult to determine the precise contribution that PDL mechanoreceptors make to such reflexes. In recent experiments, Bonte *et al.* (1993) have attempted to overcome these reservations by placing osseointegrated implants into the bone of cats in which one of the maxillary canine teeth had previously been present. The response of motor units in the temporalis muscle in response to forces applied to the implant was then compared with the response to forces applied to the maxillary canine tooth on the opposite side. Experiments of this kind allowed the effects of stimulating the PDL mechanoreceptive neurones to be separated out from the effects of stimulating receptors situated in more distant sites. To avoid the problems of applying a transient force (which is also likely to be able to stimulate rate sensitive mechanoreceptors distant to the periodontium), a ramp increase in force, which was then held stable, was considered to be the most appropriate for the study. In the first part of the study recordings were made from the trigeminal ganglion and peripheral nerves in response to forces applied to the implants and the maxillary teeth. Neurones were identified which responded to forces applied to the maxillary teeth but none were found which responded to forces applied to the implant. Taken together with the fact that the implants are immobile in the bone, the observations provided convincing evidence that forces applied to implants do not stimulate primary afferent mechanoreceptive neurones in the tissues in their immediate environment.

However, there is little doubt that mechanoreceptors distant from the tissues that invest and support the implant can be stimulated when a force is applied to it. Forces applied to the natural teeth can also be expected to stimulate distant mechanoreceptors in a similar manner to implants but, in addition, mechanoreceptors in the PDL itself would be stimulated. This difference made it possible to investigate the role of the PDL mechanoreceptors in the reflexes of jaw opening. The activity of motor units in the temporalis muscles was studied in response to ramp plateau forces up to 1 N applied to the maxillary canine tooth and the maxillary implant using peri-stimulus time histograms and cusum analysis. A small amount of inhibition of the motor units was observed in response to the applied forces to the implant (*Fig. 7.17*). However, the inhibition was much more profound when similar forces were applied to the tooth (see *Fig. 7.17*). The observations in this series of experiments therefore provide good evidence that mechanoreceptors in the PDL are involved in evoking reflex inhibitions of motor unit activity in the temporalis muscle.

These experiments call into question the relative importance of PDL mechanoreceptors in jaw reflexes. It has generally been thought that they have a significant role in controlling activity during mastication in the muscles that close the jaw. Dessem *et al.* (1988) suggested that they could be expected to provide negative feedback control of forces exerted on the teeth during mastication and related tasks. However, the mechanical thresholds of PDL mechanoreceptors are well documented and they range from 10–800 mN (reviewed in Linden, 1990). It is apparent that a force as low as 1 N would be sufficient to evoke a response from the vast majority of PDL mechanoreceptors, some even at maximal frequency. During mastication, the magnitude of bite force generated is obviously much higher than this. Since it was shown that forces of 1 N or lower applied to the implant itself (which is immobile in the bone and was shown not to have any innervation) can stimulate neurones that result in an inhibition of temporalis motor unit activity, it is very likely that, with the sizes of the bite forces that occur in mastication, a large number of mechanoreceptive neurones would be stimulated. Many of these would not be situated in the periodontium but may affect the activity of motor neurones in the jaw-closing muscles. The results of the study provide clear evidence that stimuli to PDL mechanoreceptive neurones do evoke reflex inhibitions of activity in the temporalis motor units. Nevertheless, such stimuli appear not to be vital for evoking such inhibitions, since mechanoreceptive neurones situated distant to the periodontium can also evoke reflex inhibitions to certain stimuli, and it is probable that these are also stimulated in mastication.

The relative contribution of the different groups of mechanoreceptors involved in mastication in the control of jaw-closing muscles clearly requires further study. Jaw opening is the principal somatic reflex evoked by intraoral stimulation. In man, the reflex involves depressions of activity in the jaw-closing muscles and can consist of at least two periods of inhibition with latencies of approximately 12 ms and 40 ms. The pattern of such responses depends on the nature and location of the stimulus. Mechanical stimuli applied to teeth can result in both the short and the long latency inhibitory periods, and it has been suggested

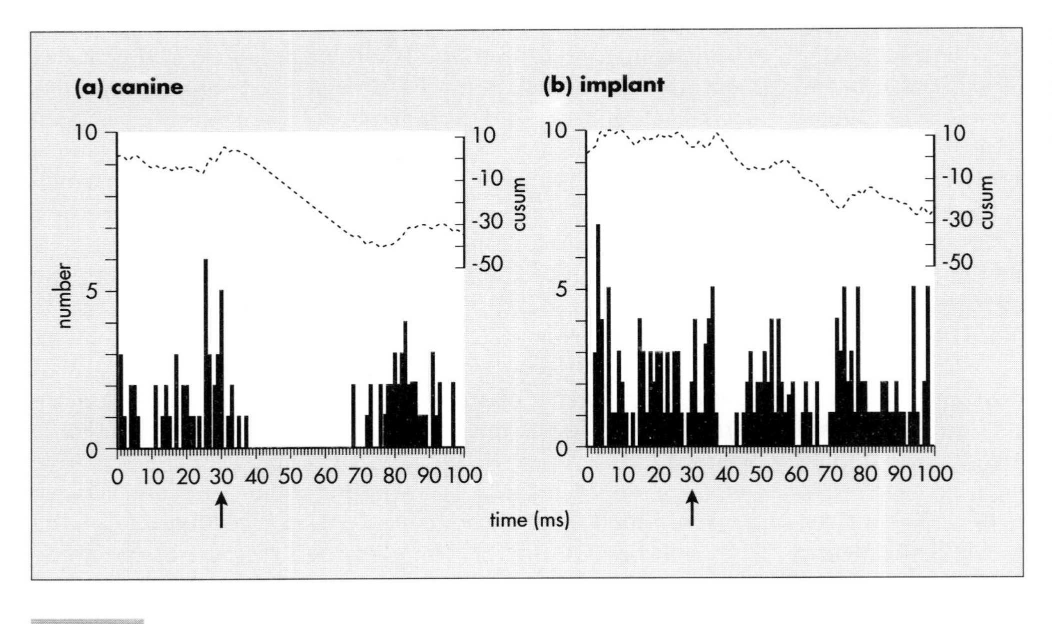

Fig. 7.17 Peri-stimulus time histograms and cusum analysis to show the response of a single motor unit in the left temporalis muscle when a 1 N force is applied to (A) a maxillary cat canine tooth and to (B) a maxillary implant. (From Bonte *et al.*, 1993.)

that PDL mechanoreceptors play a role in evoking these responses. However, the evidence is incomplete and most of the forces applied are fast transient or tapping forces, any of which are likely to affect receptors distant from, as well as within, the PDL. Observations made on the response characteristics of PDL mechanoreceptors in the cat suggest that ramp-plateau stimuli are more likely to excite exclusively these types of receptors and that a force of 1 N is sufficient to evoke responses from most PDL mechanoreceptors. Recent preliminary experiments in which discrete controlled mechanical stimuli have been applied to human teeth suggest that PDL mechanoreceptors may contribute to only the short latency inhibitory reflex in jaw-closing muscles (Louca *et al.*, 1994).

THE EFFECT OF TREATMENT AND DISEASE ON THE INNERVATION OF THE PDL

There has been only one physiological study in the cat in which the response characteristics of periodontal mechanoreceptors have been studied during orthodontic loading. Loescher *et al.* (1993) investigated these neurones after orthodontic forces had been applied for either 3 days or 12 weeks, and also 8 weeks after the tooth had been moved into a new position and the tissues allowed to recover. Recordings were made from single neurones dissected from the inferior alveolar nerve. It was found that some of the receptor characteristics of the neurones altered both during and after the tooth had been moved into a new position. It was suggested that the altered receptor characteristics resulted from a combination of disorganization of the collagen matrix and direct injury to the nerve terminals.

Schnorpfeil *et al.* (1991) have shown that chronic inflammatory periodontal disease resulted in signs of neuropathy of the autonomic part of the nervous system. There have been no reported studies on the physiological properties of PDL mechanoreceptors in periodontal disease.

Kvinnsland *et al.* (1992) studied the morphological changes in sensory nerves in the periodontium by means of immunohistochemistry (using antibodies to protein gene product) following occlusal trauma. The responses after unilateral induced traumatic occlusion in the first maxillary molar of the rat remained localized to cervical and apical tissues throughout the experiment.

Damage by trauma to the neurones that innervate the PDL could occur either as a result of restorative procedures (e.g. endodontics or surgical procedures involving the tooth apex) or as a result of damage to a nerve trunk. The effects of injury and inflammation to periapical nerves has been reviewed by Byers *et al.* (1990). Holland (1991) found that pulpectomy did not affect the incidence or distribution pattern of nerves in the PDL. However, Holland (1992) investigated the effect of pulpectomy on the periapical innervation of the ferret canine tooth and described a proliferation of periapical nerves within an area of chronic inflammation. This persisted over 12 months, perhaps owing to the irritation caused by the endodontic material.

Loescher and Robinson (1989b) investigated the properties of the PDL mechanoreceptors after crushing or sectioning injuries to the inferior alveolar nerve. They found that the PDL had been reinnervated as early as 12 weeks after the injury, but there were changes in some of the properties of the neurones. Loescher and Holland (1991) found that 12 weeks after section of the inferior alveolar nerve, the total number of axons innervating the PDL was half that found in the controls. In later work, Loescher and Robinson (1991a) looked at the properties of neurones that had reinnervated the PDL 1 year after nerve section injuries. They found that even after this long recovery period, the characteristics of mechanoreceptors do not return to normal, and they thought it probable that these changes are permanent. The same authors studied the characteristics of neurones that had reinnervated the PDL following the reimplantation of teeth in the cat and concluded that again the characteristics did not return to normal 1 year after surgical intervention (Loescher and Robinson, 1991b).

After tooth loss, the remnants of the PDL break down and disappear (reviewed by Simpson, 1969). Neurones that innervate the PDL could respond to this by:

- regenerating to the periosteum or oral mucosa covering the alveolar process;
- forming a neuroma in the bone; or
- degenerating completely (especially if traumatized by a tooth extraction) (Hansen 1980).

The only electrophysiological study that recorded from neurones known to have innervated the PDL before the teeth were extracted was performed by Linden and Scott (1989b) in the cat. They found that at least some of the mesencephalic nucleus neurones that previously innervated the PDL of the mandibular canine and incisor teeth were still present in the inferior alveolar nerve up to 2 years after tooth extraction. The majority of these neurones were situated in the edentulous ridge of the mandible where they could be stimulated electrically. However, it was not possible to stimulate them mechanically despite the use of large forces. A small number had reinnervated new soft tissue sites where they could be mechanically stimulated. It was concluded, however, that since the majority did not reinnervate new tissues in which they could be mechanically stimulated, it is unlikely that they have any functional role after tooth loss. There is no reason to suspect that the neurones with their cell bodies in the trigeminal ganglion would be any different after tooth extraction.

It is noteworthy that reflexes of masticatory muscles and salivation can still be observed as a result of artificial tooth contact in edentulous patients wearing full dentures (Matthews and Yemm, 1970; Bellwood and Heath, 1987). These reflexes, as already discussed, have generally been attributed to PDL mechanoreceptors. The reasons for these findings are not known although, as discussed earlier, it is likely that receptors other than those in the periodontium also contribute to such reflexes.

CONCLUSIONS

Since the first edition of this book, there have been considerable advances in our understanding of the innervation of the PDL. In this review, we have concentrated on the recent advances. From the morphological point of view we have little doubt that PDL mechanoreceptors are unencapsulated Ruffini nerve endings, with projections into the surrounding connective tissues. Using comparisons with Ruffini nerve endings in other structures, it is suggested that these projections (along with the Schwann cell sheath) have a role in the transduction process. Furthermore, when a force is applied to a tooth crown, the physiological response characteristics of an individual PDL mechanoreceptor are dependent on the position (relative to the fulcrum) of the Ruffini nerve ending within the PDL and its relation to the surrounding tissues.

The central connections of the larger diameter neurones that innervate the PDL are now more clearly defined, but we are still unsure of the precise roles of these receptors in mastication and salivation. There is little doubt as to their role in sensation. There is still very little known about the smaller diameter neurones represented in the periodontal ligament. Studies on the effects of disease states on the neurones and their functions are very much in their infancy.

REFERENCES

Aars H (1978) Adrenergic receptors in periodontal vessels. Acta Physiol Scand 102, 34–35A (abstract).

Aars H, Brodin P and Bjørnland T. (1988) Sympathetic modulation of the jaw opening reflex in anaesthetized rabbits. Acta Physiol Scand 134, 319–325.

Aars H and Linden RWA (1982) The effects of sympathetic trunk stimulation on the position and mobility of the canine tooth of the cat. Arch Oral Biol 27, 399–404.

Amano N and Iwasaki T (1982) Response characteristics of primary periodontal mechanoreceptive neurones in the trigeminal mesencephalic nucleus to trapezoidal mechanical stimulation of a single tooth in the rat. Brain Res 237, 309–323.

Anderson D, Hector MP and Linden RWA (1985) The possible relation between mastication and parotid secretion in the rabbit. J Physiol 364, 19–29.

Appenteng K, Lund JP and Séguin JJ (1982) Intraoral mechanoreceptor activity during jaw movement in the anaesthetised rabbit. J Neurophysiol 48, 27–37.

Bae YC, Nagase Y, Yoshida A, Shigenaga Y and Sugimoto T (1993) Synaptic connections of a periodontal primary afferent neuron within the subnucleus oralis of the cat. Brain Res 606, 175–179.

Balogh K and Csiba A (1967) Die Nerveenversorgung des Zahnfleisches. Dtsch Zahn Mund Kieferheilkd 49, 299–305.

Beaudreau DE and Jerge CR (1968) Somatotopic representation in the gasserian ganglion of tactile peripheral fields in the cat. Arch Oral Biol 13, 247–256.

Beertsen W, Everts V and van den Hooff A (1974) Fine structure and possible function of cells containing leptomeric organelles in the periodontal ligament of the rat incisor. Arch Oral Biol 19, 1099–1100.

Bellwood P and Heath MR (1987) A study of the masticatory–salivary reflex in complete denture users. J Dent Res 66, 858 (abstract).

Berkovitz BKB (1990) The structure of the periodontal ligament: an update. Eur J Orthod 12, 51–76.

Berkovitz BKB and Shore RC (1978) High mitochondrial density within periodontal nerve fibres of the periodontal ligament of the rat incisor. Arch Oral Biol 23, 207–213.

Berkovitz BKB, Shore RC and Moxham BJ (1983) The occurrence of a lamellated nerve terminal in the periodontal ligament of the rat incisor. Arch Oral Biol 28, 99–101.

Berkovitz BKB and Sloan P (1979) Attachment tissues of the teeth in Caiman sclerops (Crocodilia). J Zool Lond 187, 179–194.

Bernick S (1952) Innervation of the primary tooth and surrounding supporting tissues of monkeys. Anat Rec 113, 215–237.

Bernick S (1956) The innervation of the teeth and periodontium of the rat. Anat Rec 125, 185–206.

Bernick S (1957) Innervation of teeth and periodontium after enzymatic removal of collagenous elements. Oral Surg Oral Med Oral Pathol 10, 323–332.

Bernick S (1959) Innervation of the teeth and periodontium. Dent Clin North Am 503–514.

Bernick S (1966) Vascular and nerve supply to the molar teeth of guinea pigs. J Dent Res 45, 249–260.

Bernick S and Levy BM (1968) Studies on the biology of the periodontium of marmosets: innervation of the periodontal ligament. J Dent Res 47, 1158–1165.

Biemesderfer D, Munger BL, Binck J and Dubner R (1978) The pilo-Ruffini complex : a non-sinus hair and associated slowly adapting mechanoreceptor in primate facial skin. Brain Res 142, 197–222.

Bonte B, Linden RWA, Scott BJJ and van Steenberghe D (1993) Role of periodontal mechanoreceptors in evoking reflexes in the jaw-closing muscles of the cat. J Physiol 465, 581–594.

Boyd IA (1954) The histological structure of the receptors in the knee-joint of the cat correlated with their physiological response. J Physiol 124, 476–488.

Bradlaw R (1939) The innervation of teeth. Proc R Soc Med 32, 1040–1053.

Brashear AD (1936) The innervation of the teeth. An analysis of nerve fibre components of the pulp and peridental tissues and their probable significance. J Comp Neurol 64, 169–185.

Brodin P, Turker KS and Miles TS (1993) Mechanoreceptors around the tooth evoke inhibitory and excitatory reflexes in the human masseter muscle. J Physiol 464, 711–723.

Byers (1984) Dental sensory receptors. Int Rev Neurobiol 25, 39–94.

Byers MR (1985) Sensory innervation of periodontal ligament of rat molars consists of unencapsulated Ruffini-like mechanoreceptors and free nerve endings. J Comp Neurol 231, 500–518.

Byers MR (1990) Segregation of NGF receptor in sensory receptors, nerves and local cells of teeth and periodontium demonstrated by EM immunocytochemistry. J Neurocytol 19, 765–775.

Byers MR and Dong WK (1989) Comparison of trigeminal receptor location and structure in the periodontal ligament of different types of teeth from the rat, cat, and monkey. J Comp Neurol 279, 117–127.

Byers MR and Holland GR (1977) Trigeminal nerve endings in gingiva, junctional epithelium and periodontal ligament of rat molars as demonstrated by autoradiography. Anat Rec 188, 509–524.

Byers, MR and Matthews B (1981) Autoradiographic demonstration of ipsilateral and contralateral sensory nerve endings in cat dentin, pulp and periodontium. Anat Rec 201, 249–260.

Byers MR, O'Connor TA, Martin RF and Dong WK (1986) Mesencephalic trigeminal sensory neurons of cat: axon pathways and structure of mechanoreceptive endings in periodontal ligament. J Comp Neurol 250, 181–191.

Byers MR, Taylor PE, Khayat BG and Kimberly CL (1990) Effects of injury and inflammation on pulpal and periapical nerves. J Endod 16, 78–84.

Capra N, Anderson KV, Pride JB and Jones TE (1984) Simultaneous demonstration of neuronal somata that innervate the tooth pulp and adjacent periodontal tissues, using two retrogradely transported anatomic markers. Exp Neurol 86, 165–170.

Cash RM and Linden RWA (1982a) Effects of sympathetic nerve stimulation on intra-oral mechanoreceptor activity in the cat. J Physiol 329, 451–463.

Cash RM, and Linden RWA (1982b) The distribution of mechanoreceptors in the periodontal ligament of the mandibular canine tooth of the cat. J Physiol 330, 439–447.

Chambers MR, Andres KH, von Duering M and Iggo A (1972) The structure and function of the slowly adapting type II mechanoreceptor in hairy skin. Q J Exp Physiol 57, 417–445.

Cody F, Lee RWH and Taylor A (1972) A functional analysis of the components of the mesencephalic nucleus of the fifth nerve in the cat. J Physiol 226, 249–261.

Corbin KB and Harrison F (1940) Function of mesencephalic root of fifth cranial nerve. J Neurophysiol 3, 423–435.

Corporon RE, Avery JK, Leeds SD and Cox CF (1974) Ultrastructure of nerve endings in the periodontal ligament of mice. J Dent Res 53, 75 (abstract).

Darian-Smith I (1966) Neural mechanisms of facial sensation. Int Rev Neurobiol 9, 301–395.

De Lange A, Hannam AG and Matthews B (1969) The diameters and conduction velocities of fibres in the terminal branches of the inferior dental nerve. Arch Oral Biol 14, 513–519.

Dependorf T (1913) Nervenverteilung in der Zahnwurzelhaut des Menschen. Dtsch Monatsschr Zahnheilkd 31, 853–864.

Dessem D, Iyadurai OD and Taylor A (1988) The role of periodontal receptors in the jaw opening reflex in the cat. J Physiol 406, 315–330.

Dixon AD (1961) Sensory nerve terminations in the oral mucosa. Arch Oral Biol 5, 105–114.

Dong WK, Chudler EH and Martin RF (1985) Physiological properties of intradental mechanoreceptors. Brain Res 334, 389–395.

Dong WK, Shiwaku T, Kawakami Y and Chudler EH (1993) Static and dynamic responses of periodontal ligament mechanoreceptors and intradental mechanoreceptors. J Neurophysiol 69, 1567–1582.

Dubner R and Sessle BJ (1971) Presynaptic excitability changes of primary afferent and corticofugal fibres projecting to trigeminal brain stem nuclei. Exp Neurol 30, 223–238.

Edwall L and Kindlova M (1971) The effect of sympathetic nerve stimulation on the rate of disappearance of tracers from various oral tissues. Acta Odont Scand 29, 385–400.

Eisenman J, Landgren S and Novin D (1963) Functional organisation in the main sensory trigeminal nucleus in the rostral subdivision of the nucleus of the spinal trigeminal tract in the cat. Acta Physiol Scand 59 (suppl 214), 1–44.

Elias SA, Taylor A and Somjen G (1987) Direct and relayed projection of periodontal receptor afferents to the cerebellum in the ferret. Proc R Soc Lond [Biol] 231, 199–216.

Everts V, Beertsen W, van den Hoof A (1977) Fine structure of an end organ in the periodontal ligament of the mouse incisor. Anat Rec 189, 73–90.

Falin LI (1958) The morphology of receptors of the tooth. Acta Anat (Basel) 35, 257–276.

Freezer SR and Sims MR (1987) A transmission electron-microscope stereological study of the blood vessels, oxytalan fibres and nerves of mouse periodontal ligament. Arch Oral Biol 32, 407–412.

Freezer SR and Sims MR (1989) Morphometry of neural structures in the mouse periodontal ligament mesial to the mandibular first molar. Aust Orthod J 11, 30–37.

Fujita Y (1987) Response properties of single sensory units innervating human periodontal ligament to force stimuli. J Stomatol Soc Jpn 54, 676–691.

Gairns FW and Aitchison JA (1950) A preliminary study of the multiplicity of nerve endings in the human gum. Dent Res 70, 180–194.

Goldberg LJ (1971) Masseter muscle excitation induced by stimulation of periodontal and gingival receptors in man. Brain Res 32, 369–381.

Goodwin GM and Luschei ES (1975) Discharge of spindle afferents from jaw-closing muscles during chewing in alert monkeys. J Neurophysiol 38, 560–571.

Griffin CJ (1972) The fine structure of end-rings in the human periodontal ligament. Arch Oral Biol 17, 785–797.

Griffin CJ and Harris R (1968) Unmyelinated nerve endings in the periodontal membrane of human teeth. Arch Oral Biol 13, 1207–1212.

Griffin CJ and Harris R (1974a) Innervation of human periodontium. I. Classification of periodontal receptors Aust Dent J 19, 51–56.

Griffin CJ and Harris R (1974b) Innervation of the human periodontium. III. Fine structure of compound receptor. Aust Dent J 19, 255–260.

Griffin CJ and Malor R (1974) An analysis of mandibular movement. In: Frontiers of Oral Physiology: Physiology of Mastication (Kawamura Y, ed), pp 159–198, Karger, Basel.

Griffin CL and Spain H (1972) Organisation and vasculature of human periodontal mechanoreceptors. Arch Oral Biol 17, 913–921.

Grigg P (1986) Biophysical studies on mechanoreceptors. J Appl Physiol 60, 1107–1115.

Grigg P and Hoffmann AH (1984) Ruffini mechanoreceptors in isolated joint capsule responses correlated with strain energy density. Somatosensory Res 2, 149–162.

Hada R (1990) [Difference in responses of free nerve endings and Ruffini-type endings innervating the cat mandibular periosteum-to square wave pressure stimuli, ramp mechanical stimuli and triangular vibrations.] Shikwa Gakuho 90, 161–80.

Halata Z (1977) The ultrastructure of the sensory nerve endings in the articular capsule of the knee joint of the domestic cat (Ruffini corpuscles and Pacinian corpuscles). J Anat 124, 717–729.

Halata Z (1988) Ruffini corpuscle – a stretch receptor in the connective tissue of the skin and locomotion apparatus. In: Progress in Brain Research (Hamann W and Iggo A, eds), Volume 74, pp 221–229, Elsevier, Amsterdam

Halata Z and Munger BL (1980) The sensory innervation of primate eyelid. Anat Rec 198, 657–670.

Halata Z and Munger BL (1985) The terminal myelin segments of afferent axons to cutaneous mechanoreceptors. Brain Res 347, 177–182.

Halata Z, Rettig T and Schulze W (1985) The ultrastructure of sensory nerve endings in the human knee joint capsule. Anat Embryol 172, 265–273.

Hannam A (1968) The conduction velocity of nerve impulses from dental mechanoreceptors in the dog. Arch Oral Biol 13, 1377–1383.

Hannam A (1969a) The response of periodontal mechanoreceptors in the dog to controlled loading of the teeth. Arch Oral Biol 14, 781–791.

Hannam A (1969b) Spontaneous activity in dental mechanosensitive units in the dog. Arch Oral Biol 14, 793–801.

Hannam AG (1970) Receptor fields of periodontal mechanosensitive units in the dog. Arch Oral Biol 15, 971–978.

Hannam AG (1982) The innervation of the periodontal ligament. In: The Periodontal Ligament in Health and Disease (Berkovitz BKB, Moxham BJ and Newman HN, eds), pp 173–196, Pergamon Press, Oxford.

Hannam AG and Farnsworth TJ (1977) Information transmission in the trigeminal mechanosensitive afferents from teeth in the cat. Arch Oral Biol 22, 181–186.

Hannam AG and Matthews B (1969) Reflex jaw opening in response to stimulation of periodontal mechanoreceptors in the cat. Arch Oral Biol 14, 415–419.

Hannam, A. Matthews B and Yemm R (1969) Changes in the activity of the masseter muscle following tooth contact in man. Arch Oral Biol 14, 1401–1406.

Hannam A. Matthews B and Yemm R (1970) Receptors involved in the response of the masseter muscle to tooth contact in man. Arch Oral Biol 15, 17–24.

Hansen HJ (1980) Neuro-histological reactions following tooth extractions. Int J Oral Surg 9, 411–426.

Harris R and Griffin CJ (1974a) Innervation of the human periodontium. II. Fine structure of simple mechanoreceptors. Aust Dent J 19, 174–181.

Harris R and Griffin CJ (1974b) Innervation of the human periodontium. IV. Fine structure of the complex mechanoreceptors and free nerve endings. Aust Dent J 19, 326–331.

Hattyasy D (1959) Zur Frage der Innervation der Zahnwurzelhaut. Z Mikrosk Anat Forsch 65, 413–433.

Hector MP and Linden RWA (1987) The possible role of periodontal mechanoreceptors in the control of parotid secretion in man. Q J Exp Physiol 72, 285–301.

Held AJ and Baud CA (1955) Surgical anatomy and physiology. The innervation of the dental organ studied by new techniques. Oral Surg Oral Med Oral Pathol 8, 1262–1269.

Holland GR (1988) The periapical innervation of the ferret canine and the local retrograde neural changes after pulpectomy. Anat Rec 220, 318–327.

Holland GR (1991) The effect of pulpectomy on the longitudinal distribution of nerve fibres in the periodontal ligament of the ferret. Arch Oral Biol 36, 161–164.

Holland GR (1992) Periapical innervation of the ferret canine one year after pulpectomy. J Dent Res 71, 470–474.

Itoh K, Wakita M and Kobayashi S (1981) Innervation of the periodontium in the monkey. Arch Histol Jpn 44, 453–466.

Jerge C (1963a) Organisation and function of the trigeminal mesencephalic nucleus. J Neurophysiol 26, 379–392.

Jerge CR (1963b) The function of the nucleus supratrigeminalis. J Neurophysiol 26, 393–402.

Johansson RS and Olsson KA (1976) Microelectrode recordings from human oral mechanoreceptors. Brain Res 118, 307–311.

Jurjiewa E (1913) Die Nervenendingungen im Zahnfleisch des Menschen und der Saugetiere. Folia Neurobiol Lpz 7, 772–780.

Kadanoff D (1929) Die Nerven und Nervenendigungen in der Zahnwurzelhaut des Menschen. Verh Physikal Medizin Ges 54, 27–32.

Kadanoff D (1967) Zur Frage der Innervation der Zahne beim Menschen. Novo Acta Leopoldina 33, 143–160.

Kannari K (1990) Sensory receptors in the periodontal ligament of hamster incisors with special reference to the distribution, ultrastructure and three-dimensional reconstruction of Ruffini endings. Arch Histol Cytol 53, 559–573.

Kannari K, Sato O, Maeda T, Iwanaga T and Fujita T (1991) A possible mechanism of mechanoreception in Ruffini endings in the periodontal ligament of hamster incisors. J Comp Neurol 313, 368–576.

Karita K, Izumi H, Tabata T, Kuriwada S, Sasano T and Sanjo D (1989) The blood flow in the periodontal ligament regulated by the sympathetic and sensory nerves in the cat. Proc Finn Dent Soc 85, 289–924.

Karita K and Tabata T (1985) Response fields of the periodontal mechanosensitive units in the superior alveolar nerve of the cat. Exp Neurol 90, 558–565.

Karita K and Tabata T (1991) Response properties of periodontal mechanosensitive units in the cat's thalamus. Exp Brain Res 86, 341–346.

Kato J, Tanne K, Ichikawa H, *et al.* (1992) Distribution of calcitonin gene-related peptide and substance P-immunoreactive nerve fibers and their correlation in the periodontal ligament of the mouse incisor. Acta Anat (Basel) 145, 101–105.

Kawamura Y and Nishiyama T (1966) Projection of dental afferent impulses to the trigeminal nuclei of the cat. Jpn J Physiol 16, 584–597.

Kerebel B (1965) Innervation of the human periodontium. Actual Odont 71, 289–312.

Kerr AC (1961) The physiological regulation of salivary secretions in man. International Series of Monographs on Oral Biology, Volume 1, Pergamon Press, Oxford.

Kerr FWL and Lysak WR (1964) Somatotopic organization of trigeminal ganglion neurones. Arch Neurol Psychiatr 11, 593–602.

Kirkpatrick DB and Kruger L (1975) Physiological properties of neurons in the principal sensory trigeminal nucleus of the cat. Exp Neurol 48, 664–690.

Kizior JE, Cuozzo JW and Bowman DC (1968) Functional and histologic assessment of the sensory innervation of the periodontal ligament of the cat. J Dent Res 47, 59–64.

Kolmer W (1925) Dienen die Zahne der Krokodilier einer speziellen Tastfunktion? Z Anat 76, 315–319.

Kruger L (1988) Mechanoreceptors and structural aspects of receptor function: Summary. Prog Brain Res 74, 291–293.

Kruger L and Michel F (1962) A single neurone analysis of buccal cavity representation in the sensory trigeminal complex of the cat. Arch Oral Biol 7, 491–503.

Kruger L, Perl ER and Sedivec MJ (1981) Fine structure of myelinated mechanical nociceptor endings in cat hairy skin. J Comp Neurol 198, 137–154.

Kubota K and Osanai K (1977) Periodontal sensory innervation of the dentition of the Japanese shrew-mole. J Dent Res 56, 531–537.

Kvinnsland I, Heyeraa KJ and Byers MR (1992) Effects of dental trauma on pulpal and periodontal nerve morphology. Proc Finn Dent Soc 88 (suppl 1), 125–32.

Lambrichts I, Creemers J and van Steenberghe D (1992) Morphology of neural endings in the human periodontal ligament: an electron microscopic study. J Periodont Res 27, 191–196.

Lambrichts I, Creemers J and van Steenberghe D (1993) Periodontal neural endings intimately relate to epithelial rests of Malassez in humans. A light and electron microscope study. J Anat 182, 153–162.

Lashley KS (1916) Reflex secretion of the human parotid gland. J Exp Psychol 1, 461–493.

Lavigne G, Kim JS, Valiquette C and Lund JP (1987) Evidence that periodontal pressoreceptors provide positive feedback to jaw closing muscles during mastication. J Neurophysiol 58, 342–358.

Lee VM and Linden RWA (1992a) An olfactory–submandibular salivary reflex in humans. Exp Physiol 77, 221–224.

Lee VM and Linden RWA (1992b) The effect of odours on stimulated parotid salivary flow in humans. Physiol Behav 52, 1121–1125.

Lewinsky W and Stewart D (1936) The innervation of the periodontal membrane. J Anat 71, 98–102.

Lewinsky W and Stewart D (1937a) The innervation of the periodontal membrane of the cat, with some observations on the function of the end-organs found in that structure. J Anat 71, 232–235.

Lewinsky W and Stewart D (1937b) A comparative study of the innervation of the periodontal membrane. Proc R Soc Med 30, 1355–1369.

Lewinsky W and Stewart D (1938) Innervation of the human gum. J Anat 72, 232–235.

Linden RWA (1975) Touch thresholds of vital and nonvital human teeth. Exp Neurol 48, 387–390.

Linden RWA (1978) Properties of intraoral mechanoreceptors represented in the mesencephalic nucleus of the fifth nerve of the cat. J Physiol 279, 395–408.

Linden RWA (1984) Periodontal mechanoreceptors. In: Sensory Receptor Mechanisms (Hamann W and Iggo A, eds), pp 179–191, World Scientific Press, Singapore.

Linden RWA (1990) Periodontal mechanoreceptors and their functions. In: Neurophysiology of the Jaws and Teeth (Taylor A, ed), pp 52–95, Macmillan, London.

Linden RWA, Millar B J and Halata Z (1994) A comparative physiological and morphological study of periodontal ligament mechanoreceptors represented in the trigeminal ganglion and mesencephalic nucleus of the cat. Anat Embryol 190, 127–135.

Linden RWA and Millar BJ (1988a) The response characteristics of mechanoreceptors related to their position in the cat canine periodontal ligament. Arch Oral Biol 33, 51–56.

Linden RWA and Millar BJ (1988b) The effect of rate of force application on the threshold of periodontal mechanoreceptors in the cat canine tooth. Arch Oral Biol 33, 715–719.

Linden RWA and Millar BJ (1989) Effect of vibration on the discharge of periodontal mechanoreceptors to controlled loading of the cat canine tooth. Arch Oral Biol 34, 275–281.

Linden RWA and Millar BJ (1992) The relation between the response properties and the position of reinnervated periodontal ligament mechanoreceptors in the cat. J Biol Buccale 20, 203–206.

Linden RWA and Millar BJ (1994) The effect of temperature on the discharge of periodontal ligament mechanoreceptors in the cat canine tooth. J Perio Res 29, 283–289.

Linden RWA and Scott BJJ (1988) The site and distribution of mechanoreceptors in the periodontal ligament of the cat represented in the mesencephalic nucleus and their possible regeneration following tooth extraction. Progr Brain Res 74, 231–236.

Linden RWA and Scott BJJ (1989a) Distribution of mesencephalic nucleus and trigeminal ganglion mechanoreceptors in the periodontal ligament of the cat. J Physiol 410, 35–44.

Linden RWA and Scott BJJ (1989b) The effect of tooth extraction on periodontal ligament mechanoreceptors represented in the mesencephalic nucleus of the cat. Arch Oral Biol 34, 937–941.

Lisney SJW and Matthews B (1978) Branched afferent nerves supplying tooth-pulp in the cat. J Physiol 279, 509–517.

Loescher AR, Al-Emram S, Sullivan PG and Robinson PP (1993) Characteristics of periodontal mechanoreceptors supplying cat canine teeth which have sustained orthodontic forces. Arch Oral Biol 38, 663–669.

Loescher AR and Holland GR (1991) Distribution and morphological characteristics of axons in the periodontal ligament of the cat canine tooth and the changes observed after reinnervation. Anat Rec 230, 57–72.

Loescher AR and Robinson PP (1989a) Response characteristics of periodontal mechanosensitive units supplying the cat's lower canine. J Neurophysiol 62, 971–978.

Loescher AR and Robinson PP (1989b) Properties of reinnervated periodontal mechanoreceptors after inferior alveolar nerve injuries in cats. J Neurophysiol 62, 979–983.

Loescher A and Robinson PP (1991a) Properties of periodontal mechanoreceptors supplying the cats lower canine at short and long periods after reinnervation. J Physiol 444, 85–97.

Loescher AR and Robinson PP (1991b) Characteristics of periodontal mechanoreceptors supplying reimplanted canine teeth in cats. Arch Oral Biol 36, 33–40.

Loewenstein WR and Rathkamp R (1955) A study on the pressoreceptive sensibility of the tooth. J Dent Res 34, 287–294.

Loewenstein WR (1971) Mechano-electric transduction in the Pacinian corpuscle. Initiation of sensory impulses in mechanoreceptors. In: Principles of Sensory Physiology (Lowenstein WR, ed), pp 269–290, Springer-Verlag, Berlin.

Louca C, Cadden SW and Linden RWA (1994) The role of periodontal ligament mechanoreceptors in jaw reflexes in man. J Physiol 475, 4–5P.

Lund JP (1990) Specialization of the reflexes of the jaws. In: Neurophysiology of the Jaws and Teeth. (Taylor A, ed), pp 142–161, Macmillan, London.

Lund JP and Sessle BJ (1974) Oral–facial and jaw muscle afferent projections to neurons in cat frontal cortex. Exp Neurol 45, 314–331.

Maeda T (1987) Sensory innervation of the periodontal ligament in the incisor and molar of the monkey, *Macaca fuscata*. An immunohistochemical study for neurofilament protein and glial-specific S-100 protein. Arch Histol Jpn 50, 437–454.

Maeda T, Iwanaga T, Fujita T, Takahashi Y and Kobayashi S (1987) Distribution of nerve fibres immunoreactive to neurofilament protein in rat molars and periodontium. Cell Tissue Res 249, 18–23.

Maeda T, Kannari K, Sato O and Iwanaga T (1990a) Nerve terminals in human periodontal ligament as demonstrated by immunohistochemistry for neurofilament protein (NFP) and S-100 protein. Arch Histol Cytol 53, 259–265.

Maeda T, Kannari K, Sato O, Kobayashi S, Iwanaga T and Fujita T (1990b) Cholinesterase activity in terminal Schwann cells associated with Ruffini endings in the periodontal ligament of rat incisors. Anat Rec 228, 339–344.

Maeda T, Sato O, Kannari K, Takagi H and Iwanaga T (1991) Immunohistochemical localization of laminin in the periodontal Ruffini endings of rat incisors: a possible function of terminal Schwann cells. Arch Histol Cytol 54, 339–348.

Maeda T, Sato O, Kobayashi S, Iwanaga T and Fujita T (1989) The ultrastructure of Ruffini endings in the periodontal ligament of rat incisors with special reference to the terminal Schwann cells (K-cells) Anat Rec 223, 95–103.

Marfurt CF and Turner DF (1983) Sensory nerve endings in the rat oro-facial region labelled by the anterograde and transganglionic transport of horseradish peroxidase: a new method for tracing peripheral nerve fibres. Brain Res 261, 1–12.

Matthews B (1965) Action potentials from dental mechanoreceptors in the dog. J Dent Res 44, 1167 (abstract 32).

Matthews B (1975) Mastication. In: Applied Physiology of the Mouth (Lavelle C, ed), pp 199–240, Wright, Bristol.

Matthews B (1986) Responses of intradental nerves to mechanical stimulation of teeth in the cat. J Dent Res 65, 506 (abstract).

Matthews B and Yemm R (1970) A silent period in the masseter electromyogram following tooth contact in subjects wearing full dentures. Arch Oral Biol 15, 531–535.

Mei N, Hartmann F and Aubert M (1977) Periodontal mechanoreceptors involved in pain. In: Pain in the Trigeminal Region (Anderson DJ and Matthews B, eds), pp 103–110, Elsevier, Amsterdam.

Mei N, Hartmann F and Roubien R (1970) Répartition des terminaisons sensibles du territoire trigéminal. Etude microphysiologique du ganglion de Gasser. Comptes Rendus Séance Soc Biol 164, 2575–2578.

Mei N, Hartmann F and Roubien R (1975) Caractéristiques fonctionnelles des mécanorécepteurs des ligaments dentaires chez le chat. J Biol Buccale 3, 29– 39.

Mengel MKC, Jyvasjarvi E and Kniffki KD (1992) Identification and characterisation of afferent periodontal C fibres in the cat. Pain 48, 413–420.

Mengel MKC, Jyvasjarvi E and Kniffki K D (1993) Identification and characterisation of afferent periodontal A delta fibres in the cat. J Physiol 464, 393–405.

Millar BJ, Halata Z and Linden RWA (1989) The structure of physiologically located periodontal ligament mechanoreceptors of the cat canine tooth. J Anat 167, 117–127.

Millar BJ, Halata Z and Linden RWA (1994) A possible explanation for the response characteristics of multi-tooth periodontal ligament mechanoreceptors in the cat. Anat Embryol 190, 445–452.

Miyake S (1990) An experimental study on regeneration of periodontal mechanoreceptors after alveolar segmental osteotomy in the cat. Shikwa Gakuho 90, 555–605.

Moxham BJ (1979) The effects of some vaso-active drugs on the eruption of the rabbit mandibular incisor. Arch Oral Biol 24, 681–688.

Moxham BJ (1981) The effects of section and stimulation of the cervical sympathetic trunk on eruption of the rabbit mandibular incisor. Arch Oral Biol 26, 887–891.

Munger BL (1971) The comparative ultrastructure of slowly and rapidly adapting mechanoreceptors. In: Oral–Facial Sensory and Motor Mechanisms (Dubner R, Kawamura Y, eds), pp 83–103, Appleton–Century–Crofts, New York.

Munger BL and Halata Z (1984) The sensorineural apparatus of the human eyelid. Am J Anat 170, 181–204.
Nakamura TK, Hanai H and Nakamura M (1982) Ultrastructure of encapsulated nerve terminals in human periodontal ligaments. Jpn J Oral Biol 24, 126–132.
Nakamura K , Nakamura M, Yoshikawa M, Kiyomura H and Hannai H (1986) Fine structure and probable sensory nerve endings in human periodontal ligaments. Okajimas Folia Anat Jpn 63, 323–380.
Ness AR (1954) The mechanoreceptors of the rabbit mandibular incisor. J Physiol 126, 475–493.
Nomura S and Mizuno N (1985) Differential distribution of cell bodies and central axons of mesencephalic trigeminal nucleus neurons supplying the jaw-closing muscles and periodontal tissue: a transganglionic tracer study in the cat. Brain Res 359, 311–319.
Okabe K (1940) A study of the neural endings in the dog periodontal membrane. J Jpn Stomatol Soc 14, 341–354.
Olsson KA, Lund JP, Valiquette C and Veilleux D (1988) Activity during mastication of periodontal mechanosensitive neurons of the trigeminal subnucleus oralis of the rabbit. J Neurophysiol 59, 341–357.
Olsson KA, Sasamoto K and Lund JP (1986) Modulation of transmission in rostral trigeminal sensory nuclei during chewing. J Neurophysiol 55, 56–75.
Passatore M and Filippi GM (1983) Sympathetic modulation of periodontal mechanoreceptors. Arch Ital Biol 121, 55–65.
Passatore M, Lucchi ML, Filippi GM, Manni E and Bortolami R (1983) Localisation of neurons innervating masticatory muscle spindle and periodontal receptors in the mesencephalic trigeminal nucleus and their reflex actions. Arch Ital Biol 121, 117–130.
Pfaffmann C (1939a) Afferent impulses from the teeth due to pressure and noxious stimulation. J Physiol 97, 207–219.
Pfaffmann C (1939b) Afferent impulses from the teeth resulting from a vibratory stimulus. J Physiol 97, 220–232.
Pimenidis MZ and Hinds JW (1977) An autoradiographic study of the sensory innervation of teeth. II. Dental pulp and periodontium. J Dent Res 56, 835–840.
Plenk H and Raab H (1970) Die Nerven der menschlichen Gingiva. Z Mikrosk Anat Forsch 81, 473–491.
Rapp R, Kirstine WD and Avery JK (1957) A study of neural endings in the human gingiva and periodontal membrane. J Can Dent Assoc 23, 637–643.
Robinson PP (1979) The course, relations and distribution of the inferior alveolar nerve and its branches in the cat. Anat Rec 195, 265–272.
Sachs F (1988a) Biophysics of mechanoreception. Membr Biochem 6, 173–195.
Sachs F (1988b) Mechanical transduction in biological systems. Crit Rev Biomed Eng 16, 121–169.
Sakada S (1971) Response of Golgi–Mazzoni corpuscles in the cat periostea to mechanical stimuli. In: Oral–Facial Sensory and Motor Mechanism (Dubner R and Kawamura Y, eds), pp 105–122, Appleton–Century–Crofts, New York.
Sakada S (1974) Mechanoreceptors in fascia, periosteum and periodontal ligament. Bull Tokyo Med Dent Univ 21 (suppl), 11–13.
Sakada S (1983) Physiology of mechanical senses of the oral structures. In: Frontiers of Oral Physiology: Oral Sensory Mechanisms, (Kawamura Y, ed), pp 1–32, Karger, Basel.
Sakada S and Aida H (1971) Localization and shape of Golgi–Mazonni corpuscles in the facial bones periosteum of the cat. Bull Tokyo Dent Coll 12, 235–258.
Sakada S and Kamio E (1970) Fiber diameters and responses of single units in the periodontal nerve of the cat mandibular canine. Bull Tokyo Dent Coll 11, 223–234.
Sakada S and Kamio E (1971) Receptive fields and directional sensitivity of single sensory units innervating the periodontal ligaments of the cat mandibular teeth. Bull Tokyo Dent Coll 12, 25–43.
Sakada S and Onodera K (1974a) On the specificity of spontaneously discharging units in cat inferior alveolar nerve. Bull Tokyo Dent Coll 15, 7–22.
Sakada S and Onodera K (1974b) Response of spontaneously discharging units to thermal stimulations. Bull Tokyo Dent Coll 15, 23–36.
Sato O, Maeda T, Iwanaga T and Kobayashi S (1989) Innervation of the incisors and periodontal ligament in several rodents: an immunohistochemical study of neurofilament protein and glia-specific S-100 protein. Acta Anat (Basel) 134, 94–99.
Sato O, Maeda T, Kannari K, Kawahara I, Iwanga T and Takano Y (1992) Innervation of the periodontal ligament in the dog with special reference to the morphology of ruffini endings. Arch Histol Cytol 55, 21–30.
Sato O, Maeda T, Kobayashi S, Iwanaga T, Fujita T and Takahashi Y (1988) Innervation of periodontal ligament and dental pulp in the rat incisor: An immunohistochemical investigation of neurofilament protein and glia-specific S-100 protein. Cell Tissue Res 251, 13–21.
Schnorpfeil S, Lang H, Eifinger FF and Addicks K (1991) Neuropathie des autonomen Nervensystems in der Gingiva bei entzundlichen Parodontopathien. Eine ultrastrukturelle Analyse. Dtsch Zahnarztl Z 46, 303–305.
Schoultz TW and Swett JE (1972) The fine structure of the Golgi tendon organ. J Neurocytol 1, 1–26.
Schroeder HE (1986) Blood supply and innervation. In: Handbook of Microscopic Anatomy, Volume 5, The Periodontium, pp 208–221, Springer-Verlag, Berlin.
Schulze C, Spaethe A and Halata Z (1993a) The sensory innervation of the gingiva and mucosa in *Monodelphis domestica*. Acta Anat (Basel) 146, 36–41.
Schulze C, Spaethe A and Halata Z (1993b) The sensory innervation of the periodontium of the third premolar in Monodelphis domestica. Acta Anat (Basel) 146, 42–45.
Sessle B and Schmitt A (1972) Effects of controlled tooth stimulation on jaw muscle activity in man. Arch Oral Biol 17, 1597–1607.
Shigenaga Y, Yoshida A, Mitsurhiro Y, Doe K and Suemune S (1988) Morphology of single mesencephalic trigeminal neurons innervating the periodontal ligament of the cat. Brain Res 448, 331–338.
Simpson HE (1966) The innervation of the periodontal membrane as observed by the apoestic technique. J Periodont Res 37, 374–376.
Simpson HE (1969) The healing of extraction wounds. Br Dent J 126, 550– 557.
Sims MR (1981) The periodontal ligament – new concepts. Ann R Australas Coll Dent Surgeons 7, 71–80.
Sims MR (1983a) The microvascular venous pool and its ultrastructural associations in mouse molar periodontal ligament – periodontal microvasculature and nerves. Aust Orthod J 8, 21–27.
Sims MR (1983b) Electron-microscopic affiliations of oxytalan fibres, nerves and the microvascular bed in the mouse periodontal ligament. Arch Oral Biol 28, 1017–1024.
Smith RD and Marcarian HQ (1968) Centripetal localization of tooth and tongue tension receptors. J Dent Res 47, 616–621.
Smith RD, Marcarian HQ and Niemer WT (1967) Bilateral relationships of the trigeminal mesencephalic nuclei and mastication. J Comp Neurol 131, 79–92.
Spencer PS and Schaumburg HH (1973) An ultrastructural study of the inner core of the Pacinian corpuscle. J Neurocytol 2, 217–235.
Stella A (1975) Contribucion al conocimiento de la neuroarquitectura del ligamento periodontal dentario y su significacion functional. Zentralbl Veterinarmed 4, 223–231.
Stewart D (1927) Some aspects of the innervation of teeth. Proc R Soc Med 20, 1675–1686.
Tabata T and Karita K (1986) Response properties of periodontal mechanosensitive fibres in the superior dental nerve of the cat. Exp Neurol 94, 469–478.

Tabata T and Karita K (1991a) Response properties of periodontal mechanosensitive neurons in the trigeminal spinal tract nucleus of the cat. Somatosens Mot Res 8, 261–269.

Tabata T and Karita K (1991b) Response properties of the periodontal mechanosensitive neurons in the thalamus of the cat: a comparison between the slowly adapting and rapidly adapting neurons. Jpn J Physiol 41, 429–441.

Tabata T and Karita K (1991c) Response properties of the periodontal mechanoreceptive neurons in the trigeminal main sensory nucleus of the cat. Exp Brain Res 84, 583–590.

Tabata T and Karita K (1992) Response field of cat trigeminal sensory complex neurons responsive to mechanical stimulation of the canine tooth. Jpn J Physiol 42, 159–164.

Tabata T and Karita K (1993) Effect of tooth temperature on activities of slowly adapting periodontal mechanoreceptors during or after long-lasting strong pressure applied to the cat upper canine tooth. Arch Oral Biol 38, 529–531.

Tabata T, Suzuki T and Watanabe M (1994) Physiological characteristics of periodontal mechanosensitive neurones in the inferior alveolar nerve of the cat. Arch Oral Biol 39, 63–70.

Tabata T, Watanabe M and Karita K (1986) Responses of somatosensory coritcal neurones to tooth pressure and their modulation by transient mouth opening in the cat. Arch Oral Biol 31, 735–740.

Taira K (1987a) The representation of the oral structures in the first somatosensory cortex of the cat. Brain Res 409, 41–51.

Taira K (1987b) Characteristics of periodontal mechanosensitive neurons in the first somatosensory cortex of the cat. Brain Res 409, 52–61.

Takagi S (1982) Conduction velocities of touch fibers and pain fibers in the inferior alveolar nerve in man. Gakuho 82, 781–798.

Taylor A and Elias SA (1984) Interaction of periodontal and jaw elevator spindle afferents in the cerebellum – sensory calibration. Brain Behav Evol 25, 157–165.

Tokumitsu Y (1956) On the innervation, especially the sensory innervation of the periodontal membrane, the dental pulp and periodontium of the lower alveolus in dog. Arch Histol Jpn 10, 123–140.

Trulsson M (1993) Multiple-tooth receptive fields of single human periodontal mechanoreceptive afferents. J Neurophysiol 69, 474–481.

Trulsson M, Johansson RS and Olsson KA (1992) Directional sensitivity of human periodontal mechanoreceptive afferents to forces applied to the teeth. J Physiol 447, 373–389.

van der Glas HW, de Laat A and van Steenberghe D (1985) Oral pressure receptors mediate a series of inhibitory and excitatory periods in the masseteric post-stimulus EMG complex following tapping of a tooth in man. Brain Res 337, 117–125.

van der Sprenkel HB (1936) Microscopical investigation of the innervation of the tooth and its surroundings. J Anat 70, 233–241.

van Steenberghe D, van der Glas HW, De Laat A, Weytjens J, Carels C and Bonte B (1989) The masseteric EMG complex (PSEC) in man: methodology, underlying reflexes and clinical perspectives. In Electromyography of Jaw Reflexes in Man (van Steenberghe D and de Laat A, eds), pp 269–287, Leuven University Press, Belgium.

Wagers PW and Smith CM (1960) Responses in dental nerves of dogs to tooth stimulation and the effects of systemically administered procaine, lidocaine and morphine. J Pharmacol and Exp Ther 130, 89–105.

Wakisaka S, Nishikawa S, Ichikawa H, Matsuo S, Takano Y and Akai M (1985) The distribution and origin of substance P-like immunoreactivity in the rat molar pulp and periodontal tissues. Arch Oral Biol 30, 813–818.

Wall PD and McMahon SB (1985) Microneuronography and its relation to perceived sensation. A critical review. Pain 21, 209–229.

Watanabe S and Dawes C (1988) A comparison of the effects of tasting and chewing foods on the flow rate of whole saliva in man. Arch Oral Biol 33, 761–764.

Watanabe M, Tabata T and Karita K (1991) Facilitatory effect of jaw opening on somatosensory (SI) cortical neurones sensitive to tooth pressure in the cat. Arch Oral Biol 36, 899–903.

Weill R, Bensadoun R and de Tourniel F (1975) Démonstration autoradiographique de l'innervation de la dent et du paradonte. Comptes Rendus Acad Sci Paris 281 (series D), 647–650.

Woda A, Azerad J and Albe-Fessard D (1983) The properties of cells in the cat trigeminal main sensory and spinal subnuclei activated by mechanical stimulation of the periodontium. Arch Oral Biol 28, 419–422.

Yamada M (1967) Interactions between the tactile sense and the mobility of the tooth. J Dent Res 46, 1256 (abstract 13).

Yamada M, Sakada S, Murata Y and Ueyama M (1961) Physiologic studies on the mechano-receptors of periodontal membrane. J Dent Res 40, 225 (abstract 1).

Yamamoto T and Sakada S (1983) Morphology and distribution of sensory nerve endings in the mouse labial mucosa. Bull Tokyo Dent Coll 24, 13–22.

Yamamoto T and Sakada S (1986) Sensory innervation of gingival and alveolar mucosa of the house musk shrew (*Suncus murinus*). Tohoku J Exp Med 150, 327–336.

Yamamura C and Shimada K (1992) Excitatory and inhibitory controls of the masseter and temporal muscles elicited from teeth in the rat. Jpn J Physiol 42, 283–297.

Yamazaki J (1948) On the sensory innervation of human periodontal membrane. Tohoku Igaku Zasshi (Sendai) 38, 7–14.

Yakota T, Koyama N, Nishikawa Y and Hasegawa A (1988) Dual somatosensory representation of the periodontium in nucleus ventralis posteromedialis of the cat thalamus. Brain Res 475, 187–191.

Zimny ML, Schutte M and Dabezies E. (1986) Mechanoreceptors in the human anterior cruciate ligament. Anat Rec 214, 204–209.

Chapter 8
Development of the Periodontal Ligament

BJ Moxham and DA Grant

THE DENTAL FOLLICLE

All the periodontal tissues that support a tooth in the jaw are derived from the dental follicle (alternatively termed the dental sac). In turn, this follicle seems to originate (at least in part) from the dental papilla – a component of the tooth germ that is usually thought of as being responsible for the formation of dentine and the dental pulp. It has also been proposed that the mesenchyme deriving the periodontium may have two differentiation compartments – an 'alveolar clade', which produces fibroblasts and osteoblasts; and a 'cement clade', which generates fibroblasts and cementoblasts (Osborn, 1984; Osborn and Price, 1988; Cho and Garant, 1989). Thus, the fibroblasts of the periodontal ligament (PDL) may be derived from different mesenchymal 'compartments'.

The dental follicle is first recognized as a condensation of mesenchymal tissue surrounding the developing tooth anlage at the cap stage. By the bell stage, the mesenchymal tissue between the enamel organ and the wall of the alveolar crypt appears to consist of three layers (Tonge, 1963) (*Fig. 8.1*). The inner layer is a vascular, fibrocellular condensation, three to four cells thick.

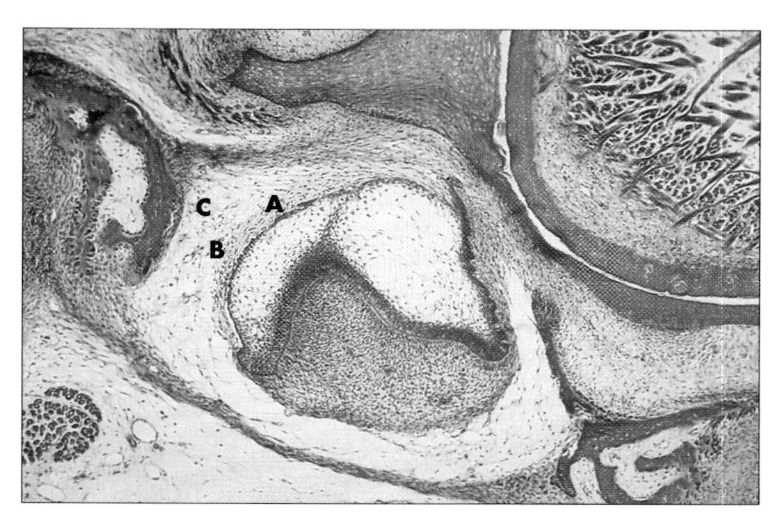

Fig. 8.1 Developing tooth germ at the 'bell' stage illustrating that the dental follicle surrounding the anlage is comprised of inner or investing (A), middle (B) and outer (C) layers. The middle and outer layers are sometimes referred to as the perifollicular mesenchyme. (Masson's trichrome; magnification × 60.)

The outer layer lining the developing alveolus is also composed of a vascular mesenchyme. Between these two layers is a loose connective tissue, which is relatively avascular. For the developing mouse molar, Palmer and Lumsden (1987) reported that the inner and outer layers are highly cellular compared with the intermediate zone, but that these three layers became indistinct by birth. That there is some anatomical basis for separation between inner and outer layers of the follicle is indicated by the observation that tooth germs dissected from the jaw are surrounded by the inner layer but not by the outer layer (Ten Cate *et al.*, 1971). The term 'dental follicle' has been used by different authors to mean different things (Tonge, 1963; Ten Cate, 1969; Schroeder, 1986). For example, Ten Cate (1969, 1972) is of the opinion that the term should be reserved for the inner (investing) layer in contact with the tooth germ, since transplantation studies (Ten Cate *et al.*, 1971; Ten Cate and Mills, 1972) suggest the inner layer alone can give rise to all the major components of the periodontium. Ten Cate terms the remaining tissue 'perifollicular'. Schroeder (1986) recognizes two mesenchymal layers surrounding the tooth germ. He uses the term 'dental follicle proper' to describe the layer of cells that appears from the base of the dental papilla and envelops the tooth, and the term 'perifollicular mesenchyme' to describe the remaining mesenchyme positioned near the developing alveolar bone. The experiments of Palmer and Lumsden (1987) and Cho and Garant (1989) generally support the view that the inner (investing) layer is the dental follicle proper responsible for the development of the periodontium (see also pages 174–5). However, Cho and Garant (1989) provide evidence that all layers contribute to the pool of periodontal fibroblasts.

There has also been debate about the precise origin of the cells that make up the dental follicle. Traditionally, it is held that the cells are derived from mesoderm near the site of the developing tooth, but Ten Cate (1969) believes they originate, at least in part, from neural crest cells that have migrated to the region of the developing jaws. The assertion that the tooth-related part of the dental follicle originates from the dental papilla (Osborn and Price, 1988) may also be considered evidence that some of the follicle is ectomesenchymal in origin.

Morrison *et al.* (1990) have started to characterize the cells of the dental follicle by assessing attachment properties and protein composition in culture. They showed that bone sialoprotein-I and fibronectin (but not laminin) promote attachment but not laminin. This contrasts completely with the properties of PDL cells in culture. It may be tempting, therefore, to conclude that such differences reflect the fact that the timed expression of integrins may be important in differentiation of PDL cells from follicle cells. However, care must be taken in the extrapolation of the results of *in vitro* experiments using PDL cells to the *in vivo* situation (see Chapter 1).

THE ROLE OF THE DENTAL FOLLICLE IN TOOTH ERUPTION

Cahill and Marks (1980) initially presented evidence for the involvement of the dental follicle in eruption, and this topic is fully reviewed in Chapter 9. Marks *et al.* (1983) and Wise *et al.* (1988) reported that there is a marked influx of monocytes into the follicle just before eruption begins. These monocytes subsequently form osteoclasts needed to produce an eruptive pathway (Wise *et al.*, 1988; Wise and Fan, 1989). At the same time, the collagen content of the follicle is significantly increased as it develops into the PDL (Gorski *et al.*, 1988). Partanen and Thesleff (1987) and Thesleff *et al.* (1987) have shown that epidermal growth factor (EGF) binds to the cells of the dental follicle, with the implication that this might have importance in terms of controlling the timing of developmental events in the tissue. Cho *et al.* (1991) have also attempted to relate the occurrence of EGF-binding sites on follicular mesenchymal cells and on developing and mature PDL fibroblasts with eruption (see page 173). Lin *et al.* (1992a,b) have recently added to the discussion concerning the regulation of development of the follicle and the PDL (including eruption) by proposing a role for electron-dense granules within the follicle cells, which are supposedly unique to the dental follicle. Indeed, they discovered that these granules can have an inhibitory effect on eruption, and they speculated on the possible interaction of EGF with the granules in the control of eruption. More information is awaited on this topic and, although it is known that the major components of the granules are 167 kDa and 200 kDa proteins, biochemical characterization is necessary.

FORMATION OF THE PERIODONTAL LIGAMENT

The formation and organization of the PDL from the dental follicle has been studied primarily by histological and transplantation techniques. Autoradiographical studies have also provided some information relating to turnover and remodelling in the developing PDL.

HISTOLOGICAL AND BIOCHEMICAL STUDIES

Root formation commences with the appearance of the epithelial root sheath (Hertwig, 1874; Diamond and Applebaum, 1942) (*Fig. 8.2*). This is thought to induce the adjacent cells of the dental papilla to differentiate into odontoblasts and to form root dentine. With root development, the epithelial cells lose their continuity, become separated from the surface of the forming root dentine, and later become the epithelial cell rests in the PDL. Mesenchymal cells of the dental follicle adjacent to root dentine differentiate into cementoblasts, which begin cementogenesis. Following the onset of root formation, changes become apparent within the dental follicle that are associated with the development of the principal fibre groups of the PDL. However, at the growing root apex, the dental follicle retains the layered appearance seen at the bell stage (Tonge, 1963; Ten Cate, 1969; Grant and Bernick, 1972).

Epithelial cells are routinely noted in the periodontal ligament (Reeve and Wentz, 1962). Their distribution, close to cementum in the young and closer to bone in the older individual has been noted (Reeve and Wentz, 1962; Simpson, 1965; Grant and Bernick, 1972). Rather than consisting of isolated remnants of the epithelial root sheath, they form a net-like structure (Simpson, 1967), which in porcine specimens may be continuous with the junctional epithelium (Grant and Bernick, 1969). With increasing age the epithelial aggregates become enlarged. The network character is lost and the aggregates are seen close to bone, in mid-ligament and as mineralised fragments (Grant and Bernick, 1972).

Species differences in root formation do exist. Lester (1969) has noted that, during root formation in molar teeth of rats, cells of the epithelial root sheath are embedded *en masse* between the forming cementum and dentine. Furthermore, he suggested that the epithelial cells may have a role to play in information transfer. Although it has been generally assumed that cementum is a product of cementoblasts, there is evidence in dogs (Owens, 1974), cats (Sloan and Beynon, 1981) and humans (Owens, 1974; Sloan and Beynon, 1981) that the innermost layer of cementum may be odontoblastic in origin. The possibility also exists that the cells of the epithelial root sheath may secrete material incorporated into the surface of the first-formed root dentine (Slavkin *et al.*, 1989).

Formation of the principal collagen fibres of the periodontal ligament

This has been described for the deciduous teeth of the marmoset (Levy and Bernick, 1968) and cat (Tonge, 1963), for the rodent molar (Sicher, 1923; Eccles, 1959; Bernick, 1960; Trott, 1962; Magnusson, 1968; Atkinson, 1972; Yamamoto and Wakita, 1991, 1992), the rodent incisor (Eccles, 1964), the ferret canine (Berkovitz and Moxham,

1990), for the permanent molars of the dog (Orban, 1927), marmoset (Grant *et al.*, 1972), macaque monkey (Magnusson, 1968), and human (Noyes *et al.*, 1943; Orban, 1957), and for the premolars of the squirrel monkey (Grant and Bernick, 1972) and the marmoset (Grant *et al.*, 1972). The information that follows is based on detailed studies of the sequential histogenesis of the PDL in squirrel monkey premolar teeth by Grant and Bernick (1972) and in marmoset premolar and molar teeth by Grant *et al.* (1972).

Formation of premolar periodontal ligament

Pre-emergence stage

Prior to eruption into the oral cavity, the premolars are enclosed in a bony crypt. PDL formation proceeds in a corono-apical sequence. When approximately one-third of the root has formed, the developing PDL appears to consist of loosely structured collagenous elements. Near the enamel–cement junction (*Fig. 8.3*), fibres arising from the cementum are demonstrable as an organized entity. They course coronally and follow the outline of the crown. In sections impregnated with silver nitrate (*Fig. 8.4*), fine argyrophilic fibres can be traced, originating from the cementum just below the enamel-cement junction and coursing occlusally around the contour of the enamel surface. Although numerous osteoblasts line the margin of the adjacent crestal bone, no fibres can be seen emerging from the bone.

In the midroot region (*Fig. 8.5*), fine, short, closely spaced fibres can be seen emerging from cementum. In the middle three-quarters of the developing PDL, there are loosely arranged fibres aligned parallel to the long axis of the root. Osteoblasts line the alveolar surface and only an occasional fibre can be seen emerging from bone.

In the periapical region (*Fig. 8.6*), fine collagenous fibres extend into the central third of the PDL and pass in an occlusal direction, parallel to the long axis of the root. Near the cementum, the fibres are densely packed and oriented in a superior–oblique direction from cementum toward the middle third of the PDL. Near the alveolar bone, fibre bundles emerging from the periapical zone course in a superior–oblique direction toward bone, in an alignment parallel to that of the fibres near cementum. They become more densely packed as they approach the osteoblast-lined bony margin, with the orientation changing to a coronal direction. The bundles finally become oriented in a superior—oblique direction from bone toward the broad central core of the developing PDL.

Emergence into the oral cavity

The direction of the fibres during this period appears to be influenced by the precise stage of eruption of the emerging tooth and by its positional relationship to the adjacent teeth. Consider the situation where the third premolar of the squirrel monkey is emerging into the oral cavity (*Fig. 8.7*) (with the neighbouring first permanent molar in functional occlusion and the second premolar in a pre-eruptive stage of development).

With respect to the cervical region of the emerging third molar, *Figs 8.7* and *8.8* show that organized fibre groups can be readily identified. Well-formed dentogingival fibres can be seen emanating from the tooth. These course occlusally to terminate in the lamina propria of the interproximal gingiva. On the mesial surface, developing transseptal fibres appear beneath the dentogingival fibres to extend obliquely in an apical direction over the alveolar crest toward the enamel–cement junction of the adjacent, unerupted premolar. On the distal surface, the developing transseptal fibre group can be traced as it emanates from cementum to extend in a superior–oblique direction over the forming alveolar crest toward the first molar. Midway, there is an intermediate zone separating these fibres from the inferior, obliquely oriented transseptal fibres of the adjacent first molar (*Fig. 8.9*).

Further apically, the forming PDL is not so well organized into fibre bundles. In the region of the cervical third of the root of the emerging third premolar, fibres extend apically in an oblique direction from cementum toward the alveolar bone. In the middle third of the root (*Fig. 8.10*), organized fibre groups that are continuous from cementum to bone cannot be demonstrated. Widely spaced, argyrophilic fibres protrude from the surface of the alveolar bone and extend for a short distance toward the tooth. These are separated from the closely spaced, short, brush-like, cemental fibres by a wide zone of loosely arranged connective tissue elements. Although this appearance is in accord with Sicher's observation in the guinea pig (Sicher, 1923), it is not supportive of Sicher's (1942b) and Orban's (1957) so-called 'intermediate plexus' in humans. In the region of the developing root apex of the third premolar, loosely organized collagenous elements like those seen in the pre-emergent premolar (see *Fig. 8.6*) are evident. These fibres arise from the apical area of the tooth and course into the PDL space.

First occlusal contacts

At this stage, fibre organization is further advanced. *Fig. 8.11* shows two premolars in closely successive stages of eruption from first occlusal contact to full articulation. Between the premolars, the dentogingival and transseptal fibre groups are well developed and easily discerned. The alveolar crest and horizontal fibres can also be identified. However, they are less distinct than the more coronal fibre groups. More apically in the PDL, fibre development is less advanced in the tooth that has erupted less.

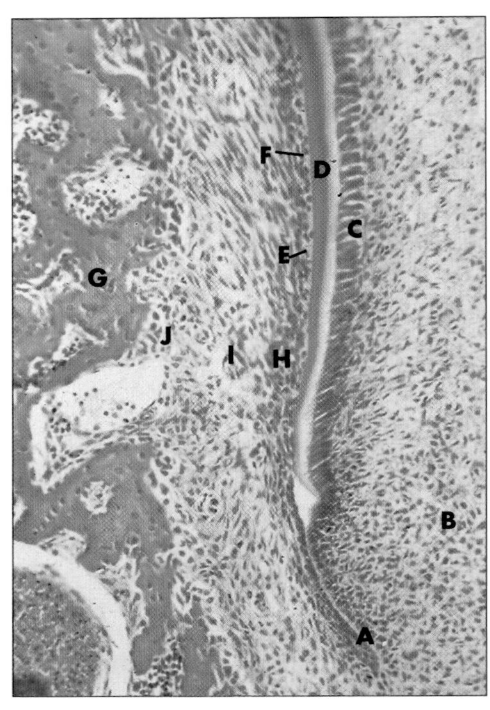

Fig. 8.2 The epithelial root sheath and root formation. A – epithelial root sheath outlining the shape of the future root; B – dental papilla; C – odontoblasts secreting root dentine (D); E – cementoblasts secreting root cementum (F); G – developing alveolar bone; H – inner or investing layer of dental follicle; I – middle layer of dental follicle; J – outer layer of dental follicle. (Haematoxylin and eosin; magnification × 150.)

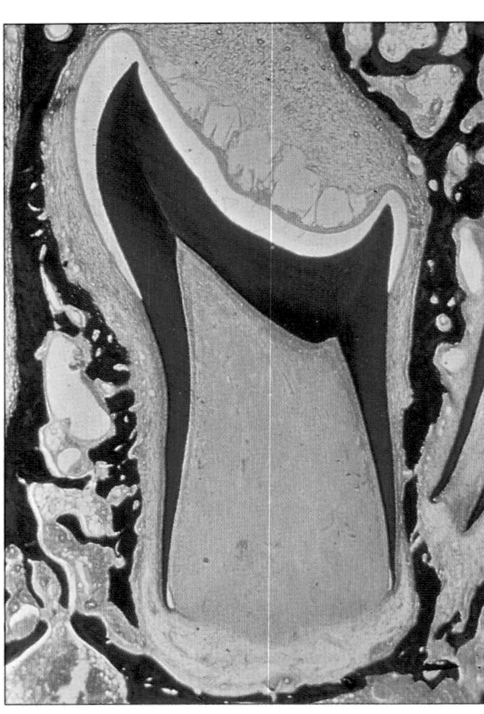

Fig. 8.3 The erupting permanent premolar is enclosed within a bony crypt. Predentogingival fibres are demonstrable, while more apically the periodontal ligament is composed of unorganized connective tissue elements. (Mallory's connective tissue stain; magnification × 30.) (Grant and Bernick, 1972.)

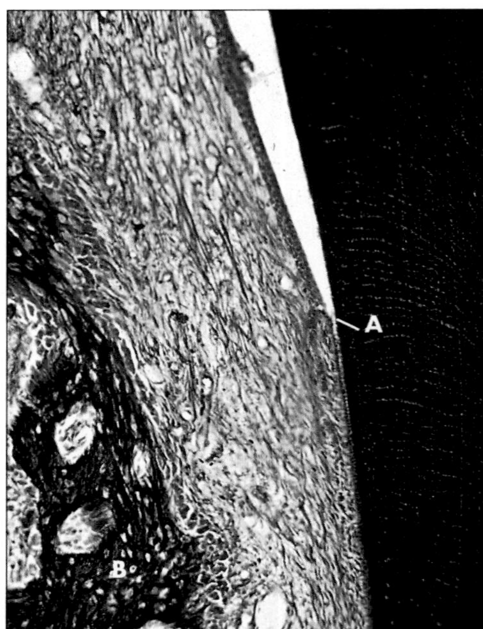

Fig. 8.4 At the cementoenamel junction of the tooth shown in Fig. 8.3, organized fibres can be observed emanating from cementum. These fibres course occlusally as they follow the outline of the crown. Intense osteoblastic activity is apparent at the bony margin. No fibres are seen emanating from bone. Apical to the cementoenamel junction, the periodontal ligament is occupied by loose, unorganized fibres. A – cementoenamel junction; B – alveolar bone. (Silver nitrate impregnation; magnification × 110.) (Grant and Bernick, 1972.)

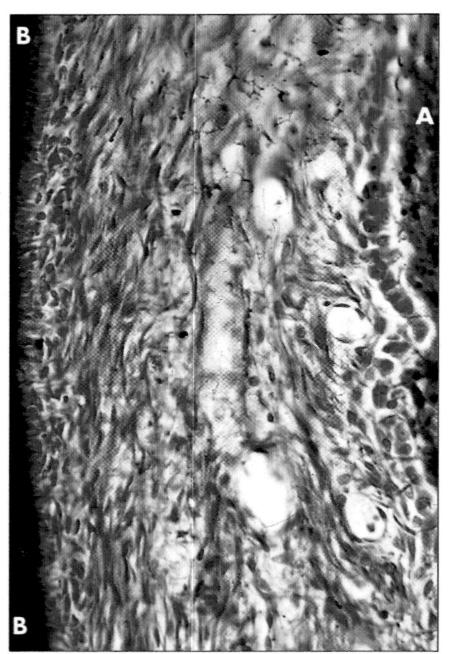

Fig. 8.5 At the midroot region of the tooth shown in Fig. 8.3, brush-like fibres are seen emanating from cementum. The central zone is very wide and is occupied by loosely arranged collagenous elements. Osteoblasts line the bony margin which is almost devoid of fibre extrusions. A – bone; B – cementum. (Silver nitrate impregnation; magnification × 200.) (Grant and Bernick, 1972.)

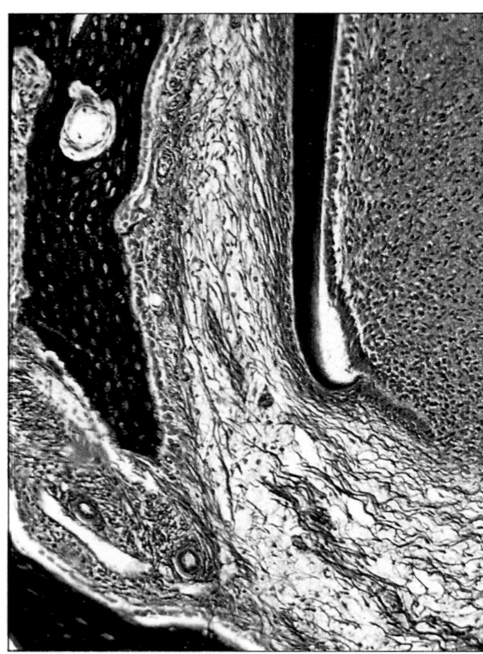

Fig. 8.6 Apically, fibres arising from beneath the tooth course into the periodontal ligament. They are orientated parallel to the long axis of the tooth. (Silver nitrate impregnation; magnification × 110.) (Grant and Bernick, 1972.)

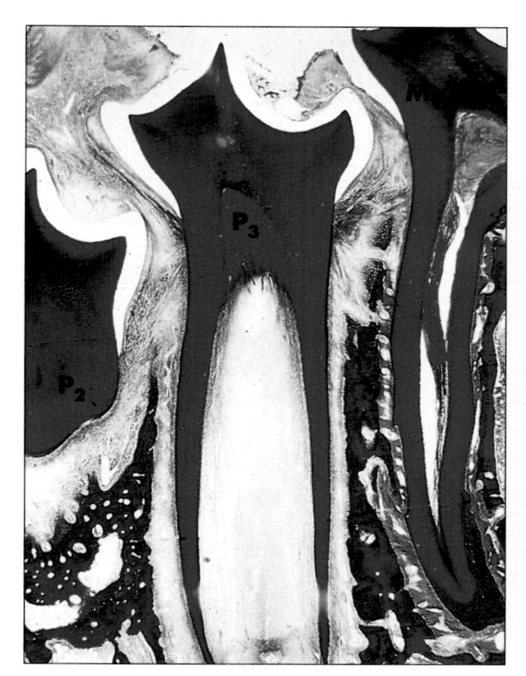

Fig. 8.7 Section showing the emergence into the oral cavity of the third premolar (P_3). As the tooth emerges, organized fibres are evident in the coronal and cervical areas. No principal fibres are demonstrable more apically in the periodontal ligament. Distally, the erupted first molar (M_1) shows a classically organized attachment apparatus. P_2 – second premolar. (Mallory's connective tissue stain; magnification × 30.) (Grant and Bernick, 1972.)

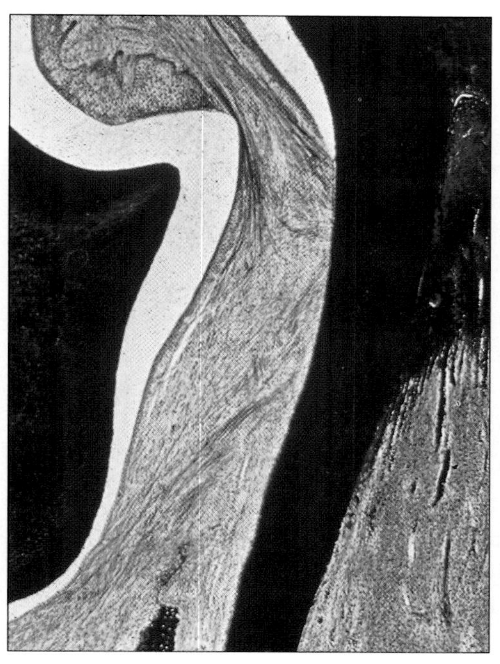

Fig. 8.8 At higher magnification of the mesial surface of the emerging tooth (P_3), well-formed dentogingival fibres course occlusally to follow the outline of the enamel surface. Less distinct, obliquely oriented fibres course apically over the forming alveolar crest toward the cervical area of the unerupted second premolar (P_2). (Silver nitrate impregnation; magnification × 90.) (Grant and Bernick, 1972.)

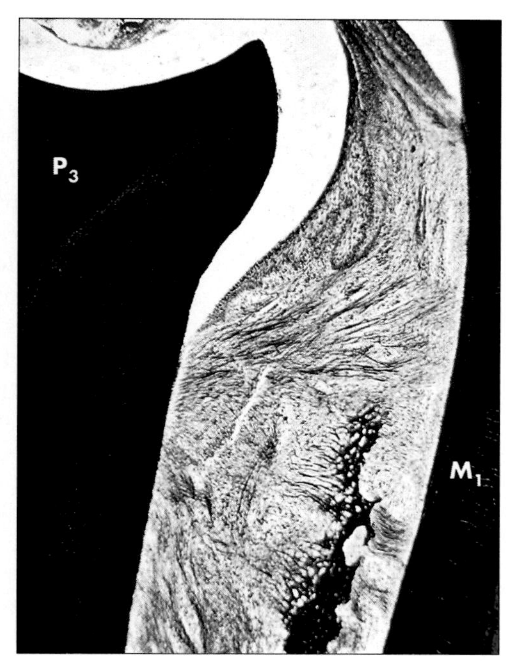

Fig. 8.9 On the distal surface of the erupting tooth (P_3), the developing transseptal fibres can be traced as they emanate from cementum to extend over the forming alveolar crest toward the first molar (M_1). More apically, fibres from cementum are separated from those from bone by an ever-narrowing intermediate zone. (Silver nitrate impregnation; magnification × 90.) (Grant and Bernick, 1972.)

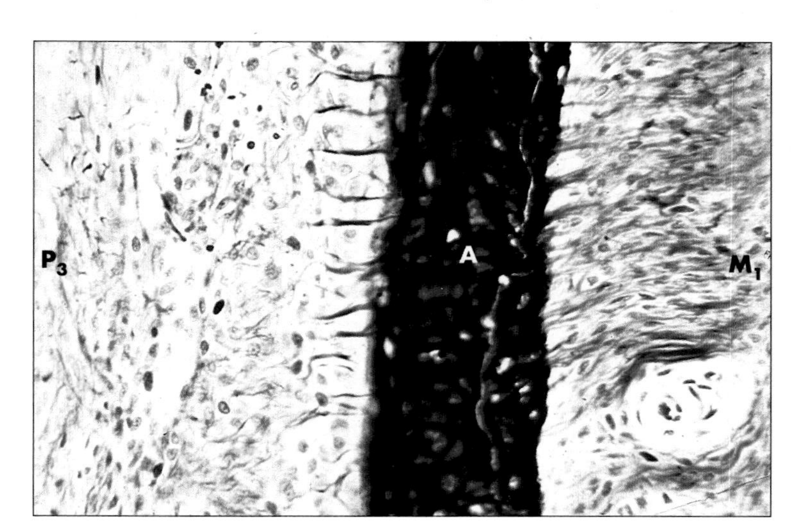

Fig. 8.10 At the midroot region of the teeth illustrated in Fig. 8.7, the classically organized and apparently continuous principal fibres of the functioning first molar (M_1) contrast with the still developing fibres of the third premolar (P_3). On the premolar, fine, short, brush-like fibres line the cemental surface and are separated from the longer, more widely spaced bony fibres by a broad zone of loosely structured collagenous elements. A – interdental bone. (Silver nitrate impregnation; magnification × 280.) (Grant and Bernick, 1972.)

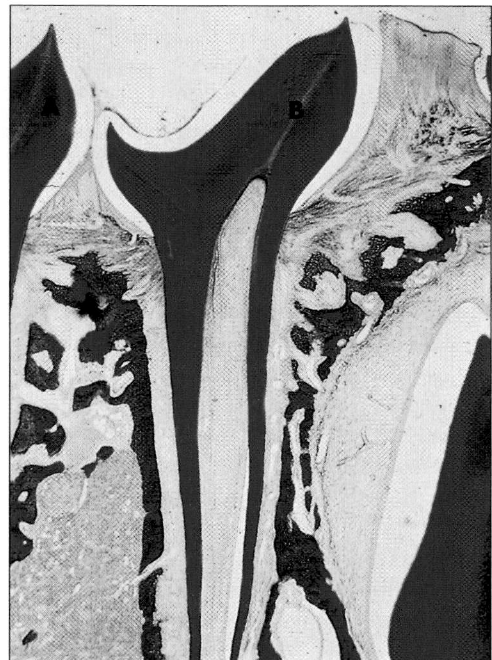

Fig. 8.11 Section showing two premolars in closely succeeding stages of eruption from first occlusal contact (tooth B) to full articulation (tooth A). The dentogingival and transseptal fibre groups are well developed on tooth A. On tooth B, obliquely oriented fibres course from cementum to bone at the cervical third of the root, while more apically the ligament becomes progressively less mature. (Mallory's connective tissue stain; magnification × 35.) (Grant and Bernick, 1972.)

At higher magnification in a section of this latter tooth impregnated with silver nitrate (*Fig. 8.12*), the features of the development of the PDL near the alveolar crest can be seen. A well-developed system of dense, intact, closely approximated transseptal fibres is present. The alveolar crestal group of fibres passes from the cementum obliquely downwards towards the alveolar bone. In the cervical third of the PDL proper, the cemental fibres appear to join with thicker, more widely spaced fibres that emerge from the alveolar bone. *Fig. 8.13* shows this area at higher magnification. Note the joining of the fibres from cementum with those from bone, and the thick fibre bundles that emerge from the bone. Such fibres seem to 'unravel' as they arborize to join the less dense groups from cementum. In the midroot region of the premolar that has erupted less (*Fig. 8.14*), the fibres lose their continuity across the periodontal space. Extensions of Sharpey fibres emerge from bone and project into the central zone. Separated from these fibres by the central zone, the diminutive cemental fibres are less perceptible as they emanate from the root into the developing PDL. By comparison, the periodontal fibres of the more erupted premolar show a more advanced stage of development in the midroot region (*Fig. 8.15*). Here, the fibres adjacent to alveolar bone are thicker and exhibit extensive branching as they appear to intertwine with the thinner fibres from cementum.

Full occlusal function

Once the premolars become functional, all the classically described principal fibre groups become demonstrable (*Fig. 8.16*). A detailed description of fibres of the functional PDL is given in Chapter 2. At the functional stage, no central zone can be seen in the PDL, as the fibre bundles form a network passing directly from cementum to alveolar bone (*Figs 8.16, 8.17*). Furthermore, the fibre bundles appear to thicken with function. This feature has also been reported in rat molars (Bernick, 1960; Trott, 1962) and incisors (van Bladeren, 1971), though it was not confirmed by Atkinson (1972) for mouse molars.

The development of periodontal fibres for the monkey premolar is summarized diagrammatically in *Figs 8.18, 8.19*.

Formation of permanent molar periodontal ligament

PDL formation in deciduous teeth and in teeth without primary predecessors (i.e. permanent molars) differs in several respects from that in secondary succedaneous teeth (Grant *et al.*, 1972), and these are illustrated in *Fig. 8.20*. The main difference is the earlier appearance of the principal collagen fibres and the lack of an intermediate zone in the erupting molar teeth. In teeth without primary predecessors, PDL fibres are formed before eruption and are seen to emanate from bone and cementum (*Fig. 8.21*). Upon eruption, their obliquity appears lessened. Grant *et al.* (1972) showed the rapidity of principal fibre formation in two closely successive pre-eruptive stages in marmosets.

The differences between teeth with and without predecessors may be explained by a chronological variation in the sequence of deposition of alveolar bone. In permanent molars, deposition of alveolar bone is completed mainly before the crown emerges into the oral cavity. In contrast, the developing permanent premolars are completely enclosed by a bony crypt and erupt from a position lingual to the deciduous molars. During eruption, resorption of the bony roof and the lateral bony walls (as well as the overlying root) must await the subsequent deposition of alveolar bone, which is deposited on the residual cryptal bone. Thus, principal fibre formation must await the deposition of alveolar bone. The late appearance of the obliquely oriented group of dentoalveolar fibres in the succedaneous teeth is of relevance when considering the collagen-contraction hypothesis of tooth eruption (see Chapter 9).

Berkovitz and Moxham (1990) investigated the development of the PDL within the mandibular dentition of the ferret (*Figs 8.22, 8.23*). As with the studies of Grant and Bernick (1972), Grant *et al.* (1972), and Bernick and Grant (1982) for monkey teeth (see pages 163–166), both succedaneous and non-succedaneous teeth were studied; however, in comparison to the findings for monkey teeth, similarities were seen in both types of tooth. No significant amounts of alveolar bone were observed being deposited beneath the erupting root apices (see *Fig 9.7*; page 192), and periodontal collagen fibres were seen attached to the walls of the sockets just before the emergence of the crown into the oral cavity. Compared to the condition several days after eruption, the collagen fibres at the time of eruption and just before eruption were thinner, had a more limited area of attachment, and were more randomly oriented. For the succedaneous teeth of monkeys, organized fibres appeared around the alveolar crest only at the time of emergence into the oral cavity. Indeed, Berkowitz and Moxham (1990) showed that, even when the teeth first reached the occlusal plane, principal fibres still did not insert into alveolar bone for the bulk of the PDL. Cahill and Marks (1982) also have reported that fibres did not attach into alveolar bone in dog premolars until the teeth reach the occlusal plane.

Major differences between the PDLs of erupting and erupted non-succedaneous ferret teeth were also reported by Berkovitz and Moxham (1990). During the early phases of eruption, the fibre bundles appeared thinner, had a less extensive attachment to the walls of the sockets, and exhibited a more random orientation. Thickening of the fibres occurred as the tooth erupted, a finding consistent with the reports of Bernick (1960), Trott (1962), and Yamamoto and Wakita (1991, 1992) for rat molars. However, Atkinson (1972) did not record it for mouse molars. In the ferret, the change from an immature ligament to a mature ligament for non-succedaneous teeth appeared to take place within the very short time of just a few days. Thus, the findings concerning the ontogeny of fibre development in the PDL indicate the existence of important species differences. These findings may also indicate the existence of differences even between teeth of the same succedaneous dentition. The reason for the apparent differences between groups as closely related as the ferret and dog is not known. However, it could possibly relate to the more rapid rate of eruption that occurs in the ferret, or to the length of the eruptive pathway. It is of course assumed that the development of the PDL in the human dentition is most likely to accord with the descriptions available for the monkey dentition. However, this assumption must not be entirely taken for granted, and detailed studies on the human periodontium are awaited.

Other features of the developing periodontal collagen fibres

The 'bundling mechanism', whereby the principal fibres of the PDL are formed, has been studied by Yamamoto and Wakita (1991, 1992) for the rat molar. They observed that, for the fibres close to the tooth (cementum) surface, the principal fibres increase in thickness with root development. They suggested that this change occurs by aggregation of fibre bundles. Initially, when root dentine calcification begins, the fibres appear as fibril aggregates in 'narrow intercellular spaces in a densely packed population of PDL cells'. With a change in cell shape and position, the intercellular spaces widen and the fibril aggregates subsequently become thicker. As root development proceeds, the PDL cells show extensive cell processes between the bundles, and these processes form distinct compartments within the tissue. These compartments seem to provide a sheath-like arrangement and the 'loose' fibril bundles develop into 'tight' fibril bundles.

Berkovitz *et al.* (1984) have studied the changes that take place in the collagen fibrils of the developing PDL. They reported that, for the mandibular first molar of the rat, the collagen fibril diameters became slightly larger as the tooth erupted into occlusion.

With respect to the periodontal connective tissue directly beneath the root apex, particular attention has been focused on the so-called 'cushion hammock ligament'. This ligament was first described by Sicher (1942a), who, because of the supposed attachments of the ligament to alveolar bone, considered that it provided a fixed, resistant base for the resolution of the forces produced by the growing root into an eruptive force. The ligament was said to be composed of a fibrous network with fluid-filled interstices. Though Sicher (1942b) was unable to observe a cushion hammock ligament beneath multirooted teeth, its presence here was reported by Scott (1953). Although subsequent authors (e.g. Hunt, 1959; Ness and Smale, 1959; Eccles, 1961; Ten Cate, 1969; Atkinson, 1972) have described the existence of a collagenous membrane beneath the developing root, it is not attached to the alveolar wall, but merges with fibres of the PDL more coronally (see *Fig. 8.6*). For this reason, it is more satisfactorily termed the 'pulp-limiting membrane'. As for its function in eruption, root resection, and transection, studies in continuously growing incisors (e.g. Berkovitz and Thomas, 1969; Moxham and Berkovitz, 1974) show that root growth is not responsible for generating eruptive forces (see Chapter 9).

The intermediate plexus is thought to be a central zone in the PDL that separates the osseous and cemental fibres. It has attracted considerable attention and much controversy. The appearance and significance of the plexus in the functioning tooth is discussed in Chapter 2. In the developing tooth, it has been suggested that an intermediate plexus might permit eruptive and migratory tooth movements. In view of the controversies surrounding the very existence of this plexus, concepts relating to its functional significance and developmental origin are merely speculative.

It has been reported that, as in marmoset molars, in the molars of the mouse (Atkinson, 1972), rat (Bernick, 1960; Thomas, 1965) and human (Thomas, 1965), periodontal fibres are present with an oblique orientation before the tooth erupts. However, Magnusson (1968) reported that a considerable portion of the root is formed before there is evidence of obliquely oriented fibres in the PDL of *Macaca irus* molars. Magnusson (1968) also noted that the inclination of the periodontal fibres decreased during eruption.

The mechanisms responsible for initiating and then maintaining the alignment of the different periodontal principal fibre groups are not known. However, it has been suggested that oblique fibre orientation is a reflection of lines of stress set up as a result of inward and upward growth of bone against the downward, and usually inward, root growth (Thomas, 1967). The oblique orientation of the fibroblasts, and hence the fibres, may be facilitated by their parallel alignment to the fibres of the pulp-limiting membrane (Atkinson, 1972). It is conceivable that the orientation of the developing principal fibre bundles relates to the arrangement of the collagen in the developing root. Owens (1979) has suggested that the basal lamina of the epithelial root sheath may play a role in orienting the first-formed dentine collagen. The initial collagen fibres produced by cementoblasts are oriented at right angles to the root surface. The odontogenic and cementogenic fibres are then mineralized, the mineralization front proceeding outwards. This perpendicular arrangement of the collagen may play a role in orienting the developing principal fibre bundles. Subsequent development of cementum is controversial (for review see Formicola *et al.*, 1971), but it involves entrapment of the principal fibres. Scanning electron micrograph studies of developing periodontal attachment surfaces (Boyde and Jones, 1968; Jones and Boyde, 1974) showed that, as the fibres are entrapped, microcalcospherites form around them. The mineralization front of the Sharpey fibre is concave and lags behind that of the surrounding collagen.

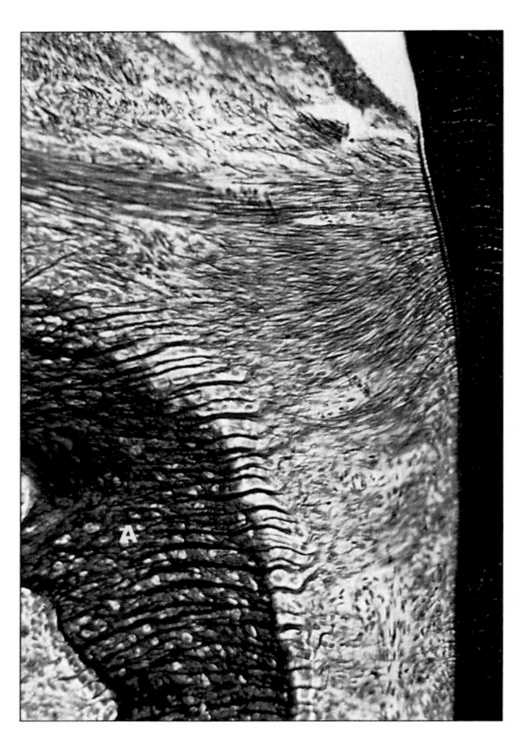

Fig. 8.12 At higher magnification of tooth B seen in Fig. 8.11, dense transseptal fibres extend from cementum over the alveolar crest. Apical to these, closely approximated fibres emerge from cementum to extend obliquely downward toward the alveolar bone. Near bone, these fibres appear to be joined with heavier, more widely spaced, Sharpey fibres. Note the depth of penetration of the Sharpey fibres into bone. A – alveolar bone. (Silver nitrate impregnation; magnification × 190.) (Grant and Bernick, 1972.)

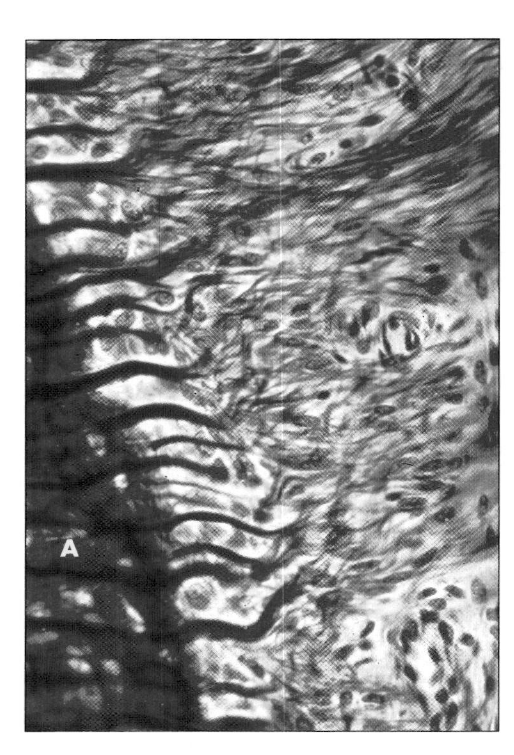

Fig. 8.13 A high-power view of Fig. 8.12 showing the joining of the cemental and osseous fibres. The heavier osseous fibres appear to 'unravel' as they splay out and they are apparently joined with the more closely spaced, finer fibres that extend toward cementum. A – alveolar bone. (Silver nitrate impregnation; magnification × 350.) (Grant and Bernick, 1972.)

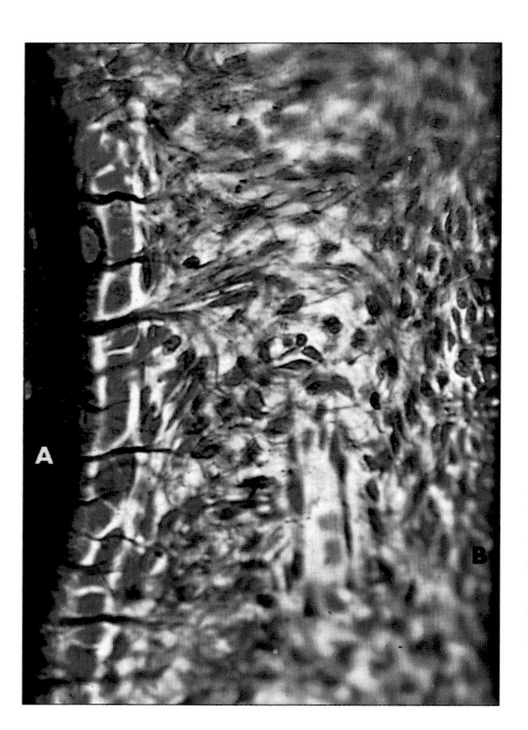

Fig. 8.14 At midroot, the ligament of the emerging premolar (shown as tooth B in Fig. 8.11) is poorly developed. Thick fibres project from bone and extend between osteoblasts into the periodontal ligament. These fibres splay outward, as if to unravel. The broad central zone of the ligament is occupied by loose collagenous elements. At the cemental surface, short, closely spaced fibres present a brush-like appearance. A – alveolar bone; B – cementum. (Silver nitrate impregnation; magnification × 200.) (Grant and Bernick, 1972.)

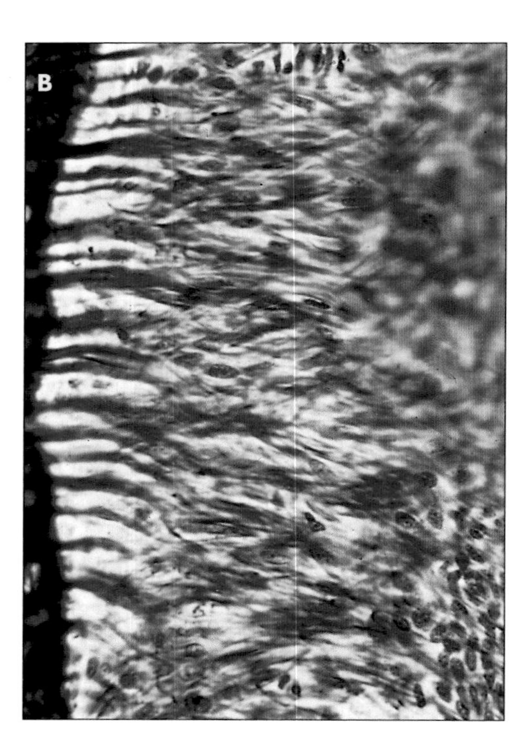

Fig. 8.15 In contrast with Fig. 8.14, fibres of the midroot periodontal ligament of the more functional premolar (tooth A in Fig. 8.11) appear continuous from bone to cementum, as the branching Sharpey's fibres are intertwined with fibres from cementum. B – alveolar bone. (Silver nitrate impregnation; magnification × 160.) (Grant and Bernick, 1972.)

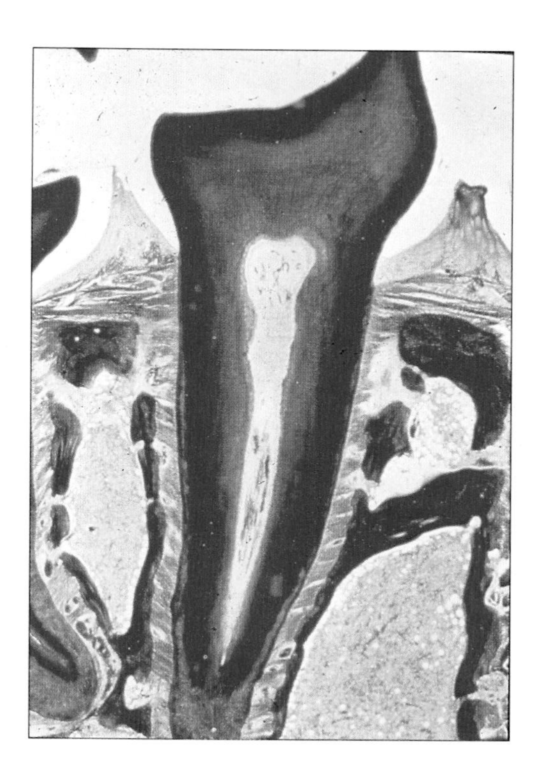

Fig. 8.16 With function, the thick, classically oriented, principal fibres are demonstrable. (Mallory's connective tissue stain; magnification × 30.) (Grant and Bernick, 1972.)

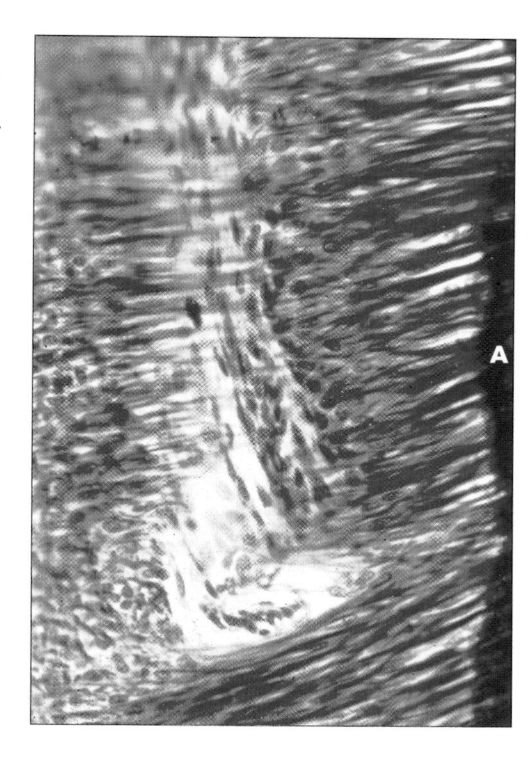

Fig. 8.17 A higher magnification of the principal fibres of the functioning tooth shows thick fibres that appear to pass from bone to tooth. A – alveolar bone. (Silver nitrate impregnation; magnification × 250.) (Grant and Bernick, 1972.)

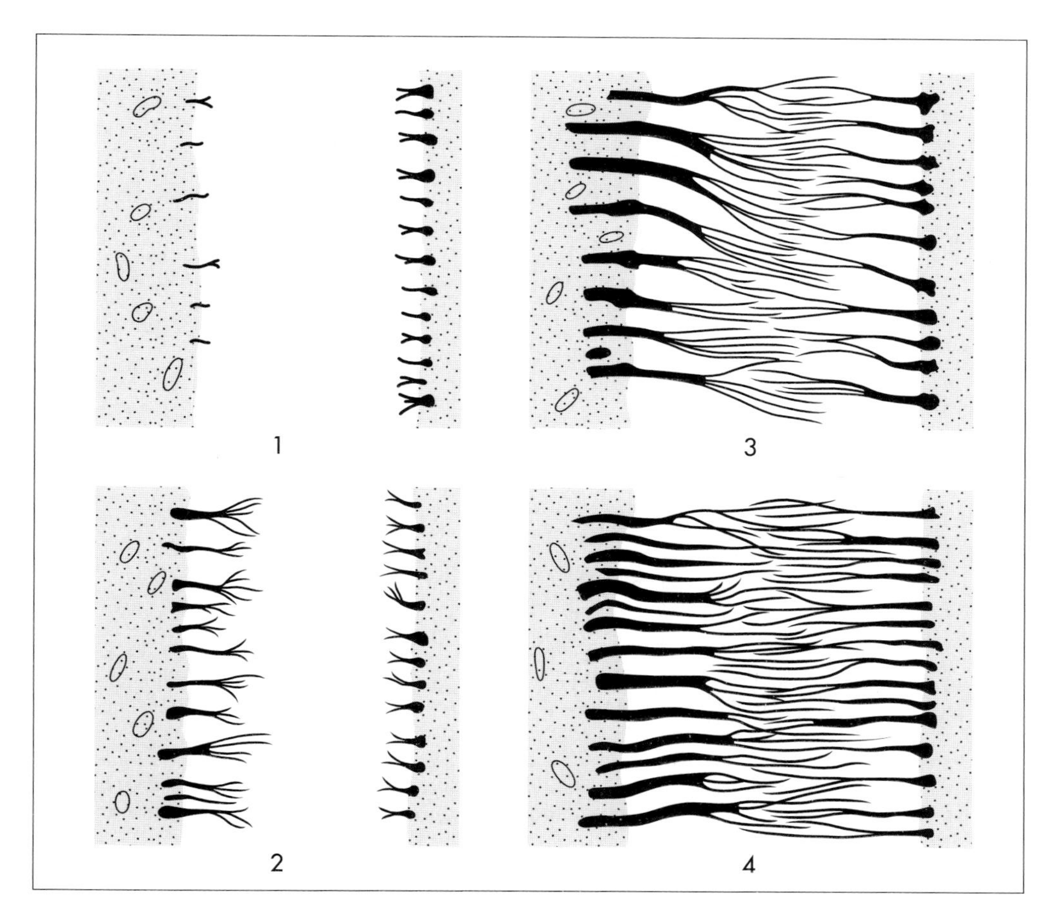

Fig. 8.18 A summary of alveolodental fibre formation. (1) Fine, brush-like fibres are first seen emanating from cementum. Only a few fibres project from the osteoblast-lined alveolar bone and extend into the non-organized, collagenous elements that occupy the broad central zone of the developing periodontal ligament. (2) Sharpey fibres, thicker and more widely spaced than those from cementum, emerge from bone to extend toward the tooth and appear to unravel as they arborize at their ends. The closely spaced, cemental fibres are still short, giving the root a brush-like appearance. (3) The alveolar fibres extend further into the central zone to join the lengthening cemental fibres. (4) With occlusal function, the principal fibres become classically organized, thicker, and apparently continuous between bone and cementum. (Grant and Bernick, 1972.)

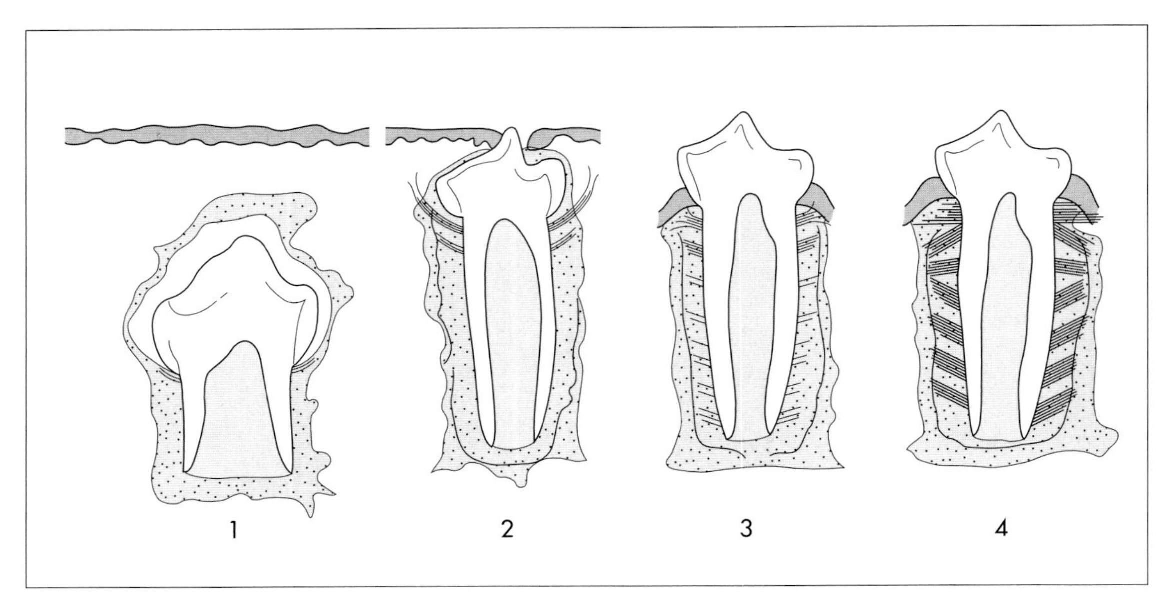

Fig. 8.19 Summary of the development of the principal collagen fibres of the periodontal ligament for the monkey premolar. (1) Pre-emergence. (2) Emergence into the oral cavity. (3) First occlusal contact. (4) Full occlusal function. (Grant *et al.*, 1972.)

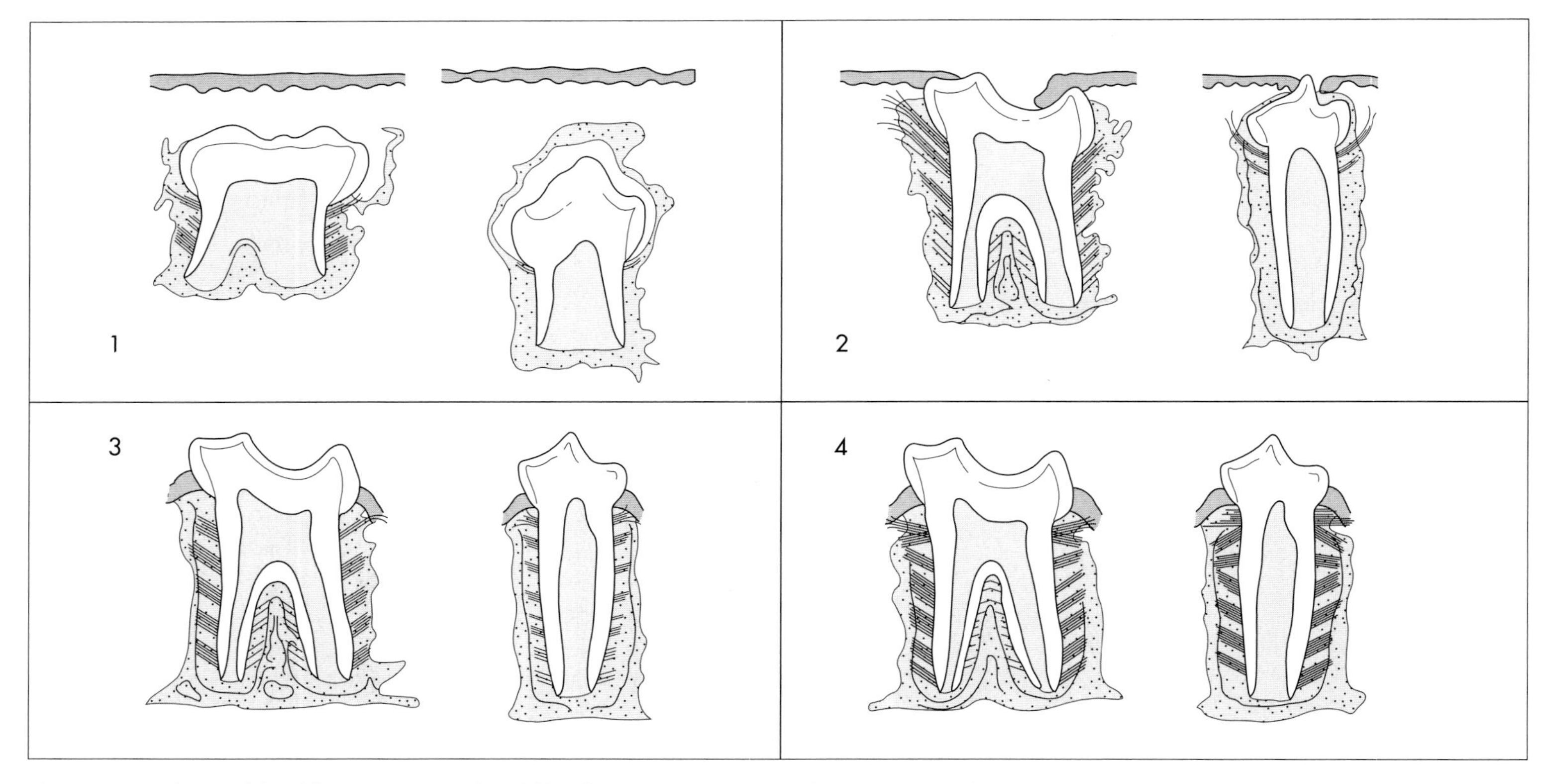

Fig. 8.20 A schema of the differences in periodontal fibre formation in primary and secondary (monkey) succedaneous teeth. Stage 1 – with root formation well advanced, the permanent molar (tooth without a predecessor) shows principal fibres extending from bone to cementum. The permanent premolar (tooth with a predecessor) shows only predentogingival fibres as an organized group. Stage 2 – upon emergence into the oral cavity, the permanent molar shows advanced fibre formation with apparently continuous principal fibres. The premolar shows organized fibres only at the alveolar crest. More apically, the periodontal ligament becomes progressively less organized. Stage 3 – with occlusal function, the molar shows complete periodontal fibre apparatus. The premolar shows apparently continuous principal fibres, except near the apex where an intermediate zone is still demonstrable. Stage 4 – with continued function, both molar and premolar show classically aligned, and apparently continuous, principal fibre groups. (Grant *et al.*, 1972.)

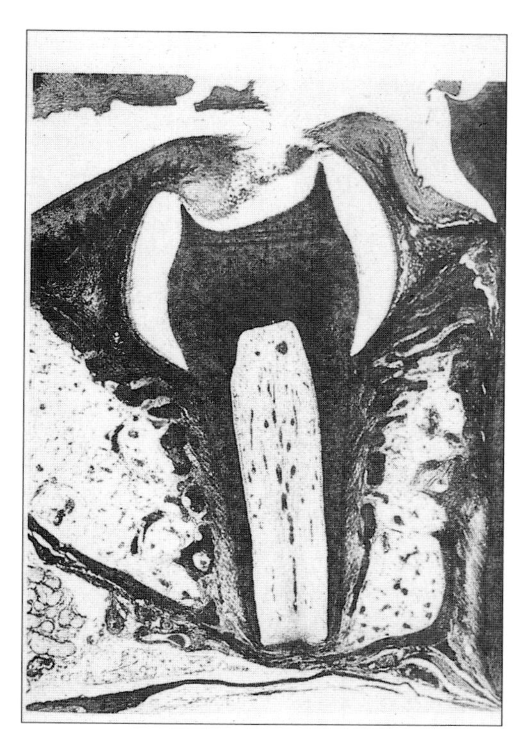

Fig. 8.21 The permanent second molar (a tooth without a predecessor) is just emerging into the oral cavity. The alveolar crest on both mesial and distal surfaces is at the midpoint of the crown. The periodontal ligament is composed of well-formed principal fibres that are oriented in a superior oblique direction from cementum to bone. (Mallory's connective tissue stain; magnification × 15.) (Grant *et al.*, 1972.)

Huang *et al.* (1991) have studied the distribution of types I and III collagens in the developing murine PDL, using immunofluorescent and immunoelectron microscopic techniques. They reported that the developing PDL principal fibres stained homogeneously for both collagen types whereas the Sharpey fibres in the alveolar bone stained heterogeneously. This contrasts with the earlier findings of Wang *et al.* (1980) who reported that the Sharpey fibres consist of a core of type I collagen with a surrounding of type III collagen. Using immunofluorescence and microfluorometry, Hou *et al.* (1993) have also investigated the expression of collagens I and III and fibronectin within gingival and PDL fibroblasts in culture. When these fibroblasts were co-cultured with cells derived from the epithelial root sheath, the fibroblasts appeared to show increased intracellular fluorescence for collagen type I and fibronectin, but no change for collagen type III. For co-cultures of gingival fibroblasts with gingival epithelial cells, there was enhanced fluorescence for type I collagen with a decrease for fibronectin. Co-culturing PDL fibroblasts with gingival epithelial cells, however, produced reduced intracellular fluorescence for both type I collagen and fibronectin. These investigations therefore provide some clues to the interactions between epithelial cells and fibroblasts in the periodontium, and it is to be hoped that similar studies will be undertaken using material from the developing periodontium.

Although considerable data are available concerning turnover of extracellular protein for functioning teeth of continuous growth and non-continuous growth (see Chapters 2 and 3), few data are available for developing teeth. It has been reported that, for developing rat and monkey molars, the uptake of ^{3}H-proline and ^{35}S is evenly distributed across the entire periodontal space (Magnusson, 1968; Kameyama, 1973). Kameyama (1973) also reported that a change in the labelling pattern with ^{3}H-proline occurs first in the cervical region of the developing PDL when the tooth emerges into the oral cavity. This change might correspond to the observation that the periodontal collagen fibres first become organized cervically (Grant and Bernick, 1972). Minkoff *et al.* (1981) have compared protein turnover (with ^{3}H-proline) in the gingival and PDL connective tissues in the developing mouse periodontium. The rate of turnover in both regions was much faster in the developing tissues than for mature tissues (Minkoff and Engstrom, 1979). Furthermore, the rate was faster in the developing oblique fibres of the PDL than in the gingival fibres studied. They also reported that 'stable core fibres', which are not metabolized, are not present in the developing periodontium. Perera and Tonge (1981a) studied the turnover of collagen in the mouse molar PDL during its eruptive phase. Prior to the emergence of this tooth into the oral cavity, the turnover rate was high, and it varied according to site. The rate in the mid-root region and near the apex appeared to be quicker than it was near the alveolar crest (half lives 4.5 days, 2.5 days, and 6 days respectively). Regardless of site, collagen turnover occurred throughout the whole thickness of the PDL and there was no evidence of a metabolically active intermediate plexus (see page 167). Perera and Tonge (1981a) also claimed that the rates varied according to stage of eruption, although their published data do not appear to bear this out.

Recently, Wise *et al.* (1992) have reported that TGF-β_1 (perhaps arising from the stellate reticulum of the enamel organ) affects the dental follicle cells so that they are stimulated to secrete more extracellular matrix proteins. In culture, dental follicle cells increased secretion of some procollagen chains by 66 per cent and of fibronectin by 7 per cent. Wise *et al.* (1992) proposed that the increased protein secretion in turn signals the development of the PDL from the connective tissues of the follicle.

Development of oxytalan fibres

The development of these fibres has been described by Fullmer (1959, 1967) for human teeth. Oxytalan fibres are first demonstrable in connective tissues destined to become PDL when about 2 mm of dentine (measured in an apico-occlusal direction) has been produced in the developing root. Oxytalan fibres also form in the connective tissues of the oral mucosa superior to developing teeth. As the epithelial root sheath loses its continuity, oxytalan fibres are first incorporated into cementum at the cervical margin and then they gradually progress toward the root apex. With further development, and after functional demands are

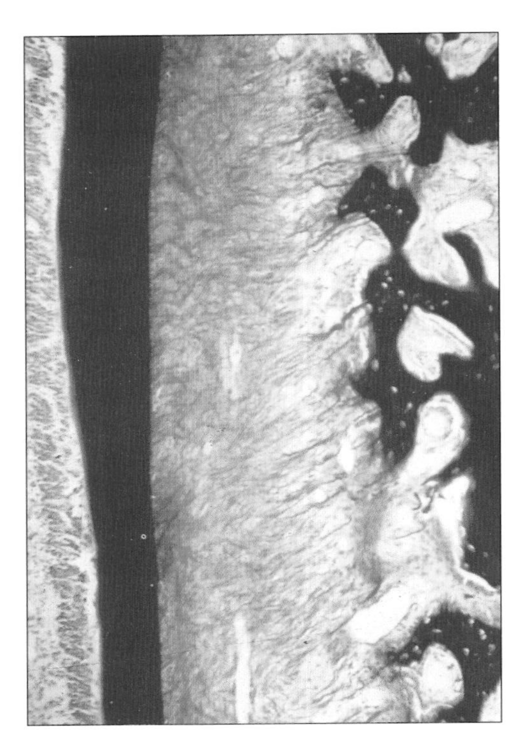

Fig. 8.22 Micrograph of longitudinal section of periodontal ligament of the permanent canine tooth of the ferret (*Mustela putorius*) just as the tooth is erupting into the oral cavity. Collagen fibre bundles can be seen passing from tooth to bone, but are not well organized in terms of thickness and orientation. (Van Giesen; magnification × 120.)

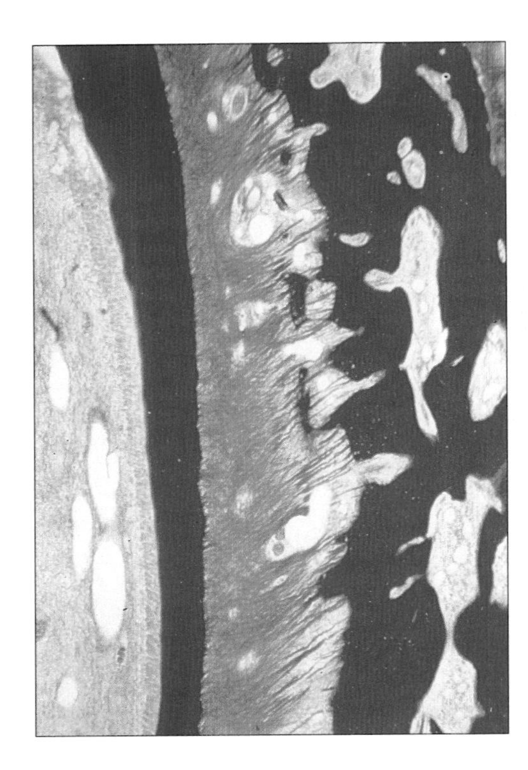

Fig. 8.23 Micrograph of longitudinal section of periodontal ligament of the permanent canine tooth of the ferret after the tooth has erupted. Compared with Fig. 8.22, the principal collagen fibre bundles are thicker and well organized. (Van Giesen; magnification × 120.)

placed upon the teeth, oxytalan fibres undergo a rearrangement and increase in size. When oxytalan fibres are first seen, they are of a size approaching the limit of resolution of the light microscope (less than 0.5 μm in diameter). In the adult, oxytalan fibres are larger than when first formed and larger in the transseptal area than in any other area about the tooth. As the vascular system becomes established in the periodontium, some oxytalan fibres extend from the adventitia and become attached to the tooth.

As is evident from the above account, much more needs to be known about the development of oxytalan fibres.

Development of the cells of the periodontal ligament

Ten Cate (1972) and Perrera and Tonge (1981b, c) have reported that the periodontal fibroblasts originate from the apical region of the developing PDL. Osborn (1984) and Osborn and Price (1988) claim that there are two differentiation compartments within the primitive mesenchyme surrounding the tooth germ: an 'alveolar clade', which gives rise to fibroblasts and osteoblasts, and a 'cement clade', which produces fibroblasts and cementoblasts. Osborn and Price (1988) have also provided evidence that the cells associated with the inner part of the dental follicle are derived from the dental papilla and that, therefore, the papilla contributes not just to the formation of dentine and the pulp but also to the periodontium.

From an ultrastructural study of the developing PDL of mouse first molars, Freeman and Ten Cate (1971) observed that, prior to root formation, the cells of the inner part of the dental follicle have the characteristics of undifferentiated or 'young' fibroblasts. Such cells were seen to contain dense accumulations of glycogen and few cytoplasmic organelles. At this time, the extracellular compartment is relatively structureless. With the onset of root formation, the cells show an increase in cytoplasmic organelles (particularly those associated with protein synthesis and secretion), a progression being seen such that the cells near the developing root apex have fewer organelles than the more coronal cells. Indeed, the evidence suggests that the cells are transformed into both cementoblasts and periodontal fibroblasts.

In developing roots of mouse molars, the transition from a loose connective tissue containing young fibroblasts and minimal extracellular collagen to a highly organized connective tissue consisting of actively functioning fibroblasts and dense extracellular bundles of collagen appears to be abrupt (Freeman and Ten Cate, 1971). In addition to the investing layer of the dental follicle, Ten Cate (1972) has provided evidence that periodontal fibroblasts are derived by proliferation from perivascular cells located in the connective tissue immediately in advance of its organization into PDL. Cho and Garant (1989) have also provided evidence that the outer layers of the follicular mesenchyme contribute to the pool of periodontal fibroblasts.

Using tritiated proline as a marker for bone formation, Ten Cate (1975) has shown that osteoblasts lining the alveolar bone surface become organized and deposit new bone at the same time as organization of the PDL. The findings from sections impregnated with silver nitrate are in accord with this observation (Bernick and Grant, 1982).

Berkovitz *et al.* (1984) conducted a quantitative ultrastructural investigation of cellular features within the developing PDL of the rat molar. They found that fibroblasts in both erupting and erupted teeth exhibited features characteristic of highly active secreting cells and not those of migrating or contracting cells. Furthermore, there were no differences in the data with regard either to the degree of cellularity of the PDL or to the fibroblast organelles.

There is little information concerning the ontogeny of other types of connective tissue cells in the PDL (see Chapter 1). However, Cho and Garant (1988) have observed that cementoblasts have a precementoblast precursor that migrates to the root surface from the dental follicle. Using ^{3}H-mannose to record the events in the development of the acellular cementum and PDL fibres in the rat, Cho and Garant (1989) have reported that 'during the formation of acellular cementum, the cementoblast phenotype is expressed for a short period of time, after which cementoblasts appear to mix with the fibroblasts of the PDL'. Thus, there are phases of cell migration from the follicle or developing PDL, cell attachment and cementum deposition, and cell detachment and redifferention into a fibroblast-like morphotype.

To begin to study the controlling mechanisms responsible for these events, Cho *et al.* (1991) assessed the occurrence of EGF-binding sites on the cementoblasts and periodontal fibroblasts of the rat molar. Earlier studies by Thesleff and co-workers had reported that ^{125}I-EGF-binding sites are located in apical follicular tissues *in vitro* (Thesleff *et al.*, 1987; Partanen and Thesleff, 1987). Cho *et al.* (1991) reported that there was a low incidence of binding sites on the follicular cells during cementoblast differentiation, but a high incidence was detected for differentiating periodontal fibroblasts located in perivascular regions and in the mesenchyme close to the alveolar bone (i.e. the perifollicular mesenchyme). Mature PDL fibroblasts also displayed numerous EGF-binding sites. These findings seem to confirm the differences between the dental follicle proper and the perifollicular mesenchyme, and they support the view that the major source of PDL fibroblast precursor cells is in the perifollicular region (Cho and Garant, 1988, 1989). Although the functional significance of EGF on the PDL remains unclear, it is conceivable that it has a mitogenic effect on the PDL fibroblast precursor cells (Thesleff *et al.*, 1987; Topham *et al.*, 1987). Cho *et al.* (1991) tried to relate EGF to eruption, since EGF administration can result in precocious emergence of the rodent incisor (e.g. Cohen, 1962; Klein, 1994). However, EGF has no effect on the emergence of the rodent molar (e.g. Moxham and Berkovitz, 1991; Klein, 1995) and the evidence against the involvement of the PDL fibroblasts in the generation of eruptive forces is at present poor (see Chapter 9).

Development of the ground substance of the periodontal ligament

Little is known about changes in the ground substance during development. Using bovine PDL from molars at varying stages of development, Pearson *et al.* (1975) reported that the content of insoluble, non-collagenous glycoproteins and collagen hexoses was higher in developing PDL than in mature PDL and that hyaluronan progressively decreased relative to chondroitin sulphate on eruption and maturation. This subject is considered further in Chaper 4.

Development of the neurovascular elements within the periodontal ligament

There is little information concerning the development of the nerve supply of the PDL. In the early bell stage of development of human teeth, there is a particularly rich innervation associated with small blood vessels in the inner, investing layer of the dental follicle (Fearnhead, 1967). Preliminary studies suggest that similar nerves in the mouse molar are adrenergic (Atkinson and Al-Takriti, 1980). Fearnhead (1967) also reported that the nerve fibres and the vessels associated with the external enamel epithelium disappeared when enamel formation was near to completion. Prior to eruption, nerve fibres could be demonstrated in the pulp but not in the PDL. With root formation and eruption, the nerves adjacent to the bone were seen to establish the periodontal innervation by growing into the developing PDL (most of them accompanying periodontal vessels). In the teeth of the marmoset (Levy and Bernick, 1968), and also in rat molars (Bernick, 1960), no sensory innervation was established until the PDL had become fully organized at the time of tooth eruption.

Few studies have been undertaken to investigate the vascular supply of the developing PDL. Kindlovà (1970) has described the development of the vasculature associated with the gingiva of rat molars. She noted that it was derived from vascular networks associated with the enamel organ and the alveolar mucosa. From this region, vessels spread apically to supply the developing PDL. Before eruption, the vascular bed of the PDL was found to be more uniform than in teeth subjected to masticatory loads, suggesting its pattern is influenced by function.

Cutright (1970) reported on the development of the vasculature of the PDL for permanent monkey teeth. The first indication of vascular development was the presence of a small, round plexus of vessels derived from vessels in the adjacent alveolar bone. This plexus was found to have direct connections with the periodontal plexus of the overlying deciduous tooth. The encircling plexus gave rise both to pulp vessels and to the periodontal plexus. This latter plexus arose by a 'thinning and compression of the vessels of the encircling plexus, forming a dense network of flattened vessels within the periodontal membrane'. Direct vascular connections were noted between the periodontal plexuses of neighbouring teeth.

Observations on the developing rodent PDL (Bernick and Grant, 1982) indicate that the vascular supply is derived from two sources. Blood vessels enter the periapical area of the PDL and pass occlusally to anastomose with perforating vessels that have coursed into, and through, the interseptal bone. As these vessels pass gingivally, their course is mainly in the alveolar-related part of the PDL. Terminal loops could not be demonstrated in the cemental part of the PDL in the rat. With eruption into functional occlusion, the vascular pathways through the PDL are not changed in the rat.

In the young adult spider monkey, Grant and Bernick (1972) observed vessels entering the periapical area of the PDL and also entering the interdental alveolar septum. The septal vessels arborized to enter and anastomose with ligament vessels. The vessels in the PDL formed two or more parallel ascending and descending channels with interconnecting loops (Grant *et al.*, 1979). In the transseptal region, a rich anastomosing plexus is formed by branches from the mesial surface of one tooth, the distal surface of the adjacent tooth, and the crestal branches of the lingual and buccal gingival vessels. From this anastomosis, arborizations arise that proceed into the lamina propria of the gingiva to form terminal loops in the connective tissue papillae.

Although Berkovitz *et al.* (1984) could not discern marked differences between the developing PDL in the erupting rat molar and the PDL in the fully erupted tooth as far as the ultrastructural features of the PDL fibroblasts were concerned, Moxham *et al.* (1987) reported that there are differences for the PDL vasculature. Although both erupting and erupted teeth showed fenestrated capillaries, there were significantly more in the erupting tooth (approximately 30×10^6 per mm^3 of PDL) compared with the fully erupted tooth (12×10^6 per mm^3 of PDL).

TRANSPLANTATION STUDIES

The important role played by the inner (investing) layer of the dental follicle in the formation of the PDL has been shown by experiments in which developing tooth germs were transplanted from the jaw to other sites. Such tooth germs continued to develop in ectopic sites to produce a root, PDL, and alveolar bone in the hamster (Hoffman, 1960) and the mouse (Ten Cate *et al.*, 1971; Ten Cate and Mills, 1972). By labelling mitotic cells with tritiated thymidine to allow the transplanted cells to be recognized, Ten Cate *et al.* (1971) presented evidence that the inner layer of the dental follicle gives origin to cementoblasts and fibroblasts of the PDL. The presence of lymphocytes around the bone produced in the vicinity of subcutaneously transplanted tooth germs suggests that such 'alveolar' bone also arises from donor tissue (Ten Cate and Mills, 1972). Further evidence in support of this has been derived from studies in which developing first molar tooth germs from mice were implanted into holes prepared in the parietal bones of adult mice (Freeman *et al.*, 1975). It has been shown that a defect created in the rodent parietal bone is effected with fibrous tissue instead of new bone (Pritchard, 1946; Melcher, 1969). However, following implantation into the parietal defect, the tooth germs continued development with the formation of roots, PDL, and new bone. This new bone fused with the old parietal bone and was presumably derived from cells of the investing layer associated with the original implant (Freeman *et al.*, 1975).

Although the above experiments suggest that, under certain conditions, cells of the investing layer of the dental follicle give rise to all the tooth-supporting tissues, this does not preclude a contribution to the PDL from the outer layers of the dental follicle during normal development. Indeed, Cho *et al.* (1991) have provided evidence that paravascular cells and the perifollicular mesenchymes are the major sources of PDL fibroblast precursor cells.

Yoshikawa and Kollar (1981) have shown that isolated mouse dental papilla, follicle, and enamel organ can form teeth with periodontal tissues when recombined in ocular grafts. Since this ability was retained by the papillary mesenchyme until day 19 of gestation, the findings indicate that their model may be of considerable use in the study of the development of the PDL. Consequently, Palmer and Lumsden (1987) have investigated the effects of tissue recombinations taken from day 16 of gestation to 10 days after birth. Their findings appeared to confirm earlier transplantation studies that the inner layer of the dental follicle could produce all the tissues of the periodontium (including bone). They also found that recombinations of enamel organ and dental papilla (without follicle) could result in regeneration of the investing layer of the follicle and development of a root-related PDL, but without bone formation. This potential appears to be retained by the papilla at least until birth. However, it was not possible to show whether the pulp retained this potential, since recombinations of enamel organ and pulp did not produce proper tooth development in the experimental model used. It was also impossible to study this potential before day 16 of gestation, because distinct mesenchymes could not be obtained at the bud and early cap stages of tooth development.

More recently, MacNeil and Thomas (1993a) have assessed the role of the epithelial root sheath in the development of the PDL by means of recombination experiments that involved the mouse tooth germ and ocular grafting. Earlier hints that the epithelium was required for PDL formation came from the tooth reimplantation experiments of Löe and Waerhaug (1961), Andreasen and Kristerson (1981) and Lindskog *et al.* (1988). Furthermore, MacNeil and Thomas (1993b) had shown that basement membrane components on the forming root surface were implicated in PDL development. Their subsequent recombination experiments showed that the formation of a PDL with fibrous attachment to bone and root requires not just the presence of dentine and follicular mesenchyme but also the epithelial root sheath. They therefore concluded that PDL development involves epithelio-mesenchymal interactions.

The scientific value of some of the transplantation studies has been questioned by Osborn and Price (1988). They point out that the evidence for the view that the investing layer of the dental follicle is the initial source of the periodontal tissues is poor, since many of the transplantation studies have not assessed whether the few remaining mesenchymal cells of the follicle or the dental pulp generate the periodontium in the transplants. From their studies (and from reinterpretation of the results of previous recombination studies), they concluded that most of the periodontium is derived from the dental papilla.

Hewage and Heaney (1990) have also criticized the transplantation studies on the basis that many components of the periodontium (e.g. dentogingival junction, alveolar bone) are rarely or never formed in such experiments. They proposed that this disadvantage might be overcome by creating a chimaeric periodontium in which connective tissue cells of odontogenic and oral mucosal origin might be identified. This was accomplished by transplanting rat maxillary first molar tooth germs with their follicles into evacuated dental crypts of histocompatible recipients of the same strain. For 71 transplants, Hewage and Heaney (1990) reported that 22 teeth erupted and formed periodontal tissues that were histologically similar to controls. By incubating tooth germs *in vitro* with ^{3}H-thymidine before grafting, they also reported that the labelled cells in the erupted teeth subsequent to grafting were randomly distributed within the PDL but were close to the junctional epithelium in the gingival connective tissues. This finding accords with the follicular origin of the PDL and also suggests a similar origin for only a specific part of the gingival connective tissue. Future studies may permit an assessment of the fate of discrete cell lineages during development of the periodontium.

In some experiments, the PDL of transplants show organization of the principal collagen fibre groups, and this suggests that there might be adaptation to later function (Atkinson and Lavelle, 1970; Ten Cate *et al.*, 1971).

THE PERIODONTAL LIGAMENT AS A MESENCHYME

There have been only a few attempts to improve our knowledge of the PDL by comparing this connective tissue with other fibrous connective tissues. When this has been attempted, the results have been inconclusive; they have indicated that, compared to other fibrous connective tissues in adult animals, the PDL in some respects resembles a connective tissue that in normal function is placed under tension, but that in other respects it resembles a tissue that is subjected to compression (Moxham, 1986). However, when the PDL is compared with fetal connective tissues (Moxham *et al.*, 1984), many of the features of the PDL, otherwise regarded as specialized features of these tissue, are more characteristic of mesenchymes. For example:

1. Fetal connective tissues have high rates of turnover (e.g. Nakamura and Nagai, 1980). High turnover rates for PDL collagen have been reported in studies based upon measurement of uptake of tritiated proline and tritiated glycine (see Chapter 3).

2. Fetal connective tissues show sharp, unimodal size–frequency distributions of small collagen fibrils (25–50 nm diameter) (e.g. Greenlee and Ross, 1967; Torp *et al.*, 1975; Parry *et al.*, 1978; Hickey and Hukins, 1981). It has been reported that collagen fibrils in the PDL show unimodal distributions with a mean diameter of 40–50 nm (see Chapter 2, *Fig. 2.7*).

3. It has been reported that the content of type III collagen in adult connective tissues is normally low, but that in fetal tissues it is present in significant amounts. Epstein (1974) and Pierard and Lapiere (1976) found that human fetal skin contained approximately 30 per cent type III collagen, with type I collagen gradually increasing in amount as the tissue developed. Butler *et al.* (1975) have demonstrated that up to 20 per cent of the collagen in bovine PDL is type III (see also Chapter 3, page 56).

4. The major reducible crosslink in the collagen of the PDL is dehydrodihydroxylysinonorleucine (Pearson *et al.*, 1975). Several workers have shown that this is also the predominant crosslink in embryonic connective tissue (e.g. Bailey and Robins, 1972; Barnes *et al.*, 1974).

5. The collagens of adult and fetal connective tissues seem to differ in their responses to lathyrogens. It has been reported that collagen fibrils in the skin of chick embryos treated with β-aminopropionitrile show increased diameters and a bimodal distribution compared with the unimodal distribution in untreated skin (van den Hooff *et al.*, 1959). Aminoacetonitrile also affects periodontal collagen by increasing the mean fibril diameter and altering the distribution (Shore *et al.*, 1984).

6. Using published micrographs of fetal connective tissues, Moxham *et al.* (1984) have calculated that the volume of ground substance is large (70 per cent of the matrix). The volume is also large in the PDL (Shore and Berkovitz, 1979; Berkovitz *et al.*, 1981; Shore *et al.*, 1982).

7. Fetal connective tissues have a high content of glucuronate-rich proteoglycans relative to L-iduronate-rich proteoglycans (dermatan sulphate) (e.g. Pearson *et al.*, 1975; Nakamura and Nagai, 1980; Scott *et al.*, 1981; Smith *et al.*, 1982). The D-glucuronate-rich CS (DS) hybrid proteoglycan found in the PDL is suggestive of fetal tissue (e.g. Gibson and Pearson, 1982; Pearson and Gibson, 1982).

8. Oxytalan fibres within the PDL may be immature elastin (pre-elastin) (see Chapter 2). In other connective tissues, the pre-elastin fibres mature to elastin during the perinatal period (e.g. Greenlee *et al.*, 1966; Bradamante and Svajger, 1977). Therefore, the presence of oxytalan can also be considered as a fetal characteristic of the PDL.

9. The fibroblasts of the PDL have characteristics that resemble fibroblasts in fetal connective tissues. Firstly, fetal tissues appear to be highly cellular (e.g. Ross and Greenlee, 1966; Greenlee and

Ross, 1967; Ippolito *et al.*, 1980). It has been shown that the fibroblasts in the PDL occupy 45 per cent of the tissue (see Chapter 1). Secondly, the fibroblasts in both fetal connective tissues and the PDL possess numerous intercellular contacts (see Chapter 1).

10. The stress–strain curve for the PDL resembles that for fetal tendon.

Thus, the PDL appears to have more in common with fetal connective tissue than with adult connective tissues, and this has important biological and clinical significance. For the clinician, it may have implications for the study of the biological mechanisms involved in orthodontic tooth movements, for the pathobiology of the PDL, for the healing potential of the PDL, and for the search for connective tissue substitutes for the PDL.

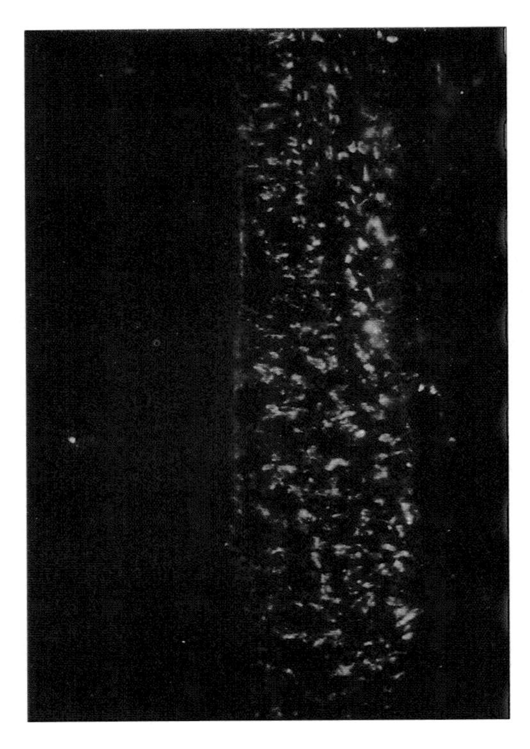

Fig. 8.24
Immunocytochemical labelling for cytokeratin 19 within the fibroblasts of the periodontal ligament of the aged rat incisor tooth (2-year-old animal). In the periodontal ligament of the mature animal vimentin and not cytokeratins are expressed. (Webb *et al.*, 1993.)

AGEING OF THE PERIODONTAL LIGAMENT

Despite the obvious importance (both biologically and clinically) of investigating the effects of ageing on the PDL, our understanding of this subject is at present poor and the literature was last reviewed by van der Velden in 1984. There have been remarkably few studies concerned with the changing composition and functions of the PDL. Indeed, the effects of ageing upon the turnover rates of the PDL extracellular matrix have yet to be assessed. Furthermore, most of the studies concerned with the structural aspects of the aged PDL have been at the light microscope level and are merely qualitative.

Concerning cellular age changes, a decrease in cellularity has been reported within the human PDL (Grant and Bernick, 1972; Severson *et al.*, 1978). Grant and Bernick (1972) described the decrease in cellularity following examination of post-mortem material from four humans aged 55, 72, 76, and 92 years, and both Grant and Bernick (1972) and Severson *et al.* (1978) relied upon qualitative assessments with no presentation of quantitative data. However, decreases in PDL cellularity have also been reported in animal studies – in the premolars of dogs (Berglundh *et al.*, 1991) and in the molars of rats (Klingsberg and Butcher, 1960; Jenson and Toto, 1968; Toto *et al.*, 1975), mice (Toto and Borg, 1968), hamsters (Klingsberg and Butcher, 1960), and monkeys (Klingsberg and Butcher, 1960; Levy *et al.*, 1972). Some quantification of the changes caused by ageing has been provided by Toto *et al.* (1975). They studied the mesial roots of rat first molars and found the cell density decreased from 93±9 cells per 110 μm^3 at 1 month to 69±7 cells per 110 μm^3 at 15 months. However, most investigators using aged rats consider the aged animal to be in excess of 24 months old.

In addition to a reduction in cell density, a decrease in the mitotic index has also been described in the aged PDL (Jensen and Toto, 1968; Toto and Borg, 1968; Toto *et al.*, 1975). From autoradiographic studies, Toto *et al.* (1975) found that the labelling index of periodontal fibroblasts decreased from 104±3 per 1000 cells at 1 month to 44±1.5 per 1000 cells at 15 months for rat molars. The suggestion was also made by these authors that the fibroblasts in ageing tissues had longer 'lives' than those in younger tissues. This awaits confirmation by, for example, tissue culture studies.

The effects of ageing on the fibroblasts of the rat PDL have been studied by Evans and Moxham (1994). They characterized quantitatively the ultrastructural features of the cells within the molar PDLs of rats aged 2 years, and the data obtained were compared with data for mature rats aged 8 weeks. In contrast to earlier qualitative studies, statistically significant differences in the PDL cellularity were not discerned. In terms of the cellular organelles, however, the fibroblasts of the aged rats differed in three respects: the areas occupied by endoplasmic reticulum were significantly less; the areas occupied by intracellular collagen profiles were also less; both the numbers and sizes of intercellular contacts were significantly different. Thus, the aged periodontal fibroblasts appeared to have diminished protein synthesis and collagen degradative capabilities. Furthermore, the nature of cell–matrix and cell–cell interactions were markedly changed.

A recent immunocytochemical investigation of the cytoskeletal components of PDL fibroblasts (Webb *et al.*, 1993) has shown that, in the PDL of the incisor of the aged rat (2–2.5 years old), the cells express cytokeratin 19 (*Fig. 8.24*). In the mature rat, only vimentin is expressed. This intermediate filament of the cytoskeleton was also seen during the most active phase of tooth eruption. Its appearance in the aged PDL may be related to the increased rates of eruption reported by Moxham (1994), or it may reflect the diminished cell–matrix and cell–cell interactions deduced from quantitative electron microscopy (Evans and Moxham, 1994)

Severson *et al.* (1978) reported that fat cells appeared within the aged human PDL. Cho and Garant (1984) have also described cell types not usually seen in the mature tissue. They found large, multinucleated fibroblastic cells in aged mouse supra-crestal periodontal connective tissues. Indeed, these cells accounted for more than 17% of the cells in aged mice. The multinucleated fibroblastic cells differ from osteoclasts at the electron microscope level in that they have considerable amounts of rough endoplasmic reticulum, a conspicuous Golgi complex, and intracellular collagen profiles. More recently, Sasaski and Garant (1993) reported that these cells also possess multiple centrioles. They concluded, therefore, that these cells arise by cell fusion. That the cells are fibroblastic was thought to be shown by their uptake of tritiated proline and by acid phosphatase activity associated with phagolysosomes. Unlike neighbouring (mononuclear) fibroblasts, however, the cell membranes did not show the presence of alkaline phosphatase. Multinuclear fibroblastic cells were not detected in the aged PDLs studied by Evans and Moxham (1994).

For the extracellular matrix of the PDL, changes due to ageing have been reported for both the collagen fibres and the ground substance. The earliest studies suggested that the amounts of soluble collagen and of 'acid mucopolysaccharides' decrease with age (Paunio, 1969; Levy *et al.*, 1972).

From histological examination of the aged human PDL, Grant and Bernick (1972) found that the main change due to age appears to be increased collagen fibrosis. They reported that the principal collagen fibre bundles were thicker; that the fibre groups were broader and more highly organized; that there were areas of hyalinization; that there was decreased argyophilia, increased fuchsinophilia, and a reduction in areas staining positive with alcian blue; and that some of the fibres were mineralized. In contrast, the number of PDL fibres is said to decrease in aged primates (Grant *et al.*, 1973]) and in human post-mortem tissues (Severson *et al.*, 1978). In line with these observations is the finding that the number of synthesizing connective tissue cells decreases in the ageing PDL (Toto and Borg, 1968; Jensen and Toto, 1968) and that there may be an age-dependent decrease in the rate of collagen synthesis (Stahl and Tonna, 1977).

For the Sharpey fibre insertions, Severson *et al.* (1978) found that the alveolar bone surface changed from smooth and regular with evenly distributed insertions of PDL fibres in younger tissue into jagged and uneven with irregular fibre insertions in aged tissue.

An important feature of the ageing of a connective tissue relates to the changes that occur in collagen fibril diameters (e.g. Happey *et al.*, 1974; Schwartz, 1987). For the PDL, however, there is disagreement as to the fate of the collagen fibrils with age. Gathercole and Keller (1982) claim that the mean fibril diameter within the human PDL decreases by nearly 50 per cent over the life span. However, these results must be carefully scrutinized since the source of information is not revealed and neither is the experimental protocol provided. This contrasts with the findings from quantitative electron microscopy of the aged rat PDL. Berkovitz *et al.* (1983) and Tasker *et al.* (1992) have shown that there is little change in fibril diameters with age. The first study showed that collagen fibrils for both the incisors and molars were not significantly different at 8 weeks and 56 weeks. The more recent investigation compared fibril diameters of the mandibular right first molars of 2-year-old rats with 8-week-old rats. Again, no significant differences were detected and, in both the young and the aged samples, a unimodal distribution of small collagen fibrils was obtained (mode approximately 42 nm). These findings are supported by the work of Luder *et al.* (1988) on the human PDL. By analysing 25, 000 periodontal fibrils at three periodontal levels of 28 freshly extracted human teeth (using 10 to 75-year-old subjects), they concluded that the average diameter of the collagen fibril (54–59 nm) remains essentially constant throughout the human lifespan.

Although in many connective tissues ageing effects can be attributed to alterations in elastin (rather than to the collagen – Rosenbloom, 1993), there is very little information concerning the effects of ageing on the elastic network of the PDL (including oxytalan). Furthermore, little is known about the changes that occur in the neurovascular elements of the PDL as a result of ageing. Grant and Bernick (1972) and Levy *et al.* (1972) reported that degenerative vascular changes can be discerned. This clearly needs further study (both at the structural and functional levels), for some of the age changes reported for the PDL may be attributed not to physiological ageing but indirectly to changes brought about by factors such as vascularity and function. Unfortunately, however, there is almost no information concerning the effects of age upon the function of the PDL. Mühlemann (1951) has shown that human teeth become less mobile with age. This change might be related to increases in length of the root or to changes in the number and diameters of the principal fibres of the PDL. Recently, Moxham (1994) has reported that the eruption rates of the rat incisor (both impeded and unimpeded, see page 187) are markedly increased with age, the mechanism whereby the eruptive force is generated being a property of the PDL (see pages 189–191).

Other studies on the effects of ageing on the periodontium have been concerned with the influence of inflammatory periodontal disease. Indeed, differentiation between age change and pathological change is imprecise and provides one of the fundamental problems in studying the pathogenesis of periodontal disease. It is well established that the prevalence of periodontitis increases with age (e.g. van der Velden, 1991). However, Johnson *et al.* (1989) have questioned whether periodontal changes were due to a disease process or an ageing process. Socransky *et al.* (1970) found that periodontal age-related changes in gnotobiotic rats occurred in the absence of inflammatory periodontal disease. In particular, gradual recession of alveolar bone occurs with increasing age (e.g. Socransky *et al.*, 1970). On the other hand, Abelatif and Burt (1987) are of the opinion that oral hygiene is the most influential factor in periodontal destruction and that the effect of age is negligible when good oral hygiene is maintained. Winkel *et al.* (1987) have shown, however, that many aged persons have considerable quantities of plaque yet do not develop periodontal destruction. On this basis, they claim that there is probably a multifactorial basis to the disease such that the influence of ageing cannot be overruled. The ageing of the PDL may have a bearing on other clinical problems. For example, orthodontic treatment is most often undertaken within the dentitions of teenagers or young adults, and it is probable that age is influential in the response of the periodontium to orthodontic loads.

Overall, the evidence suggests that there is some degeneration of the PDL with age. However, some features (e.g. the lack of change for collagen fibril diameters) indicate that the reactions and mechanisms of this degeneration may differ markedly from other fibrous connective tissues. The relative paucity of studies on this topic is therefore to be regretted.

REFERENCES

Abelatif HM and Burt BA (1987) An epidemiological investigation into the relative importance of age and oral hygiene status as determinants of periodontitis. J Dent Res 66, 13–88.

Andreasen JO and Kristerson L (1981) Evaluation of different types of auto-transplanted connective tissues as potential periodontal ligament substitutes. Int J Oral Surg 10, 189–201.

Atkinson ME (1972) The development of the mouse periodontium. J Periodont Res 7, 255–260.

Atkinson ME and Al-Takriti S (1980) A histochemical study of the innervation of developing teeth. J Dent Res 59, special issue D, 1807.

Atkinson ME and Lavelle CLB (1970) Experimental tooth transplantation in the mouse. J Anat 106, 180.

Bailey AJ and Robins SP (1972) Embryonic skin collagen. Replacement of the type of aldimine crosslinks during the early growth period. FEBS Lett 21, 330–334.

Barnes MJ, Constable BJ, Morton LF and Royce PM (1974) Age related variations in hydroxylation of lysine and proline in collagen. Biochem J 139, 461–468.

Berglundh T, Lindhe J and Sterrett JD (1991) Clinical and structural characteristics of the periodontal tissues in young and old dogs. J Clin Periodont 18, 616–623.

Berkovitz BKB and Moxham BJ (1990) The development of the periodontal ligament with special reference to collagen fibre ontogeny. J Biol Buccale 18, 227–236.

Berkovitz BKB, Shore RC and Moxham BJ (1983) Age changes of the periodontal ligament in the rat dentition. J Dent Res 62, 434.

Berkovitz BKB, Shore RC and Moxham BJ (1984) Ultrastructural studies on the developing periodontal ligament. INSERM 125, 545–556.

Berkovitz BKB and Thomas NR (1969) Unimpeded eruption in the root-resected lower incisor of the rat with a preliminary note on root transection. Arch Oral Biol 14, 771–780.

Berkovitz BKB, Weaver ME, Shore RC and Moxham BJ (1981) Fibril diameters in the extracellular matrix of the periodontal connective tissues of the rat. Connect Tissue Res 8, 127–132.

Bernick S (1960) The organization of the periodontal membrane fibres of the developing molars of rats. Arch Oral Biol 2, 57–63.

Bernick S and Grant DA (1982) Development of the periodontal ligament. In: The Periodontal Ligament in Health and Disease (Berkovitz BKB, Moxham BJ and Newman HN, eds), pp 197–213, Pergamon Press, Oxford.

Boyde A and Jones SJ (1968) Scanning electron microscopy of cementum and Sharpey fibre bone. Z Zellforsch 92, 536–548.

Bradamante Z and Svajger A (1977) Pre-elastic (oxytalan) fibres in the developing elastic cartilage of the external ear of the rat. J Anat 123, 735–743.

Butler WT, Birkedal-Hansen H, Beegle WF, Taylor RE and Chung E (1975) Proteins of the periodontium. Identification of collagens with the $\alpha(I)_2$, $\alpha2$ and $\alpha(III)_3$ structures in bovine periodontal ligament. J Biol Chem 250, 8907–8912.

Cahill DR and Marks SC Jr (1980) Tooth eruption: evidence for the central role of the dental follicle. J Oral Path 9, 189–200.

Cahill DR and Marks SC Jr (1982) Chronology and histology of exfoliation and eruption of mandibular premolars in dogs. J Morphol 171, 213–218.

Cho MI and Garant PR (1984) Formation of multinucleated fibroblasts in the periodontal ligaments of old mice. Anat Rec 208, 185–196.

Cho MI and Garant PR (1988) Ultrastructural evidence of directed cell migration during initial cementoblast differentiation in root formation. J Periodont Res 23, 268–276.

Cho MI and Garant PR (1989) Radioautographic study of [^{3}H]mannose utilization during cementoblast differentiation, formation of acellular cementum and development of periodontal ligament principal fibres. Anat Rec 223, 209–222.

Cho MI, Lin WIL and Garant PR (1991) Occurrence of epidermal growth factor-binding sites during differentiation of cementoblasts and periodontal ligament fibroblasts of the young rat: a light and electron microscopic radioautographic study. Anat Rec 231, 14–24.

Cohen S (1962) Isolation of a mouse submaxillary gland extract accelerating incisor eruption and eyelid opening in the new-born animal. J Biol Chem 237, 1555–1562.

Cutright DE (1970) The morphogenesis of the vascular supply to the permanent teeth of *Macaca rhesus*. Oral Surg 30, 284–291.

Diamond M and Applebaum E (1942) The epithelial sheath: Histogenesis and function. J Dent Res 21, 403–411.

Eccles JD (1959) The development of the periodontal membrane: the principal fibres of the molar teeth. Dent Practr Dent Rec 10, 31–35.

Eccles JD (1961) Studies in the development of the periodontal membrane: The apical region of the erupting tooth. Dent Practr Dent Rec 11, 153–157.

Eccles JD (1964) The development of the periodontal membrane in the rat incisor. Arch Oral Biol 9, 127–133.

Epstein EH (1974) $\alpha I(III)_3$ human skin collagen. Release by pepsin digestion and preponderance in foetal life. J Biol Chem 249, 3225–3231.

Evans IL and Moxham BJ (1994) The effects of ageing on the fibroblasts of the connective tissues comprising the rat periodontal ligament. J Anat 184, 198–199.

Fearnhead RW (1967) Innervation of dental tissues. In: Structural and Chemical Organization of Teeth, volume 1 (Miles AEW, ed), pp 247–281, Academic Press, London.

Formicola AJ, Krampf JI and White EG (1971) Cementogenesis in developing rat molars. J Periodontol 42, 766–773.

Freeman E and Ten Cate AR (1971) Development of the periodontium: an electron microscope study. J Periodontol 42, 387–395.

Freeman E, Ten Cate AR and Dickenson J (1975) Development of a gomphosis by tooth germ implants in the parietal bone of the mouse. Arch Oral Biol 20, 139–140.

Fullmer HM (1959) Observations on the development of oxytalan fibres in the periodontium of man. J Dent Res 38, 510–518.

Fullmer HM (1967) The development of oxytalan fibres. In: The Mechanism of Tooth Support (Anderson DJ, Eastoe JE, Melcher AH and Picton DCA, eds), pp 72–75, Wright, Bristol.

Gathercole LJ and Keller A (1982) Biophysical aspects of the fibres of the periodontal ligament. In: The Periodontal Ligament in Health and Disease (Berkovitz BKB, Moxham BJ and Newman HN, eds), pp 197–213, Pergamon Press, Oxford.

Gibson GJ and Pearson CH (1982). Sulphated galactosaminoglycans of bovine periodontal ligament. Connect Tissue Res 10, 161–167.

Gorski JP, Marks SC Jr, Cahill DR and Wise GE (1988) Developmental changes in the extracellular matrix of the dental follicle during tooth eruption. Connect Tissue Res 18, 175–190.

Grant DA and Bernick S (1967) A possible continuity between epithelial attachment and epithelial rests in miniature swine. J Periodontol 40, 87

Grant DA and Bernick S (1972) The periodontum of ageing humans. J Periodontol 43, 660.

Grant DA and Bernick S (1972) The formation of the periodontal ligament. J Periodontol 43, 17–25.

Grant DA, Bernick S, Levy BM and Dreizin S (1972) A comparative study of periodontal ligament development in teeth with and without predecessors in marmosets. J Periodontol 43, 162–169.

Grant DA, Chase J and Bernick S (1973) Biology of the periodontium in primates of the *Galago* species. I. The normal periodontium in young animals. II. Inflammatory periodontal disease. III Lability of cementum. IV Changes in ageing. Ankylosis. J Periodontol 44, 540–550.

Grant DA, Stern I and Everett F (1979) Periodontics, p 84, Mosby, St Louis.

Greenlee TK and Ross R (1967) The development of the rat flexor digital tendon. A fine structure study. J Ultrastruct Res 18, 354–376.

Greenlee TK, Ross R and Hartman JL (1966). The fine structure of elastic fibers. J Cell Biol 30, 59–71.

Happey F, Naylor A, Palframan J, Pearson CH and Turner RL (1974) Variations in the diameter of collagen fibrils, bound hexose and associated glycoproteins in the intervertebral disc. In: Connective Tissues – Biochemistry and Pathophysiology (Fricke R and Hartman F, eds), pp 67–70, Springer-Verlag, Berlin.

Hertwig O (1874) Über das Zahnsystem der Amphibien und seine Bedeutung für die Genese des Skelets der Munhole. Arch Mikrosk Anat 11 (suppl), 55–56.

Hewage S and Heaney TG (1990) Creation of a chimaeric periodontium in the rat by isotopic tooth germ transplantation. Arch Oral Biol 35, 681–684.

Hickey DS and Hukins DWL (1981). Collagen fibril diameters and elastic fibres in the annulus fibrosus of human fetal intervertebral disc. J Anat 133, 351–357.

Hoffman RL (1960) Formation of periodontal tissues around subcutaneously transplanted hamster molars. J Dent Res 39, 781–789.

Hou LT, Kollar EJ and Yaeger JA (1993) Epithelial cell-fibroblast interactions: modulation of extracellular matrix proteins in cultured oral cells. J Periodont Res 28, 102–114.

Huang YH, Ohsaki Y and Kurisu K (1991) Distribution of type I and type III collagen in the developing periodontal ligament of mice. Matrix 11, 25–35.

Hunt AM (1959) A description of the molar teeth and investing tissues of normal guinea-pigs. J Dent Res 38, 216–231.

Ippolito E, Natali PG, Postacchini F, Accinni L and De Martino C (1980) Morphological, immunochemical, and biochemical study of rabbit achilles tendon at various ages. J Bone Joint Surg 62, 583–598.

Jensen JL and Toto PD (1968) Radioactive labelling index of the periodontal ligament in ageing rats. J Dent Res 47, 149.

Johnson BD, Mulligan K, Kiyak KA and Marder M (1989) Aging or disease – periodontal changes and treatment considerations in the older dental patient. Gerodontology 8, 109–118.

Jones SJ and Boyde A (1974) The organization and gross mineralization patterns of the collagen fibres in Sharpey fibre bone. Cell Tissue Res 148, 83–96.

Kameyama U (1973) An autoradiographic investigation of the developing rat periodontal membrane. Arch Oral Biol 18, 473–480.

Kindlovà M (1970) The development of the vascular bed of the marginal periodontium. J Periodont Res 5, 135–140.

Klein RM (1995) Growth factors and tooth eruption. In: Biological Mechanisms of Tooth Eruption, Resorption and Replacement by Implants (Davidovitch Z, ed), EBSCO Media, Birmingham, Alabama. (In press.)

Klingsberg J and Butcher EO (1960) Comparative histology of age change in oral tissues of rat, hamster and monkey. J Dent Res 39, 158.

Lester KS (1969) The unusual nature of root formation in molar teeth of the laboratory rat. J Ultrastruct Res 28, 481–506.

Levy BM and Bernick S (1968) Development of organization of the periodontal ligament of deciduous teeth in marmosets (*Callithrix jacchus*). J Dent Res 47, 27–33.

Levy BM, Dreizen S and Bernick S (1972) Effect of aging on the marmoset periodontium. J Oral Pathol 1, 61–65.

Lin F, Fan W and Wise GE (1992a) Isolation of granule proteins from cells of the dental follicle and stellate reticulum of rat mandibular molars. Arch Oral Biol 37, 831–840.

Lin F, Fan W and Wise GE (1992b) Granule proteins of the dental follicle and stellate reticulum inhibit tooth eruption and eyelid opening in postnatal rats. Arch Oral Biol 37, 841–847.

Lindskog S, Blomlof L and Hammarstrom L (1988) Evidence for a role of odontogenic epithelium in maintaining the periodontal ligament space. J Clin Periodontol 15, 371–373.

Löe H and Waerhaug J (1961) Experimental reimplantation of teeth in dogs and monkeys. Arch Oral Biol 3, 176–184.

Luder HU, Zinmerli I and Schroeder HE (1988) Do collagen fibrils of the periodontal ligament shrink with age? J Periodont Res 23, 46–52.

MacNeil RL and Thomas HF (1993a) Development of the murine periodontium. II. Role of the epithelial root sheath in formation of the periodontal attachment. J Periodontol 64, 285–291.

MacNeil RL and Thomas HF (1993b) Development of the murine periodontium. I. Role of basement membrane in promoting mineralized tissue attachment to the developing root surface. J Periodontol 64, 95–102.

Magnusson B (1968) Tissue changes during molar tooth eruption. Trans R Schs Dent Stockh Umea 13, 1–122.

Marks SC Jr, Cahill DR and Wise GE (1983) The cytology of the dental follicle and adjacent alveolar bone during tooth eruption in the dog. Am J Anat 168, 277–289.

Melcher AH (1969) Role of the periosteum in repair of wounds of the parietal bone of the rat. Arch Oral Biol 14, 1101–1109.

Minkoff R and Engstrom TG (1979) A long-term comparison of protein turnover in subcrestal vs supracrestal fibre tracts in the mouse periodontium. Arch Oral Biol 24, 817–824.

Minkoff R, Stevens CJ and Karon JM (1981) Autoradiography of protein turnover in subcrestal versus supracrestal fibre tracts of the developing mouse periodontium. Arch Oral Biol 26, 1069–1073.

Morrison G, Sauk J, Shroff B, Thomas HF, Foster R and Somerman M (1990) Characterization of dental sac cells in vitro. J Dent Res 69, 275.

Moxham BJ (1986) Studies on the mechanical properties of the periodontal ligament. In: Current Topics in Oral Biology (Matthews B and Lisney SJW, eds), pp 73–82, University of Bristol Press, Bristol.

Moxham BJ (1994) The effects of ageing upon the eruption of the rat mandibular incisor J Dent Res 73, 837.

Moxham BJ and Berkovitz BKB (1974) The effects of root transection on the unimpeded eruption rate of the rabbit mandibular incisor. Arch Oral Biol 19, 903–909.

Moxham BJ and Berkovitz BKB (1991) The effects of epidermal growth factor (EGF) on the eruption of the mouse dentition. J Dent Res 70, 717.

Moxham BJ, Berkovitz BKB and Shore RC (1984) Is the periodontal ligament a foetal connective tissue? INSERM 125, 557–564.

Moxham BJ, Shore RC and Berkovitz BKB (1987) Fenestrated capillaries in the periodontal connective tissues of the erupting and erupted rat molar. Arch Oral Biol 32, 477–481.

Mühlemann HR (1951) Periodontometry: a method for measuring tooth mobility. Oral Surg 4, 1220–1228.

Nakamura T and Nagai Y (1980). Developmental changes in the synthesis of glycosaminoglycans and collagen in embryonic chick skin. J Biochem 87, 629–637.

Ness AR and Smale DE (1959) The distribution of mitoses and cells in the tissues bounded by the socket wall of the rabbit mandibular incisor. Proc R Soc Lond [Biol] 151, 106–128.

Noyes FB, Schour I and Noyes HJ (1943) In: Oral Histology and Embryology, p 170, Lea and Febiger, Philadelphia.

Orban BJ (1927) Embryology and histogenesis. In: Fortschritte Zahnheilkunde (Mische J, ed) 3, 749. Cited in Orban BJ (1944) Oral Histology and Embryology, 1st edition, Mosby, St Louis.

Orban BJ (1957) Oral histology and embryology, 4th edition, p 185, Mosby, St Louis.

Osborn JW (1984) From reptile to mammal: evolutionary considerations of the dentition with emphasis on tooth attachment. Symp Zool Soc Lond 52, 549–572.

Osborn JW and Price DG (1988) An autoradiographic study of periodontal development in the mouse. J Dent Res 67, 455–461.

Owens PDA (1974) A light microscopic study of the development of the roots of premolar teeth in dog. Arch Oral Biol 19, 528–538.

Owens PDA (1979) A light and electron microscopic study of the early stages of root surface formation in molar teeth in the rat. Arch Oral Biol 24, 901–907.

Palmer RM and Lumsden AGS (1987) Development of periodontal ligament and alveolar bone in homografted recombinations of enamel organs and papillary, pulpal and follicular mesenchyme in the mouse. Arch Oral Biol 32, 281–289.

Parry DAD, Barnes GRG and Craig AS (1978). A comparison of the size distribution of collagen fibrils in connective tissues as a function of age and a possible relation between fibril size distribution and mechanical properties. Proc Roy Soc Lond [Biol] 203, 305–321.

Partanen AM and Thesleff I (1987) Localization and quantitation of I-125-epidermal growth-factor binding in mouse embryonic tooth and other embryonic tissues at different developmental stages. Dev Biol 120, 186–197.

Paunio K (1969) Periodontal connective tissue. Biochemical studies of disease in man. Suomen Hammaslaariseuran 65, 250–290.

Pearson CH and Gibson GJ (1982). Proteoglycans of bovine periodontal ligament and skin. Biochem J 201, 27–37.

Pearson CH, Wohllebe M, Carmichael DJ and Chovelon A (1975) Bovine periodontal ligament. An investigation of the collagen, glycosaminoglycan and insoluble glycoprotein components at different stages of tissue development. Connect Tissue Res 3, 195–206.

Perera KAS and Tonge CH (1981a) Metabolic turnover of collagen in the mouse molar periodontal ligament during tooth eruption. J Anat 133, 359–370.

Perera KAS and Tonge CH (1981b) Fibroblast cell proliferation in the mouse molar periodontal ligament. J Anat 133, 77–90.

Perera KAS and Tonge CH (1981c) Fibroblast cell population kinetics in the mouse molar periodontal ligament and tooth eruption. J Anat 133, 281–300.

Pierard GE and Lapiere CM (1976). Microanatomy and mechanical properties of the dermis in bovine foetus and newborn calves. Arch Int Physiol Biochem 84, suppl fasc 3, abstract 91.

Pritchard JJ (1946) Repair of fractures of the parietal bone in rats. J Anat 80, 55–60.

Reeve CM Wentz FJ (1962) The prevalence, morphology and distribution of the epithelial cell rests in the human periodontal ligament. Oral Surg 15, 785.

Rosenbloom J (1993) Elastin. In: Connective tissue and its heritable disorders (Royce PM and Steinmann B, eds), pp 167–188, Wiley–Liss, New York.

Ross R and Greenlee TK (1966). Electron microscopy: Attachment sites between tissue cells. Science 153, 997–999.

Sasakai T and Garant PR (1993) Multinucleated fibroblastic cells in the periodontal ligaments of aged rats. J Periodont Res 28, 65–71.

Schroeder HE (1986) The Periodontium. Springer Verlag, Berlin.

Schwartz W (1987) Morphology and differentiation of the connective tissue fibres. In: Connective Tissue. (Tunbridge RE *et al.*, eds) pp 144–156. Blackwells, Oxford.

Scott JE, Orford CR and Hughes EW (1981). Proteoglycan–collagen arrangements in developing rat tail tendon. Biochem J, 195, 573–581.

Scott JH (1953) How teeth erupt. Dent Practr Dent Rec 3, 345–350.

Severson JA, Moffett BC, Kokich V and Seplipsky H (1978) A histologic study of age changes in the adult human periodontal joint (ligament). J Periodontol 49, 189–200.

Shore RC and Berkovitz BKB (1979) An ultrastructural study of periodontal ligament fibroblasts in relation to their possible role in tooth eruption and intracellular collagen degradation in the rat. Arch Oral Biol 24, 155–164.

Shore RC, Moxham BJ and Berkovitz BKB (1982). A quantitative comparison of the ultrastructure of the periodontal ligaments of impeded and unimpeded rat incisors. Arch Oral Biol 27, 423–430.

Shore RC, Moxham BJ and Berkovitz BKB (1984) Changes in collagen fibril diameters in a lathyritic connective tissue. Connect Tissue Res 12, 249–255.

Sicher H (1923) Bau und Funktion des Fixationsapparates der Meerschweinenmolaren. Z Stomat 21, 580. Cited in Orban BJ (1944) Oral Histology and Embryology, 1st edition, Mosby, St Louis.

Sicher H (1942a) Tooth eruption: the axial movement of continuously growing teeth. J Dent Res 21, 201–210.

Sicher H (1942b) Tooth eruption: axial movement of teeth of limited growth. J Dent Res 21, 395–402.

Simpson HE (1965) The degeneration of the rests of Malassez with age as observed by the apoxestic technique. J Periodontol 36, 288.

Simpson HE (1967) A three-dimensional approach to the microscopy of the periodontal membrane. Proc Roy Soc Med 60, 537.

Slavkin HC, Bringas P Jr, Bessem C, *et al.* (1989) Hertwig's epithelial root sheath differentiation and initial cementum and bone formation during long term culture of mouse mandibular first molars using serumless, chemically defined medium. J Periodont Res 24, 28–40.

Sloan P and Beynon AD (1981) Development and structure of the cementum–dentine junction in man and cat. J Dent Res 60, 1135.

Smith LT, Holbrook KA and Byers PH (1982). Structure of the dermal matrix during development and in the adult. J Invest Derm 79 (suppl 1), 93S–104S.

Socransky SS, Hubersak C and Propas D (1970) Induction of periodontal destruction in gnotobiotic rats by the human oral strain of *Actinomyces naeslundii*. Arch Oral Biol 15, 993–995.

Stahl SS and Tonna EA (1977) H^3–proline study of ageing periodontal ligament matrix formation. Comparison between matrices adjacent to either cemental or bone surfaces. J Periodont Res 12, 318–322.

Tasker H, Moxham BJ and Symons D (1992) Ultrastructural study of the collagen in the periodontal ligaments of aged rats. J Dent Res 71, 643.

Ten Cate AR (1969) The development of the periodontium. In: Biology of the Periodontium (Melcher AH and Bowen WH, eds), pp 53–89, Academic Press, London.

Ten Cate AR (1972) Developmental aspects of the periodontium. In: Developmental Aspects of Oral Biology (Slavkin HC and Bavetta LA, eds), pp 309–324, Academic Press, London.

Ten Cate AR (1975) Formation of supporting bone in association with periodontal ligament organization in the mouse. Arch Oral Biol 20, 137–138.

Ten Cate AR and Mills C (1972) The development of the periodontium. The origin of the alveolar bone. Anat Rec 173, 69–78.

Ten Cate AR, Mills C and Solomon G (1971) The development of the periodontium. An autoradiographic and transplantation study. Anat Rec 170, 365–380.

Thesleff I, Partanen AM and Rihtniemi L (1987) Localization of epidermal growth-factor receptors in mouse incisors and human premolars during eruption. Eur J Orthod 9, 24–32.

Thomas NR (1965) The process and mechanism of tooth eruption. PhD thesis, Bristol University.

Thomas NR (1967) The properties of collagen in the periodontium of an erupting tooth. In: The mechanism of tooth support (Anderson DJ, Eastoe JE, Melcher AH and Picton DCA, eds), pp 102–106. Wright, Bristol.

Tonge CH (1963) The development and arrangement of the dental follicle. Trans Eur Orthod Soc 118–126.

Topham RT, Chiego DJ, Gattone VH, Hinton DA and Klein RM. (1987) The effect of epidermal growth-factor on neonatal incisor differentiation in the mouse. Dev Biol 124, 532–543.

Torp S, Baer E and Friedman B (1975). Effects of age and mechanical deformation on the ultrastructure of tendon. In: Structure of Fibrous Biopolymers (Atkins EDT and Keller A, eds), pp 223–250, Butterworths, Londons.

Toto PD and Borg M (1968) Effects of age changes of the premitotic index in the periodontium of mice. J Dent Res 47, 70.

Toto PD, Rubenstein and Garguilo AW (1975) Labelling index and cell density of aging rat oral tissues. J Dent Res 54, 553–556.

Trott JR (1962) The development of the periodontal attachment in the rat. Acta Anat (Basel) 51, 313–328.

van Bladeren TPM (1971) Tooth eruption and the development of the periodontal fibres. Trans Eur Orthod Soc 427–437.

van den Hooff A, Levene CI and Gross J (1959). Morphologic evidence for collagen changes in chick embryos treated with β–aminopropionitrile. J Exp Med 110, 1017–1027.

van der Velden U (1984) Effect of age on the periodontium. J Clin Periodontol 11, 281–294.

van der Velden U (1991) The onset age of periodontal destruction. J Clin Periodontol 18, 380–383.

Wang HW, Nanda V, Rao LG, Melcher AH, Heersche JNM and Sodek J (1980) Specific immunohistochemical localization of type III collagen in porcine periodontal tissues using the peroxidase–antiperoxidase method. J Histochem Cytochem 28, 1215–1223.

Webb PP, Benjamin M, Moxham BJ and Ralphs JR (1993) Age-related changes in intermediate filament expression in the periodontium of rats. J Anat 84, 198.

Winkel EG, Abbas F, van der Velden U, Vroom TM, Scholte G and Hart AAM (1987) Experimental gingivitis in relation to age in individuals not susceptible to periodontal destruction. J Clin Periodontol 14, 499–507.

Wise GE and Fan W (1989) Changes in the tartrate-resistant acid-phosphatase cell population in dental follicles and bony crypts of rat molars during tooth eruption. J Dent Res 68, 150–156.

Wise GE, Lin F and Fan W (1992) Effects of transforming growth factor-β_1 on cultured dental follicle cells from rat mandibular molars. Arch Oral Biol 37, 471–478.

Wise GE, Marks SC Jr, Cahill DR and Gorski JP (1988) Ultrastructural features of the dental follicle and enamel organ prior to and during tooth eruption. In: The Biological Mechanisms of Tooth Eruption and Root Resorption (Davidovitch Z, ed), pp 243–249, EBSCO Media, Birmingham, Alabama.

Yamamoto T and Wakita M (1991) The development and structure of principal fibers and cellular cementum in rat molars. J Periodont Res 26, 129–137.

Yamamoto T and Wakita M (1992) Bundle formation of principal fibers in rat molars. J Periodont Res 27, 20–27.

Yoshikawa DK and Kollar EJ (1981) Recombination experiments on the odontogenic roles of mouse dental papilla and dental sac tissues in ocular grafts. Arch Oral Biol 26, 303–307.

Chapter 9

The Periodontal Ligament and Physiological Tooth Movements

BJ Moxham, BKB Berkovitz

INTRODUCTION

Physiological tooth movements are those movements that a tooth makes to attain, and then to maintain, its functional position. Such movements include axial and non-axial movements during both the developmental stages of a tooth within the jaw and the functional stages within the oral cavity. They are associated with the processes of tooth growth, eruption, and drift and with movements produced by (and following) the application of physiological external forces to the tooth. As will be shown, the periodontal tissues are involved in the generation of, or resistance to, many of these movements. This chapter is concerned primarily with eruption and drift. Chapters 10 and 11 deal with the effects on the periodontal tissues of external forces.

Tooth eruption and drifting can be described in relation to three phases in the development of a tooth: the pre-eruptive phase, the eruptive phase, and the intraoral phase (*Fig. 9.1*). The pre-eruptive phase starts with the formation of the tooth bud and ends with the initiation of root formation. The eruptive phase starts with the onset of root development and ends when the crown penetrates the mucosa to appear in the oral cavity. After this, the tooth is in its intraoral phase. It must be emphasized that eruption appears to be continuous, not phasic, and the use of the above schema does not necessarily imply that different mechanisms might be operating during the different phases to produce similar tooth movements (e.g. Steedle and Proffit, 1985; Cahill *et al.*, 1988). As yet, there is little evidence to assess such a view. Despite these caveats, the schema does provide a convenient method for describing the various patterns of physiological tooth movement. For further discussion about the patterns and control of eruptive movements at different stages, the reader is referred to a detailed review by Steedle and Proffit (1985).

PRE-ERUPTIVE PHASE

Throughout the pre-eruptive phase, the tooth remains in its developmental, intraosseous location. During this phase there is concentric growth of the tooth within its follicle, any convergence of the occlusal surface of the developing tooth and the occlusal plane being attributed not to active bodily movement of the tooth but to growth of the tooth germ (Thomas, 1965; Darling and Levers, 1975, 1976; Steedle and Proffit, 1985).

However, human teeth can show some axial movement towards the occlusal plane during the pre-eruptive phase (Darling and Levers, 1976). Similar conclusions have been drawn from studies of the development of rat molar teeth (O'Brien *et al.*, 1958; Thomas 1965). Studies of bone activity on the walls of the alveolar crypts suggest that there is drifting and tilting of the teeth during the pre-eruptive stage. For cat molars, bone deposition on the lingual walls and resorption on the buccal walls of the dental crypts is associated with a backward relocation of the teeth (Manson, 1968). Distolingual deposition of bone within the crypts of monkey mandibular permanent incisors is associated with a forward and

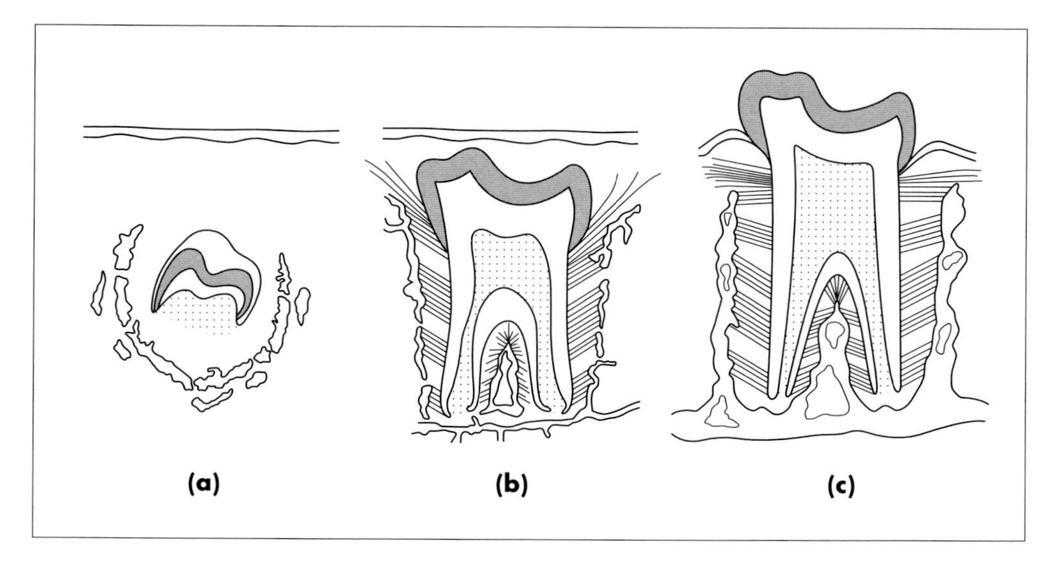

Fig. 9.1 Diagram illustrating the three phases in the development of a tooth. (a) pre-eruptive phase; (b) eruptive phase; (c) intraoral phase.

outward relocation (Baume, 1953). Madder-feeding experiments using the pig indicate a considerable range of drifting movements during the pre-eruptive phase (Brash, 1928).

Whether the bone activity observed in the above studies caused the tooth movements or whether it was the response to movement produced by another agency has not been established. Drifting and tilting of human teeth prior to their eruption have also been observed (Logan, 1935; Ooe, 1968).

ERUPTIVE PHASE

The eruptive phase is characterized by an axial migration of the tooth that involves its active bodily movement (Carlson, 1944; Thomas, 1965; Bjork and Skieller, 1972; Darling and Levers, 1975; Steedle and Proffit, 1985). During this phase, there are significant changes leading to the development of the periodontal ligament, and such changes are described in Chapter 8.

It is usually claimed that, as the forming root grows towards the floor of the crypt, there is resorption of bone in this location. With the onset of eruption, space is created for the developing root, and resorption is no longer seen at the fundus. Where the distance moved by the tooth is greater than the amount of root formed, bone is deposited on the crypt floor (Ten Cate, 1976). More recently, it has been reported that, under the control of the dental follicle, an eruptive pathway is created for dog premolars with bone resorption above the erupting tooth and bone deposition below the tooth (e.g. Cahill and Marks, 1980, 1982; Marks and Cahill, 1984, 1986; Gorski and Marks, 1992; Marks, in press). However, study of the postnatal growth of the mandible in the rat, guinea pig, and cat indicates that bone resorption predominates in the floors of the molar crypts throughout the period of root formation (Manson, 1968). Where bone deposition was seen, it was thought to be related to relocation of the crypt within the growing mandible rather than to eruption.

Darling and Levers (1976) measured the axial movement of some types of human mandibular teeth during the eruptive phase using the mandibular canal as a reference feature. The calculated rates of eruption showed much variation, ranging from 1.2 mm per year for the permanent mandibular third molar to 3.5 mm per year for the permanent mandibular second premolar. Darling and Levers also noted that eruption commenced once the roots began to form. However, experiments on erupting dog premolars suggest that the commencement of root formation is not a critical event. When the developing crown was removed and replaced by a metal or silicone replica, the replica erupted in the absence of a root and an attached periodontal ligament (Marks and Cahill, 1984) (see *Fig. 9.11*).

Little is known about tilting and drifting movements of teeth during the eruptive phase. From a cephalometric appraisal of the eruption of human permanent maxillary incisors, evidence has been obtained to show that they erupt along the path of least resistance (Fletcher, 1963). Fletcher suggested that three elements offered resistance:

- the cortical bone of the outer and inner plates of the alveolus;
- neighbouring developing permanent teeth; and
- deciduous predecessors (or fragments of such teeth).

Teeth were seen to be deflected in their eruptive path by such structures, showing tilting movements. Di Biase (1976) studied delayed eruption of human permanent maxillary incisors associated with supernumerary teeth. Following removal of the supernumerary he observed that, where there was space in the dental arch greater than the width of the crown of the permanent incisor, significant changes in the inclination of the incisor often occurred during its subsequent eruption. He also claimed that the eruptive path of the incisor through the bone was straight if it was upright in the alveolus, but that its path was curved in cases in which it was initially inclined mesially or distally.

INTRAORAL PHASE

During the intraoral phase, the tooth, having emerged into the oral cavity, continues to erupt to attain its functional position. However, the emergence may be facilitated by recession of the mucosa around the erupting tooth. Picton (1989) reported that, for a monkey tooth emerging into the mouth, although extrusion was a progressive feature manifesting as eruption, the rates of extrusion were inconsistent and were substantially higher than expected eruption rates. He concluded by reaffirming that the position a tooth adopts in the mouth is determined by the interplay of the opposing sets of greatly differing forces associated with mastication, tooth support, and eruption.

Measurements of the rates of emergence of human teeth into the oral cavity before they reach the occlusal plane have been made by Burke and Newell (1958), Burke (1963), Berkovitz and Bass (1976), Smith (1980), and Proffit (in press). Burke and Newell (1958) reported that the rates of eruption of the permanent maxillary central incisors of one of their patients were greatest at the time of crown emergence, and decreased thereafter. During the first month of their emergence, the teeth were seen to erupt by approximately 1 mm. Burke (1963) recorded the eruption of a large number of human permanent maxillary central incisors whose eruption was delayed. After surgical exposure, their initial rates of eruption were about 2 mm per month. Smith (1980) has measured eruption of human canine and premolar teeth. He found that the most rapid rate of movement was for a mandibular second premolar (4.5 mm in 14 weeks). Smith (1978) also recorded the changing depths of the gingival crevice during eruption. The crevices of teeth that had just penetrated the mucosa were found to exceed 7 mm in depth, but became more shallow as eruption continued. This reduction, he claimed, was associated partly with the eruptive movements and partly with gingival 'recoil'. The patterns of eruption and of gingival 'recoil' were characterized by rapid changes initially followed by slower ones (though considerable variations were found).

The studies of Burke and Newell (1958), Burke (1963), and Smith (1978) used the occlusal plane as a datum for measurements. Because of the young age of the participants in these studies, however, the occlusal plane may not be stable. Berkovitz and Bass (1976) have determined the rates of emergence of human permanent maxillary third molars for a group of students with an average age of 19 years. They also employed the occlusal plane for measurements, believing that it was more stable for the older age group as evidenced by data from Darling and Levers (1976). Where space was available, the maximum rate of eruption was found to be 1 mm per 3 months. In crowded dentitions, the rate was less than 1 mm per 6 months. This study also indicated that exposure of the crown was the result of gingival recession as well as eruption of the tooth (i.e. passive eruption) (*Fig. 9.2*).

Proffit (in press) used video microscopes to monitor the emergence of 23 maxillary second premolars in 21 children aged approximately 11.5 years (range 9.4–13.4). He reported that there is a diurnal variation in eruptive behaviour. Eruption rates in excess of 3 μm per hour were recorded during the night while there was intrusion during the day, presumably as a result of masticatory loading. Proffit (1994) also observed that eruption is greatest when the body is supine during the evening.

Burke and Newell (1958), Berkovitz and Bass (1976), Smith (1978), and Proffit (1994) have reported that human teeth show decreases in eruption as they approach the occlusal plane. Indeed, a similar pattern has been observed as the mandibular canine tooth of the ferret emerges and reaches its functional position (Moxham and Berkovitz, 1988). It has not been established whether the changes in eruption as the tooth nears occlusion are due to a fundamental change in the eruptive mechanism, whether they are due to the retarding action of occlusal forces, whether they are due to structural or biomechanical changes within the periodontium, or whether they are due to a combination of these mechanisms. Steedle and Proffit (1985) suggest that there might be changes in the metabolic activities of the periodontal ligament (PDL). Quantitative electronmicroscopic analysis of the various components of the PDLs of erupting and newly erupted rat molars show that, although there is little change in the connective tissue components of the ligament, there are major changes in the periodontal vasculature (Berkovitz *et al.*, 1985; Moxham *et al.*, 1987).

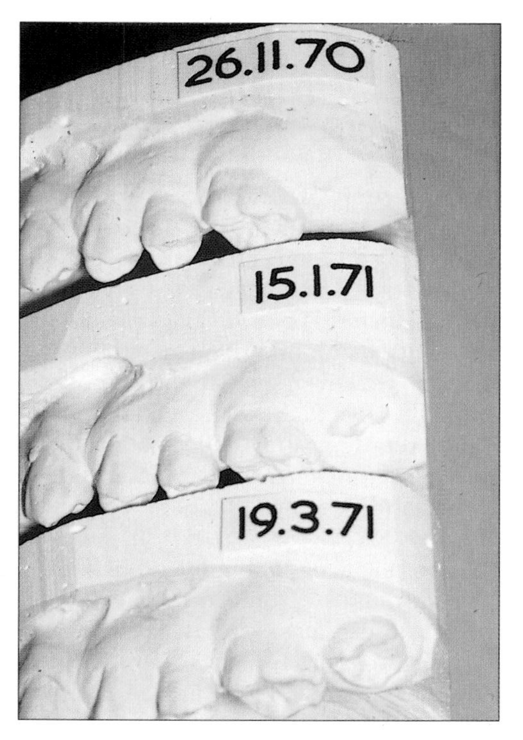

Fig. 9.2 Three successive plaster models of a patient showing the entry of the crown of the third maxillary molar into the oral cavity. Measurements indicated that there has been no active occlusal movement of this tooth, whose crown has therefore become uncovered by recession of the overlying mucosa. (The first permanent molar has been extracted.) (Berkovitz and Bass, 1976.)

That axial, eruption-like movements are possible after the establishment of a tooth's functional position in the dental arch has been established in horizontal studies of human material (Murphy, 1959; Levers and Darling, 1983; Whittaker *et al.*, 1982, 1985). A common enough example is provided by the case when an unopposed tooth overerupts (Boyle, 1955; Cohn, 1966; Moss and Picton, 1967; Pihlstrom and Ramfjord, 1971). Although an increase in dental cement formation around the root apex has been observed in these situations (Boyle, 1955; Pihlstrom and Ramfjord, 1971), the small amount of movement involved and the difficulty of distinguishing cause from effect have prevented identification of the mechanisms responsible. Cohn (1966) has studied the behaviour of molar teeth in mice following the extraction of varying combinations of opposing teeth. He concluded that the degree of overeruption depended upon; the position of the tooth with respect to the missing opposing molars; the degree of non-function to which the tooth was subjected; and the length of time the tooth remained out of function. In a study using macaque monkeys, Moss and Picton (1967) observed that the mandibular cheek teeth of adult animals overerupted at a rate of approximately 75 μm per week following the extraction of opposing teeth.

The ability of incisor teeth to overerupt after they have reached the occlusal plane has been studied in rhesus monkeys by Schneiderman (1989), who placed a bite-raising splint over the molar teeth to open the bite interincisally by 15 mm. Schneiderman reported that, over a period of 48 weeks, the maxillary incisors in adult animals erupted on average a further 2.2 mm and the mandibular incisors erupted 1.5 mm.

Even in the presence of opposing teeth, eruption-like movements may be observed. Darling and Levers (1976) have reported that, although eruption stops once a tooth reaches occlusion, a second phase of axial movement in an occlusal direction may occur at about 14–16 years of age. They suggested that such movements are a response to condylar growth, which effectively separates the jaws and produces disturbance of the occlusal 'equilibrium' and 'release' of the eruptive forces. Siersbaek-Nielsen (1971) has obtained similar results from studies using the analysis of jaw growth and tooth eruption with respect to metallic implants. The findings indicate that incisor eruption rate shows a distinct spurt coincident with spurts of growth at puberty. Such axial movements have also been reported to occur in mouse molars (Dreyer and Sampson, 1984). It is often stated that eruption-like movements may also be seen in the mature human to compensate for occlusal wear of the teeth and to prevent excessive loss of facial height (e.g. Murphy, 1959). However, Ainamo and Talari (1976) suggested that vertical growth within the alveolar processes occurs independently of both attrition and masticatory function. This claim is supported by the finding that, where the food is mainly non-abrasive, the lower facial height for adults may increase by 0.4 mm per year (Thompson and Kendrick, 1964). Furthermore, with a highly abrasive diet, the amount of compensatory alveolar growth and eruption may be insufficient, leading to a reduction of the lower facial height (Murphy, 1959).

In addition to axial movements during the intraoral phase, there may be tilting movements (e.g. Berkovitz and Bass, 1976) and movements of a tooth in the horizontal plane – approximal (mesial and distal) drift and lateral drift. Mesial drift has been the phenomenon to which most attention has been paid. It is assumed that mesial drift occurs as a response to approximal wear. As a consequence, mutual support of the teeth under masticatory loads is said to be enhanced and the interdental tissues protected from trauma. From studies on skulls of Australian Aborigines, Begg (1954) and Murphy (1959) have reported that contact with neighbouring teeth was maintained in both the deciduous and permanent dentitions despite progressive loss of approximal enamel and dentine. Modern Australian Aborigines show less interproximal wear (Corruccini, 1990). The existence of mesial drift in humans has been confirmed by studies reporting reduction in dental arch length with age (Goldstein and Stanton, 1935; Black, 1936; Cohen, 1940; Brown and Daugaard-Jensen, 1950; Speck, 1950; Barrow and White, 1952; Begg, 1954; Sved, 1955; Lysell, 1958; Moorrees, 1959; Knott, 1961; Vego, 1962; Sillman, 1964; Lammie and Posselt, 1965; Lundström, 1969; Yilmaz, 1973, 1976). However, Baume (1950), Clinch (1951), Sillman (1951), and Henriques (1953) failed to show any reduction. Using plaster casts with the palatal rugae as reference landmarks, Lebret (1967) has shown mesial drifting of the permanent maxillary first molar and canine from the time of their emergence into the oral cavity.

Considerable variations in rates of mesial drift in humans have been reported. From the studies involving measurement of dental arch length in modern humans, the rates range from about 0.05 mm per year (Lammie and Posselt, 1965) to 0.7 mm per year (Moorrees, 1959). It is conceivable that the variation in rates relates to such factors as age, diet, dimensions of the various types of teeth studied and methods of measurement. The data also suggest that the rates for mandibular teeth are greater than for maxillary teeth.

Mesial drift has been observed not only in humans but also in monkeys (Baume and Becks, 1950; Latham and Scott, 1960; Moss and Picton, 1967), pigs (Brash, 1927; Yilmaz, 1976), and the elephant, manatee, and dugong (Brash, 1927). However, Sicher and Weinmann (1944), Myers and Wyatt (1961), Kronman (1971), and Dreyer and Sampson (1984) have shown that approximal migration of rodent molars occurs in a distal direction and King *et al.* (1991) reported a rate of distal drift of nearly 8 μm per day in adult rats.

Lateral drift is usually associated with changes in the dimensions of the dental arch of the growing child. Study of plaster casts suggests that the well-documented labial drifting of the erupting permanent incisors as the deciduous teeth become exfoliated is a change in angulation rather than whole bodily drift (Picton, 1976). Many studies have been undertaken to determine the rates and timing of lateral expansion of the dental arches (e.g. Friel, 1945; Moorrees, 1964; Sillman, 1964). It seems that little increase in arch dimension occurs after the eruption of the permanent teeth. The final arch width in the canine, premolar, and molar regions is achieved by the age of 12 or 13 years, although growth of other oral tissues continues for several years. However, labiolingual changes are said to occur in the heavily worn dentition. Begg (1954) described a progressive trend to an edge-to-edge occlusion of the incisors in Australian Aborigines. Little information is available concerning lateral drift in animals.

Finally, a word of caution needs to be given about interpreting tooth movements. Bjork and Skieller (1972), using amalgam implants to provide reference features for studying movements of human permanent teeth, found that developmental rotation of the facial skeleton was associated with compensatory movements of the teeth. Thus, the growth of the jaws may be responsible for tooth movements which, to the unwary, might seem to be attributable to another cause.

THE MECHANISMS OF TOOTH ERUPTION

Among recent reviews on this topic are those by Moxham and Berkovitz (1982), Jacobson (1983), Picton (1989), Burn-Murdoch (1990), Gorski and Marks (1992), and Sandy (1992). It is clear from such reviews that the controversies that have raged around the nature of the eruptive mechanism have been due, in no small part, to the desire to establish a single factor or system responsible for generating the eruptive force. However, even the most cursory glance through the literature shows that the search for a prime mover has been in vain and accordingly (and indeed almost from desperation) the eruptive mechanism is often described as multifactorial (e.g. Melcher and Beertsen, 1978; Moxham and Berkovitz, 1982).

The overall process of eruption is undoubtedly multifactorial. For a tooth to erupt, there must not only be a mechanism responsible for generating the forces causing tooth extrusion, but also a process whereby such forces are translated into eruption by movements through the surrounding tissues. Indeed, there are considerable changes in the tissues overlying an erupting tooth before its emergence into the mouth (e.g. Melcher, 1967; Ten Cate, 1971; Cahill and Marks, 1980, 1982; Marks *et al.*, 1983; Gorski *et al.*, 1988), and eruption can be affected by factors related to the resistance of the surrounding tissues (Moxham and Berkovitz, 1981; Burn-Murdoch, 1990). There must also be a process whereby eruptive movements are sustained as a result of the tooth being supported in its new position, and there must be remodelling of the periodontal tissues to maintain the functional integrity of the system. While many of these processes are at present poorly understood, it is important to realize that a change in eruption may thus be due to a change in the eruptive force, to a change in the resistance to eruption, to a change in the remodelling characteristics of the supporting tissues, or indeed to more than one of these factors.

Recent evidence indicates that the mechanism for generating the eruptive force may itself be multifactorial. Many different drugs and hormones are able to change eruptive behaviour and it might be expected that agents having different effects might be influencing different factors. Thus, experiments involving different combinations of drugs could be of value in assessing whether eruption is multifactorial. Three drug combinations have been considered in this context (Moxham and Berkovitz, 1983). Firstly, when thyroxine and hydrocortisone, drugs that accelerate eruption, were given in combination, the subsequent acceleration was greater than that of the individual drugs alone. This could support a multifactorial concept if the two hormones were considered to have different actions on the eruptive process (although the cause of their actions is unknown). However, it is possible that the hormones merely affect the same factor and we are simply observing a dose-related phenomenon. Administration of cyclophosphamide, a drug known to inhibit eruption (Adatia and Berkovitz, 1981; Burn-Murdoch, 1988), combined with hydrocortisone caused no difference compared with the administration of cyclophosphamide alone. The findings with this combination of cyclophosphamide and hydrocortisone seem to support a multifactorial basis for eruption because, whereas cyclophosphamide is capable of preventing a reaction to hydrocortisone, the tooth still shows some eruption, albeit at a rate much lower than controls. Therefore, there could be a factor partly responsible for eruption that is sensitive to hydrocortisone and that is abolished by cyclophosphamide, whereas a different factor not so sensitive to hydrocortisone remains to allow some eruption (Moxham and Berkovitz, 1983).

Aladdin and Burn-Murdoch (1985b) have also suggested that two mechanisms are responsible for the eruption of the resected rat incisor (i.e. continuously growing incisors whose proliferative basal tissues have been removed). They reported that the unimpeded eruption rates for the resected tooth showed a slow first phase after surgery and then a faster phase with normal rates after a few days. Procedures to alter tissue fluid pressures in sockets of resected teeth had their effects during the second phase of normal eruption. Subsequently, Burn-Murdoch (1988) reported that the mechanism for the eruption of the resected tooth during its initial slow phase is insensitive to cortisone whereas the mechanism during the later faster phases is sensitive to cortisone. Indeed, he found that corticosteroids accelerated and cyclophosphamide slowed the eruption during the later phases of normal eruption, but neither drug had any effect during the early, slow phase of eruption following root resection. He concluded that the findings supported the hypothesis that there is a mechanism present in resected incisors during their phase of normal eruption that is not operable during their slow phases.

More recently, Burn-Murdoch (1988, 1989) reinterpreted earlier results to offer an explanation not related to the multifactorial basis for the eruptive mechanism. He claimed that cyclophosphamide imposes a maximum rate upon eruption by changes within the PDL and that corticosteroids in combination could therefore not be expected to increase eruption. The possible 'rate limitation properties' of cyclophosphamide do not preclude interpretation of findings in terms of a multifactorial basis to the mechanism generating the force(s) of eruption unless there are significant changes in the resistance or remodelling features of the tissues as a result of this drug. This has yet to be assessed and, even if it were the case, it seems to us doubtful that the changes in resistance or remodelling would be such as to abolish completely the effects of corticosteroids instead of merely diminishing the responses.

Before reviewing the various studies that have been undertaken to assess the factors or systems implicated in the generation of the forces of eruption, it is necessary to describe the pattern and measurement of eruption of the continuously growing incisor and its relevance as a model for the study of the eruptive mechanism of a tooth of limited growth. This course of action is appropriate since so many of the investigations into the eruptive mechanism have used the continuously growing incisors of rodents and lagomorphs. The reader is referred to reviews by Schour and Massler (1942) and Ness (1964) for accounts of the structure of the continuously growing incisor.

Much early research involved determining eruption rates of continuously growing incisors in occlusion (i.e. impeded eruption rates). Since there appears to be some relationship between eruption and attrition (Ness, 1964), impeded eruption rates cannot always be considered a proper expression of eruption. Indeed, experimentally induced changes in impeded eruption rates may be more a reflection of changes in biting behaviour than of changes in the eruptive mechanism. To obviate variables associated with attrition, eruption rates of incisors which have been cut out of occlusion (i.e. unimpeded eruption rates) have been monitored. Unimpeded eruption rates are consistently greater than impeded eruption rates (Ness, 1964) – for the rat the unimpeded eruption rate is about 1 mm per day, and the impeded eruption rate is approximately 0.4 mm/day. Although unimpeded eruption rates are generally considered to be a full expression of the eruptive potential that is 'released' with the removal of occlusal stresses, an unimpeded tooth may still have to bear some, if not considerable, loads.

There is also evidence that suggests that normal unimpeded eruption rates are not realized immediately. Chiba *et al.* (1973) found that the unimpeded eruption rates of rat mandibular incisors were not fully reached until 12–16 hours after the teeth were removed from the bite. Using a technique for the continuous recording of eruption of the rabbit mandibular incisor, Moxham (1979a) calculated that 3 hours after the teeth became unimpeded the eruption rates were only equivalent to approximately 700 μm per day. Five days after becoming unimpeded, however, the rates were equivalent to approximately 1200 μm per day. A factor that needs to be considered when studying the unimpeded tooth is the possibility of fundamental changes in the periodontal tissues, which may affect eruption. However, Beertsen and Everts (1977) and Shore *et al.* (1982) could not discern any marked structural and ultrastructural differences between the PDLs of impeded and unimpeded teeth. Nevertheless, some information is available to suggest the possibility of biomechanical changes, the chronically unimpeded incisor of the rabbit showing greater mobility with axially directed extrusive loads (Moxham and Berkovitz, 1981; Chiba and Komatsu, 1988).

Two approaches have been adopted to study the behaviour of a tooth during its eruption. The most favoured approach relies upon the determination of eruption rates from measurements of changes in tooth position. Alternatively, the forces of eruption can be measured.

Tooth movements may be determined from periodic measurements of tooth position or they may be recorded continuously. Various techniques have been used for detecting periodic changes in the eruption of a continuously growing incisor (Schour and van Dyke, 1932; Ness, 1954, 1956, 1965; Bryer, 1957; Adams and Main, 1962; Main and Adams, 1965; Michaeli and Weinreb, 1968; Chiba *et al.*, 1973; Robins, 1979). These have relied on measurements made by direct vision using calipers, measurements made by vision using a dissecting microscope incorporating a calibrated eyepiece, or measurements made from standardized radiographs or photographs. Various anatomical features are used as reference points (e.g. the occlusal plane, alveolar crest, and gingival margin) in association with marks on the teeth. Only the methods of Michaeli and Weinreb (1968) and Chiba *et al.* (1973) have been used to determine eruption rates at intervals of less than 24 hours.

Recently, a series of investigations by Burn-Murdoch and colleagues has highlighted some of the problems of recording eruption from periodic measurements of tooth position (Aladdin and Burn-Murdoch, 1984, 1985a; Burn-Murdoch, 1988, 1992, 1994; Burn-Murdoch and Light, 1992). Details of a technique employing a variable capacitance displacement transducer to allow the continuous recording of eruption of rabbit incisors have been published by Matthews and Berkovitz (1972) and by Moxham (1979a). The sensitivity of the system is such that a change of 1 μm between the plates can produce a movement of 10 mm on a pen recorder (*Figs 9.3* and *914*). Because of its sensitivity, the continuously recording technique has the advantage of being able to assess the immediate and short-term effects of experimental interference with eruption. Using this technique, Moxham (1979a) has shown that eruption of a rabbit mandibular incisor is continuous, though there is considerable variation in the rates (even from minute to minute).

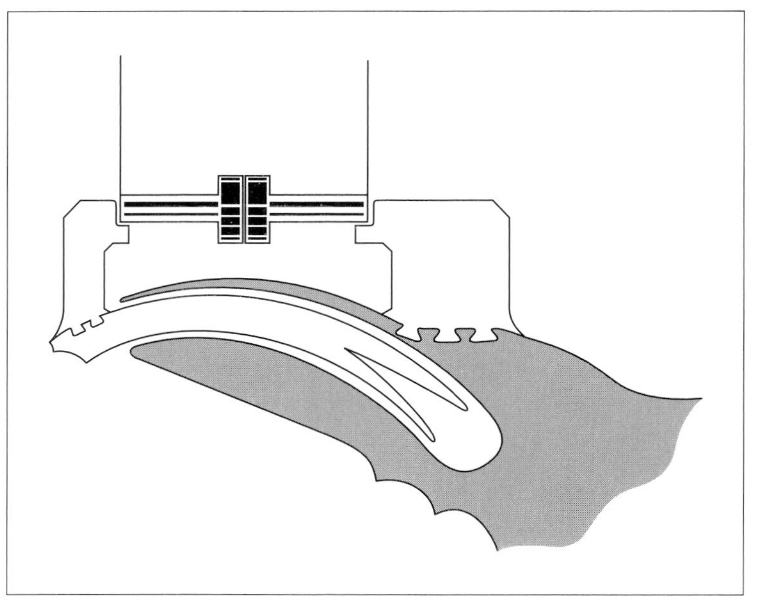

Fig. 9.3 Diagram showing the variable capacitance displacement transducer. One plate is mounted on the tooth, while the reference plate is fixed to adjacent bone. With movement of the tooth relative to bone, there is a separation of the plates and a change in capacitance of the transducer. The plates are part of a circuit whose output may be displayed on a pen recorder.

In addition, an ultrasonic transit-time technique has been described by Aars (1976), Myhre *et al.* (1979), and Leendertz *et al.* (1986) to record the axial position of teeth, and this could be modified to monitor eruption. More recently, continuous recordings of eruption have been accomplished using video microscopes (Proffit *et al.*, 1991) and other precision optical devices (Paterson *et al.*, 1991). Using such instruments, Proffit (in press) has reported that there is diurnal variation in the eruptive behaviour of the human maxillary second premolar.

Measurement of forces exerted by erupting teeth has been undertaken by many researchers. Taylor and Butcher (1951) and Miura and Ito (1968) used similar techniques of elastic traction to oppose the eruption of continuously growing incisors over periods of up to 3 weeks. Taylor and Butcher (1951) reported that a force of 0.05 N was sufficient to stop the eruption of rat mandibular incisors. Miura and Ito (1968) found that 0.07 N was required to prevent eruption of rabbit maxillary incisors. In both studies, it was reported that the teeth were intruded into their sockets if the tension exceeded that required to arrest eruption. For erupting dog canines and rat incisors, Thomas (1976) recorded ‘eruptive forces’ of between 0.005 N and 0.025 N. Steigman *et al.* (1981) reported that the force necessary to oppose the eruption of the rat incisor was between 0.08 N and 0.095 N, and Burn-Murdoch (1981) claims that a load as low as 0.001 N can result in the cessation of eruption of the rat incisor.

Steedle *et al.* (1983) have also reported that loads between 0.002 N and 0.004 N are sufficient to stop the eruption of the rabbit mandibular incisor, and that a load above 0.025 N produces intrusion. However, Proffit and Sellers (1986) later found that the duration of the forces has more important effects on eruption than force magnitude, loads having to be present on the tooth for 50 per cent of the time before eruption ceases and the tooth intrudes. Furthermore, for many of these studies, the extent to which the continuous application of forces to the teeth over long periods might unduly disturb the periodontal tissues and their functioning was not assessed, and it remains a matter of conjecture as to whether physiological values for the forces that an erupting tooth can exert can be derived from techniques that physically prevent the tooth from erupting. Clearly, the reported values for the forces preventing eruption reflect the difference between the 'true' eruptive force and the resistant forces of the tissues through which the tooth erupts. For information concerning the long-term effects of orthodontic-type loads upon the eruptive potential and upon the PDL, see Steigman *et al.* (1983), Steigman *et al.* (1987), and Steigman *et al.* (1991) (see also Chapter 11).

There is, of course, much debate concerning the validity of extrapolating results from the study of the eruption of the continuously growing incisor to the mechanisms responsible for the eruption of teeth of limited growth (see Burn-Murdoch, 1988). Since only teeth of limited growth are found in the earliest mammals, teeth of continuous growth have probably evolved from teeth of limited growth. It has been argued, therefore, that continuous eruption is based upon the exploitation of mechanisms already present in teeth of limited growth (Ness, 1956). This argument is supported by the finding that continuous eruption has appeared in the teeth of mammals in widely divergent orders, and that both continuously and non-continuously growing teeth may be found in the same dentition.

As yet, however, there is little experimental evidence to show that the eruptive mechanism in teeth of continuous growth is similar to that in teeth of limited growth. To support the view that similar processes underlie eruption of both types of teeth, it has been reported that propylthiouracil retards the appearance in the oral cavity of molars in newborn rats (Paynter, 1954) and reduces the impeded eruption rates of adult rat incisors (Garren and Greep, 1955). However, other drugs are known to have different effects on the eruptive behaviour of the two tooth types (e.g. Moxham and Berkovitz, 1988; Lin *et al.*, 1992). Marks *et al.* (1983) and Cahill *et al.* (1988) claim that their observations on the pattern and control of the eruption of teeth of limited growth question the value of eruption studies employing the rodent incisor. However, various investigations using both tooth types have shown that:

- the tooth itself is not an agent effecting its eruption, being instead a property of the connective tissues of the dental follicle/PDL (see pages 189–191);
- that non-tractional forces are involved (see page 191); and
- that the periodontal vasculature may have some role (see pages 198–204).

Furthermore, experimental evidence has been presented that indicates that newly erupted teeth of monkey erupt in a similar manner to rodent incisors (Picton, 1989). Thus, when comparing the eruption of the two tooth types, it is as well to remember their similarities as to dwell on their differences.

THE ROLE OF THE PERIODONTAL LIGAMENT IN THE GENERATION OF THE ERUPTIVE FORCE

Eruption has been attributed to a variety of causative agents. These may be broadly classified into those that are associated with the periodontal connective tissues and those that are not. In the first category are hypotheses related to contraction of periodontal collagen, to traction generated by periodontal fibroblasts, and to pressure exerted by vascular or fluid elements around or beneath the tooth. In the second category are hypotheses associated with alveolar bone growth, root growth, and pulp cell proliferation.

From experiments that have eliminated factors listed in the second category, there is now evidence that the mechanism responsible for generating the eruptive force resides in the PDL. That root growth and pulp cell proliferation are not essential for eruption of teeth of limited growth is evident from studies where root growth was prevented following either surgery (Cahill and Marks, 1980) (*Fig. 9.4*) or irradiation (Gowgiel, 1961). In both

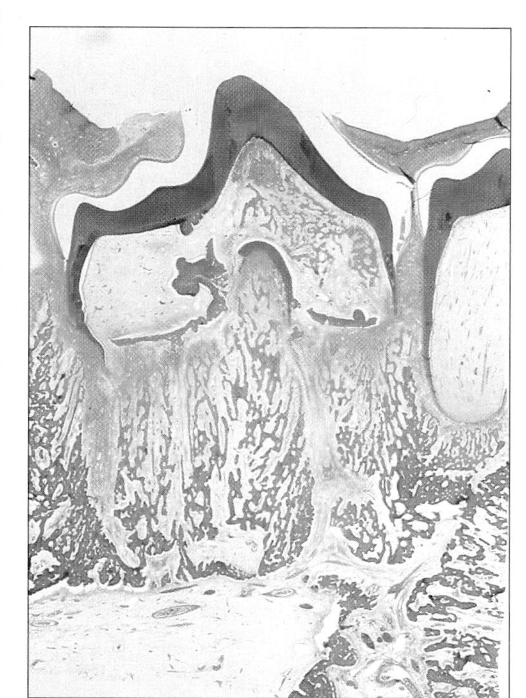

Fig. 9.4
Photomicrograph illustrating successful eruption of a dog premolar tooth whose roots were surgically removed soon after they started to develop when the crown still lay deep within the jaws. Note the bone deposition filling in the region beneath this 'rootless' tooth. (Toluidine blue, magnification × 7.) (Cahill and Marks, 1980.)

situations, the rootless teeth erupted. Similarly, for the continuously growing rodent incisor, the tooth continues to erupt following surgical removal of the basal proliferative zone (root resection), the remaining tooth fragment eventually being exfoliated from the socket (*Fig. 9.5*) (Bryer, 1957; Kostlàn *et al.*, 1960; Berkovitz and Thomas, 1969; Pitaru *et al.*, 1976; Burn-Murdoch, 1988). In addition, following surgical transection of the continuously growing incisor, the distal segment continues to erupt in the absence of any contribution from the remaining fragment containing the proliferative basal zone (Berkovitz, 1971; Moxham and Berkovitz, 1974) (*Fig. 9.6*). Although it might be argued that the 'eruption' of the resected or transected tooth is an artificial exfoliation, because many agents and drugs (e.g. hydrocortisone, thyroxine, demecolcine, triethanomelamine, and aminoacetonitrile) have the same effects on the eruption of the normal tooth and the resected tooth (Berkovitz, 1972; Berkovitz *et al.*, 1972; Chiba and Ohshima, 1985; Burn-Murdoch, 1988), the mechanism of eruption of the surgically altered tooth is considered to be similar to that of a normal tooth.

The fact that alveolar bone deposition beneath an erupting tooth cannot be responsible for tooth eruption is evident from studies that report its absence during the main eruptive phase (O'Brien, *et al.*, 1958; Manson, 1967, 1968; Kameyama, 1973; Berkovitz and Moxham, 1990) (*Fig. 9.7*). Indeed, the predominant activity in the fundus of the alveolar crypt during this phase is bone resorption (Manson, 1967, 1968). There are differences between species and differences between sites for alveolar bone activity; this is clearly evident from the work of Cahill (1969, 1970), Marks (1987), Cahill and Marks (1980, 1982), Wise *et al.* (1985) and Marks and Cahill (1986, 1987), who observed considerable amounts of bone deposition beneath the roots of erupting premolar teeth in dogs (*Figs 9.8, 9.9*). Where present, fundic bone deposition may be related to the distance the tooth has to erupt. If this distance is greater than the length of the root, then some fundic bone deposition is obviously necessary to maintain the normal dimensions of the periodontal space in this region (Thomas, 1965; Kenney and Ramfjord, 1969). Clearly, alveolar bone deposition cannot account for eruption in the continuously growing incisor or following root resection and root transection when the socket beneath the erupting tooth fragment is simply filled with a fluid (Berkovitz, 1971) (*Fig. 9.10*).

The studies of Cahill and Marks (1980, 1982), Marks and Cahill (1984) and Marks *et al.* (1983) also confirm the importance of the precursor of the PDL, the dental follicle, in the eruptive process. These authors demonstrated that, if the developing crown of a dog premolar, together with its surrounding dental follicle, was first removed and then replaced, the tooth erupted. When the crown was replaced without the follicle, there was no eruption. When the tooth alone was removed without major disturbance of the dental follicle, an eruptive pathway was still created and the empty socket was translocated in an occlusal direction. Furthermore, when the crown was replaced by a metal or silicone replica, the replica 'erupted' (*Fig. 9.11*). These studies led Cahill and Marks to conclude that the dental follicle (together possibly

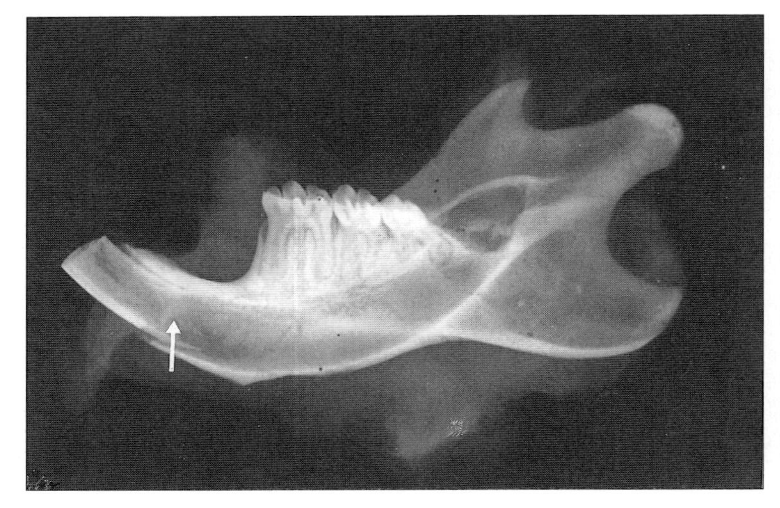

Fig. 9.5 Radiograph of rat mandible showing the effects of removing the proliferating basal tissues (i.e. root resection). Eruption of the remaining tooth segment has continued. The arrow indicates the base of the resected tooth, which is about to be exfoliated.

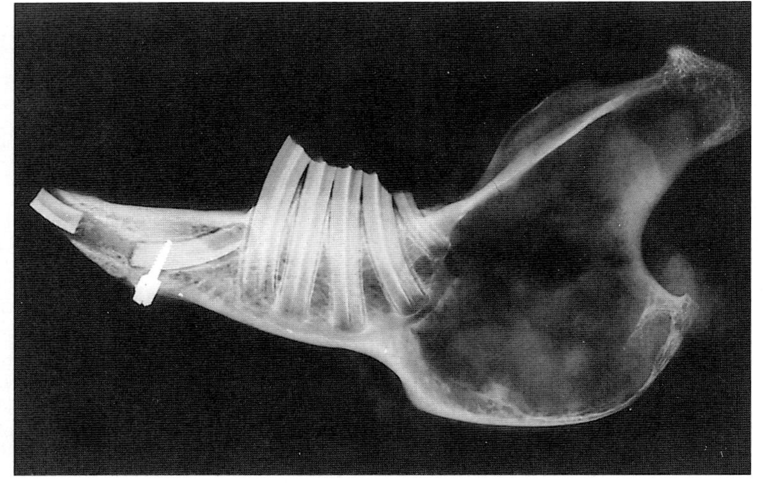

Fig. 9.6 Radiograph of a rabbit mandible in which the incisor tooth has been transected and a metal pin placed in the proximal segment to ensure it does not erupt. The distal segment has continued to erupt and has reached the level of the alveolar crest. (Moxham and Berkovitz, 1974.)

with the reduced enamel epithelium) was responsible for eruption by coordinating the polarized activity of bone resorption and deposition around an erupting tooth.

Subsequently, the cell biology of bone remodeling during eruption has been investigated (Marks *et al.*, 1983; Wise *et al.*, 1985; Wise and Fan, 1989, 1991; Wise *et al.*, 1992), and the developmental changes in the extracellular matrix of the dental follicle have been reported by Gorski *et al.* (1988). For a full review of bone activity during eruption, see Gorski and Marks (1992). Most recently, Gorski (in press) has described a protein within the dental follicle (but also within the cardiac connective tissues) called DF-95, which appears to be selectively degraded at the onset of eruption. It is as yet unclear whether this protein influences the eruptive mechanism *per se* (for example, by affecting the fibroblast cells, the osteoblasts, and osteoclasts that are remodelling the dental crypt or producing the eruptive pathway, or by affecting the vasculature in the dental follicle); it is also unclear whether this protein remains in the follicular–periodontal connective tissues throughout the eruptive process (both before and after tooth emergence).

Even though the evidence favours the involvement of the dental follicle–PDL in the generation of the force or forces of eruption, all available evidence, whether obtained from teeth of continuous growth or from teeth of limited growth, demonstrates unequivocally that the force or forces are not tractional and do not work through an attached collagen fibre network; rather, they are related to pressures within these tissues. It has long been known that rootless teeth can erupt (Gowgiel, 1961; Carl and Wood, 1980; Brin *et al.*, 1985). Related to these findings, experimental studies using the premolar teeth of dogs show that such teeth can also erupt without roots (Cahill and Marks, 1980; see *Fig. 9.4*) and without attachment of the PDL fibres (Cahill and Marks, 1982). Furthermore, provided the dental follicle remains intact, a rootless, unattached metal or silcone replica of the tooth will also erupt (see *Fig. 9.11*). Further evidence against a tractional force is provided by histological observations on the developing PDL (see Chapter 8): in some monkey teeth an organized system of periodontal fibres does not appear until after the teeth have emerged and attained their functional occlusal positions. Finally, experiments using the continuously growing rodent incisor show that such teeth can erupt at normal rates even though the periodontal collagen network has been disrupted by lathyrogens (see pages 191–192).

Part of the problem of assessing a biological process invoked to explain the mechanism or mechanisms responsible for eruption resides in the belief that there is always a 'definitive' experiment to provide proof or disproof. That this is highly unlikely can be easily gleaned from the great number and variety of experiments, using wholly different techniques, that have been employed to study eruption, and also from the obvious difficulties of studying precisely the biology of the periodontal connective tissues, which are never present in large, easily accessible amounts and which display complex interactions between their various components. Consequently, the evidence relating to any biological system proposed as the source of eruptive forces can only be judged by accepting that there are at present technological and scientific limitations, and by reviewing the totality of the evidence from all the various sources. To do this, we propose that the evidence should be judged according to the following five criteria:

1. The proposed system must be capable of producing a force under physiological conditions which is sufficient to move a tooth in a direction favouring eruption.
2. Experimentally induced changes to the system should cause predictable changes in eruption.
3. The system requires characteristics that enable it to sustain eruptive movements over long periods of time.
4. The biochemical characteristics of the system should be consistent with the production of an eruptive force.
5. The morphological features associated with the system should be consistent with the production of an eruptive force.

Using such criteria, we will now review the three major hypotheses of eruption which involve the periodontal connective tissues: the periodontal collagen contraction hypothesis, the periodontal fibroblast traction hypothesis, and the vascular–periodontal tissue hydrostatic pressure hypotheses.

THE PERIODONTAL COLLAGEN CONTRACTION HYPOTHESIS

This hypothesis, originally conceived by Shrimpton (1960), was developed by Thomas (1965, 1976). It involves a tractional force being developed within the PDL, and considerable evidence against this idea has already been presented (see above).

First criterion

There is as yet no evidence that, under physiological conditions, collagen can contract. Indeed, the biochemical mechanisms proposed to account for the contraction of collagen *in vivo* (see criterion 4 above) would seem to be untenable (Bailey, 1968, 1976).

Second criterion

In relation to the second criterion, in order to induce changes experimentally to the proposed collagen contraction system, drugs that interfere with collagen maturation have been administered with the aim of retarding eruption. One such group of substances, commonly referred to as the lathyrogens, can specifically inhibit the formation of crosslinks. As might be expected, lathyritically affected teeth have 'weakened' PDLs and exhibit increased mobility (Berkovitz *et al.*, 1972; Ohshima, 1982; Moxham and Berkovitz, 1984; Ohshima *et al.*, 1989). Understandably, therefore, lathyritic teeth maintained in occlusion show a retarded eruption rate because of the occlusal loads impinging upon the weakened PDL (e.g. Sarnat and Sciaky, 1965; Berkovitz *et al.*, 1972). However,

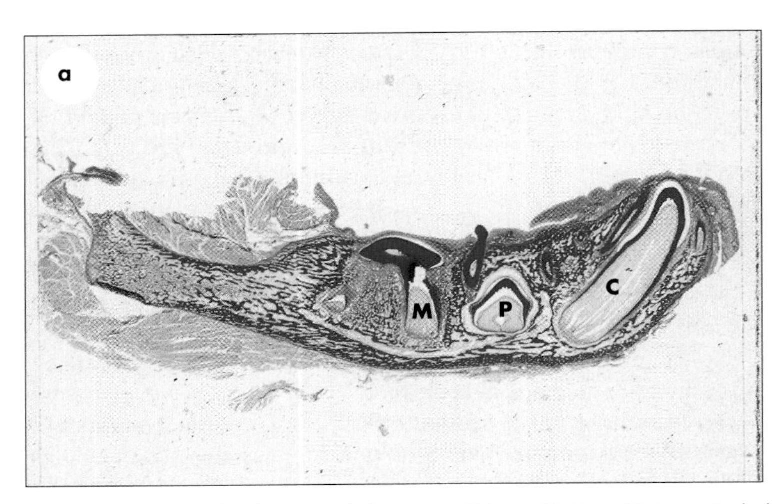

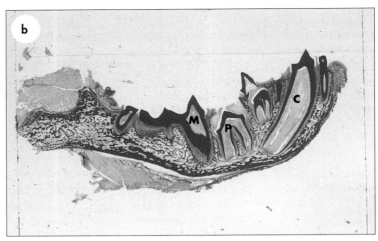

Fig. 9.7 (a) Longitudinal section of ferret mandible at 42 days. Note particularly the position of the root apices of the unerupted permanent teeth in relation to the lower border of the mandible. (b) Longitudinal section of ferret mandible at 66 days. Compared with (a), the permanent teeth have erupted a considerable distance, yet the root apices have the same relationship to the lower border of the mandible, indicating an absence of alveolar bone deposition in relation to eruptive movements. C – permanent canine; P – third premolar; M – first permanent molar. (Van Gieson, magnification × 4.) (Berkovitz and Moxham, 1990.)

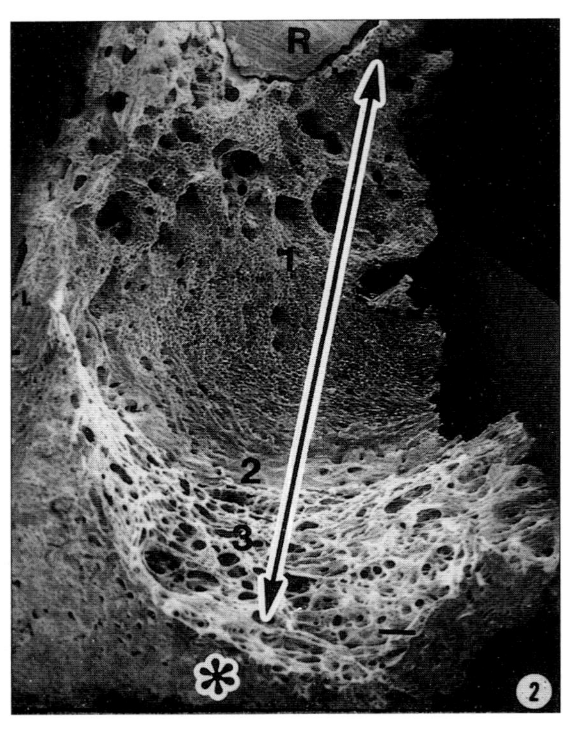

Fig. 9.8 Low-power scanning elctron microscopy of the crypt of the left third permanent mandibular premolar from a 16-week-old beagle dog. The crypt has been sectioned transversely and this view shows the mineralized anterior (mesial) surface of the crypt after removal of all soft tissues with NaOCl. The arrow indicates the long axis of the crown of the permanent tooth. Bone surfaces early in eruption exhibit three morphologically distinct appearances (numbered 1, 2, and 3 from coronal to apical). L – lateral cortical plate of mandible; R – root of deciduous third premolar. * – roof of mandibular canal. Region 1 shows resorbing bone, region 2 resting bone and region 3 bone deposition. Bar = 200 μm. (Marks, 1987.)

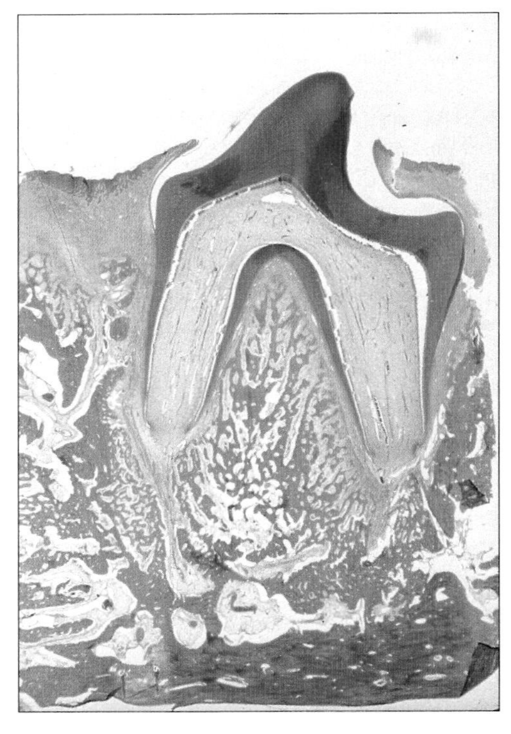

Fig. 9.9 Section of erupting premolar in the dog. There is evidence of considerable bone deposition beneath the roots and in the interradicular region. (Haematoxylin and eosin, magnification × 6.) (Cahill and Marks, 1980.)

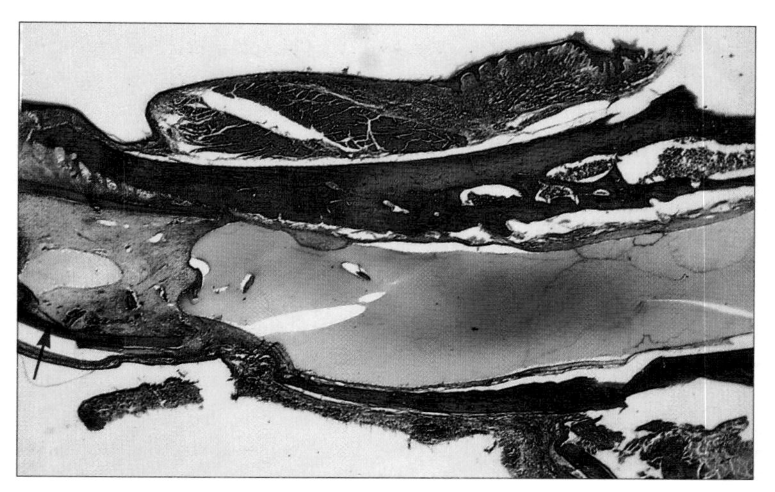

Fig. 9.10 Longitudinal section through a rat mandible following root transection. The tooth fragment (arrowed) has erupted to the region of the alveolar crest and is about to be exfoliated. The socket beneath the tooth contains no organized tissue and *in vivo* it is filled with fluid. (Masson's trichrome; magnification × 9.)

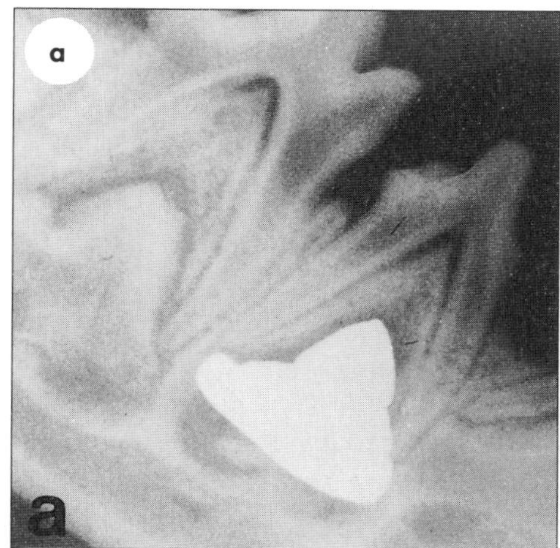

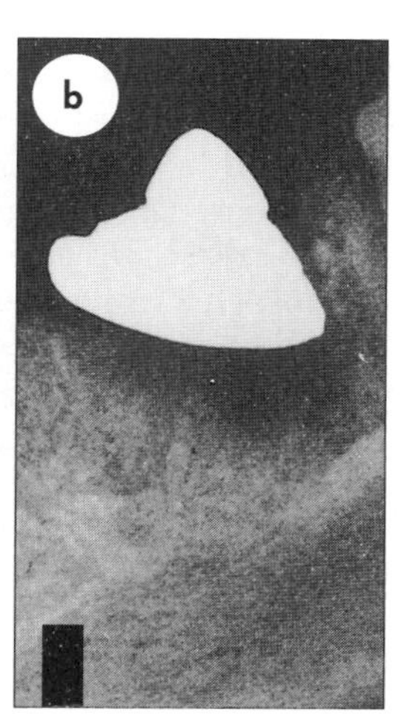

Fig. 9.11 (a) Radiograph showing developing premolar crown having been surgically removed and a silicone replica replaced in the same crypt with the dental follicle remaining intact. (b) A later radiograph when the overlying deciduous molar tooth has been shed and the silicone replica has 'erupted' into the oral cavity. (Marks and Cahill, 1984.)

despite one contrary study (Thomas, 1967), the lathyritically affected rodent incisor erupts at normal rates when maintained free of the bite in the unimpeded state (Berkovitz *et al.*, 1972; Tsuruta *et al.*, 1974; Michaeli *et al.*, 1975).

Collagen metabolism may be affected experimentally in other ways. Gould (1968) and Barnes and Kodicek (1972) have shown that ascorbic acid plays an important role in the formation of collagen, either at the step that involves the hydroxylation of proline to hydroxyproline or at the step that involves the hydroxylation of an unhydroxylated precursor to the hydroxylated compound. In scorbutic animals, the synthesis of collagen is depressed (e.g. Ten Cate *et al.*, 1976), as is collagen degradation (Prockop and Kivirikko, 1968). There is little or no new collagen formation in wounds, and this deficiency may account for a loss of tensile strength (Harkness, 1968). It has been shown that both impeded eruption rates (Dalldorf and Zall, 1930; Berkovitz, 1974) and unimpeded eruption rates (Berkovitz, 1974) are retarded in scorbutic guinea pigs. Although these findings may be regarded as providing evidence for the contraction of collagen hypothesis, care must be taken in interpreting the results, as other systems that might contribute to eruption (such as the vascular system) may also be severely affected in the scorbutic animal (e.g. Chattergee, 1967; Kutsky, 1973).

Third criterion

Our third criterion, which requires the system to have features that enable eruption to be sustained chronically, has been satisfied to a considerable extent. Firstly, in order to sustain eruptive movements over long periods, periodontal collagen would have to exhibit high turnover rates. High rates have been reported by all authors who have studied turnover in the PDL (e.g. Sodek and Limeback, 1979; Sodek, 1983; van den Boss and Tonino, 1984; Sodek and Ferrier, 1988; see also Chapter 3).

Nevertheless, there does not seem to be any direct relationship between eruption rate and turnover rate of collagen – some workers report that the rates within fully erupted rat molars are greater than those within the continuously growing incisor (Sodek, 1978; Sodek and Ferrier, 1988), others report the reverse (Taverne *et al.*, 1986), and still others report no change in turnover rates when eruption rates are increased by making incisors unimpeded (van den Boss and Tonino, 1984). Furthermore, periodontal fibroblasts in incisors that have been experimentally immobilized have the same numbers of intracellular organelles as those that erupt normally (Shore *et al.*, 1985).

Secondly, it is necessary to provide some specialized remodelling mechanism within the PDL in order to allow contraction of periodontal collagen to be sustained while maintaining new tooth positions resulting from previous contractions. It was once thought that the intermediate fibre plexus within the PDL might provide such a remodelling mechanism. However, this fibre plexus, along with an associated concept known as the 'zone of shear', is the subject of considerable controversy (see Chapter 2). Certainly, autoradiographic studies show that there is a rapid and uniform uptake of (and subsequent uniform loss of) label across the entire width of the PDL (e.g. Rippin, 1976a,b, 1978; Beertsen and Everts, 1977; Perera and Tonge, 1981).

Fourth criterion

With reference to this criterion, Thomas (1965, 1976) has suggested a variety of biochemical mechanisms for the contraction of collagen, including:

- a decrease in entropy during electrostatic attraction of disordered tropocollagen macromolecules and alignment along lines of stress;
- a linear polymerization producing a decrease in length of macromolecules;
- a shrinkage associated with dehydration;
- a system analogous to the sliding of actomyosin filaments;
- an interfibrillar repulsion produced by the interaction of adjacent electrical double layers;
- the formation of intermolecular crosslinks.

However, all the explanations offered for the underlying cause of collagen contraction are considered to be biochemically untenable (Bailey, 1968, 1976).

Fifth criterion

The fifth criterion, which relates the morphological features of the periodontal collagen to eruption, is not satisfied either, as there is evidence that, for some teeth (e.g. some succedaneous teeth), the oblique fibres either are not present or are poorly organized during the main phase of eruption (e.g. Grant *et al.*, 1972; Cahill and Marks, 1982; Pearson, 1982; Berkovitz and Moxham, 1990; see also Chapter 8). Thus, overall the evidence against the notion that periodontal collagen contraction is responsible for generating eruptive forces is so strong that the hypothesis appears to be disproved.

A variation on the collagen contraction hypothesis has recently appeared in the work of Katona and colleagues (Katona *et al.*, 1987, 1988, 1989, 1990). It is proposed, mainly from theoretical considerations, that eruption results 'from intermittent alveolar bone deformations resulting from occlusal function and the accompanying effect on the periodontal ligament fibres'. A 'supraosseous' element is suggested, which is attributed to passive traction in the periodontal fibres as they are pulled by the deforming walls of the tooth socket. Putting aside the lack of experimental research to assess the proposals, and the hypothetical basis without recourse to periodontal biology to explain the maintenance of a new position following eruptive movements, sufficient evidence can already be provided to argue against a tractional eruptive force, whether actively or passively derived (see page 191).

THE PERIODONTAL FIBROBLAST TRACTION HYPOTHESIS

According to this hypothesis, the eruptive force is a tractional force developed by the periodontal fibroblasts. A fibroblast, adherent to a substratum, pulls itself forward by an actin-based contractile mechanism. As action and reaction are equal and opposite, a force is exerted on the substratum, tending to put it into compression in the region between the ends of the cell and into tension beyond them (Aubin and Opas, 1989). In a wider context, fibroblast traction may be important in connective tissue morphogenesis (Bellows *et al.*, 1981; Stopak and Harris, 1982; Oster *et al.*, 1983; Lewis, 1984).

Fibroblast 'traction' in the PDL as a cause of eruption was suggested by Ness (1967) from an appreciation that wound contraction may be mediated by fibroblast-like cells in granulation tissue (James, 1964). It has been shown that 'fibroblasts' from granulation tissue resemble smooth muscle cells morphologically (e.g. Gabbiani *et al.*, 1971; Gabbiani, 1979) and antigenically (Hirschel *et al.*, 1971); such cells have been termed myofibroblasts.

The properties of the cell associated with the development of traction are cell adhesion, motility, and contractility (Stopak and Harris, 1982; Aubin and Opas, 1989). With respect to the eruptive process, it has still not been made clear as to whether any force generated by the periodontal fibroblasts is transmitted directly to the tooth via the cells (and, if so, how), or whether the forces are transmitted indirectly via the collagen fibres. The most readily accepted notion is that fibroblasts migrate up the PDL (i.e. occlusally), pulling the erupting tooth along behind. A variant of this would be for the cells to generate an equal and opposite force by migrating rootwards (Harris and Dmytryk, 1989); however, no one has yet formulated a working hypothesis around this latter interpretation. Presumably tension could also be developed by contraction of the fibroblasts without necessitating much migratory activity of the fibroblasts, but again such a view has not been properly elaborated to account for continuous eruption. Of course, all of this may merely be conjecture, bearing in mind that there is strong evidence against the idea that the eruptive force is a tractional force.

First criterion

With regard to our first criterion, there is as yet no evidence that periodontal fibroblasts generate significant traction *in vivo*. Majno *et al.* (1971) have shown that wound granulation tissue (like smooth muscle) contracts with 5-OH tryptamine, adrenaline, bradykinin, and angiotensin, the contraction being mediated by myofibroblasts. However, van den Brenk and Stone (1974) were unable to demonstrate any effect of smooth-muscle agents on uninjured connective tissue, and such demonstrations have not been undertaken on normal periodontal connective tissues *in vivo*.

There is undoubted evidence that fibroblasts *in vitro* can generate tensional forces. This can be observed when the cells are cultured on silicone rubber substrata. The locomotion of the cells is accomplished by the exertion of shearing forces, which are directed tangentially to the plasma membrane of the cells. The rubber is thrown into compression wrinkles beneath the cells while tension wrinkles radiate from the ends of the cells (Harris *et al.*, 1980; Harris *et al.*, 1981). The strength of the cellular traction varied considerably between cell types (Harris *et al.*, 1981). Bellows *et al.* (1981) demonstrated that periodontal fibroblasts incorporated into three-dimensional collagen gels produced contraction of the gels. Subsequently, these authors also showed that sufficient tension could be generated to bring together fragments of tooth and bone initially placed some distance apart within the gel (Bellows *et al.*, 1982a). However, it might be straining credulity too far to assume that such activity observed *in vitro* can be easily extrapolated to the situation *in vivo* (see Chapter 1).

Second criterion

There is little evidence directly relating to experimentally produced changes in eruption rate. This is because of the difficulty of specifically affecting cell traction, whether by inhibiting cell motility, cell contractility, or both, without influencing other systems. For example, drugs that disrupt microtubules, such as colchicine and demecolcine, significantly retard eruption (Berkovitz, 1972; Chiba *et al.*, 1980; Beertsen *et al.*, 1984; Chiba and Ohshima, 1985). However, such findings cannot simply be interpreted as evidence for the cell tractional hypothesis, since an antimicrotubular agent such as colchicine also affects all proliferating cells in the body, increases viscosity of hyaluronan *in vitro* (Castor and Prince, 1964), reduces collagen synthesis (Bornstein, 1974; Garant and Cho, 1979), affects the contractility of granulation tissue (van den Brenk and Stone, 1974), and raises blood pressure by causing arterial constriction (Fergusson, 1952). *In vitro* studies demonstrate that the contraction associated with periodontal fibroblasts described with the first criterion above can be inhibited by colcemid and cytochalasin D, suggesting that microtubules and microfilaments are involved in the contractile mechanism (Bellows *et al.*, 1982a). An injection of cytochalasin B (15 mg/kg body weight), a drug that disrupts microfilaments *in vitro*, did not affect unimpeded eruption rates (Chiba *et al.*, 1983), although the drug's precise effect *in vivo* awaits clarification.

Third criterion

With regard to this criterion, the advocates of the fibroblast traction hypothesis regard as important the fact that cell motility occurs in an occlusal direction, a feature that might allow eruption to be sustained by fibroblasts. Autoradiographic studies indicate that periodontal fibroblasts move occlusally at a rate equal to that of eruption. Furthermore, when the eruption rate of the rodent incisor is increased by rendering the tooth unimpeded, there is a concomitant increase in the rate of migration of the cells in the cement-related part of the PDL (Beertsen, 1975; Beertsen and Everts, 1977; Michaeli *et al.*, 1988). Conversely, when eruption is prevented by pinning, cell migration ceases (Beertsen and Hoeben, 1987). Ness (1970) claimed that fibroblasts are 'born' near the root apex of the tooth, from where they move upwards with the erupting tooth towards the gingival part of the ligament, where they eventually die. Zajicek (1974) even reported evidence of a velocity gradient, with cells near the tooth surface moving at twice the speed of the erupting tooth (though this has yet to be corroborated). Although providing evidence of a shift in the position of the periodontal fibroblasts, such work does not in itself indicate whether the cells are moving actively to generate the eruptive force or are merely being transported passively within the ligament as a response to an eruptive force produced elsewhere. In this context, the site of the zone of shear in the PDL as the tooth erupts is still a contentious issue (see Chapter 2).

Fourth criterion

For eruption to occur as a result of fibroblast motility, one has to postulate that periodontal fibroblasts are migrating at rates at least equal to eruption rates. In the unimpeded rodent incisor, this rate can be over 1 mm per day. Can fibroblasts achieve such rates *in vivo*? Under the most carefully controlled conditions *in vitro*, fibroblasts reach speeds of about 60 μm per hour (Bard and Hay, 1975). For PDL fibroblasts *in vitro*, rates of about 12 μm per hour have been recorded (equivalent to nearly 300 μm per day) (Brunette *et al.*, 1977). If periodontal fibroblasts do generate the eruptive force, an explanation still needs to be found as to how the fibroblasts migrate at such a rapid rate and in one direction through the dense fibrous connective tissue, and how they migrate in such a coordinated manner. Furthermore, bearing in mind the high cellularity of the tissue, does this have any implications for the concept of contact inhibition (e.g. Abercrombie and Heaysman, 1953)? There is also evidence of an indirect relationship between the force of cell traction and the migration rate of the cell, very motile cells exerting the weakest traction (Harris, *et al.*, 1981). Further aspects of this subject are considered below in relation to our fifth criterion.

Fifth criterion

Although it is not yet easy to evaluate the fibroblast traction hypothesis with regard to the fourth criterion, more information exists with relevance to the fifth criterion. Indeed, most of the studies concerning this hypothesis have attempted to relate the morphological features of periodontal fibroblasts to their proposed tractional properties. Whilst the study of fibroblast morphology would not in itself make it possible to 'prove' that the cells generate tension *in vivo*, the structure of the periodontal fibroblast should at least be compatible with its proposed function.

Beertsen *et al.* (1974) and Melcher and Beertsen (1977) suggested that the presence of microtubules and microfilaments in periodontal fibroblasts provided a structural basis for the motile properties necessary to generate tension. Fibroblasts migrating in tissue culture exhibit marked polarity of shape and also possess polarized arrays of microfilament bundles and microtubules, particularly in the tail region (Wessels *et al.*, 1973;

Table 9.1 (Moxham *et al.*, 1991).

Structure		Enamel-related connective tissue (Mean ± SE)	Periodontal ligament (Mean ± SE)	Significance or difference
Cells	Vv Sv	0.40 ± 0.08 2.06 ± 0.45	0.43 ± 0.04 1.84 ± 0.12	NS NS
Endoplasmic reticulum	Vvc Svc	0.051 ± 0.002 2.030 ± 0.113	0.057 ± 0.002 2.151 ± 0.143	NS NS
Mitochondria	Vvc	0.020 ± 0.001	0.018 ± 0.002	NS
Microfilament bundles	Vvc	0.047 ± 0.007	0.042 ± 0.005	NS
Microtubules (transverse section)	Nac	6.19 ± 0.60	2.95 ± 0.30	p<0.01
Microtubules (longitudinal section)	Nac	5.56 ± 0.64	2.92 ± 0.54	p<0.05
Lysosomes	Vvc	0.0060 ± 0.0020	0.0061 ± 0.0010	NS
Collagen profiles	Vvc	0.0015 ± 0.0002	0.0008 ± 0.0002	NS

Vv = Volume fraction, i.e. volume of structure per unit volume of tissue -
Sv = Surface area of structure per unit volume of tissue - Vvc = Volume of structure per unit volume of cell -
Svc = Surface area of structure per unit volume of cell -
Nac = Number of profiles of structure per μm² of cell profile.

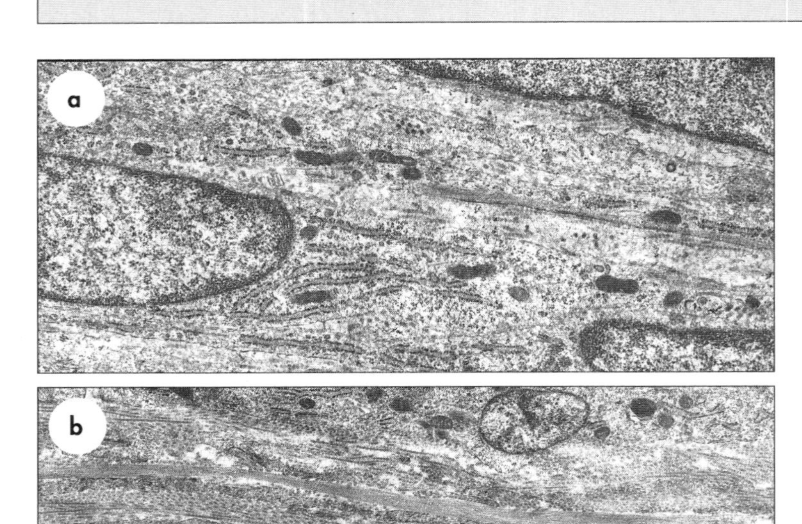

Fig. 9.12 Electron micrograph of (a) periodontal fibroblasts and (b) fibroblasts associated with the enamel-related connective tissue. The overall morphology and intracellular organelle content are similar. (Magnfication × 9000.)

Goldman *et al.*, 1976; Vasiliev and Gelfand, 1976; Hay, 1982). However, Tomasek *et al.* (1982), on examining the contractile proteins of cultured fibroblasts, came to the opinion that the microfilament bundles (stress fibres) were not essential for efficient movement of cells within collagen lattices. Microfilaments and microtubules are found in all cells and in association with basic functions such as intracellular transport, cytoskeletal support, endocytosis, and exocytosis. Thus, the mere presence of these organelles in periodontal fibroblasts may not be significant in terms of understanding eruption. The quantity and orientation of such organelles may be of greater importance, although there is little quantifiable information available (see Chapter 1). Shore and Berkovitz (1979) found that microfilament bundles were not especially prominent in the fibroblasts of the rat incisor PDL and the microfilaments were not preferentially aligned (a feature which might be expected if the cells were specifically migrating in an occlusal direction).

Azuma *et al.* (1975) claimed to be able to distinguish a subpopulation of fibroblasts in the PDL that resembled smooth-muscle cells, the so-called myofibroblasts (e.g. Gabbiani *et al.*, 1971; Gabbiani, 1979). Such cells have specific morphological characteristics (see this page) and the findings of Azuma *et al.* (1975) are not supported by other workers who have studied the ultrastructure of the cells of the PDL (e.g. Ten Cate, 1972; Beertsen *et al.*, 1974; Garant, 1976; Shore and Berkovitz, 1979; Yamasaki *et al.*, 1987).

One approach to relate structure with function, and thereby to assess the possibility of fibroblast traction occurring *in vivo*, is to analyse the structure of the periodontal fibroblasts in teeth exhibiting different eruptive behaviours. For example, there may be differing energy requirements (and thus differences in mitochondrial volume) or variations in the amounts of microfilaments and microtubules present. However, on comparing PDL fibroblasts in erupting and erupted rat molars (Berkovitz *et al.*, 1984), normal and unimpeded incisors (Shore *et al.*, 1982), and normal and immobilized incisors (Shore *et al.*, 1985), few differences were found between any of the groups and none were found that appeared consistent with the view that fibroblasts generate the eruptive force. Also significant from the data was the lack of differences between fibroblasts from the continuously growing incisor and the fully erupted molar.

Further comparisons are possible between the two distinct periodontal connective tissues around the continuously growing rodent incisor (i.e. the PDL proper and the enamel-related connective tissue on the labial aspect). The latter has no attachment to the tooth or to the bone and its fibroblasts have never been implicated in generating an eruptive force. When quantitative, ultrastructural comparisons of various cellular elements were made (Moxham *et al.*, 1991), it was evident that the two cell populations were virtually indistinguishable (*Table 9.1* and *Fig. 9.12*). One noteworthy detail relates to the quantification of microtubules. Beertsen *et al.* (1984) reported that there is a direct correlation between the number of microtubules and the eruption rate. Thus, with increasing amounts of colchicine, there was a greater reduction in eruption rate and a greater disruption of the microtubules. Furthermore, Shore *et al.* (1982) found more microtubules in periodontal fibroblasts from unimpeded incisors than from impeded incisors. However, in the case of immobilized (pinned) incisors where fibroblasts showed no eruption (Beertsen and Hoeben, 1987), there were no significant differences in microtubules compared with normal controls (Shore *et al.*, 1985). Another argument against a relationship between microtubules and eruption is the observation that there are significantly more microtubules in the enamel-related fibroblasts than in the periodontal fibroblasts (see *Table 9.1*). Additionally, the numbers of microtubules seen in transverse and longitudinal sections of the rat incisor ligament were found to be similar, implying that there is no polarity for this organelle within periodontal fibroblasts in the direction of expected eruption (Moxham *et al.*, 1991).

Much of the evidence relating to the generation of fibroblast traction depends on a consideration of *in vitro* studies, and the relevance of such work to the *in vivo* state must be considered very carefully. The most detailed morphological studies of periodontal fibroblasts during gel contraction have been carried out by Bellows *et al.* (1982a,b). At the stage of gel contraction, the cells appear elongated and spindle-shaped. Ultrastructurally, although lacking a basal lamina, they show features characteristic of myofibroblasts in possessing thick cell coats, numerous structures that resemble gap junctions, occasional crenulated nuclei, only small amounts of endoplasmic reticulum, and considerable amounts of microfilamentous material dispersed throughout the cytoplasm. In exhibiting these features, tension-generating fibroblasts differ from periodontal fibroblasts *in vivo*, which (at least in the case of the rat incisor) have an irregular disc shape (Shore and Berkovitz, 1979), a cytoplasm containing considerable amounts of rough endoplasmic reticulum, and less microfilamentous material, primarily in the form of stress fibres beneath the cell membrane (see Chapter 1). Gap junctions are infrequent *in vivo*, where the more common type of intercellular contact is the simplified desmosome (Shore *et al.*, 1981). Significantly, as contraction of the collagen gel *in vitro* ceased, the morphology of the cultured fibroblasts changed to resemble PDL fibroblasts *in vivo*. Indeed, if PDL fibroblasts become transformed when initially placed in tissue culture conditions *in vitro*, then great care must be taken before extrapolating to the *in vivo* situation.

Bellows *et al.* (1981) observed that PDL fibroblasts incorporated into three-dimensional collagen gels produced greater compaction of the gel than other types of cell did. However, Murphy and Daniel (1987) observed that the amount of compaction depended on how many passages the cells had been passed through before being utilized, and they also found that the amount of contraction did not differ significantly between periodontal fibroblasts and fibroblasts derived from human sclera or foreskin; human gingival fibroblasts produced most contraction. In a preliminary communication, Hughes and Issberner (1988) also report that periodontal fibroblasts contract collagen gels less than fibroblasts from oral mucosa and the attached gingiva. Another obvious complication relating to *in vitro* studies is that the nature of the substratum can significantly affect the morphology of the cells (Hay, 1982; Aubin and Opas, 1989). Further consideration of periodontal fibroblasts *in vitro* is given in Chapter 1.

Overall, therefore, the evidence for the periodontal fibroblast hypothesis at present remains poor. Future work will have to ascertain whether periodontal fibroblast motility and contractility can occur via a periodontal element other than the collagen fibres (or even in the absence of a tooth root) since the evidence against a tractional eruptive force is strong (see page 191). That cellular features may provide developmental markers for changes in eruptive behaviour is shown by immunocytochemical study of the proteins that make up the intermediate filaments (IF) of the cytoskeleton within the fibroblasts of the rat molar PDL (Webb *et al.*, 1994; Moxham, in press). In addition to expressing vimentin (type III IF characteristic of mesenchymal cells; Kreis and Vale, 1993), the fibroblasts can also express cytokeratins (type I and II IF polypeptides, said to be characteristic of epithelial cells; Kreis and Vale, 1993). In particular, the cytokeratins appear at the time of maximum eruption of the rat molar (i.e. just as the tooth emerges into the mouth) but are no longer expressed once the tooth has reached occlusion. Further work which involves experimental alteration of eruption will be necessary to confirm that these cytoskeletal proteins are markers of eruption and, even then, it is likely that their appearance relates indirectly to the mechanism by which the eruptive force is generated (*see Fig. 1.13*)

THE VASCULAR AND PERIODONTAL TISSUE HYDROSTATIC PRESSURE HYPOTHESES

Constant (1900) and Carne (1924) were the first to suggest that the eruptive force was related to blood pressures. Ness and Smale (1959) developed this idea in terms of the Starling hypothesis (1909), the eruptive force being deemed to be derived from the hydrostatic pressure of the dental connective tissues (and therefore only indirectly from vascular pressures). Whether acting directly or indirectly, the vasculature of the pulp or the PDL or both may be involved, even though experiments on the resected continuously growing incisor implicate the PDL as the source of the eruptive mechanism (see pages 189–191). Recent reviews concerning the vascular hypotheses of eruption have been written by Sutton and Graze (1985), by Moxham (1988), and by Burn-Murdoch (1988, 1990). Aspects of vascular physiology are also discussed in Chapter 6.

The vascular hypotheses of eruption differ from many other hypotheses in that it is not necessary to invoke a tractional mode of activity within the periodontal tissues. Indeed, the evidence against the eruptive force being a tractional force acting on the collagen fibres of the PDL is very strong.

First criterion

In terms of our first criterion, there have been many studies reporting that teeth at rest show small pulsatile movements that are synchronous with the arterial pulse (e.g. Korber, 1970; Ng *et al.*, 1981). Thus, vascular pressures can produce forces sufficient to move a tooth under physiological conditions.

Two observations on the eruptive behaviour of the rabbit mandibular incisor may also be pertinent here. Moxham (1979a) reported that significant changes in eruption could occur following spontaneous drops in arterial blood pressure that were not induced experimentally. In addition, after death, the rabbit incisor ceases to erupt with the sudden drop in arterial blood pressure and the cessation of the heart beat, the tooth gradually intruding once the arterial blood pressure drops to zero. Myhre *et al.* (1979) have also reported that the rabbit incisor is markedly influenced by arterial blood pressures and they have confirmed the events of death. Recently, Chiba (in press) has also reported that extrusive forces for the erupting rat incisor were markedly reduced at death and in association with the fall of arterial blood pressures. Furthermore, Proffit (in press), while monitoring the eruptive behaviour of human maxillary premolars, observed that body position has an influence, and this might be related to cardiovascular changes with posture.

Second criterion

Experiments directed towards altering blood flow and pressures in the vessels of a tooth have relied either on the administration of drugs with vasoactive properties or on section and stimulation of the vasomotor nerve supply (see also Chapter 6).

Main and Adams (1966) reported that daily intramuscular doses of the hypotensive agents guanethidine and hydrallazine over 8 days to normotensive rats did not affect the rates of unimpeded eruption of their incisors. Litvin and de Marco (1973) reported that twice-daily intramuscular injections of the diuretic furosemide to rabbits over 8 days did not affect the unimpeded eruption of the incisors. However, twice-daily intramuscular injections of the antidiuretic vasopressin over 8 days increased the unimpeded eruption rates. Main and Adams (1966) and Litvin and de Marco (1973) used techniques for determining eruption rates which required an assessment of changes in tooth position at intervals of 2 days and 4 days respectively. As changes in the vasculature may only be short term, their techniques may not be sufficiently sensitive to monitor changes in eruptive behaviour. The increase in eruption rate following the administration of pitressin reported by Litvin and de Marco (1973) may be less reliable because their method of measurement (with calipers from the interdental papilla) is crude.

The immediate and short-term effects of a variety of drugs with vasoactive properties have been investigated using the rabbit mandibular incisor (Moxham, 1979b). Intravenous administration of the hypotensive agents hexamethonium, hydrallazine, and guanethidine produced short-term but significant increases in eruption rates (*Fig. 9.13*). Although main arterial blood pressure falls with the hypotensive agents, for the periodontal microcirculation there is likely to be an increase in vascular pressures, which – arguing from Starling's hypothesis – should result in an increase in tissue fluid pressures and hence an increase in eruption. The initial response with guanethidine was a marked intrusive movement of the tooth. This can be explained by recourse to the known pharmacological properties of the drug. Guanethidine acts by depleting noradrenaline at the nerve terminals (e.g. Boura and Green, 1965; Nickerson, 1970). Therefore, the initial intrusion is probably a response to the noradrenaline. Indeed, infusions of noradrenaline into the subclavian artery were found to have significant intrusive effects on tooth movements (*Fig. 9.14*). Increased eruption with hexamethonium has also been reported by Lisney *et al.* (1972), and Myhre *et al.* (1979) have observed intrusive movements of the rabbit maxillary incisor with intravenous noradrenaline. The latter further reported that intravenous papaverine induced marked extrusive movements. Aars (1982b) has shown that β-adrenoceptor blockers (propanolol and the β_2-adrenoceptor antagnoists ICI 118 551 and H 35/25) can produce tooth extrusion, and that this is reversed or prevented by isoprenaline. Chiba (in press) has confirmed (for the rat incisor) that vasoactive drugs such as adrenaline, noradrenaline, isoprenaline, hexamethonium, and PG_2 affect the periodontal vasculature, extrusive movements and extrusive forces. Of particular significance is the fact that the responses to vasoactive drugs were found to be dose dependent.

Studies on the effects of sympathectomy using techniques for measuring eruption at discrete intervals of more than 24 hours are inconclusive. Increased impeded eruption rates have been recorded after sympathectomy for the incisors of rats (Breitner

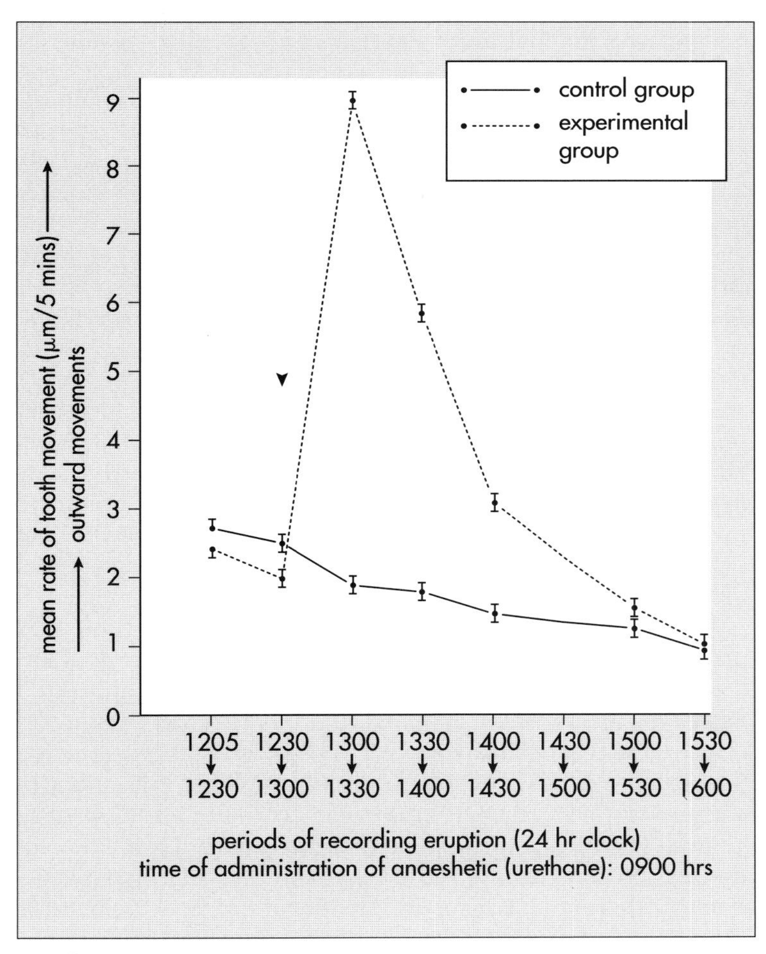

Fig. 9.13 Graphs showing group mean rates of movements (in μm per 5 min) of erupting rabbit mandibular incisors for a control group of animals and an experimental group where a single dose of hexamethonium (10 mg/kg) was administered intravenously at 1300 h (arrow) to each animal. (Moxham, 1979b.)

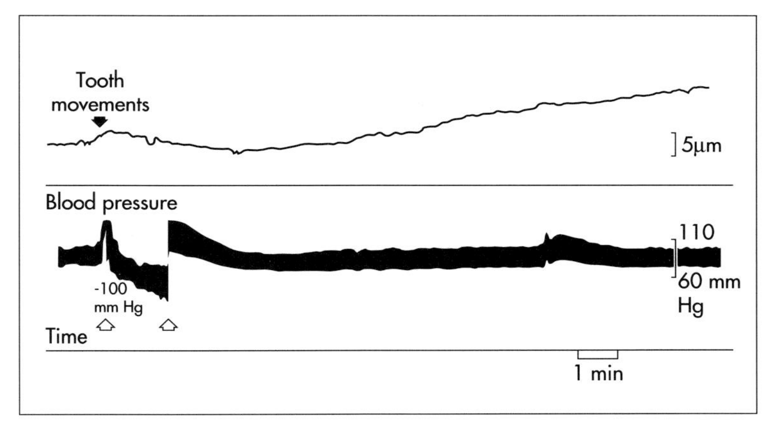

Fig. 9.14 Record of the movements of a rabbit mandibular incisor showing the immediate effects of a close arterial injection of noradrenaline (0.003 mg/kg) (arrow). Note that eruption-like movements ceased on injecting the noradrenaline, the incisor intruding into its socket (by about 8 μm) for a period of approximately 5 minutes. Thereafter, eruption-like movements recommenced. The marker arrows on the blood pressure trace indicate the use of an offsetting device. (Moxham, 1979b.)

and Leist, 1927), guinea pigs (Leist, 1927), and rabbits (King, 1937). Unimpeded eruption rates of rat incisors were reported to increase following sympathectomy (Bryer, 1957). However, similar experiments using rat incisors produced no effects on impeded eruption rates (Taylor and Butcher, 1951; Miller, 1957; Moss and Crikelair, 1960), and Klein *et al* (1981) found only a minimal influence on the timing of the emergence of teeth in neonatal mice.

Thus, the failure to establish any consistent change in eruption following sympathectomy may argue against the vascular hypotheses of eruption. There is no certainty, however, that nerve section caused the change in vascular–tissue pressures that one might have expected. First, because sympathetic section not only reduces arteriolar tone but can also reduce venomotor tone, it may not cause a rise in filtration pressure. Second, even though capillary filtration is increased, the tissue pressure may not rise, because of tissue compliance. In the dog leg, Guyton *et al.* (1971) have shown that the volume of fluid can rise by nearly 100 per cent with only a small change in tissue hydrostatic pressure. (Since the tooth and its supporting tissues are housed in a bony socket, it seems unlikely that there is such compliance.) Third, there is the possibility of the blood vessels re-establishing their calibre soon after sympathectomy (eg. Barcroft and Swan, 1953). However, using a transducer to produce a continuous recording of the eruption of a rabbit incisor, Moxham (1981) has shown that section of the cervical sympathetic trunk was associated with an increase in the extrusive (eruption-like) rates of the ipsilateral incisor during the first 90 minutes after sympathectomy (*Fig. 9.15*). Similar results have been reported by Aars (1982a) with bilateral sympathectomy. Stimulation of the peripheral cut end of the sympathetic trunk was associated with intrusive movements of the incisor (*Fig. 9.16*). Similar findings have been described by Aars (1982a,b, 1983) and by Aars and Linden (1982). They also found that the intrusion induced by sympathetic nerve stimulation could be markedly reduced by both α-adrenoceptor antagonists (phentolamine) and by β-adrenoceptor blockade (Aars, 1982a,b, 1983; Aars and Linden, 1982).

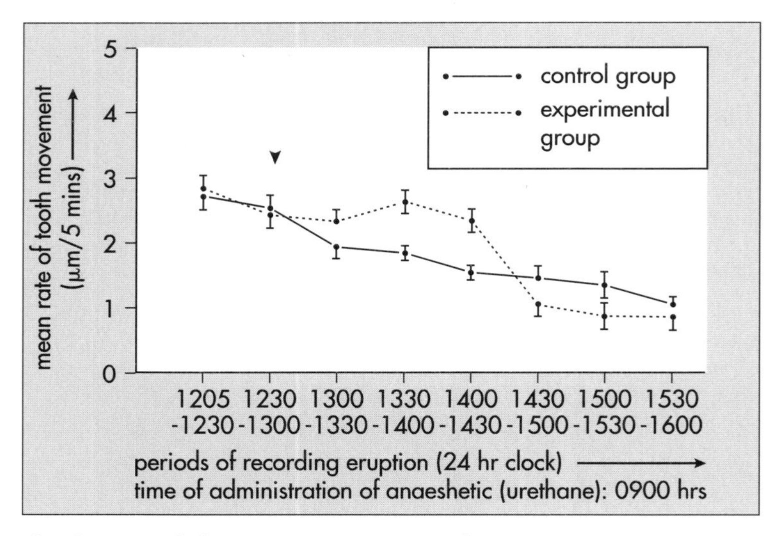

Fig. 9.15 Graph showing group mean rates of movement (in μm per 5 min) of erupting rabbit mandibular incisors for a control group of animals and an experimental group where the ipsilateral cervical sympathetic trunk was sectioned. These data were obtained using a variable capacitance displacement transducer measuring eruption over a 4-hour period (1200–1600 h). The marker arrow indicates that sympathectomy was undertaken in each animal of the experimental group at 1300 h. (Moxham, 1981.)

Third criterion

With regard to this criterion, if vascular–tissue pressures affect eruption then, in order to maintain an eruptive force, there must be a high-pressure system within and around the tooth either with free mobility of fluid or with differential pressures between the basal and coronal parts of the erupting tooth.

The possible role of tissue pressures in eruption has been reviewed by Burn-Murdoch (1988, 1990). It is clear that the various techniques for measuring tissue hydrostatic pressures are often difficult and can produce disparate results. In the main, the tissue pressures recorded in and around the tooth have been high, considering the low, and sometimes even negative, values (in relation to atmospheric pressure) that have been recorded from other connective tissues (e.g. Guyton, 1963, 1976). Pressures in the dental pulp of about 20 mm Hg above atmospheric pressure (and up to 60 mm Hg) have been reported (Wynn *et al.*, 1963; Beveridge *et al.*, 1964; Brown and Yankowitz, 1964; Brown and Beveridge, 1966; Brown *et al.*, 1969; van Hassel and Brown, 1969; van Hassel, 1971; Stenvik *et al.*, 1972; van Hassel and McMinn, 1972). Within the PDLs of dog canines, pressures of about 10 mm Hg above atmospheric pressure have been recorded (Lamb and van Hassel, 1972; Palcanis, 1973), although Walker *et al.* (1978) claim that the pressures are below atmospheric pressure. Aladdin and Burn-Murdoch (1987) and Burn-Murdoch (1988) have also reported negative pressures in the pulps of erupting rat incisors. More recently, Kristiansen and Heyeraas (1989) seemed to have developed a reliable technique for measuring PDL interstitial pressures directly and have reported that, for the rat PDL, the pressures average 15 mm Hg above atmospheric pressure (see Chapter 6).

It can be argued that, if pressure in or around the tooth is to produce eruptive movements, there must be a pressure gradient, the direction of which favours axial movement of the tooth out of its socket. Ness (1964) suggested that this pressure acts in, and is restricted to, the basal region of the root. With the exception of periapical effusions said to be of vascular origin and described by Magnusson (1968), there is little evidence to support these ideas. Thomas (1976) is of the opinion that the results of resection and transection experiments argue against the vascular hypotheses. It was his belief that the surgical treatment prevents the build up of pressure by 'opening the system'. However, it has been reported that fluid fills the space beneath the erupting resected tooth (Berkovitz, 1971) (see *Fig. 9.10*). The possibility that this fluid can attain a pressure that is sufficiently great to be responsible for the

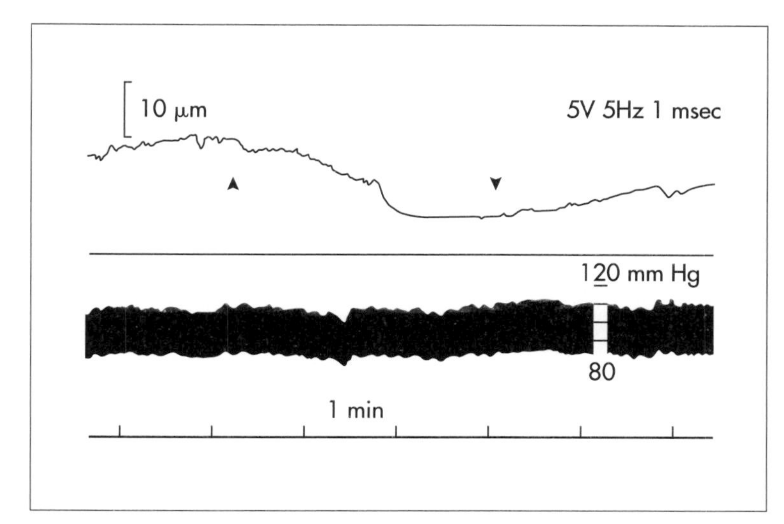

Fig. 9.16 Movements of a rabbit mandibular incisor recorded using a variable capacitance displacement transducer when the peripheral cut end of the ipsilateral cervical sympathetic trunk was stimulated. In this case, the stimulus strength was 5 V, the frequency of the impulses was 5 Hz, and the duration of each impulse was 1 ms. The period of stimulation was 3 minutes, as indicated by the marker arrowhead. (Moxham, 1981.)

eruption of the resected tooth cannot be dismissed. Indeed, Aladdin and Burn-Murdoch (1985b) and Burn-Murdoch (1988) have reported that daily irrigation of the base of the resected socket with isotonic saline (to prevent pressure developing in the socket, or to reduce it) and maintaining the sockets of resected incisors open to the oral cavity significantly reduced the unimpeded eruption rates. When hypertonic solutions were placed in the pulp cavity (to withdraw fluid from the resected base and hence to lower pressures) eruption was again slowed.

A differential between the pressures in the tissues above and below an erupting tooth has been demonstrated by van Hassel and McMinn (1972). They showed that the average tissue pressure above erupting teeth in young dogs was 10 mm Hg above atmospheric pressure. The average pressure within the pulps of the erupting teeth was 23 mm Hg above atmospheric pressure. In every case, the pressure differential favoured eruptive movements (the mean differential being 13±4 mm Hg). Assuming the tissue pressure at the base of the tooth to be the same as that for the coronal pulp tissue from which pressure recordings were monitored, the authors calculated that an average force of 15 g could be generated by the tissue fluid at the base of the tooth. It has yet to be determined, however, whether a force of this magnitude is sufficient to cause a tooth to erupt, since the nature and magnitude of the forces resisting eruption are unknown. The mechanism responsible for maintaining these pressure gradients is also not known.

Fourth criterion

For this criterion, recent reviews of the biochemistry of the dental connective tissues have been provided by Carmichael (1982), Gathercole and Keller (1982), Pearson (1982), Rahmetulla (1992), and Mariotti (1993), and these reviews provide some information pertinent to the vascular hypotheses of eruption (see also Chapter 4). Hydrostatic pressures in connective tissues may be exerted either by fluid that is free in the tissues or by fluid which is bound to fibres or ground substance. The ground substance, through its hyaluronate and sulphated proteoglycans, appears to be the major water-binding constituent of a connective tissue (Schubert and Hamerman, 1968; Bentley, 1970; Melcher and Walker, 1976; Bettelheim and Brady, 1979; Pearson, 1982). Glycosaminoglycan chains in dilute solutions are known to extend segmentally away from the central core protein, creating a water entrapping domain. In tissue such as cartilage, proteoglycans can attain concentrations of 10 per cent or more as their wet weight in the matrix, such that they occupy volumes of 10 mg/ml or less. In this state, the glycosaminoglycan chains have been demonstrated by ^{13}C-NMR studies still to be segmentally mobile (Torchia *et al.*, 1977) and to have a high anionic charge density. It is by this method that the glycosaminoglycans exert a swelling pressure that is resisted by the rigid collagenous network. This process allows tissues such as cartilage to withstand compressive loads with minimal deformation. Guyton (1972) has shown that interstitial gel removed from a tissue and placed in an electrolyte medium can swell considerably (up to 50 per cent) and will exert much pressure against any physical barrier that attempts to prevent its swelling. The PDL, and tooth position, may be affected by electrolyte balance; this is indicated by the work of Tyler and Burn-Murdoch (1976). Using incisor teeth in dissected rat mandibles, they reported that solutions of varying electrolyte content, when perfused into the PDL, produced predictable intrusive and extrusive tooth movements depending upon whether the solutions were hypertonic or hypotonic. This work has recently been developed to study the effects of such solutions *in vivo* (see page 201).

Pearson (1982), reviewing the work of Gibson (1979), reported that the composition of the ground substance in the PDLs of bovine incisors changed at various stages of tooth eruption (*Fig. 9.17*). If proteoglycans are involved in the mechanism of tooth eruption, it seems more likely to be proteoglycan-1 than proteodermatan sulphate because of the quantitative changes and the probable locations of the proteoglycans in the tissue. An interfibrillar location of proteoglycan-1 would allow a fuller expression of its ability to influence the osmotic pressure and swelling of the tissue compared with proteodermatan sulphate, which is more intimately associated with collagen fibrils (e.g. Pearson, 1982). The latter association might partly 'tie up' the dermatan sulphate chains and reduce their effect on tissue swelling, in a manner similar to that observed when glycosaminoglycans in umbilical cord or cornea are allowed to interact with polycations (Gelman and Silberberg, 1976; Comper and Laurent, 1978). Hyaluronate, like proteoglycan-1, will be less affected by interactions with collagen. However, the content of this glycosaminoglycan is almost constant during eruption. Thus, proteoglycan-1 may control the internal osmotic pressure of the PDL during tooth eruption. Furthermore, small changes in concentration of glycosaminoglycans and proteoglycans may have a considerable effect on osmotic pressures because their behaviour is 'non-ideal' (Comper and Laurent, 1978; Urban *et al.* 1979). Any physical swelling of the tissue is likely to be opposed by the elastic contribution of the collagen fibres (Comper and Laurent, 1978). However, the development of the collagen fibres shows considerable variation in erupting teeth (see Chapter 8). Komatsu and Chiba (1987) have measured the colloid osmotic pressure of the dental pulp fluid in the rat incisor after pulpotomy. They reported that the osmotic pressures decreased with decreases in eruption rates. Care must be taken in interpretation, however, because long-term changes in osmotic pressure might have important influences not only on the interstitial fluids but also on the morphology and behaviour of the cells (as suggested for chondrocytes by Ogston, 1970).

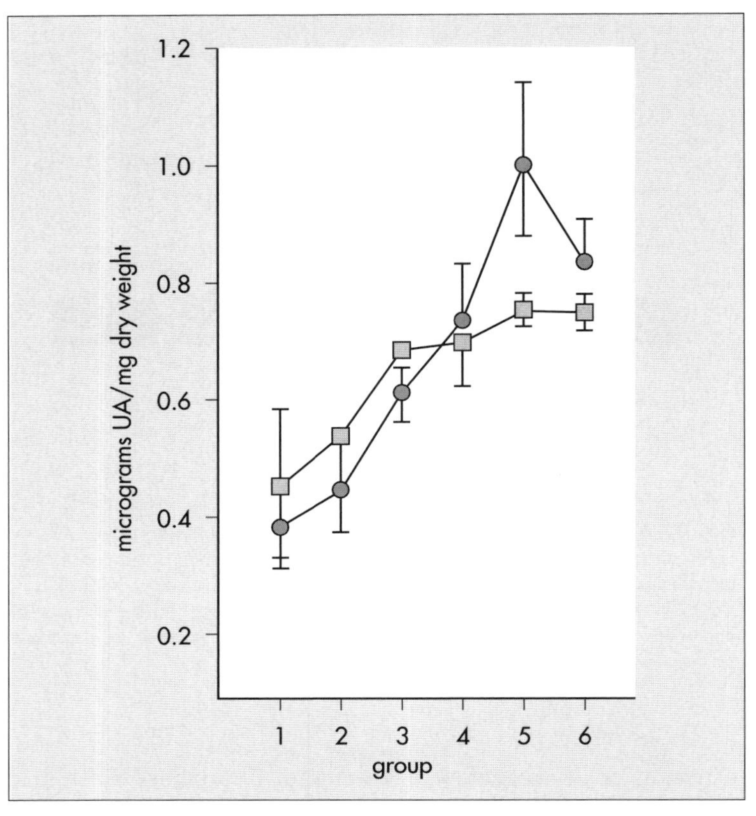

Fig. 9.17 Glycosaminoglycans in the developing PDL. Unerupted and erupted bovine incisors were divided into six groups according to size, wet weight, root formation, position in the jaw, and attrition. Follicle and ligaments were dissected for histological examination and isolation of glycosaminoglycan fractions. Group 1 specimens consisted of dental follicle. A recognizable periodontal ligament had developed in group 2 specimens. Sharpey fibres were discerned in group 3 onwards. Average root length increased from groups 2 to 4, but no significant lengthening was observed in group 5 or 6. The typical obliquely oriented collagen fibres were first observed in group 5 specimens (at which stage the tooth had just erupted into the oral cavity), and such fibres were predominant in group 6 specimens from fully erupted teeth. Note the significant increase in one of the glycosaminoglycan fractions during the stage of active eruption. The closed circles represent proteoglycan 1. The squares represent dermatan sulphate. (Courtesy Dr CH Pearson.)

The effect of rate of eruption on PDL glycosylaminoglycan (GAG) content has recently been reported by Kirkham *et al.* (1993). Experiments were conducted in which the rate of eruption of rat incisors was either increased by making the tooth unimpeded or eliminated by means of pinning. Sulphated GAG content increased fourfold during accelerated eruption, and it decreased correspondingly in the absence of eruption. The data are consistent with the view that the ground substance of the PDL plays a role in the generation of the eruptive force. Another possibility is that the changes reflect changes in turnover of the extracellular matrix in response to changes in eruption rate. This is unlikely, however, because both collagen and sulphated GAG turnover rates in the PDL of unimpeded teeth do not appear to change (Slootweg, 1976; van den Bos and Tonino, 1984) nor do they change when eruption is prevented (Taverne, 1989). Another explanation may be found in relation to the recent findings that cell motility is influenced by the GAG composition of the ground substance within a connective tissue (see Chapter 4). Thus, the data may be interpreted as being consistent with the fibroblast traction hypothesis of eruption. However, this still assumes that the eruptive force is a tractional force, an assumption that is not borne out by the available evidence (see page 191). Furthermore, although a particular GAG (e.g. chondroitin sulphate) may promote cell motility in some situations, in other tissues the same GAG inhibits motility.

Fifth criterion

Histological and ultrastructural studies provide some information about the role of the vasculature during tooth eruption. Bryer (1957) studied the effects of nutritional disturbances and surgical interference on the eruption of the rodent incisor, relating the resulting changes in vascularity of the PDL to eruption rate. He reported that a reduction in eruption (following vitamin A deficiency, rickets, vitamin D toxicity, cobalt administration, and various surgical interferences with the tissues and blood supply to the teeth) was associated with a reduced vascularity. An increase in eruption (during semistarvation and after localized sympathectomy) appeared to be associated with an increased vascularity. However, Bryer's studies relied upon a subjective assessment of vascularity without quantification. Furthermore, although vitamin C deficiency reduces eruption rates (Berkovitz, 1974), it is associated with hyperaemia and oedema of the pulp (Hojer and Westin, 1925; Key and Elphick, 1931; McLean *et al.*, 1939).

Magnusson (1968, 1973) observed what he called 'periapical effusions' beneath the molars of rats and monkeys. He claimed these effusions were induced by changes in the permeability of the periapical vessels. He further suggested that the effusions separated the tooth from the bone and thereby created the eruptive migration. However, the precise nature of such effusions awaits clarification, as does the question of whether they can generate a force sufficient to effect tooth eruption.

Several papers have been published which assessed quantitatively the ultrastructural features of the periodontal tissues in the rat dentition under different stages of eruption. Firstly, the tissues of the unimpeded and impeded rat incisor were compared, there being no major changes with respect to fibroblast morphology and the extracellular matrix (Shore *et al.*, 1982). In another study, the erupting and the erupted rat molar were studied, but again no differences were discerned for the cellular and extracellular components (Berkovitz *et al.*, 1984). Subsequently, Moxham *et al.* (1985) assessed quantitatively the ultrastructural features of the periodontal vasculature for the rat incisor at different locations along the PDL and for the fully erupted rat molar. Since there had been reports that the capillaries might be fenestrated (Corpron *et al.*, 1976; Frank *et al.*, 1976), Moxham *et al.* (1985) counted the number of fenestrations per mm^2 of endothelium and the number of fenestrations per mm^3 of tissue (*Table 9.2*). For the incisor PDL, the differences in the numbers of fenestrations along the length of the tooth could provide some basis for explaining differential vascular behaviour within the PDL, which might have a bearing on the eruptive mechanism. However, the distribution could be related to the high metabolic activity of the ligament (particularly in the proliferative basal region). This study also showed that the fully erupted rat molar (a tooth of limited growth) had almost four times as many fenestrations for its periodontal vasculature as the incisor. This suggested that the presence of fenestrations in the PDL might not be related directly to the eruptive mechanism. To assess this further, Moxham *et al.* (1987) compared the periodontal vasculatures of the erupting and the erupted rat molar. It was discovered that, whereas the PDL of the erupted molar contains a greater volume of capillaries, the ligament of the erupting tooth has a greater percentage of its capillary surface area occupied by fenestrations and contains a greater number of fenestrations per

Table 9.2
Data relating to the capillaries and fenestrations in the connective tissue of the periodontal ligaments of the incisor and first molar of the rat (Moxham *et al.*, 1985).

Tissue		Approximate distance from alveolar crest	Capillaries as percentage of tissue	Capillary surface area per mm^3 of tissue (μm^{2}x10^6)	Fenestrations per μm^2 of endothelium	Fenestrations per mm^3 of tissue (x10^6)
Incisor	segment 1	3 mm	6.7 ± 1.6	12.6 ± 1.6	0.078 ± 0.027	0.98 ± 0.31
	segment 2	8 mm	41.8 ± 7.6	25.0 ± 3.2	0.115 ± 0.029	2.87 ± 0.44
	segment 3	12 mm	52.0 ± 6.7	38.8 ± 1.7	0.105 ± 0.031	4.07 ± 1.38
Molar			22.1 ± 5.6	31.8 ± 7.6	0.370 ± 0.030	11.76 ± 3.01

unit volume of tissue (*Table 9.3*). Thus, unlike the connective tissue elements within the PDL, the periodontal vasculatures do at least demonstrate marked morphological changes that are related to the eruptive phase of the tooth.

CONCLUSIONS FROM APPLICATIONS OF THE FIVE CRITERIA

Several conclusions concerning the eruptive mechanism may be drawn from this section of the review.

1. Despite morphological and developmental differences between teeth of continuous and limited growth, there is information suggesting that the eruptive mechanisms are similar.
2. There is both experimental and theoretical evidence indicating that the eruptive process (including the mechanism for generating eruptive forces) is multifactorial.
3. The evidence showing that the eruptive forces are generated within the PDL or its developmental precursor (the dental follicle) is strong.
4. For teeth of both limited and continuous growth, the eruptive forces are not produced by tractional forces acting through the collagen framework of the PDL and do not necessarily require the development of the tooth root.
5. There is much evidence against the notion that collagen contraction within the PDL generates an eruptive force.
6. There is as yet little evidence to support the view that fibroblast migration or contraction is responsible for the eruptive force.
7. Evidence from various types of experiment suggests that at least one of the factors responsible for eruption is related to tissue hydrostatic pressures in the connective tissues around (and within) the tooth, moderated by the activity of the periodontal vasculature.

THE MECHANISMS OF MESIAL DRIFT

Although approximal drift in both mesial and distal directions has been reported (see page 186), most attention has been paid to mesial drift, since this is the main direction for human teeth. Consequently, this section is concerned with mechanisms of mesial drift. It is possible, however, that similar kinds of mechanisms are responsible for distal drift. Mesial drift can allow contact to be maintained between teeth after approximal wear. This will lead to a shortening of the dental arch (for review see Yilmaz *et al*., 1980), which may have relevance when considering the space requirements for the successful eruption of the third mandibular molars (e.g. Tait, 1982, 1984). Mesial drift can be visualized as affecting the dentition as a whole, or as a more localized movement affecting individual teeth. Furthermore, the movement may be a bodily one or a tilt.

The hypotheses that have been proposed to explain the mechanisms by which the forces producing drift are generated can be classified broadly into those that invoke external loads being placed upon the teeth and those in which forces are generated in the periodontium. In the first category are factors related to the anterior component of occlusal force, to oral soft-tissue pressures, and to erupting molars. In the second category are hypotheses relating to the deposition and resorption of alveolar bone and to contraction of the transseptal fibre system. Most of the research described has been undertaken on monkeys.

THE ANTERIOR COMPONENT OF OCCLUSAL FORCE

According to this hypothesis, when the teeth occlude, part of the force is transmitted in a forward direction because the teeth are inclined mesially. It is well known that the long axes of most human teeth are inclined mesially (e.g. Dewel, 1949). Stallard

Table 9.3
Data relating to the capillaries and fenestrations in the periodontal ligaments of erupted and erupting first molars of the rat (Moxham *et al.*, 1987).

Tissue	Capillaries as per cent of tissue	Capillary surface area ($\mu m^2 \times 10^6$) per mm^3 of tissue	Fenestrations per μm^2 of endothelium	Fenestrations per mm^3 of tissue ($\times 10^6$)
Erupted molar	22.1 ± 5.6	32.4 ± 7.8	0.37 ± 0.03	11.76 ± 3.01
Erupting molar	4.8 ± 1.0	14.8 ± 1.2	2.16 ± 0.54	30.45 ± 5.60
Significance of difference	$p < 0.05$	NS	$p < 0.05$	$p < 0.05$

(1923), Osborn (1961), Picton (1962) and Southard *et al.* (1989) have all demonstrated the reality of the anterior component of force in humans. Southard *et al.* (1989) used frictional force measurements and observed that distribution and dissipation of force at the contact points approximated to an exponential function. They found that for an occlusal load of 20 lb (9 kg), a force of 5 lb (2.25 kg) against the molars, and 11 lb (5 kg) against the canine was recorded. In some subjects, the force crossed the mid-line (up to the canine of the contralateral side) but did not progress across interdental spaces. Southard *et al.* (1990) and Southard *et al.* (1991) also found that interdental contact tightness was not a static feature of occlusion, but varied as a function of posture, a decrease being recorded in the supine position. However, whether an anterior component of occlusal force can be translated into the forward migration of mesial drift has not been clarified. It must also be remembered that occlusal loads are normally generated on the teeth for only relatively short periods (only a few minutes during the day; Graf, 1969).

Some evidence in favour of this hypothesis could be derived from the observations of Anders (1971), who prevented mesial tilting by rigidly splinting together posterior teeth and concluded that this decreased their tendency to migrate mesially.

Moss and Picton (1967) measured the approximal drift of the cheek teeth of *Macaca irus* monkeys with and without their antagonists, contact points being disked away to encourage movement. It was observed that teeth without antagonists continued to drift mesially. Indeed, they moved at faster rates, even leading to the suggestion that interlocking of opposing molars actually retards drift. Moss and Picton (1970) again showed that teeth migrated mesially in the absence of occlusal loads. Although these results argue against the anterior component of occlusal force, overeruption of the unopposed teeth did occur and the direction of overeruption may have contributed towards the drift (i.e. the molars, being inclined mesially, drifted mesially; the premolars, being inclined distally, drifted distally). Thus, it might also be concluded that teeth tend to drift in the direction in which they are aligned. However, Picton and Moss (1974) reported no significant correlation between the angulation of the roots of the cheek teeth of *Macaca irus* monkeys and the direction or distance of approximal drift of these teeth. They therefore concluded that the inclination of the roots was not an important factor contributing to drift. Picton and Moss (1978) also examined the effects of reducing cusp height on the rate of drift. They found that drift was significantly more rapid on the side with reduced cusps during the first 2–3 weeks (although less evident after longer periods), and they again concluded that interdigitation of cusps during normal function retards drift.

Unlike Moss and Picton (1967) and Picton and Moss (1978), van Beek and Fidler (1977) observed that the interdental spaces created between the cheek teeth of *Macaca irus* closed faster when the opposing teeth were in occlusion than when the teeth were out of occlusion (an average of 16.5 μm per week compared with 6.5 μm per week, the rates slowing down with time). The rate of space closure was an exponential rather than a linear one. In addition to grinding away the occlusal surfaces, these authors also disked the interproximal surfaces of both the mandibular and the opposing maxillary cheek teeth so that, in occlusion, the molars could move in pairs. They concluded that functional occlusion does play an important role in the mechanism of mesial tooth migration. These views were supported by van Beek (1979) who found mesial drift of first molars was reduced when the contact with the second molar was removed.

Picton and Moss (1980) reshaped the occlusal surfaces of teeth such that, in occlusion, the sloping of the cusps either favoured or opposed mesial drift. Although drift occurred in both situations, because it was greater where the slopes favoured drift, these authors conceded that an occlusal factor was at least partly involved in drift, but that it was not the most important factor (see page 207).

SOFT-TISSUE PRESSURES

Wallace (1904) first suggested that drift might be produced by forces exerted by the cheeks and the tongue. Winders (1962), Gould and Picton (1964) and Lear *et al.* (1965) have demonstrated the reality of such forces on buccal and lingual surfaces of human teeth. Weinstein (1967) showed that if the morphology of buccal or lingual surfaces of teeth was altered by inlays, the balance of soft-tissue pressures was disturbed and resulted in the teeth drifting.

To assess this hypothesis, Moss and Picton (1970) eliminated forces from the cheeks and tongue by placing an acrylic dome over the cheek teeth on one side of the arch. The opposing teeth were also extracted. After periods varying from 6–17 weeks, the molars covered by the dome were found to have drifted towards each other at approximately the same rate as the control teeth, suggesting that forces from the cheeks and tongue do not play a significant part in producing drift.

Yilmaz *et al.* (1980) studied drift occurring anterior to ankylosed deciduous mandibular molars. By a process of elimination, they concluded that drift of the anterior teeth might be due to pressure from the tongue.

THE ERUPTIVE FORCE OF MOLARS

It has been proposed that erupting molars exert a force against the distal aspect of the teeth immediately anterior, thereby producing mesial migration (Trauner, 1912; Korkhaus, 1938). Some evidence for this stems from the observation that space produced by extraction of premolars for orthodontic purposes is closed by drift of molars more rapidly in patients who have third molars than in patients where third molars had been previously extracted

(Schwarze, 1972, 1973). Further support for this view has been forwarded by van Beek (1979). He showed that mesial drifting of maxillary and mandibular first molars was reduced in *Macaca irus* if the interproximal contacts between first and second molars were removed.

To assess the possible forces from unerupted human third mandibular molars, Southard *et al.* (1991) measured contact tightness following unilateral removal of this tooth. If the hypothesis were true, then one might expect a decrease in the value of contact tightness on the operated side, while no change would indicate these teeth exerted no force. However, these authors reported a bilateral decrease on both sides following unilateral removal of an unerupted third molar. The cause of this unexpected result appeared to be the significant effect of posture on contact tightness.

The fact that forces from erupting molars are not essential for mesial drift is evident from observations that drift occurs:

- after the dentition has fully developed (e.g. Begg, 1954; Moss and Picton, 1967, 1970);
- in front of ankylosed teeth (Yilmaz *et al.*, 1980); and
- in teeth where there are no contacts with adjacent teeth (Moss and Picton, 1967, 1970).

THE DEPOSITION AND RESORPTION OF ALVEOLAR BONE

Mesial drifting of teeth has been attributed to bone deposition distal to the tooth with resorption mesially (Sicher and Weinmann, 1944). Although such histological changes are well documented (e.g. Moss and Picton, 1967; Robinson and Schneider, 1992), these may be the result rather than the cause of the migration. Furthermore, it is difficult to separate bone activity related to tooth movements from that related to jaw growth (e.g. Manson, 1968).

Apart from a consideration of alveolar bone involvement in drift, Dastmalchi *et al.* (1990) reported that cementum was significantly thicker on the distal surfaces of teeth and that the size of the difference increased with age. What the functional significance of this difference is remains unknown. The questions as to whether it is related to possible tensional forces generated on the distal root surface during drift, whether the amount deposited can account for the rates of drift reported and whether, like bone, it may be an effect rather than a cause, await clarification.

CONTRACTION OF THE TRANSSEPTAL FIBRE SYSTEM

Scott (1967) suggested that transseptal fibres might maintain contact between the teeth. Thompson *et al.* (1958), Boese (1969), Edwards (1970), Strahan and Mills (1970), and Pinson and Strahan (1974) have reported that the relapse of teeth moved orthodontically could be reduced when gingivectomy was undertaken. Murphey (1970) reported that, following extraction of the mandibular first molars in a young adult monkey, the adjacent premolars migrated distally once transseptal fibres developed across the healing socket. Such findings indicate that the gingival fibres may play a role in stabilizing tooth position and in restoring the position of displaced teeth. However, movement of teeth in association with extraction sites may relate to the presence of granulation tissue, which is not homologous to the normal state (see page 194).

On the basis of experiments that indicated that approximal drift could occur in the absence of forces from the tongue, cheeks, and opposing teeth, Moss and Picton (1967, 1970) concluded that the principal cause of drift lies in or around the roots of the teeth. Initially, these authors implicated contraction of the transseptal fibre system as the mechanism generating the force, but fibroblasts within the region have also been implicated in generating the tensional force (Moss, 1976; Picton and Moss, 1980). To assess this hypothesis, Picton and Moss (1973) measured the migration of the cheek teeth in monkeys after the interdental soft tissues were scraped away or cut vertically to interrupt the continuity of the transseptal fibre system. They reported a significant reduction in drift compared with teeth with non-traumatized gingivae in the same animal. (Significantly, even the surgically treated teeth drifted approximately 20 μm per week, compared with 55 μm per week for control teeth.) It is possible, of course, that inflammatory changes influenced the results, perhaps by increasing the resistance to drift. However, in two animals where there was repeated surgical removal of interdental papillae without apparent effects on the deeper transseptal fibres, the rates of drift were not reduced, suggesting that inflammation alone was not a significant factor in retarding drift.

Moss and Picton (1974) surgically divided first and second mandibular molars into mesial and distal fragments. Where the interdental tissues were not damaged, the mesial and distal fragments of a tooth moved apart. Where the interdental tissues were scraped away, mesial and distal fragments initially remained stationary (though they later moved together), providing some evidence of a tensional system in the interdental region. Using a movement transducer to provide a continuous recording of tooth position, Moss and Picton (1982) demonstrated a sustained approximation of pairs of adjacent teeth during a recording period of 2 hours; this occurred immediately after tooth contacts were removed. They proposed that removal of the approximal tooth contact allowed the transseptal fibre system to contract and produce approximation of the adjacent teeth. Removal of tooth contacts with teeth adjacent to the test pairs of teeth caused separation of the latter, the underlying basis again being interpreted as contraction of the transseptal fibres.

Using lead acetate as a bone marker in rats, Robinson and Schneider (1992) found that, following the surgical removal of the transseptal fibre region (supracrestal fibrotomy), there was a significant decrease in both horizontal and vertical bone deposition, indicating a decrease both in drift and in vertical tooth movements compared with controls.

Although admitting a contribution by occlusal forces to drift, 205) concluded that a greater contribution was provided by the transseptal fibres for, when the interdental soft tissues were surgically removed, the teeth whose reshaped occlusal forces favoured drift still moved very slowly together, whereas those whose reshaping did not favour drift moved apart.

Yilmaz *et al.* (1980) studied patients with a unilateral ankylosis affecting the deciduous molar. Forward movement of the teeth still occurred anterior to the ankylosed tooth in association with the presence of interdental spacing. In addition to providing evidence against the eruptive force of molars, these observations would also appear to argue against contraction of the transseptal fibres as causing mesial drift, because of the appearance of spacing during the forward movement of the anterior teeth. Whereas in humans all the teeth seemed to drift forwards at the same rate, different tooth types in the pig (where diastemata are present as a normal feature) drifted at different rates (Yilmaz *et al.*, 1981).

In summary, the mechanism causing mesial drift needs to be considered in the same critical way as that described for the eruptive mechanism. As for tooth eruption, no one hypothesis concerning a prime mover is supported by the experimental evidence, and likewise, the mechanism can be regarded as multifactorial. In terms of involvement of the periodontium, only the interdental gingiva has been considered. However, if the PDL is implicated (if only as a secondary factor whose remodelling is necessary to allow for movement), then the factors relating to the role of the ligament in eruption (see page 00) are relevant to a discussion on mesial drift. To date, there is insufficient basic information to enable us to define the characteristics of the system necessary to produce drift. For example, what is the magnitude of the force necessary to produce drift, and what is the resistive force that has to be overcome to produce movement? And, is drift a continuous or an intermittent process?

REFERENCES

Aars H (1976) Sympathetic nervous control of axial position of the rabbit incisor tooth. Acta Physiol Scand Suppl 440, 131.

Aars H (1982a) The influence of sympathetic nerve activity on axial position of the rabbit incisor tooth. Acta Physiol Scand 116, 417–421.

Aars H (1982b) The influence of vascular β-adrenoceptors on the position and mobility of the rabbit incisor tooth. Acta Physiol Scand 116, 423–428.

Aars H (1983) Effects of sympathetic nerve activity on changes in the position of the rabbit incisor tooth evoked by acute alterations in arterial blood pressure. Arch Oral Biol 28, 497–500.

Aars H and Linden RWA (1982) The effects of sympathetic trunk stimulation on the position and mobility of the canine tooth of the cat. Arch Oral Biol 27, 399–404.

Abercrombie MA and Heaysman JEM (1953) Observations on the social behaviour of cells in tissue culture. 1. Speed of movement of chick heart fibroblasts in relation to their mutual contacts. Exp Cell Res 5, 111–131.

Adams D and Main JHP (1962) A radiographic method of measuring unimpeded eruption rates in the rat incisor. J Physiol 160, 1–2.

Adatia AK and Berkovitz BKB (1981) The effects of cyclophosphamide on eruption of the continuously growing mandibular incisor of the rat. Arch Oral Biol 26, 607–613.

Ainamo J and Talari A (1976) Eruptive movements of teeth in human adults. In: The Eruption and Occlusion of Teeth (Poole DF and Stack MV, eds), pp 97–107, Butterworths, London.

Aladdin QI and Burn-Murdoch RA (1984) From where should eruption rates be measured? J Dent 63, 512.

Aladdin QI and Burn-Murdoch RA (1985a) Techniques for choosing reference points from which to measure eruption rates of rat incisors. Arch Oral Biol 30, 531–537.

Aladdin QI and Burn-Murdoch RA (1985b) The effect of procedures intended to alter the interstitial fluid pressure in the sockets of resected rat incisors on their eruption rates. Arch Oral Biol 30, 525–530.

Aladdin QI and Burn-Murdoch RA (1987) Interstitial fluid pressure in the pulp of the rat incisor. Arch Oral Biol 32, 307–309.

Anders I (1971) Use of the curved laminographic technique to study mesial migration due to functional forces. J Dent Res 50, p 704.

Aubin JE and Opas M (1989) Cell adhesion and contractility. In: Biological Mechanisms of Tooth Eruption and Root Resorption (Davidovitch Z, ed), pp 43–51, EBSCO Media, Birmingham, Alabama.

Azuma M, Enlow D, Fredrickson RG and Gaston LG (1975) A myofibroblastic basis for the physical forces that produce tooth drift and eruption, skeletal displacement of sutures, and periosteal migration. In Determinants of Mandibular Form and Growth (McNamara JD, ed), pp 179–207, University of Michigan, Ann Arbor.

Bailey AJ (1968) The nature of collagen. Comp Biochem Physiol [B] 26, 297–423.

Bailey AJ (1976) In: The Eruption and Occlusion of Teeth (Poole DFG and Stack MV, ed), pp 306–307, Wrights, Bristol.

Barcroft H and Swan HJC (1953) Sympathetic control of human blood vessels. Monogr Physiol Soc 1.

Bard JBL and Hay ED (1975) The behaviour of fibroblasts from developing avian cornea. J Cell Biol 67, 400–418.

Barnes JM and Kodicek E (1972) Biological hydroxylations and ascorbic acid with special regard to collagen metabolism. Vitam Horm 30, 1–43.

Barrow CG and White JR (1952) Developmental changes of the maxillary and mandibular dental arches. Angle Orthodont 22, 41–46.

Baume LJ (1950) Physiologic tooth migration and its significance for the development of occlusion. J Dent Res 29, 331–337.

Baume LJ (1953) The development of the lower permanent incisors and their supporting bone. Am J Orthod 39, 526–544.

Baume LJ and Becks H (1950) Development of the dentition of *Macaca mulatta*. Am J Orthod 36, 723–748.

Beertsen W (1973) Tissue dynamics in the periodontal ligament of the mandibular incisor of the mouse: a preliminary report. Arch Oral Biol 18, 61–66.

Beertsen W (1975) Migration of fibroblasts in the periodontal ligament of the mouse incisor as revealed by autoradiography. Arch Oral Biol 20, 659–666.

Beertsen W and Everts V (1977) The site of remodelling of collagen in the periodontal ligament of the mouse incisor. Anat Rec 189, 479–498.

Beertsen W and Hoeben KA (1987) Movement of fibroblasts in the periodontal ligament of the mouse incisor is related to eruption. J Dent Res 66, 1006–1010.

Beertsen W, Everts V, Hoeben KA and Niehof J (1984) Microtubules in periodontal ligament cells in relation to tooth eruption and collagen degradation. J Periodont Res 19, 489–500.

Beertsen W, Everts V and Van Den Hooff A (1974) Fine structure of fibroblasts in the periodontal ligament of the rat incisor and their possible role in tooth eruption. Arch Oral Biol 19, 1087–1098.

Begg PR (1954) Stone Age man's dentition with reference to anatomically correct occlusion, the etiology of malocclusion, and a technique for its treatment. Am J Orthodont 40, 298–312, 373–383, 462–475, 517–531.

Bellows CG, Melcher AH and Aubin JE (1981) Contraction and organization of collagen gels by cells cultured from periodontal ligament, gingiva and bone suggest functional differences between the cell types. J Cell Sci 50, 299–314.

Bellows CG, Melcher AH and Aubin JE (1982a) Association between tension and orientation of periodontal ligament fibroblasts and exogenous collagen fibres in collagen gels in vitro. J Cell Sci 58, 125–138.

Bellows CG, Melcher AH, Bhargava U and Aubin JE (1982b) Fibroblasts contracting three-dimensional collagen gels exhibit ultrastructure consistent with either contraction or protein secretion. J Ultrastruct Res 78, 178–192.

Bentley JP (1970) The biological role of the ground substance mucopolysaccharides. Adv Biol Skin 10, 103–121.

Berkovitz BKB (1971) The effect of root transection and partial root resection on the unimpeded eruption rate of the rat incisor. Arch Oral Biol 16, 1033–1043.

Berkovitz BKB (1972) The effect of demecolcine and of triethanomelamine on the unimpeded eruption rate of normal and root resected incisor teeth in rats. Arch Oral Biol 17, 937–947.

Berkovitz BKB (1974) The effect of vitamin C deficient diet on eruption rates for the guinea pig lower incisor. Arch Oral Biol 197, 807–814.

Berkovitz BKB and Bass TB (1976) Eruption rates of human upper third molars. J Dent Res 55, 460–464.

Berkovitz BKB, Migdalski A and Solomon M (1972) The effect of the lathyritic agent aminoacetonitrile on the unimpeded eruption rate in normal and root-resected rat lower incisors. Arch Oral Biol 17, 1755–1763.

Berkovitz BKB and Moxham BJ (1984) The mobility of the lathyritic rabbit incisor in response to axially directed extrusive loads. Arch Oral Biol 29, 773–778.

Berkovitz BKB and Moxham BJ (1990) The development of the periodontal ligament with special reference to collagen fibre ontogeny. J Biol Buccale 18, 227–236.

Berkovitz BKB, Shore RC and Moxham BJ (1984) Ultrastructural studies on the developing periodontal ligament. In: Tooth Morphogenesis and Differentiation 125 (Ruch JV and Belcourt AB, eds), pp 545–556, Colloquium of the Institut National de la Santé et de la Recherche Médicale.

Berkovitz BKB, Shore RC and Moxham BJ (1985) Ultrastructural studies on the developing periodontal ligament. INSERM 125, 545–556.

Berkovitz BKB and Thomas NR (1969) Unimpeded eruption in the root-resected lower incisor of the rat with a preliminary note on root transection. Arch Oral Biol 14, 771–780.

Bettelheim FA and Brady E (1979) Hydration and proteoglycan content of rat skin. In: Glycoconjugates (Schauer R *et al.*, eds) pp 662–664, Georg Thieme, Stuttgart.

Beveridge E, Gross R, Yankowitz D and Brown AC (1964) The relation between dental pulp tissue pressure and systemic arterial blood pressure. J Dent Res 43, 805.

Bjork A and Skieller V (1972) Facial development and tooth eruption. An implant study at the age of puberty. Am J Orthod 62, 339–383.

Black GV (1936) Operative Dentistry, volume 1, Medico-Dental, Chicago.

Boese LR (1969) Increased stability of orthodontically rotated teeth following gingivectomy in *Macaca nemestrina*. Am J Orthodont 56, 273–290.

Bornstein P (1974) The biosynthesis of collagen. Ann Rev Biochem 43, 567–603.

Boura ALA and Green AF (1965) Adrenergic neurone blocking agents. Ann Rev Pharmacol 5, 183–212.

Boyle, PE (1955) Kronfeld's Histopathology of the Teeth and their Surrounding Structures, 4th edition, Kimpton, London.

Brash JC (1927) The growth of the alveolar bone and its relation to the movement of teeth, including eruption. Part II. Dent Rec 27, 1–27.

Brash JC (1928) The growth of the alveolar bone and its relation to the movements of the teeth including eruption. Int J Orthod 14, 196–223, 283–293, 398–405, 487–494, 494–504.

Breitner C and Leist M (1927) Über den Einfluss des vegetativum Nervensystems auf die Zähne. Z Stomatol 25, 772–776.

Brin I, Zilberman Y, Galili D and Fuks A (1985) Eruption of rootless teeth in congenital renal disease. Oral Surg Oral Med Oral Pathol 60, 61–64.

Brown AC and Beveridge EE (1966) The relation between tooth pulp pressure and systemic arterial pressure. Arch Oral Biol 11, 1181–1193.

Brown VP and Daugaard-Jensen I (1950) Changes in the dentition from the early teens to the early twenties. Acta Odont Scand 9, 177–192.

Brown AC and Yankowitz D (1964) Tooth pulp tissue pressure and hydraulic permeability. Circ Res 15, 42–50.

Brown AC, Barrow BL, Gadd GN and Van Hassel HJ (1969) Tooth pulp transcapillary osmotic pressure in the dog. Arch Oral Biol 14, 491–502.

Brunette DM, Kanoza RJ, Marmary Y, Chan J and Melcher AH (1977) Interactions between epithelial and fibroblast-like cells in cultures derived from monkey periodontal ligament. J Cell Sci 27, 127–140.

Bryer LW (1957) An experimental evaluation of the physiology of tooth eruption. Int Dent J 7, 432–478.

Burke PH (1963) Eruptive movements of permanent maxillary central incisor teeth in the human. Proc R Soc Med 56, 513–515.

Burke PH and Newell DJ (1958) A photographic method of measuring eruption of certain human teeth. Am J Orthod 44, 590–602.

Burn-Murdoch RA (1981) The effect of applied forces on the eruption of rat maxillary incisors. Arch Oral Biol 26, 939–943.

Burn-Murdoch RA (1988) The effects of corticosteroids and cyclophosphamide on the eruption of resected incisor teeth in the rat. Arch Oral Biol 33, 661–667.

Burn-Murdoch RA (1989) Does interstitial pressure have a role in tooth eruption? In: Biological Mechanisms of Tooth Eruption and Root Resorption (Davidovitch Z, ed), pp 225–232, EBSCO Media, Birmingham, Alabama.

Burn-Murdoch RA (1990) The role of the vasculature in tooth eruption. Eur J Orthod 12, 101–108.

Burn-Murdoch RA (1992) The effect of consistency of the diet and shortening incisor teeth in rats on the eruption rates and intraoral lengths of the shortened incisors. J Physiol 446.

Burn-Murdoch RA (in press) In: The Biological Mechanisms of Tooth Eruption, Resorption and Replacement by Implants (Davidovitch Z, ed), EBSCO Media, Birmingham, Alabama.

Burn-Murdoch RA and Light L (1992) Assessing the stability of reference points used for recording movements by discontinuing measurements of position. J Physiol 446, 477P.

Cahill DR (1969) Eruptive pathway formation in the presence of experimental tooth impaction in puppies. Anat Rec 164, 67–78.

Cahill DR (1970) The histology and rate of tooth eruption with and without temporary impaction in the dog. Anat Rec 166, 225–238.

Cahill DR and Marks SCJr. (1980) Tooth eruption: evidence for the central role of the dental follicle. J Oral Pathol 9, 189–200.

Cahill DR and Marks SCJr. (1982) Chronology and histology of exfoliation and eruption of mandibular premolars in dogs. J Morphol 171, 213–218.

Cahill DR, Marks SC Jr, Wise GE and Gorski JP (1988) A review and comparison of tooth eruption systems used in experimentation – a new proposal on tooth eruption. In: Biological Mechanisms of Tooth Eruption and Root Resorption (Davidovitch Z, ed), pp 1–7, EBSCO Media, Birmingham,Alabama.

Carl W and Wood R (1980) Effects of irradiation on the developing dentition and supporting bone. J Am Dent Asooc 101, 646–648.

Carlson H (1944) Studies on the rate and amount of eruption of certain human teeth. Am J Orthod 30, 575–588.

Carmichael DJ (1982) Biochemistry of the fibres of the periodontal ligament. In: The Periodontal Ligament in Health and Disease (Berkovitz BKB, Moxham BJ and Newman HN, eds), pp 197–213, Pergamon Press, Oxford.

Carne DF (1924) A new theory of the eruption of the teeth. Br Dent J 45, 624–632.

Castor CW and Prince RK (1964) Modulation of the intrinsic viscosity of hyaluronic acid formed by human fibroblasts *in vitro*: the effects of hydrocortisone and colchicine. Biochim Biophys Acta 83, 165–177.

Chattergee GC (1967) Effects of ascorbic acid deficiency in animals. In: The Vitamins, volume 1 (Sebrell WH and Harris RS, eds), pp 407–437, Academic Press, London.

Chiba M (in press).

Chiba M and Komatsu K (1988) *In vitro* estimation of the resisting force of tooth eruption and the zone of shear in the rat incisor. In: Biological Mechanisms of Tooth Eruption and Root Resorption. (Davidovitch Z, ed), pp 193–205, EBSCO Media, Birmingham, Alabama.

Chiba M, Tsuruta M and Eto K (1973) A photographic method of measuring eruption rates of rat mandibular incisors. Arch Oral Biol 18, 1003–1010.

Chiba M and Ohshima S (1985) Effects of colchicine and hydrocortisone on unimpeded eruption rates of root-resected mandibular incisors of rats. Arch Oral Biol 30, 147–153.

Chiba M, Ohshima S and Takizawa K (1983) The effect of a microfilament-disrupting drug, chytochalasin B, on 6-hourly and daily eruption rates of the rat mandibular incisor. Arch Oral Biol 28, 651–653.

Chiba M, Takizawa K and Ohshima S (1980) Dose-response effects of colchicine and vinblastine on unimpeded eruption rates of the rat mandibular incisor. Arch Oral Biol 25, 115–119.

Clinch L (1951) An analysis of serial models between three and eight years of age. Dent Rec 71, 61–72.

Cohen JT (1940) Growth and development of the dental arches in children. J Am Dent Assoc 27, 1250–1260.

Cohn SA (1966) Disuse atrophy of the periodontium in mice following partial loss of function. Arch Oral Biol 11, 95–105.

Comper WD and Laurent TC (1978) Physiological function of connective tissue polysaccharides. Physiol Rev 58, 255–315.

Constant TE (1900) The eruption of the teeth. Int Dent Congr 2, 180–192.

Corpron KE, Avery JK, Morawa AP and Lee SD (1976) Ultrastructure of capillaries in mouse periodontium. J Dent Res 55, 551.

Corruccini RS (1990) Australian aboriginal tooth succession, interproximal attrition and Begg's theory. Am J Orthod Dentofacial Orthop 97, 349–357.

Dalldorf G and Zall C (1930) Tooth growth in experimental scurvy. J Exp Med 52, 57–63.

Darling AI and Levers BGH (1975) The pattern of eruption of some human teeth. Arch Oral Biol 20, 89–96.

Darling AI and Levers BGH (1976) The pattern of eruption. In: The Eruption and Occlusion of Teeth (Poole DFG and Stack MV, eds), pp 80–96, Butterworths, London.

Dastmalchi R, Polson A, Bouwsma O and Proskin H (1990) Cementum thickness and mesial drift. J Clin Periodont 17, 709–713.

Dewel BF (1949) Clinical observations on the axial inclination of teeth. Am J Orthodont 35, 98–115.

Di Biase DD (1976) Dental abnormalities affecting eruption. In: The Eruption and Occlusion of Teeth. (Poole DFG and Stack MV, eds), pp 156–168, Butterworths, London.

Dreyer CW and Sampson WJ (1984) Effects of lathyrism on mouse molar migration. J Periodont Res 19, 424–433.

Edwards JG (1970) A surgical procedure to eliminate rotational relapse. Am J Orthodont 57, 35–46.

Fergusson FC Jr (1952) Colchicine. 1. General pharmacology. J Pharmacol Exp Therapy 106, 261–270.

Fletcher GGT (1963) A cephalometric appraisal of the development of malocclusion. Trans Br Soc Study Orthod 124–154.

Frank RM, Fellinger E and Steurer P (1976) Ultrastructure du ligament alveolodentaire du rat. J Biol Buccale 4, 295–313.

Friel S (1945) Migrations of teeth following extractions. Proc R Soc Med 38, 456–462.

Gabbiani G (1979) The role of contractile proteins in wound healing and fibrocontractive diseases. Methods Achiev Exp Pathol 9, 187–206.

Gabbiani G, Ryan GB and Majno G (1971) Presence of modified fibroblasts in granulation tissue and their possible role in wound contraction. Experientia 27, 549–550.

Garant PR (1976) Collagen resorption by fibroblasts. J Periodont 47, 380–390.

Garant PR and Cho MI (1979) Cytoplasmic polarisation of periodontal ligament fibroblasts. J Periodont Res 14, 95–106.

Garren L and Greep RO (1955) Effects of thyroid hormone and propylthiouracil on eruption rate of upper incisor teeth in rats. Proc Soc Exp Biol Med 90, 652–655.

Gathercole LJ and Keller A (1982) Biophysical aspects of the fibres of the periodontal ligament. In: The Periodontal Ligament in Health and Disease (Berkovitz BKB, Moxham BJ and Newman HN, eds), pp 197–213, Pergamon Press, Oxford.

Gelman RA and Silberberg A (1976) The effect of a strongly interacting macromolecular probe on the swelling and exclusion properties of loose connective tissue. Conn Tissue Res 4, 79–90.

Gibson (1979) Proteoglycans of the periodontal ligament. PhD thesis, University of Alberta.

Goldman RD, Schloss JA and Starger JM (1976) Organizational changes of actin-like microfilaments during animal cell movements. In Cell Motility Book (Goldman AR, Pollard T and Rosenbaum J, eds), pp 217–245, Cold Spring Harbour Laboratory.

Goldstein MS and Stanton FL (1935) Changes in dimension and form of the dental arches with age. Int J Orthod 21, 357–380.

Gorski JP (in press) In: The Biological Mechanisms of Tooth Eruption, Resorption and Replacement by Implants. EBSCO Media, Birmingham, Alabama.

Gorski JP, Marks SC Jr, Cahill DR and Wise GE (1988) Developmental changes in the extracellular matrix of the dental follicle during tooth eruption. Conn Tissue 18, 175–190.

Gorski JP and Marks SC Jr (1992) Current concepts of the biology of tooth eruption. Oral Biol Med 3, 185–206 (critical review).

Gould BS (1968) The role of certain vitamins in collagen formation. In: Treatise on Collagen (Gould BS, ed), pp 323–365, Academic Press, London.

Gould MSE and Picton DCA (1964) A study of pressures exerted by the lips and cheeks on the teeth of subjects with normal occlusion. Arch Oral Biol 9, 469–478.

Gowgiel JM (1961) Eruption of irradiation-produced rootless teeth in monkeys. J Dent 40, 538–547.

Graf H (1969) Bruxism. Dent Clin North Am 13, 659–665.

Grant D, Bernick S, Levy BM and Dreizin S (1972) A comparative study of periodontal ligament developed in teeth with and without predecessors in marmosets. J Periodont 43, 162–169.

Guyton AC (1963) A concept of negative interstitial pressure based on pressures in implanted capsules. Circulation 12, 399–414.

Guyton AC (1972) Compliance of the interstitial space and the measurement of tissue pressure. Pflugers Arch 336 (suppl), S1–S20.

Guyton AC (1976) Textbook of Medical Physiology, 5th edition, Saunders, Philadelphia.

Guyton AC, Granger HJ and Taylor AE (1971) Interstitial fluid pressure. Physiol Rev 51, 527–563.

Harkness RD (1968) Mechanical properties of collagenous tissues. In: Treatise on Collagen, volume 2, Biology of Collagen (Gould BS, ed), pp 248–310, Academic Press, London.
Harris AK and Dmytryk JJ (1989) Cell traction: implications for the mechanism of tooth eruption. In: Biological Mechanisms of Tooth Eruption and Root Resorption (Davidovitch Z, ed), pp 181–186. EBSCO Media, Alabama.
Harris AK, Stopak D and Wild PW (1981) Fibroblast traction as a mechanism for collagen morphogenesis. Nature 290, 249–251.
Harris AK, Wild PW and Stopak D (1980) Silicone rubber substrata: a new wrinkle in the study of cell locomotion. Science 208, 177–179.
Hay ED (1982) Interaction of embryonic cell surface and cytoskeleton with extracellular matrix. Am J Anat 165, 1–12.
Henriques AC (1953) The growth of the palate and the growth of the face during the period of the changing dentition. Am J Orthod 39, 836–858.
Hirschel BJ, Gabbiani G, Ryan GB and Majno G (1971) Fibroblasts of granulation tissue: immunofluorescent staining with antismooth muscle serum. Proc Soc Exp Biol Med 138, 466–469.
Hojer A and Westin G (1925) Jaws and teeth in scorbutic guinea pigs. Dental Cosmos 67, 1–24.
Hughes FJ and Issberner JP (1988) Phenotypic variations in contraction of fibroblasts derived from the periodontal tissues. J Dent Res 67, 646 (abstract).
Jacobson A (1983) The physiology of tooth eruption. Birth defects – original article series 19, 67–82.
James DW (1964) Wound contraction – a synthesis. In: Advances in Biology of Skin, volume 5. (Montagna W and Billingham RE, eds), pp 216–230, Pergamon, Oxford.
Kameyama Y (1973) The pattern of alveolar bone activity during development and eruption of the molar in the rat. J Periodont 8, 179–191.
Katona TR (1990) Engineering considerations in the design of abutments. The Compendium of Continuing Education in Dentistry 11, 382–388.
Katona TR, Boyle AM, Curcio FB, Keates JK, Mazzara RJ and Tackney VM (1987) Mechanisms of tooth eruption in a computer-generated analysis of functional jaw deformations in man. Arch Oral Biol 32, 367–369.
Katona TR, Boyle AM, Keates JK and Tackney VM (1989) An engineering model of tooth eruption in man. In: The Biological Mechanisms of Tooth Eruption and Root Resorption (Davidovitch Z, ed), pp 269–275 EBSCO Media, Birmingham, Alabama.
Katona TR, Tackney VM and Keates JK (1988) A computer model of the periodontal ligament space in man. Arch Oral Biol 33, 839–844.
Kenney EB and Ramfjord SP (1969) Patterns of root and alveolar bone growth associated with development and eruption of teeth in rhesus monkeys. J Dent Res 48, 251–256.
Key KM and Elphick GK (1931) A quantitative method for the determination of vitamin C. Biochem J 25, 888–897.
King JD (1937) Dietary deficiency, nerve lesions and the dental tissues. J Physiol 88, 62–77.
King GJ, Keeling SD, McCoy EA and Ward TH (1991) Measuring dental drift and orthodontic tooth movement in response to various initial forces in adult rats. Am J Orthod Dentofacial Orthop 99, 456–465.
Kirkham J, Robinson C, Phull JK, Shore RC, Moxham BJ and Berkovitz BKB (1993) The effect of rate of eruption on periodontal ligament glycosylaminoglycan content and enamel formation in the rat incisor. Cell Tissue Res 274, 413–419.
Knott VB (1961) Size and form of the dental arches in children with good occlusion studied longitudinally from age 9 years to late adolescence. Am J Phys Anthropol 19, 263–284.
Komatsu K and Chiba M (1987) Preliminary measurements of colloid osmotic pressure of the dental pulp fluid in the rat mandibular incisor after pulpotomy. In: Microcirculation – an Update, volume 2 (Tsuchiya *et al.*, eds), pp 121–122, Elsevier, Amsterdam.
Korber KH (1970) Periodontal pulsation. J Periodont 41, 686–708.
Korkhaus G (1938) Clinical studies of the ontogenetic development of the dentition. Dent Rec 58, 641–654.
Kostlàn J, Thorová J and Skach M (1960) Erupce llodavého zubu po resekei jeho rustové zony. Cslka Stomat 6, 401–410.
Kreis T and Vale R (1993) Guidebook to the Cytoskeletal and Motor Proteins. Oxford University Press, Oxford.
Kristiansen AB and Heyeraas KJ (1989) Micropuncture measurements of interstitial fluid pressure in the rat periodontal ligament. Proc Finn Dent Soc 85, 295–300.
Kronman JH (1971) Tissue reaction and recovery following experimental tooth movement. Angle Orthod 41, 125–132.
Kutsky RJ (1973) Handbook of Vitamins and Hormones. Van Nostrand Reinhold, New York.
Lamb RE and van Hassel HJ (1972) Tissue pressure in the periodontal ligament. J Dent 51 (abs), 240.
Lammie GA and Posselt U (1965) Progressive changes in the dentition of adults. J Periodont 36, 443–454.
Latham RA and Scott JH (1960) Mesial movement of the teeth in the Rhesus monkey. Eur Orthod Soc 199–203.
Lear CSG, Catz J, Grossman RC, Flanagan JB and Moorrees CFA (1965) Measurement of lateral muscle forces on the dental arches. Arch Oral Biol 10, 669–689.
Lebret LML (1967) Tooth migration. In: The Mechanisms of Tooth Support (Anderson DJ, Eastoe JE, Melcher AH and Picton DCA, eds), pp 120–125, Wright, Bristol.
Leendertz JA, Moxham BJ and Berkovitz BKB (1986) Computer-controlled force transducer and ultrasonic displacement transducer to continously record movement of tooth during loading. Med Biol Eng Comput 24, 216–218.
Leist M (1927) Über den Einfluss des vegetativum Nervensystems auf die Zähne. Z Stomat 25, 765–771.
Levers BJH and Darling AI (1983) Continuous eruption of some adult human teeth of ancient populations. Arch Oral Biol 28, 401–408.
Lewis J (1984) Morphogenesis by fibroblast traction. Nature 307, 413–444.
Lin F, Fan W and Wise GE (1992) Granule proteins of the dental follicle and stellate reticulum inhibit tooth eruption and eyelid opening in post-natal rats. Arch Oral Biol 37, 841–847.
Lisney SJW, Matthews B and Sharp SE (1972) Observations on eruption with use of a continuous recording technique. J Dent Res 51, 1265.
Litvin PE and De Marco TJ (1973) The effect of a diuretic and antidiuretic on tooth eruption. Oral Surg 35, 294–298.
Logan WHG (1935) A histologic study of the anatomical structures forming the oral cavity. J Am Dent Assoc 22, 3–30.
Lundström A (1969) Changes in crowding and spacing of the teeth with age. Dent Practr Dent Rec 19, 218–223.
Lysell L (1958) Qualitative and quantitative determination of attrition and the ensuing tooth migration. Acta Odont Scand 16, 267–292.
McLean DL, Sheppard M and McHenry EW (1939) Tissue changes in ascorbic acid deficient guinea pigs. Br J Expt Pathol 20, 451–457.
Magnusson B (1968) Tissue changes during molar tooth eruption. Trans R Schs Dent Stochk Umea 13, 1–122.
Magnusson B (1973) Autoradiographic study of erupting teeth in rats after intracardial injection of 131 1-fibrinogen. Scand J Dent 81, 130–134.
Main JHP and Adams D (1965) Measurement of the rate of eruption of the rat incisor. Arch Oral Biol 10, 999–1008.
Main JHP and Adams D (1966) Experiments on the rat incisor into the cellular proliferation and blood pressure theories of tooth eruption. Arch Oral Biol 11, 163–179.
Majno G, Gabbiani G, Hirschel BJ, Ryan GB and Statkov PR (1971) Contraction of granulation tissue *in vitro*: similarity to smooth muscle. Science 173, 548–550.
Manson JD (1967) Bone changes associated with tooth eruption. In: The Mechanism of Tooth Support (Anderson DJ, Eastoe JE, Melcher AH and Picton DCA, eds), pp 98–101, Wright, Bristol.

Manson JD (1968) A Comparative Study of the Postnatal Growth of the Mandible. Kimpton, London.

Mariotti A (1993) The extracellular matrix of the periodontium. Periodontology 2000 1, 39–63.

Marks SC Jr (1987) Tooth eruption: the regulation of a localized, bilaterally symmetrical metabolic event in alveolar bone. Scan Microsc 1, 1125–1133.

Marks SC Jr (in press) In: Biological Mechanisms of Tooth Eruption, Resorption and Replacement by Implants (Davidovitch Z, ed). EBSCO Media, Birmingham, Alabama.

Marks SC Jr and Cahill JR (1984) Experimental study in the dog of the non-active role of the tooth in the eruptive process. Arch Oral Biol 29, 311–322.

Marks SC Jr and Cahill JR (1986) Ultrastructure of alveolar bone during tooth eruption in the dog. Am J Anat 177, 427–438.

Marks SC Jr and Cahill JR (1987) Regional control by the dental follicle of alterations in alveolar bone metabolism during tooth eruption. J Oral Pathol 16, 164–169.

Marks SC Jr, Cahill JR and Wise GE (1983) The cytology of the dental follicle and adjacent alveolar bone during tooth eruption in the dog. Am J Anat 168, 277–289.

Massler M and Schour J (1941) Studies on tooth development. Am J Orthod 27, 552–576.

Matthews B and Berkovitz BKB (1972) Continuous recording of tooth eruption in the rabbit. Arch Oral Biol 17, 817–820.

Melcher AH (1967) Remodelling of the periodontal ligament during eruption of the rat incisor. Arch Oral Biol 12, 1649–1652.

Melcher AH and Beertsen W (1977) The physiology of tooth eruption. In: The Biology of Occlusal Development. Monographs in Craniofacial Growth, number 7 (McNamara JA, ed), pp 1–23, University of Michigan, Ann Arbor.

Melcher AH and Walker TW (1976) The periodontal ligament in attachment and as a shock absorber. In: The Eruption and Occlusion of Teeth (Poole DPG and Stack MV, eds), pp 183–192, Butterworths, London.

Michaeli Y, Pitaru S, Zajicek G and Weinreb MM (1975) Role of attrition and occlusal contact in the physiology of the rat incisor: IX Impeded and unimpeded eruption in lathyritic rats. J Dent Res 54, 891–898.

Michaeli Y, Steigman S, Barad A and Weinreb M Jr (1988) Three dimensional presentation of cell migration in the periodontal ligament of the rat incisor. Anat Rec 221, 584–590.

Michaeli Y and Weinreb MM (1968) Role of attrition and occlusal contact in the physiology of the rat incisor: II Diurnal rhythm in eruption and attrition. J Dent Res 47, 486–491.

Miller BG (1957) Investigations of the influence of vascularity and innervation on tooth resorption and eruption. J Dent Res 36, 669–676.

Miura F and Ito G (1968) Eruptive force of rabbit's upper incisors. Trans Eur Orthod Soc, 121–126.

Moorrees CFA (1959) The Dentition of the Growing Child. Harvard University Press.

Moorrees CFA (1964) Dental development – a growth study based on tooth eruption as a measure of physiologic age. Trans Eur Orthod Soc 92–105.

Moss JP (1976) A review of the theories of approximal migration of teeth. In: The Eruption and Occlusion of Teeth (Poole DFG and Stack MV, eds), pp 205–212, Butterworths, London.

Moss JP and Picton DCA (1967) Experimental mesial drift in adult monkeys (*Macaca irus*). Arch Oral Biol 12, 1313–1320.

Moss JP and Picton DCA (1970) Mesial drift of teeth in adult monkeys (*Macaca irus*) when forces from the cheeks and tongue have been eliminated. Arch Oral Biol 15, 979–986.

Moss JP and Picton DCA (1974) The effect on approximal drift of cheek teeth of dividing mandibular molars of adult monkey (*Macaca irus*), Arch Oral Biol 19, 1211–1214.

Moss JP and Picton DCA (1980) The effects on approximal drift of altering the horizontal component of biting force in adult monkeys (*Macaca irus*). Arch Oral Biol 25, 45–48.

Moss JP and Picton DCA (1982) Short term changes in mesiodistal position of teeth following removal of approximal contacts in the monkey, *Macaca fascicularis*. Arch Oral Biol 27, 273–278.

Moss ML and Crikelair GF (1960) Progressive facial hemiatrophy following cervical sympathectomy in the rat. Arch Oral Biol 1, 254–258.

Moxham BJ (1979a) Recording the eruption of the rabbit mandibular incisor using a device for continuously monitoring tooth movements. Arch Oral Biol 24, 889–899.

Moxham BJ (1979b) The effects of some vaso-active drugs on the eruption of the rabbit mandibular incisor. Arch Oral Biol 24, 681–688.

Moxham BJ (1981) The effects of section and stimulation of the cervical sympathetic trunk on eruption of the rabbit mandibular incisor. Arch Oral Biol 26, 887–891.

Moxham BJ (1988) The role of the periodontal vasculature in tooth eruption. In: Biological Mechanisms of Tooth Eruption and Root Resorption (Davidovitch Z, ed), pp 207–224. EBSCO Media, Birmingham, Alabama.

Moxham BJ (in press) What the structure and biochemistry of the periodontal ligament tell us about the mechanisms of tooth eruption. In: Biological Mechanisms of Tooth Eruption, Root Resorption and Dental Implants (Davidovitch Z, ed), EBSCO Media, Birmingham, Alabama.

Moxham BJ and Berkovitz BKB (1974) The effects of root transection on the unimpeded eruption rate of the rabbit mandibular incisor. Arch Oral Biol 19, 903–909.

Moxham BJ and Berkovitz BKB (1981) A quantitative assessment of the effects of axially directed extrusive loads on displacement of the impeded and unimpeded rabbit mandibular incisor. Arch Oral Biol 26, 208–215.

Moxham BJ and Berkovitz BKB (1982) The periodontal ligament and physiological tooth movements. In: The Periodontal Ligament in Health and Disease, 1st edition (Berkovitz BKB, Moxham BJ and Newman HN, eds), pp 215-247, Pergamon Press, Oxford.

Moxham BJ and Berkovitz BKB (1983) Interactions between thyroxine, hydrocortisone and cyclophosphamide in their effects on the eruption of the rat mandibular incisor. Arch Oral Biol 28, 1083–1087.

Moxham BJ and Berkovitz BKB (1984) The mobility of the lathyritic rabbit mandibular incisor in response to axially directed extrusive loads. Arch Oral Biol 29, 773–778.

Moxham BJ and Berkovitz BKB (1988) Continuous monitoring of the movements of erupting and newly erupted teeth of limited growth (ferret mandibular canines) and their responses to hexamethonium. Arch Oral Biol 33, 919–923.

Moxham BJ, Shore RC and Berkovitz BKB (1985) Fenestrated capillaries in the connective tissues of the periodontal ligament. Microvasc Res 30, 116–124.

Moxham BJ, Shore RC and Berkovitz BKB (1987) Fenestrated capillaries in the periodontal connective tissues of the erupting and erupted rat molar. Arch Oral Biol 32, 477–481.

Moxham BJ, Shore RC and Berkovitz BKB (1991) A quantitative study of the ultrastructure of fibroblasts within the enamel-related connective tissue of rat incisor. J Biol Buccale 19, 135–140.

Murphey WH (1970) Oxytetracycline microfluorescent comparison of orthodontic retraction into recent and healed extraction sites. Am J Orthod 58, 215–239.

Murphy KG and Daniel JC (1987) Human periodontal ligament in vitro: cell culture passage effect on collagen gel contraction. J Periodont 22, 342–347.

Murphy T (1959) Compensatory mechanisms in facial height adjustment to functional tooth attrition. Aust Dent J 4, 312–323.

Myers HI and Wyatt WP (1961) Some histopathologic changes in the hamster as the result of a continuously acting orthodontic appliance. J Dent 40, 846–856.

Myhre L, Preus HR and Aars H (1979) Influences of axial load and blood pressure on the position of the rabbit's incisor tooth. Acta Odont Scand 37, 153–159.

Ness AR (1954) Measuring the continuous eruption of the rabbit mandibular incisor. J Physiol 124, 13–15.

Ness AR (1956) The response of the rabbit mandibular incisor to experimental shortening and to the prevention of its eruption. Proc R Soc Lond [Biol] 146, 129–154.

Ness AR (1964) Movement and forces in tooth eruption. In: Advances in Oral Biology, volume 1 (Stable PH, ed), pp 33–75, Academic Press, London.

Ness AR (1965) Eruption rates of impeded and unimpeded mandibular incisors of the adult laboratory mouse. Arch Oral Biol 10, 439–451.

Ness AR (1967) Eruption – a review. In: The Mechanisms of Tooth Support (Anderson DJ, Eastoe JE, Melcher AH and Picton DCA, eds), pp 84–88. Wright, Bristol.

Ness AR (1970) Eruption '70. Apex J Univ Coll Hosp Dent Soc 4, 23–27.

Ness AR and Smale DE (1959) The distribution of mitoses and cells in the tissues bounded by the socket wall of the rabbit mandibular incisor. Proc R Soc Lond 151, 106–128.

Ng GC, Walker, TW Zing, W and Burke PS (1981) Effects of tooth loading on the periodontal vasculature of the mandibular fourth premolar in dogs. Arch Oral Biol 26, 189–195.

Nickerson M (1970) In: The Pharmacological Basis of Therapeutics, 4th edition (Goodman LS and Gilman A, eds), Macmillan, London.

O'Brien C, Bhaskar SN and Brodie AG (1958) Eruptive mechanism and movement in the first molar of the rat. J Dent Res 37, 467–484.

Ogston AG (1970) The biological functions of glycosaminoglycans. In: Chemistry and Molecular Biology of the Intercellular Matrix, volume 3 (Balazs EA, ed), pp 1231–1240, Academic Press, London.

Ohshima S (1982) Effects of lathyrogens on the mechanical properties of the periodontium in the rat mandibular incisor. Tsurumi Univ J Dent Res 8, 345–356.

Ohshima S, Nakamura G and Chiba M (1989) Effects of lathyrogens on the mechanical strength of the periodontal ligament in the rat mandibular first molar. J Periodont 24, 343–350.

Ooe T (1968) Human Tooth and Dental Arch Development. Ishiyakn, Japan.

Osborn JW (1961) An investigation into the interdental forces occurring between the teeth of the same arch during clenching of the jaws. Arch Oral Biol 5, 202–211.

Oster GF, Murray JD and Harris AK (1983) Mechanical aspects of mesenchymal morphogenesis. J Embryol Exp Morphol 78, 83–125.

Palcanis KG (1973) Effect of occlusal trauma on interstitial pressure in the periodontal ligament. J Dent Res 52, 903–910.

Paterson RL, Maddox RA, Proffit WR and Wright DC (1987) A technique for real time measurement of human tooth eruption. Proceedings IEEE Symposium on Engineering in Biology and Medicine, Boston.

Paynter KJ (1954) The effect of propylthiouracil on the development of molar teeth of rats. J Dent Res 33, 364–376.

Pearson CH (1982) The ground substance of the periodontal ligament. In: The Periodontal Ligament in Health and Disease (Berkovitz BKB, Moxham BJ and Newman HN, eds), pp 119–149, Pergamon Press, Oxford.

Perera KAS and Tonge CH (1981) Metabolic turnover of collagen in the mouse molar periodontal ligament during tooth eruption. J Anat 133, 359–370.

Picton DCA (1962) Tilting movements of teeth during biting. Arch Oral Biol 7, 151–159.

Picton DCA (1976) Tooth movement as mesial and lateral drift. In: The eruption and occlusion of teeth (Poole DFG and Stack MV, eds), pp 108–119, Butterworths, London.

Picton DCA (1989) The periodontal enigma: eruption versus tooth support. Eur J Orthod 11, 430–439.

Picton DCA and Moss JP (1973) The part played by the trans-septal fibre system in experimental approximal drift of the cheek teeth of monkeys (*Macaca irus*). Arch Oral Biol 18, 669–680.

Picton DCA and Moss JP (1974) The relationship between the angulation of the roots and the rate of approximal drift of cheek teeth in adult monkeys. Br J Orthod 1, 105–110.

Picton DCA and Moss JP (1978) The effect of reducing cusp height on the rate of approximal drift of cheek teeth in adult monkeys (*Macaca irus*). Arch Oral Biol 23, 219–223.

Picton DCA and Moss JP (1980) The effect on approximal drift of altering the horizontal component of biting force in adult monkeys. Arch Oral Biol 25, 45–48.

Pihlstrom BL and Ramfjord SP (1971) Periodontal effect of nonfunction in monkeys. J Periodont 42, 748–756.

Pinson RR and Strahan JD (1974) The effect on the relapse of orthodontically rotated teeth of surgical division of the gingival fibres – pericision. Br J Orthod 1, 87–91.

Pitaru S, Michaeli Y, Zajicek G and Weinreb MM (1976) Role of attrition and occlusal contact in the physiology of the rat incisor. IX. The part played by the periodontal ligament in the eruptive process. J Dent Res 55, 819–824.

Prockop DJ and Kirivikko KI (1968) Hydroxyproline and the metabolism of collagen. In: Treatise on Collagen (Gould BS, ed), pp 215–246, Academic Press, London.

Proffit WR (1994) in press.

Proffit WR, Prewitt JR, Baik HS and Lee CF (1991) Video microscope observations of human premolar eruption. J Dent Res 70, 15–18.

Proffit WR and Sellers KT (1986) The effect of intermittent forces on eruption of the rabbit incisor. J Dent 65, 118–122.

Rahmetulla F (1992) Proteoglycans of oral tissues. Crit Rev Oral Biol Med 3, 135–162.

Rippin JW (1976a) Collagen turnover in the periodontal ligament under normal and altered functional forces. I Young rat molars. J Periodont 11, 101–107.

Rippin JW (1976b) Collagen turnover in rat molar periodontal ligament. In: The eruption and occlusion of teeth (Poole DFG and Stack MV, eds), pp 304–305, Butterworths, London.

Rippin JW (1978) Collagen turnover in the periodontal ligament under normal and altered functional forces. II Adult rat molars. J Periodont 13, 149–154.

Robins MW (1979) A photographic method of measuring eruption rates of the mandibular incisors of the mouse. J Dent 58 (special issue C), 1273.

Robinson JA and Schneider BJ (1992) Histological evaluation of the effect of transseptal fibre resection on the rate of physiological migration of rat molar teeth. Arch Oral Biol 37, 371–375.

Sandy JR (1992) Tooth eruption and orthodontic tooth movement. Br Dent J 172, 141–149.

Sarnat H and Sciaky I (1965) Experimental lathyrism in rats: effect of removing incisal stress. Periodontics 3, 128–134.

Schneiderman ED (1989) A longitudinal cephalometric study of incisor supra-eruption in young and adult rhesus monkeys (*Macaca mulatta*). Arch Oral Biol 34, 137–141.

Schour I and Massler M (1942) The teeth. In: The Rat in Laboratory Investigation, 2nd edition (Farris EJ and Griffith JQ, eds), pp 104–165, Lippincott, London.

Schour I and Van Dyke HB (1932) Changes in the teeth following hypophysectomy. I Changes in the incisor of the white rat. Am J Anat 50, 397–433.

Schubert M and Hamerman D (1968) A Primer on Connective Tissue Biochemistry. Lea and Febiger, Philadelphia.

Schwarze CW (1972) Langzeitstudie über das sagittale Positionsverhalten der ersten Molaren. Forstschr Kieferorthop 33, 93–102.

Schwarze CW (1973) Hat die Keimentfernung der Weisheitszähne Einfluss auf Spatform des Zahnbogens? Forstschr Kieferorthop 34, 387–400.

Scott JH (1967) Dento-facial Development and Growth. Pergamon Press, Oxford.
Shore RC and Berkovitz BKB (1979) An ultrastructural study of periodontal ligament fibroblasts in relation to their possible role in tooth eruption and intracellular collagen degradation in the rat. Arch Oral Biol 24, 155–164.
Shore RC, Berkovitz BKB and Moxham BJ (1981) Intercellular contacts between fibroblasts in the periodontal connective tissues of the rat. J Anat 133, 67–76.
Shore RC, Berkovitz BKB and Moxham BJ (1985) The effects of preventing movement of the rat incisor on the structure of its periodontal ligament. Arch Oral Biol 30, 221–228.
Shore RC, Moxham BJ and Berkovitz BKB (1982) A quantitative comparison of the ultrastructure of the periodontal ligaments of impeded and unimpeded rat incisors. Arch Oral Biol 27, 423–430.
Shrimpton BA (1960) Dynamics of eruption. NZ Dent J 56, 122–124.
Sicher H (1942) Tooth eruption: the axial movement of continuously growing teeth. J Dent Res 21, 201–210.
Sicher H and Weinmann JP (1944) Bone growth and physiologic tooth movement. Am J Orthod 30, 109–132.
Siersbaek-Nielsen S (1971) Rate of eruption of central incisors at puberty: an implant study on eight boys. Tandlaegebladet 75, 1288–1295.
Sillman JH (1951) Serial study of good occlusion from birth to 12 years of age. Am J Orthod 37, 481–507.
Sillman JH (1964) Dimensional changes of the dental arches: longitudinal study from birth to 25 years. Am J Orthod 50, 824–842.
Slootweg RN (1976) Changes in collagenous and non-collagenous proteins in the periodontal ligament during acceleration of eruption. A biochemical and histological investigation in different sectors of the periodontal ligament in the guinea pig incisor. PhD thesis, University of Utrecht, Netherlands.
Smith RG (1978) A clinical study into the depth of the so-called gingival crevice of some erupting teeth of humans. MDS thesis, Bristol University.
Smith RG (1980) A clinical study into the rate of eruption of some human permanent teeth. Arch Oral Biol 25, 675–681.
Sodek J (1978) A comparison of collagen and non-collagenous protein metabolism in rat molar and incisor periodontal ligaments. Arch Oral Biol 23, 977–982.
Sodek J (1983) Periodontal ligament: metabolism. In: CRC Handbook of Experimental Aspects of Oral Biochemistry (Lazzari P, ed), pp 183–193, CRC Press, Florida.
Sodek J and Ferrier J (1988) Collagen remodelling in rat periodontal tissues: Compensation for precursor reutilization confirms rapid turnover of collagen. Collagen Rel Res 8, 11–21.
Sodek J and Limeback H (1979) Comparison of the rates of synthesis, conversion and maturation of type I and type III collagen in rat periodontal tissues. J Biol Chem 154, 10496-10502.
Southard TE, Behrents RG and Tolley EA (1989) The anterior component of force. Am J Orthod Dentofacial Orthop 97, 41–44.
Southard TE, Southard KA and Tolley EA (1990) Variation of approximal tooth contact tightness with postural change. J Dent Res 69, 1776–1779.
Southard TE, Southard KA and Weedon (1991) Mesial force from unerupted third molars. Am J Orthod Dentofacial Orthop 99, 220–225.
Speck NT (1950) A longitudinal study of developmental changes in human lower dental arches. Angle Orthod 20, 215–228.
Stallard H (1923) The anterior component of the force of mastication and its significance to the dental apparatus. Dent Cosmos 65, 457–474.
Starling EH (1909) The fluids of the body. Keener, Chicago.
Steedle JR and Proffit WR (1985) The pattern and control of eruptive tooth movements. Am J Orthod 87, 56–66.
Steedle JR, Proffit WR and Fields HW (1983) The effects of continuous axially directed intrusive loads on the erupting rabbit mandibular incisor. Arch Oral Biol 28, 1149–1153.
Steigman S, Harari D and Michaeli Y (1983) Long-term effect of intrusive loads of varying magnitude upon the eruptive potential of rat incisors. Am J Orthod 84, 254–259.
Steigman S, Michaeli Y, Yitschaky M and Schweizer B (1991) Dynamics of tissue changes found after mechanical loading of the rat incisor. 1. A three dimensional longitudinal study of the morphologic aspects. Am J Orthod Dentofacial Orthop 99, 533–542.
Steigman S, Michaeli Y and Weinreb M (1987) Structural changes in the dental and periodontal tissues of the rat incisor following application of orthodontic loads. Am J Orthod Dentofacial Orthop 91, 49–56.
Steigman S, Michaeli Y and Zajicek G (1981) The influence of calibrated loads upon the rate of eruption of mandibular rat incisors. Arch Oral Biol 26, 327–331.
Stenvik A, Iversen J and Mjör IA (1972) Tissue pressure and histology of normal and inflamed tooth pulps in Macaque monkeys. Arch Oral Biol 17, 1501–1511.
Stopak D and Harris AK (1982) Connective tissue morphogenesis by fibroblast traction. 1. Tissue culture observations. Dev Biol 90, 383–398.
Strahan JD and Mills JRE (1970) A preliminary report on the severing of gingival fibres following rotation of teeth. Dent Practit 21, 101–103.
Sutton PRN and Graze HR (1985) The blood-vessel thrust theory of tooth eruption and migration. Medical Hypotheses 18, 289–295.
Sved A (1955) The mesial drift of teeth during growth. Am J Orthod 41, 539–553.
Tait RV (1982) Mesial migration and lower third molar tilt. Br J Orthod 9, 41–47.
Tait RV (1984) Further observations on third molar tilt. Br J Orthodont 11, 200–204.
Taverne AAR (1989) Study of the role of collagen in tooth eruption. PhD thesis, University of Utrecht, Netherlands.
Taverne AAR, Lemmens IG and Tonino GJM (1984) Lathyrogens and the role of collagen in the eruption of the rat incisor. Arch Oral Biol 31, 127–131.
Taylor AC and Butcher EO (1951) The regulation of eruption rate in the incisor teeth of the white rat. J Exp Zool 117, 165–188.
Ten Cate AR (1971) Physiological resorption of connective tissue associated with tooth eruption. J Periodont Res 6, 168–181.
Ten Cate AR (1972) Morphological studies of fibrocytes in connective tissue undergoing rapid remodelling. J Anat 112, 401–414.
Ten Cate AR (1976) Tooth eruption. In: Orban's Oral Histology and Embryology, 8th edition (Bhaskar SN, ed), p 365, Mosby, St Louis.
Ten Cate AR, Deporter DA and Freeman E (1976) The fate of fibroblasts in the remodelling of periodontal ligament during physiologic tooth movement. Am J Orthod 69, 155–168.
Thomas NR (1965) The Process and Mechanism of Tooth Eruption. PhD thesis, University of Bristol.
Thomas NR (1967) The properties of collagen in the periodontium of an erupting tooth. In: The Mechanisms of Tooth Support (Anderson DJ, Eastoe JE, Melcher AH and Picton DCA, eds), pp 102–106, Wright, Bristol.
Thomas NR (1976) Collagen as the generator of tooth eruption. In: The Eruption and Occlusion of Teeth (Poole DFG and Stack MV, eds), pp 290–301, Butterworths, London.
Thompson HE, Myers HI, Waterman JM and Flanagan VD (1958) Preliminary macroscopic observations concerning the potentiality of supra-alveolar collagenous fibres in orthodontics. Am J Orthod 44, 485–497.
Thompson JL Jr and Kendrick GS (1964) Changes in the vertical dimensions of the human male skull during the third and fourth decades of life. Anat Rec 150, 209–213.
Tomasek JJ, Hay ED and Fujiwara K (1982) Collagen modulates cell shape and cytoskeleton of embryonic corneal and fibroma fibroblasts: distribution of actin, actinin and myosin. Dev Biol 92, 107–122.

Torchia DA, Hasson MA and Hascall VC (1977) Investigation of molecular motion of proteoglycans in cartilage by 13-C magnetic resonance. J Biol Chem 251, 3617–3625.

Trauner F (1912) The causes of progressive movement of the teeth towards the front. Am J Orthod 3, 144–158.

Tsurata M, Eto K and Chiba M (1974) Effect of daily or 4-hourly administrations of lathyrogens on the eruption rates of impeded and unimpeded mandibular incisors of rats. Arch Oral Biol 19, 1221–1226.

Tyler DW and Burn-Murdoch RA (1976) Tooth movements in an in vitro model system. In: The Eruption and Occlusion of Teeth. (Poole DFG and Stack MV, eds), pp 302–304, Butterworths, London.

Urban JPG, Maroudas A, Bayliss, MT and Dillon J (1979) Swelling pressure of proteoglycans at the concentrations found in cartilaginous tissues. Biorheology 16, 447–464.

van Beek H (1979) The transfer of mesial drift potential along the dental arch in Macaca irus: an experimental study of tooth migration rate related to horizontal vectors of occlusal forces. Eur J Orthodont 1, 125–129.

van Beek H and Fidler VJ (1977) An experimental study of the effect of functional occlusion on mesial tooth migration in macaque monkeys. Arch Oral Biol 22, 269–271.

van den Bos T and Tonino GJM (1984) Composition and metabolism of the extracellular matrix in the periodontal ligament of impeded and unimpeded rat incisors. Arch Oral Biol 29, 893–897.

van den Brenk HA and Stone MG (1974) Actions and interactions of colchicine and cytochalasin B on contraction of granulation tissue and on mitosis. Nature 251, 327–329.

van Hassel HJ (1971) Physiology of the human dental pulp. Oral Surg 32, 126–134.

van Hassel HJ and Brown AC (1969) Effect of temperature changes on intrapulpal pressure and hydraulic permeability in dogs. Arch Oral Biol 14, 301–315.

van Hassel HJ and McMinn RG (1972) Pressure differential favouring tooth eruption in the dog. Arch Oral Biol 17, 183–190.

Vasiliev JM and Gelfand IM (1976) Effects of colcemid on morphogenetic processes and locomotion of fibroblasts. In: Cell Motility Book (Goldman AR, Pollard T and Rosenbaum J, eds), pp 279–304, Cold Spring Harbour Laboratory.

Vego L (1962) A longitudinal study of the mandibular arch perimeter. Angle Orthod 32, 187–192.

Walker TW, Ng GC and Burke PS (1978) Fluid pressures in the periodontal ligament of the mandibular canine tooth in dogs. Arch Oral Biol 23, 753–765.

Wallace JS (1904) General outline of the causes of irregularities of the teeth (chapter 1), Dental Manufacturing, London.

Webb PP, Benjamin M, Moxham BJ and Ralphs JR (1994) Age-related changes in intermediate filament expression in the periodontium of rats. J Anat 184, 198.

Weinstein S (1967) Minimal forces in tooth movement. Am J Orthod 53, 881–903.

Wessels NK, Spooner BS and Ludvena MA (1973) Surface movements, microfilaments and cell locomotion. In: Locomotion of Tissue Cells. CIBA Symposium 14, pp 53–77, Elsevier, Amsterdam.

Whittaker DK, Parker JH and Jenkins C (1982) Tooth attrition and continuing eruption in a Romano-British population. Arch Oral Biol 27, 405–409.

Whittaker DK, Molleson T, Daniel AT, Williams JT, Rose P and Resteghini R (1985) Quantitative assessment of tooth wear, alveolar crest height and continuing eruption in a Romano-British population. Arch Oral Biol 30, 493–501.

Winders RV (1962) Recent findings in myometric research. Angle Orthod 32, 38–44.

Wise GE and Fan W (1989) Changes in the tartrate-resistant acid-phosphatase cell population in dental follicles and bony crypts of rat molars during tooth eruption. J Dent Res 68, 150–156.

Wise GE and Fan W (1991) Immunolocalization of transforming growth-factor-Beta in rat molars. J Oral Pathol Med 20, 74–80.

Wise GE, Lin F and Fan W (1992) Culture and characterisation of dental follicle cells from rat molars. Cell Tissue Res 267, 483–492.

Wise GE, Marks SC Jr and Cahill DR (1985) Ultrastructural features of the dental follicle associated with formation of the tooth eruption pathway in the dog. J Oral Pathol 14, 15–26.

Wynn W, Haldi J, Hopf MA and John K (1963) Pressure within the pulp chamber of the dog's tooth relative to arterial blood pressure. J Dent Res 42, 1169–1177.

Yamasaki A, Rose GG, Pirero GJ and Mahan CJ (1987) Ultrastructural and morphometric analyses of human cementoblasts and periodontal fibroblasts. J Periodont 58, 192–201.

Yilmaz RS (1973) Mesial drift of the teeth. MSc thesis, Bristol University.

Yilmaz RS (1976) Horizontal tooth movement and jaw growth. PhD thesis, Bristol University.

Yilmaz RS, Darling AI and Levers BGH (1980) Mesial drift of human teeth assessed from ankylosed deciduous molars. Arch Oral Biol 25, 127–131.

Yilmaz RS, Darling AI and Levers BGH (1981) Experimental tooth ankylosis and horizontal tooth movement in the pig. Arch Oral Biol 26, 41–47.

Zajicek G (1974) Fibroblast cell kinetics in the periodontal ligament of the mouse. Cell Tissue Kinet 7, 479–492.

Chapter 10
The Effects of External Forces on the Periodontal Ligament

BJ Moxham and BKB Berkovitz

INTRODUCTION

External forces of a physiological nature impinge upon a tooth mainly axially (i.e. along the long axis of the tooth and in an intrusive or extrusive direction) or horizontally. The significance of studying the responses to physiological loading relates not only to our understanding of the tooth support mechanism but also extends clinically to an appreciation of the loss of support occurring with periodontal pathology and to the reactions of the tooth to orthodontic loading. Until the early 1980s, there had been many investigations into the tooth support mechanism, much of the research being centred around Picton and co-workers. Sadly, little research has been undertaken in recent years, and therefore our earlier reviews of the topic (Moxham and Berkovitz, 1982a,b) still remain essentially valid. Nevertheless, what has been produced since 1982 has served to confirm that the commonly believed notion of the periodontal ligament (PDL) behaving as a 'suspensory ligament' is a gross simplification of the complex mechanical and biological reactions occurring when external forces are placed upon the teeth.

The majority of studies concerned with the physiological forces impinging upon the teeth relate to those associated with mastication. Far less is known about the forces derived from other sources (e.g. the forces generated during speech and swallowing). The reader is referred to our previous reviews (Moxham and Berkovitz, 1982a,b) for detailed accounts of the sources and nature of physiological external loads. For a review of the nature of orthodontic loads, see Proffit and Fields (1993).

THE EFFECTS OF PHYSIOLOGICAL EXTERNAL LOADS UPON TOOTH POSITION (TOOTH MOBILITY STUDIES)

Picton (1990) has defined tooth mobility as 'the relationship between a short-acting force and the resulting horizontal or vertical displacement'. The study of tooth mobility following the application of defined loads to teeth whose periodontal tissues are regarded as physiologically normal has provided important and general information concerning the mechanical properties of the periodontium, and so in essence helps to determine whether the periodontium behaves as an elastic, viscoelastic, or thixotropic system.

INTRUSIVE TOOTH MOBILITY

Research on the effects of axial intrusive loads on tooth mobility was pioneered by Parfitt (1960). His experiments utilized devices for simultaneously recording tooth movement and applied force on human maxillary incisors. Intrusive loads were applied manually as an increasing force at various rates until the desired peak force was obtained. Parfitt reported that, if the intrusive force was gradually and evenly increased, the displacement of the tooth showed an initial rapidly rising phase with loads up to about 1 N. With greater loads, the displacement appeared to fade in a logarithmic manner (*Fig. 10.1*). To illustrate this point, Parfitt calculated that the mean displacement for a thrust of 1 N was approximately 20 μm, while an increase from 1 N to 10 N produced an additional movement of only 8 μm. Parfitt's findings show that the first phase of tooth mobility changes gradually to the second

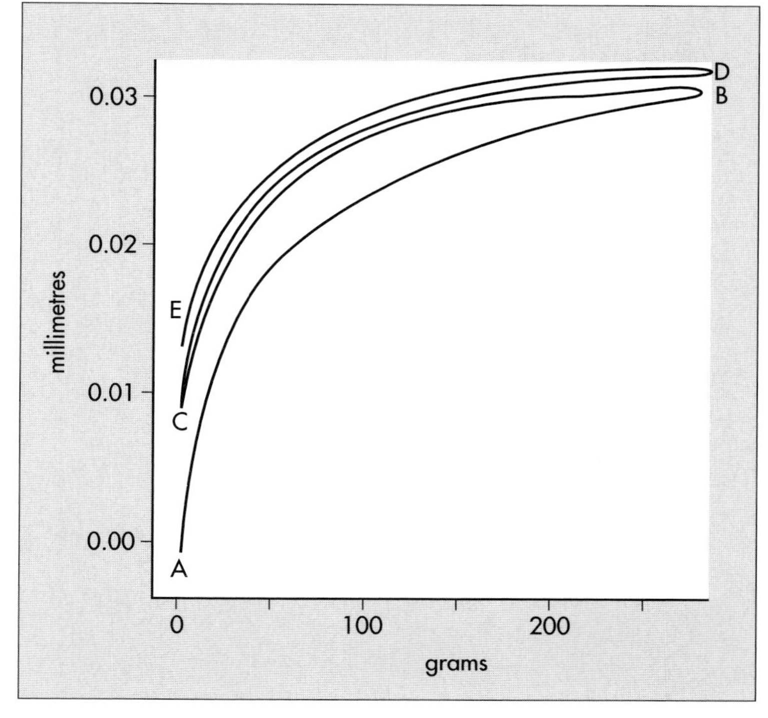

Fig. 10.1 The axial load–mobility curve for a human maxillary incisor. A – initial position; B – position at peak force on the first application; C – return point on removal of force; D – position at peak force on the second application; E – return point after the second removal. (Parfitt, 1960.)

phase, although the change can first be detected at about 0.3 N. When 5 N peak-loads were maintained on the tooth, intrusion continued by a regular amount with each period of time (approximately 2 µm per minute) until a point was reached where no further displacement could be recorded. With repeated intermittent forces of the same order, however, intrusive movements took place beyond the limit reached with the maintained force. The mobility appeared to be influenced by the rate of application of the load and the interval between loads. Less displacement of the tooth was produced if the load was applied rapidly. Where a series of intrusive loads of approximately 5 N was applied with intervals of 2–5 seconds, the tooth did not have sufficient time to return to its original position before the application of the next load (*Fig. 10.2*). Indeed, after each successive load the tooth returned slightly less far. Furthermore, the intrusive mobility of the tooth was gradually reduced with each successive load, and the tooth appeared to be intruded progressively into the socket as the series continued.

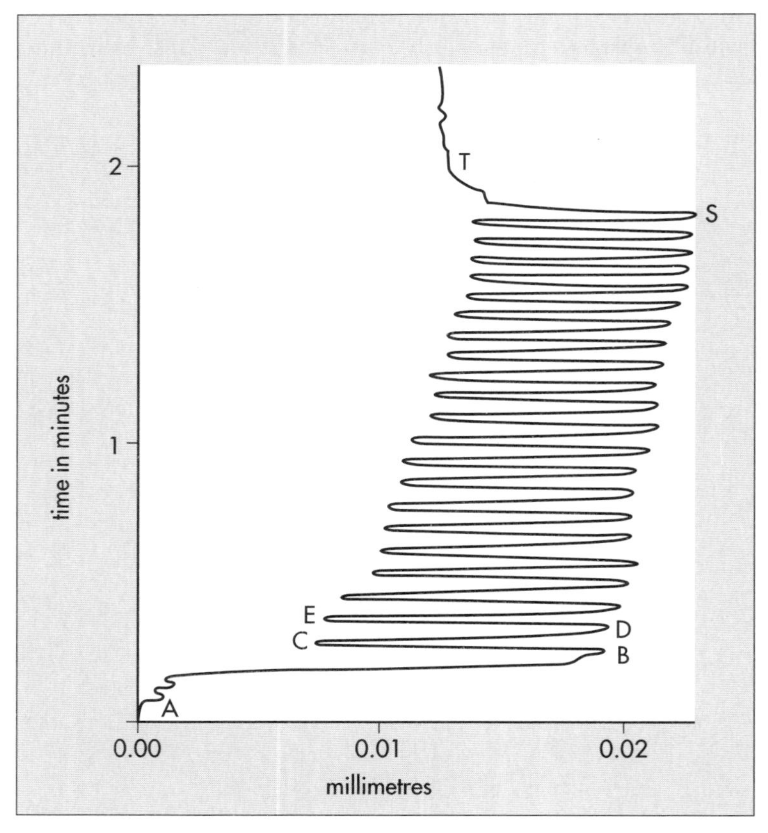

Fig. 10.2 The axial movement–time curve of a human maxillary incisor tooth. A – initial position; B – position at 5 N peak force on the first application; C – first return on removal of force; D – position at 5 N peak force on the second application; E – second return on removal of force; S – position at 5 N peak force on the 22nd application; T – return point after the final removal of force. (Parfitt, 1960.)

On removing an intrusive load, Parfitt (1960) demonstrated that the tooth recovered its original position in two phases. The first recovery phase showed a rapid return towards its original position in an almost linear manner with time. The second phase involved a slower recovery, there being an apparent logarithmic relationship between movement and time. Full recovery was found to take 1–2 minutes with an intermittent load. Recovery took longer where the load had been maintained.

In discussing his results, Parfitt was of the opinion that, contrary to the belief at that time, the tooth could not be supported simply by tension through inelastic fibre bundles. He suggested that 'several distinct and independently variable systems' were involved in tooth support. Though it was not possible to demonstrate the precise mechanisms that underly the patterns of tooth displacements, Parfitt suggested that the tooth was supported by fluids related to both the vascular and tissue fluid systems in the PDL. This interpretation was based partly upon his observation that tooth movements occurred in synchrony with the arterial pulse wave with intrusive loads less than 0.15 N.

The work of Parfitt has been developed extensively, particularly by Picton and co-workers. Picton (1962b, 1963a) published the results of studies on tooth mobility in human maxillary incisors, mandibular first premolars and maxillary first molars during biting. His apparatus at this time consisted of two movement transducers incorporating resistance-wire strain gauges soldered to the wings of a rubber dam clamp which was placed on the test tooth (*Fig. 10.3a*). Metal pointers from the transducers were rested on the teeth immediately adjacent to the test tooth to provide reference points. Biting forces up to 20 N were applied to the test tooth via a dynamometer anchored to teeth in the opposing jaw. Three thrusts were made to each tooth studied, the time interval between thrusts being 30 seconds to 1 minute. Picton claimed that tilting of the teeth during the biting thrusts could be accounted for. However, he emphasized that, since the adjacent reference teeth were also probably displaced by the thrusts, the values obtained for tooth mobility were not to be regarded as absolute. Although considerable variation was sometimes found between consecutive thrusts, the pattern and amount of intrusive tooth movements were similar to those obtained by Parfitt (1960) (*Fig. 10.3b*). Thus, the load–tooth mobility curves revealed an initial phase of relatively free movement followed by a second phase of less movement. However, the changeover between the two phases appeared to be rather variable, and tended to occur at the higher load of approximately 4 N.

In contrast to the early findings of Parfitt (1960), the relationship between intrusive force and displacement is not simply logarithmic. Using more reliable techniques for monitoring tooth displacement, Wills *et al.* (1974, 1976, 1978) showed that, on plotting log displacement versus log force for macaque monkey teeth, there was a two-phase parabolic relationship with discontinuity occurring within the force range 0.5–0.8 N (*Fig. 10.4*).

In view of Parfitt's (1960) assertion that tooth mobility is influenced by the rate of loading and the time interval between thrusts, further investigations concerning this have been conducted by Picton (1963b, 1964a,b) and Wills *et al.* (1978). The first of these studies (Picton, 1963b) was motivated by the need to standardize techniques by reducing the sources of variation observed in previous research (Picton, 1962b, 1963a). Techniques similar to those used for his earlier experiments were employed. However, the next but one teeth on each side of the test tooth were now used as reference teeth. This was done since the teeth immediately adjacent may show movements when force is applied to the test tooth (Picton, 1962a). Axial loads rising from 0–20 N were applied manually to the test tooth, and graphic records of the force were used to enable the rate of thrust to be controlled. Picton emphasized the need to take care to stabilize the point of application of the dynamometer on the test tooth and to ensure that the direction of thrust was axial. Variation in the rate of thrust (in the range 0.5–25 second rise-time) produced no consistent effect on the load–mobility curves. Variation of the time interval between thrusts, however, did have an effect. Using standard rise-times, 2 second or 5 second intervals between thrusts caused progressive reduction in mobility, and the tooth failed to return to its initial position on removing the load – a finding similar to that observed by Parfitt (1960). Variable effects were seen with longer time intervals between thrusts of 1–2 minutes. In six out of 10 teeth studied, with 1 minute intervals between thrusts, there was no change (or a slight decrease) in mobility. In seven out of eight teeth studied, no change or a slight increase in mobility was recorded with 1.5 minute intervals. With 2 minute intervals, all 10 teeth showed a progressive increase in mobility. Picton concluded

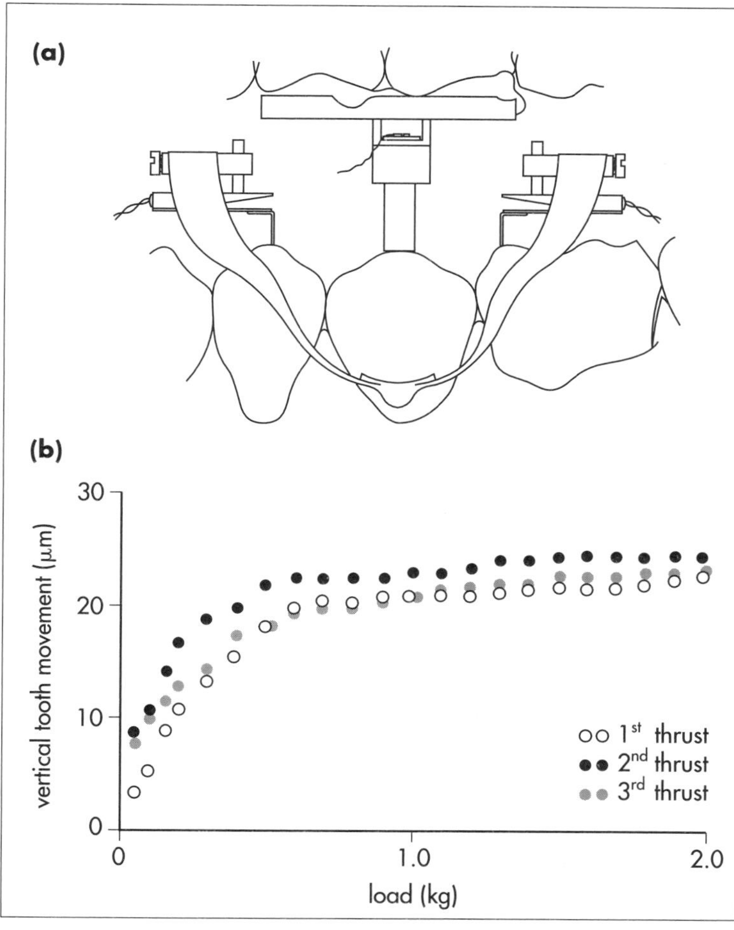

Fig. 10.3 (a) Diagrammatic representation of apparatus used by Picton to study tooth mobility. Two transducers of movement are fixed to the wings of a rubber dam clamp which is mounted on the tooth to be studied and free from adjacent teeth. A dynamometer fixed to the opposing teeth is used to measure the force applied to the test tooth. (Picton, 1962b.) (b) Vertical mobility curves obtained for a human maxillary first permanent molar. (Picton, 1963a.)

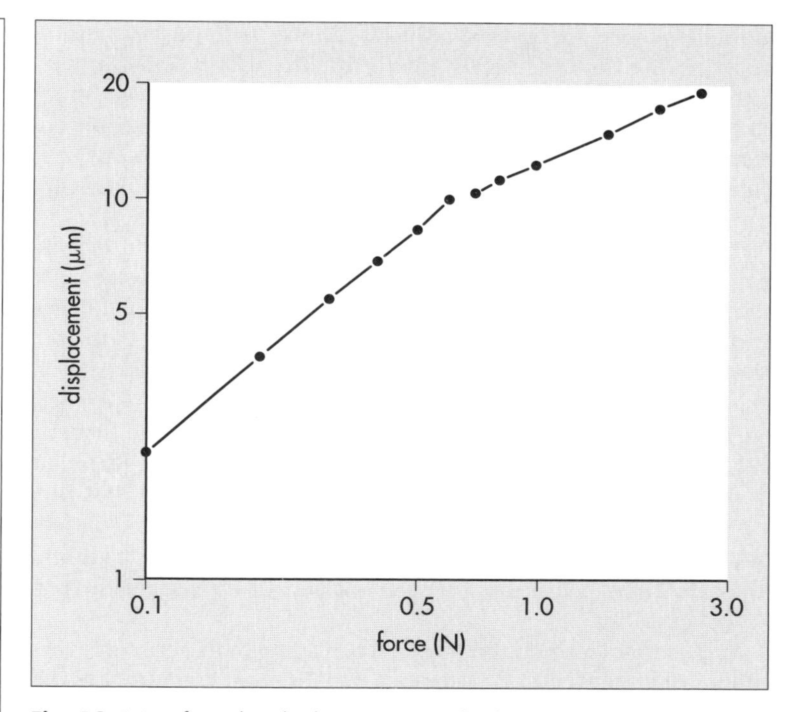

Fig. 10.4. Log force–log displacement curve for force applied to a maxillary central incisor of a macaque monkey at a rate of 4 N per second^{-1}. (Wills *et al.*, 1978.)

that a time interval of 1–1.5 minutes between thrusts is necessary to ensure repeatable load–mobility curves. Variation of the time interval between thrusts, however, had an effect. Picton interpreted the increased mobility seen with 2 minute intervals as the consequence of the tooth adopting an extruded position in the interval between thrusts.

Picton's 1964a experiments generally confirm his 1963b study. However, he observed that, whilst there was a gradual increase in mobility of human maxillary incisors when thrusts of 2 N or 20 N were applied at 2 minute intervals, there was a more abrupt increase in mobility in the 2 minutes following 20 thrusts applied with 5 second intervals. He claimed that rapidly repeated thrusts may thus act as a stimulus for increase in mobility and extrusion. Picton suggested that the possibility that the increase in mobility was the result of passive extrusion (owing to lack of restraining forces) was countered by the finding that a series of thrusts applied with intervals of 2 minutes still produced a gradual increase in mobility where there was a 30–60 minute rest period before applying the thrusts, during which the bite was propped open. Although his previous experiments (Picton, 1963b) showed that 20 N thrusts applied at 5 second and 2 minute intervals resulted respectively in a reduction and an increase in tooth mobility, this difference could not be discerned where a 20 N load was maintained on the tooth for up to 5 minutes prior to experimentation.

The effects of applying axial intrusive thrusts with intervals approximating to those observed during mastication were also studied by Picton (1964b). From the findings of Anderson (1956a) and Graf (1963), he calculated that the mean interval between chewing thrusts is 412 ms. Using this estimate, the degree of recovery was studied for some human maxillary central incisors during a series of 20 N loads applied at rates of 10 or 60 thrusts per minute. The pattern of recovery had characteristics similar to those reported by Parfitt (1960). Picton calculated that the initial linear phase of recovery would have been completed within 412 ms in only five of the 10 teeth studied. This implies that a tooth tends to remain in a depressed position in its socket during normal chewing.

In contrast to the findings of Picton's 1963b experiment, the studies of Wills *et al.* (1978) suggest that different loading rates do have a significant effect on tooth mobility. They reported that the rapid application of loads rising to 4 N caused less tooth displacement than with loads applied more gradually. Apart from differences in the apparatus used to record tooth displacement, a number of differences exist between the 1963b and 1978 experiments:

1. Human teeth were studied in 1963, the teeth of macaque monkeys in 1978.
2. In the 1963 experiment, peak thrusts of 20 N were applied, the rate of thrust varying from 0.5 seconds to 24 seconds rise-time. In the 1978 experiment, three rates of loading were applied. The force was applied as a linear ramp function at rates of 4 N per second or 12 N per second. The third type of loading was sufficiently rapid to approximate to a step function, the load being applied within 0.01 of a second.
3. In 1978, six preconditioning thrusts of 4 N were applied at 10 second intervals and the tooth allowed to recover for 2 minutes.

In discussing their results, Wills *et al.* (1978) did not refer to Picton's 1963b paper and therefore did not reconcile the contrasting results.

Picton (1984) studied axial mobility in relation to changes in rest position. Teeth undisturbed for 3 hours became extruded and subsequently exhibited a marked reduction in axial displacement to loads. Teeth that had been intruded for 3 hours showed:

- a decreased mobility when intruded a distance equivalent to less than 800 mN force and
- an increased mobility when intruded a distance greater than 800 mN.

In discussing the possible biological mechanisms involved, Wills and Picton (1981) and Picton (1984) hypothesized that the explanation for behaviour of this sort lay in the degree of aggregation of proteoglycans in the ground substance.

The experiments so far described show that the relationship between intrusive force and tooth mobility is 'non-Hookean' and the possibility was raised that the periodontium might have viscoelastic properties. Further studies by Bien and Ayers (1965), Bien (1966), Wills *et al.* (1972), Picton and Wills (1978), Coehlo and Moxham (1989), Moxham and Coehlo (1989) and Picton (1989) have been undertaken to assess this.

The experiments of Bien and Ayers (1965) and Bien (1966) were conducted on rat maxillary incisors using loads ranging from 0.35–15 N. Measurement of the displacement of the test tooth was made relative to the adjacent unloaded incisor by means of a microscope fitted with a vernier micrometer eyepiece. Unlike most experiments on tooth mobility up to that time, their method involved the sudden application of a deadweight load, which was maintained for several minutes and then suddenly removed. Thus, the relationship between tooth displacement and time could be investigated. Their findings showed a biphasic intrusive response and a biphasic recovery response, the first phase in both showing more rapid displacement (*Fig. 10.5*). Bien (1966) believed the results demonstrated that the PDL behaved as a viscoelastic gel. He compared the behaviour of the periodontal tissues to various arrangements of mechanical springs and dampers. The dimensional changes that would be produced on loading and unloading a variety of mechanical models are described in *Fig. 10.6*. Bien suggested that the intrusive and recovery responses of the tooth under load could be represented by a Maxwell element.

Wills *et al.* (1972) analysed the displacement–time curves obtained following the sudden removal of axial intrusive loads of 2.5 N to the incisors of monkeys. Using a technique of exponential curve fitting, they claimed to be able to discern three (occasionally four) phases in the recovery of a tooth. They also suggested that their results showed that the periodontium is not analogous to a simple Maxwell element, but should be represented by a series of Voigt elements. The use of graphical techniques for curve fitting is open to criticism. For example, because the exact contour of a curve may be difficult to delineate in the face of expected observational errors, the exact number of separate exponential components which comprise it cannot always be established with confidence (Shipley and Clark, 1972). Furthermore, one must have *a priori* grounds for suggesting that the curve consists of a series of exponentials, since other mathematical models can be made to fit. In view of such criticisms, we believe that the more reliable mathematical techniques devised for the analysis – Draper and Smith (1966) – are to be preferred to graphical techniques.

Picton and Wills (1978) illustrated records of the pattern of displacement and recovery of a monkey incisor with an intrusive load applied as a ramp function (*Fig. 10.7*), likening the response to the force–displacement relationship of a Voigt element. They also listed five other characteristics of the stressed PDL which they claimed identified this tissue as viscoelastic:

1. Loads sustained for many seconds or minutes cause creep.
2. There is an inverse relationship between the rate of loading and displacement.
3. The higher the rate of loading, the less is the distinction between early and late phases of displacement.
4. If loadings are repeated at intervals of less than 1.5 minutes, the recovery becomes progressively more incomplete.

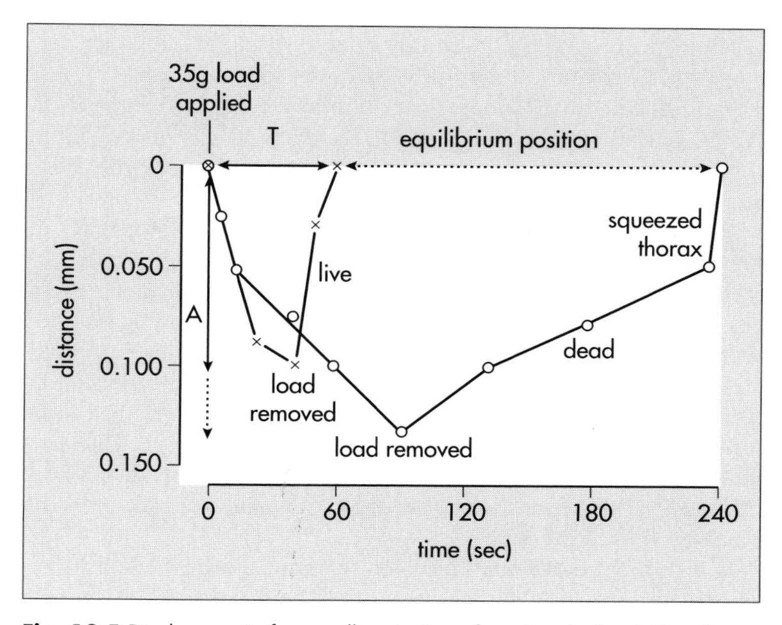

Fig. 10.5 Displacement of a maxillary incisor of a rat under load. The plottings are diagrammatic representations of the intrusion of the tooth into its socket under load, and its restoration to the equilibrium level after removal of the load. A complete cycle is the period T (abscissa) while the magnitude of the intrusion from the point of equilibrium is the amplitude A (ordinate). (Bien, 1966.)

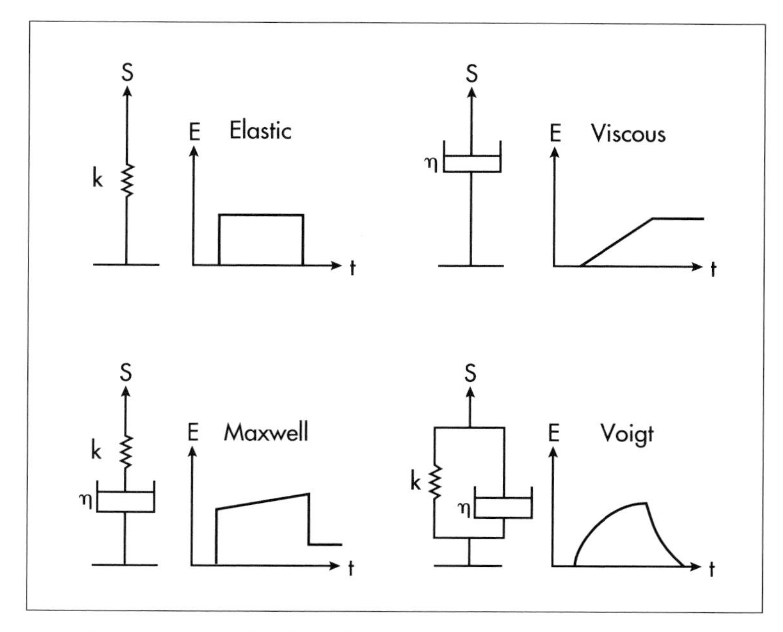

Fig. 10.6 Four simple rheological analogues and schematic representations of the dimensional changes with time which would be produced on loading and unloading each model. (Picton *et al.*, 1974.)

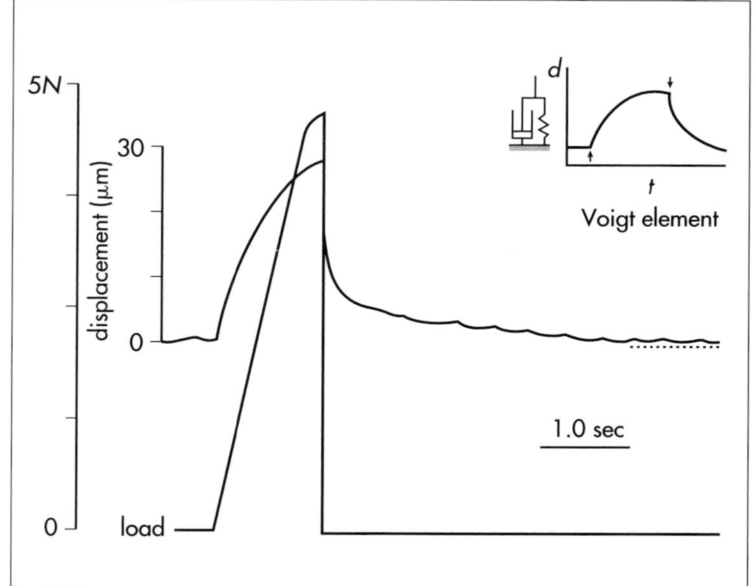

Fig. 10.7 Record showing the axial load to the maxillary central incisor of a macaque monkey in the lower trace and the intrusion in the upper record. The inset shows how the pattern of displacement and recovery in the upper record can be likened to that of a viscoelastic Voigt element. (Picton and Wills, 1978.)

5. The rate of recovery is directly related to the loading rate and indirectly related to the duration of the load.

In addition to the models described by Bien (1966), Wills *et al.* (1972) and Picton and Wills (1978), Ross *et al.* (1976) have suggested that the most suitable model is a three-parameter non-linear spring.

Coehlo and Moxham (1989) studied the intrusive mobility of the guinea pig incisor and concluded that the pattern of mobility was consistent with the view that the periodontal tissues are viscoelastic. This conclusion was reached when a significant time dependency of the response was observed. In a later report, however, Moxham and Coehlo (1989) claimed that, if the loads were held on the teeth for short durations equivalent to those reported during mastication in humans (Anderson, 1956a,b; Bearn, 1973), then more nearly elastic responses are produced (*Fig. 10.8*). This latter finding has been confirmed for the teeth of monkeys by Picton (1989).

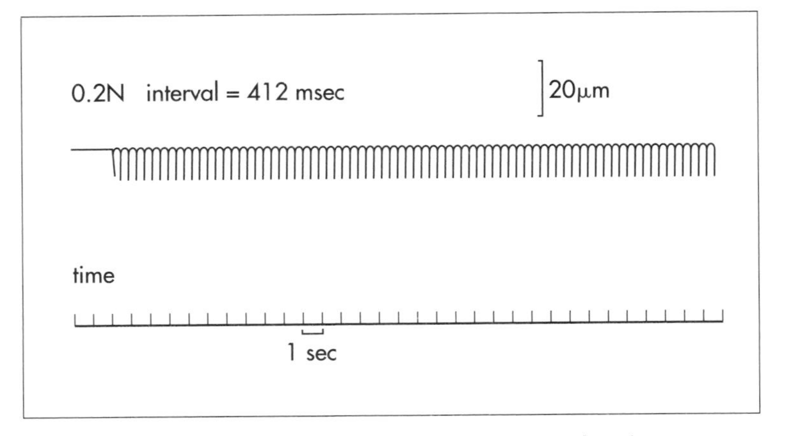

Fig. 10.8. Record illustrating the effects on tooth position of applying an intrusive 'vibrational' load of 0.2 N (10 ms duration, 412 ms interval) to a guinea pig mandibular incisor. (Moxham and Coehlo, 1989.)

It is conceivable that physical characteristics other than viscoelasticity could account for the patterns of tooth displacement observed. For example, the possibility that the periodontal tissues are thixotropic should be considered. A thixotropic material is one which can undergo gel/sol/gel transformations (Pryce-Jones, 1936). In general, a thixotropic system has the following rheological characteristics:

- an isothermal change in viscosity brought about by pressure alone;
- the system undergoes a time-dependent recovery and maintains its contours when the pressure is removed.
- the flow curve (i.e. the shear stress versus the shear rate) has a hysteresis loop.

Kardos and Simpson (1979, 1980) attempted to explain the mechanisms associated with the passage of an erupting tooth through the jaws, orthodontic tooth movement, and tooth support on the basis of the PDL being thixotropic. They reinterpreted the data from the experiments of Parfitt (1960), claiming that the behaviour of a tooth with axial intrusive loads was consistent with the properties of a thixotropic material. However, care should be taken not to overspeculate since a radical change in our ideas concerning the structure, biochemical composition and function of the PDL would be necessary if it is thixotropic and, even in unfixed tissue, collagen fibres can still be easily discerned (see Chapter 2).

There have in recent times been several studies concerned with applying intrusive loads onto erupting teeth in order to try to ascertain the magnitude of the force of eruption. These studies have been more fully described in Chapter 9. Here, it need only be re-emphasized that the low forces needed to stop a tooth erupting merely reflect the difference between the force of eruption and the force resisting eruption. That there is a relationship between the eruptive mechanism and the tooth support mechanism is clear. Firstly, Picton (1989) has pointed out that 'the position a tooth adopts is determined by the interplay of these two opposing sets of greatly differing forces'. Secondly, extrusive movements may be related to eruption and to recovery movements following the removal of intrusive loads. Thirdly, the eruptive and tooth support mechanisms are both properties of the PDL; indeed, it is most unlikely that one can physiologically 'microdissect' the PDL since, in such a connective tissue, all components must act in a concerted manner to maintain tissue function and integrity.

EXTRUSIVE TOOTH MOBILITY

Parfitt (1960) reported that tractional forces of approximately 0.15 N and 0.3 N caused a human maxillary central incisor to extrude by 6 μm and 8 μm respectively. Heners (1974) claimed that human maxillary central incisors extruded by about 20 μm with 5 N loads. Although some preliminary reports have been published using holographic techniques to measure with great accuracy movements of human teeth in three dimensions with extrusive loads (Every *et al.*, 1978, 1979), the promise of these initial reports has not been subsequently fulfilled by substantial, published research.

The pattern of tooth mobility during, and following, the sustained application of an extrusive load has been described by Moxham and Berkovitz (1979) for the rabbit mandibular incisor. The method of applying loads and the displacement transducer used to monitor tooth position continuously is illustrated diagrammatically in *Fig. 10.9*. The typical responses of a rabbit incisor to the sudden application of an extrusive load which is maintained for 5 minutes and then suddenly removed is shown in *Fig. 10.10*. On applying the load, a biphasic response is seen. During the first phase, there is a rapid, instantaneous extrusion of the tooth. The second phase involves a more gradual extrusion. A similar, but intrusive, biphasic recovery response is observed on removing the load. The amount of displacement of the tooth during the first phase of both the extrusive and recovery cycles is similar. However, the second phase of the extrusive cycle is generally greater than that of the recovery cycle. Thus, the tooth does not return to its resting position but shows a slightly extruded position. Similar biphasic responses to extrusive loads have been observed for teeth of non-continuous growth, i.e. ferret mandibular canines (Moxham and Berkovitz, 1983), and for rat maxillary incisors (Burn-Murdoch, personal communication).

A quantitative assessment of the effects of extrusive loads on the rabbit mandibular incisor was undertaken by Moxham and Berkovitz (1981) (*Fig. 10.11*). The results show that, while both first and second phases of the extrusive and recovery cycles are force dependent,

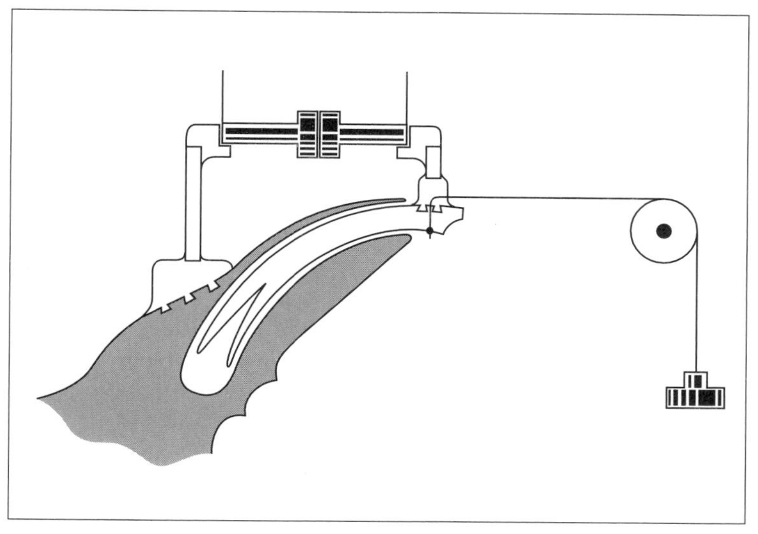

Fig. 10.9 Diagrammatic representation showing an extrusive load being applied over a pulley to a rabbit mandibular incisor on to which a variable capacitance displacement transducer has been placed. (Moxham and Berkovitz, 1979.)

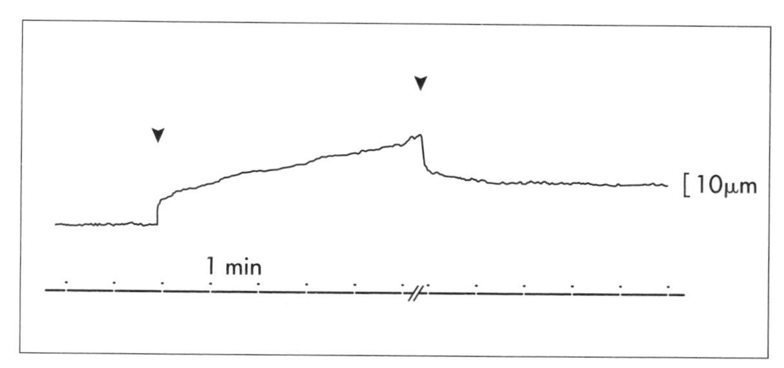

Fig. 10.10 Pen recorder trace illustrating the effects on tooth position of applying an extrusive load to a rabbit mandibular incisor. The first arrow indicates application and the second arrow indicates removal of the load. In this instance a load of 0.05 N was applied. Note that, for both the loading and recovery cycles, biphasic tooth movements occur. (Moxham and Berkovitz, 1979.)

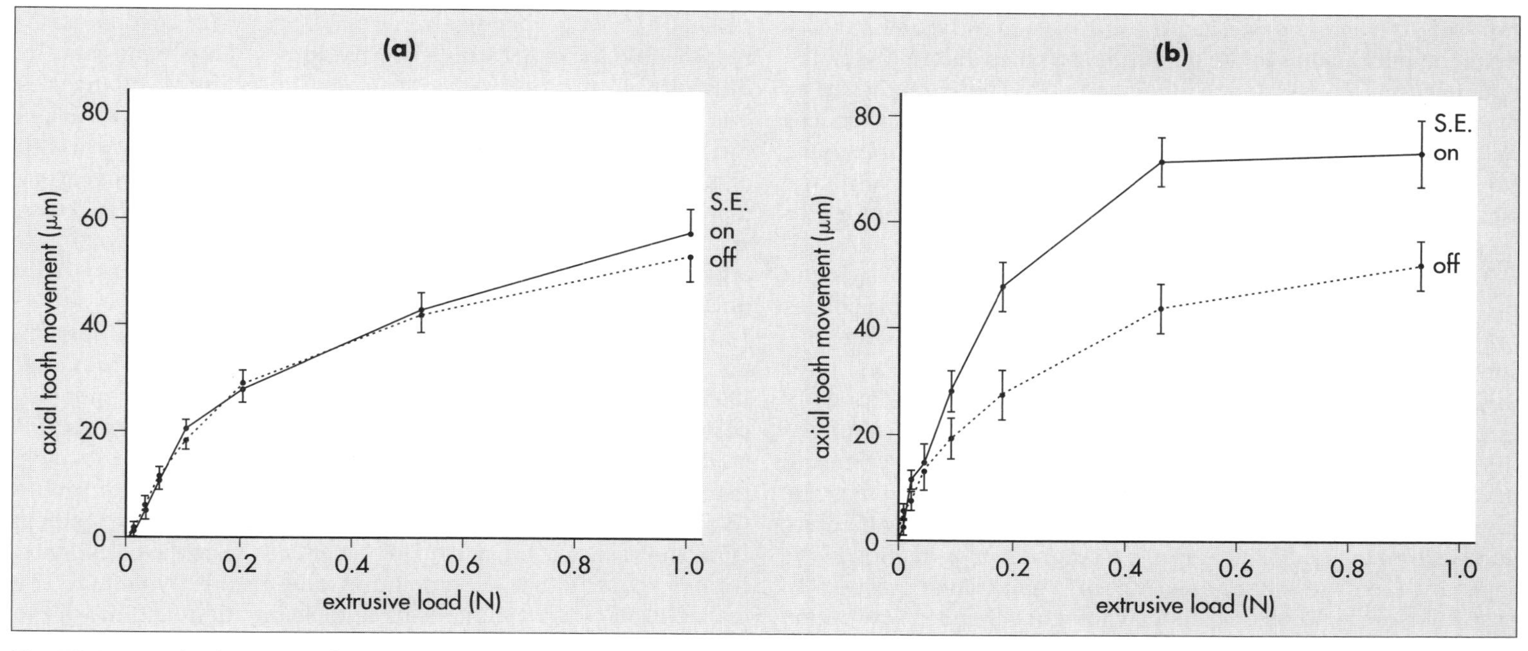

Fig. 10.11 Graphs showing axial movements of rabbit mandibular incisors (right) in response to extrusive loads. Each point represents the mean movement for the incisors of twelve animals (±1 SE). (a) First phase of movement with load on and off. (b) Second phase of movement with load on and off. See *Fig. 10.10* for demonstration of the phases. (Moxham and Berkovitz, 1981.)

they are not linearly graded. This indicates that the responses do not have Hooke-type characteristics, and it may support the view that the periodontal tissues behave as a viscoelastic system.

Moxham and Berkovitz (1989) have also compared the response to extrusive loading of ferret mandibular canines that were either erupting or erupted. Although qualitatively a similar biphasic, viscoelastic response followed both the application and removal of loads in both types of teeth, significantly more mobility for all phases of the loading and recovery cycles was observed in the erupting teeth (*Fig. 10.12*).

Comparing the reactions of the rabbit mandibular incisor to extrusive loads (Moxham and Berkovitz, 1979, 1981) with the reactions of the rat maxillary incisor to intrusive loads (Bien and Ayers, 1965; Bien, 1966), the following differences are notable:

- whereas an instantaneous elastic displacement of the rabbit incisor to the sudden application of an extrusive load was observed, the first response of the rat incisor to an intrusive load was more gradual;
- whereas the rat incisor returned to its original resting position within minutes of the intrusive load being removed, at the end of the extrusive recovery cycle the rabbit incisor showed a slightly extruded position; and
- the responses of the rat incisor to intrusive loads changed significantly after death, the tooth only returning to its resting position after the load had been removed when the thorax was squeezed. However, in both live and dead rabbits it was possible to observe similar reactions to extrusive loads.

Thus, although there are some similarities in the responses of a continuously growing incisor to intrusive and extrusive loads, the differences suggest that these loads may be resisted by different mechanisms in the periodontal tissues. Alternatively, the differences may be related to differences in the periodontal tissues of the experimental animals used. Evidence of further differences between extrusive and intrusive loading of the same tooth come from comparisons of the degree of displacement with loads of the same magnitude, the data showing that the displacement is less for extrusive loads (Picton 1986, 1990).

Experiments involving the application of extrusive loads can provide information not only about the biomechanical properties of the PDL but also about other characteristics of this tissue (e.g. the eruptive mechanism). Moxham and Berkovitz (1981) have investigated differences in the reactions to extrusive loads of impeded and unimpeded rabbit mandibular incisors erupting at different rates. The unimpeded teeth were cut out of the bite and maintained so for 5 days before experimentation, whereas the impeded teeth were left in occlusion. The results obtained are summarized in *Fig. 10.13*. They show a significant reduction in the resistance of the unimpeded rabbit mandibular incisor to extrusive forces. Thus, it is conceivable that changes in eruption rates may be associated with changes in resistance to eruption

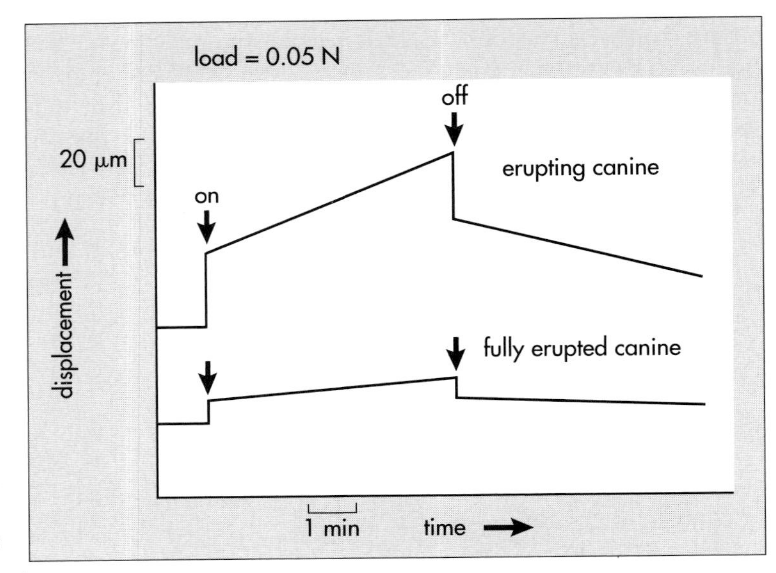

Fig. 10.12 A diagrammatic representation of the pattern of mobility of the erupting and erupted ferret mandibular canine obtained from the group mean axial displacements for 0.05 N loads. Note that biphasic responses occur following both the sudden application of a load and its sudden removal. The amount of displacement is greater for all phases for the erupting tooth. (Moxham and Berkovitz, 1989.)

rather than with changes in the mechanism (or mechanisms) responsible for generating eruptive forces. This highlights the difficulty of interpreting experimentally produced changes in eruption rates. Investigations have also been undertaken to assess the effects of lathyrogens upon the PDLs of rabbit incisors with extrusive loads (Moxham and Berkovitz, 1984). Since lathyrogens markedly disrupt the collagen framework of the PDL, mobility was, not unexpectedly, significantly increased for the lathyritically affected tooth, but the pattern of mobility remained essentially unchanged (see also page 231, *Fig. 10.23* and Chapter 9).

The lack of change in the pattern of mobility (for both loading and recovery cycles) for the lathyritic PDL (Moxham and Berkovitz, 1984) indicates the difficulty of interpreting mobility patterns in terms of the biology of the PDL. Similarly, Wills and Manderson (1977) have reported responses to static intrusive loading of the palates of macaque monkeys similar to the responses of the periodontal tissues following extrusive loading. Since the tissues of the palate differ markedly from the periodontal tissues in structure, composition and tissue dynamics, the explanation of the mechanisms underlying the reactions of the periodontal tissues to loading may be elusive.

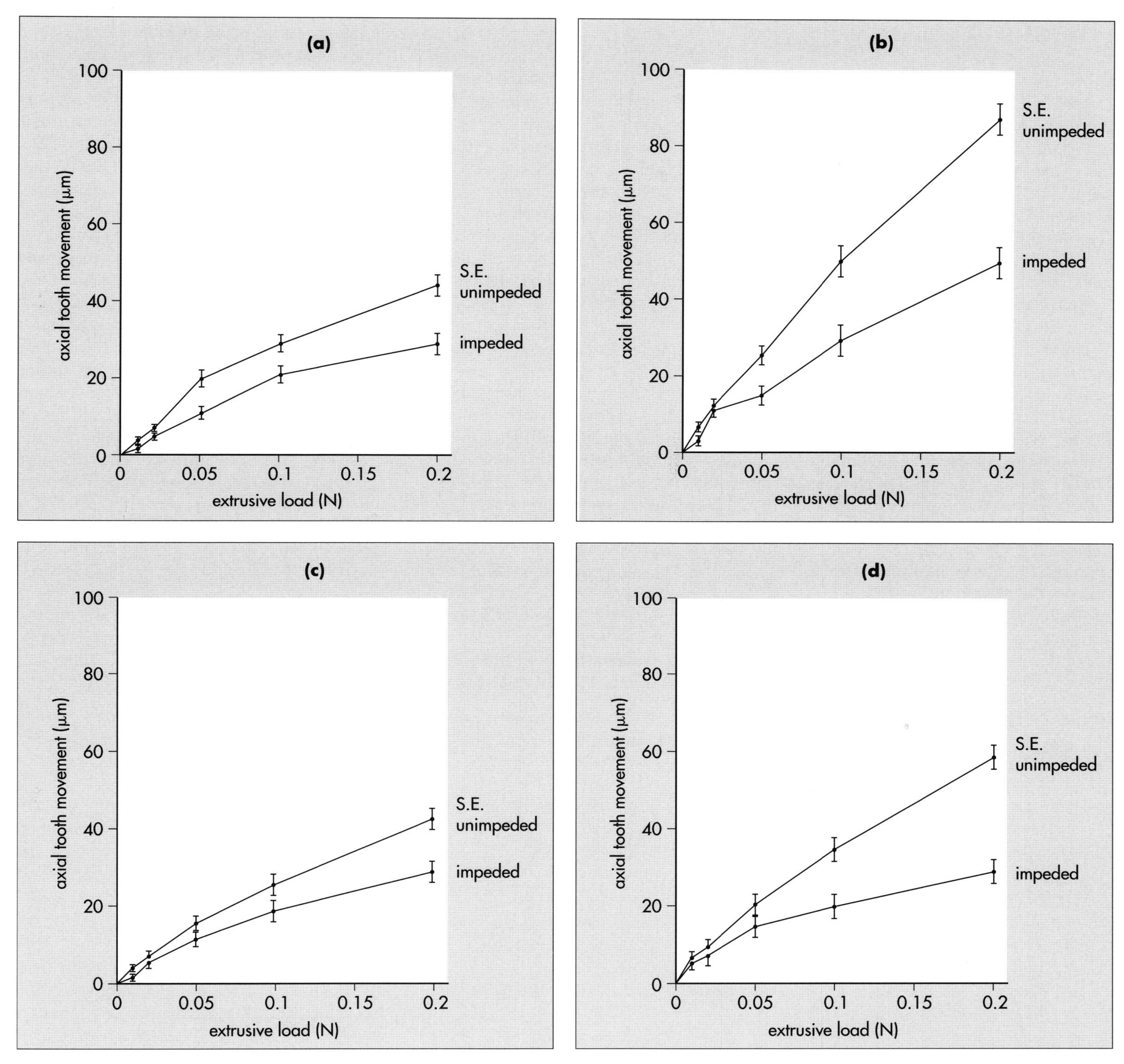

Fig. 10.13 Graphs showing axial movements of impeded and unimpeded rabbit mandibular incisors in response to extrusive loads. Each point represents the mean movement for the incisors of twelve animals (±1 SE). (a) First phase of movement with load on. (b) Second phase of movement with load on. (c) First phase of movement with load off. (d) Second phase of movement with load off. See *Fig. 10.10* for demonstration of the phases. (Moxham and Berkovitz, 1981.)

HORIZONTAL TOOTH MOBILITY

Experiments on tooth mobility using horizontal loads of short duration are similar in concept and technique to those using axial intrusive loads. Most of the studies that have been conducted have used loads that are directed buccolingually and that are applied to the crowns of the teeth, producing tipping movements. In contrast with axial loads, which are of relatively large magnitude (e.g. Anderson, 1956a,b; Ahlgren, 1967) and which are likely to be of very short duration, the physiological horizontal loads generated by the lips, cheeks, and tongue are much smaller in magnitude and are usually prolonged (e.g. Gould and Picton, 1964; Evans and Sue, 1979).

In 1951, Mühlemann reported a method for measuring horizontal tooth mobility. He employed a dial indicator attached intraorally to record tooth displacement and a hand-held dynamometer to apply loads. He subsequently published a series of papers describing mobility of rhesus monkey teeth (Mühlemann, 1954a,b,c; Mühlemann and Zander, 1954). In these, loads ranging from 0.5–5 N were applied for 2 seconds. It was observed that the mobility for both single and multirooted teeth did not increase linearly with increasing load but showed a 'quasi-logarithmic' relationship (*Fig. 10.14*). Initially, there was a relatively marked change in mobility with increasing load. Above 1 N, however, a load increase did not have so great an effect. As an example, for the tooth illustrated in *Fig. 10.14*, a load of 1 N produced a displacement of approximately 150 µm. A 5 N load produced only a further 50 µm displacement. Molars seemed to show slightly less mobility than incisors. If a load was rapidly repeated or was prolonged, an increase in mobility was seen (mainly for loads in the 'initial phase'). The original load–tooth mobility curve was restored after 25 minutes' rest.

This pattern of mobility has been confirmed by other workers using a variety of teeth and techniques (e.g. Mühlemann, 1960; Parfitt, 1961; Picton, 1964b; Mühlemann *et al.*, 1965; Picton, 1965; Picton and Davies, 1967; Picton, 1967, 1969; Christiansen and Burstone, 1969; Picton and Slatter, 1972). Furthermore, as noted by Picton (1969), this pattern resembles the reactions described for axial intrusive loads. It is usually claimed, however, that axial loads induce much smaller displacements than horizontal loads (e.g. Mühlemann, 1967; Heners, 1974). Persson and Svenson (1980) and Renggli *et al.* (1984) have also provided evidence that tooth displacement is highest for horizontal forces and lowest for extrusive and rotational forces (Daly *et al.*, 1974; Picton 1986, 1990).

The recovery of a tooth on removal of a horizontal load has been described by Picton (1964b). He studied human maxillary central incisors and first premolars following horizontal thrusts of 10 N applied at rates of about 10 per minute and 60 per minute. He reported that the recovery was in two phases. Initially, there was a fast return of the tooth towards its starting position (in a linear manner with time). As the tooth approached the starting position, a second and logarithmic phase developed. The biphasic recovery response has been reported by others (e.g. Hofmann, 1963; Mühlemann *et al.*, 1965; Körber and Körber, 1967; Körber, 1971; Picton *et al.*, 1974; Ross *et al.*, 1976).

It has been established that tooth displacement during the application of a horizontal load is time dependent (e.g. Körber, 1971; Ross *et al.*, 1976; Burstone *et al.*, 1978). *Fig. 10.15* illustrates the pattern for a human maxillary central incisor following the

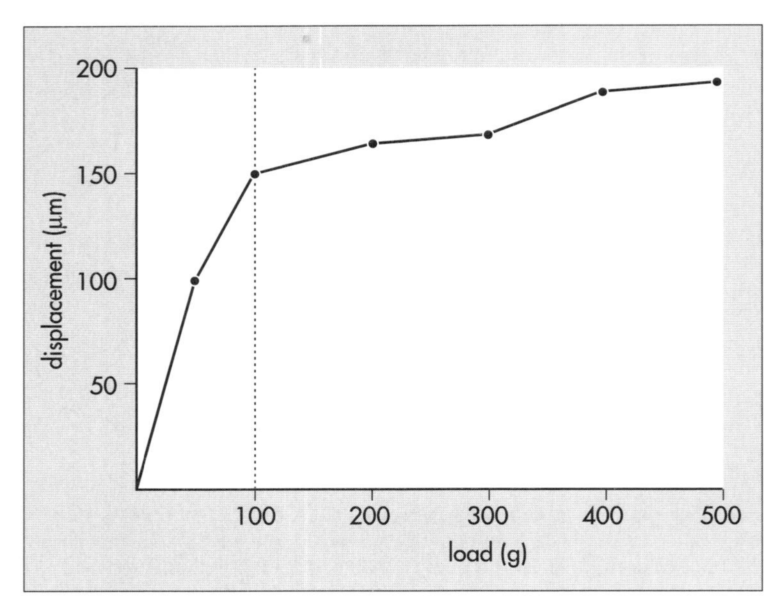

Fig. 10.14. Graph showing the relationship between horizontal tooth displacement and load for Rhesus monkey teeth. The broken vertical line delineates the initial phase of tooth mobility from the secondary phase. (Mühlemann, 1954a.)

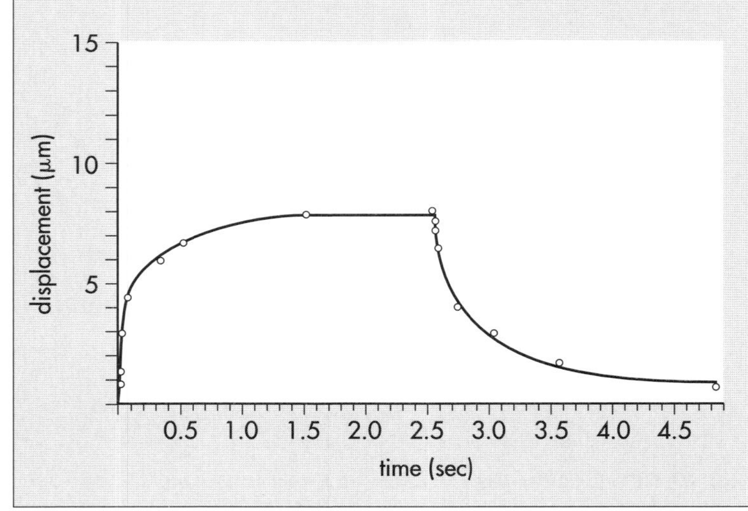

Fig. 10.15 Graph illustrating the relationship between horizontal tooth displacement and time following the sudden application (and sudden removal) of a lingually directed load of 0.05 N to a human maxillary central incisor. (Ross *et al.*, 1976.)

sudden application and sudden removal of a load observed by Ross *et al.* (1976). Thus, on applying the load there is an initial rapid displacement away from the force, followed by a phase of more gradual displacement. There is also a biphasic response on removal of the load. These responses also show similarities with those obtained with an axial load (see pages 00). As for axial loads, attempts have been made to describe the responses in terms of rheological models. The resistance of the periodontal tissues to horizontal loading cannot be explained in terms of a simple linear mechanical model. Although the pattern shown in *Fig. 10.15* might suggest a viscoelastic system composed of Maxwell or Voigt elements (springs and dampers in series or in parallel – see *Fig. 10.6*), Ross *et al.* (1976) proposed a three-parameter non-linear spring model for the periodontal tissues. As for the attempts to model responses to axial loads, however, further work is necessary to show the biological significance. Furthermore, other physical properties (e.g. thixotropy) may complicate the issue.

Lear *et al.* (1972) and Lear *et al.* (1974) investigated the threshold levels for displacement of human maxillary central incisors and first premolars in response to horizontal forces. For thrusts lasting 100 ms, the threshold was approximately 0.01 N. The thresholds, however, were related to the duration of force. When loads were applied for 25 ms, the threshold was raised to 0.03 N. It is noteworthy that to date most investigators have used horizontal loads much above threshold values.

Moxham *et al.* (1987, 1990) have described the results of loading sheep incisors linguolabially. The usual biphasic response was seen, with considerable displacement being recorded (e.g. a displacement of 1 mm for a load of 0.2 N during a 5 minute period). Compared with the initial elastic response, the second (creep) phase of mobility was smaller (*Figs. 10.16, 10.17, 10.18*).

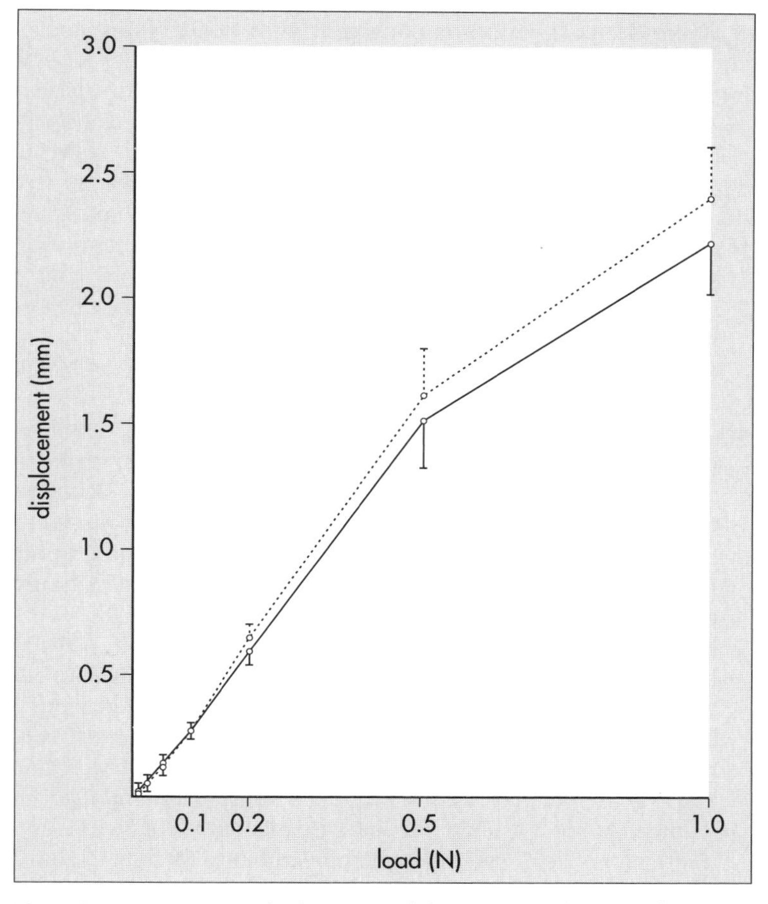

Fig. 10.17 Group mean displacements of sheep incisors during the first phases following application and removal of loads directed linguolabially. (o ——— o on, o- - - -o off). (Moxham *et al.*, 1987.)

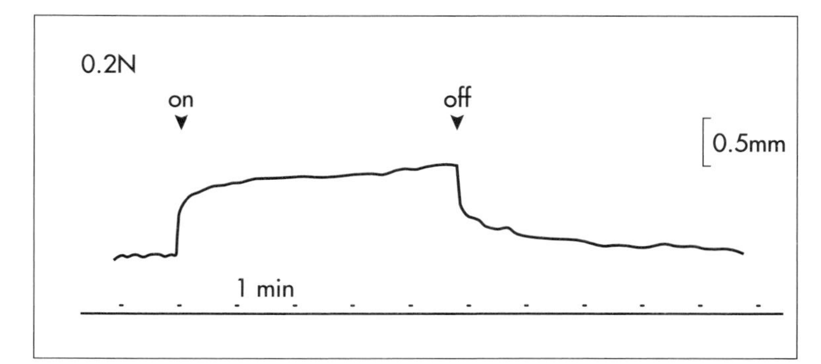

Fig. 10.16 Typical biphasic responses of the sheep incisor to the sudden application and sudden removal of a load directed linguolabially. (Moxham *et al.*, 1987.)

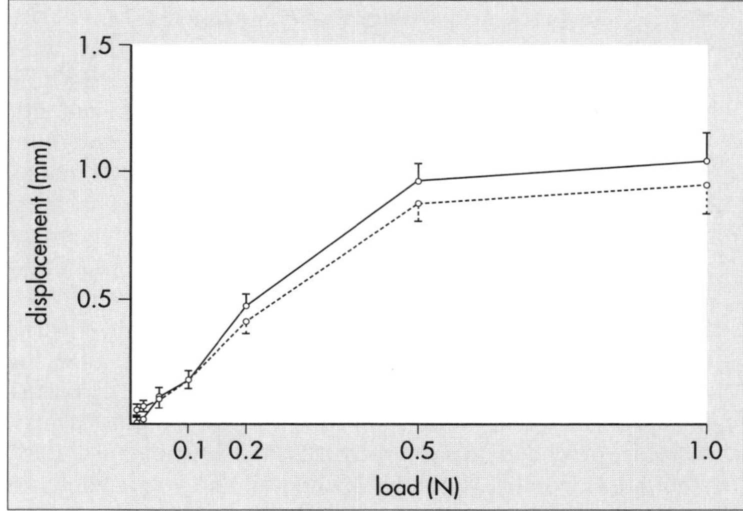

Fig. 10.18 Group mean displacements of sheep incisors during the second phases following application and removal of loads directed linguolabially. (o ——— o on, o- - - -o off). (Moxham *et al.*, 1987.)

While the pattern of displacement with horizontal loads of short duration is of significance for appreciating the general mechanical characteristics of the periodontal tissues, the amount of displacement is probably more relevant for assessing the clinical state of the periodontium. However, though there is agreement about the basic pattern, data about amounts of displacement are unreliable because of problems of comparing results from different experiments. Some of these problems are:

1. A variety of teeth and experimental animals have been used.
2. The root length and degree of tilt in the alveolus have not always been considered.
3. There has been no standard loading regime (in terms of the range of loads and duration of application).
4. Different techniques of applying loads and recording displacement have been used. The techniques differ both in terms of sensitivity and in basic principle of design. For example, Mühlemann's (1951) mechanical displacement transducer recorded in units of 10 μm, while the non-invasive, holographic technique of Burstone and Pryputniewicz (1980) had a stated accuracy of 0.5 μm.
5. As is the case for axial intrusive loads, it has been shown that horizontal mobility is influenced by the rate of loading (Körber and Körber, 1967; Körber, 1971; Lear *et al.*, 1972). Indeed, a marked change can be recorded even for small differences in rate. Körber (1971) reported that, for a human maxillary incisor, a rate of 5 N per 0.25 second produced a displacement of about 7 μm, a rate of 5 N per 1 second a displacement of 36 μm, and a rate of 5 N per 2 seconds a displacement of 58 mm. Because it is not always clear in most reports whether loading was instantaneous, complications in comparing data might arise if even slight differences in loading rate occurred.
6. Most studies have applied loads in buccolingual directions. Picton and Slatter (1972) studied the effects of mesiodistally directed loads following removal of contact points. Even with buccolingual loads, the presence of tooth contacts may influence the results. Mühlemann (1954b) reported that removal of contact points can produce an increase in mobility. Thus, the question arises: in the absence of comment about tooth contacts in most reports, should it be assumed that all the teeth were able to move in a similar unrestricted manner?
7. It is reasonable to assume that the functional state of the tooth influences mobility. It has been shown that the previous loading history affects tooth mobility. Indeed, some studies using axial intrusive loads employ a standard series of conditioning thrusts prior to the experiment proper (e.g. Wills *et al.*, 1978). The work of Mühlemann (1954b) and Körber (1971) suggests that there is also a change in mobility if experiments using horizontal loads are preceded by priming thrusts. Mühlemann (1960, 1967) stated that mobility is greater in children and young adults, in females, and during pregnancy. Himmel *et al.* (1957) and O'Leary *et al.* (1966) claim that mobility is lowest in the evening and highest in the morning on waking. O'Leary *et al.* (1966) also showed that lack of occlusal contact can affect tooth mobility. Mühlemann (1954a) has reported that erupting teeth have greater mobility than erupted teeth. In most studies on horizontal mobility, the functional state of the teeth is not considered, and it is conceivable that there could be markedly different states in different studies.
8. Since horizontal loads produce tipping movements, it is important to have a standardized point both for applying loads and for measuring displacement. Details of the placement of the apparatus are not always given, and it is unlikely that such points correspond in different studies.

Sophisticated techniques based upon the principle of holography have also been employed to study horizontal mobility (Bowley *et al.*, 1974; Pryputniewicz *et al.*, 1978; Burstone *et al.*, 1978; Pryputniewicz and Burstone, 1979; Burstone and Pryputniewicz, 1980). Because of the sensitivity and accuracy, such techniques seemed to provide the possibility of precise data about the force–displacement characteristics of human teeth. Indeed, Burstone and Pryputniewicz (1980) claimed that previous work was unreliable primarily because the experiments used techniques that were relatively inaccurate, could not measure three-dimensional displacements and, being invasive, influenced the tooth movement. *Fig. 10.19* shows an example of the relationship

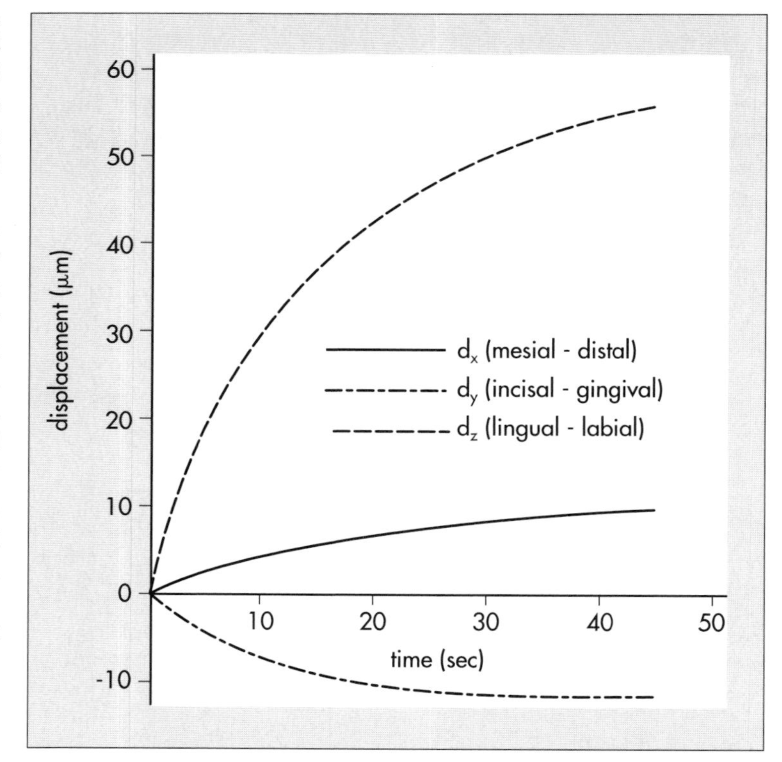

Fig. 10.19 Graph showing the relationship between displacement (in three dimensions) and time from the instant of the application of a force (3 N in a linguolabial direction, parallel to the occlusal plane) for a human maxillary central incisor. (Burstone *et al.*, 1978.)

between displacement and time observed with a labially directed 3 N load reported by Burstone *et al.* (1978). While the largest motion was, as expected, in the linguolabial direction, there was also an extrusion and displacement mesiodistally. Newer techniques that are being developed to monitor tooth mobility involving finite-element models (Anderson *et al.*, 1991), the use of an impedence head device (Oka *et al.*, 1989), and the Siemens 'Periotest' instrument (e.g. D'Hoedt *et al.*, 1985) should soon provide us with additional information.

The centre of rotation with horizontal loads

A horizontal load applied to the crown of a tooth will tip the tooth around a centre of rotation. Mühlemann (1951) suggested that this centre varied in position according to the size and angulation of the load. Mühlemann and Houglum (1954) and Mühlemann and Zander (1954) described techniques for estimating rotation centres in single-rooted teeth. The latter study indicated that the rotation centre varied with the size of the load and the type of tooth. However, Haack and Weinstein (1963) claim that a force directed at a given point in a given direction produced the same rotation centre regardless of magnitude.

Christiansen and Burstone (1969) determined the centres of rotation of human maxillary central incisors using lingual, labial, and mesial tipping loads ranging from about 0.2 N to about 7 N. They reported that the centre is related not to the magnitude of load but to the moment–force ratio. A theoretical rotation centre was calculated based upon a formula devised according to the concepts of Burstone (1962):

$$\text{moment–force ratio} = 0.068h^2/y$$

Where h is the distance between the alveolar crest and the root apex, y is the distance between the centre of rotation and the 'centoid' (a point 40 per cent of the distance apical to the distance between the alveolar crest and the root apex).

The formula assumes that the tooth is in equilibrium, that the stress distribution is uniform along the root, and that the stress—strain ratio is uniform or linear. The theoretical rotation centre was found by Christiansen and Burstone (1969) to be about 55 per cent of the distance from the apex to the alveolar crest. The theoretical centre was compared with experimentally determined centres for the incisors of six subjects. For three subjects, the experimental centre closely approximated the theoretical centre with loads above 0.5 N.

A tooth–periodontium model based upon plane elasticity theory and plane photoelasticity has been devised by Nikolai (1974) to enable determination of the location of rotation centres in single-rooted teeth with horizontal crown loading. It was assumed that the PDL is homogeneous and isotropic, that it exhibits Hookean behaviour, that it is residual stress-free, and that the crown load is transferred totally and in a continuously distributed manner across the root–PDL boundary. It was claimed that the rotation centres determined using the model were located only slightly occlusal to that predicted according to the concepts of Burstone (1962). However, this model (like Burstone's) is two-dimensional and some of the assumptions seem erroneous. Furthermore, the time-dependent behaviour of the tissues was not considered.

Using holography, Burstone *et al.* (1978) and Pryputniewicz and Burstone (1979) determined rotation centres for some human maxillary incisors with labially directed loads of 3 N or 5 N. Pryputniewicz and Burstone (1979) reported that, with a slight modification to the formula used by Christiansen and Burstone (1969), the theoretical centre fitted reasonably with the experimentally determined centre. They also reported differences in the rotation centre with 3 N and 5 N loads. However, unlike previous views that higher loads moved rotation centres coronally, the centres for the higher loads were moved apically. The results also showed that, the longer the root, the further apical the rotation centre. Despite the apparent errors or conceptual limitations involved in formulating theoretical models, it is remarkable that the experimental data from this study should still show reasonable fit. Pryputniewicz and Burstone (1979) were of the opinion that the minor discrepancies could be attributed to differences between a two-dimensional model with linear properties of the PDL and a three-dimensional *in vivo* situation with a ligament having non-linear characteristics.

The effects of horizontal orthodontic loads on tooth displacement

The histological changes and principles of cell biology occurring within the PDL following orthodontic loading are discussed in Chapters 11 and 12. Here, we will describe briefly the pattern of tooth movements in response to orthodontic loads of long duration which produce tilting. Little information is available concerning the threshold force for such movements. Bass and Stephens (1970) suggest that orthodontic movements are unlikely to occur with forces below 0.1 N. (This compares with the loads of 1.5–3 N that are necessary to move a tooth bodily – Storey and Smith, 1952.)

Crabb and Wilson (1972) determined the rate of space closure between maxillary canines and second premolars following extraction of the maxillary first premolars. The forces applied to the canines were in the range of 0.3–0.5 N. The springs were reactivated every 28 days. The results indicate a mean rate of space closure of about 1 mm per 28 days.

Reitan (1975) has described several phases associated with orthodontic tooth movement (*Fig. 10.20*). With light, continuous, orthodontic loads, it seems to take on average 5 days before the periodontal tissues are compressed to the point where there is a cessation of tooth movement. This period is shortened with excessive loads. There then follows a period of about 2–3 weeks during which the tooth shows only minor changes in position. However, a secondary period of tooth movement occurs after undermining of the bone. The pattern shown in *Fig. 10.20* is typical of the reactions that occur when the load is not regularly reactivated. *Fig. 10.21* shows the pattern that occurs when a load is strictly maintained with frequent reactivation.

Following the removal of an orthodontic load, there is a period of recovery or relapse. *Fig. 10.22* illustrates a case of relapse reported by Reitan (1967). Note that in this instance there was considerable relapse during the first day after the orthodontic appliances had been removed. Thereafter, relapse may be prevented for a short while by periodontal changes or new bone formation.

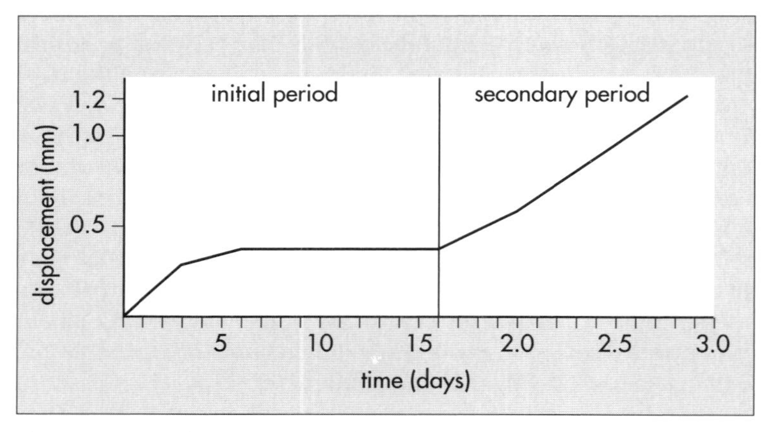

Fig. 10.20 Graph illustrating the relationship between tooth displacement and time following the application of a light orthodontic load. (Reitan, 1975.)

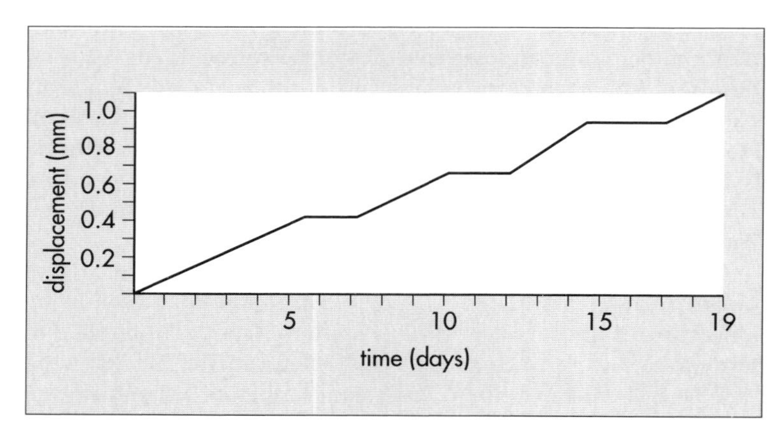

Fig. 10.21 Graph showing the relationship between tooth displacement and time following the application of an orthodontic load that was frequently reactivated. (Reitan, 1975.)

STUDIES TO DETERMINE THE ULTIMATE TENSILE STRENGTH OF THE PERIODONTAL LIGAMENT *IN VITRO*

The forces required to extract teeth from their sockets in dissected jaws have been studied for the rat molar (Chiba and Ohkawa, 1980; Kinoshita *et al.*, 1982; Tsuruta *et al.*, 1982; Ohshima *et al.*, 1989; Ohshima *et al.*, 1991; Hong *et al.*, 1992), the rat incisor (Chiba *et al.*, 1980; Chiba, Kuroda and Ohshima, 1981; Chiba *et al.*, 1981; Ohshima, 1982; Chiba and Komatsu, 1988) and the hamster molar (Yamazaki, 1992) under varying experimental and pathological conditions. Accordingly, it is assumed that such useful biomechanical parameters for the PDL as maximum shear load, maximum deformation, elastic stiffness, and failure energy in shear can be obtained by breaking the ligament with high extrusive loads (Chiba and Ohkawa, 1980; Chiba *et al.*, 1982; Hong, 1990). In the earliest studies, the velocity of loading was arbitrarily fixed at 5 mm per minute (e.g. Chiba *et al.*, 1980, 1981; Chiba, Kuroda and Ohshima, 1981; Ohshima, 1982). However, with velocities between 1 and 25 mm per minute, the ultimate tensile strengths of the PDL in the rat molar do not appear to be affected (Chiba *et al.*, 1982) nor are the reactions of human teeth to velocities of 0.05–0.5 mm per minute (Ralph, 1982). Significant effects are seen for the rat incisor (Chiba and Komatsu, 1988) if the range of velocity of loading is wide enough. In particular, marked differences were found when the velocities of loading corresponded to impeded and unimpeded eruption rates (*Table 10.1*).

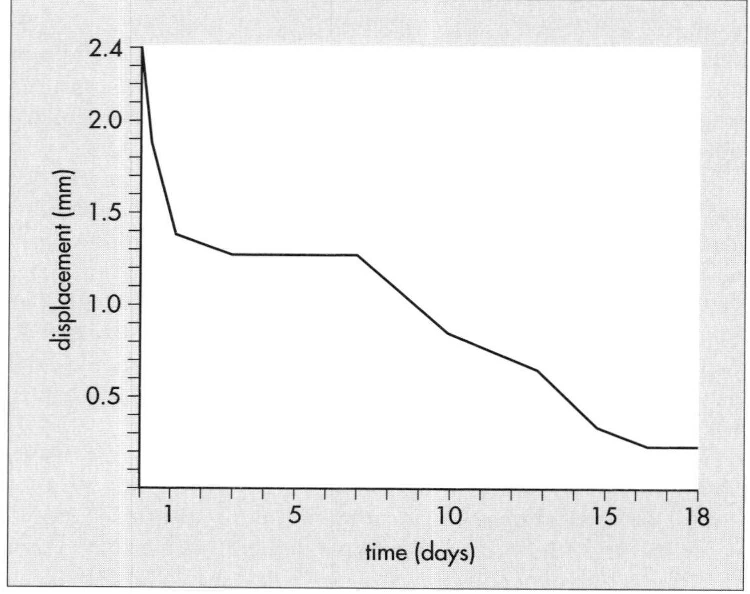

Fig. 10.22 Graph showing the relationship between the degree of relapse and time, following labial tipping of a maxillary lateral incisor with a force of 0.4 N. (Reitan, 1967.)

Even with constraints relating to the velocity and direction of the extracting forces, experiments have been conducted to assess the effects on the ultimate tensile strengths of the PDL of altering the functional characteristics of the tissue before killing the animals. To date, the effects of different ages (Chiba *et al.*, 1980), artificial restraint of the tooth (Chiba *et al.*, 1981), adrenocorticoids (Chiba, Kuroda and Ohshima, 1981), lathyrogens (Ohshima, 1982; Ohshima *et al.*, 1989), removal of teeth from the bite (i.e. the unimpeded tooth) and hypofunction (Chiba *et al.*, 1981; Kinoshita *et al.*, 1982; Chiba and Komatsu, 1988; Komatsu, 1988; Ohshima *et al.*, 1991), orthodontic-type loading (Tsuruta *et al.*, 1982; Ohkawa, 1982; Hong, 1990; Hong *et al.*, 1992), and periodontitis of the hamster molar induced by diet (Yamazaki, 1992) have been studied. Criticisms of this experimental model (acknowledged by Chiba and his group) stem from lack of standardization, because the dimensions of the PDL were not quantified (Komatsu and Chiba, 1993), and also from the very act of studying the effects of loading in dissected jaws (such *in vitro* techniques clearly being influenced by such factors as post-mortem changes and tissue damage – Chiba *et al.*, 1982, 1990; Komatsu, 1988). Nevertheless, the data obtained hint at a possible role for the periodontal collagen in the resistance to high extracting forces in the absence of contributions from the periodontal vasculature, ground substance interactions, and fluid dynamics.

Table 10.1
Mechanical properties of the periodontal ligament calculated from load-deformation curves.

	Impeded group	Unimpeded group
Maximum load (mN)	11.16 ± 2.62	9.93 ± 2.17
Maximum deformation (μm)	333 ± 90	408 ± 78*
Failure energy (mN•mm)	2.56 — 0.97	2.80 ± 1.10
Elastic stiffness (mN/mm)	158.3 ± 46.7	81.9 ± 26.4**

Mean ± SD of 20 rats shown in each group. Impeded and unimpeded incisors were pulled at 0.5mm/day and 1.0mm/day respectively. Significant differences between impeded and unimpeded groups, * $p < 0.01$, ** $p < 0.001$. (Chiba and Komatsu, 1988.)

More recently, Chiba and co-workers have published a series of papers in which attempts were made to assess the mechanical responses of the PDL from transverse sections of the rat molar or incisor (or both). The techniques adopted stemmed from earlier studies by Ralph (1982) and Mandel *et al.* (1986). It was assumed that these techniques would allow more meaningful comparisons to be made between experiments (and at different levels of the PDL) by enabling quantification of the dimensions of the PDL. Initially, the techniques were described by Komatsu (1988) and Chiba *et al.* (1990). To date, they have studied experimentally the effects of velocity of loading on the rat molar (Komatsu and Chiba, 1993) and the rat incisor (Chiba and Komatsu, 1993), and the effects of lathyrogens (Yamaguchi, 1992). Notwithstanding the problems associated with experiments conducted *in vitro*, the overtly reductionist approach arising from investigating thin sections of tissue and not the whole tissue requires much caution in interpretation of results.

Finally, and before considering the biological basis of tooth support, two general comments should be made concerning the interpretations of the findings of the experiments on physiological tooth mobility. Firstly, we should be aware that biting loads during mastication and swallowing are more complex than the loading regimes used in any of the experiments conducted to date. Furthermore, even with a unidirectional load, complex multi-directional tooth movements in the socket are produced (e.g. Pryputniewicz and Burstone, 1979). It is perhaps for such reasons that there has been relatively little recent work on the tooth support mechanism. Secondly, some have been tempted to speculate on the significance of their findings in terms of the biology of the periodontal tissues. For example, Picton (1989) has reported that the typical load–displacement and recovery curve (see *Fig. 10.7*) can be explained biologically in the following way: 'The initial force causes fluid, mostly in the blood vessels, to be displaced together with the cells, ground substance and fibres so that the tooth moves quite freely across the ligament. As the force increases to about 1 N in man, the principal fibres progressively come under tension. In this second phase of tooth mobility, which is substantially linear, the increasing load is transmitted to the alveolar bone and supporting trabeculae causing measurable displacement of the socket and distortion of the alveolar process.' An alternative explanation might relate to the crimp morphology of the periodontal collagen (see page 233 and Chapter 2). However, we are not convinced of the efficacy of this approach and we remain of the opinion that this aspect can be elucidated best by research involving the effects of loading on experimentally altered periodontal tissues, and this is the subject of the following section.

THE PERIODONTAL LIGAMENT AND THE TOOTH SUPPORT MECHANISM

THE BIOLOGICAL MECHANISMS INVOLVED IN THE SUPPORT AGAINST AXIAL, INTRUSIVE LOADS

The role of the collagen fibres: tension versus compression within the periodontal ligament

The classical view of the tooth support mechanism holds that the PDL is a 'suspensory ligament'. Accordingly, it is envisaged that the major structures supporting the tooth are the principal oblique fibres of the PDL and that, by their Sharpey fibre attachments into the alveolar bone and the cementum of the root of the tooth, they transmit axial loads in the form of tension to the alveolar bone. The concept of a 'suspensory ligament' also implies that the tissues behave in an elastic manner and that the relationship between load and tooth displacement follows Hooke's Law.

The results of physiological tooth mobility studies (see page 215–220) do not lend full support to the suspensory ligament hypothesis. It is clear that, whilst elastic responses can be elicited under certain masticatory-like loads (Moxham and Coehlo, 1989 – see *Fig. 10.8*; Picton, 1989), in other circumstances the response is time-dependent and suggests that the periodontal tissues are viscoelastic (Bien and Ayers, 1965; Bien, 1966; Wills *et al.*, 1972; Ross *et al.*, 1976; Picton and Wills, 1978; Moxham and Berkovitz, 1979, 1981; Coehlo and Moxham, 1989). Furthermore, the tissues display the property of hysteresis. This latter, non-Hookean characteristic is seen when the path of recovery on release of a load is not along the pathway of displacement during loading (see *Fig. 10.1*). Of further importance is the fact that response patterns of tooth loading are not dependent on the orientation of the fibres of the PDL and are similar whether intrusive, extrusive, or horizontal loads are applied. When the amounts of displacement with extrusive loads are compared with the amounts of intrusive loads, the results also provide arguments against the idea of a 'suspensory ligament' for the periodontium. It might be expected that, considering the direction of obliquity of the main principal fibres in the PDL, the total displacement with an extrusive load would be greater than for an intrusive load of the same magnitude (although extrusion would be opposed by the alveolar crestal and apical groups of principal fibres). However, the converse is the case (Picton, 1986, 1990). Providing some indication of the involvement of the periodontal collagen in the resistance to large extracting forces are the studies of Chiba and co-workers on the ultimate tensile strength of the PDL (see pages 228–229).

Some early dissenting voices against the tensional hypothesis were those of Synge (1933a,b) and Gabel (1956). These authors suggested that the lengths of the fibres are too great to account for the relatively small degree of mobility. Furthermore, the inverse relationship between loading rate and displacement would not be expected to occur if simple tension were the only mechanism involved in tooth support (Körber, 1971). Subsequently, Picton (1965), Picton and Davies (1967), Picton and Picton (1988) and Picton (1988, 1989) have conducted experiments to evaluate the relative importance of tension and compression in the tooth support mechanism.

The earliest experiments involved examining the distortion of the mesial and distal alveolar margins when axial intrusive loads and horizontal loads were applied to the teeth of monkeys (Picton, 1965; Picton and Davies, 1967). It was observed that intrusive thrusts caused dilation of the socket in 80 per cent of cases, little or no distortion in 12 per cent of cases and constriction in the remaining 8 per cent. The conclusion was drawn that the periodontal tissues act, at least in part, as a compressive system in resisting axial loads, since convergence of the alveolar margins was predicted if a tensional system had been involved. However, it is unlikely that a rigid structure such as the alveolar margin could be pulled in around its whole circumference even if tension was exerted upon it. Furthermore, the experiments do not disprove the notion that collagen fibres in the PDL are placed under tension, especially since no direct observations of the tissue under load were made. Picton and Wills (1981) have tried to visualize the principal fibres of the PDL *in vivo* when the tooth is loaded, but the results were inconclusive when applied to the question of whether they straightened sufficiently to generate tension.

The possibility that a tooth might be supported by both compressive and tensional reactions in different parts of the PDL was considered by Picton (1965, 1989). That tension may be of importance was shown by the finding that application of horizontal force to a tooth displaced the alveolar crest a similar distance whether the force was directed towards or away from the palate (Picton, 1965). Furthermore, Picton and Slatter (1972) observed that cutting the gingiva and PDL with a thin steel blade produced a similar increase in horizontal mobility when the tooth was pushed towards or away from the site of the trauma.

One criticism that may be levelled at the experiments of Picton (1965) and Picton and Davies (1967) is that surgical trauma of the periodontium, produced in order to expose the alveolar margins, may have caused disturbance to the tooth support mechanism. Whilst this possibility was acknowledged, Picton and Davies (1967) claimed that the trauma was minimal. Indeed, Picton (1967) reported that axial tooth mobility was only slightly increased by surgical trauma to the mesial and distal regions of the periodontium.

In a later experiment, Picton and Picton (1987) investigated the effects on the mobility of monkey teeth of removing the apical half of the tooth supporting tissues (i.e. apicectomy). They reported that, despite such major surgical interference, tooth mobility was unimpaired. The conclusion that was reached initially was that the experiment provided evidence against a compressive mode of activity for the PDL since the apical part of the PDL was considered to be the only part which could provide a 'cushion' during intrusive loading. This experiment confirmed an earlier study on the effects of apicectomy upon porcine molars *in vitro* (Gathercole, 1987). Subsequently, however, Picton (1988) has shown that removal of the PDL surrounding the coronal area of the root to a depth of 4–5 mm and consisting of about one-third of the ligament (i.e. that which is thought to provide the main region put into tension with intrusive loads) also did not significantly affect the intrusive mobility of the monkey teeth. These experiments therefore do not provide definitive evidence for or against tension or compression in the periodontal tissues, and we should only conclude that it is possible for quite extensive areas of the healthy PDL to be 'traumatized' without gross disturbance to the support mechanism.

In experimental studies of tooth mobility, specific components of the periodontal connective tissues must be changed (or experimental surgery must be performed) in order to ascertain the possible role of that component in tooth support. To date, few experiments have been conducted to assess how experimental changes to the collagen fibres affect the reactions of teeth to loading. Parfitt (1967) claimed to have shown that collagenases altered the characteristics of the movement of teeth *in vitro* with intrusive loads. However, it is not possible to assess this work properly since details of the experiment were not published. That collagen does play a role in the tooth support mechanism can also be deduced from experiments in which collagen cross-linking was inhibited by the administration to rats of lathyritic agents. Berkovitz *et al.* (1972) reported that there was considerable dilaceration of the roots of maxillary incisor teeth maintained in occlusion, whereas teeth relatively free of the occlusion showed no such disturbance. The ease with which teeth could be manually extracted provided evidence that the lathyrogen had produced an effect on the collagen of the PDL. Moxham and Berkovitz (1984) assessed the mobility of rabbit incisors with lathyritically affected PDLs to axially directed extrusive loads. It was reported that, compared with control, non-lathyritically affected tissues, there was a considerable increase in the amount of tooth mobility on loading. However, the precise mechanism by which this occurred proved elusive since, whether considering the loading or recovery cycles, the patterns of mobility were unaltered (*Fig. 10.23*). Experiments involving the assessment of the forces required to extract rat mandibular incisors and molars *in vitro* confirm that lathyrogens significantly reduce the mechanical strength of the PDL (Ohshima, 1982; Ohshima *et al.*, 1989; Yamaguchi, 1992).

Berkovitz and Moxham (1990) related the development of the PDL to the increased mobility to extrusive loading seen in erupting, as opposed to erupted, teeth (Moxham and Berkovitz, 1989) (see *Fig. 10.12*). Although Berkovitz and Moxham (1990) reported that the collagen fibres of newly erupting teeth were poorly organized and that this may be a factor related to the increased tooth mobility, the authors also stated that other factors, as yet unrecognized, may also be associated with the change in mobility. For example, differences in the vasculature have been reported between erupting and erupted rat molars (Moxham *et al.*, 1987).

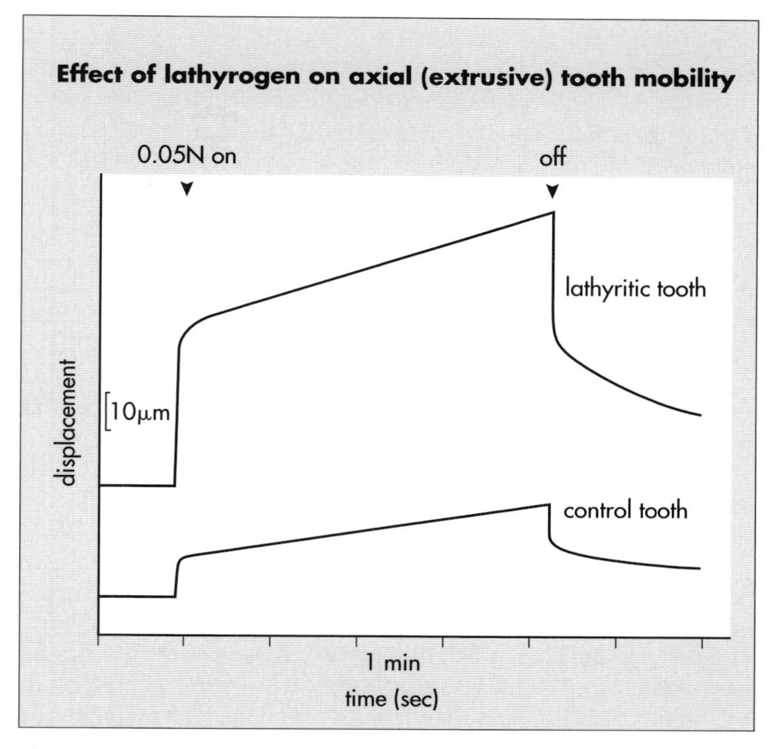

Fig. 10.23 The pattern of mobility of the rabbit mandibular incisor in lathyritic and pair-fed control animals with extrusive loading. Note that biphasic responses occur after both the sudden application of the load and its sudden removal, although the amount of displacement is greater for all phases in the lathyritic animal. (Moxham and Berkovitz, 1984.)

Picton (1990) studied intrusive displacement before and within 3 minutes after tooth reimplantation following extraction in monkeys (*Macaca fascicularis*). He found a substantial increase in intrusion with recovery, and he concluded that tension was an important mechanism of support in the intact periodontal ligament.

Morphological studies and biochemical studies on the periodontal connective tissues also provide evidence against the 'suspensory ligament' hypothesis. Morphologically, there have been quantitative electron microscopy studies that have been conducted with the purpose of ascertaining whether the PDL has the features of a connective tissue placed in tension or a tissue under compression. Indeed, there is evidence suggesting that the ultrastructure of a connective tissue is dictated by the mechanical demands placed upon the tissue (e.g. Parry *et al.*, 1978; Merrilees and Flint, 1980; Postacchini and de Martino, 1980; Flint *et al.*, 1984). Differences in collagen fibril diameters have been reported for connective tissues under tension or compression. Merrilees and

Flint (1980) found that the fibrils in areas of compression are small (approximately 30 nm diameter) and have sharply unimodal distributions. For tissues in tension, on the other hand, many of the fibrils are large and the distribution is bimodal (approximately 30 nm and 150 nm). The distribution of collagen fibrils in the PDL is unimodal, with a mode of between 40 and 50 nm (e.g. Berkovitz *et al.*, 1981; Svoboda *et al.*, 1983; Luder *et al.*, 1988) (see *Fig. 2.7*). Merrilees and Flint (1980) also reported differences in the axial periodicity of the collagen. The periodicity is approximately 62 nm in areas of tension and 54 nm in areas of compression. For the PDL, the axial periodicity is approximately 57 nm (Moxham, 1985).

Where the tissues are in tension, the fibroblasts are elongated parallel to the collagen fibres and have long, thin processes, which occasionally branch. Their membranes are also indented by the surrounding collagen. In regions of compression, the fibroblasts appear chondrocyte-like, with round profiles, and the adjacent fibrils do not indent the membranes (Merrilees and Flint, 1980). For the PDL, the fibroblasts are similar to those in regions of tension, possessing large flattened processes. However, the membranes are smooth and without indentations.

Merrilees and Flint (1980) have reported that connective tissues in compression contain considerably more ground substance within the fibre bundles than tissues in tension (50 per cent and 27 per cent respectively). Berkovitz *et al.* (1981) calculated that the fibre bundles in the PDL contain large volumes of ground susbtance (approximately 65 per cent). Not only the volume of ground substance but also the type of glycosaminoglycans seems to vary between connective tissues under tension and compression. Gillard *et al.* (1979) claimed that dermatan sulphate is the predominant glycosaminoglycan in tissues under tension, whereas chondroitin sulphate predominates in tissues under compression. Pearson (1982) reported that dermatan sulphate is the major component of the sulphated galactosaminoglycans in bovine PDL and that the proteoglycans are proteodermatan sulphate and a proteoglycan containing CS (DS) hybrids (PG_1). Indeed, a fully sulphated, authentic chondroitin sulphate was not detected for the proteoglycans. Further evidence supporting the view that the PDL is similar to a connective tissue placed in compression comes from the reactions of the tissue to Masson's trichrome histological stain. Flint *et al.* (1975) provided evidence that collagen in tissues under tension stains red with Masson's trichrome whereas collagen under compression stains green. Indeed, they reported that the stretched connective tissue of skin changed from staining green to red. The collagen fibres of the PDL stain green with Masson's trichrome.

Table 10.2 summarizes the above morphological and biochemical findings and shows that the PDL has features resembling both connective tissues placed in tension and connective tissues subjected to compression (although the weight of evidence perhaps favours compression). A note of caution needs to be introduced when comparing such morphological and biochemical characteristics of the PDL with other adult tendons, particularly since the former is loaded only intermittently. However, to help elucidate the apparent contradiction between tension and compression within the PDL, the ultrastructure of the PDL has been examined when the mechanical demands placed upon the tissue were altered experimentally. In the rat incisor maintained free of the bite (i.e. the unimpeded incisor) for 3 weeks, the only differences observed were an increase in number of microtubules and simplified desmosomes in the fibroblasts and a decrease in the amount of ground substance within the collagen bundles (Shore *et al.*, 1982). For the rat incisor immobilized by pinning for

Table 10.2
Relationship between the morphological and biochemical features of the periodontal ligament and mechanical properties.

Features of the periodontal ligament suggesting tension	Features of the periodontal ligament suggesting compression
Sharpey fibre structure	Small collagen fibril diameters Unimodal collagen size/frequency distribution
The flattened, disc shape of the fibroblasts	
Dermatan sulphate-rich composition of ground substance	Distribution of Sharpey fibres to socket
	Smooth surface of fibroblast membrane
	Large amounts of ground substance
	Masson trichrome staining

3 weeks, there was a slight decrease in collagen fibril diameters and an increase in amount of ground substance (Shore *et al.*, 1985). It might be concluded, therefore, that major changes in mechanical demand are associated with only minor changes in PDL ultrastructure. This is confirmed by the study of Schellens *et al.* (1982), who pinned rat incisors for 6 months and found few apparent changes in the structure of the PDL.

Undoubtedly, there are morphological characteristics of the collagen within the PDL which highlight their importance in the tooth support mechanism. In Chapter 2, Sloan argues that the organization of the periodontal collagen reflects the magnitude and direction of the masticatory forces. Indeed, the overlapping arrangement of the periodontal collagen fibres seen by scanning electron microscopy and polarizing microscopy could help resist intrusive loads and compress blood vessels, some fibres always being placed in tension regardless of the direction of the force. Further evidence relates to the Sharpey fibre insertions and to collagen crimps. The collagen bundles of the PDL insert into alveolar bone in a similar manner to tendon inserting into bone (i.e. in the form of mineralized Sharpey fibres). Jones and Boyde (1972) found that, where the periodontal fibres inserted obliquely, mineralization of the Sharpey fibre occurs at approximately right angles to the long axis of the fibres. Furthermore, the mineralized parts of the fibre are concave relative to the matrix and are studded with mineral clusters. This arrangement is said to indicate that the fibres are subjected to tensional forces. However, studies on the distribution of Sharpey fibres into the alveolar bone indicate that, whereas the crestal one-third of the socket is almost entirely covered with Sharpey fibre insertions, the remaining two-thirds has very few (Sloan, 1981; see also Chapter 2). Indeed, many of the oblique fibres of the ligament could terminate not in the bone but around (or close to) the blood vessels lining the tooth socket.

Harkness (1968) observed that unstressed collagen fibres are wavy, and thus it can be envisaged that the collagen fibres gradually straighten out with intrusive loads. In addition, examination of the PDL in polarized light has shown that, as for many connective tissues elsewhere in the body, the collagen is crimped (see Chapter 2), and it has been proposed that this may confer special mechanical properties to the ligament, enabling the tissue to absorb tensile loads without extending the collagen fibrils and generating heat (Diamant *et al.*, 1972; Keller and Gathercole, 1976; Trelstad and Silver, 1981; Gathercole and Keller, 1982).

The role of the periodontal vasculature and interstitial fluid

Boyle (1938) initially implicated the vascular system in the tooth support mechanism. Parfitt (1960) attempted to interpret his findings on physiological tooth mobility in terms of fluid movements in both the blood vessels and ground substance of the PDL. From experiments conducted by Bien and Ayers (1965), Bien (1966) proposed a haemodynamic hypothesis of tooth support. This was based upon the pattern of recovery of a rat maxillary incisor after the removal of an intrusive load before and immediately after death. It was reported that complete recovery to the preloading position was not spontaneous but required thoracic massage (see *Fig. 10.5*). (Note, however, that Moxham and Berkovitz (1983) have reported that the response of teeth of both continuous and non-continuous growth to extrusive loads was similar before and immediately after death.) Furthermore, Picton (1990) has shown that the viscoelastic response is still present in dissected jaws fixed in formal saline, although reduced in magnitude (*Fig. 10.24*).

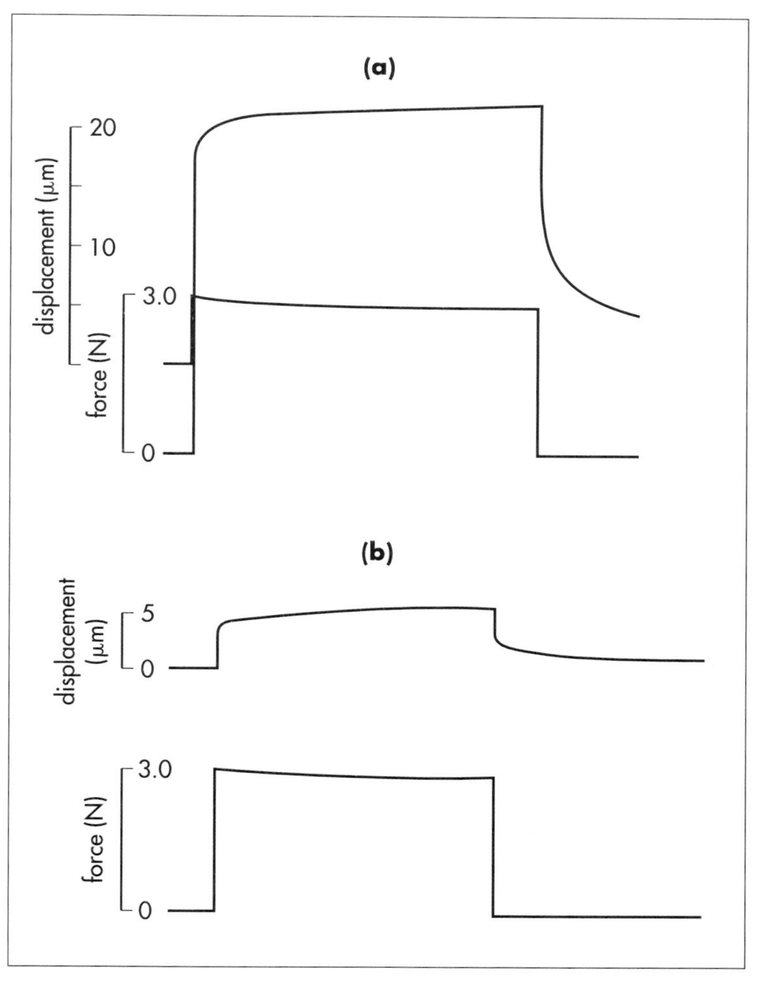

Fig. 10.24 (a) Intrusive load sustained on the tooth *in vivo* for 10 seconds. Creep is evident with a delay in recovery in the upper trace. (b) This shows the same experimental arrangement as in (a) but on the dissected maxilla. The specimen had been placed in formal saline for 6 weeks, but it still shows a biphasic response. (Picton, 1990.)

Because of the biphasic response to axial loading, Bien (1966) claimed that two fluid-damping effects were implicated in the tooth support mechanism. The first damping effect was thought to involve a squeeze film. This is analogous to a thin film of lubricant between load-bearing surfaces in which the fluid under pressure is squeezed to the edges of the plate in order to cushion the load. The second damping effect was thought to involve vascular changes within the periodontal tissues. Ballooning of small blood vessels to produce cirsoid aneurysms was said to occur as a result of constriction of the vessels by intervening fibres of the ligament. Bien claimed that cirsoid aneurysms, as flexible-walled sacs of fluid, act as minute springs. He further considered that they replenish the squeeze film, dissipating kinetic energy by forcing fluid through the vessel walls. Interesting as these concepts are, there is little evidence to support them. With regard to the role of periodontal fluid in tooth support, we know too little about its distribution and behaviour within the PDL to enable us to predict the effects of loading upon it. For example, is the distinction between bound and unbound water of significance? Furthermore, movement of water between the vascular and extravascular components, between one part of the ligament and another, and even between the PDL and alveolar bone seems likely to influence the behaviour of the tooth under loading. With regard to the contribution of the cirsoid aneurysms, there is no evidence to support their formation. Despite these criticisms, the work of Bien and Ayers (1965) and Bien (1966) demonstrates the importance of the vascular system in the tooth support mechanism by providing a mechanism by which there is recovery of position after intrusive loads are removed.

Several investigations have shown that tooth position is influenced by the periodontal vasculature. Parfitt (1960), Hofmann and Diemer (1963), Körber and Körber (1967), Körber (1970, 1971), Slatter and Picton (1972), Packman *et al.* (1977) and Burn-Murdoch and Picton (1978) have observed that teeth show pulsatile movements that are synchronous with the arterial pulse. Parfitt (1960) noted that systemically administered atropine given to a human subject resulted in slight extrusion of a maxillary incisor. Wills and Picton (1978) reported changes in the resting position of incisor teeth in macaque monkeys following submucosal injections of saline and water. In nearly every case, water caused an extrusion, but there was a more frequent intrusion following saline injection. Moxham (1979, 1981), in studying the influence of the vascular system on tooth eruption in rabbit incisors, has reported that hypotensive drugs (noradrenaline, acetylcholine) and section and stimulation of the sympathetic trunk have marked effects on tooth position (see also Chapter 9). Chiba (1995) has reported similar results for the rat incisor.

Investigations have been undertaken to assess the influence of vascular–fluid systems of the periodontium on tooth mobility. Wills *et al.* (1976) have observed that the intravenous administration of angiotensin resulted in a reduced displacement with intrusive loads in the teeth of macaque monkeys. Similar changes in mobility have been observed following the submucosal injection of noradrenaline at sites both near and at a distance from the test tooth (Slatter and Picton, 1972; Wills *et al.*, 1976). A consistent pattern was not seen, however, when the noradrenaline solution was injected near the test tooth. It was suggested that in these circumstances there might be distinct vasoconstrictor and volume effects of the carrier solution. Wills *et al.* (1976) also reported a reduction in mobility following exsanguination. A trend towards a return to normal mobility was observed after exsanguination when the thorax was squeezed. Wills and Picton (1978) found that submucosal injection of water caused an increased mobility with intrusive loads. However, conflicting effects have been reported with saline. Wills *et al.* (1976) claimed that submucosal injections of saline gave a considerable increase in displacement, while Wills and Picton (1978) have shown that a decrease in mobility can result.

Although the experiments involving submucosal injections of solutions seem to confirm the importance of the vasculature and fluids of the PDL in the tooth support mechanism, care must be taken in interpreting the findings. Firstly, we know too little of the physical, chemical, and biological properties of the PDL to be able to predict with confidence the effects of such solutions. Secondly, injected solutions may have more than one effect. For example, it has already been mentioned that noradrenaline may have a vasoconstrictor effect and an effect related to the carrier solution. In addition, Wills and Picton (1978) suggest that saline and water may not only produce volume changes within the periodontal tissues but also affect the biochemistry of the collagen and ground substance.

Another approach to study the role of the vasculature in the tooth support mechanism involves assessing the effects of loading on blood flow through the PDL (see Chapter 5). Packman *et al.* (1977) attempted to investigate the effects of both axial and horizontal loads on the periodontal microcirculation using photoelectric plethysmography. Although they reported that significant changes in blood flow could be discerned during loading, it is not possible to evaluate how much of the change also related to circulatory changes in the alveolar bone and gingiva. Aars and Linden (1982) and Aars (1983a,b) have shown that the acute mobility of the tooth to some degree depends upon vascularly mediated changes in resting position of the tooth, and sudden changes in tooth displacement require an immediate shift in vascular volumes within the PDL. Packman *et al.* (1977), Ng *et al.* (1981), Gangler and Merte (1983) and Sasano *et al.* (1992) have all provided evidence that blood is shunted from compression zones (or in and out of the alveolar bone) during loading. Gangler and Merte (1983), using a vital microscopic technique, also reported that both compression and tension in the PDL led to ischaemic areas, beginning in the venules and capillaries and ending in the arteries. In terms of blood flow in the loaded PDL,

Kvinnsland *et al.* (1989) and Kvinnsland *et al.* (1992) reported that, for the rat molar, the flow was increased by orthodontic-type forces sustained over several days. In the human maxillary central incisor, Hertrich and Raab (1990) found that intrusive forces between 0.1 and 0.5 N could reduce blood flow, but this rapidly returned to control levels when the force was sustained.

Periodontal tissue pressures have also been reported to change during loading. Schärer and Hayashi (1969) were the first to record such changes. Walker *et al.* (1978) have recorded changes in fluid pressures in the PDLs of the canine teeth of dogs during and following the application of loads up to 5 N. They reported that, on applying a load, there was an immediate increase in pressure, which decayed rapidly (halving time less than 1 second). Removal of the load produced an inverse pattern (but with a reduced peak pressure and a longer halving time). However, since the pressure changes were small compared with the loads applied, they concluded that the free fluids of the PDL make only minor contributions to tooth support. They stated that the major contributions are provided by 'the solid (collagen fibres) and semi-solid (ground substance) compartments of the ligament, acting in conjunction with the periodontal vasculature'. In considering the significance of their findings, the well-known difficulties of recording tissue fluid pressures reliably (e.g. Guyton, 1963; Brown, 1968; Stromberg and Wiederhielm, 1977; van Hassel and McMinn, 1972; Walker *et al.*, 1978) must be borne in mind.

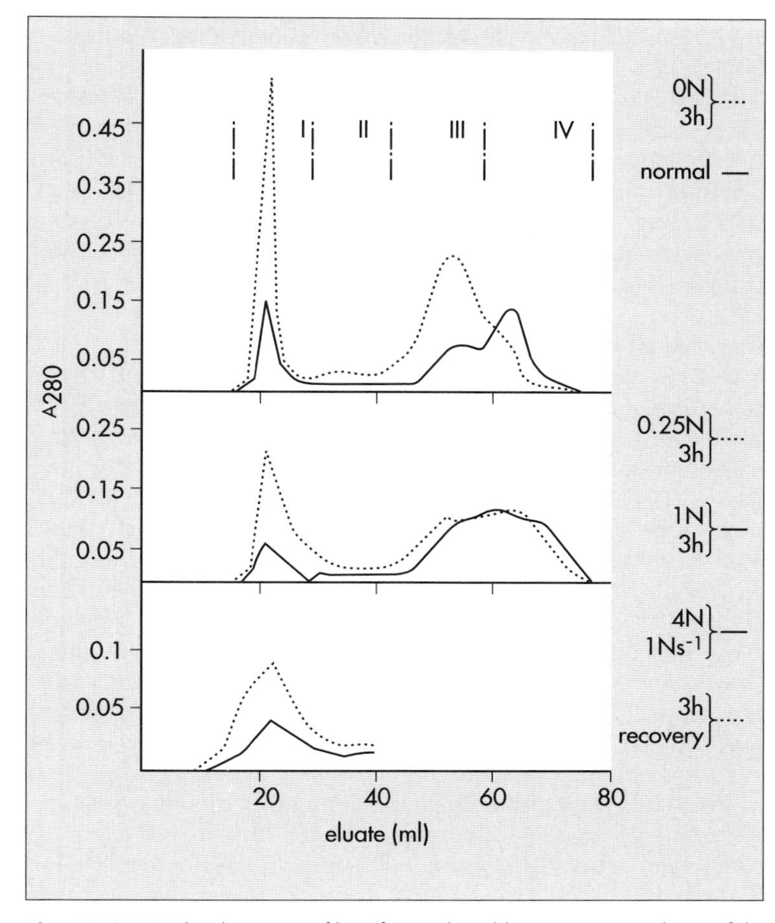

Fig. 10.25 Molecular-size profiles of periodontal ligament proteoglycans following various degrees of intrusive loadings of macaque monkey teeth. (top) High molecular weight fraction (peak-i) increased when the periodontal ligament is undisturbed for 3 hours. (middle) Decrease in peak-i size between 0.25 N and 1 N loads. (bottom) Further decrease in peak-i size with 4 N loads followed by an increase during a 3 hour undisturbed recovery phase. (Embery *et al.*, 1987.)

The role of the periodontal ground substance

As indicated in Chapter 4, a proper understanding of the ground substance of the PDL is only just beginning to emerge. However, two major constituents are water (bound and free) and sugar–protein complexes (e.g. proteoglycans). Experiments designed to determine the significance of periodontal fluids in the tooth support mechanism have already been described. Wills and Picton (1980) have studied the effect on axial tooth mobility of submucosal injections of hyaluronidase in macaque monkeys. The solvent used was water. They reported that injections of water alone produced a transient increase in mobility within 30 minutes; this was still apparent at 1 hour. Following injections of hyaluronidase, there was a marked increase in mobility after 20 minutes for a single thrust, with a subsequent rapid return towards the mobility of control teeth. No such increase in mobility was recorded when a sixteen-thrust regimen was used. Previous work had indicated a reduction in mobility following injections of hyaluronidase with saline (Picton, 1976). However, the precise effects of such injections on the PDL need to be established before any observations can be correctly interpreted.

Biochemically, Embery *et al.* (1987) have shown that the ground substance components of the PDL have an important role in the tooth support mechanism (*Fig. 10.25*). Their experiments were based upon an hypothesis derived from earlier studies, which suggested that the degree of aggregation of proteoglycans in the PDL could explain aspects of physiological tooth mobility (Wills and Picton, 1981; Picton, 1984). Proteoglycan-like fractions were isolated by Embery *et al.* (1987) from the PDLs of the teeth of macaque monkeys after intrusive loading. In a 'non-functioning' state, when the teeth were unloaded for a period of 3 hours, a high molecular weight fraction (minimum 2×10^6 Da) was increased by 70 per cent compared with the normally functioning ligament. On the other hand, with loads between 0.25 N and 1 N, this fraction was reduced by approximately 70 per cent. Loads of 4 N were associated with a further decrease, followed by an increase during a 3 hour undisturbed recovery phase. Thus, it is conceivable that the pattern of aggregation and disaggregation of proteoglycans in the PDL could explain changes in tooth mobility (see also Picton, 1989).

Shore *et al.* (1985) have reported from quantitative electron-microscopy that there is an increase in the volume of ground substance in the PDL where the rat incisor is prevented from moving (by pinning) for 3 weeks. Furthermore, Kirkham *et al.* (1993) have recorded marked decreases in the sulphated glycosylaminoglycan content of the PDL when the rat incisor was pinned.

The role of alveolar bone

It has been demonstrated that forces applied to teeth cause distortion of adjacent bone, which tends to spread to the rest of the jaw (e.g. Jung, 1952; McDowell and Regli, 1961; Picton, 1962c). Using horizontal loads on macaque monkey teeth, Picton and Davies (1967) noted that displacement of the bone of the tooth socket was mainly in the same direction as the thrust. However, with some thrusts the bone was seen to be displaced in the direction opposite to the root. This might suggest that distortion of the bone was produced by the spread of stress from elsewhere in the alveolus (Picton, 1969). Picton (1965) and Picton and Davies (1967) have observed that the alveolar margins are dilated under axial loads. Picton (1969) and Picton *et al.* (1974) have suggested that the fast initial phase of recovery following removal of an intrusive load may be accounted for by recoil of bone.

Taken together with studies indicating that mobility patterns are not significantly affected following loss of the cervical component of the PDL (Picton, 1988) or the fundus of the alveolus (Gathercole, 1987; Picton and Picton 1987), one can conclude that the alveolar bone does not have a simple 'either/or' role in participating in the generation of tension or compression during the tooth support mechanism.

THE BIOLOGICAL MECHANISMS INVOLVED IN THE SUPPORT AGAINST HORIZONTAL LOADS

Since the pattern of mobility with horizontal loads has similarities to that for axial loads, it is likely that the mechanisms involved in the resistance of the periodontal tissues to these loads are also similar.

Mühlemann (1951) noted that the biphasic pattern of mobility was lost in human ankylosed teeth. He concluded that the normal pattern for horizontal mobility was a function of the PDL. From light microscopic observations, Mühlemann (1954a) and Mühlemann and Zander (1954) claimed that the amount of initial tooth mobility was related to the degree of organization of the PDL. A loosely structured ligament appeared to show more mobility than one with densely organized collagen fibres. Mühlemann and Zander (1954) stated that the first phase of mobility with loads below 1 N is due to an intra-alveolar tipping of the tooth with reorientation of the fibre bundles. With a load at the transition between the first and second phase (1 N), they claimed that the already stretched fibre bundles on the tension side resisted any further root displacement and prevented a further increase of the periodontal width on that side. Higher loads were thought to lead to distortion and compression of the periodontium with deformation of the alveolar bone. For a description of the histological changes following orthodontic tooth movement, the reader is referred to Chapter 11.

The role of the periodontal tissues in resisting horizontal loads has been evaluated further by observations of the displacement of the alveolar margins (Picton, 1965) and by tooth-mobility studies following surgical trauma to the gingival and periodontal tissues (Picton, 1967, Picton and Slatter, 1972). All three investigations were conducted on monkey teeth. Picton (1965) reported that, with loads of 2.5 N applied labially or lingually, the lingual and labial alveolar margins were usually displaced in the same direction as the applied force. The amount of displacement was similar for both margins. He thus confirmed that horizontal loads produced a combination of compression and tension in different regions of the periodontium. Unlike Mühlemann and Zander (1954), Picton noted that bone distortion occurred with loads less than 1 N (often with loads as low as 0.5 N).

Picton (1967) studied the effects of traumatizing the periodontal tissues on the mesial and distal surfaces of maxillary incisor teeth subjected to loads in labiopalatal directions. Little change in tooth mobility was seen (though forces applied labially seem to show a slight increase). He concluded that limited areas of the PDL tangential to the load may be traumatized without gross disturbance of the mechanisms of tooth support.

Picton and Slatter (1972) assessed the effects of traumatizing the periodontal tissues on the mesial or distal surfaces of incisors subjected to loads applied in mesial and distal directions. They reported an increase in mobility whether the tooth was displaced towards or away from the site of trauma. They again concluded that tension and compression operate when a horizontal load is applied to a tooth, both appearing to be of equal importance.

As for axial loads, we believe that a biological interpretation of the patterns of horizontal mobility is speculative unless supported by experiments involving observations of the consequences of imposing selective changes to the periodontium. However, little work has been conducted using this approach. Mühlemann (1954c) studied the effects of heat or formalin treatment on teeth in dissected monkey jaws. He claimed that these treatments abolished the initial phase of tooth mobility and reduced the amount of secondary mobility. He suggested that these results could be explained in terms of an alteration in the periodontal fibres. The unphysiological nature of these *in vitro* experiments cast doubt on their relevance to the *in vivo* situation, especially since it has been shown that tissue fluids and vasculature play a role in the tooth support mechanism (see pages 233–235). Indeed, Körber (1962) reported that hyperaemia and the local injection of vasoconstrictors influenced horizontal tooth mobility. Furthermore, the experiments of Packman *et al.* (1977) suggest that horizontal loading can affect blood flow in the PDL (see Chapter 5).

SUMMARY

By reviewing the totality of the evidence, the following general conclusions about the tooth support mechanism can be drawn from experiments involving the placement of loads on normal and experimentally altered periodontal tissues:

1. The relationship between force and displacement is 'non-Hookean' (being non-linear and multiphasic) and the characteristics of physiological tooth mobility are consistent with the view that, under some loading conditions, the periodontal tissues behave as a viscoelastic system.
2. There is evidence that the PDL is placed under both tension and compression during loading, although the weight of evidence indicates that morphologically and biochemically the ligament more closely resembles a connective tissue under compression.
3. Neither the results of physiological or experimental tooth-mobility studies nor the results of morphological or biochemical studies support the view that tooth support mechanism is mediated principally by the collagen fibres of the PDL acting as a 'suspensory ligament'. Indeed, biologically there is evidence suggesting that many of the components of the periodontal connective tissues are involved in tooth support. Therefore, we can avoid a reductive dilemma by concluding that the tooth support mechanism is a property or function of the PDL as a whole.

REFERENCES

Aars H (1983a) Effects of sympathetic nerve activity on changes in the position of the rabbit incisor tooth evoked by acute alterations in arterial blood pressure. Arch Oral Biol 28, 497–500.

Aars H (1983b) Effects of sympathetic nerve activity on acute mobility of the rabbit incisor tooth. Acta Odont Scand 41, 287–292.

Aars H and Linden RWA (1982) The effects of sympathetic trunk stimulation on the position and mobility of the canine tooth of the cat. Arch Oral Biol 27, 399–404.

Ahlgren J (1967) Patterns of chewing and malocclusion of teeth. A Clinical study. Acta Odont Scand 25, 3–13.

Anderson DJ (1956a) Measurement of stress in mastication. I. J Dent Res 35, 664–670.

Anderson DJ (1956b) Measurement of stress in mastication II. J Dent Res 35, 671–673.

Anderson KL, Pederson EH and Melson B (1991) Material parameters and stress profiles within the periodontal ligament. Am J Orthod Dentofacial Orthop 99, 427–440.

Bass TP and Stephens CD (1970) Some experiments with orthodontic springs. Dent Practr 21, 21–36.

Bearn M (1973) Effect of different occlusal profiles on the masticatory forces transmitted by complete dentures. Br Dent J 134, 7–10.

Berkovitz BKB and Moxham BJ (1990) The development of the periodontal ligament with special reference to collagen fibre ontogeny. J Biol Buccale 18, 227–236.

Berkovitz BKB, Weaver ME, Shore RC and Moxham BJ (1981) Fibril diameters in the extracellular matrix of the periodontal connective tissues of the rat. Conn Tissue Res 8, 127–132.

Berkovitz BKB, Migdalski A and Solomon M (1972) The effect of the lathyritic agent amino-acetonitrile on the unimpeded eruption rate in normal and root-resected rat lower incisors. Arch Oral Biol 17, 1755–1763.

Bien SM (1966) Fluid dynamic mechanisms which regulate tooth movement. In: Advances in Oral Biology, volume 2 (Staple PH, ed), pp 173–201, Academic Press, London.

Bien SM and Ayers HD (1965) Responses of rat maxillary incisors to loads. J Dent Res 44, 517–520.

Bowley WW, Burstone CJ, Koenig HA and Slatkowski R (1974) Prediction of tooth displacement using laser holography and finite element technique. Proceedings of the Symposium of Commission V, International Society for Photogrammetry, Washington, pp 241–273.

Boyle PE (1938) Tooth suspension. A comparative study of the paradental tissues of man and of the guinea pig. J Dent Res 20, 87–92.

Brown AC (1968) Pulp tissue pressure and blood flow. In: Biology of the dental pulp organ (Finn SB, ed), pp 381–395, University of Alabama Press, Alabama.

Burn-Murdoch RA and Picton DCA (1978) A technique for measuring eruption rates in rats of maxillary incisors under intrusive loads. Arch Oral Biol 23, 563–566.

Burstone CJ (1962) The biomechanics of tooth movement. In: Vistas in Orthodontics (Kraus BS and Riedel RA, eds), pp 197–213, Lea and Febiger, Philadelphia.

Burstone CJ and Pryputniewicz RJ (1980) Holographic determination of centers of rotation produced by orthodontic forces. Am J Orthod 77, 396–409.

Burstone CJ, Pryputniewicz RJ and Bowley WW (1978) Holographic measurement of tooth mobility in three dimensions. J Periodont Res 13, 283–294.

Chiba M (1995) The possible role of the periodontal ligament and vasculature in axial movements of the rat incisor. In: Biological Mechanisms of Tooth Eruption, Resorption and Replacement by Implants (Davidovitch Z, ed), EBSCO Media, Birmingham, Alabama (in press).

Chiba M and Komatsu K (1988) *In vitro* estimation of the resisting force of tooth eruption and the zone of shear in the rat incisor periodontal ligament. In: The Biological Mechanisms of Tooth Eruption and Root Resorption (Davidovitch Z, ed), pp 193–205, EBSCO Media, Birmingham, Alabama.

Chiba M and Komatsu K (1993) Mechanical responses of the periodontal ligament in the transverse section of the rat mandibular incisor at various velocities of loading in vitro. J Biomech 26, 561–570.

Chiba M and Ohkawa S (1980) Measurement of the tensile strength of the periodontium in the rat mandibular first molar. Arch Oral Biol 25, 569–572.

Chiba M, Ohshima S, Kuroda T and Ohkawa S (1981) Effects of repeated shortenings and of artificial restraint on the tensile strength of the periodontium of the rat mandibular incisor. Arch Oral Biol 26, 135–141.

Chiba M, Kinoshita Y, Nakamura G, Ohshima S, Ishikawa S, Tsuruta M and Ozawa M (1982) Effects of storage of jaws in saline and of velocity of loading on the force required to extract rat mandibular first molars. Arch Oral Biol 27, 905–907.

Chiba M, Yamane A, Ohshima S and Komatsu K (1990) In vitro measurement of regional differences in the mechanical properties of the periodontal ligament in the rat mandibular incisor. Arch Oral Biol 35, 153–161.

Chiba M, Kuroda T and Ohshima S (1981) Effects of adrenocorticoids on impeded and unimpeded eruption rates and on the mechanical properties in the rat mandibular incisor. Arch Oral Biol 26, 577–583.

Chiba M, Ohshima S and Takizawa K (1980) Measurement of the force required to extract the mandibular incisor of rats of various ages. Arch Oral Biol 25, 683–687.

Christiansen RL and Burstone CJ (1969) Centers of rotation within the periodontal space. Am J Orthod 55, 353–369.
Coehlo A and Moxham BJ (1989) Intrusive mobility of the incisor tooth of the guinea pig. Arch Oral Biol 34, 383–386.
Crabb JJ and Wilson HJ (1972) The relation between orthodontic spring force and space closure. Dent Practr 22, 233–240.
D'Hoedt B, Lukas D, Muhlbradt L, *et al.* (1985) Das Periotestverfahren – Entwicklung und klinische Prüfung. Dtsch Zahnarztl Z 40, 113–125.
Daly CH, Nichols JI, Kydd WL and Nansen PD (1974) The response of the human periodontal ligament to torsional loading. J Biomech 7, 517–522.
Diamant J, Keller A, Baer E, Litt M and Arridge RGC (1972) Collagen: Ultrastructure and its relation to mechanical properties as a function of ageing. Proc R Soc Lond [Biol] 180, 293–315.
Draper NR and Smith H (1966) Applied Regression Analysis, Wiley, New York.
Embery G, Picton DC and Stanbury JB (1987) Biochemical changes in periodontal ligament ground substance associated with short-term intrusive loading in adult monkeys (*Macaca fasicularis*). Arch Oral Biol 32, 545–549.
Every TW, Burstone CJ and Pryputniewicz RJ (1978) Holographic measurement of incisor extrusion. J Dent Res 57 (special issue A), 164 (abstract).
Every TW, Burstone CJ and Pryputniewicz RJ (1979) Holographic analysis of tooth movement resulting from known axial loads. J Dent Res 58 (special Issue A), 1243 (abstract).
Flint MH, Lyons MF, Meaney MF and Williams DE (1975) The Masson staining of collagen – an explanation of an apparent paradox. Histochem J 7, 529–546.
Flint MH, Craig AS, Reilly HC, Gillard GC and Parry DAD (1984) Collagen fibril diameters and glycosaminoglycans content of skins – indices of tissue maturity and function. Conn Tissue Res 13, 69–81.
Gabel AB (1956) A mathematical analysis of the function of the fibres of the periodontal membrane. J Periodont 27, 191–198.
Gangler P and Merte K (1983) Effects of force application on periodontal blood circulation. J Periodont Res 18, 86–92.
Gathercole LJ (1987) *In vitro* mechanics of intrusive loading in the porcine cheek teeth with intact and perforated root apices. Arch Oral Biol 32, 249–255.
Gathercole LJ and Keller A (1982) Biophysical aspects of the fibres of the periodontal ligament. In: The Periodontal Ligament in Health and Disease, 1st edition (Berkovitz BKB, Moxham BJ and Newman HN, eds) pp 103–117, Pergamon Press, Oxford.
Gillard GC, Reilly HC, Bell-Booth PG and Flint MH (1979) The influence of mechanical forces on the glycosaminoglycan content of the rabbit flexor digitorum profundus tendon. Conn Tissue Res 7, 37–46.
Gould MSE and Picton DCA (1964) A study of pressures exerted by the lips and cheeks on the teeth of subjects with normal occlusion. Arch Oral Biol 9, 469–478.
Graf H (1963) Occlusal Contact Patterns in Mastication. MS Thesis, University of Rochester, New York (quoted by Picton DCA, 1964b).
Guyton AC (1963) A concept of negative interstitial pressure based on pressures in implanted capsules. Circ Res 12, 399–414.
Haack DC and Weinstein S (1963) Geometry and mechanics as related to tooth movement studied by means of two-dimensional model. J Am Dent Assoc 66, 157–164.
Harkness RD (1968) Mechanical properties of collagenous tissues. In: Treatise on Collagen, volume 2: Biology of Collagen, Part A (Gould BS, ed), pp 248–310, Academic Press, London.
Heners M (1974) Syndesmotic limiting movement of the periodontal ligament. Int Dent J 24, 319–327.
Hertrich K and Raab WHM (1990) Reaktive Änderung der parodontalen Mikrozirkulation bei kieferorthopädischen Kräften. Fortschr Kieferorthop 51, 253–258.
Himmel GK, Marthaler TM, Rateitschak KH and Mühlemann HR (1957) Experimental changes of diurnal periodicity in the physiological properties of periodontal structures. Helv Odont Acta Zur 1, 16–22.
Hofmann M (1963) Zahnbeweglichkeit – Bestimmung und Analyse. Dtsch Zahnarztl Z 18, 924–933.
Hofmann M and Diemer R (1963) Die Pulsation des Zahnes. Dtsch Zahnarztl Z 18, 1268–1274.
Hong RK (1990) The effects of orthodontic forces on the mechanical properties of the periodontal ligament in the rat maxillary molar. Am J Orthod Dentofacial Orthop 98, 533–543.
Hong RK, Yamane A, Kuwahara Y and Chiba M (1992) The effect of orthodontic retention on the mechanical properties of the periodontal ligament in the rat maxillary first molar. J Dent Res 71, 1350–1354.
Jones SJ and Boyde A (1972) A study of human root cemental surfaces as prepared for and examined in the SEM. Z Zellforsch 130, 318–337.
Jung F (1952) Die Elastizitat der Skeletteile des Gebis-systems. Stoma 5, 74–93.
Kardos TB and Simpson LD (1979) A theoretical consideration of the periodontal membrane as a collagenous thixotropic system and its relationship to tooth eruption. J Periodont Res 14, 444–451.
Kardos TB and Simpson LD (1980) A new periodontal membrane biology based upon thixotropic concepts. Am J Orthod 77, 508–515.
Keller A and Gathercole LJ (1976) Biophysical and mechanical properties of collagen in relation to function. In: The Eruption and Occlusion of Teeth (Poole DFG and Stack MV, eds), pp 262–266, Butterworths, London.
Kinoshita Y, Tonooka K and Chiba M (1982) The effect of hypofunction on the mechanical properties of the periodontium in the rat mandibular first molar. Arch Oral Biol 27, 881–885.
Kirkham J, Robinson C, Phull JK, Shore RC, Moxham BJ and Berkovitz BKB (1993) The effect of rate of eruption on periodontal ligament glycosylaminoglycan content and enamel formation in the rat incisor. Cell Tissue Res 274, 413–419.
Komatsu K (1988) *In vitro* mechanics of the periodontal ligament in impeded and unimpeded rat mandibular incisors. Arch Oral Biol 33, 783–791.
Komatsu K and Chiba M (1993) The effect of velocity of loading on the biomechanical responses of the periodontal ligament in transverse sections of the rat molar *in vitro*. Arch Oral Biol 38, 369–375.
Körber KH (1962) Elektronisches Messen der Zahnbe-weglichkeit. Dtsch Zahnarztebl 16, 605.
Körber KH (1970) Periodontal pulsation. J Periodont 41, 686–708.
Körber KH (1971) Electronic registration of tooth movements. Int Dent J 21, 466–477.
Körber KH and Körber E (1967) Patterns of physiological movement in tooth support. In: Mechanisms of Tooth Support (Anderson DJ, Eastoe JE, Melcher AH and Picton DCA, eds), pp 148–153, Wright, Bristol.
Kvinnsland S, Heyeraas KJ and Ofjord ES (1989) Effects of experimental tooth movement on periodontal and pulpal blood flow. Eur J Orthod 11, 200–205.
Kvinnsland S, Kristiansen AB, Kvinnsland I and Heyeraas KJ (1992) Effect of experimental traumatic occlusion on periodontal and pulpal blood flow. Acta Odont Scand 50, 211–219.
Lear CSC, Decou RE and Ng DHP (1974) Threshold levels for displacement of human maxillary central incisors in response to lingually directed forces. J Dent Res 53, 942.
Lear CSC, Mackay JS and Lowe AA (1972) Threshold levels for displacement of human teeth in response to laterally directed forces. J Dent Res 51, 1478–1482.
Luder HV, Zimmerli I and Schroeder HE (1988) Do collagen fibrils of the periodontal ligament shrink with age? J Periodont Res 23, 46–52.
Mandel U, Dalgaard P and Viidik A (1986) A biomechanical study of the human periodontal ligament. J Biomech 9, 637–645.

McDowell JA and Regli CP (1961) A quantitative analysis of the decrease in width of the mandibular arch during forced movements of the mandible. J Dent Res 40, 1183–1185.

Merrilees MJ and Flint MH (1980) Ultrastructural study of tension and pressure zones in a rabbit flexor tendon. Am J Anat 157, 87–106.

Moxham BJ (1979) The effects of some vaso-active drugs on the eruption of the rabbit mandibular incisor. Arch Oral Biol 24, 681–688.

Moxham BJ (1981) The effects of section and stimulation of the cervical sympathetic trunk on eruption of the rabbit mandibular incisor. Arch Oral Biol 26, 887–891.

Moxham BJ (1985) Studies on the mechanical properties of the periodontal ligament. In: Current Topics in Oral Biology (Lisney SJW and Matthews B, eds), pp 73–82, University of Bristol Press, Bristol.

Moxham BJ and Berkovitz BKB (1979) The effects of axially directed extrusive loads on movements of the mandibular incisor of the rabbit. Arch Oral Biol 24, 759–763.

Moxham BJ and Berkovitz BKB (1981) A quantitative assessment of the effects of axially directed extrusive loads on displacement of the impeded and unimpeded rabbit mandibular incisor. Arch Oral Biol 26, 209–215.

Moxham BJ and Berkovitz BKB (1982a) The effects of external forces on the periodontal ligament – the response to axial loads. In: The Periodontal Ligament in Health and Disease, 1st edition (Berkovitz, BKB, Moxham, BJ and Newman, HN, eds), pp 249–268, Pergamon Press, Oxford.

Moxham BJ and Berkovitz BKB (1982b) The effects of external forces on the periodontal ligament – the response to horizontal loads (section A). In: The Periodontal Ligament in Health and Disease, 1st edition (Berkovitz, BKB, Moxham, BJ and Newman, HN, eds), pp 269–275, Pergamon Press, Oxford.

Moxham BJ and Berkovitz BKB (1983) Continuous monitoring of the position of the ferret mandibular canine tooth to enable comparisons with the continuously growing rabbit incisor. Arch Oral Biol 28, 477–481.

Moxham BJ and Berkovitz BKB (1984) The mobility of the lathyritic rabbit mandibular incisor in response to axially directed extrusive loads. Arch Oral Biol 29, 773–778.

Moxham BJ and Berkovitz BKB (1989) A comparison of the biomechanical properties of the periodontal ligaments of erupting and erupted teeth of non-continuous growth (ferret mandibular canines). Arch Oral Biol 34, 763–766.

Moxham BJ, Berkovitz BKB, Shore RC and Spence JA (1987) A laboratory method for studying tooth mobility of the mandibular central incisor of the sheep. Res Vet Sci 42, 61–64.

Moxham BJ and Coehlo A (1989) Intrusive mobility of the guinea pig incisor with vibrational loading. J Dent Res 68, 596.

Moxham BJ, Shore RC and Berkovitz BKB (1987) Fenestrated capillaries in the periodontal connective tissues of the erupting and erupted rat molar. Arch Oral Biol 32, 477–481.

Moxham BJ, Shore RC and Berkovitz BKB (1990) The effects of inflammatory periodontal disease (broken mouth) on the mobility of the sheep incisor. Res Vet Sci 48, 99–102.

Mühlemann HR (1951) Periodontometry; a method for measuring tooth mobility. Oral Surg Oral Med Oral Pathol 4, 1220–1233.

Mühlemann HR (1954a) Tooth mobility: The measuring method. Initial and secondary tooth mobility. J Periodont 25, 22–29.

Mühlemann HR (1954b) Tooth mobility (II). Role of interdental contact points and of activation on tooth mobility. J Periodont 25, 125–128.

Mühlemann HR (1954c) Tooth mobility (IV) Tooth mobility changes through artificial alterations of the periodontium. J Periodont 25, 198–202.

Mühlemann HR (1960) Ten years of tooth mobility measurements. J Periodont 31, 110–122.

Mühlemann HR (1967) Tooth mobility: a review of clinical aspects and research findings. J Periodont 36, 686–708.

Mühlemann HR and Houglum MW (1954) The determination of the tooth rotation center. Oral Surg Oral Med Oral Pathol 7, 392–394.

Mühlemann HR, Savdir S and Rateitschak KH (1965) Tooth mobility – Its causes and significance. J Periodont 36, 148–153.

Mühlemann HR and Zander HA (1954) Tooth mobility (III). The mechanism of tooth mobility. J Periodont 25, 128–137.

Ng GC, Walker TW, Zingg W and Burke PS (1981) Effects of tooth loading on the periodontal vasculature of the mandibular fourth premolar in dogs. Arch Oral Biol 26, 189–195.

Nikolai RJ (1974) Periodontal ligament reaction and displacement of a maxillary central incisor subjected to transverse crown loading. J Biomech 7, 93–99.

O'Leary TJ, Rudd KD and Nabers CL (1966) Factors affecting horizontal tooth mobility. Periodontics 4, 308–315.

Ohkawa S (1982) Effects of orthodontic forces and anti-inflammatory drugs on the mechanical strength of the periodontium in the rat mandibular first molar. Am J Orthod 81, 498–502.

Ohshima S (1982) Effects of lathyrogens on the mechanical properties of the periodontium in the rat mandibular incisor. Tsurumi Univ Dent J 8, 345–356.

Ohshima S, Komatsu K, Yamane A and Chiba M (1991) Prolonged effects of hypofunction on the mechanical strength of the periodontal ligament in rat mandibular molars. Arch Oral Biol 36, 905–911.

Ohshima S, Nakamura G and Chiba M (1989) Effects of lathyrogens on the mechanical strength of the periodontal ligament in the rat mandibular first molar. J Periodont Res 24, 343–350.

Oka H, Yamamoto T, Saratari K and Kawaoe T (1989) Application of mechanical mobility of periodontal tissues to tooth mobility examination. Med Biol Eng Comput 27, 75–81.

Packman H, Shoher I and Stein RS (1977) Vascular responses in the human periodontal ligament and alveolar bone detected by photoelectric plethysmography: the effect of force application to the tooth. J Periodontol 48, 194–200.

Parfitt GJ (1960) Measurement of the physiological mobility of individual teeth in an axial direction. J Dent Res 39, 608–618.

Parfitt GJ (1961) The dynamics of a tooth in function. J Periodont 32, 102–107.

Parfitt GJ (1967) The physical analysis of the tooth-supporting structures. In: Mechanisms of Tooth Support (Anderson DJ, Eastoe JE, Melcher AH and Picton DCA, eds), pp 154–156, Wright, Bristol.

Parry DAD, Barnes GRG and Craig AS (1978) A comparison of the size distribution of collagen fibrils in connective tissues as a function of age and a possible relation between fibril size distribution and mechanical properties. Proc R Soc London [Biol] 203, 305–321.

Pearson CH (1982) The ground substance of the periodontal ligament. In: The Periodontal Ligament in Health and Disease, 1st edition (Berkovitz BKB, Moxham BJ and Newman HN, eds), pp 119–149, Pergamon Press, Oxford.

Persson R and Svenson A (1980) Assessment of tooth mobility using small loads I. J Clin Periodont 7, 259–275.

Picton DCA (1962a) Tilting movements of teeth during biting. Arch Oral Biol 7, 151–159.

Picton DCA (1962b) A study of normal tooth mobility and the changes with periodontal disease. Dent Practr 12, 167–173.

Picton DCA (1962c) Distortion of the jaws during biting. Arch Oral Biol 7, 573–580.

Picton DCA (1963a) Vertical movement of cheek teeth during biting. Arch Oral Biol 8, 109–118.

Picton DCA (1963b) The effect on normal vertical tooth mobility of the rate of thrust and time interval between thrusts. Arch Oral Biol 8, 291–299.

Picton DCA (1964a) The effect of repeated thrusts on normal axial tooth mobility. Arch Oral Biol 9, 55–63.

Picton DCA (1964b) Some implications of normal tooth mobility during mastication. Arch Oral Biol 9, 565–573.

Picton DCA (1965) On the part played by the socket in tooth support. Arch Oral Biol 10, 945–955.

Picton DCA (1967) The effect on tooth mobility of trauma to the mesial and distal regions of the periodontal membranes in monkeys. Helv Odont Acta 11, 105–112.

Picton DCA (1969) The effect of external forces on the periodontium. In: Biology of the Periodontium (Melcher AH and Bowen WH, eds), pp 363–419, Academic Press, London.

Picton DCA (1976) Discussion in: The eruption and occlusion of teeth (Poole DFG and Stack MV, eds), pp 224, Butterworths, London.

Picton DCA (1984) Changes in axial mobility of undisturbed teeth and following sustained intrusive forces in adult monkeys (*Macaca fascicularis*). Arch Oral Biol 29, 959–964.

Picton DCA (1986) Extrusive tooth mobility in adult monkeys. Arch Oral Biol 30, 369–372.

Picton DCA (1988) The effect of intrusive tooth mobility of surgically removing the cervical periodontal ligament in monkeys (*Macaca fascicularis*). Arch Oral Biol 33, 301–304.

Picton DCA (1989) The periodontal enigma: eruption versus tooth support. Eur J Orthodont 11, 430–439.

Picton DCA (1990) Tooth mobility – an update. Eur J Orthodont 12, 109–115.

Picton DCA and Davies WIR (1967) Dimensional changes in the periodontal membrane of monkeys (*Macaca irus*) due to horizontal thrusts applied to the teeth. Arch Oral Biol 12, 1635–1643.

Picton DCA, Johns RB, Wills DJ and Davies WIR (1974) The relationship between the mechanisms of tooth and implant support. In: Oral Science Review, 5 (Melcher AH and Zarb GA, eds), pp 3–22, Munksgaard, Copenhagen.

Picton DCA and Picton HM (1987) The effects of excision of the root apex on the intrusive mobility of anterior teeth in adult monkeys. Arch Oral Biol 32, 323–327.

Picton DCA and Slatter JM (1972) The effect on horizontal tooth mobility of experimental trauma to the periodontal membrane in regions of tension or compression in monkey. J Periodont Res 7, 35–41.

Picton DCA and Wills DJ (1978) Viscoelastic properties of the periodontal ligament and mucous membrane. J Prosthet Dent 40, 263–272.

Picton DCA and Wills DJ (1981) Visualisation by scanning electron microscopy of the periodontal ligament *in vivo* in the macaque monkey. Arch Oral Biol 26, 821–825.

Postacchini F and De Martino C (1980) Regeneration of rabbit calcaneal tendon maturation of collagen and elastic fibers following partial tenotomy. Conn Tissue Res 8, 41–47.

Proffit WR and Fields HW (1993) Contemporary Orthodontics. Mosby, St Louis.

Pryce-Jones J (1936) Some fundamental aspects of thixotropy. J Oil Colour Chem Assoc 19, 295–337.

Pryputniewicz RJ and Burstone CJ (1979) The effect of time and force magnitude on orthodontic tooth movement. J Dent Res 58, 1754–1764.

Pryputniewicz RJ, Burstone CJ and Bowley WW (1978) Determination of arbitrary tooth displacements. J Dent Res 57, 663–674.

Ralph WJ (1982) Tensile behaviour of the periodontal ligament. J Periodont Res 17, 423–426.

Reitan K (1967) Clinical and histologic observations on tooth movement during and after orthodontic treatment. Am J Orthod 53, 721–745.

Reitan K (1975). Biomechanical principles and reactions. In: Current orthodontic concepts and techniques, volume l, 2nd edition (Graber TM and Swain BF, eds), pp 111–229, Saunders, Philadelphia.

Renggli HH, Allet B and Spanauf AJ (1984) Splinting of teeth with fixed bridges. J Oral Rehab 11, 535–537.

Ross GG, Lear CS and Decou R (1976) Modeling the lateral movement of teeth. J Biomech 9, 723–734.

Sasano T, Kuriwada S, Sanjo D, Izumi H, Tabata T and Karita K (1992) Acute response of periodontal ligament blood flow to external force application. J Periodont Res 27, 301–304.

Schärer P and Hayashi Y (1969) A qualitative study on intraperiodontal pressure. Parodontologie 23, 3–10.

Schellens JPM, Everts V and Beertsen W (1982) Quantitative analysis of connective tissue resorption in the supra-alveolar region of the mouse incisor ligament. J Periodont Res 17, 407–422.

Shipley RA and Clark RE (1972) Tracer Methods for In Vitro Kinetics, p 72, Academic Press, London.

Shore RC, Berkovitz BKB and Moxham BJ (1985) The effects of preventing movement of the rat incisor on the structure of its periodontal ligament. Arch Oral Biol 30, 221–228.

Shore RC, Moxham BJ and Berkovitz BKB (1982) A quantitative comparison of the ultrastructure of the periodontal ligaments of impeded and unimpeded rat incisors. Arch Oral Biol 27, 423–430.

Slatter JM and Picton DCA (1972) The effect on intrusive tooth mobility of noradrenaline injected locally in monkeys. J Periodont Res 7, 144–150.

Sloan P (1981) Some observations on the distribution and form of alveolar Sharpey fibres in the rat, rabbit, macaque and man. J Dent Res 60, 1193.

Storey E and Smith R (1952) Force in orthodontics and its relations to tooth movement. Aust Dent J 56, 11–18.

Stromberg DD and Wiederhielm CA (1977) Intravascular and tissue space oncotic and hydrostatic pressure. In: Microcirculation (Kaley G and Altura BM, eds), pp 187–196, University Park Press, Baltimore.

Svoboda EL, Howley TP and Deporter DA (1983) Collagen fibril diameter and its relation to collagen turnover in three soft tissues. Connective tissues in the rat. Conn Tissue Res 12, 43–48.

Synge JL (1933a) The lightness of teeth, considered as a problem concerning the equilibrium of a thin incompressible elastic membrane. Philos Trans R Soc Lond [Biol] 231A, 435–477.

Synge JL (1933b) The equilibrium of a tooth with a general conical root. Philos Mag 15, 969–973.

Trelstad RL and Silver FH (1981) Matrix assembly. In: Cell biology of extracellular matrix (Hay ED, ed), pp 179–215, Plenum Press, New York.

Tsuruta M, Ohkawa S, Nakatani Y, Kuwahara Y and Chiba M (1982) Effect of experimental tooth movement on the mechanical strength of the periodontium in the rat mandibular first molar. Arch Oral Biol 27, 875–879.

Van Hassel HJ and McMinn RG (1972) Pressure differential following tooth eruption in the dog. Arch Oral Biol 17, 183–190.

Walker TW, Ng GC and Burke PS (1978) Fluid pressures in the periodontal ligament of the mandibular canine tooth in dogs. Arch Oral Biol 23, 753–765.

Wills DJ and Manderson RD (1977) Biomechanical aspects of the support of partial dentures. J Dent 5, 310–318.

Wills DJ and Picton DCA (1978) Changes in the mobility and resting position of incisor teeth in macaque monkeys. Arch Oral Biol 23, 225–229.

Wills DJ and Picton DCA (1980). The effect on apical tooth mobility of submucosal injections of hyaluronidase in adult *Macaca irus* monkeys. J Dent Res 59 (special Issue D), 1841.

Wills DJ and Picton DCA (1981) Changes in the force–extrusion relationship of the teeth with its resting position in macaque monkeys. Arch Oral Biol 26, 827–829.

Wills DJ, Picton DCA and Davies WIR (1972) An investigation of the viscoelastic properties of the periodontium in monkeys. J Periodont Res 7, 42–51.

Wills DJ, Picton DCA and Davies WIR (1974) The effect of the rate of application of force on the intrusion of central incisors in adult monkeys (*Macaca irus*). J Dent Res 53, 1054.

Wills DJ, Picton DCA and Davies WIR (1976) A study of the fluid systems of the periodontium in macaque monkeys. Arch Oral Biol 21, 175–185.

Wills DJ, Picton DCA and Davies WIR (1978) The intrusion of the tooth for different loading rates. J Biomech 11, 429–434.

Yamaguchi S (1992) Analysis of stress–strain curves at fast and slow velocities of loading *in vitro* in the transverse section of the rat incisor periodontal ligament following the administration of Beta-aminopropionitrile. Arch Oral Biol 37, 439–444.

Yamazaki Y (1992) Effects of destructive periodontitis, induced by diet, on the mechanical properties of the periodontal ligament of the mandibular first molar in golden hamsters. J Periodont Res 27, 149–158.

Chapter 11

The Histological Responses of the Periodontal Ligament to Horizontal Orthodontic Loads

P Rygh, P Brudvik

INTRODUCTION

Our knowledge of the effects of orthodontic loading on the periodontal ligament (PDL) has been based largely on empirical observations and trial-and-error clinical treatment. Our understanding of this topic will undoubtedly be improved by new advances in cell biology and, as a corollary, the information thus obtained should influence clinical treatment.

For physiological tooth movement, the tooth moves mainly in a buccal direction into cancellous bone or, owing to growth, into cortical bone. This is a slow process. For orthodontic tooth movement in the labiolingual direction, teeth may be moved rapidly into, and through, a cortical bone plate if compensating apposition of bone does not occur. It is the orthodontic force per area of the PDL that is important. The total force applied to a tooth is not decisive.

The transformation of mechanical stimuli into cellular reactions will be briefly outlined, even though orthodontic reactions reflect basic cellular response mechanisms. (For a more detailed description of this topic, see Chapter 12).

This presentation will focus on general tissue reactions to tooth movement and mechanisms related to one of the most unwanted sequelae to orthodontic treatment: root resorption. The inflammatory reactions seen in response to orthodontic strain that is felt to be locally too high by tissues in the PDL will be emphasized in this chapter, since the recognition of these aspects and identification of reacting cells have altered our current outlook on the mechanisms involved.

A load acting more or less perpendicular to the longitudinal axis of a tooth produces wide areas of pressure on one side of the root and corresponding areas of tension on the other. If the force could be placed near the centre of the root (through its centre of resistance) a translation or bodily movement of the tooth would be produced, with a relatively uniform distribution of pressure on one side of the root and of tension on the other (*Fig. 11.1a*). In practice, to produce translation for orthodontic treatment, forces have to be applied against the crown of the tooth via some system that will ensure a two-point contact (e.g. as seen in the 'edge-wise' technique, in which brackets or tubes allow closely fitting rectangular arches to produce the necessary couple). A tipping movement can easily occur as a result of the application of a horizontal force unless special precautions are taken. The point of rotation for such movement varies, depending on the site of force application, the shape of the tooth, and the architecture of the tooth's supporting system. The result is that crown and root tip in opposite directions (*Fig. 11.1b*), producing pressure and tension zones on either side of the root and a varying distribution of stress. This means that the load produced is concentrated in localized areas of the PDL.

There are two major advantages in using, for orthodontic purposes, horizontal forces that produce bodily movement of the tooth as opposed to forces that produce tipping movements. First, the end result appears to be more stable (Reitan and Rygh, 1994). Secondly, since in producing translation, loads are dissipated over the entire side of the tooth, there is greater control of the applied forces. On the other hand, the magnitude of the force is difficult to control with tipping because of the localized concentration of stresses in the PDL.

By applying horizontal forces to a tooth, pressure and tension zones are induced along the root surfaces. In such zones, it is reasonable to assume that the fibrous part of the PDL and the 'viscoelastic' shock-absorbing system are not being activated uniformly and that the resulting morphological changes within the PDL will differ where the tooth is pressed against the alveolar wall and where it is drawn away from it.

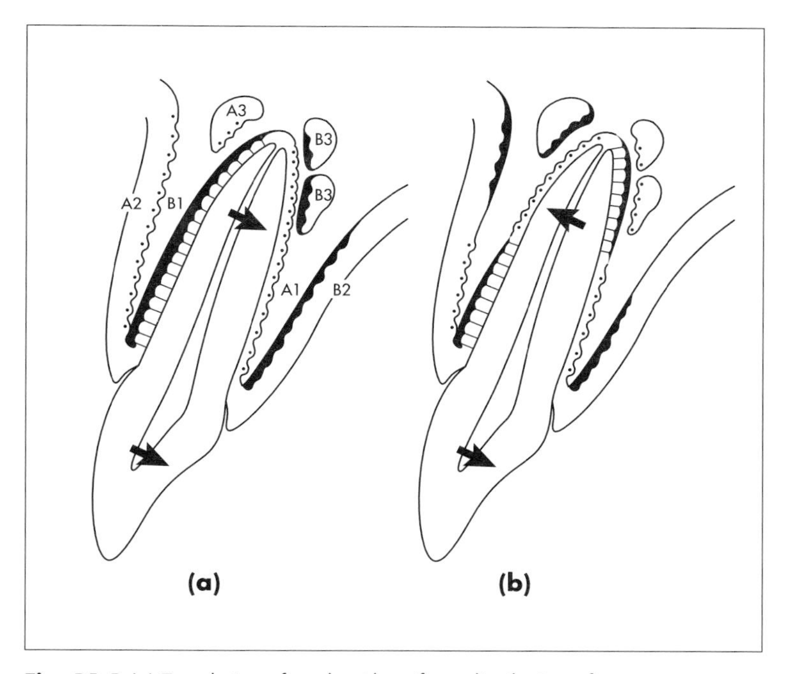

Fig. 11.1 (a) Translation of tooth with uniform distribution of pressure on one side of the root. Bone resorption occurs along the alveolar surface (A1) on the pressure side, on the labial surface of the alveolar process (A2), and in marrow spaces (A3). Bone deposition occurs along the alveolar surface (B1) on the tension side, on the lingual surface of the alveolar process (B2), and in marrow spaces (B3). (b) Tipping of tooth with pressure and tension zones on both sides of the root.

RESPONSES ON THE TENSION SIDE

When a continuous horizontal force of 0.15 N or more is applied to the crown of a tooth, the periodontal space will become wider on the side where the tooth is drawn away from the alveolar bone. Bundles of fibres are stretched and the alveolar crest is pulled in the same direction (see *Fig. 11.1a*).

A number of cellular processes are activated within the PDL. There is an increase in the number of connective tissue cells by cell division. For young humans, incipient cell proliferation is seen after 30–40 hours, particularly near the socket wall. Osteoid tissue will be deposited on the wall shortly after (*Fig. 11.2*). Where the fibrous bundles are thick, new bone appears to be deposited along them. If the bundles are thin, a more uniform layer is deposited along the root surface (Reitan, 1951). Calcification in the deeper layers of the osteoid starts shortly afterwards, while the superficial part remains uncalcified.

Metabolic activity during experimental tooth movement has been studied autoradiographically. Crumley (1964) observed that incorporation of ^{3}H-proline was increased slightly on the tension side of rat molars, while Baumrind and Buck (1970) found an initial decline in the uptake of this labelled amino acid.

The blood vessels appear to be distended. In longitudinal sections of the tooth, fibroblasts in the PDL are oriented in the same direction as the principal fibres: in the direction of strain. The fibroblasts appear spindle-shaped. The cells adjacent to the alveolar wall often appear more spherical (*Fig. 11.3*).

It has been thought that PDL fibres at the alveolar bone surface became entrapped passively by the advancing front of new bone formation to form Sharpey fibres (e.g. Kraw and Enlow, 1967). However, more recent findings suggest that new Sharpey fibres are secreted simultaneously with new bone deposition. As the fibroblasts migrate with the bone, they may deposit either entirely new Sharpey fibres or new fibrils, which are incorporated into existing fibres (Garant and Cho, 1979) (*Fig. 11.4*). Whilst part of the newly synthesized collagen will be incorporated into the new osteoid, some will be incorporated into the PDL (*Fig. 11.5*), perhaps associated with the increase in width on the tension side (Rygh, 1976). Lengthening of fibres seems also to occur by incorporation of new fibrils into existing fibres (even at some distance from the alveolar bone wall).

The observation by Ten Cate (1972) that fibroblasts were able both to break down and to produce collagen fibrils led to the assumption that, in the healthy PDL, all collagen degradation was intracellular (Ten Cate and Deporter, 1975) (see also Chapter 1), and that rapid remodelling of the periodontal tissue during experimental or therapeutic tooth movement would be characterized by a very high ratio of internalized collagen or fibroblast

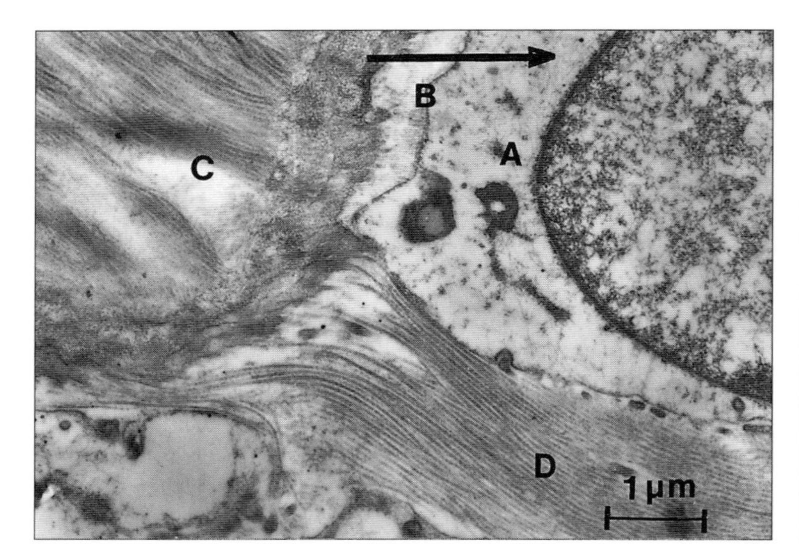

Fig. 11.2 Electron micrograph of the PDL on the tension side of a rat first molar following experimental movement in the direction of the arrow for 7 days. Osteoblast (A) deposits osteoid (B) on the surface of the alveolar bone (C). Collagen fibre (D) inserts into the new bone. (Magnification × 9000.)

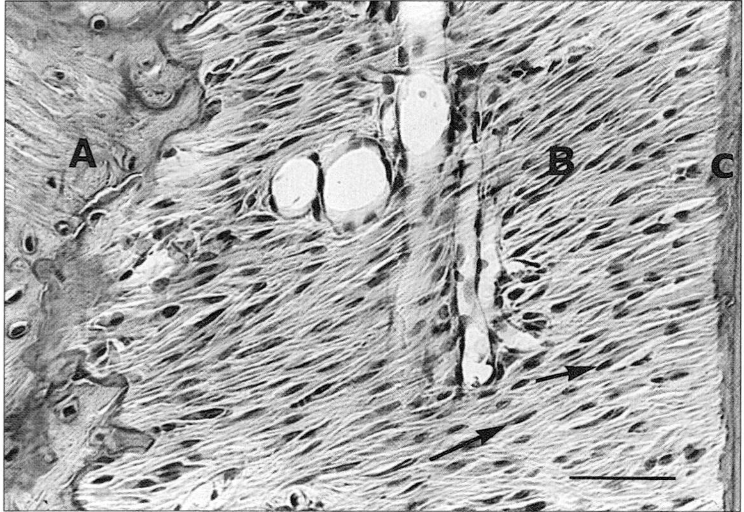

Fig. 11.3 Longitudinal section of PDL under tension on the distal side of a rat first molar moved by continuous force for 7 days. The region is close to the alveolar crest. A – alveolar bone; B – periodontal ligament; C – cementum. In this plane, the fibroblasts are spindle-shaped and oriented in the direction of pull (arrow), while the cells adjacent to the alveolar wall are more rounded. (Bar = 50 μm.)

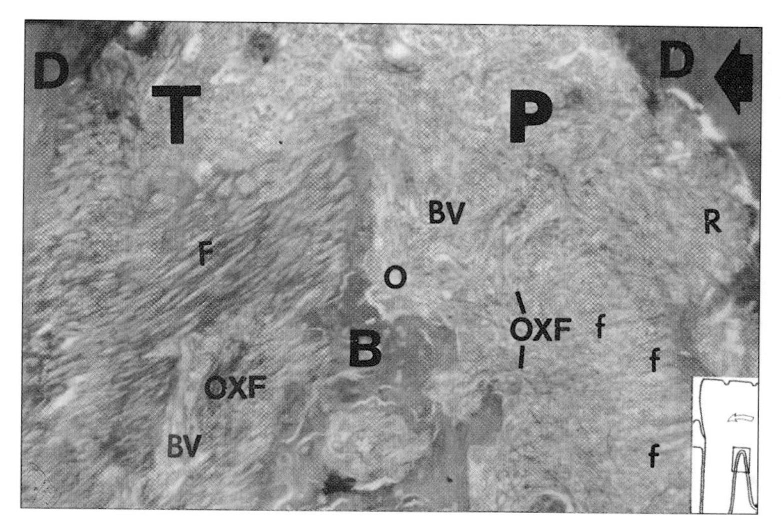

Fig. 11.4 Mesial movement (arrow) of first maxillary molar for 21 days. B – interradicular bone, D – dentine. Stretched collagen fibres (stained dark green) are shown in area of tension (T). Behind a chain of osteoclasts (O), the majority of Sharpey fibres in the pressure area (P) seem to have disappeared. Only thin fibrils (f) persist in the mid-region fibres (OXF). R – root resorption, BV – blood vessel. (Aldehyde–fuchsin–Halmi stain × 440). (From Rygh P *et al.*, 1986.)

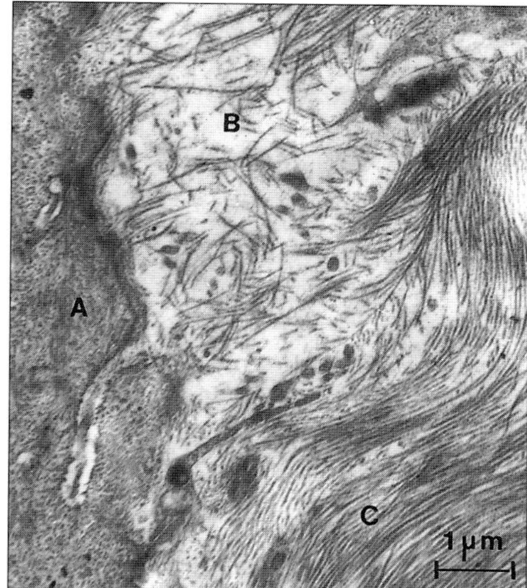

Fig. 11.5 Electron micrograph of the tension side of the rat PDL adjacent to alveolar bone (A) 15 days after being moved experimentally by a continuous force. Note the loosely arranged unoriented collagen fibrils (B) as well as the fibre bundle (C). (Magnification × 9000.)

volume. Freeman and Ten Cate (1978) did not discern any localized concentration of fibroblasts with intracellular collagen profiles on the tension side of the PDL of rat molars.

Investigations on the vascular and inflammatory-like reactions in the PDL of experimentally moved teeth have contributed to a better understanding of fibre remodelling. In areas of experimental tension of the PDL, a great increase in vascular activity could be observed (Rygh *et al.*, 1986) (see *Fig. 11.4*). This was indicated by an increase in the space occupied by the blood vessels, most commonly seen in the middle of the PDL and towards the alveolar bone. Khouw and Goldhaber (1970), using light microscopy, had reported vasodilatation in areas of tension, so this was not a new observation. Transmission electron microscopy, however, permitted identification of a great number of cells paravascularly, concomitant with the vascular infiltration. Macrophages (*Fig. 11.6*), and other leucocytes that migrate out of the PDL blood vessels simultaneously with proteins and fluids, are known to be capable of producing and releasing a variety of factors. The introduction of leucocytes into the PDL during the early stages of

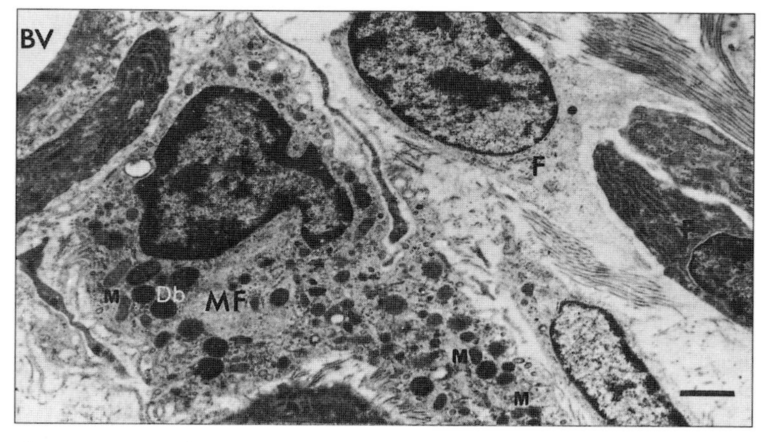

Fig. 11.6 Area of tension in the middle of the periodontal ligament: experimental time – 14 days. Macrophage (MF) shown with many dense bodies (Db) of varying size and stainability and mitochondria (M) near blood vessel (BV); F – fibroblast. (Bar = 1 μm; magnification × 10 000.) (From Rygh P *et al.*, 1986.)

orthodontic treatment was noted by Rygh and Selvig (1973), Rygh (1974, 1976), and Storey (1973). The significance of this finding far exceeds the early observation that cells of the immune system participate actively in phagocytosing necrotic tissues in compressed zones of the PDL. In fact, these cells are not only active removers of tissues that have been altered by pathological conditions, but, most importantly, they are producers of numerous signal molecules that perform a myriad of functions, from chemoattraction to stimulation of mitogenesis and cytodifferentiation (see Chapter 12).

The reactions that occur where the PDL is overstressed are the typical efforts by the body to counteract noxious stimuli and to repair or replace damaged tissue. Storey (1973) emphasized the development of an inflammatory process in the stressed PDL even when light forces are being used.

Laboratory experiments revealed that, in local areas of tension, the volume of the collagen fibres running from tooth to alveolar bone was reduced as the volume of blood vessels increased. In transmission electron microscopy, collagen fibrils and other formed structures appear more sparse in the intercellular spaces in areas of tension after 5 days (Rygh *et al.*, 1986) (*Fig. 11.7*). Since the extensive breakdown and remodelling of fibres that was observed on rapid experimental tooth movement was not reflected by a concomitant increase in phagocytic activity by PDL fibroblasts, other mechanisms seem more likely; extracellular breakdown of collagen by collagenases possibly produced through macrophage–fibroblast interaction.

Pettigrew *et al.* (1980) recognized a tissue-derived collagenase inhibitor, and other observations indicated that collagenase is present on the surface of collagen fibrils. The possibility therefore arises that resorption of periodontal connective tissue is influenced because collagenase-inhibitor production is changed under certain circumstances. It is of note that, in the physiological situation of tooth shedding in kittens, the removal of collagen from the PDL occurs extracellularly and does not, to any great degree, involve phagocytic activity (Ten Cate and Anderson, 1986).

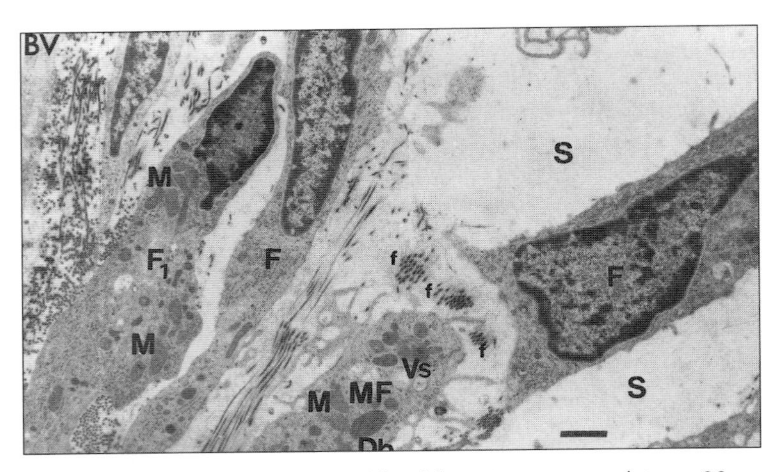

Fig. 11.7 Area of tension in the middle of the PDL; experimental time – 28 days. Macrophage (MF) shown with pseudopodia, dense bodies (Db), and vesicles (Vs) surrounded by sparse, granular fibrous elements (f). Wide intercellular spaces (S) without formed elements surround fibroblasts (F). Mitochondria (M) abound in fibroblast (F) near blood vessel (BV). (Bar = 1 μm; magnification × 8000.) (From Rygh P *et al.*, 1986.)

REACTIONS TO HEAVY LOADS IN AREAS OF TENSION

Although haemorrhage and the presence of osteoclasts in areas of tension was reported by Oppenheim (1944), it seems likely, in most therapeutic parallel movement of teeth, that there is little (or only localized) overstretching of the PDL in areas of tension. During continuous tipping, however, such a reaction may occur (*Fig. 11.8*). Experimental tipping of first molars in rats (for periods varying from 6 hours to 28 days) in order to study reactions to heavy, continuous loads, indicated a pattern in the reaction of PDL and bone to tensional stress (Rygh *et al.*, 1986). Up to a certain level of stress duration, the reactions mainly occur in the PDL and involve increasing vascularization, cell proliferation, fibre formation, and osteoid apposition to the bone surface (see *Fig. 11.8a*). Beyond a certain level of stress–duration, there is decreased vascular supply in the PDL, with cell death occurring between stretched fibres. Scarcity of fibroblasts (responsible for adequate matrix remodelling) was also reported by Michaeli and Everts (1988). It is of note that reactions at this stage mainly occcur within the alveolar bone, probably to compensate for the failing remodelling of the PDL due to overstretching. Vascular invasion into the bone and ensuing removal/resorption of the alveolar bone wall occurs from adjacent narrow spaces. This in turn permits vascular invasion, bringing cells into the PDL from the alveolar bone. Resorption of parts of the alveolar bone may occur from both sides of the alveolar lamina (see *Fig. 8b*). With prolonged high force, there is a temporary increase in PDL width. A vertical reduction in the height of the approximal alveolar bone may also occur. There is reason to assume that pressure on the alveolar crest from the stretched transseptal fibre system contributes to resorption of bone. A tipping tooth movement accentuates the vertical reduction. In the normal periodontium, the reduction of bone height is temporary.

Apposition of new bone is considerable during 21 days of tooth movement. Along the root surface the cells may be pulled away from the cementum surface, at least in the cervical area (*Fig. 11.9*).

RESPONSES OF THE PERIODONTAL LIGAMENT ON THE PRESSURE SIDE

On the side of the PDL towards which a tooth is being moved, the periodontal space becomes narrower. The crest of the alveolar bone is slightly deformed. Assuming that the applied force is sufficiently strong and is maintained for long enough, certain cellular mechanisms will occur within the PDL and on the surfaces of the alveolar bone.

Similarities exist between changes elicited by experimental, orthodontic-like forces and the remodelling changes of the supporting tissues of teeth with physiological migration. Histological studies of the PDL of such teeth show resorption of the alveolar bone surface on the side towards which the tooth is moving (e.g. Reitan, 1951; Kraw and Enlow, 1967). In physiological tooth movement (where tartrate-resistant acid phosphatase – TRAP – is used to identify osteoclasts), a few osteoclasts can be observed resorbing the alveolar bone wall. Vascular activity is low and few leucocytes and macrophages are seen. (Brudvig and Rygh, 1993a) (*Fig. 11.10*). However, whereas with physiological migration the number of osteoclasts is usually low (indicating a rather slow process), orthodontic-like forces elicit more dramatic changes. Such changes can be categorized broadly into 'direct resorption', where the pressure is relatively light, and 'hyalinization', where the pressure is large enough to produce degenerative changes.

DIRECT RESORPTION

Some hours after the application of a horizontal orthodontic force of the order of 0.3–1 N to a human premolar, osteoclasts can be seen in the PDL along the alveolar bone surface. In children aged between 10 and 13 years, Reitan (1951) found occasional evidence of resorption after 12 hours, and resorption was invariably seen by 40 hours. With optimum force after 3–4 days, numerous osteoclasts are present along the alveolar wall. While in clinical orthodontics an initial phase of overcompression of the PDL is nearly always unavoidable (*Fig. 10.11c*), experimental movement of the first molar in rats and mice has shown that the second molar is also pulled forward, possibly through the intermediary of the transseptal fibres (see also Chapter 9). This force is evidently ideal for movement by direct resorption of the bone septum (*Figs 10.11a,b*). The use of TRAP staining for the identification of osteoclasts and osteoclast precursors never revealed positive staining of cells on alveolar bone surfaces away from which the teeth physiologically migrated (see *Fig. 11.10b*). Along the alveolar bone surface in areas of experimental tension, positive TRAP staining was frequent, which indicates either resorption due to the pressure from the second molar being pulled positively in a mesial direction through the supra-alveolar fibres when the first molar was actively moved by a spring or local damage of the alveolar bone surface (see *Fig. 10.11b*).

In light microscopical sections, a clear zone often separated resorbing cells from the bone (*Fig. 11.12*). This artefact appears to be related to the destruction of both alveolar bone and Sharpey fibres. With the electron microscope, however, the ruffled border of osteoclasts is seen to be in close contact with the resorbing bone surface (*Fig. 11.13*) and both crystals and collagen fibres may be found between the cell processes. Garant (1976) has observed fibroblasts with increased amounts of intracellular collagen profiles near osteoclasts in the PDL of rat molars, and the question remains as to whether such fibroblasts also play a role in bone resorption. There is extensive remodelling of collagen throughout the PDL (with the possible exception of Sharpey fibres at the root surface) (see *Figs 11.4, 11.12*). At the same time, there is formation of new collagen, which becomes attached to the alveolar bone by localized bone apposition (*Fig. 11.14*). Collagen detached from alveolar bone during resorptive activity may become reattached to bone or to pre-existing periodontal collagen fibres by the local activity of osteoblasts or fibroblasts respectively (Beertsen *et al.*, 1979).

The precise pathway by which degraded collagen is removed has still to be determined. Freeman and Ten Cate (1978) implicate periodontal fibroblasts because of the presence within many of these cells of intracellular collagen profiles (see also Chapter 1). Extracellular breakdown by fibroblast-like cells occurs locally in some situations in the PDL (e.g. in the removal of surface cementum within the pressure zone – Brudvik and Rygh, 1993b). However, compressed necrotic tissue in hyalinized zones is removed to a considerable extent by macrophages (Kvam, 1972a,b; Rygh, 1974) (see *Fig. 11.19*).

During physiological migration, resorption of collagen may occur in a selective manner. It is possible that this ensures that, at any given time, most of the supporting apparatus of the tooth remains intact (see *Fig. 11a*).

Little is known about the reaction of the ground substance of the PDL in areas subjected to pressure of long duration. The ground substance appears to be the major water-binding constituent of connective tissues (Schubert and Hammerman, 1968;) (see also Chapter 4). Even though it is presumed that both bound and unbound water are present in the PDL, it is not known whether there is movement of water between the vascular and extravascular compartments during loading and unloading of a tooth (Melcher and Walker, 1976). The question of whether ground substance will flow (and under what conditions) is still unanswered.

The rich blood supply to the PDL may play a role in the mechanisms of tooth eruption and tooth support (see Chapters 9 and 10), although little is known concerning the reactions of the periodontal vasculature to moderate pressure. However, unless an adequate vascular supply is present, the differentiation of specialized cells will not take place. The periodontal vasculature ought to be capable, therefore, of compensating for any increased pressure associated with the initial narrowing of the PDL.

The width of the periodontal space seems to be important in determining the reactions of the PDL to load and is itself directly related to the functional state of the tooth. Recently erupted teeth in children have a wider PDL than those in adults (and particularly those not in function, such as impacted teeth, where the width of the ligament may be only one-third of that seen in erupted teeth (Coolidge, 1937). This may help explain why children's teeth are more easily moved orthodontically than adult's teeth (see page

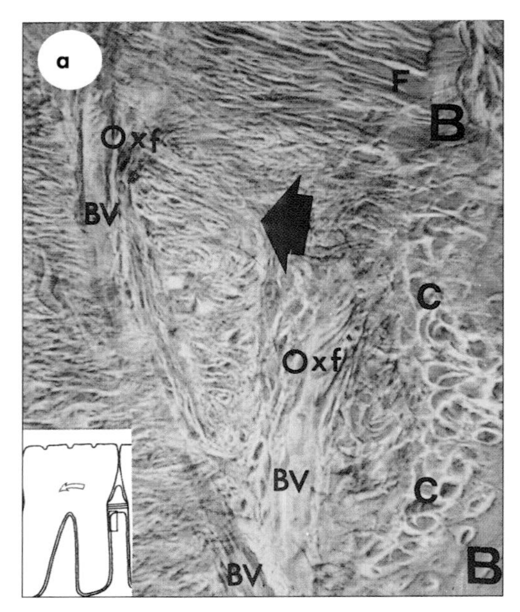

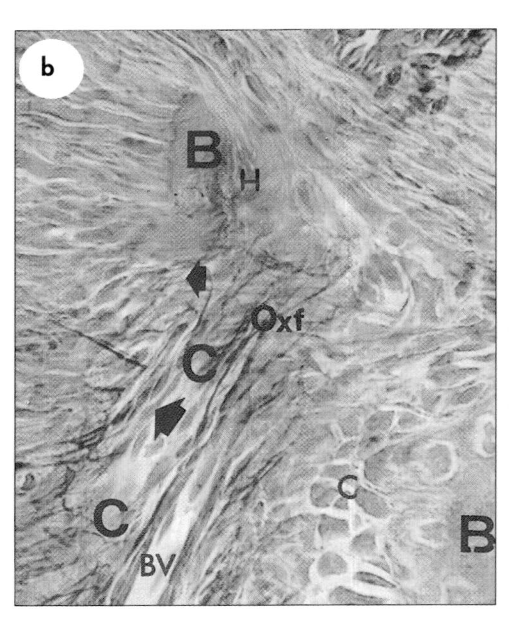

Fig. 11.8 Area of tension after 28 days of mesial movement (arrow). (a) There is marked vascular activity with dilated blood vessels (BV) and oxytalan fibres (OXF) in the middle of PDL and near the alveolar bone wall (B), where a high number of cells (C) are seen. Persisting Sharpey fibrils (F) are present near the part of alveolar bone (B) without vascular infiltration. Sharpey fibrils disappear in areas near bone with vascular infiltration. (b) Same specimen, sections 6 μm apart. Blood vessels (BV) are proliferated inside the alveolar bone (B) behind bone plate. Cells (C) surrounding the blood vessel seem to have infiltrated the alveolar bone plate from behind and broken down parts of the alveolar bone plate and its inserting Sharpey fibres (arrow). OXF – oxytalan fibres; H – hyalinization-like zone. (Aldehyde–fuchsin–Halmi stain; magnification × 900.) (From Rygh P *et al.*, 1986.)

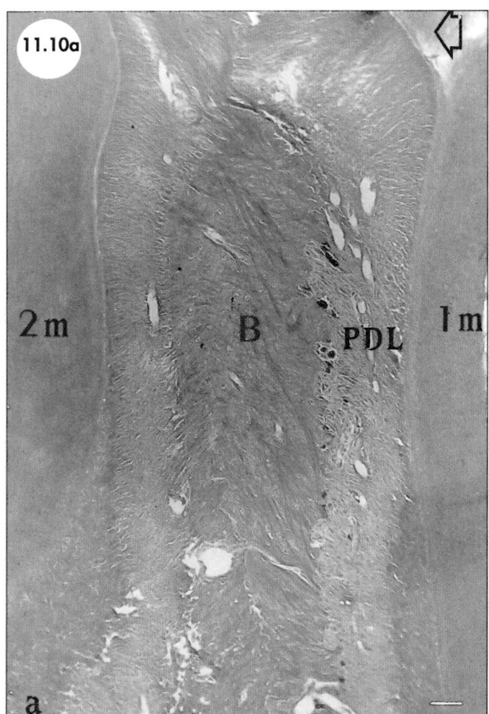

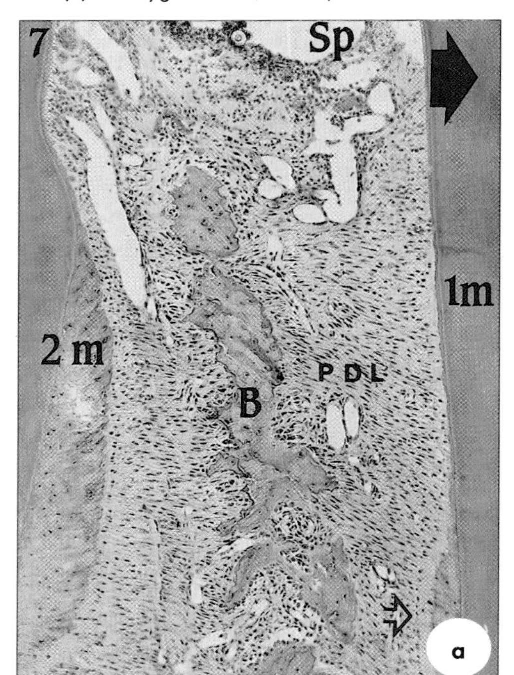

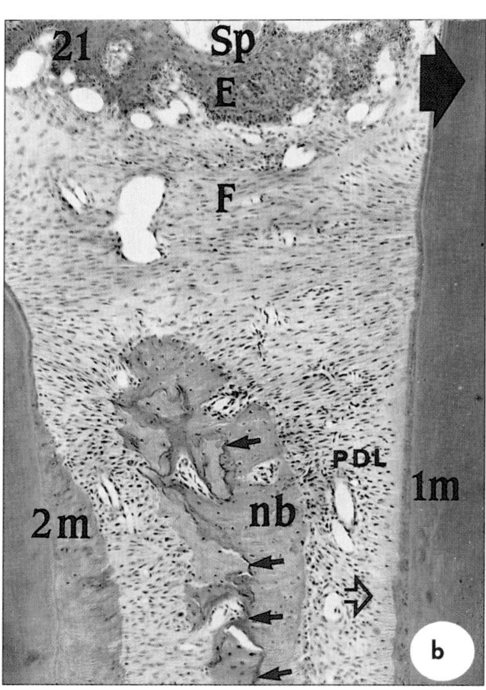

Fig. 11.9 (a) Interradicular alveolar septum between first rat molar (1M) moved in direction of large arrow spring (Sp) for 7 days. Inflammatory breakdown of supra-alveolar epithelium and fibres is seen. PDL is widened in area of tension where cells occur at some distance from unmineralized cementum (open arrow). (b) After 21 days intact supra-alveolar epithelium (E) and transseptal fibres (F). New bone apposition (nb). Thickened cementum (open arrow). (Haematoxylin and eosin.) (Bar = 50 μm.)

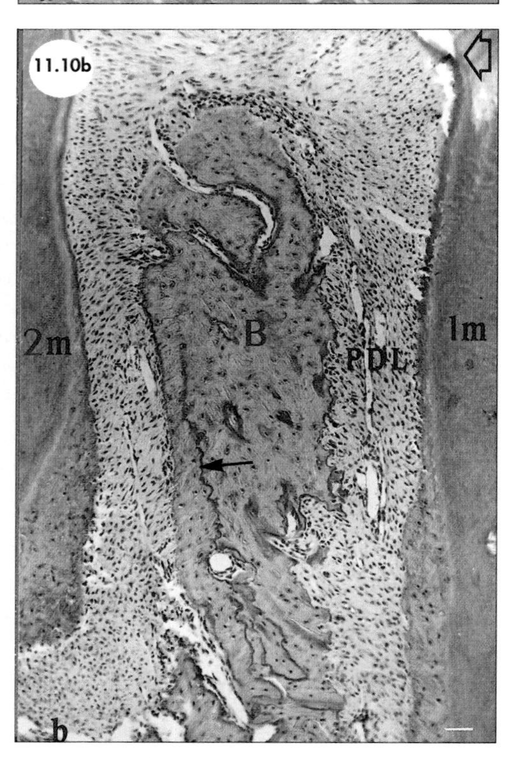

Fig. 11.10 Physiological tooth migration of the first (1m) and second (2m) molar (rat) in direction of open arrows. (a) Scattered osteoclasts stained red on interradicular bone (B) (TRAP). (b) Neighbouring section with demarcation line in B indicating apposition (Haematoxylin and eosin.) (Bars = 50 μm.)

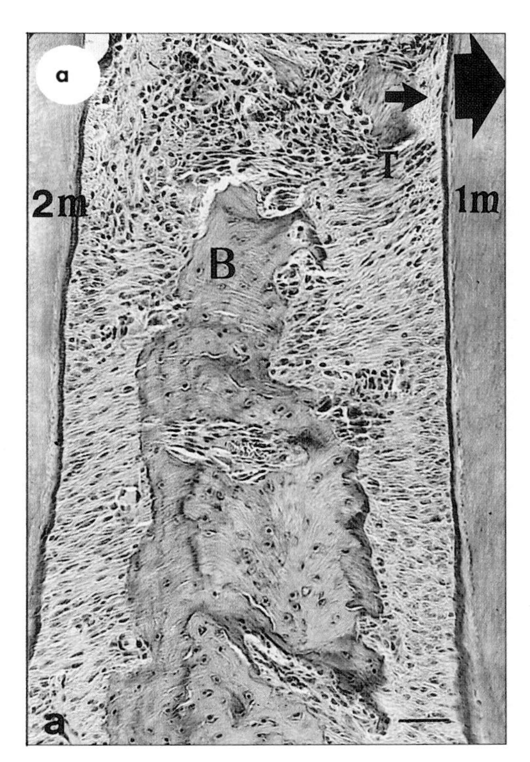

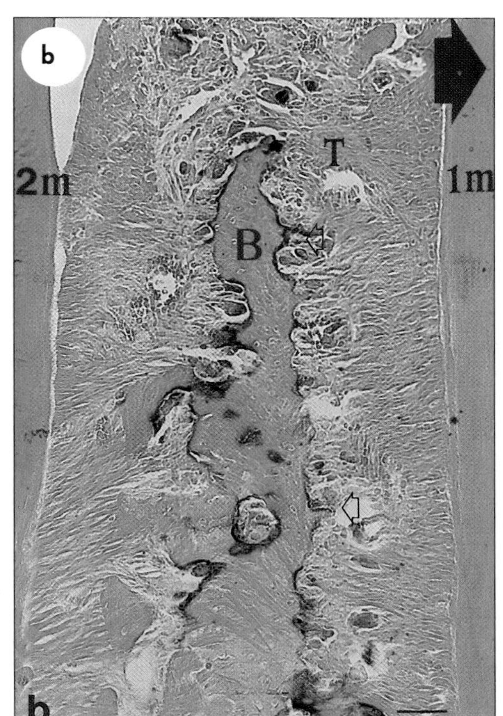

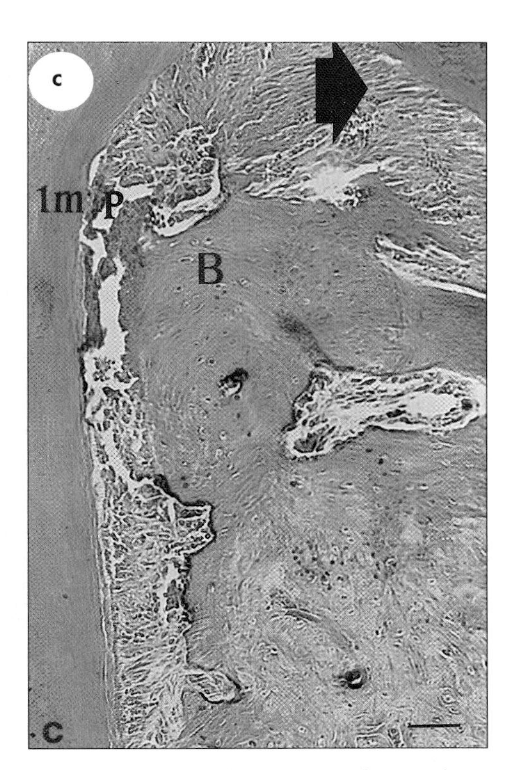

Fig. 11.11 Experimental movement of the first mouse molar (1m) in mesial direction (large arrows) for 6 days. (a and b) Second molar (2m) moved passively through tension of transseptal fibre system with direct resorption of bone (B) by osteoclasts (stained red by TRAP). In area of tension (T), overstretched fibres on cervical root surface (small arrow in (a)) can be seen; these stain positively with TRAP along alveolar bone (open arrows). (c) In area of pressure (P), overcompression of PDL is seen. Osteoclasts (red stain) along alveolar bone and in marrow spaces. (a – haematoxylin and eosin; b, c – TRAP.) (Bar = 50 μm.)

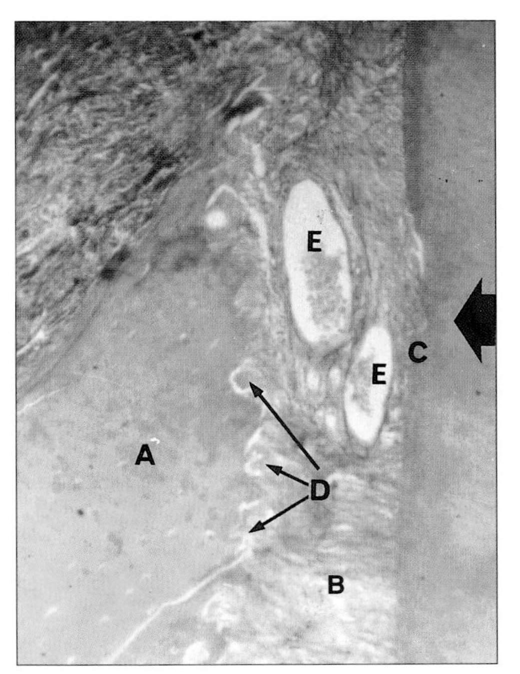

Fig. 11.12 Longitudinal section of the pressure (mesial) side of the PDL of a rat first molar moved experimentally by a continuous force for 3 weeks, near the alveolar crest region. The arrow shows the direction of force. A – alveolar bone; B – periodontal ligament (note width); C – cementum; D – direct resorption by osteoclasts; E – blood vessels. Note the clear zone between the osteoclasts and the surface of the alveolar bone. (Aldehyde–fuchsin–Halmi after oxidation; magnification × 230.)

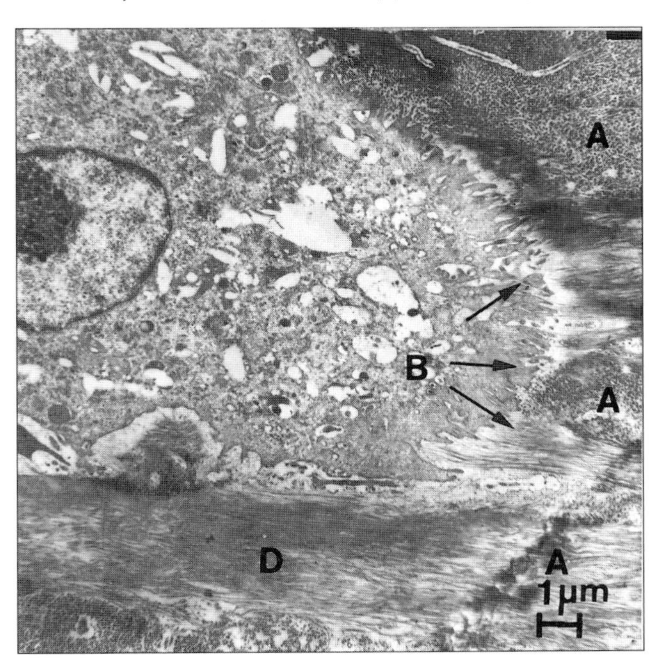

Fig. 11.13 Detail of pressure area corresponding to *Fig. 11.12.* Alveolar bone (A) is resorbed by osteoclast (B). Note intimate contact between bone and the osteoclast's ruffled border area (arrows). The adjacent Sharpey fibre (D) does not seem to be affected by the osteoclast. (Electron micrograph of demineralized section; magnification × 2800.)

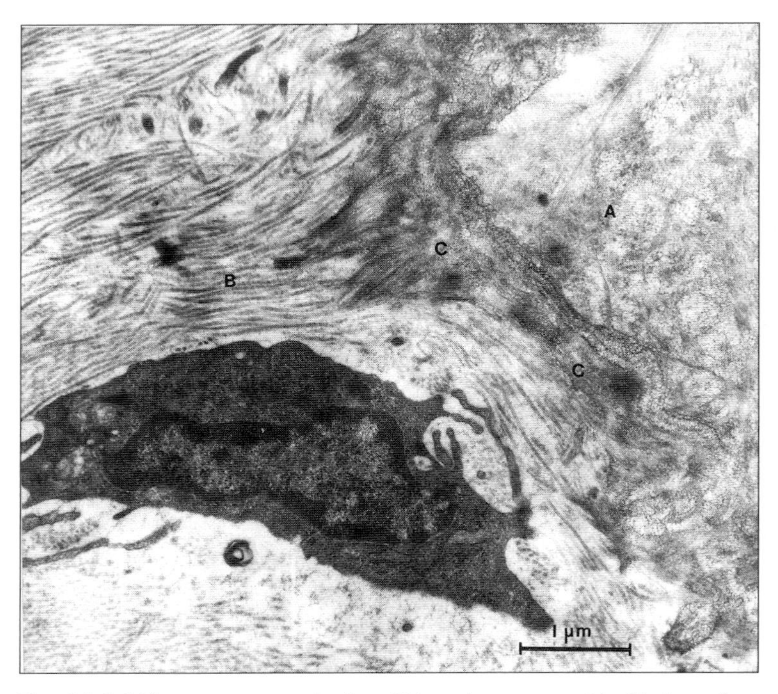

Fig. 11.14 Electron micrograph of rat PDL on the pressure side 21 days after being moved experimentally by continuous force. A – alveolar bone; B – new periodontal collagen fibrils becoming attached by deposition of new bone (C). (Decalcified section.; magnification × 18,000.)

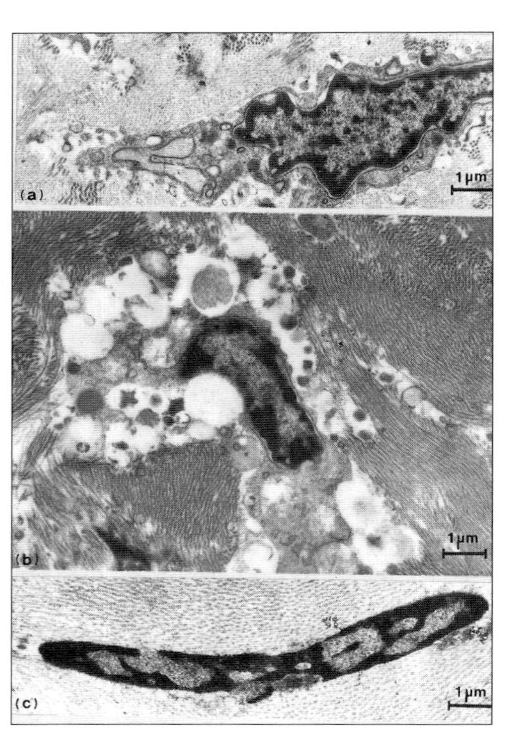

Fig. 11.15 Electron micrograph showing degenerative changes within periodontal fibroblasts during hyalinization of the PDL following application of continuous force of 10 g. (a) Swelling of endoplasmic reticulum (duration of force 30 minutes). (b) Advanced swelling with formation of vacuoles (duration of force 2 hours). (c) Cell nucleus during breakdown (duration of force 2 hours). (Magnification × 9000.)

255). Under non-pathological conditions, the width of the PDL will give an indication of its capacity for remodelling during the initial phase of increased loading of the tooth. With extensive direct resorption of the socket wall as the result of the application of orthodontic forces, the width of the PDL is increased (see *Fig. 11.11b*). Only during the initial phase of orthodontic tooth movement and reactivation of an applied force is there a narrowing of the PDL on the pressure side.

HYALINIZATION

Increased pressure in a localized region of the PDL can easily exceed the optimum and inhibit the differentiation of osteoclasts. As a result, the direct resorption of alveolar bone, which would 'relieve' the pressure in the PDL, cannot occur. Instead, a series of degenerative tissue reactions take place, commencing within a few hours. The term 'hyalinization' is used to describe these tissue reactions, owing to the fact that the degenerated tissue has a glassy appearance in routine histological sections (see *Fig. 10.11c*). The presence of hyalinization has been interpreted by Kardos and Simpson (1980) as representing a change in consistency of the collagenous matrix rather than its degeneration, and as providing evidence that the PDL has the properties of a thixotropic gel (see Chapter 2).

With experimental labial tipping of, for example, a human incisor or premolar, a pronounced pressure zone is seen in the PDL after 2 days (Rygh, 1973a). Tissue changes within the PDL (see *Figs 10.11a,b*) are characterized by oedema, gradual obliteration of blood vessels, and the breakdown of walls of veins. The vascular changes are followed by leakage of blood constituents into the extravascular space. Changes in the fibroblasts are also seen. These often begin with moderate swelling of the endoplasmic reticulum (*Fig. 11.15a*). More extensive swelling and the formation of vacuoles occur later (*Fig. 11.15b*), followed by rupture of the cytoplasmic membrane and loss of cytoplasm (Rygh, 1972b). This leaves isolated nuclei, which undergo lysis over a period of several weeks (*Fig. 11.15c*). Rygh (1973b) has shown that, after 3–5 weeks, some of the collagen fibrils undergo a longitudinal splitting. However, most collagen retains its typical banded appearance and is altered less than was assumed previously (e.g. Kvam, 1972a). Hyalinized areas in the lathyritic PDL contain normal collagen fibrils (Shore *et al.*, 1984).

It is not known what happens to the ground substance in a hyalinized zone. It is possible that, as long as ground substance remains in the PDL, the tissue will show its glassy appearance. With long-acting, heavy compression, the ground substance and tissue fluid can be squeezed out of the compressed zone, reducing the distance between the tooth and alveolar wall to 5–10 μm (Rygh, 1977).

The degenerative processes of the different tissue components persist as long as the pressure is maintained and, by so doing, they prevent recolonization of the damaged tissue by cells from the adjacent, undamaged PDL (Rygh, 1972a). With time,

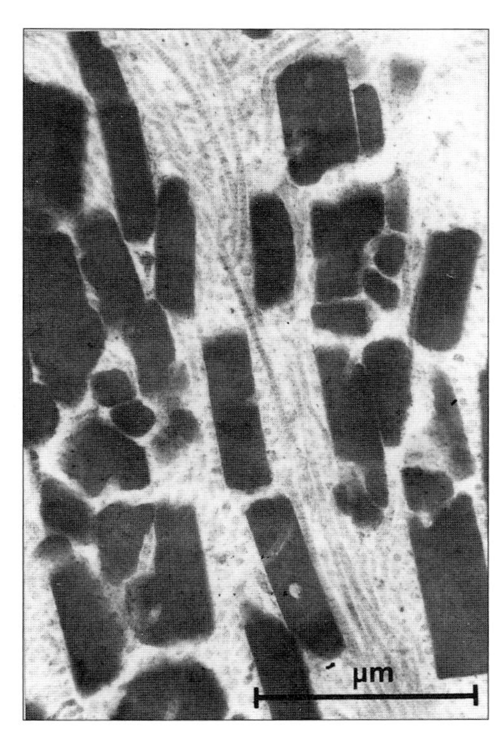

Fig. 11.16 Electron micrograph of PDL showing formation of crystals during breakdown of erythrocytes in hyalinized zone following application of continuous force for 2 days. (Magnificaton × 29,000.)

accumulated erythrocyte breakdown products in the pressure region may undergo crystallization (*Fig. 11.16*).

All tooth movement stops until the adjacent bone is resorbed by cells that differentiate on spongiosa surface of the bone or subperiosteally, where there is no cancellous bone between the lamina dura and the external cortical bone (see *Fig. 10.11c*). This indirect ('undermining') resorption occurs at the same time as the invasion of phagocytosing cells from the peripheral undamaged ligament and from the bone marrow spaces (*Fig. 11.17*). All tissue components (including collagen) damaged during compression are eventually removed (*Fig. 11.18*). Extracellular breakdown by fibroblast-like cells occurs locally in some situations in the PDL, e.g. in removal of surface cementum in pressure zones (Brudvik and Rygh, 1993b). However, compressed necrotic tissue in hyalinized zones is to a considerable extent removed by macrophages (Kvam, 1972b; Rygh, 1974) (*Fig. 11.19*). During tipping movements, an area of compression (as seen in the alveolar crestal regions) can act as a fulcrum (see *Fig. 11.17*).

Hyalinized areas are normally removed after a 3–5 week period, provided that, if any further force is to be applied, there is only gentle reactivation. The 'post-hyalinized' PDL under pressure is markedly wider than before, perhaps in order to withstand the greater mechanical influences. If the orthodontic loads are now removed, the original width is rapidly attained (Rygh, 1973a,b).

Reitan (1961) has studied the behaviour of epithelial cell rests in teeth subjected to orthodontic loads. He observed that there was no regeneration of the epithelial cells following regeneration of hyalinized connective tissue. This has not been substantiated by Brice *et al.* (1991) and Brudvik and Rygh (in press).

With the moderate orthodontic forces now used clinically, hyalinized zones are usually confined to a localized area of the PDL, and are about 1–2 mm in length (Reitan, 1951).

ROOT RESORPTION

This is probably the most unwanted sequela to orthodontic tooth movement. Statistically, root resorption is negligible, the mean reduction of tooth length having been reported to be between 0.7 and 1.6 mm (Sjölien and Zachrisson, 1973; Linge and Linge, 1984). Root resorption with severe loss of substance and reduction of tooth length occurs in about 5% of the treated patients. The aetiology of individual susceptibility is not known. Systemic disease, endocrine disturbances, hypocalcaemia (Engström, 1988), immune response (King and Courts, 1988, 1989), and abnormal root function may be factors that lower the protection of the root surface against insults.

Accumulating evidence indicates that generally there is an association between orthodontic root resorption and the presence and removal of necrotic hyalinized PDL tissue (see *Fig. 11.17*). The initial attack of root resorption follows a consistent pattern: starting in the periphery (zone 1) of the main hyalinized zone and occurring some days later beneath the main hyalinized zone (zone 2) (*Fig. 11.20*) (Brudvik and Rygh, 1993a,b; 1994a,b). The cell populations involved during the initial phase of removal/ resorption of the root surface in zone 1 are different from those involved during the later phase in Zone 2 (see *Fig. 11.22*).

1. At the periphery, the cells invading and removing the necrotic, overcompressed tissue (as well as those that resorb the most superficial layer of the root surface) originate from the adjacent healthy PDL. Negative staining by TRAP indicates that these cells are not osteoclasts or osteoclast precursors (see *Fig. 11.17*). At the ultrastructural level these cells are fibroblast-like.
2. The cells that remove the central parts of the necrotic PDL spend a considerable time on the task and only after several days does any viable cell reach the root surface. These cells seem to originate from the marrow spaces of the alveolar bone, situated behind the hyalinized zone. The cells enter the PDL either through bone channels connecting the bone marrow spaces and the PDL or after having resorbed the bone wall of the alveolar socket from the marrow aspect. The latter process has often been termed 'indirect resorption' (*Figs 11.21, 11.22*).

Many mononucleated macrophage-like cells in the PDL remove necrotic tissue by phagocytosis (see *Fig. 11.19*). The early findings of Rygh (1974) showed that these cells dominated the situation. It is not known whether macrophages are involved with the penetration into the root surface, although previous ultrastructural studies indicate that there is tissue removal of surface layers (Rygh, 1974). On the other hand, more recent studies (Brudvik and Rygh, 1994a,b) have shown that multinucleated cells, staining very strongly with TRAP and having a non-ruffled border surface characterized by cup-like filopodia, are engaged in the

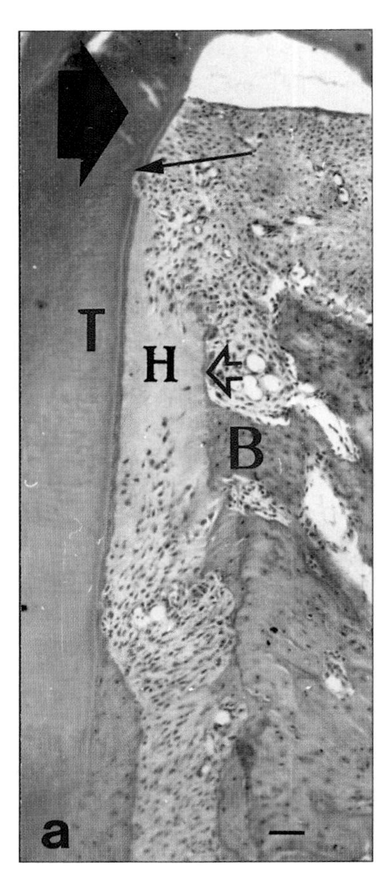

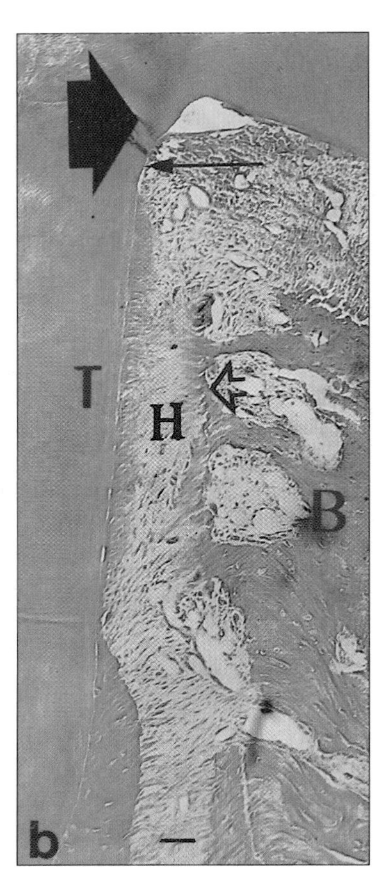

Fig. 11.17 First molar (T) of rat moved for 3 days in direction of large arrows. Hyalinized zone (H). The small arrow indicates initial root resorption by TRAP-negative cells in cervical periphery; the open arrow in (a) indicates TRAP-stained (red) cells in marrow spaces, which have resorbed bone (B), and which in PDL remove necrotic tissue. (a – Haematoxylin and eosin; b – TRAP.) (Bars = 50 μm.)

Fig. 11.18 Electron micrograph showing a blood vessel (A) invading a hyalinized zone and occupying the entire space between the alveolar bone (B) and cementum (C) 5 days following application of continuous force. All periodontal structures have been removed. (Magnification × 8000.)

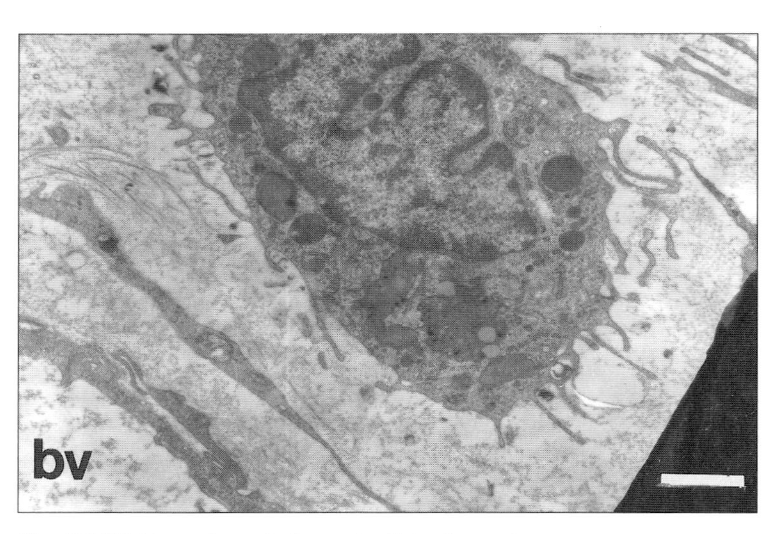

Fig. 11.19 Macrophage in former hyalinized zone in pressure area near blood vessel (BV) after 28 days of tooth movement. (Original magnification × 24,000.) (Bar = 1 μm.)

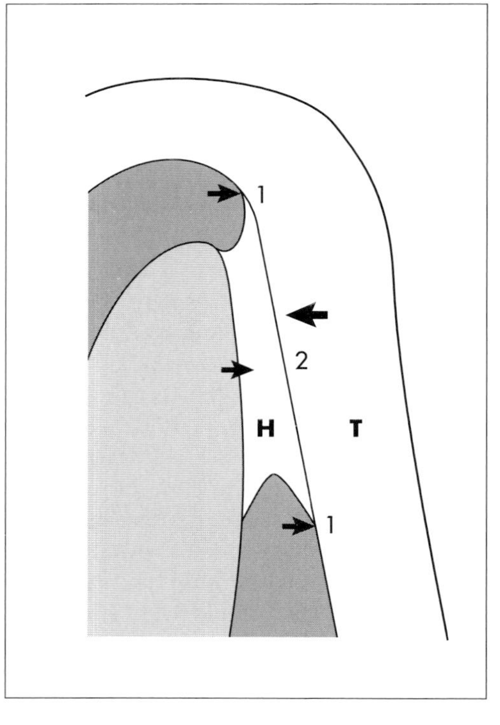

Fig. 11.20 Initial root resorption starts in periphery (zones 1) and occurs later beneath main hyalinized tissue (H) in zone 2. T = tooth.

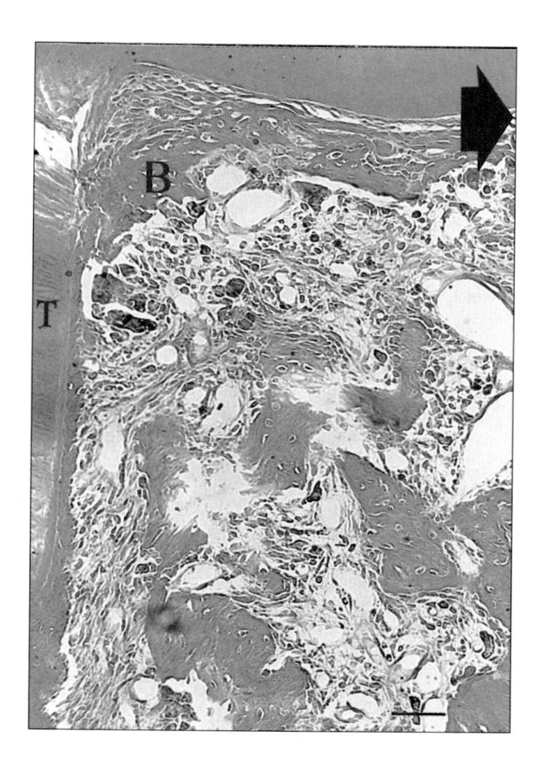

Fig. 11.21 First molar (T) of rat moved for 3 days in direction of the arrow. Multinucleated TRAP-positive cells with open relationship to former marrow space remove necrotic overcompressed PDL tissue and resorb bone (B). (Bar = 50 μm.)

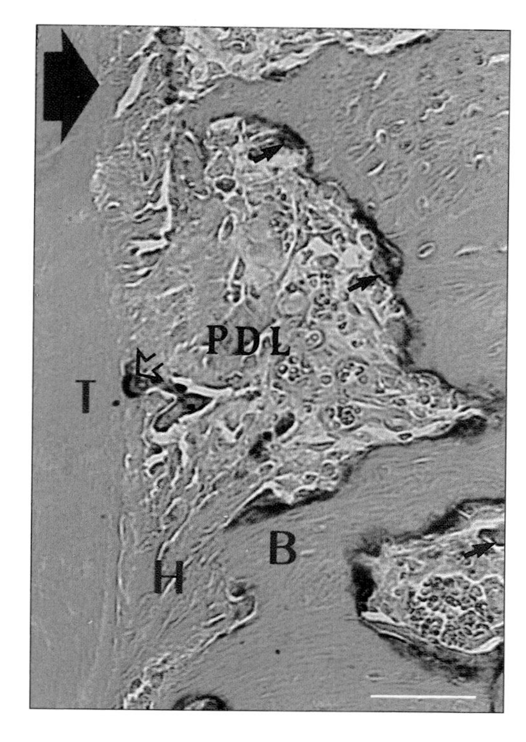

Fig. 11.22. Experimental tooth movement for 8 days (mouse). Initial root resorption beneath partly removed hyalinized tissue (H) by TRAP-positive multinucleated cell. Heavy stain of ruffled border area (open arrow). Neighbouring multinucleated cell near necrotic tissue. Osteoclasts resorb bone (B) in marrow spaces (small arrows). (TRAP.) (Bar = 50 μm.)

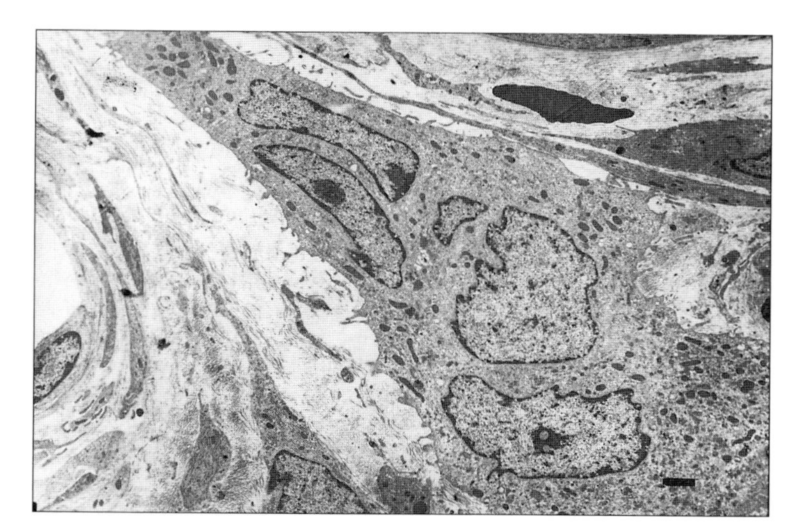

Fig. 11.23 Electron micrograph of multinucleated cell with non-ruffled surface border characterized by cup-like filopodia, associated with removal of necrotic tissue. (Magnification × 2000.) (Bar = 1 μm.)

removal of necrotic tissue (*Fig. 11.23*). These cells are presently believed to be multinucleated giant cells belonging to the mononuclear phagocytic system. The intense staining by TRAP indicates that the tartrate-resistant phosphatase enzyme is of great importance for the removal of both the necrotic PDL tissue and the root surface. It is assumed that the multinucleated giant cells, having a major contribution to the removal of necrotic tissue of the hyalinized zone, would perceive (on reaching the root surface) the outer unmineralized layer of the surface cementum as being contaminated mineral and as another damaged tissue to be removed (Brudvik and Rygh, 1994b).

Our recent research reveals that the extent of the hyalinized zone at 3–4 days corresponds well with the extent of the resorbed root surface after three weeks (*Fig. 11.24*). This indicates that the extent of root surface damage – which is closely associated with the applied force to a certain locality of the PDL – decides the extent of root resorption, provided that the applied force is of sufficient duration.

REACTIONS ON OTHER ROOT SURFACES

In addition to the pressure and tension sides of the root, there are two lateral root surfaces of the tooth to consider. *Fig. 11.25* shows diagrammatically the changes occurring in these regions during tooth movement. In the areas of the PDL corresponding to such lateral surfaces, extensive reorientation of collagen fibres occurs. Furthermore, the insertion of these fibres into alveolar bone (and presumably the arrangement of the ground substance) is undergoing restructuring and reorientation (Rygh, 1973b). Such remodelling may be needed to ensure stability after orthodontic tooth movement. It is likely that this point has been underestimated with regard to the tendency for relapse.

SOME REACTIONS IN OTHER REGIONS OF THE PERIODONTIUM

The remodelling of the PDL is only one aspect of the alteration of the tooth-supporting tissues under load. The pattern of reactions in the PDL is dependent on the architecture of the surrounding structures and must therefore be seen in relation to the response in these tissues. When a tooth moves into a new position in response to a change in its environment, the supporting structures move with it. The architecture of the supporting structures (i.e. gingiva, PDL, and the alveolar bone) is under continuous adjustment, according to functional needs.

ALVEOLAR BONE

On both the pressure and tension sides, resorption and deposition processes occur on both the endosteal and the periosteal aspects.

Generally, direct resorption of the alveolar wall is accompanied by deposition of bone on the opposite surface. In this way, constant dimensions of the alveolar bone are maintained (see *Fig. 11.25*). The alveolar wall adjacent to a hyalinized area of PDL is resorbed from the spongiosa aspect. In marrow spaces, resorption occurs on the side away from the tooth if the PDL and alveolar bone wall are intact. Behind the alveolar bone wall adjacent to a hyalinized zone, resorption occurs on the marrow space surface towards the tooth (undermining resorption) (see *Figs 11.11c, 11.17, 11.22*). However, if the bone is of a more compact nature, it resorbs directly from its external surface. At the same time, osteoclasts differentiate from the relatively normal PDL tissue at the periphery of the hyalinized zone (Reitan, 1951; Rygh, 1973a). Such osteoclasts resorb alveolar bone and allow some relocation of the tooth.

Since remodelling of bone by resorption and deposition is mediated by cells situated on bone surfaces, the architecture of the bone has an important bearing on the rate of tooth movement following loading. Thus, in cancellous bone with thin trabeculae and a large number of osteogenic cells, the greater cell surface area will provide a favourable environment for rapid remodelling, and therefore rapid tooth movement. This is especially evident with teeth that are moved into new extraction sites. In the cell-rich tissue that establishes and fills the alveolus, orthodontic remodelling occurs very quickly. For example, under optimal conditions, a maxillary canine can be moved by translation a full tooth's breadth into the extraction space of a first premolar within 100 days.

In compact (cortical) bone, resorption must occur either from the inner alveolar or outer periosteal surfaces (see *Fig. 11.1b*). If the endosteal surface of cortical bone bordering a hyalinized zone is thick, direct resorption from the outer alveolar side can take a considerable time (Reitan, 1951). In this situation, compensatory bone deposition may not occur, and the overall result is a loss of some alveolar bone. Such a problem arises with labial movement or extrusion of teeth when using large forces. More often the problem is associated with poor local hygiene, particularly in adult patients. It has been claimed that compensatory deposition does not occur on the bony aspect adjacent to hyalinized areas (Melcher, 1976). Nevertheless, such deposition of bone may be observed close to compressed areas in rats (*Fig. 11.26*).

In orthodontic treatment where a pronounced horizontal tooth movement is desired, one ought to use moderate forces that will be distributed as evenly as possible over the pressure side. This will ensure that direct resorption can occur. During treatment planning, the means by which the force is to be applied (as well as the amount of force to be applied) should be considered carefully with respect to the shape of the tooth and to the structure of the surrounding supporting tissues. It is often possible to move a tooth through cancellous bone instead of cortical bone by first moving teeth from the cortical into the middle part of the alveolar process .

GINGIVA

In certain types of orthodontic tooth movement, relapse to the original position is thought to involve the supra-alveolar structures. Reitan (1959) found that after rotation of maxillary lateral incisors in the dog, the gingival fibre bundles remained stretched and displaced 33 weeks later. However, the principal fibres of the PDL readjusted very rapidly. Furthermore, it has been shown that gingivectomy and surgical circumferential incision of gingival fibres may reduce relapse to a considerable extent (e.g. Edwards, 1968). Pinson and Strahan (1974) reduced relapse after rotation by approximately 50 per cent following surgical division of the gingival fibres. Edwards (1968) implicated oxytalan fibres as a cause for relapse because they become larger and more numerous during orthodontic treatment. More recent research (Bowling and Rygh, 1988) showed that there was no increase of oxytalan within the transseptal fibre bundles, although in the PDL deep to the transseptal fibres a slight increase occurred. The oxytalan fibres were nearly always seen in close proximity to blood vessels. It has been shown that vascular activity and blood vessel proliferation increase in the periodontium incident to tooth movement. It is unlikely, however, that this plays a role in relapse of orthodontic movement (Bowling and Rygh, 1988).

It has been suggested that the slower remodelling of gingival structures is due to slower collagen turnover in gingival connective tissue than in the PDL, although the turnover in gingiva is still rapid (Skougaard, Levi and Simpson, 1969; Sodek, 1977). The reasons for such differences remain unknown. One possibility may relate to the fact that many gingival fibres are not attached to alveolar bone. Among the important groups of gingival fibres are the transseptal fibres, which, by some as yet unknown mechanism, have been implicated in the process of approximal drift. Row and Johnson (1990) have studied remodelling of the transseptal fibres following release of orthodontic forces using tritiated proline. They found that transseptal fibres adjust their length by rapid remodelling in regions experiencing a tensile force, and that collagenous protein turnover within the middle third of the transseptal fibres is more rapid subsequent to release of orthodontic force than during normal physiologic drift. They concluded that transseptal fibres were unlikely to be a factor in relapse of orthodontically treated cells.

INFLUENCING VARIABLES

NATURE OF THE LOAD

The duration of the force seems to be of paramount importance. Observations suggest that long-acting small forces may summate over a certain period and produce similar reactions to large forces that act for only brief periods (Reitan, 1951). It is difficult, however, to characterize the tissue responses elicited by very small intermittent forces as the number of osteoclasts is small and the rate of bone deposition is slow.

All natural stimuli are intermittent in character. The interrelationship between the force, its duration, and its frequency determines whether tooth movement or compensatory strengthening of the supporting apparatus will occur. It has been claimed that no orthodontic movement will take place if the force duration does not exceed 6 hours per day (Proffit, personal communication).

If one applies a very small, but continuous, horizontal force to a tooth, the normal stimuli from occlusal function (swallowing, chewing, etc.) will cause an additional intermittent force. When this continuous force is increased beyond a certain limit, the tooth will be unable to recoil from the alveolar wall against which it is being pressed. In the case of intermittent loads, each time the application of a force is interrupted the tooth tends to return to its original position. On the pressure side, the vasculature is disturbed less easily and hyalinization occurs to a lesser degree and over a smaller area than with a continuous force. One sees large numbers of cells associated with an increased width of the PDL, on both the pressure and tension sides. In relation to the maintenance or even the increase of functional stimuli, as seen with certain removable appliances (such as activators, monoblocs, Bimler plates, etc.), the number of cells in the PDL will also increase. These cell numbers are greater than those seen in response to continuous forces of the same magnitude (e.g. Reitan, 1951).

Bone deposition on the tension side is dependent on the length of time the force is applied, and it occurs faster during an active stretching period. If the rest periods between force application are too long (or too frequent), bone deposition is limited (Reitan and Rygh, 1994). When bodily tooth movement is required over a considerable distance, therefore, a continuous force (or a continuous force interrupted only by short intervals) is advantageous.

AGE OF THE PATIENT

Age is an important determinant of the periodontal response to forces. The capacity for adaptation is greatest during the period of active growth. It is stated that there are more fibroblasts and less collagen in the PDL of a child than in the PDL of an adult (see also Chapter 8), and that the alveolar bone surface in children is lined with osteoblasts, in contrast to their more sparse distribution in adults (Reitan, 1954). Alveolar bone in a young person contains more marrow spaces than in an adult. In young dogs, a considerable increase in the number of cells is seen on the tension side after 12 hours (Gottlieb and Orban, 1931). In children, fibroblast proliferation is seen on the tension side 30–40 hours after applying a horizontal load (Reitan, 1951). On the other hand, in adults it occurs only after several days (Reitan, 1954). Indeed, perhaps it is the delayed cellular response in adults that is

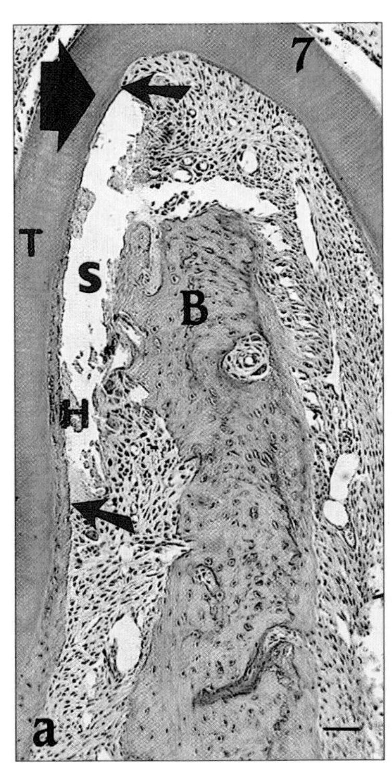

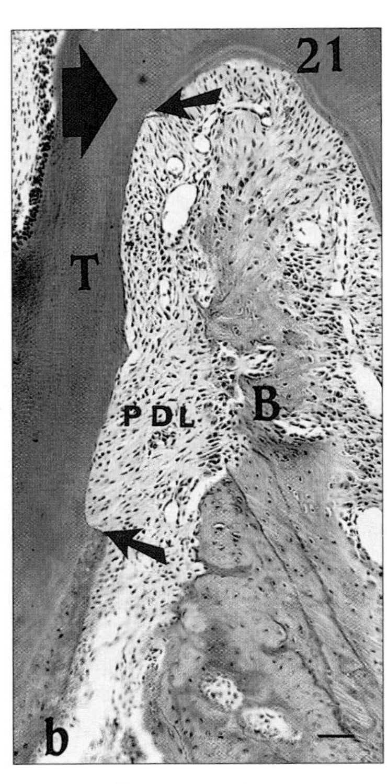

Fig. 11.24 (a) Hyalinized zone (between two small arrows) with empty space (S) as artefact after tooth movement for 7 days (rat). (b) Root resorption area (between two small arrows) after 21 days of tooth movement corresponds with previous hyalinized zone. (Large arrows indicate direction of tooth movement; Haematoxylin and eosin.) (Bar = 50 μm.)

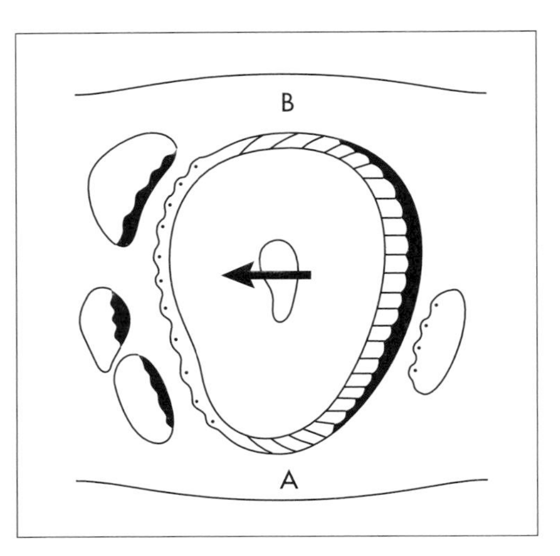

Fig. 11.25 Diagram illustrating the extensive reorientation of fibrous and other elements on the lingual (A) and buccal (B) aspects of the PDL during tooth movement.

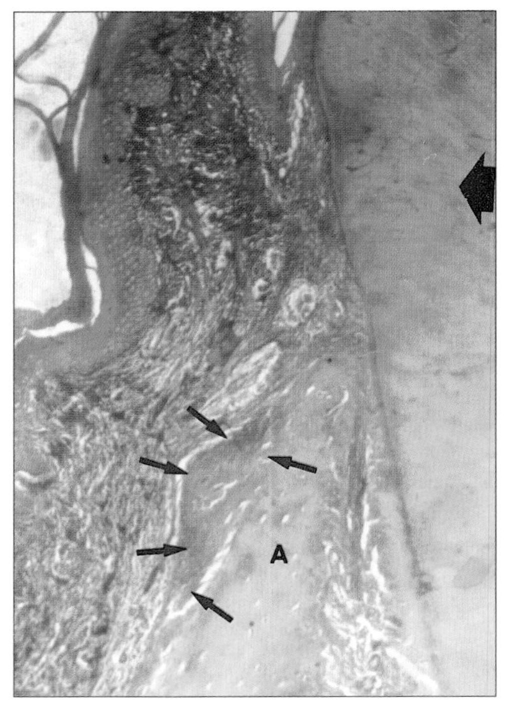

Fig. 11.26. Longitudinal section of PDL of rat first molar near the alveolar crest 14 days after application of continuous force in the direction indicated by large arrow. Note the compensatory bone deposition (arrows) on the external surface of the buccal alveolar bone (A). (Aldehyde–fuchsin–Halmi oxidation; magnification × 180.)

associated with the greater stability of adult teeth. During orthodontic treatment, growth may be utilized by inhibiting the sagittal development of the jaws and stimulating the vertical development of the jaws to reduce or eliminate any discrepancy between upper and lower dental arches; in such cases little tooth movement may be needed.

The healthy supporting tissues of an adult tooth provide resistance to changing occlusal loads. In the aged patient, however, the periodontium appears to undergo some degenerative changes (see Chapter 8). For example, the amount of newly formed bone per unit time is less in the elderly (Frost, 1994). The effect of these changes might be thought to reduce the ability of the periodontium to resist displacement of the tooth under occlusal loads. However, Mühlemann (1951) has shown that human teeth become less mobile with age. This change might be related to an increase in the length of the root or to changes in the number and diameter of the principal fibres in the PDL.

THE ARCHITECTURE OF THE PERIODONTIUM

This varies from individual to individual, even in children. For example, bone density and the nature of the fibre system may produce varying degrees of resistance to given environmental forces. Perhaps such variation may account for the different tendencies of the teeth in different patients to relapse after orthodontic treatment.

HORMONAL BALANCE

The hormonal balance and related factors – such as medication (e.g. cortisone), the presence of an allergy or general disease (e.g. osteomalacia, epilepsy) – may influence the tissue response to orthodontic tooth movement (Melsen *et al.*, 1976). However, the precise mechanisms remain unknown, though it is conceivable that altered rates of turnover of the tooth-supporting tissues or factors relating to bone metabolism may be involved.

REFERENCES

Baumrind S and Buck DL (1970) Rate changes in cell replication and protein synthesis in the periodontal ligament incident to tooth movement. Am J Orthodont 57, 109–131.

Beertsen W, Brekelmans M and Everts V (1979) The site of collagen resorption in the periodontal ligament of the rodent molar. Anat Rec 192, 305–317.

Bowling K and Rygh P (1988) A quantitative study of oxytalan fibres in the transseptal region and tension zones of rat molars following orthodontic movement. Eur J Orthod 10, 13–26.

Brice GL, Sampson WJ and Sims MR (1991) An ultrastructural evaluation of the relationship between epithelial rests of Malassez and orthodontic root resorption and repair in man. Aust J Orthod 12, 90–94.

Brudvik P and Rygh P (1993a) The initial phase of orthodontic root resorption incident to local compression of the periodontal ligament. Eur J Orthod 15, 249–263.

Brudvik P and Rygh P (1993b) Non-clast cells start orthodontic root resorption in the periphery of hyalinized zones. Eur J Orthod 15, 467–480.

Brudvik P and Rygh P, (1994a) Root resorption beneath the main hyalinized zone. Eur J Orthod 16, 249-263.

Brudvik P and Rygh P (1994b) Multinucleated cells remove the hyalinized tissue and start resorption of adjacent root surfaces. Eur J Orthod 16, 265–273.

Brudvik P and Rygh P. The repair of orthodontic root resorption. Eur J Orthod (in press).

Coolidge ED (1937) The thickness of the human periodontal membrane. J Am Dent Ass Cosmos 24, 1260–1270.

Crumley PJ (1964) Collagen formation in the normal and stressed periodontium. Periodontics 2, 53–61.

Edwards JG (1968) A study of the periodontium during orthodontic rotation of teeth. Am J Orthodont 54, 441–459.

Engström C (1988) Root resorptions during orthodontic tooth movement and bone remodelling dynamics during hypocalcaemia and treatment with biphosphonate. In: The Biological Mechanism of Tooth Eruption and Root Resorption (Davidovitch Z, eds), pp391–397. EBSCO Media, Birmingham, Alabama.

Freeman E and Ten Cate AR (1978) Early ultrastructural changes in the periodontal ligament during orthodontic tooth movement. J Dent Res 57 (special issue A), 138.

Frost HF (1994) Wolff's Law and bone's structural adaptations to mechanical usage: an overview for clinicians. Angle Orthod 64, 175–188.

Garant PR (1976) Collagen resorption by fibroblasts. J Periodontol 47, 380–390.

Garant PR and Cho MI (1979) Autoradiographic evidence of the coordination of the genesis of Sharpey's fibres with new bone formation in the periodontium of the mouse. J Periodont Res 14, 107–114.

Gottlieb B and Orban B (1931) Die Veränderungen der Geurche bei Übermässigen Beanspruchung der Zähne. Thieme, Leipzig.

Kardos TB and Simpson LO (1980) A new periodontal membrane biology based upon thixotropic concepts. Am J Orthod 77, 508–515.

Khouw FE and Goldhaber P (1970) Changes in vasculature of the periodontium associated with tooth movement in the rhesus monkey and dog. Arch Oral Biol 15, 1125–1132.

King GJ and Courts FJ (1988) Changes in titer of tooth rot antibodies accompanying traumatic root resorption. In: Biological Mechanisms of Tooth Eruption and Root Resorption (Davidovitch, Z, ed), pp 365–370, EBSCO Media, Birmingham, Alabama.

King GJ and Courts FJ (1989) Humoral immune response to active root resorption. In: Biological Basis of Tooth Movement (Norton LA and Burstone CJ, eds), pp 275–285, CRC Press, Boca Raton, Florida.

Kraw AG and Enlow DH (1967) Continuous attachment of the periodontal membrane. Am J Anat 120, 133–148.

Kvam E (1972a) Scanning electron microscopy of tissue changes on the pressure surface of human premolars following experimental tooth movement. Scand J Dent Res 80, 357–368.

Kvam E (1972b) Cellular dynamics on the pressure side of the rat periodontium following experimental tooth movement. Scand J Dent Res 80, 369–383.

Linge BO and Linge L (1984) Apical root resorption in the upper front teeth during orthodontic treatment: a longitudinal radiographic study of incisor root length. In: Malocclusion and the Periodontium, Monograph 15, Craniofacial Growth Series (McNamara JA Jr and Ribbens K, eds), pp165–185. University of Michigan, Ann Arbor.

Melcher AH (1976) Biological processes in tooth eruption and tooth movement. In: Scientific Foundations of Dentistry (Cohen H and Kramer IRH, eds), pp417–425. Heinemann, London.

Melcher AH and Walker TW (1976) The periodontal ligament in attachment and as a shock absorber. In: The Eruption and Occlusion of Teeth (Poole DGF and Stack MV, eds), pp 183–192, Butterworth, London.

Melsen B, Melsen F and Mosekilde K (1976) Bone changes of importance in the orthodontic patient with epilepsy. Trans Eur Orthodont Soc 227, 233.

Michaeli W and Everts V (1988) Three-dimensional presentation of cell migration in the periodontal ligament of the rat incisor. Anat Rec 221, 584–590.

Mühlemann HR (1951) Periodontometry: a method for measuring tooth mobility. Oral Surg Oral Med Oral Pathol 4, 1220–1223.

Oppenheim A (1944) Possibility for orthodontic physiologic movement. Am J Orthodont 30, 277.

Pettigrew DW, Sodek J, Wang HW and Brunette DM (1980) Inhibitors of collagenolytic enzymes synthesized by fibroblasts and epithelial cells from porcine and macaque periodontal tissues. Arch Oral Biol 25, 269–274.

Pinson RR and Strahan HD (1974) The effect on the relapse of orthodontically rotated teeth of surgical division of the ginvigal fibres. Br J Orthodont 1, 87–91.

Proffit WR (personal communication).

Reitan K (1951) The initial tissue reaction incident to orthodontic tooth movement as related to the influence of function. Acta Odont Scand, suppl 6, 1–240.

Reitan K (1954) Tissue reaction as related to the age factor. Dent Rec 74, 271–278.

Reitan K (1959) Tissue rearrangement during retention of orthodontically rotated teeth. Angle Orthod 29, 105–113.

Reitan K (1961) Behaviour of Malassez epithelial rests during orthodontic tooth movement. Acta Odont Scand 19 443–468.

Reitan K and Rygh P (1994). Biomechanical principles and reactions. In: Current Orthodontic Concepts and Techniques, 2nd edition (Graber TM and Vanarsdalljr RL, eds), pp 96–112. Mosby, St Louis.

Reitan K and Rygh P (1979) Vevsreaksjoner ved ortodontisk terapi. In: Nordisk Klinisk Odontologi (Holst JJ, ed), Chapter 15, III, 3.

Row KL and Johnson RB (1990) Distribution of 3H-proline within transeptal fibres of the rat following release of orthodontic fibres. Am J Anat 189, 179–188.

Rygh P (1972a) Ultrastructural vascular changes in pressure zones of rat molar periodontium incident to orthodontic tooth movement. Scand J Dent Res 80, 307–321.

Rygh P (1972b) Ultrastructural cellular reactions in pressure zones of rat molar periodontium incident to orthodontic tooth movement. Acta Odont Scand 30, 575–593.

Rygh P (1973a) Ultrastructural changes in pressure zones of human periodontium incident to orthodontic tooth movement. Acta Odont Scand 31, 109–122.

Rygh P (1973b) Ultrastructural pressure changes in the periodontal fibres and their attachment in rat molar periodontium incident to orthodontic tooth movement. Scand J Dent Res 81 467–480.

Rygh P (1974) Elimination of hyalinized periodontal tissues associated with orthodontic tooth movement. Scand J Dent Res 82 57–73.

Rygh P (1976) Ultrastructural changes in tension zones of rat molar periodontium incident to orthodontic tooth movement. Am J Orthod 70 269–281.

Rygh P (1977) Orthodontic root resorptions studied by electron microscopy. Angle Orthod 47 1–16.

Rygh P and Selvig KA (1973) Erythrocyte crystallization in rat molar periodontium incident to tooth movement. Scand J Dent Res 81 62–73.

Rygh P, Bowling K, Hovlandsdal L and Williams S (1986) Activation of the vascular system: a main mediator of periodontal fibre remodelling in orthodontic tooth movement. Am J Orthod 89, 453–468.

Schubert M and Hammerman D (1968) A Primer on Connective Tissue Histochemistry. Lea and Febiger, Philadelphia.

Shore RC, Berkovitz BKB and Moxham BJ (1984) Histological study, including quantification, of the periodontal ligament in the lathyritic rat mandibular dentition. Arch Oral Biol 29, 263–273.

Sjölien T and Zachrisson BU (1973) Periodontal bone support and tooth length in orthodontically treated and untreated persons. Am J Orthod 64, 28–37.

Skougaard MR, Levi BM and Simpson J (1969) Collagen metabolism in skin and periodontal membrane of the marmoset. J Periodont Res 4 28–29.

Sodek J (1977) A comparison of the rates of synthesis and turnover of collagen and non-collagen proteins in adult rat periodontal tissues and skin using a microassay. Arch Oral Biol 22, 655–666.

Storey E (1973) The nature of tooth movement. Am J Orthodont 63, 292–314.

Ten Cate AR (1972) The role of fibroblasts in the remodelling of the periodontal ligament during physiologic tooth movement. Am J Orthod 69, 155–168.

Ten Cate AR and Anderson RD (1986) An ultrastructural study of tooth resorption in the kitten. J Dent Res 65, 1087–1093.

Ten Cate AR and Deporter DA (1975) The degradative role of the fibroblast in the remodelling and turnover of collagen in soft connective tissue. Anat Rec 182, 1–14.

Chapter 12
Cell Biology Associated with Orthodontic Tooth Movement

Zeev Davidovitch

INTRODUCTION

Orthodontic tooth movements are facilitated by the transmission of mechanical forces from the dental roots to the surrounding tissues, where cells are stimulated to remodel the matrices that engulf them. In the early years of the twentieth century, histologic observations revealed extensive cellular activities in the mechanically stressed periodontal ligament (PDL), involving fibroblasts, endothelial cells, and alveolar bone surface cells (Sandstedt, 1904, 1905), as well as osteocytes and endosteal cells (Oppenheim, 1911).

Although tissue and cellular responses are now known to be evoked immediately following force application, orthodontic treatment is a lengthy and intermittent procedure, often lasting 2 years or more, and consisting of frequent applications of force to most of the teeth.

Hence, the paradental cells of orthodontic patients are subjected to repeated exposures to mechanical forces of various magnitudes, frequencies, and durations. Many cell types are involved in this lengthy tissue remodeling process. For the PDL, the main cell types are fibroblasts, sensory nerves, endothelial cells, and epithelial rests of Malassez. Bordering the PDL are root surface cells (cementoblasts) and alveolar bone surface cells (osteoblasts and osteoclasts). Entering the PDL from its vascular network are cells of the immune system (including macrophages, lymphocytes, and polymorphonuclear cells), whose molecular products stimulate and modulate the activity of the paradental cells. The initial effect of appliance activation is physical, consisting of gradual movement of tissue fluids (Bien, 1966), accompanied by increasing distortion of extracellular matrix and cells (Storey, 1973). This distortion evokes a rapid cellular response by all mechanosensitive cell types. Among these cell types are sensory nerve fibres that release vasoactive neuropeptides from their endings, and capillary endothelial cells that facilitate migration of leucocytes into the PDL. Hence, the initial effect of orthodontic force is physical, followed closely by a biologic response.

In the review that follows, it will be seen that much of what we surmise about the cell biology associated with orthodontic tooth movement has been gleaned from knowledge obtained from similar tissues elsewhere in the body or from *in vitro* studies. Problems of extrapolating to the PDL *in vivo* are obvious, but fortunately much of the knowledge is now being confirmed by appropriate studies of the PDL, particularly from immunocytochemistry.

CELL–MATRIX INTERACTIONS

Mechanical stresses alter the structural and functional properties of cells at the cellular, molecular, and genetic levels, leading to both rapid responses in the neighboring tissues, and slower adaptive changes. Cellular responses to mechanical stresses involve an interplay between structural elements and biochemical second messengers. The extracellular matrix (ECM) and cell surface proteins are linked to the cytoskeleton, and activate ion channels and enzymes by mechanical deformation. As a result of force-induced fluid movement, the extracellular concentration of bioactive ligands at the cell surface is altered, indirectly transducing force effects to cells.

The ECM molecules that transduce mechanical forces to cells are collagen, proteoglycans, laminin, and fibronectin, which surround all anchorage-dependent cells. This transduction occurs by matrix binding to integrins and other cell surface receptors. Adhesion of cells to matrix induces reorganization of the cytoskeleton, which controls cell surface receptors, secretion of cytokines, ribosome function, and gene transcription (Nathan and Sporn, 1991). It can also affect the response of cell surface receptors to various signal molecules, such as cytokines.

Stress is force per unit area, which may be expressed as pressure acting inward upon a cell, frictional shear at the surface, and tensile reactive forces acting outwards. When cells are subjected to shear stress or mechanical stretching, a diverse set of responses is evoked; some are extremely fast, while others develop over many hours. Stress causes strain, defined as the change in length per unit length (one strain is a change in length of 100 per cent).

In osteoblast-like cells, the first measured response to physiological levels of strain is an increase of intracellular free Ca^{2+} within 100 ms and an increase in membrane potential through activation of K^+ channels (Jones and Bingmann, 1991). The elevated Ca^{2+} levels persist for the duration of the strain, while the membrane potential declines, suggesting that the Ca^{2+} source is intracellular. This increase in Ca^{2+} concentration is probably related to the activation of phospholipase C (PLC) which releases inositol triphosphate (IP_3) within 10 seconds. Elevated levels of PLC further increase the concentrations of intracellular Ca^{2+}, probably by stimulating K^+ channels. Activation of PLC can account for many of the effects of strain, such as the activation of protein kinase C (PKC) by diaglycerol (DAG) 3–4 minutes after force application (Jones *et al.*, 1991). Phospholipase A (PLA) is activated shortly thereafter, acting on stores of arachidonic acid in the plasma membrane, leading to the detection of prostaglandin E_2 (PGE_2) at about 10 minutes, followed by products of lipoxigenase, and significant elevations in intracellular levels of adenosine 3',5'-monophosphate (cyclic AMP, cAMP) and guanosine 3',5'-monophosphate (cyclic GMP, cGMP). Cyclic nucleotide-mediated phosphorylation reactions in the cytoplasm and nucleus lead to cellular synthetic and secretory activities.

FORCE TRANSDUCTION BY THE CYTOSKELETON

There is compelling evidence to suggest that the mechanism of transduction of physical force to anchorage-dependent cells is a combination of force transmission through cytoskeletal elements, and transduction of the force to biochemical signals at mechanotransducer sites, where F-actin microfilaments appear to play a pivotal role. In several cell types, disruption of actin inhibits the stimulation of adenylate cyclase and stretch-activated ion channels in response to deformation (Watson, 1991). Actin filaments are anchored in the plasma membrane at several sites, predominantly associated with focal adhesions to the ECM, integral membrane proteins (integrins), and the nuclear membrane (Davis and Tripathi, 1993). Several ECM proteins are recognized by integrins, which are proteinaceous molecules that traverse the plasma membrane, extending to the cytoplasm on one side and the ECM on the other (*Fig. 12.1*). In the cytoplasm, integrins do not bind directly to microfilaments, but rather they bind indirectly through other proteins such as talin, vinculin, and α-actinin (Burridge *et al.*, 1988). Likewise, outside the cell, integrin attaches to the matrix by association with fibronectin or vitronectin.

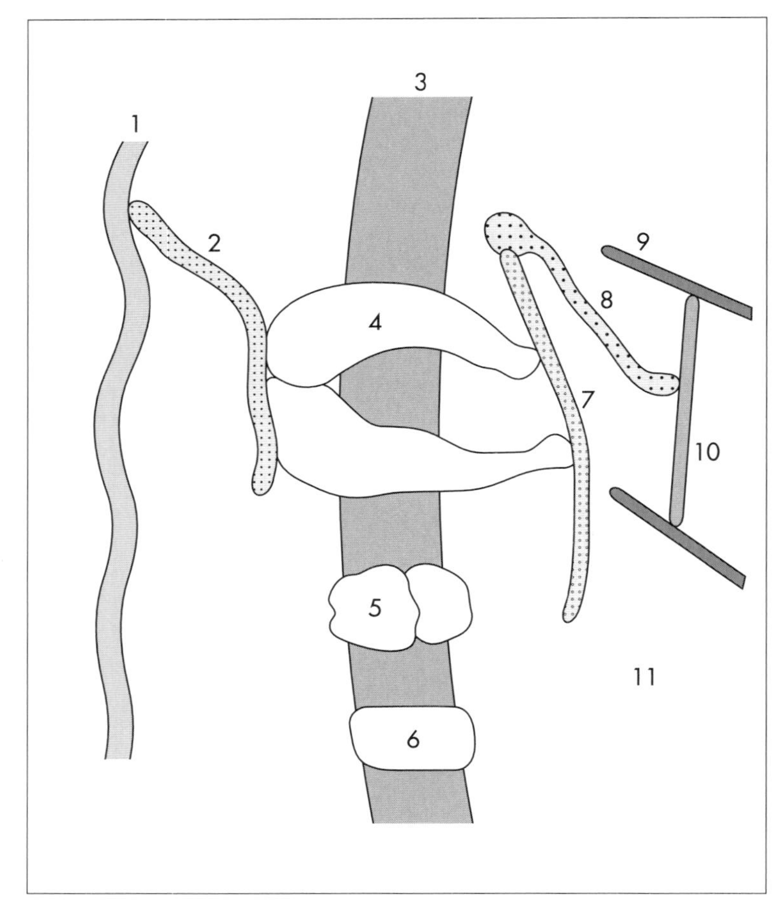

Fig. 12.1 Diagrammatic presentation of some of the cellular and extracellular components associated with cell contact to ECM and its response to physicochemical stimuli. 1 – collagen fibre in the ECM; 2 – fibronectin; 3 – plasma membrane; 4 – integrin; 5 – receptor complex; 6 – ion channel; 7 – talin; 8 – vinculin; 9 – F-actin; 10 – α-actinin; 11 – cytoplasm.

Alterations in the shape of cells or ECM can cause profound changes in the attachment mechanism and cellular phenotypic expression. In mammary epithelium, cell rounding is usually associated with inhibition of cell growth and promotion of cytodifferentiation (Emerman and Pitelka, 1977). Hence, cells that assume a round shape may expose specific parts of their genome and become more sensitive to certain external stimuli.

MECHANOSENSITIVE ION CHANNELS

There is strong evidence that most cells have ion channels capable of regulating cellular mechanics. These channels appear to be mechanosensitive (Morris, 1990), as their open state probably depends on stress at the plasma membrane. Such channels were postulated long ago as a means of mechanoelectrical transduction in nerve and muscle cells. However, it is evident that most other cell types have such channel components in their membranes. These channels are ubiquitous: they are found in every cell at a uniform density of the order of 1 per mm^2 (Brezden *et al.*, 1986; Moody and Bosma, 1989; Sachs, 1988). Calcium ions may enter cells in significant amounts through these channels (Christensen, 1987, Cooper *et al.*, 1986; Lansman *et al.*, 1987). Tensions generated in patch electrodes to activate stretch sensitive channels are of the same order of magnitude as those recorded in migrating fibroblasts (Harris *et al.*, 1980; Morris and Sigurdson, 1989).

FORCE-CELL FUNCTION INTERACTIONS THROUGH THE EXTRACELLULAR MATRIX

Tension in the cellular plasma membrane can be generated by contraction of cytoskeletal elements, intracellular osmotic changes, or alterations in the physical state of the ECM. Ingber and Jamieson (1985) constructed three-dimensional cell models consisting of a discontinuous array of compression-resistant struts, pulled open by connection with tension elements. The stability of such a structure depends on maintenance of tensional integrity. Based on these models, and cellular behaviour *in vitro*, it was concluded that important functions are regulated by the integrity and composition of the ECM, which can connect with the cell nucleus through the continuous system of cytoskeletal filaments and plasma membrane receptors. Hence, physical forces generated by the cytoskeleton or the ECM can be important regulators of cell and tissue growth. Such interactions between force and cell function have been reported to occur in lymphocytes, myotubes, endothelial cells (Davies and Tripathi, 1993), osteoblasts and osteocytes, and arterial smooth muscle cells (Leung *et al.*, 1976).

The mechanism of mechanochemical stimuli is likely transduced into chemical information through local changes in thermodynamic parameters (Ingber and Jamieson, 1985), where activation energy of a reaction is produced by pressure and volume alterations, and chemical reactions and macromolecular polymerization processes can be selectively promoted or inhibited as a result of mechanical perturbation of the cell surface. In neurites, cytoskeletal polymerization can be modulated by mechanical forces applied to the cell surface (Joshi *et al.*, 1985). Similar changes can be caused by interactions of cells with growth factors. For example, alterations in the distribution of actin and vinculin occur in fibroblasts in response to exposure to platelet-derived growth factor (PDGF) (Herman and Pledger, 1985; Hedberg *et al.*, 1993). Treatment of mouse osteoblasts with transforming growth factor β (TGF-β) increases DNA synthesis and cell respreading, in association with increased polymerization of actin, a-actinin, and tubulin (Lomri and Marie, 1990). Likewise, the arrangement and function of steroid hormone receptors may be very sensitive to mechanical perturbation because they are associated physically with the nuclear protein matrix (Barrak and Coffey, 1982).

It is, therefore, evident that mechanical forces can affect cellular function by either deforming the cells or the ECM, leading to polymerization of cytoskeletal elements and modification of receptor availability. However, force application to teeth can also evoke electric potentials in the strained tissues (Cochran *et al.*, 1967; Zengo *et al.*, 1973, 1974), and these potentials can activate cells by altering their membrane potential. The origin of this piezoelectric potential appears to be the collagen portion of the ECM (Marino and Becker, 1971).

BIOELECTRIC SIGNALS IN MECHANICALLY STRESSED TISSUES

The bendability of the alveolar bone during orthodontic tooth movement was first suggested by Farrar (1888), and later confirmed in rats (Baumrind, 1969) and humans (Grimm, 1972). A mechanism by which force-evoked electric potentials may reach the surface of bone cells was proposed by Pollack *et al.* (1984). According to this hypothesis, bone is surrounded by an electric double layer in which electric charges flow in coordination with stress-related fluid flow. This stress-generated potential may affect the charge of cell membranes, as well as that of macromolecules in their neighborhood. Endogenous ionic currents are evoked in intact and damaged mouse bones (Borgens, 1984). These currents can probably be attributed to streaming potentials rather than to piezoelectricity, owing to their long decay period, suggesting that in mechanically stressed bone the source of current is cells rather than matrix.

Measurements of electric potentials in dog alveolar bone *in vivo* and *in vitro* (Zengo *et al.*, 1973, 1974) have demonstrated that the concave (compressed) side of the orthodontically treated bone is electronegative with respect to the convex (tension) side, suggesting that negative potentials during bone bending can facilitate osteogenesis, while positive potentials will cause bone resorption. However, measurements in fracture sites (Borgens, 1984) did not disclose such a correlation, but rather showed that as current enters the lesion its dispersion (pathway and density) is unpredictable, owing to the complexity of the distribution of the mineralized and non-mineralized matrices.

OPTIMAL LOADS FOR OSTEOGENIC RESPONSE AND THEIR TARGET CELLS

While it is evident that bone cells are sensitive to applied mechanical loads, it is unclear what are the optimal magnitudes, frequencies, and durations of such loads. Experimenting *in vivo* with turkey and rooster ulnas, Lanyon *et al.* (1982), Lanyon and Rubin (1984), Lanyon (1987), Rubin and Lanyon (1985), and Skerry *et al.* (1990) freed the bones from muscle attachments without severing the nervous and vascular supplies. Mechanical loads were applied to the bones by inserting metallic pins at the ends of the bones and attaching the pins to an external loading apparatus. Bone mass was gradually lost after this procedure, but the loss was prevented by 4 cycles per day of 10,000–12,000 μ-strain, 0.5 Hz, for 42 days. When the number of cycles was increased to 36 per day, bone formation increased significantly. Continuous (static) loads had no effect on bone remodelling, whereas similar loads applied intermittently for a total of a few minutes daily increased bone mass substantially (Lanyon and Rubin, 1984). The magnitude of strain in the loaded bone seems to be directly associated with the nature and degree of the remodeling response. Peak longitudinal strains below 0.001 are associated with bone loss, whereas peak strains above this level are related to marked enhancement of periosteal and endosteal bone formation (Rubin and Lanyon, 1985). To achieve a maximal osteogenic response, only 72 seconds of load bearing per day were required.

Based on the above observations, it was hypothesized that the most likely candidate cell to sense the distribution, rate of change, and magnitude of strain in the bone matrix is the osteocyte (Lanyon, 1987). The important feature of strain is its unusual distribution rather than merely a large magnitude. Osteocytes apparently respond not only to the transient effects of mechanical strain, but also to the persistent effects on the matrix. The ECM molecule most likely to be sensitive to strain is proteoglycan (Skerry *et al.*, 1990), a large, highly charged structure, which may be induced by strain to attach to cell surface receptors or cytoskeletal components. Since proteoglycan reorientation lasts 1–2 days, it can provide a physical basis for 'strain memory' in bone. Hence, this model proposes that mechanical loads distort bone ECM, and that the resulting deformation persists, affecting osteocytes, which are the prime targets for the applied load. Bone surface cells, mainly osteoblasts, are activated through cell–cell communications with adjacent osteocytes.

Extrapolated into an orthodontic situation, the above hypothesis may imply that mechanical forces should not be applied to teeth continuously, but rather for short periods of time and intermittently. An experiment in rats, to test this hypothesis, was conducted by Gibson *et al.* (1992). Rats whose molars were subjected to only 1 hour of force application demonstrated continuous tooth movement for 2 weeks. These results demonstrate that the ECM of the alveolar bone PDL complex behaves in a manner similar to that proposed by Lanyon and his associates. Clinically, this observation implies that remodelling of paradental tissues can be evoked by force applications of very short durations.

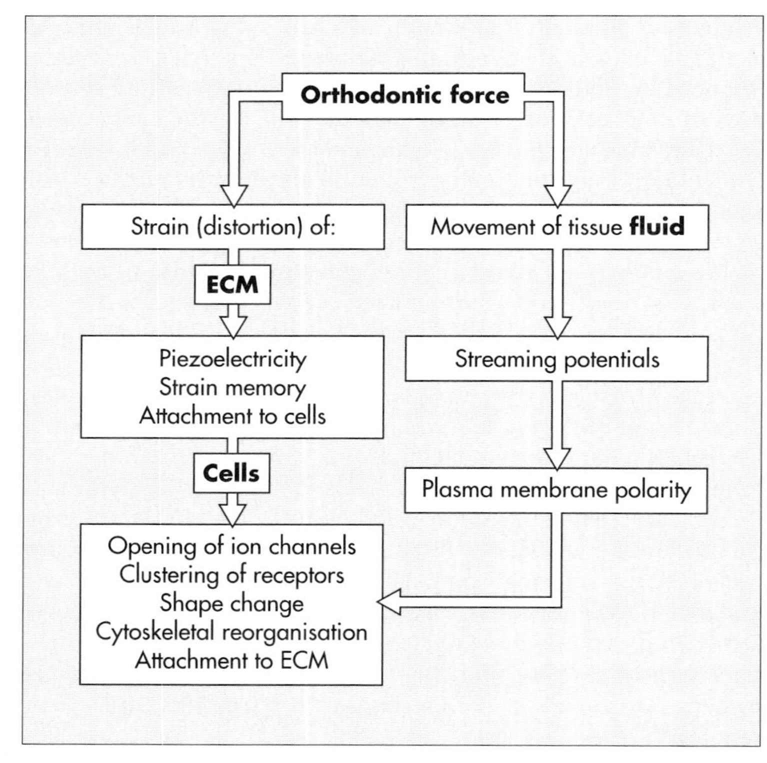

Fig. 12.2 A schematic outline of the general effects of orthodontic forces on paradental tissues. Initially, the applied force causes movement of tissue fluids, which allows development of strain (distortion) of ECM and cells. Bioelectric phenomena occur, owing to the motion of fluid ions and charged macromolecules, and the developing strains in cells and ECM. In cells, shape changes are associated with opening of ion channels, relocation of receptors, reorganization of cytoskeletal elements, and changes in the attachment (anchorage) status between cells and ECM.

In summary, the initial physical outcome of mechanical force application to teeth is gradual distortion of the PDL, alveolar bone, and gingival tissues. Both ECM and cells are strained as fluids are caused to move (*Fig. 12.2*). Bone strains persist for 24–48 hours, owing to slow reorientation of proteoglycans, maintaining a strained environment in the vicinity of the enclosed cells. The motion of the extracellular fluids may approximate ions and charged macromolecules to the cell surface, causing electrophysical interactions, changes in plasma membrane polarity, and ion movement through membrane channels. Most alveolar bone and PDL cells are anchorage dependent – hence the distortion of the ECM alters their shape. This shape change signifies introduction of strains to the cytoskeletal system, thereby transmitting physical signals from the ECM directly to the nucleus, evoking responses by each major component of the cellular unit – the plasma membrane, the cytoplasm, and the nucleus.

In the plasma membrane, mechanosensitive ion channels are activated by mechanical perturbations, facilitating temporal fluxes of ions such as Ca^{2+} and K^{+}, leading to enzymatic activation which results in elevation of the cellular IP_3, PGE_2 synthesis, and cytoplasmic cAMP and cGMP.

EFFECTS OF TISSUE DISTORTION ON THE SYNTHESIS AND RELEASE OF SIGNAL MOLECULES

NEUROTRANSMITTERS

Beyond this general scheme of cell stimulation by mechanical perturbations lies the realization that following the initial activation stage is the response stage, which may vary widely according to the cell type. As the ECM fluids in the mechanically stressed PDL shift, sensory nerve endings in the PDL release their contents, which include vasoactive neuropeptides such as substance P (SP) (Nicolay *et al.*, 1990), vasoactive intestinal polypeptide (VIP) (Davidovitch *et al.*, 1988), and calcitonin gene-related peptide (CGRP) (Kvinnsland and Kvinnsland, 1990; Davidovitch, 1991). Localization of these molecules in dental and paradental tissues is facilitated by immunohistochemistry.

Increased immunoreactivity for SP in the PDL in the early phases of orthodontic treatment is demonstrated in *Figs 12.3, 12.4*. The effects of SP in peripheral tissues include vasodilation and increased capillary permeability. These effects may contribute to the plasma extravasation and increased local blood flow that accompany inflammation. SP has been identified as a stimulator of bone resorption, particularly in arthritis (Levine *et al.*, 1984; Lotz *et al.*, 1987). Injection of interleukin-1α (IL-1α) into rabbit knees (O'Byrne *et al.*, 1990) caused increases of SP and PGE_2 in joint fluids at 4 hours, 24 hours, and 48 hours. In the rat PDL, SP-containing nerves were localized along blood vessels, primarily in the middle and apical regions (Wakisaka *et al.*, 1985). In cats, SP is distributed sparsely in the PDL, but during tooth movement its immunoreactivity is markedly intensified in nerve fibres, as well as in PDL fibroblasts and alveolar bone osteoblasts, suggesting that these cells are capable of binding SP that has been released from nerve endings (Nicolay *et al.*, 1990). Moreover, administration of SP to human PDL fibroblasts *in vitro* significantly increased the concentration of cAMP in the cells and of PGE_2 in the medium within 1 minute (Davidovitch *et al.*, 1988).

During orthodontic tooth movement in cats, intense staining for VIP was localized in the compressed PDL near sites of bone resorption and in the pulp of moving teeth (Motakef *et al.*, 1990). This peptide of 28 amino acids (first isolated from porcine duodenum – Said and Mutt, 1970) was found to be a potent stimulator of bone resorption *in vitro*, in a mechanism independent of PGE_2 (Hohmann *et al.*, 1983). It is localized in periosteal nerve fibres of porcine rib, tibia, and vertebra (Hohmann *et al.*, 1986), and is also localized in the mouse PDL, mainly around blood vessels in the apical segment (Harness, 1989). High-affinity receptors for VIP were found in binding studies on human osteosarcoma cells (Hohmann and Tashjian, 1984).

Another neurotransmitter that may be an important regulator of paradental tissue remodelling during orthodontic tooth movement is CGRP, which seems to coexist with SP in small- to medium-diameter sensory ganglion neurons (Rosenfeld *et al.*, 1983). In cats, local intra-arterial infusion of SP or CGRP caused a concentration-dependent increase in nasal blood flow (Stjärne *et al.*, 1989). In the cat pulp, CGRP-like immunoreactivity was observed in nerves along blood vessels as well as in the subodontoblastic zone (Wakisaka *et al.*, 1987). It was also localized in the mouse PDL (Kata *et al.*, 1990) and the rat mandibular periosteum (Hill and Elde, 1988). Intra-arterial infusion of CGRP and SP in the cat dental pulp produced vasodilation, which was 10 times greater when CGRP was administered after SP than before it (Gazelius *et al.*, 1987).

During tooth movement in rats, Kvinnsland and Kvinnsland (1990) localized CGRP in the dental pulp and PDL. In untreated teeth, CGRP was found in nerves surrounding blood vessels. After 5 days of molar movement, CGRP immunoreactivity intensified, especially in PDL tension sites, where fibroblasts appeared to contain this neuropeptide. A similar pattern of increased cellular staining for CGRP was observed in cats following orthodontic force application to maxillary canines for 1 h, 2 days, 7 days, and 28 days (Okamoto *et al.*, 1991). After 1 hour of treatment, CGRP immunoreactivity was intensified at PDL tension sites (*Figs 12.5, 12.6*), but it was especially intense after 28 days in compressed PDL adjacent to areas of necrosis.

Hence, neurotransmitters such as SP, VIP, and CGRP may play a dual role in the mechanically stressed PDL. On the one hand, these signal molecules may act upon capillary endothelial cells, promoting vasodilation, and facilitating migration of leucocytes out of the capillaries into the extravascular space. On the other hand, diffusion of these neuropeptides in the PDL after their release from sensory nerve endings may introduce them to specific receptors on various cell types in the PDL, thereby contributing to the regulation of their activities.

CYTOKINES

Introduction of leucocytes into the PDL during the early stages of orthodontic treatment was noted by Rygh and Selvig (1973), by Rygh (1974), and by Storey (1973). The significance of this finding exceeds by far the early observation that cells of the immune system participate actively in phagocytosing necrotic tissues in compressed zones of the PDL. In fact, these cells are not only active removers of tissues altered by pathological conditions, but most importantly they are producers of numerous signal molecules that perform a myriad of functions (from chemoattraction to stimulation of mitogenesis and cytodifferentiation).

The products of these cells may be classified in different categories, such as cytokines, growth factors, colony stimulating factors, and cell adhesion molecules. Each of these ligands may act as an autocrine, as well as a paracrine, in causing activation of target cells. However, monocytes, macrophages, and T and B lymphocytes are not the only producers of these molecules. Osteoblasts, fibroblasts, epithelial cells, endothelial cells, and platelets have all been found to be capable of synthesizing and secreting many of these factors, thus adding to the complexity of the overall scheme of cell-mediated remodelling of the mechanically stressed periodontium. Confounding this complexity is evidence that immune cells bind neurotransmitters (Lotz *et al.*, 1988; Laurenzi *et al.*, 1989; Hafström *et al.*, 1989; Roscetti *et al.*, 1988; Marotti *et al.*, 1990), while cells of the nervous system respond to products of immune cells (Fagarasan *et al.*, 1990; Fagarasan and Axelrod, 1990).

Cytokines were once thought to be signal molecules produced exclusively by leucocytes. However, cytokine-like molecules were later discovered to be synthesized by many cell types, including osteoblasts, fibroblasts, endothelial cells, and nerve cells, and to function as autocrines and paracrines. Cytokines that were found to affect bone metabolism are interleukin 1 (IL-1), interleukin 2 (IL-2), interleukin 3 (IL-3), interleukin 6 (IL-6), tumor necrosis factor α (TNF-α), and gamma interferon (IFN-γ). The most potent stimulator of bone resorption *in vitro* among these cytokines is IL-1. Secretion of IL-1 is triggered by various stimuli, including other cytokines, bacterial products, neurotransmitters, and mechanical forces. IL-1 has two forms, α and β, which are coded by different genes, but which have similar biological actions, systemically and locally – they attract leucocytes, stimulate fibroblasts and endothelial cells to proliferate, and enhance bone resorption (Gowen *et al.*, 1985; Boyce *et al.*, 1989; Sabatini *et al.*, 1988; Feige *et al.*, 1989).

Osteoblasts are apparently the target cells for IL-1 in bone (Thomson *et al.*, 1986), conveying a message to osteoclasts to

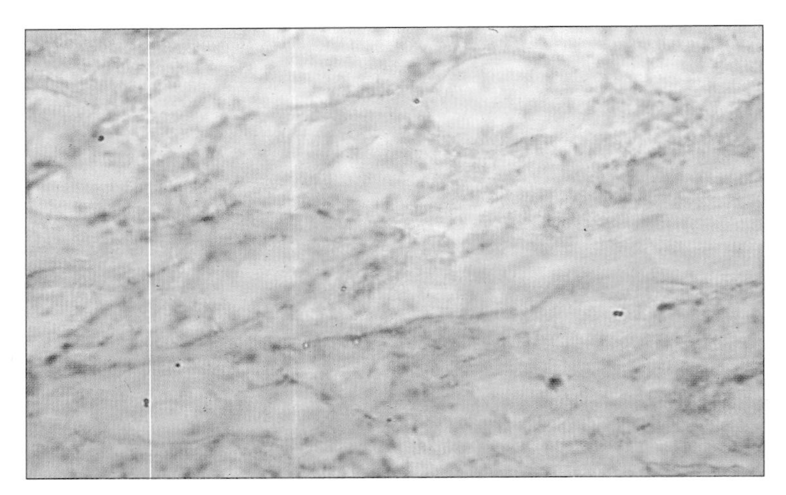

Fig. 12.3 SP immunoreactivity in unstressed cat maxillary canine PDL. Faint brown diaminobenzidine (DAB) deposits depict SP localization. (Magnfication × 1480.)

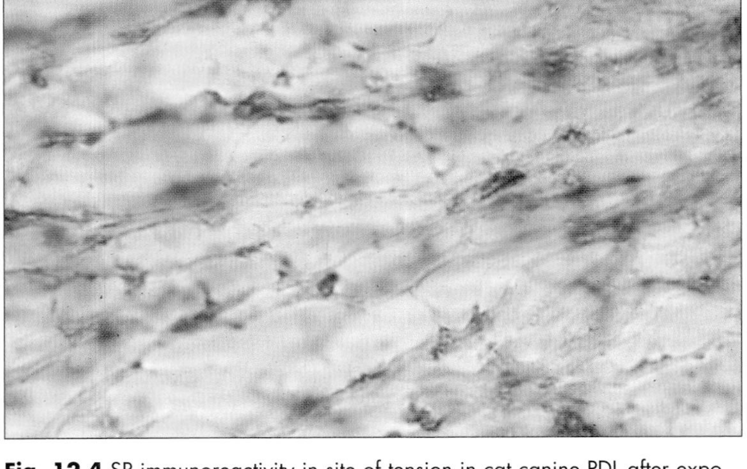

Fig. 12.4 SP immunoreactivity in site of tension in cat canine PDL after exposure to 12 hours of distal moving force of 80 g. Dark DAB deposits suggest a marked increase of SP bound to cells and ECM. (Magnification × 1480.)

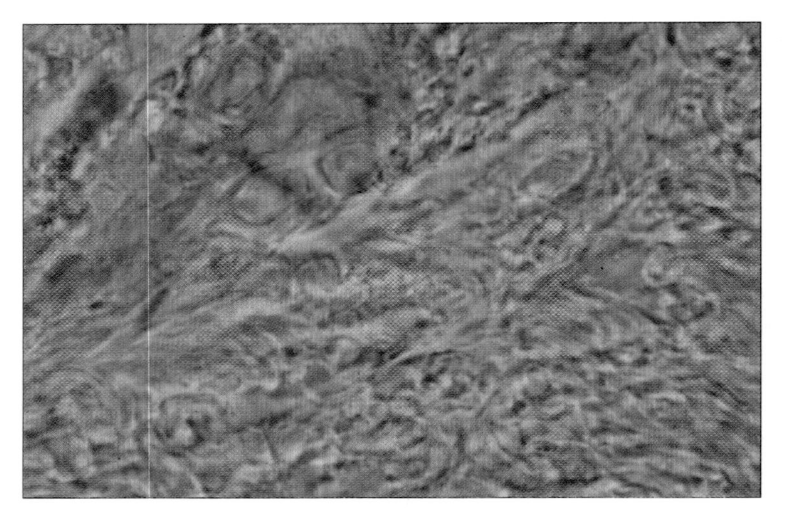

Fig. 12.5 CGRP immunoreactivity in unstressed cat maxillary canine PDL. Light brown DAB deposits are seen over PDL cells. (Magnification × 1480.)

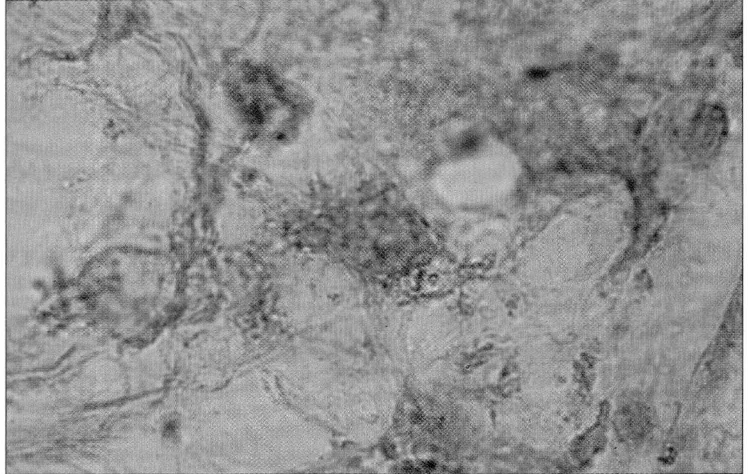

Fig. 12.6 CGRP immunoreactivity in site of tension in cat canine PDL after 1 hour exposure to an 80 g distal driving force. DAB deposits over PDL cells are darker than in *Fig. 12.5*, suggesting enhanced binding of CGRP by PDL cells. (Magnification × 1480.)

resorb bone. When fetal rat long bones were incubated with IL-1a or IL-1β and with PTH, a synergistic effect on ^{45}Ca release was recorded when both cytokine and hormone were introduced simultaneously. Minimal amounts of these agents were required for causing this synergistic effect. Human PDL *in vitro* fibroblasts apparently react similarly to exposure to cytokines. When incubated with graded doses of IL-1α, IL-1β, TNF-α, and IFN-g for 15, 30, and 60 minutes or for 2, 4, 24, 48, and 72 hours, the cells responded with dose- and time-related increases in the levels of PGE and cAMP (Saito *et al.*, 1990a). When added to the cell-containing media simultaneously, the effects of these cytokines varied in degree, depending on the particular combinations of cytokines (Saito *et al.*, 1990b). In this case, the administration of cytokine combinations was found to be additive, synergistic, subtractive, or inhibitory on the production of PGE, depending on the length of incubation time. For example, 24 hours after the simultaneous administration of IL-1β and TNF-α, the level of PGE in the medium increased synergistically, but at 72 hours it was lower than that produced by control cells. In most cases, the addition of IFN-γ with IL-1 or TNF-α reduced the level of PGE in the medium.

When human PDL fibroblasts were stretched *in vitro* by the use of convex templates for 2–60 minutes, significant elevations occurred in PGE and cAMP within 15 minutes, and the addition of IL-1β caused synergistic, additive, or even subtractive effects, depending on the length of the incubation period (Ngan *et al.*, 1990). Conditioned media derived from PDL cells stimulated by mechanical stress in the presence of IL-1β caused significantly more bone resorption than conditioned media obtained from cells that had been treated by either factor alone (Saito *et al.*, 1991).

During orthodontic tooth movement in cats, immunoreactivity for IL-1β is markedly intensified in areas of PDL tension (*Figs 12.7, 12.8, 12.9, 12.10*), but especially in sites of PDL compression (*Fig 12.11*). In the latter sites, necrotic PDL zones are surrounded by

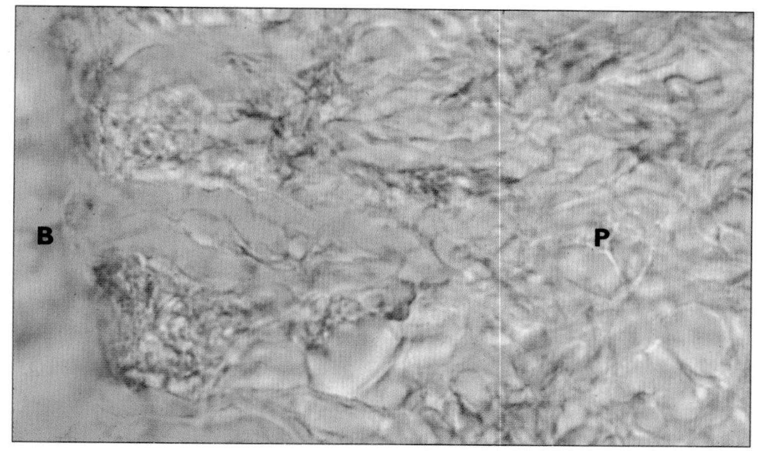

Fig. 12.7 IL-1β immunoreactivity in stressed PDL and alveolar bone of cat maxillary canine. B – alveolar bone; P – periodontal ligament. Note the light brown DAB deposits over osteoblasts and adjacent PDL cells. (Magnification × 1480.)

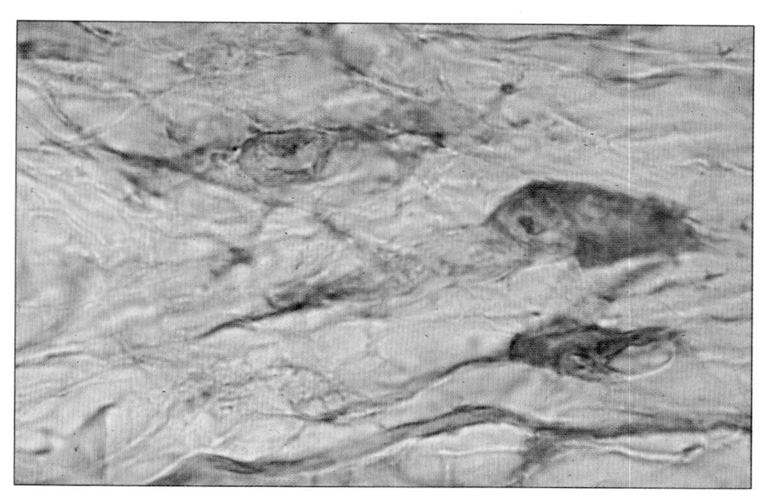

Fig. 12.8 IL-1β immunoreactivity in PDL tension site mesial to cat maxillary canine after 3 hours of orthodontic treatment. Dark brown DAB deposits over PDL cells suggest increased 1L-1β content. (Magnification × 1480.)

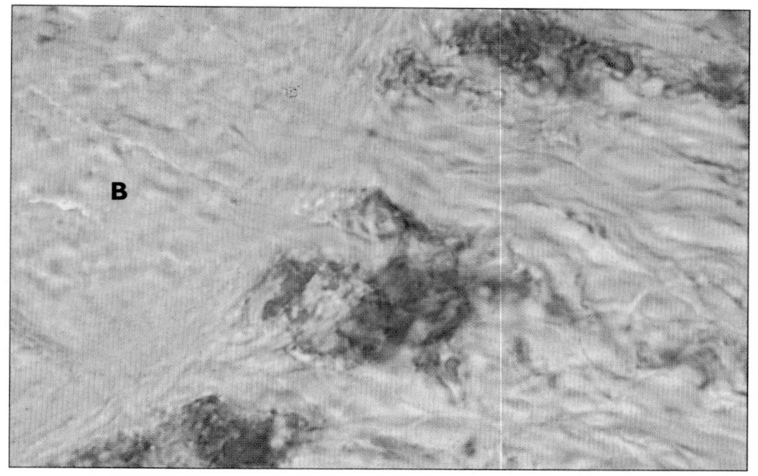

Fig. 12.9 IL-1β immunoreactivity in alveolar bone osteoblasts in PDL tension site after 14 days of orthodontic treatment. B – alveolar bone. Dark brown DAB deposits over osteoblasts. (Magnification × 1480.)

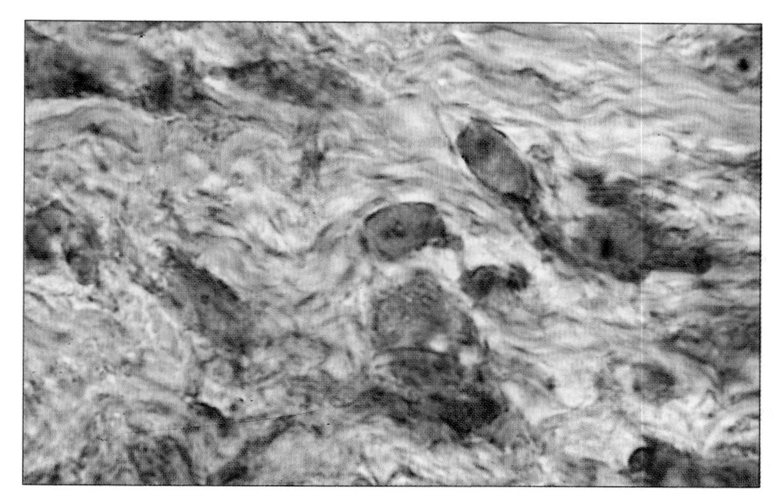

Fig. 12.10 IL-1β immunoreactivity in PDL tension site mesial to cat maxillary canine after 14 days of orthodontic treatment. Dark brown deposits are seen over PDL cells. (Magnification × 1480.)

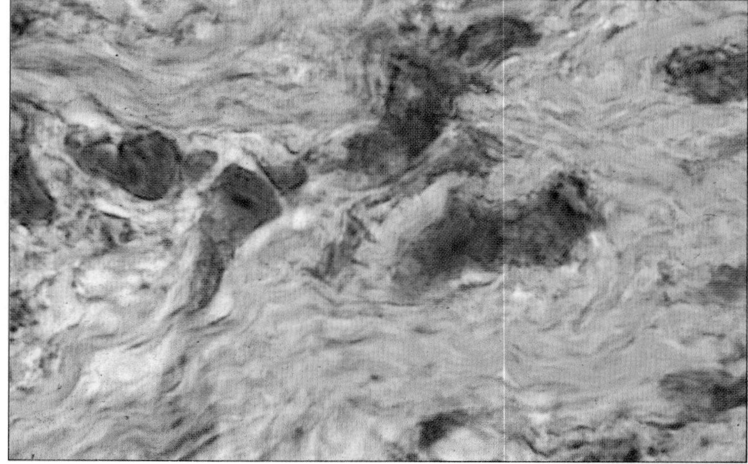

Fig. 12.11 IL-1β immunoreactivity in PDL compression site distal to cat maxillary canine after 14 days of orthodontic treatment. PDL cells in the zone bordering the necrotic compressed PDL are stained intensely for IL-1b (dark brown DAB deposits). (Magnification × 1480.)

multiple mononucleated cells, probably a mixture of macrophages or fibroblasts, and these cells stain particularly darkly for IL-1β (see *Fig. 12.11*). Alveolar bone marrow cells usually stain mildly for this cytokine, but near orthodontically treated teeth this cell population displays a marked increase of staining intensity (*Figs 12.12, 12.13*). Likewise, PDL cells and alveolar bone osteoblasts display intense staining for TNF-α during orthodontic force application to teeth, both in areas of PDL tension and in areas of PDL compression (*Figs 12.14, 12.15, 12.16*). This 17 kDa molecule is synthesized mainly by monocytes and macrophages, and is a major participant in inflammation. It stimulates endothelial cells to secrete IL-1 (Bevilacqua *et al.*, 1986) and increases their adhesion to leucocytes (Gamble *et al.*, 1985). In terms of enhancement of bone resorption *in vitro*, IL-1 is much more potent that TNF-α (Stashenko *et al.*, 1987) but suboptimal concentrations of IL-1 in combination with suboptimal concentrations of TNF-a, synergistically stimulate the formation of osteoclast-like cells from human marrow cells (Pfeilschifer *et al.*, 1989).

In contrast to IL-1 and TNF-α, which enhance bone resorption *in vivo* and *in vitro*, IFN-γ was found to interfere with this process. This cytokine is a lymphocytic product that antagonizes the effects of other cytokines and growth factors. It was found to abolish completely the resorptive effects of IL-1 and TNF-α in mouse calvaria, but not those of PTH or vitamin D_3 (Gowen *et al.*, 1986). Human osteoblast-like cells are stimulated by TNF-α to proliferate and to produce PGE_2, while their alkaline phosphatase activity and osteocalcin release are inhibited. However, the effects of IFN-γ on this cell population is exactly the opposite (Gowen *et al.*, 1988). In general, IFN-γ is believed to limit inflammation and to favour tissue repair. Melin *et al.* (1989) reported that it stimulates proliferation of human dental pulp fibroblasts, while inhibiting synthesis of types I and III collagen and of fibronectin. During tooth movement in cats, very faint IFN-γ immunoreactivity was found in unstressed PDL fibroblasts, while intense straining was observed in cells in compressed PDL, near sites of bone resorption (*Figs 12.17, 12.18*). Here, IFN-γ may promote fusion of osteoclast progenitor cells (Vignery *et al.*, 1990) while modulating the effects of resorption-promoting cytokines on these cells.

GROWTH FACTORS

Among the most abundant growth factors in bone is transforming growth factor β (TGF-β). This small polypeptide is produced by several cell types, including fibroblasts and osteoblasts. It is deposited in the ECM in a latent form, and is activated by proteases as a 25 kDa peptide of 112 amino acids (TGF-β1). There are several isoforms of TGF-β, and the subunits of these isoforms share a high degree of homology with those of TGF-β1 (TGF-β2–5). The richest source of TGF-β are platelets and bone (Assoian *et al.*, 1983; Seyedin *et al.*, 1985). It attracts monocytes and fibroblasts, and stimulates angiogenesis *in vitro* (Merwin *et al.*, 1990). Receptors for TGF-β1 are ubiquitous (Wakefield *et al.*, 1987), emphasizing its potential significance as a regulatory molecule. In a normal response to injury, platelet aggregation and degranulation trigger the release of numerous inflammatory mediators, including TGFβ from the a granules (Assoian *et al.*, 1983). At the onset of inflammation, TGF-β may provide a potent chemotactic ligand for peripheral blood monocytes (Wahl *et al.*, 1987). Monocytes exposed to TGF-β *in vitro* show augmented gene expression for IL-1, TNF-α, and other growth factors (Wahl *et al.*, 1987; Wiseman *et al.*, 1988; Chantry *et al.*, 1988). In tissue repair, TGF-β is a potent attractant of fibroblasts and a regulator of their growth (Postlethwaite *et al.*, 1987). It also upregulates transcription and translation of matrix components such as types I, III, and V collagen, and fibronectin (Ignoz and Massague, 1986; Raghow *et al.*, 1987). Associated with the increased matrix synthesis is the ability of TGF-β to decrease secretion of matrix-specific proteases, while increasing the production of their inhibitors (Edwards *et al.*, 1987; Overall *et al.*, 1991).

Isoforms of TGF-β are abundant in bone matrix, mainly in their latent form (Centrella *et al.*, 1991). In osteoblast-rich cultures from fetal rats, TGF-β1, β2, and β3 increased DNA synthesis in low concentrations, but reduced it at higher levels (Centrella *et al.*, 1987; Ten Dijke *et al.*, 1990). All three isoforms also enhance synthesis of collagen and non-collagenous protein. TGF-β in bone cells also causes enhanced alkaline phosphatase activity, osteoblastic chemotaxis, and osteopontin levels. It stimulates osteoblast-like cells to produce PGE_2 (Marusic *et al.*, 1991), and this effect is increased synergistically in the presence of IL-2. Daily injections of TGF-β1 and TGF-β2 into the parietal periosteum of neonatal rats resulted in a two-fold increase in bone thickness (Noda and Camilliere, 1989). While promoting bone apposition, TGF-β inhibits rat bone resorption, and formation of osteoclast-like cells from human marrow cells (Chenu *et al.*, 1988; Pfeilschifter *et al.*, 1988). However, osteoclasts are capable of activating latent forms of TGF-β derived from bone (Oreffo *et al.*, 1989), and this activation is apparently performed at an acidic pH.

During orthodontic tooth movement in cats, both PDL cells and alveolar bone osteoblasts display enhanced TGF-β1 immunoreactivity (*Figs 12.19, 12.20, 12.21*). This enhancement is seen as early as 1 hour after the application of force to teeth, and it is widespread throughout the PDL. In contrast, unstressed paradental cells are usually devoid of staining for TGF-β1.

Other growth factors that may participate in regulating the activities of paradental cells during orthodontic tooth movement are platelet-derived growth factor (PDGF), fibroblast growth factors (FGF), and insulin-like growth factor (IGF). All have been found to affect endothelial cells, fibroblasts, and bone cells.

Of particular interest in this regard is PDGF, because mechanical damage is virtually always caused by orthodontic forces to the periodontal vasculature, resulting in migration of platelets into the extravascular space of the PDL (Rygh and Selvig, 1973; Storey, 1973). Each time an orthodontic appliance is reactivated, trauma is reintroduced to the PDL. Hence, platelets may be one of the most important cells governing the remodelling of the strained dental support tissues. Platelets are highly adaptive for haemostasis and wound healing. They contain and release adhesive proteins and proteases, enhance vascular permeability, alter vascular tone, and take up, store, or metabolize vasoactive substances (Packham *et al.*, 1968). Platelets provide a major source of growth factors for mesenchymal cells, particularly vascular cells, in the form of PDGF (Deuel and Huang, 1984). In addition, platelets interact with circulating leucocytes and with vascular endothelium to modulate inflammatory activities of phagocytes and of the vascular surface.

Originally, PDGF was isolated from platelets, but was subsequently found to be synthesized by various cell types (including those of bone). It is a 30 kDa dimer, the product of two genes, with resulting three isoforms. The PDGF A and B genes are expressed by normal and malignant cells, while bone cells seem to express exclusively the PDGF A gene (Graves *et al.*, 1989; Rydziel *et al.*, 1992). Wound healing is characterized by early migration into the injured area by platelets and leucocytes, followed by endothelial cells and fibroblasts. This migration is promoted by PDGF, which serves as a chemoattractant (Pierce *et al.*, 1991; Deuel and Kawahara, 1991) and which is a potent mitogen for mesenchymally derived cells (Ross *et al.*, 1974; Kohler and Lipton, 1974). Along with the expression of genes that mediate mitogenic signals, PDGF induces the transcription of genes that encode various cytokines, such as IL-6, TGF-β1, and M-CSF (Pierce *et al.* 1989a; Pierce *et al.*, 1989b; Cochran *et al.*, 1983; Kohase *et al.*, 1987; Rollins *et al.*, 1988).

In bone, as in other tissues, PDGF increases DNA synthesis, as well as collagen synthesis and degradation (Canalis *et al.*, 1989; Centrella *et al.*, 1989; Hanks *et al.*, 1986; Piché and Graves, 1989), perhaps by increasing production of collagenase by osteoblasts or by decreasing synthesis of collagenase inhibitors. However, there could be a direct effect of PDGF on cells capable of degrading bone matrix – incubation of peripheral blood monocytes with bone particles resulted in release of ^{45}Ca into the medium, and this was enhanced by PDGF in a dose-dependent manner (Lyndon Key *et al.*, 1983).

During orthodontic treatment, a process that extends over many months, PDGF may enter the PDL after each activation of the orthodontic appliance, as mechanical damage to capillaries occurs. As an agent that promotes tissue healing, it may act on PDL fibroblasts and endothelial cells, as well as on alveolar bone surface cells. During the healing periods, as platelets are depleted from the strained PDL, additional amounts of PDGF may be synthesized by cells of the PDL and alveolar bone, and may then act locally as autocrines or paracrines in concert with other signal molecules or ions.

Other growth factors that may function similarly in the PDL are FGF and IGF. FGF is mitogenic for most non-terminally differentiated cells of mesodermal and neuroectodermal origin. In addition to fibroblasts and endothelial cells, target cells include myoblasts, chondrocytes, and osteoblasts. Two forms of FGF were found, one in acidic pI (αFGF), the other in basic pI (βFGF). Within the context of inflammation, βFGF has an angiogenic potential. It is stored in the ECM, bound to heparin sulphate proteoglycan (Folkman *et al.*, 1988) and it is mobilized by plasminogen-activator-mediated proteolytic activity, or by heparanases and collagenases. Basic FGF can be released by endothelial cell cytosolic storage sites through physiological and pathological plasma membrane wounds (Muthukrishnan *et al.*, 1991), and it then promotes tissue repair. Since αFGF and βFGF lack a signal sequence, they are thought to be sequestered within the cells responsible for their synthesis and to be released only after damage to their plasma membrane. Bone cells are capable of synthesizing βFGF *in vitro* and of secreting it into their surrounding ECM, where it may act as an autocrine or a paracrine signal (Globus *et al.*, 1989). Treatment of rat bone marrow cells *in vitro* with bFGF caused an increase in DNA synthesis, alkaline phosphatase activity, and the formation of bone-like nodules (Noff *et al.*, 1989). However, in fetal rat long bones, αFGF increased the rate of resorption, as the target cells seemed to be osteoblasts (Shen *et al.*, 1989).

IGFs are a family of peptides that promote cell proliferation and differentiation and that have insulin-like metabolic effects. The two major forms of IGF, IGF-I (7.6 kDa) and IGF-II (7.4 kDa) are single chain peptides, with 65 per cent homology. The production of IGF-I is regulated by factors such as growth hormone, oestrogen, and insulin, and also by fasting. Serum IGF-I is low in the neonatal period, rises to peak values during puberty, then slowly declines with ageing (Hall and Sara, 1983). The liver is the main organ producing IGF-I in humans and rodents. In bone, a variety of systemic and local factors regulate the action of IGF-I. These factors include growth hormone, PTH, vitamin D_3, corticosteroids, TGF-β1, IL-1, and PGF_{2a}. In mouse osteoblast-like cultures, both IGF-I and and IGF-II increased c-fos mRNA levels 25–28-fold in 15–30 minutes (Merriman *et al.*, 1990). Rat calvaria secrete detectable amounts of IGF-II, and this secretion can be reduced significantly by cortisol and bFGF (Canalis *et al.*, 1991). In newborn lambs, a single intravenous injection of IGF-II caused a rapid and sustained increase of serum osteocalcin, indicating a direct stimulation of osteoblastic function (Coxam *et al.*, 1992). When IGF-I was added to PDL cells in culture, it caused a dose-related increase in DNA synthesis (Blom *et al.*, 1992).

COLONY STIMULATING FACTORS

Orthodontic tooth movement is facilitated by removal by osteoclasts of alveolar bone in sites of PDL compression. These multinucleated cells are formed by fusion of progenitor cells that enter the PDL through the vascular system, or that migrate into it from adjacent alveolar bone marrow spaces through channels connecting these non-mineralized entities. Colony stimulating

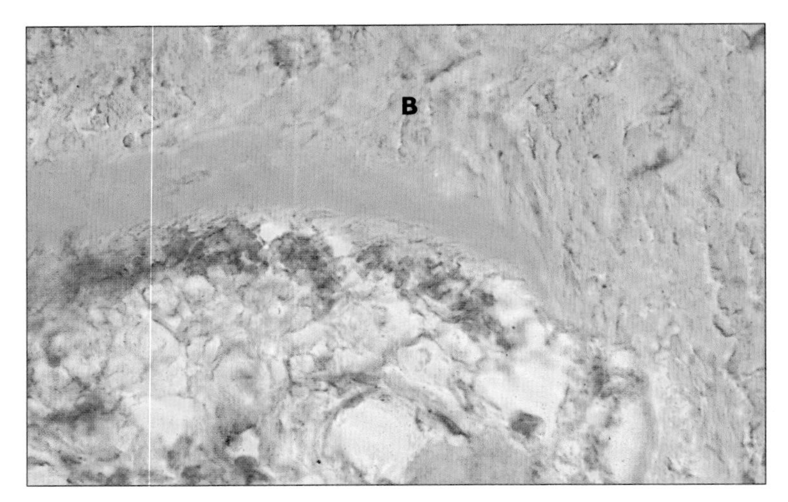

Fig. 12.12 IL-1β immunoreactivity in cat alveolar bone (B) marrow cells near unstressed maxillary canine. Light brown DAB deposits over marrow cells and endosteal osteoblasts. (Magnification × 660.)

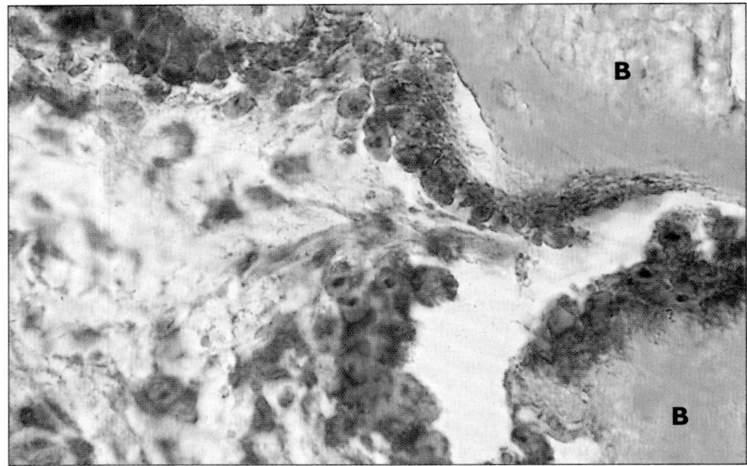

Fig. 12.13 IL-1β immunoreactivity in cat alveolar bone (B) marrow cells distal to maxillary canine after 14 days of orthodontic treatment. This marrow cavity is localized adjacent to a zone of necrotic, compressed PDL. The endosteal osteoblasts and many marrow cells display dark DAB deposits, suggesting increased IL-1β content. (Magnification × 660.)

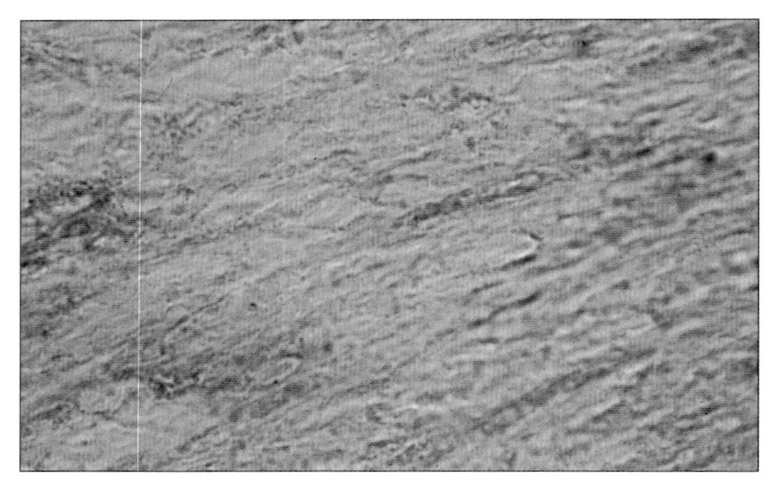

Fig. 12.14 TNF-α immureactivity in unstressed cat maxillary canine PDL. Light brown DAB deposits are seen over PDL cells. (Magnification × 1480.)

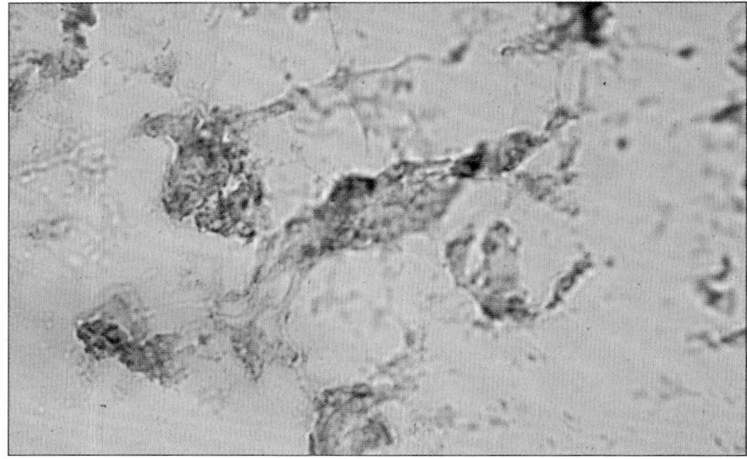

Fig. 12.15 TNF-α immunoreactivity in PDL compression site distal to cat maxillary canine after 56 days of orthodontic treatment. Dark brown DAB deposits cover cells that appear to be invading the compressed, necrotic PDL zone. (Magnification × 1480.)

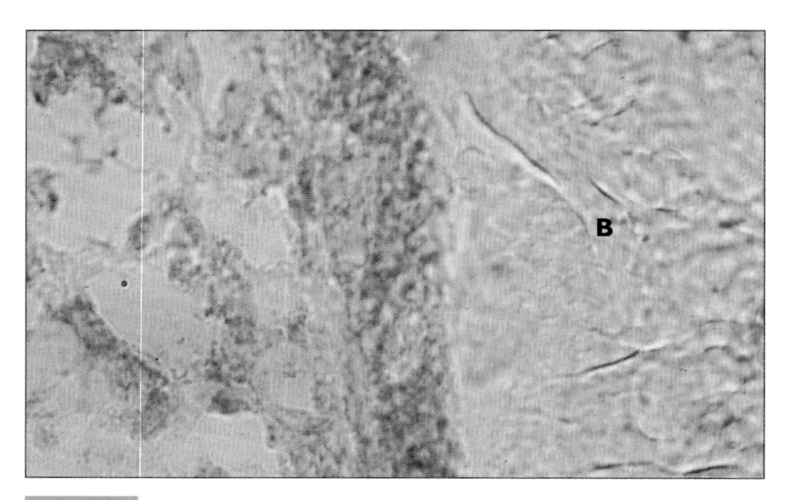

Fig. 12.16 IL-α immunoreactivity in alveolar bone (B) osteoblasts at a site of PDL compression after 56 days of force-induced distal movement of a cat maxillary canine. The osteoblasts stain mildly for TNF-α, as do adjacent PDL cells. (Magnification × 1480.)

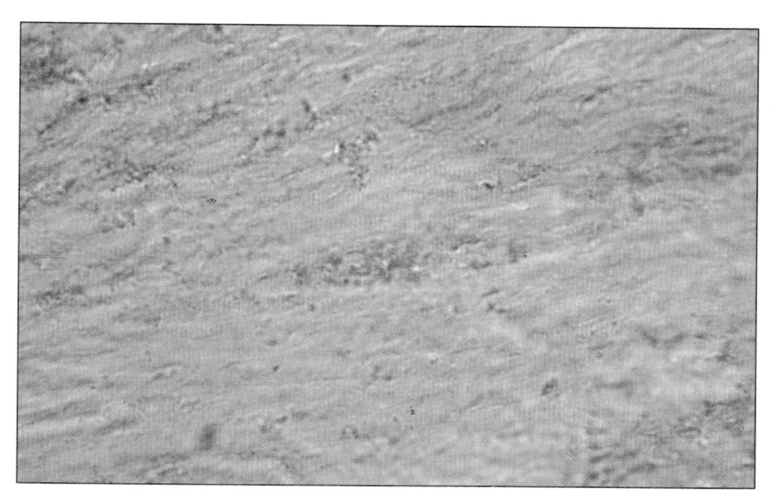

Fig. 12.17 IFN-γ immunoreactivity in unstressed maxillary canine PDL. Very light brown DAB deposits cover PDL cells. (Magnification × 1480.)

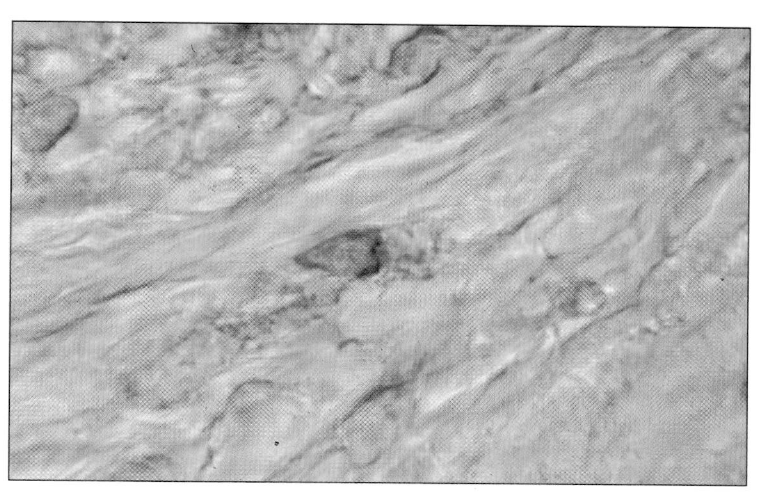

Fig. 12.18 IFN-γ immunoreactivity in PDL compression site distal to cat maxillary canine after 48 hours of orthodontic treatment. Distinct brown DAB deposits are seen over PDL cells at the edge of the necrotic, compressed PDL. (Magnification × 1480.)

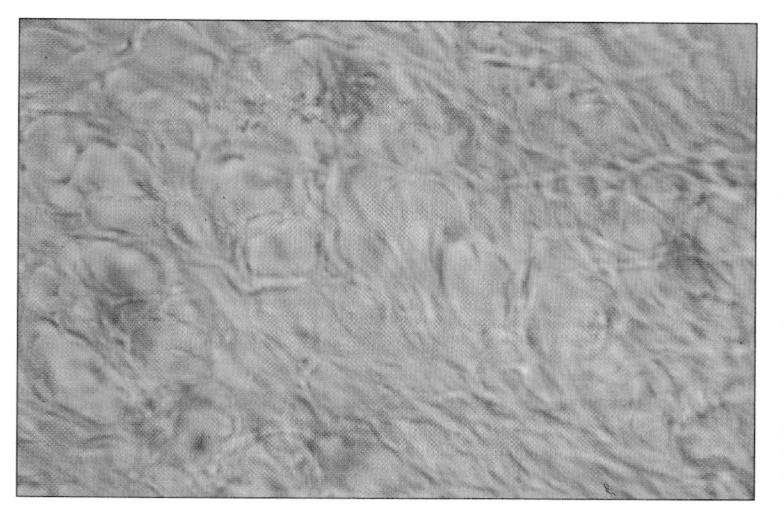

Fig. 12.19 TGF-β1 immunoreactivity in unstressed cat maxillary canine PDL. Light brown DAB deposits are seen over PDL cells. (Magnification × 1480.)

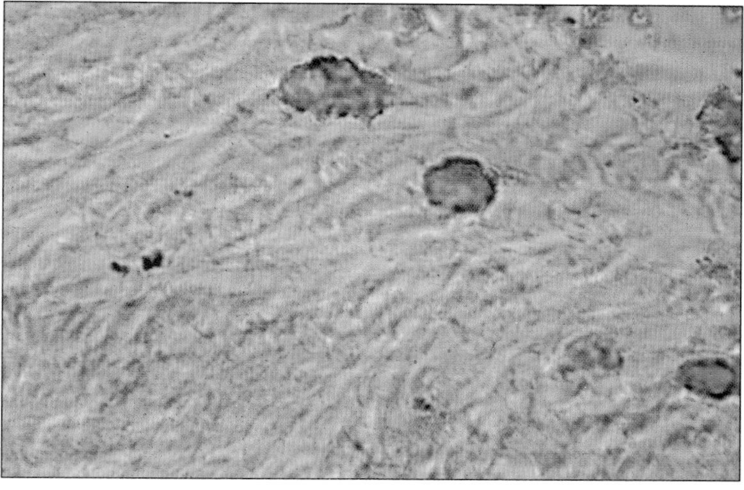

Fig. 12.20 TGF-β1 immunoreactivity in PDL tension site mesial to cat maxillary canine, 1 hour after the onset of orthodontic treatment. Dark brown deposits are visible over PDL cells. (Magnification × 1480.)

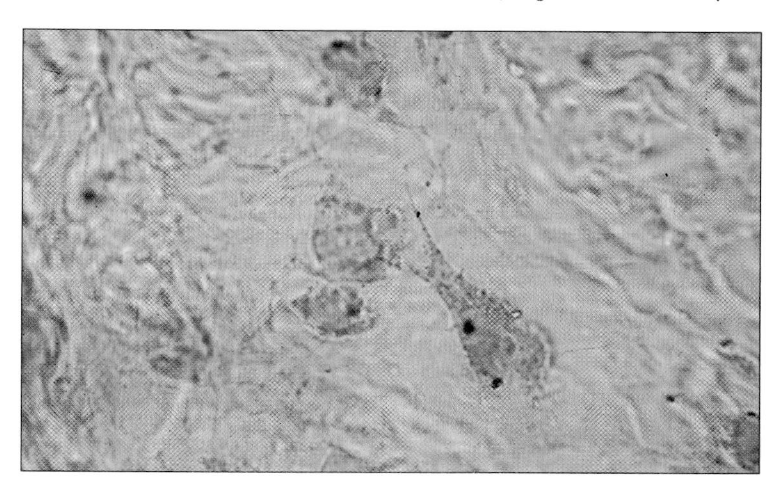

Fig. 12.21 TGF-β1 immunoreactivity in PDL compression site distal to cat maxillary canine, 1 hour after the onset of orthodontic treatment. PDL cells in the compression zone stain mildly for TGF-b1. (Magnification × 1480.)

factors (CSF), specifically those related to granulocytes (G-CSF), macrophages (M-CSF), or to both cell types (GM-CSF), may be of particular importance in this process. These molecules are specific glycoproteins, which interact to regulate the production, maturation, and function of granulocytes and monocytes–macrophages. At least two classes of growth factors appear to modulate haematopoiesis and mature blood cells: class I factors act on pluripotent early committed bone marrow cell progenitors (IL-6, IL-3, and GM-CSF); and class II factors which act on later stage committed cells (G-CSF, M-CSF, and erythropoietin). Fibroblasts and endothelial cells synthesize M-CSF and it can be found in normal serum. G-CSF is found in about 10 per cent of normal sera, but GM-CSF is undetectable in serum, although it can be found in the ECM of bone marrow. Activation of monocytes and phagocytes by inflammatory mediators can evoke synthesis of large amounts of these factors.

Osteoclasts can form as a result of culturing bone marrow cells with M-CSF for 10 days, then with bone rudiments (Kahn and Simmons, 1975). Multinucleated cells can also form in the absence of bone after prolonged incubations of marrow cells with M-CSF or GM-CSF (MacDonald *et al.*, 1986). Colony stimulating activity can also be produced by osteoblast-like cells in the absence of marrow (Elford *et al.*, 1987). While M-CSF may be an active regulator of osteoclast differentiation, it appears to inhibit resorption by mature osteoclasts (Hattersley *et al.*, 1988). In osteopetrosis, however, where fibroblasts do not secrete M-CSF and macrophages are absent from the bone marrow, administration of M-CSF restores these defects, including defects caused by the absence of bone resorption (Marks *et al.*, 1992). Quiescent fibroblasts show little expression of M-CSF, but stimulation with factors that induce proliferation (such as EGF, PDGF, and FGF or IL-1) increase M-CSF expression by these cells (Falkenburg *et al.*, 1990). Human M-CSF was originally purified from urine and was shown to be a glycosylated, 85 kDa homodimer. However, another M-CSF molecule (150–200 kDa) has been reported to be produced by osteoblasts (Ohtsuki *et al.*, 1992).

Mouse calvaria and calvarial cells synthesize and secrete CSFs in response to bacterial products and cytokines. While M-CSF does not seem to stimulate basal bone resorption, GM-CSF does enhance this activity when allowed to be present for 5 days with bone in culture, and it also augments resorption caused by PGE_2 (Bertolini and Strassmann, 1991). Moreover, GM-CSF is produced in large quantities by synoviocytes in arthritic joints and it participates in enhancing neutrophil-mediated cartilage degradation (Kowanko and Ferrante, 1991). In terms of promoting osteoclast formation from marrow cells, M-CSF is the most potent agent, followed by GM-CSF, IL-3, and G-CSF (Takahashi *et al.*, 1991).

IL-3 is a 14–30 kDa protein, with multiple haematopoietic actions, stimulatory as well as inhibitory. It competes with GM-CSF for binding to a common receptor, stimulates proliferation and differentiation of multilineage cells (including macrophages; Oster and Schulz, 1991), induces calcitonin receptor expression in rat marrow cell cultures, and enhances bone resorption in cultures containing vitamin D_3 (Hattersley and Chambers, 1990). During orthodontic tooth movement in cats, IL-3 can be detected in the PDL after 2 days and 7 days of force application. At day 7, PDL osteoclasts and neighbouring mononucleated cells stain intensely for IL-3 (*Figs 12.22, 12.23, 12.24*).

Another cytokine with stimulatory effects on osteoclast formation is interleukin 6 (IL-6), a 26 kDa protein that mediates the acute phase response in humans (Wong and Clark, 1988). Its production by fibroblasts is stimulated by IL-1 and TNF and is inhibited by TGF-β1. Incubation of mouse calvaria and calvarial osteoblasts with PTH induces production of IL-6 and IL-1α, an effect that persists for 6 days (Li *et al.*, 1991). Cytokines, such as IL-1α and TNF-α, also enhance synthesis of IL-6 by osteoblasts *in vitro*, and IL-1 and IL-6 together increase bone resorption *in vitro*, the number of osteoclasts increasing three-fold (Ishimi *et al.*, 1990). Functionally, however, osteoblasts appear to be affected only slightly by IL-6 (in terms of proliferation, alkaline phosphatase activity, osteocalcin production, and PGE_2 release), which suggests that, although IL-6 is produced by these cells, it does not act as an autocrine. During tooth movement, IL-6 can be localized in alveolar bone osteoblasts in sites of PDL compression, in agreement with Roodman's hypothesis (1992) that IL-6 is produced by osteoblasts and acts on osteoclast progenitors.

PARATHYROID HORMONE-RELATED PROTEIN

The PDL, with its complex population of cells, sensitive and responsive to a plethora of physical and chemical stimuli, may react to one more signal molecule of great interest, parathyroid hormone-related protein (PTH-rP). This protein of 139–173 amino acids, with N-terminal homology to PTH, was initially isolated from tumours of patients with humoral hypercalcemia of malignancy. However, its expression was later found in many tissues (Ikeda *et al.*, 1988), and it is found in very high concentrations in milk. Like PTH 1–34, PTH-rP 1–34 enhances both bone formation and resorption (Kitazawa *et al.*, 1991), while its C-terminal 107–139 inhibits resorption. As in the case of most other bone-related signal molecules, target cells for PTH-rP seem to be the osteoblasts, as indicated by their increased PGE_2 release following exposure to PTH-rP (Mitnick *et al.*, 1992). Fetal rat long bones in culture release peptides that are antigenically similar to PTH-rP (Bergmann *et al.*, 1990) and that are stored in the ECM. In osteoblast-like cells, PTH and PTH-rP are potent stimulators of IGF-binding protein production (Torring *et al.*, 1991) and IL-6 synthesis (Löwik *et al.*, 1989). Inhibition of the effects of PTH-rP on bone cells is caused *in vitro* by TNF-α, and *in vivo* by IL-4. Light PTH-rP immunoreactivity is observed in the non-mechanically stimulated PDL of the cat. Following the application of orthodontic forces, however, PDL cells and osteoblasts in both sites of tension and compression display intense staining for PTH-rP, particularly in the early hours of treatment (*Figs 12.25, 12.26*), implying that this signal molecule is involved in the process of force-induced remodelling of the PDL and alveolar bone.

PROSTAGLANDINS

It may be concluded that orthodontic treatment subjects paradental cells to mechanical distortion and damage, and to physicochemical and related biochemical signals. One of the earliest results of this physicochemical perturbation of cells and ECM is the synthesis and secretion of prostaglandins by the affected cells. This event is clearly evident in cat paradental tissues, as the immunoreactivity for PGE_2 is markedly enhanced in both alveolar bone osteoblasts and PDL fibroblasts (*Figs 12.27, 12.28*). Hence, at the early moments or hours of treatment, PGE_2 may be a pivotal molecule, acting as both autocrine and paracrine signal. Within a short time, as the paradental tissues become progressively strained by the applied forces, the cells are subjected to other 'first messengers', products of cells of the nervous and immune systems. The binding of these signal molecules to cell membrane receptors leads to the enzymatic conversion of cytoplasmic ATP and GTP into cAMP and cGMP. Indeed, immunohistochemical processing of paradental tissues during orthodontic treatment reveals marked increases in the concentrations of these intracellular 'second messengers' (*Figs 12.29, 12.30, 12.31, 12.32*). It is clear that PGE_2 remains an important cause of these temporal elevations in cAMP and cGMP, as demonstrated *in vivo* and *in vitro* by the use of inhibitors of PGE_2 synthesis. However, many of the neurotransmitters, cytokines, and growth factors also utilize the cyclic nucleotide route. Therefore, it is difficult to attribute fluctuations in cAMP and cGMP to any specific single stimulating factor, but rather it has to be assumed that they are related to the simultaneous effects of a number of available signals. A vigorous clinical response may thus result from a synergistic effect of a number of factors acting simultaneously.

SUMMARY AND CONCLUSIONS

Some of the major events and interactions that occur in paradental tissues during exposure to orthodontic forces are illustrated in *Fig. 12.33*. This is a clinical procedure that may last many months. Two facts deserve attention in this regard:

- the presence of a number of cell types in paradental tissues, each with distinct characteristics; and
- the interactions among these cells and between these cells and their surrounding matrix.

In the initial phases of orthodontic treatment, especially when the applied force is continuous, PDL fluids are shifted, and a gradual strain (distortion) of the ECM and cells develops. Owing to this fluid shift, charged molecules and ions may be brought into contact with the plasma membrane of cells (stress-generated potential), as the ECM, both mineralized and non-mineralized, is distorted, creating short-lived piezoelectric spikes. These bioelectric phenomena can lead to cellular activation by changing plasma membrane polarity and ion channel activity.

In the alveolar bone, the main target cells for this initial strain may be the osteocytes, as the strain persists, either owing to continuous orthodontic force application, or to the 'strain memory' feature of the matrix proteoglycans that is implemented when intermittent forces are applied. Most paradental cells are anchorage dependent – hence their attachment to the surrounding ECM results in cellular strain and change in shape concomitant with distortion of the ECM.

This alteration in cellular shape affects cytoskeletal elements, such as F-actin, that are connected on one end to the ECM, and on the other to the cell nucleus. Hence, the cytoskeleton may transmit mechanical perturbations directly to the nucleus, as well as reaction energy to cytoplasmic enzymes. In the plasma membrane, altered tension can activate mechanosensitive ion channels, and mobilize surface receptors. In osteoblasts *in vitro*, the earliest recorded response to force application is a spike of cytoplasmic Ca^{2+}, followed by elevations in IP_3, PKC, PGE_2, and cAMP.

The situation *in vivo,* however, is very different. The PDL contains an elaborate network of nerve fibres and blood vessels. Force-induced distortion of paradental tissues causes release of neuropeptides from nerve endings in the PDL and alveolar bone marrow spaces. Some of these molecules are vasoactive, causing vasodilation, plasma extravasation, and migration of leucocytes into the extravascular space. These migratory cells of the immune system synthesize and secrete a wide array of cytokines and growth factors, which regulate the activity of endothelial cells, fibroblasts, epithelial cells, and bone cells in the affected area. These native paradental cells are also capable of producing similar signal molecules, which act as autocrines or paracrines.

In this environment, there are also endocrine molecules, and factors obtained through the individual's diet and drug consumption. Some, or all of these factors, when applied simultaneously to paradental cells, can evoke reactions that are synergistic, additive, or inhibitory. Such interactions also occur between mechanical force and cytokines such as IL-1β, and may provide the biologic foundation for paradental cell stimulation *in vivo*, where only very small concentrations of signal molecules are needed to evoke a powerful cellular response, owing to the synergistic nature of the response.

In most cases of orthodontic tooth movement, tissue damage occurs, as PDL capillaries are stretched or compressed excessively. This vascular breakdown allows whole blood to be extruded into the distorted tissues, including large amounts of platelets, which are pivotal cells in the healing process. They introduce to the PDL various cytokines and growth factors, particularly PDGF, and these factors enhance chemotaxis, cell proliferation, and bone remodelling.

Lastly, force-induced strain in the alveolar bone seems to affect cells in the marrow spaces, increasing their production of cytokines, growth factors, and colony-stimulating factors. Some

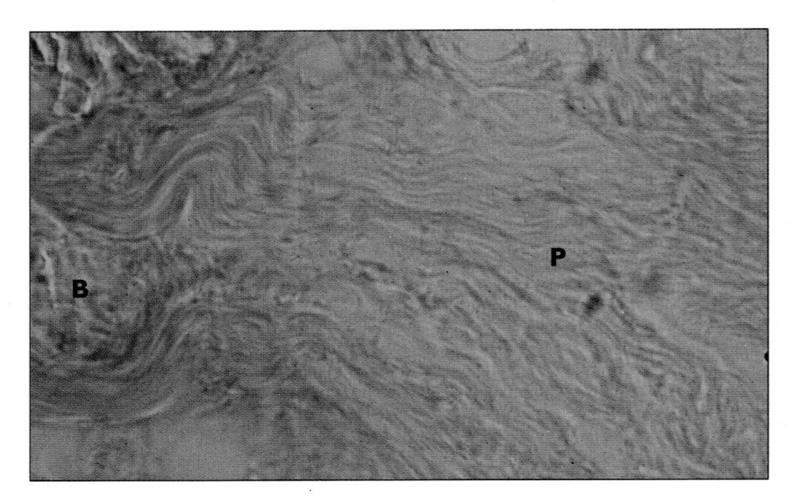

Fig. 12.22 IL-3 immunoreactivity in unstressed cat maxillary canine PDL (P) and alveolar bone (B). Very faint DAB brown deposits are visible over the bone surface cells. (Magnification × 1480.)

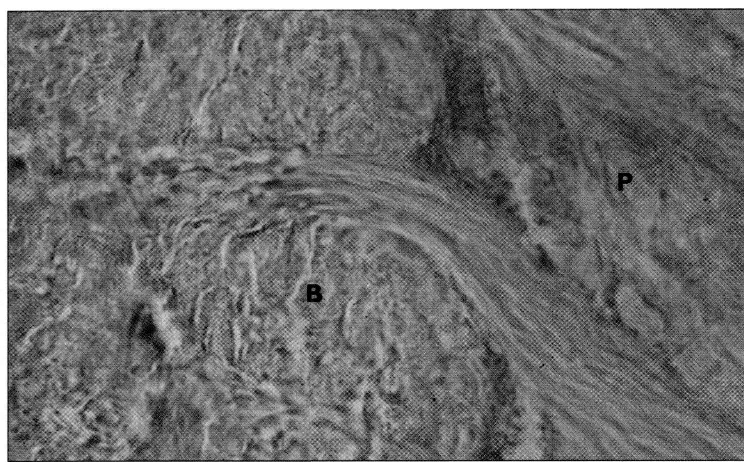

Fig. 12.23 IL-3 immunoreactivity in PDL tension site mesial to cat maxillary canine, after 7 days of orthodontic treatment. B – alveolar bone; P – PDL. Osteoblasts are stained distinctly for IL-3 (brown DAB deposits). (Magnification × 1480.)

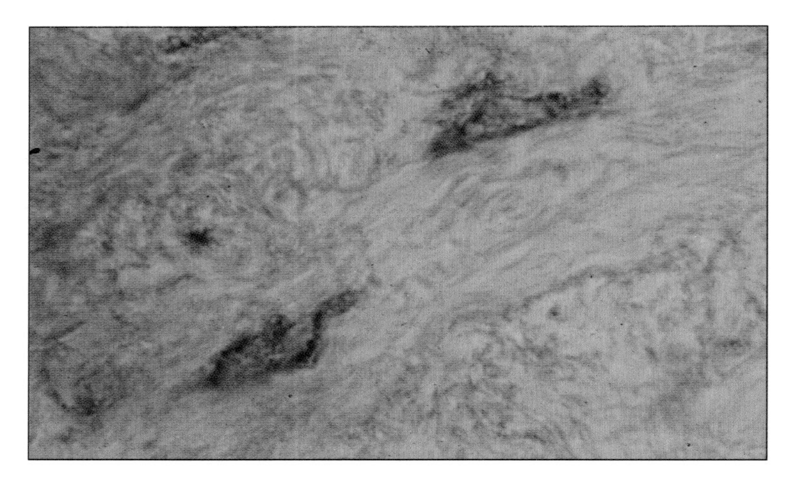

Fig. 12.24 IL-3 immunoreactivity in PDL compression site distal to cat maxillary canine, after 7 days of orthodontic treatment. Dark DAB deposits are seen over PDL cells at the edge of the necrotic, compressed PDL. (Magnification × 1480.)

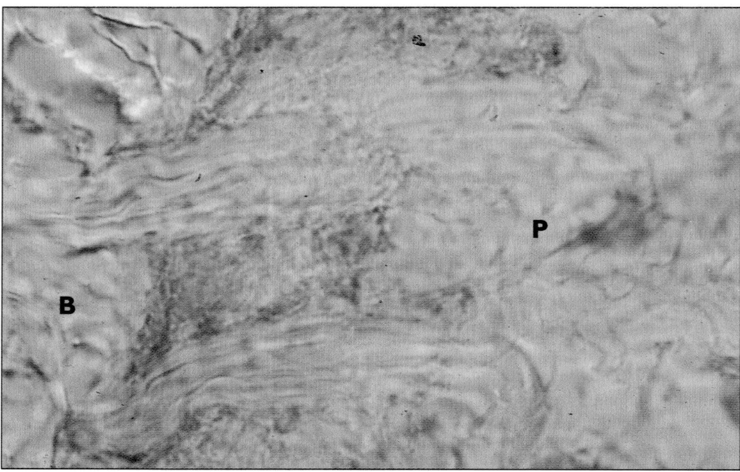

Fig. 12.25 PTH-rP immunoreactivity in unstressed cat maxillary canine alveolar bone (B) and PDL (P) cells. Light brown DAB reaction products are seen over osteoblasts and adjacent PDL cells. (Magnification × 1480.)

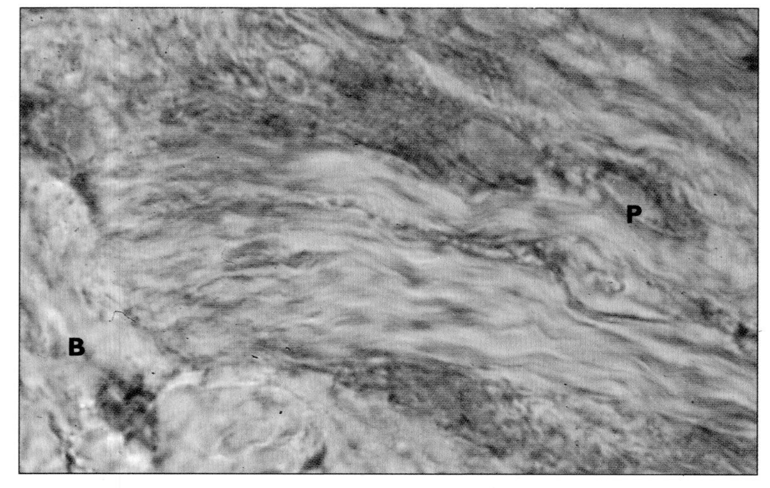

Fig. 12.26 PTH-rP immunoreactivity in PDL tension site mesial to cat maxillary canine, after 6 hours of orthodontic treatment. B – alveolar bone; P – PDL. Osteoblasts and adjacent PDL cells are covered with distinct brown deposits of DAB. (Magnification × 1480.)

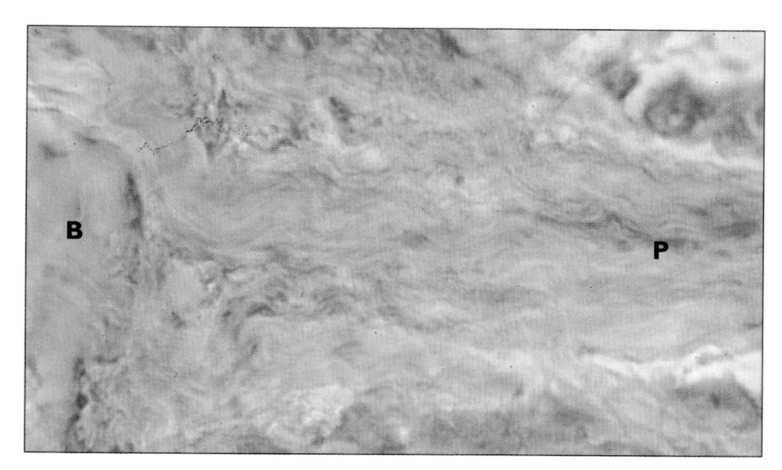

Fig. 12.27 PGE immunoreactivity in unstressed cat maxillary canine alveolar bone (B) and PDL (P). Light brown DAB deposits are seen over some of the cells, particularly the PDL cells. The osteoblasts appear flat, and contain small areas of dark DAB deposits (arrows). (Magnification × 1480.)

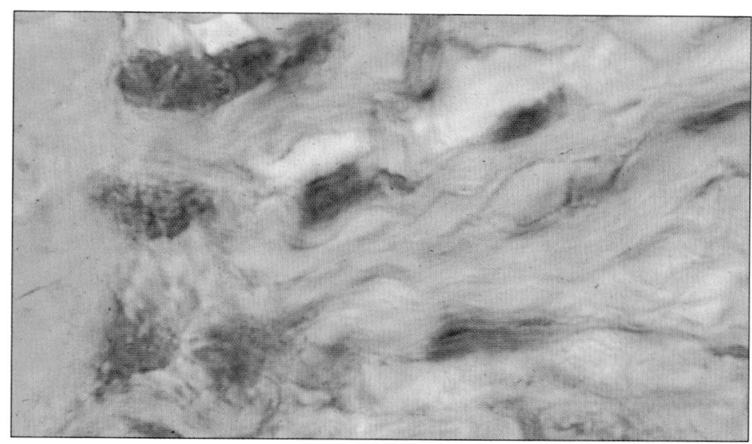

Fig. 12.28 PGE immunoreactivity in PDL tension site mesial to cat maxillary canine, after 24 hrs of orthodontic treatment. Dark brown DAB deposits are seen over the osteoblasts and neighbouring fibroblasts. The osteoblasts appear larger and rounder than their control counterparts in *Fig. 12.27*. (Magnification × 1480.)

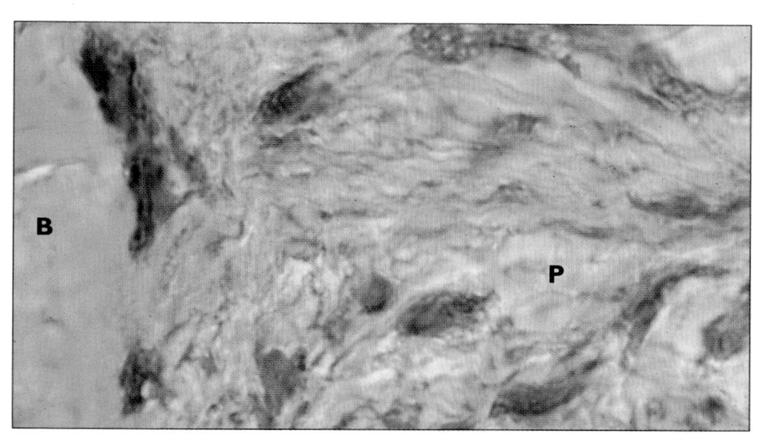

Fig. 12.29 Cyclic AMP immunoreactivity in unstressed cat maxillary canine alveolar bone (B) and PDL (P). Osteoblasts and PDL cells are both covered by distinct brown DAB deposits. The osteoblasts appear flat. (Magnification × 1480.)

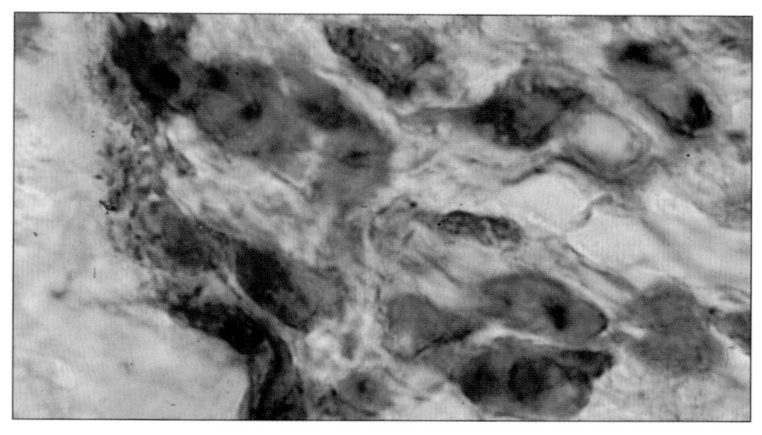

Fig. 12.30 Cyclic AMP immunoreactivity in PDL tension site mesial to cat maxillary canine, after 24 hours of orthodontic treatment. Osteoblasts and PDL cells are both intensely stained for cAMP, as the osteoblasts appear larger and round in comparison with their control counterparts in *Fig. 12.29*. (Magnification × 1480.)

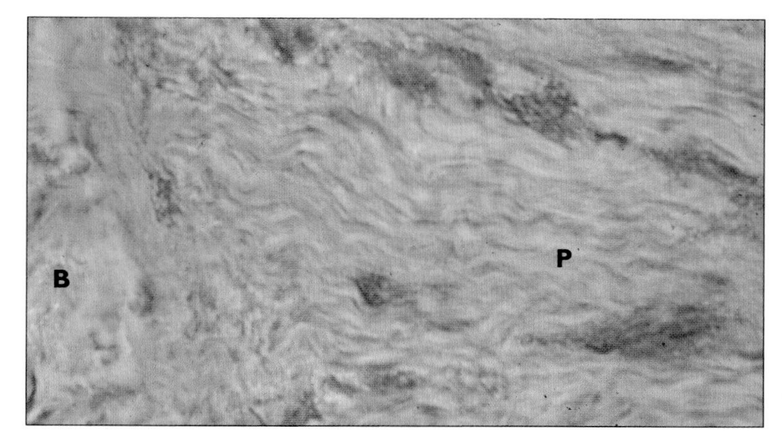

Fig. 12.31 Cyclic GMP immunoreactivity in unstressed cat maxillary canine alveolar bone (B) and PDL (P). While PDL fibroblasts are stained mildly for cGMP, osteoblasts are hardly stained. (Magnification × 1480.)

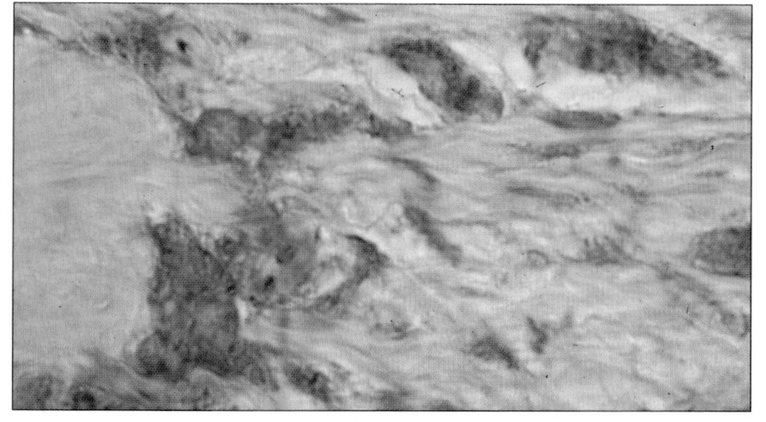

Fig. 12.32 Cyclic GMP immunoreactivity in PDL tension site mesial to cat maxillary canine after 14 days of orthodontic treatment. Both osteoblasts and PDL cells are covered with dark DAB deposits, particularly over the cytoplasm. (Magnification × 1480.)

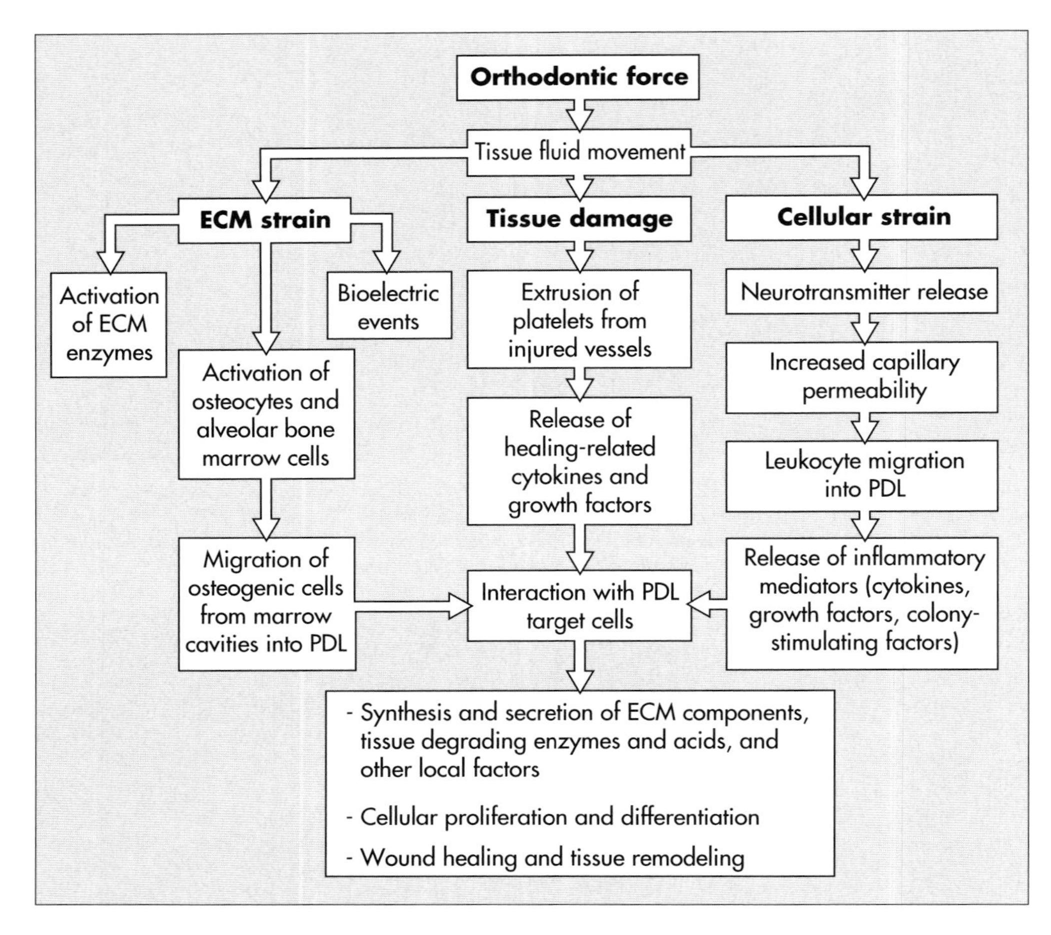

Fig. 12.33 Some events and interactions occurring in paradental tissues during exposure to orthodontic forces. The initial event is movement of tissue fluids, followed by ECM and cellular strain, and local damage to the PDL. In this scheme, target cells in the PDL and alveolar bone are exposed to bioelectric signals, as well as to signal molecules derived from sensory nerve endings, from migratory leucocytes, and from platelets. In addition, paradental cells are stimulated to produce cytokines, growth factors, and colony-stimulating factors that may function as autocrines or paracrines. The outcome of this physical and chemical perturbation of paradental cells is tissue remodelling and tooth movement.

of the latter, such as M-CSF and IL-3, stimulate progenitor cells to fuse into multinucleated osteoclasts. Since alveolar bone marrow spaces are connected through channels with the PDL, it is conceivable that marrow cell can migrate into it and participate in its remodelling.

During a typical course of orthodontic treatment, appliances are activated frequently. In this fashion, the cycle of cell stimulation by factors related to inflammation and trauma and wound healing is repeated, and tissue distortion is reintroduced. While all *in vitro* experiments on cell and tissue response to applied mechanical forces are based upon short-term trials, some *in vivo* studies have lasted 2–3 months, and their results suggest that, while many of the signal molecules, local and systemic, are present in the strained tissues, their concentrations differ from those in the initial periods, and cells in these zones appear to become increasingly refractory to the mechanical perturbation. It is therefore conceivable that, at different periods of treatment, different combinations of signal molecules come into play in these tissues, based on cycles of injury and healing, and the composition of the PDL cell populations at each period.

ACKNOWLEDGEMENT

Supported by NIDR grant no DE08428.

NOTE

Figs 12.3–12.32 all counterstained with 0.1% fast green.

REFERENCES

Assoian RK, Komoriya A, Meyers CA, Miller DM and Sporn MB (1983) Transforming growth factor-β in human platelets. Identification of a major storage site, purification and characterization. J Biol Chem 258, 7155–7160.

Barrak ER and Coffey DS (1982) Biological properties of the nuclear matrix: steroid hormone binding. Recent Prog Horm Res 38, 133–195.

Baumrind S (1969) A reconsideration of the propriety of the 'pressure–tension' hypothesis. Am J Orthod 55, 12–21.

Bergmann P, Nijs-de Wolf N, Pepersack T and Corvilain J (1990) Release of parathyroid hormone-like peptides by fetal rat long bones in culture. J Bone Min Res 5, 741–753.

Bertolini DR and Strassmann G (1991) Differential activity of granulocyte–macrophage and macrophage colony stimulating factors on bone resorption in fetal rat long bone organ cultures. Cytokine 3, 421–427.

Bevilacqua MP, Pober JS, Majeau GR, Fiers W, Cotran RS and Gimbrone L Jr (1986) Recombinant tumor necrosis factor induces procoagulant activity in cultured human vascular endothelium: characterization and comparison with the actions of interleukin 1. Proc Natl Acad Sci USA 83, 4533–4537.

Bien SM (1966) Fluid dynamic mechanisms which regulate tooth movement. Adv Oral Biol 2, 173–201.

Blom S, Holmstrup P and Dabelsteen E (1992) The effect of insulin-like growth factor-I and human growth hormone on periodontal ligament fibroblast morphology, growth pattern, DNA synthesis and receptor binding. J Periodontol 63, 960–968.

Borgens RB (1984) Endogenous ionic currents traverse intact and damaged bone. Science 225, 478–482.

Boyce BF, Yates AJP and Mundy GR (1989) Bolus injections of recombinant human interleukin-1 cause transient hypocalcemia in normal mice. Endocrinology 125, 2780–2783.

Brezden BL, Gardner DR and Morris CE (1986) A potassium-selective channel in isolated *Lymnaea stagnalis* heart muscle cells. J Exp Biol 123, 175–189.

Burridge K, Fath K, Kelly T, Nuckels T and Turner C (1988) Focal adhesions: Transmembrane junctions between the extracellular matrix and the cytoskeleton. Annu Rev Cell Biol 4, 487–527.

Canalis E, Centrella M and McCarthy TL (1991) Regulation of insulin-like growth factor-II production in bone cultures. Endocrinology 129, 2457–2462.

Canalis E, McCarthy TL and Centrella M (1989) Effects of platelet-derived growth factor on bone formation *in vitro*. J Cell Physiol 140, 530–537.

Centrealla M, McCarthy TL and Canalis E (1987) Transforming growth factor β is a bifunctional regulator of replication and collagen synthesis in osteoblast-enriched cultures from fetal rat parietal bone. J Biol Chem 262, 2869–2874.

Centrella M, McCarthy TL and Canalis E (1989) Platelet-derived growth factor enhances deoxyribonucleic acid and collagen synthesis in osteoblast-enriched cultures from fetal rat parietal bone. Endocrinology 125, 13–19.

Centrella M, McCarthy TL and Canalis E (1991) Transforming growth factor beta and remodeling of bone. J Bone Joint Surg [Am] 73–A, 1418–1428.

Chantry D, Turner M and Feldman M (1988) Regulation of interleukin 1 and tumor necrosis factor mRNA and protein by transforming growth factor-β. Lymphokine Res 7, 283.

Chenu C, Pfeilschifer J, Mundy GR and Roodman GD (1988) Transforming growth factor beta inhibits formation of osteoclast-like cells in long-term human marrow cultures. Proc Natl Acad Sci USA 85, 5683–5687.

Christensen O (1987) Mediation of cell volume regulation by Ca^{2+} influx through stretch-activated channels. Nature 330, 66–68.

Cochran GVB, Pawluk RJ and Bassett CAL (1967) Stress generated electric potentials in the mandible and teeth. Arch Oral Biol 12, 917–920.

Cochran BH, Reffel AC and Stiles CD (1983) Molecular cloning of gene sequences regulated by platelet-derived growth factor. Cell 33, 939–947.

Cogoli A, Valluchi-Morf M, Mueller M and Breigleb W (1980) Effect of hypogravity on human lymphocyte activation. Aviat Space Environ Med 51, 29–34.

Cooper KE, Tang JM, Rae JL and Eisenberg RS (1986) A cation channel in frog lense epithelia responsive to pressure and calcium. J Memb Biol 93, 259–269.

Coxam V, Davicco MJ, Pastoureau P, Delmas PD and Barlet JP (1992) Insulin-like growth factor-II increases plasma osteocalcin concentration in newborn lambs. Bone Miner 17, 177–186.

Davidovitch Z, Nicolay OF, Ngan PW and Shanfeld JL (1988) Neurotransmitters, cytokines and the control of alveolar bone remodeling in orthodontics. Dent Clin North Am 32, 411–435.

Davidovitch Z (1991) Tooth movement. Crit Rev Oral Biol Med 2, 411–450.

Davies PF and Tripathi SC (1993) Mechanical stress mechanisms and the cell: An endothelial paradigm. Circ Res 72, 239–245.

Deuel TF and Kawahara RS (1991) Growth factors and wound healing: platelet-derived growth factor as a model cytokine. Annu Rev Med 42, 567–584.

Deuel TF and Huang JS (1984) Platelet-derived growth factor: structure, function and roles in normal and transformed cells. J Clin Invest 74, 669–676.

Dewhirst FE, Ago JM, Perso WJ and Stashenko P (1987) Synergism between parathyroid hormone and interleukin 1 in stimulating bone resorption in organ culture. J Bone Min Res 2, 127–134.

Edward DR, Murphy G, Reynolds JJ, Whitman SE, Docherty AJP, Angel P and Heath JK (1987) TGF-β modulates the expression of collagenase and TIMP. J Eur Mol Biol 6, 1899–1904.

Elford PR, Felix R, Cecchini M, Trechsel U and Fleish H (1987) Murine osteoblastlike cells and the osteogenic cell MC3T3–E1 release a macrophage colony-stimulating activity in culture. Calcif Tissue Int 41, 151–156.

Emerman JT and Pitelka DR (1977) Maintenance and induction of morphological differentiation in associated mammary epithelium on floating collagen membranes. In vitro 13, 316–328.

Fagarasan MO and Axelrod J (1990) Interleukin-1 amplifies the action of pituitary secretagogues via protein kinases. Int J Neurosci 51, 311–313.

Fagarasan MO, Bishop JF, Rinaudo MS and Axelrod J (1990) Interleukin 1 induces early protein phosphorylation and requires only a short exposure for late induced secretion of β-endorphin in a mouse pituitary cell line. Proc Natl Acad Sci USA 87, 2555–2559.

Falkenburg JHF, Harrington MA, Walsh WK, Daub R and Broxmeyer HE (1990) Gene expression and release of macrophage-colony stimulating factor in quiescent and proliferating fibroblasts. Effects of serum, fibroblast growth-promoting factors, and IL-1. J Immunol 144, 4657–4662.

Farrar JN (1888) Treatise on Irregularities of the Teeth and their Correction, p 758, DeVinne Press, New York.

Feige U, Karbowski A, Rordorf-Adam C and Pataki A (1989) Arthritis induced by continuous infusion of hr-interleukin-1α into the rabbit knee joint. Int J Tissue React 11, 225–238.

Folkman J, Klagsburn M, Sasse J, Wadzinski M, Ingber D and Vlodavsky I (1988) A heparin-binding angiogenic protein-basic fibroblast growth factor is stored within basement membrane. Am J Pathol 130, 393–400.

Gamble JR, Harlan JM, Klebanoff SJ and Vadas MA (1985) Stimulation of the adherence of neutrophils to umbilical vein endothelium by human recombinant tumor necrosis factor. Proc Natl Acad Sci USA 82, 8667–8671.

Gazelius B, Edwall B, Olgart L, Lundberg JM, Hökfelt T and Fischer JA (1987) Vasodilatory effects and coexistence of calcitonin gene-related peptide (CGRP) and substance P in sensory nerves of cat dental pulp. Acta Physiol Scand 130, 33–40.

Gibson JM, King GJ and Keeling SD (1992) Long-term orthodontic tooth movement response to short-term force in the rat. Angle Orthodont 62, 211–215.

Globus KB, Plouet J and Gospodarowicz D (1989) Cultured bovine bone cells synthesize basic fibroblast growth factor and store it in their extracellular matrix. Endocrinology 124, 1539–1547.

Gowen M, MacDonald BR and Russell G (1988) Actions of recombinant human γ-interferon and tumor necrosis factor-α on the proliferation and osteoblastic characteristics of human trabecular bone cells *in vitro*. Arthritis Rheum 31, 1500–1507.

Gowen M, Nedwin GE and Mundy GR (1986) Preferential inhibition of cytokine-stimulated bone resorption by recombinant interferon gamma. J Bone Min Res 1, 479–483.

Gowen M, Wood DD and Russell GG (1985) Stimulation of the proliferation of human bone cell *in vitro* by human monocyte products with interleukin-1 activity. J Clin Invest 75, 1223–1229.

Graves DT, Valentin-Opran A, Delgado R, Valente AJ, Mundy G and Piché J (1989) The potential role of platelet-derived growth factor as an autocrine or paracrine factor for human bone cells. Tissue Res 23, 209–218.

Grimm FM (1972) Bone bending, a feature of orthodontic tooth movement. Am J Orthod 62, 384–393.

Hafström I, Gyllenhammer H, Palmblad J and Ringertz B (1989) Substance P activates and modulates neutrophil oxidative metabolism and aggregation. J Rheumatol 16, 1033–1037.

Hall K and Sara VR (1983) Growth and somatomedins. Vitam Horm 40, 175–233.

Hanks CT, Kim JS and Edwards CA (1986) Growth control of cultured rat calvarium cells by platelet-derived growth factor. J Oral Pathol 15, 476–483.

Harness MS (1989) Vasoactive intestinal peptide-like immunoreactivity in rodent taste cells. Neuroscience 33, 411–419.

Harris AK, Wild P and Stopak D (1980) Silicone rubber substrata: a new wrinkle in the study of cell locomotion. Science 208, 177–179.

Hattersley G, Dorey E, Horton MA and Chambers TJ (1988) Human macrophage colony-stimulating factor inhibits bone resorption by osteoclasts disaggregated from rat bone. J Cell Physiol 137, 199–203.

Hattersley G and Chambers TJ (1990) Effects of interleukin 3 and of granulocyte–macrophage and macrophage stimulating factors on osteoclast differentiation from mouse hemopoietic tissue. J Cell Physiol 142, 201–209.

Hedberg KM, Bengtsson T, Safiejko-Mroczka B, Bell PB and Lindroth M (1993) PDGF and neomycin induce similar changes in actin cytoskeleton in human fibroblasts. Cell Motil Cytoskeleton 24, 139–149.

Herman B and Pledger WJ (1985) Platelet-derived growth factor-induced alteration in vinculin and actin distribution in BALB/c-3T3 cells. J Cell Biol 100, 1031–1040.

Hill EL and Elde R (1988) Calcitonin gene-related peptide-immunoreactive nerve fibers in mandibular periosteum of rat: evidence for primary afferent origin. Neurosci Lett 85, 172–178.

Hohmann E, Levine L and Tashjian AH Jr (1983) Vasoactive intestinal peptide stimulates bone resorption via a cyclic adenosine 3', 5'-monophosphate-dependent mechanism. Endocrinology 112, 1233–1239.

Hohmann EL and Tashjian AH Jr (1984) Functional receptors for vasoactive intestinal peptide of human osteosarcoma cells. Endocrinology 114, 1321–1327.

Hohmann EL, Elde RP, Pysany JA, Einzig S and Gebhard RL (1986) Innervation of periosteum and bone by sympathetic vasoactive intestinal peptide-containing nerve fibers. Science 232, 868–871.

Ignoz RA and Massague J (1986) Transforming growth factor-β stimulates the expression of fibronectin and collagen and their incorporation into the extracellular matrix. J Biol Chem 261, 4337–4345.

Ikeda K, Weir EC, Mangin M, Dannies PS, Kinder B, Deftos LJ, Brown EM and Broadus AE (1988) Expression of messenger ribonucleic acids encoding a parathyroid hormone-like peptide in normal human and animal tissues with abnormal expression in human parathyroid adenomas. Mol Endocrinol 2, 1230–1236.

Ingber DE and Jamieson JD (1985) Cells as tensegrity structures: architectural regulation of histodifferentiation by physical forces transduced over basement membrane. In: Gene Expression During Normal and Malignant Differentiation (Anderson LC, Gahmberg CG and Ekblom P, eds), pp 13–32, Academic Press, Orlando, Florida.

Ishimi Y, Miyaura C, Jin CH, Akatsu T, Abe E, Nakamura Y, Yamaguchi A, Yoshiki S, Matsuda T, Hirano T, Kishimoto T and Suda T (1990) IL-6 is produced by osteoblasts and induces bone resorption. J Immunol 145, 3297–3303.

Jones DB, Nolte H, Scholuebbers JG, Turner E and Veltel D (1991) Biochemical signal transduction of mechanical strain in osteoblast-like cells. Biomaterials 12, 101–110.

Jones DB and Bingmann D (1991) How do osteoblasts respond to mechanical stimulation? Cells and Materials 1, 329–340.

Joshi HC, Chu D, Buxbaum RE and Heidermann SR (1985) Tension and compression in the cytoskeleton of PC 12 newrites. J Cell Biol 101, 697–705.

Kahn AJ and Simmons DJ (1975) Investigations of cell lineage in bone using a chimera of chick and quail embryonic tissue. Nature 258, 325–327.

Kata J, Ichikawa H, Wakisaka S, Matsuo S, Sakuda M and Akai M (1990) The distribution of vasoactive intestinal polypeptides and calcitonin gene-related peptide in the periodontal ligament of mouse molar teeth. Arch Oral Biol 35, 63–66.

Kitazawa R, Imai Y, Fukase M and Fujita T (1991) Effects of continuous infusion of parathyroid hormone and parathyroid hormone-related peptide on rat bone in vivo: comparative study by histomorphometry. Bone Miner 12, 157–166.

Kohase M, May LT, Tamm IV, Vilcek J and Sehgal PB (1987) A cytokine network in human diploid fibroblasts: interactions of beta-interferons, tumor necrosis factor, platelet-derived growth factor and interleukin-1. Mol Cell Biol 7, 273–280.

Kohler N and Lipton A (1974) Platelets as a source of fibroblast growth-promoting activity. Exp Cell Res 87, 297–308.

Kowanko IC and Ferrante A (1991) Granulocyte–macrophage colony-stimulating factor augments neutrophil-mediated cartilage degradation and neutrophil adherence. Arthritis Rheum 34, 1452–1460.

Kvinnsland I and Kvinnsland S (1990) Changes in CGRP-immunoreactive nerve fibers during experimental tooth movement in rats. Eur J Orthod 12, 320–329.

Lansman JB, Hallam TJ and Rink TJ (1987) Single stretch-activated ion channels in vascular endothelial cells as mechanotransducers. Nature 325, 811–813.

Lanyon LE (1987) Functional strain in bone tissue as an objective, and controlling stimulus for adaptive bone remodeling. J Biomech 20, 1083–1093.

Lanyon LE and Rubin CT (1984) Static vs dynamic loads as an influence on bone remodeling. J Biomech 17, 897–905.

Lanyon LE, Goodship AE, Pye CJ and MacFie JH (1982) Mechanically adaptive bone remodeling. J Biomech 15, 141–154.

Laurenzi MA, Persson MAA, Dalsgaard CJ and Rindgdén O (1989) Stimulation of human B lymphocyte differentiation by the neuropeptides substance P and neurokinin A. Scand J Immunol 30, 695–701.

Leung DYM, Glagov S and Mathews MB (1976) Cyclic stretching stimulates synthesis of matrix components by arterial smooth muscle cells *in vitro*. Science 191, 475–477.

Levine JD, Clark R, Devor M, Helms C, Moskowitz MA and Basbaum AI (1984) Intraneuronal substance P contributes to the severity of experimental arthritis. Science 226, 547–549.

Li N, Ouchi Y, Okamoto Y, Masuyama A, Kaneki M, Futami A, Hosoi T, Nakamura T and Orimo H (1991) Effect of parathyroid hormone on release of interleukin 1 and interleukin 6 from cultured mouse osteoblastic cells. Biochem Biophys Res Commun 179, 236–242.

Lomri A and Marie PJ (1990) Effects of transforming growth factor type β on expression of cytoskeletal proteins in endosteal mouse osteoblastic cells. Bone 11, 445–451.

Lotz M, Vaughn JH and Carson DA (1988) Effect of neuropeptides on production of inflammatory cytokines by human monocytes. Science 241, 1218–1221.

Lotz M, Carson DA and Vaughn JH (1987) Substance P activation of rheumatoid synoviocytes: Neural pathway in pathogenesis of arthritis. Science 235, 893–895.

Löwik CWGM, van der Pluijm G, Bloys H, Hoekman K, Bijvoet OLM, Aarden LA and Papapoulos SE (1989) Parathyroid hormone (PTH) and PTH-like protein (PLP) stimulate interleukin-6 production by osteogenic cells: A possible role of interleukin-6 in osteoclastogeneis. Biochem Biophys Res Commun 162, 1546–1552.

Lozupone E, Favia A and Grimaldi A (1992) Effect of intermittent mechanical force on bone tissue *in vitro*: preliminary results. J Bone Min Res 2, S407.

Lyndon Key L Jr, Carnes DL, Weichselbaum R and Anast CS (1983) Platelet-derived growth factor stimulates bone resorption by monocyte monolayers. Endocrinology 112, 761–762.

MacDonald BR, Mundy GR, Clark S, Wong EA, Kuehl TJ, Stanley ER and Roodman GD (1986) Effects of human recombinant CSF-GM and highly purified CSF-I on the formation of multinucleated cells with osteoclast characteristics in long-term bone marrow cultures. J Bone Min Res 1, 227–232.

Marino AA and Becker RO (1971) The origin of the piezoelectric effect in bone. Calcif Tissue Int 8, 177–180.

Marks SC Jr, Wojtowicz A, Szperl M, Urbanowska E, MacKay CA, Wiktor-Jedrzejczak W, Stanley ER and Aukerman SL (1992) Administration of colony stimulating factor-1 corrects some macrophage, dental and skeletal defects in an osteopetrotic mutation (toothless, tl) in the rat. Bone 13, 89–93.

Marotti T, Sverko V and Hrsak I (1990) Modulation of superoxide anion release from human polymorphonuclear cells by Met- and Leu-enkephalin. Brain Behav Immun 4, 13–22.

Marusic A, Kalinowski JF, Harrison JR, Centrella M, Raisz LG and Lorenzo JA (1991) Effects of transforming growth factor β and interleukin 1α on prostaglandin synthesis in serum-deprived osteoblastic cells. J Immunol 146, 2633–2638.

Melin M, Hartmann DJ, Magliore H, Falcoff E, Auriault C and Grimaud JA (1989) Human recombinant gamma-interferon stimulates proliferation and inhibits collagen and fibronectin production by human dental pulp fibroblasts. Cell Mol Biol 35, 97–110.

Merriman HL, La Tour D, Linkhart TA, Mohan S, Baylink DJ and Strong DD (1990) Insulin-like growth factor-I and insulin-like growth factor II induce c-fos in mouse osteoblastic cells. Calcif Tissue Int 46, 258–262.

Merwin JR, Anderson JM, Kocher O, Van Itallie CM and Madri JA (1990) Transforming growth factor beta 1 modulates extracellular matrix organization and cell–cell junctional complex formation during in vitro angiogenesis. J Cell Physiol 142, 117–128.

Mitnick M, Isales C, Paliwal I and Insogna K (1992) Parathyroid hormone-related protein stimulates prostaglandin E_2 release from human osteoblast-like cells: Modulating effect on peptide length. J Bone Min Res 7, 887–896.

Moody WJ and Bosma MM (1989) A nonselective ion channel activated by membrane deformation in oocytes of the ascidian Boltenia Villosa. J Memb Biol 107, 179–188.

Morris CE and Sigurdson WJ (1989) Stretch-inactivated ion channels coexist with stretch-activated ion channels. Science 243, 807–809.

Morris, CE (1990) Mechanosensitive ion channels. J Memb Biol 113, 93–107.

Motakef M, Shanfeld J and Davidovitch Z (1990) Localization of VIP at bone resorption sites *in vivo*. J Dent Res 69, 253.

Muthukrishnan L, Warder E and McNeil PL (1991) Basic fibroblast growth factor is efficiently released from a cytosolic storage site through plasma membrane disruptions of endothelial cells. J Cell Physiol 148, 1–16.

Nathan C and Sporn M (1991) Cytokines in context. Cell Biol 113, 981–986.

Ngan, P Saito S, Saito M, Shanfeld J and Davidovitch Z (1990) The interactive effects of mechanical stress and interleukin 1β on prostaglandin E and cyclic AMP production in human periodontal ligament fibroblasts *in vitro*: Comparison with cloned osteoblastic cells of mouse (MC3T3–E1). Arch Oral Biol 35, 717–725.

Nicolay OF, Davidovitch Z, Shanfeld JL and Alley K (1990) Substance P immunoreactivity in periodontal tissues during orthodontic tooth movement. Bone Miner 11, 19–29.

Noda M and Camilliere JJ (1989) In vivo stimulation of bone formation by type β transforming growth factor. Endocrinology 124, 2991–2994.

Noff D, Pitaru S and Savion N (1989) Basic fibroblast growth factor enhances the capacity of bone marrow cells to form bone-like nodules in vitro. FEBS Lett 250, 619–621.

O'Byrne EM, Blancuzzi VJ, Wilson DE, Wong M, Peppard J, Simke J and Yang JA (1990) Increased intra-articular substance P and prostaglandin E_2 following injection of interleukin-1 in rabbits. Int J Tissue React 12, 11–14.

Ohtsuki T, Suzu S, Nagata N and Motoyoshi K (1992) A human osteoblastic cell line, MG-63, produces two molecular types of macrophage-colony-stimulating factor. Biochim Biophys Acta 1136, 297–301.

Okamoto Y, Davidovitch Z and Shanfeld J (1991) CGRP in dental pulp and periodontal ligament during tooth movement. J Dent Res 70, 524.

Oppenheim A (1911) Tissue changes, particularly of the bone, incident to tooth movement. Am Orthod 3, 57–67; 113–132.

Oreffo ROC, Mundy GR, Seyedin SM and Bonewald LF (1989) Activation of the bone-derived latent TGF beta complex by isolated osteoclasts. Biochem Biophys Res Commun 158, 817–823.

Oster W and Schulz G (1991) Interleukin 3: Biological and clinical effects. Int J Cell Cloning 9, 5–23.

Overall CM, Wrana JL and Sodek J (1991) Transcriptional and post-transcriptional regulation of a 72–kDa gelatinase/type IV collagenase by transforming growth factor-β1 in human fibroblasts. J Biol Chem 266, 14064–14071.

Packham MA, Nishizawa E and Mustard JF (1968) Response of platelets to tissue injury. Biochem Pharmacol 17 (Suppl), 171–184.

Pfeilschifter J, Seyedin SM and Mundy GR (1988) Transforming growth factor beta inhibits bone resorption in fetal rat long bone cultures. J Clin Invest 82, 680–685.

Piché JE and Graves DT (1989) Study of the growth factor requirements of human bone derived cells: A comparison with human fibroblasts. Bone 10, 131–138.

Pierce GF, Mustoe TA, Altrock BW, Deuel TF and Thomason A (1991) Role of platelet-derived growth factor in wound healing. J Cell Biochem 45, 319–326.

Pierce GF, Mustoe TA, Lingelbach J, Masakowski VR, Griffin GL, Senior RM and Deuel TF (1989) Platelet-derived growth factor and transforming growth factor-beta enhance tissue repair activities by unique mechanisms. J Cell Biol 109, 429–440.

Pierce GF, Mustoe TA, Lingelbach J, Masakowski VR, Gramates P and Deuel TF (1989) Transforming growth factor beta reverses the glucocorticoid-induced wound-healing deficit in rats: possible regulation in macrophages by platelet-derived growth factor. Proc Natl Acad Sci USA 86, 2229–2233.

Pollack SR, Salzstein R and Pienkowski D (1984) The electric double layer in bone and its influence on stress-generated potentials. Calcif Tissue Int 36, S77–S81.

Postlethwaite AE, Keski-Oja J, Moses HL and Kang AH (1987) Stimulation of the chemotactic migration of human fibroblast by transforming growth factor beta. J Exp Med 165, 251–256.

Raghow R, Postlethwaite AE, Keski-Oja J, Moses HL and Kang AH (1987) Transforming growth factor beta increases steady state levels of type I procollagen and fibronectin messenger RNAs postranscriptionally in cultured human dermal fibroblasts. J Clin Invest 79, 1285–1288.

Rollins BJ, Morrison ED and Stiles CD (1988) Cloning and expression of JE, a gene inducible by platelet-derived growth factor and whose product has cytokine-like properties. Proc Natl Acad Sci USA 85, 3738–3742.

Roodman GD (1992) Interleukin 6: An osteotropic factor? J Bone Min Res 7, 475–478.

Roscetti G, Ausiello CM, Palma C, Gulla P and Roda G (1988) Enkephalin activity on antigen-induced proliferation of human peripheral blood mononucleate cells. Int J Immunopharmacol 10, 819–823.

Rosenfeld MG, Mermod JJ, Amara SG, Swanson LW, Swachenko PE, Rivier J, Vale WW and Evans RM (1983) Production of a novel neuropeoptide encoded by the calcitonin gene via tissue-specific RNA processing. Nature 304, 129–135.

Ross R, Glomset J, Kariya B and Harker L (1974) A platelet-dependent serum factor that stimulates the proliferation of arterial smooth muscle cells in vitro. Proc Natl Acad Sci USA 71, 1207–1210.

Rubin CT and Lanyon LE (1985) Regulation of bone mass by mechanical strain magnitude. Calcif Tissue Int 37, 411–417.

Rydziel S, Ladd C, McCarthy TL, Centrella M and Canalis E (1992) Determination and expression of platelet-derived growth factor-AA in bone cell cultures. Endocrinology 130, 1916–1922.

Rygh P (1974) Elimination of hyalinized periodontal tissues associated with orthodontic tooth movement. Scand J Dent Res 82, 57–73.

Rygh P and Selvig KA (1973) Erythrocytic crystallization in rat molar periodontium incident to tooth movement. Scand J Dent Res 81, 62–73.

Sabatini M, Boyce M, Aufdemorte T, Bonewald L and Mundy GR (1988) Infusion of recombinant human interleukins 1α and 1β cause hypercalcemia in normal mice. Proc Natl Acad Sci USA 85, 5235–5239.

Sachs F (1988) Mechanical transduction in biological systems. Crit Rev Biomed Eng 16, 141–169.

Said SI and Mutt V (1970) Polypeptide with broad biological activity: isolation from small intestine. Science 169, 1217–1219.

Saito S, Ngan P, Saito M, Lanese R, Shanfeld J and Davidovitch Z (1990b) Interactive effects between cytokines on PGE production by human periodontal ligament fibroblasts *in vitro*. J Dent Res 69, 1456–1462.

Saito S, Saito M, Ngan P, Shanfeld J and Davidovitch Z (1991) Interleukin 1β and prostaglandin E are involved in the response of periodontal cells to mechanical stress *in vivo* and *in vitro*. Am J Orthod Dentofacial Orthop 98, 226–240.

Saito S, Ngan P, Saito M, Kim K, Lanese R, Shanfeld J and Davidovitch Z (1990a) Effects of cytokines on prostaglandin E and cAMP in human periodontal ligament fibroblasts *in vivo*. Arch Oral Biol 35, 387–395.

Sandstedt C (1905) Einige beiträge zur theori der zahnregulierung. Nord Tandlaeg Tidskr 6, 1–18.

Sandstedt C (1904) Einige beiträge zur theori der zahnregulierung. Nord Tandlaeg Tidskr 5, 236–256.

Seyedin SM, Thomas TC, Thompson AY, Rosen DM and Piez KA (1985) Purification and characterization of two cartilage-inducing factors from bovine demineralized bone. Proc Natl Acad Sci USA 82, 2267–2271.

Shen V, Kohler G, Huang J, Huang SS and Peck WA (1989) An acidic fibroblast growth factor stimulates DNA synthesis, inhibits collagen and alkaline phosphatase synthesis and induces resorption in bone. Bone Miner 7, 205–219.

Skerry TM, Suswillo R, el Haj AJ, Ali NN, Dodds RA and Lanyon LE (1990) Load-induced proteoglycan orientation in bone tissue *in vivo* and *in vitro*. Calif Tissue Int 46, 318–326.

Stashenko P, Dewhirst FE, Peros WJ, Kent RL and Ago M (1987) Synergistic interactions between interleukin 1, tumor necrosis factor, and lymphotoxin in bone resorption. J Immunol 138, 464–468.

Stjärne P, Lundblad L, Ängård A, Hökfelt T and Lundberg JM (1989) Tachykinins and calcitonin gene-related peptide: co-existence in sensory nerves of the nasal mucosa and effects on blood flow. Cell Tissue Res 256, 439–446.

Storey E (1973) The nature of tooth movement. Am J Orthod 63, 292–324.

Takahashi N, Udagawa N, Akatsu T, Tanaka H, Shionome M and Suda T (1991) Role of colony-stimulating factors in osteoclast development. J Bone Min Res 6, 977–985.

ten Dijke P, Iwata KK, Goddard C, Pieler C, Canalis E, McCarthy TL and Centrella M (1990) Recombinant transforming growth factor type β3: biological activities and receptor binding properties in isolated bone cells. Mol Cell Biol 10, 4473–4479.

Thomson BM, Saklatvala J and Chambers TJ (1986) Osteoblasts mediate interleukin 1 stimulation of bone resorption by rat osteoclasts. J Exp Med 150, 104–112.

Torring O, Firek AF, Heath H III and Conover CA (1991) Parathyroid hormone and parathyroid hormone-related peptide stimulate insulin-like growth factor-binding protein secretion by rat osteoblast-like cells through a adenosine 3', 5'–monophosphate-dependent mechanism. Endocrinology 128, 1006–1014.

Vandenburgh HH and Kaufman S (1981) Stretch-induced growth of skeletal myotubes correlates with activation of the sodium pump. J Cell Physiol 109, 205–214.

Vignery A, Niven-Fairchild T and Shepard MH (1990) Recombinant murine interferon-γ inhibits the fusion of mouse alveolar macrophages *in vitro*, but stimulates the formation of osteoclast-like cells in implanted syngeneic bone particles in mice *in vivo*. J Bone Min Res 5, 637–644.

Wahl SM, Hunt DA, Wakefield LM, McCarthney-Francis N, Wahl LM, Roberts AB and Sporn MB (1987) Transforming growth factor type beta induces monocyte chemotaxis and growth factor production. Proc Natl Acad Sci USA 84, 5788–5792.

Wakefield LM, Smith DM, Masui T, Harris CC and Sporn MB (1987) Distribution and modulation of the cellular receptor for transforming growth factor-β. J Cell Biol 105, 965–975.

Wakisaka S, Nishikawa S, Tchikawa H, Matsuo S, Takano Y and Akai M (1985) The distribution and origin of substance P-like immunoreactivity in the rat molar pulp and periodontal tissues. Arch Oral Biol 30, 813–818.

Wakisaka S, Ichikawa H, Nishikawa S, Matsuo S, Takano Y and Akai M (1987) The distribution and origin of calcitonin gene-related peptide-containing nerve fibers in feline dental pulp. Histochemistry 86, 585–589.

Watson PA (1991) Function follows form: Generation of intracellular signals by cell deformation. FASEB J 5, 2013–2019.

Wiseman DM, Polverini PJ, Kamp DW and Leibovich SJ (1988) Transforming growth factor-beta (TGFβ) is chemotactic for human monocytes and induces their expression of angiogenic activity. Biochem Biophys Res Commun 157, 793–800.

Wong GG and Clark SC (1988) Multiple actions of interleukin 6 within a cytokine network. Immunol Today 9, 137–139.

Zengo AN, Bassett CAL, Pawluk RJ and Prountzos G (1974) *In vivo* bioelectric potentials in the dentoalveolar complex. Am J Orthodont 66, 130–139.

Zengo AN, Pawluk RJ and Bassett CAL (1973) Stress-induced bioelectric potentials in the dentoalveolar complex. Am J Orthodont 64, 17–27.

Chapter 13
Developmental Anomalies and Periodontal Diseases

AH Brook

INTRODUCTION

In discussing developmental anomalies and periodontal disease, it is necessary to consider first the evidence for a genetic component in common periodontal disease and adult periodontitis, and the mechanisms by which it is mediated. Secondly, what are the genetic factors in specific conditions confined to the periodontal ligament (PDL)? Thirdly, what conditions in the normal and abnormal development of the dentoalveolar structures predispose to or modify the development of periodontal diseases? Finally, which developmentally determined generalized diseases are frequently accompanied by periodontal pathology?

GENETIC FACTORS IN INFLAMMATORY PERIODONTAL DISEASE

The fact that genetic factors can exert a considerable influence on the periodontium is shown by several conditions that are caused by mutant single genes, e.g. acatalasia, hypophosphatasia, and cyclic neutropenia, in which severe periodontitis is a constant and striking finding. These mutant genes have their effect on periodontal structures in all environments and so illustrate the marked periodontal pathology that inherited characteristics can produce. However, these conditions are systemic diseases with a periodontal component, and they will be discussed later. First of all, the role of genetic factors in common periodontal disease must be considered.

ADULT PERIODONTITIS

Common periodontal disease clearly has a complex aetiology in which there is a genetic component (Gorlin *et al.*, 1967). Unfortunately, the data on the extent and nature of this genetic component are still limited since there have been relatively few population, family, or twin studies; indirect evidence is therefore also important.

The tendency of various racial groups to exhibit differing severity of adult periodontitis (AP) has been discussed by several authors. Zimmerman and Baker (1960) noted a higher incidence of gingival disease in Negro than in white children. Chung *et al.* (1970) carried out a genetic and epidemiological study in 9912 Hawaiian school children, aged 12–18 years. After allowance had been made for the effects of epidemiologic factors and variation in oral hygiene, they found a non-additive racial effect on periodontal disease, discernible when racial crossing was between major racial groups. Children of Hawaiian ancestry had a distinctly greater severity of disease than other racial groups. Children of mixed race had an average periodontal score that was closer to the parental race with the lower mean.

Wiktop *et al.* (1966) considered the effects of inbreeding on periodontitis in a study of 2821 people from an inbred population, the Brandy-wine Triracial isolate (Negro–white–Indian) of southern Maryland. They found that the periodontal indices by age and sex were very similar to those of Baltimore Negroes, but approximately 50 per cent higher than Baltimore whites by age. Males showed approximately 40 per cent more disease than females. Both gingivitis and periodontal pocketing increased with the degree of inbreeding. The authors considered the possibility of a socioeconomic effect, but since there was no difference between the socioeconomic scores of the three groups, the effect is more likely to have been genetic. Niswander (1975) suggests that recessive genes may be involved in the aetiology of AP. However, the results of these population and family studies are also compatible with a polygenic influence, itself part of a multifactorial aetiology.

A limited number of important bacterial components are influenced by the race and diagnosis of the group examined. Thus, Schenkein *et al.* (1993) found that *Porphyromonas gingivalis* and *Peptostreptococcus anaerobius* were significantly associated with black subjects and *Fusobacterium nucleatum* with white subjects in an adult periodontitis group.

Gunsolley *et al.* (1991) have demonstrated further that race is an important variable in certain parameters of pathogenesis of periodontal diseases, as for example in the antibody response to certain periodontal bacteria. Race also influences the chemotactic responsiveness of polymorphonuclear leucocytes from individuals with and without periodontal disease (Schenkein *et al.*, 1991).

Another method of studying the genetic basis of common disease is to investigate the incidence of the disease in groups characterized by specific genes, such as those for blood groups. If a disease occurs at a significantly higher rate in those with a particular blood group, a genetic mechanism may well be involved. Polevitzky (1929) studied AP in relation to blood grouping and found a slight increase in persons of blood group A and a slight decrease in those of blood group B. In contrast, Carmichael (1965) found no significant correlation between ABO blood groups and periodontal disease. Pradhan *et al.* (1971) suggested that Carmichael's findings could have been influenced by sample size and the fact that the groups were heterogeneous with regard to age, socioeconomic factors and oral hygiene habits. They claimed that their own study group of medical students were homogeneous in age, dietary habits, living conditions, and oral hygiene habits. They reported a broad correlation between periodontal disease and blood groups, but none with secretor status for group-specific substances in saliva. Groups O and AB were more frequently associated with severe degrees of periodontal involvement. Malena (1972) found a lower than expected number of subjects with the A blood group among gingivitis patients. The periodontitis group Kaslick *et al.* (1980) was not significantly different from either the normal study group or the general population control in terms of ABO grouping. This result agrees with those of Barros and Witkop (1963) and Carmichael (1965) but not with Polevitzky (1929) or Pradhan *et al.* (1971).

Specific immune responses are also under genetic control. It has been shown that genes responsible for specific immune responses are placed close to each other and to the histocompatibility locus. The 'histocompatibility' antigens are the expression of 'histocompatibility' genes, and certain HL-A antigens have been associated with particular diseases. Kaslick *et al.* (1980) examined the association between ABO blood groups (see above), HL-A antigens, and periodontal disease in young adults. They divided 238 Caucasians into normal, necrotizing ulcerative gingivitis, chronic gingivitis, juvenile periodontitis and periodontitis groups. Results showed that, compared to the normal group, there was a significant reduction in HL-A2 antigen frequency in the periodontitis group, a trend toward HL-A2 frequency reduction in juvenile periodontitis group and a significant reduction in HL-A2 frequency when both of these bone loss groups were combined into one group. When only those under 25 years of age were studied in the combined bone-loss group, there was more of a reduction in HL-A2 frequency.

Selective immunoglobulin A deficiency (IgAd) and common variable immunodeficiency (CVI) are both immunological diseases characterized by deficient antibody production (Rosen *et al.*, 1983). IgAd and CVI individuals lack the dominant isotype IgA in saliva, which serves as the first line of defence in the oral cavity. Bratthall and Björkander (1980) reported immunodeficient subjects with a higher level of tooth loss than immunocompetent patients. However, Robertson *et al.* (1978) did not find increased susceptibility to periodontal disease in IgAd and CVI. subjects. Engström *et al.* (1992) have found no difference in number of teeth or periodontal pocket depth when patients with IgAd and CVI were compared with age- and sex-matched controls, although lichenoid mucosal manifestations were found to be more frequent in both types of immunoglobulin deficient subjects. The impairment within these individuals is mainly in the B lymphocytes, and may not be severe enough to affect the periodontium. Alpha-antitrypsin is a serum protease inhibitor produced by the liver; it has an established role in response to destructive inflammatory disease. It exhibits inheritable genetic polymorphism (Pi types). Peterson and Marsh (1979) reported that certain Pi types appear to be related to increased susceptibility to chronic periodontitis. The periodontitis population they observed varied significantly from the control population; the presence of the Z gene in the MZ Pi type appeared to be increased in people susceptible to adult periodontitis.

Regarding genetic factors in AP as assessed from animal experiments, Baer and Lieberman (1959) found one mouse strain susceptible to AP while another two strains were relatively resistant. The trabecular pattern of the alveolar bone was said to be distinct for each strain and was not altered by diet. They concluded that the physical consistency of the diet, the width of maxilla and the weight of the mandible were not important aetiological factors in AP in these mice strains.

The study of twins by Michalowicz *et al.* (1991) indicated that a significant proportion of the variance for periodontal disease related traits is genetic in origin. Probing depth, clinical attachment loss, gingivitis, and plaque were assessed in 110 pairs of adult twins, of whom 63 monozygous and 33 dizygous pairs had been reared together and 14 monozygous pairs reared apart. A significant genetic component was demonstrated and heritability estimates were obtained for 38–82 per cent of the population variance being attributable to genetic factors.

From the above information, it is apparent that genetic factors in chronic inflammatory periodontal disease are complex and that the isolation of these factors is difficult. There does seem to be an important genetic component in common periodontal disease. but we cannot yet confidently identify the inheritance pattern.

CONDITIONS CONFINED TO THE PERIODONTAL LIGAMENT

JUVENILE PERIODONTITIS

Baer (1971) described juvenile periodontitis (JP) as 'a disease of the periodontium, occurring in an otherwise healthy adolescent, characterized by a rapid loss of alveolar bone about more than one tooth of the permanent dentition. There are two basic forms in which it occurs. In one form the teeth affected are the incisors and the first molars. In the other, more generalized form, most of the dentition can be affected. The amount of destruction manifested is not commensurate with the amounts of local irritants present.'

The role of plaque and the host response, as well as the histopathology of the ligament, are considered in Chapter 14. Here will be considered both direct and indirect evidence for the role of genetic factors in the aetiology of JP. The direct evidence relates to the familial occurrence of JP. The indirect evidence arises from a consideration of the part played in aetiology by the immune system, and the distribution of blood groups and antigen types.

In considering the more direct evidence for genetic factors, there is a suggestion that JP occurs more frequently among relatives of affected patients than in the general population. The familial occurrence of JP has been reported by Cohen and Goldman (1960); Benjamin and Baer (1967); Butler (1969); Mühlemann (1972); Jorgenson *et al.* (1975) and Kirkham (1977). Rao and Tewani (1968) also noticed a familial occurrence in 49 cases out of 89. Benjamin and Baer (1967) found JP in siblings, identical twins, 'parents-offspring', and first cousins. In Butler's (1969) family of five children, a 15-year-old boy and his sister aged 12 had JP, and a maternal aunt and grandfather had lost their teeth at an early age. A case of JP spanning three generations has been reported (Sussman and Baer, 1978). In a Danish study of about 150 cases of JP (Frandsen, 1978), there were three pairs of identical twins affected by the disease (although the bone loss was not similar in the twins).

From such evidence it seems likely that inheritance plays a considerable part in the aetiology of JP. The point to consider next is by which genetic mechanisms this is mediated.

Melnick *et al.* (1976) carried out a segregation analysis on the pedigrees already available in the literature. They claimed that a dominant trait with 78 per cent penetrance was the model that best fitted the available data. Since there was a preponderance of females among those affected, they conclude that it is an X-linked dominant trait with decreased penetrance. Melnick *et al.* (1976) also reported that several of the suggested clinical types of JP had appeared in a single family, raising the question whether there are separate types of JP or variations in the expression of a single gene.

In contrast, Fourel (1972) and Jorgenson *et al.* (1975) have suggested an autosomal recessive mode of inheritance. Each study examined only one family, although the family investigated by Fourel involved more than 20 members. In addition to the family study, both authors based their views on other reported families, on reported consanguinity, and on the higher frequency of JP in isolates. However, when Fourel refers to consanguinity, it is in relation to the Papillon–Lefèvre syndrome, which is an autosomal recessive condition (see page 288).

Saxén (1980a,b) examined the appearance of affected individuals in different generations. From a total of 62 parents of 31 propositi, all but two were examined. No affected parent was found. This is strong evidence against a dominant mode of Mendelian inheritance. Of the 64 siblings examined, 11 were affected. Saxén showed that her results were compatible with an autosomal recessive mode of inheritance. The sex ratio among the propositi, (20 females and 11 males) could be attributed either to chance or to self-selection, with females attending the dentist more frequently. This should not be reflected in the affected siblings. The small number of affected siblings (11) does not permit conclusions in any direction although the ratio (7:4) was similar to that among the propositi.

The report of Sussman and Baer (1978) on JP in three generations appears initially to be contrary to a hypothesis of recessive inheritance. They reported a 17-year-old girl, her 30-year-old mother and 50-year-old grandmother as having JP. However, bearing in mind the criteria for JP, the disease of a 50-year-old person with almost all the natural teeth remaining, and only some 2–3 mm bone loss in the maxilla, is difficult to diagnose as JP. Moreover, it is compatible with recessive inheritance for the mother and the daughter to have the disease, provided that the father was a heterozygote for this gene.

If JP is transmitted recessively, its gene frequency would be rather high, i.e. 0.03 (or 3 per cent) (Saxén, 1980a). Lack of certainty concerning the sex ratio of affected individuals is an important factor preventing agreement on the mode of inheritance.

As is the case in AP, the ABO blood groups have been analysed in JP. Kaslick, West and Chasens (1980) found many patients to be of blood group B and a smaller number than expected to be of group O. Their conclusion was that a genetic factor played a role in the aetiology of JP. Malena's (1972) results suggested that the blood phenotype A was more susceptible to the disease than phenotypes A_2, B, AB, and O.

The association between periodontal disease and HLA-A2 antigen has been investigated. Kaslick *et al.* (1975) found that only 25 per cent of patients with JP were HLA-A2 antigen positive whereas 61 per cent of the normal controls were positive. The corresponding figure for patients with adult periodontitis was 21 per cent. Reinholdt *et al.* (1977) also found a low frequency of HLA-A2 antigen in patients with JP but not in a chronic periodontitis group. These authors reported that the tissue-type specificities HLA-A9, HLA-A28, and HLA-BW15 were of significantly higher frequency in the JP group.

In view of the familial incidence and the possibility of immunological mechanisms being involved in JP, Cullinan *et al.* (1980) undertook a study to determine whether the familial susceptibility was dependent on genes within the MHC and whether it could be associated with the expression of a particular association between JP and HLA among unrelated individuals or in families. They found no such association and no support for the possibility of 'molecular mimicry' of the Gram-negative micro-organisms which could be linked with JP and a particular HLA antigen.

Data have also been reported that indicate further that the host cellular defence is impaired in individuals with JP (See Chapter 15). Deficiencies in the response of neutrophils and lymphocytes to those Gram-negative bacteria which have been associated with JP, have been described (Slots, 1976; Clark *et al.*, 1977; Liljenberg and Lindhe, 1980). A number of studies implicate the role of low responsiveness of the polymorphonuclear leucocytes in chemotaxis and phagocytosis (Cianciola *et al.*, 1977; Van Dyke *et al.*, 1980; Cogen *et al.*, 1986). Raised serum alkaline phosphatase levels in affected patients were noted by Melnick *et al.* (1976), and a defect of citric acid metabolishm has been suggested by Tsunemitsu *et al.* (1964). Reisel (1971) has suggested that JP is an early manifestation of juvenile skeletal osteoporosis. However, these suggestions await further investigation as regards possible primary bone defects in periodontitis.

Third molar germs were transplanted into sockets of freshly extracted first molars from periodontosis patients with resultant complete healing of the bone (Baer and Gamble, 1966). A similar result was reported by Borring-Møller and Frandsen (1978), who performed tooth transplantations in eight patients with JP and followed the cases for 7 years. No pocket depths over 3 mm were found, nor was there any abnormal mobility of the transplanted teeth. Both these studies make doubtful any primary role of the bone in this disease.

Turning now to consider the direct evidence concerning the genetics of JP, two basic problems have become apparent (Potter, 1990). The first is the aetiological heterogeneity, so that simple Mendelian sub-forms based solely on clinical diagnositic criteria cannot easily be defined. The second is the probable non-Mendelian nature of its aggregation within families so that simple autosomal dominant or recessive or X-linked transmission cannot elucidate the multifactorial nature of its aetiology with genetic and environmental interactions (Potter, 1989).

Dealing with the underlying clinical heterogeneity and subdividing into increasingly homogeneous sub-forms, based on laboratory parameters as well as clinical findings, is important. Rather than being a single entity, JP may be a symptom complex that includes several distinct disorders. First, early onset periodontal destruction occurs in a number of different syndromes arising from single gene mutations or from chromosomal anomalies (Saxén, 1980a,b).

Secondly, there is a wide range of estimated prevalences reported for different gender, racial, and ethnic groups (Saxén 1980a,b). If the marked preponderance of females affected is a true finding rather than a distortion produced by study methodology, then it might be that there are sub-forms in the separate genders. Within the national survery of the oral health of US children, conducted in 1986–1987, the periodontal assessment of 14–17 year olds showed blacks were at much greater risk for all forms of early onset periodontitis than whites (Löe and Brown, 1991). Moreover, whether there are differences in clinical phenotypes between ethnic groups is still unclear. Cogen *et al.* (1992) support this suggestion and consider also that the preponderance of JP among black as compared to white subjects is further evidence for the genetic component of the disease.

Thirdly, within clinical sub-forms there is evidence of heterogeneity; in the study of Genco *et al.* (1986), 70 per cent of patients with localized JP suffered from a defect in chemotaxis while others did not. Both localized and generalized JP occur in some families but not in all (Potter, 1990).

Further support for heterogeneity comes from the range of explanations offered for familial aggregation from different studies: autosomal dominant (Bixler, 1987), X-linked dominant (Melnick *et al.*, 1976), and autosomal recessive (Saxen and Nevanlinna, 1984; Long *et al.*, 1987; Boughman *et al.*, 1988). While a number of the later publications have favoured the autosomal recessive hypothesis, Potter (1990) has questioned this on the reported very low occurrence in parents compared to observed risk for siblings of probands, and she also argues that the two-fold increase in affected females as compared to males is not consistent with a simple recessive model.

However, Hart *et al.* (1992), in re-examining the published evidence on the inheritance of JP, consider that the greater number of affected females is probably a reflection of incomplete pedigree information, with under-representation of males. Hart *et al.* (1991) examined 24 families with a high density of JP (i.e. two or more affected individuals in a family), ascertained through affected probands. For these families, 80 per cent of the probands were female, but the proportions of affected male and female siblings were equal. Similar findings are reported by Saxen (1980a,b), Van Dyke *et al.* (1985) and Boughman *et al.* (1986).

It is also asserted that the reported lack of father-to-son transmision may arise from incomplete family data. Two studies of more complete data sets (Boughman *et al.*, 1986; Saxby, 1987) have demonstrated male-to-male transmission. Results of segregation analyses in some studies using more complete data sets are compatible with autosomal inheritance of JP (Long *et al.*, 1987; Beaty *et al.*, 1987).

Another aspect of recent finding is that the onset of JP may occur earlier than was generally accepted. Cogen *et al.* (1992) carried out a retrospective cross-sectional study of 4757 patients at the Children's Hospital of Alabama. For a number of systemically healthy patients, diagnosed as having JP in the permanent dentition, there were radiographs available from the deciduous and the mixed dentitions. For the majority of these patients, there was radiographic evidence of bone loss in the prepubertal years.

Thus, the current understanding of JP is that it is a complex disorder, the familial nature of which may include common family environments as well as genetic factors. Attempting to define subforms by immunological and microbial as well as clinical and genetic methods could lead to further understanding. So that independently transmissible sub-forms can be defined, a multifactorial statistical approach can be used to supplement the clinical and laboratory methods (Smith, 1976; Reich *et al.*, 1979; Potter, 1990).

ABNORMAL DEVELOPMENTS OF THE DENTOALVEOLAR COMPLEX – THEIR IMPORTANCE IN CHRONIC INFLAMMATORY PERIODONTAL DISEASE

A number of developmental factors may contribute to the initiation and progression of chronic inflammatory periodontal disease. The influence of tooth morphology and structure is discussed here.

TOOTH MORPHOLOGY

Some developmental variations of tooth morphology may provide shelter for accumulation and retention of plaque, thus predisposing the tooth to a localized periodontal lesion (Shiloah and Kopczyk, 1979).

The morphological characteristics of the periodontium are in part related to the shape of the teeth (Wheeler, 1961; Schluger *et al.*, 1977; Grant *et al.*, 1988). Morphological defects of the dentition can be regarded as a predisposing cause of periodontal disease. Buccal gingival contours, marginal ridges on the occlusal surfaces of posterior teeth, and normal contact areas all play a part in the food-shedding mechanism to protect the marginal gingiva and the gingival crevice (Lee *et al.*, 1968). Excessive contours and concavities can hamper efforts to remove plaque (Shiloah and Kopczyk, 1979).

It has been suggested that two basic forms of gingivae are found, described as 'scalloped-thin' and 'flat-thick' (Ochsenbein and Ross, 1973; Seibert and Lindhe, 1989). The scalloped-thin 'periodontal biotype' (Seibert and Linde, 1989) was described as associated with a tapering crown form and small proximal contact areas located near the incisal edge of the tooth. In contrast, flat-thick gingivae were related to a tooth with a squared labial form, a distinct cervical convexity, and relatively large, more apically placed contact areas. The thickness of alveolar bone was considered also to be related to tooth form, with the scalloped-thin gingivae accompanied by the thinner bone rather than the flat-thick type.

It has also been proposed that the severity of periodontal disease clinical features may vary with the morphology of the tissues (Ochsenbein and Ross, 1973; Seibert and Lindhe, 1989). Thus, deep periodontal pockets may be associated with plaque-related inflammation in individuals with flat-thick gingival tissues, while individuals with scalloped-thin gingivae may show recession of the gingival margin.

Olsson and Lindhe (1991) considered further the relationship of crown form and symptoms associated with periodontal disease. They reported that individuals with a long, narrow form of upper central incisors had experienced more recession at labial surfaces than subjects with a short, wide form. Animal studies, however, have indicated that an inflammatory lesion residing in thin gingival tissue may result in more gingival recession than a similar lesion in a thick gingiva (Baker and Seymour, 1976; Wennstrom *et al.*, 1982).

The relationship between the crown form of the permanent maxillary incisors and canines and the morphological characteristics and thickness of the gingivae in a group of 108 adolescents devoid of symptoms of destructive periodontal disease has been described by Olsson *et al.* (1993). They reported that individuals whose central incisors had a long narrow form, when compared to individuals having a short wide crown form, demonstrated a narrow zone of keratinized gingivae, shallow probing depth, and a pronounced scalloped contour of the gingival margin. However, there was no significant difference between these groups with respect to the thickness of the free gingivae. A given crown form of the central incisors was accompanied by a similar form in the lateral incisors and canines.

In multirooted teeth, as the pathological process advances, areas of the cement–enamel junction and of the root furcations become exposed. Furcation morphology takes many forms. Some roots are splayed; other are fused, leaving a concavity or groove but no separation of roots. Most furcations are between such extremes. The more constricted the furcation, the more difficult it is to clean. Variation in the level of the furcation may well influence the progress of the periodontal lesion, as in the condition of taurodontism (Holt and Brook, 1979).

In taurodontism, the body of the tooth is enlarged at the expense of the roots (Keith, 1913). The pulp chamber appears large and often extends below the level of the alveolar crest. The usual constriction at the level of the amelocemental junction is frequently absent (Hamner, Witkop and Metro, 1964). Depending on the level of the furcation, the affected teeth have been termed hypotaurodont, mesotaurodont, and hypertaurodont. In hypertaurodontism, the pulp chamber extends nearly to the apex with little division of the root. The more apical location of the furcation in taurodont teeth militates against their early involvement in periodontitis.

Taurodontism is seen in some patients with amelogenesis imperfecta, e.g. in the mixed type of enamel defect, in which there is both hypocalcification and hypoplasia. A similar association is present as part of the Trichodento-osseous syndrome (Witkop, 1975) where, in addition to enamel defects and taurodontism, there is also tight curly hair and sclerosis of bone. The condition has also been seen in male patients with polypoidy of the X-chromosome, e.g. Klinefelter's syndrome (XXY) (Sauk, 1980).

Taurodontism is thought to originate from a defect in Hertwig's root sheath, which fails either to invaginate at the usual horizontal level or to achieve union of the flaps which determine root morphodifferentiation (Holt and Brook, 1979).

Enamel projections are irregularities of the enamel margin of deciduous and permanent molars. They may extend from the cement–enamel junction in molars toward and, perhaps, into the furcation. This phenomenon has been correlated with furcation involvement in CIPD. Teeth with this anomaly may have a cul-de-sac of unattached gingiva, which accumulates dental plaque. They also occur on taurodont teeth. The projections have been classified into three groups:

- class 1 – a distinct change in the cement–enamel junction, with enamel projecting towards the furcation;
- class 2 – enamel projecting further towards but not involving the furcation; and
- class 3 – extending to involve the furcation.

Class 3 projections occur more often on mandibular than maxillary teeth, especially on the buccal aspect (Masters and Hoskins, 1964). Indeed, their clinical observations seemed to associate enamel projections with approximately 90 per cent of isolated bifurcational involvements (Leib *et al.*, 1967). Bissada and Abdelmalek (1973) reported a 50 per cent correlation between cervicoenamel projection and furcation involvement. In other studies, however, no statistically significant association between extensions and furcation involvements has been shown (Holt, 1976). Estimates of their frequency in the deciduous dentition are not available. Microscopic studies of extracted permanent teeth suggest a range of 6–24 per cent for the class 3 projections. There appears to be a higher prevalence in persons of Mongoloid origin than in Caucasians (Masters and Hoskins, 1964; Holt, 1976).

Enamel pearls are isolated, round, or oval deposits that are composed of enamel only or that contain a dentine core, which may also enclose an extension of pulpal tissue. They have not been found in the deciduous dentition. Most reports of pearls in the permanent dentition have been confined to molars, but they have also been seen on incisors and premolars, although not on canines. They tend to occur distally on upper molars and buccally on lower molars, often being bilaterally symmetrical. On extracted teeth examined macroscopically, the overall incidence ranged from 1–7 per cent (Holt, 1976). Pearls may occur singly or as multiples on one tooth. Kerr (1961) suggested, because of the frequency with which they occur in bifurcations, that enamel pearls may influence the development and progress of a pocket in that region. He postulated that the PDL fibres had no true attachment to the tooth in the area of the cervicoenamel projection or the enamel pearl.

Grooving of the crown and root surfaces is a structural variation in many teeth. Lee *et al.* (1968) describe developmental grooves on the palatal surface of maxillary incisor teeth, commencing at the junction of the cingulum and the lateral marginal ridges, and extending on to the root surface. They may continue for variable distances along the length of the distolingual aspect of the root. The defect is in communication with the gingival crevice. The epithelial attachment in this area is frequently diseased, forming a ready pathway for the ingress of bacterial metabolites and the formation of an infrabony periodontal pocket.

Everett and Kramer (1972) found grooves in 2 per cent of maxillary lateral incisors, while Lee *et al.* (1968) described 13 cases of palatogingival grooving in teeth of individuals of both Chinese and Indian origin. Withers *et al.* (1981) reported a prevalence of 4.4 per cent of maxillary lateral incisors having palatogingival grooves, and Kogan (1986) found a similar frequency of 4.6 per cent in both central and lateral incisors. Of the grooves in Kogan's (1986) study, over half terminated on the root surface. In lateral incisors, 43 per cent of grooves on the root extended less than 5 mm; 47 per cent extended between 6–10 mm; and 10 per cent extended for more than 10 mm. Only 4 per cent of all specimens had an enamel extension that lined at least part of the groove, and in no case did it extend more than 5 mm down the root. The extent of the groove is an important fact in the prognosis of the tooth (Gher and Vernino, 1980).

Deep lingual or buccal grooves marking the site of incomplete root bifurcations are found particularly in mandibular second molars. They have also been described in mandibular first premolars (Holt, 1976), and lingual grooves from the occlusal surface of these teeth extending towards the gingival margin have been observed by Berry (1978).

In addition to those invaginations whose primary site of origin is the tooth crown, invaginations have been described by several authors in which the apparent site of origin is the tooth root (Oehlers, 1958). Provided the opening of the invagination has no connection with the oral cavity, no complications need ensue. With loss of gingival attachment, however, infection and necrosis of the pulp could follow in the same way as with a coronal invagination.

There are instances of double teeth where adventitious furcations can form surface projections of cervical enamel and create an obvious PDL problem (Brook and Winter, 1970).

Boyde and Jones (1972) carried out a scanning electron microscope study of completed enamel surfaces of unerupted human teeth. They speculated that cervical enamel surface projections could serve as plaque-retaining features.

It may be concluded that there are a variety of crown root forms and cervical enamel projections which may predispose teeth to involvement in severe or complicated chronic inflammatory periodontal disease (CIPD).

TOOTH STRUCTURE

Many anomalies of enamel structure, both genetic and environmental, may allow plaque to accumulate, owing to surface roughness, pitting, or grooving. The poor appearance and the lack of improvement to be achieved by tooth brushing mean that there is little motivation for good hygiene. Extreme discomfort may be experienced by children with hypocalcified enamel when ingesting a wide variety of foods and drink. In some defects, the enamel may break off as large flakes to expose wide areas of sensitive dentine. Poor masticatory function and inadequate oral hygiene may result.

DENTINE DYSPLASIA (SHIELDS TYPE 1)

This condition has previously been termed rootless teeth, non-opalescent and opalescent dentine, and radicular dentine dysplasia. The teeth have clinically normal crown form but short roots, abnormal root form, and at least partial absence of pulp chamber and canals. Both dentitions are affected. The teeth are often malpositioned and very mobile and therefore easily displaced, even by minor trauma. The disease is inherited as an autosomal dominant trait with a frequency of about 1 in 100 000. Teeth affected by this condition tend to migrate and to be exfoliated early, even though there is usually little associated gingivitis (Sedano *et al.*, 1977).

SYSTEMIC DEVELOPMENTAL DISORDERS WITH PERIODONTAL LIGAMENT INVOLVEMENT

DISEASE AFFECTING TOOTH ERUPTION

Developmental disturbances to eruption of teeth may arise directly, by influencing the mechanism or mechanisms responsible for generating eruptive forces, or they may arise indirectly, by structures presenting a barrier in the pathway of the erupting tooth. Although the eruptive mechanism is as yet unknown (see Chapter 9), it is thought to reside within the PDL. Few abnormalities seem to affect the eruptive mechanism directly. Cleidocranial dysostosis results in a generalized failure of tooth eruption throughout the jaws. It is transmitted as an autosomal dominant condition (Gorlin *et al.*, 1976). Other conditions where there may be a generalized failure in tooth eruption relate to hormonal disturbances, and these are described in Chapter 21. With respect to indirect factors, Di Biase (1976) has reviewed dental abnormalities that may affect eruption. It can also be envisaged that abnormal changes within the mucosa overlying a developing tooth, as in hereditary fibromatosis gingivae, could increase the resistance to eruption, with the result that the tooth may be prevented from erupting. Since in these situations eruption will occur once the overlying tissue is surgically removed (Duckworth, 1962; Howard, 1966; Johnson, 1969; Di Biase, 1971), it may be that the PDL is unaffected.

DOWN'S SYNDROME

Many patients with Down's syndrome have CIPD (Cohen *et al.*, 1961). Dow (1951) found that over 90 per cent of 8–12-year-old 'Mongoloid' children had periodontal disease. Cutress *et al.* (1970) reported that the severe periodontal disease commonly found in subjects with trisomy 21 started at an early age – 5 years or younger – and progressed at such a rate that some teeth were lost by the age of 10–11 years. By examining patients aged 19–25 years of age, Kisling and Krebs (1963) found the prevalence of gingivitis to be 100 per cent. Cohen and Goldman (1960) observed severe periodontitis in over 90 per cent of a group of Mongoloid patients. Similar findings were reported by Johnson and Young (1963).

Periodontal disease in these patients does not seem to affect all areas of the mouth. Cohen and Goldman (1960) found radiographically that the most frequent sites of bone loss were the anterior regions of both jaws. Johnson and Young (1963) also reported that the anterior region of the mandible had more severe periodontal destruction. Although the alveolar bone loss occurs in both dentitions, it is more common around permanent teeth (Cohen and Goldman, 1960; Johnson and Young, 1963). There is some suggestion that males are affected more severely than females (McMillan and Kashgarian, 1961).

In an attempt to consider whether there is truly a systemic factor predisposing patients with Down's syndrome to CIPD, or whether the levels of disease could be attributed entirely to environmental effects, comparison has been made of trisomy 21 patients with other congenitally mentally retarded patients. Johnson and Young (1963) reported that the severity of periodontal disease in patients with Down's syndrome was about twice that in other congenitally mentally retarded patients. They found no cases with severe alveolar bone loss in non-Mongoloid children. Sznajder *et al.* (1968) found that both Mongoloid and cerebral palsy children had poor oral hygiene and similar plaque indices. However, cerebral palsy children did not have advanced periodontal disease with pocket formation, as did the Mongoloid children. Cutress *et al.* (1970) found that extractions for periodontal disease in a large group of subjects aged 10–24 years were largely confined to Down's syndrome patients. Few of the other mentally retarded subjects in his study had extractions for periodontal disease, and none of the normal subjects had required such treatment.

Swallow (1964) and Cutress *et al.* (1970) reported a higher prevalence of periodontal disease in institutionalized patients with Down's syndrome than in those living at home. This suggests that both the genetic background of the patient and the environment in which he or she lives influence the level of CIPD. The relatively low severity of CIPD in Down's syndrome patients living at home suggests that oral hygiene practices may be different. However, Cutress *et al.* (1970) reported that the oral hygiene scores for institutionalized and home groups of Down's syndrome patients did not differ significantly. Moreover, the greater severity of periodontal disease in trisomy subjects cannot be explained by the amount of calculus present, because calculus scores were similar both for Down's syndrome patients and for other mentally retarded, institutionalized subjects. Local factors, such as tongue abnormalities, dental morphological abnormalities, malocclusion, and poor masticatory function, may be important (de Grouchy and Turleau, 1990). Cohen and Goldman (1960) suggested that there was reduced resistance to 'local irritation'. No evidence has been found for differences in the microbiology of plaque samples in Down's syndrome subjects, other mentally retarded subjects, and normal subjects (Cutress *et al.*, 1970).

Regarding other factors in the periodontal problems of patients with Down's syndrome, Sobel *et al.* (1958) showed that they exhibited a lower absorption of vitamin A, lower serum calcium, and lower serum albumin. Severity of CIPD in Down's syndrome patients may therefore depend on a combination of genetic and environmental factors, although the precise nature of these is still not clear.

IMMUNODEFICIENCY DISEASES

Immunodeficient patients, characterized primarily by dysfunction of the secretory IgA system, have been reported to show less periodontal inflammation than immunocompetent subjects matched by age and Plaque Index (Robertson *et al.*, 1980). In addition, the immunodeficiency disease did not seem to predispose to acute pathology involving the gingiva or other oral soft tissues. The findings with respect to gingival inflammation agree with previous studies of immunodeficient patients (Robertson and Cooper, 1974) and studies of patients receiving immunosuppressive agents (Tollefsen *et al.*, 1978). Thus, the salivary immunoglobulins probably do not play a major protective role in the early periodontal lesion.

Diminished levels of gingival inflammation in these patients allow speculation of either a qualitative difference in oral microflora or an impairment in host ability to react to plaque. Some differences have been reported in the microbial composition of plaque obtained from patients with abnormalities of the immune system (Brown, 1978). With respect to the host response, the nature of the cellular infiltrate in the local periodontal lesions may be important (see Chapter 14).

HAEMATOLOGICAL DISEASES

Many neutrophil disorders, as well as histiocytosis, are developmental in origin. They are considered in chapter 18, which deals with blood and lymphoreticular diseases as they affect the PDL.

CONNECTIVE TISSUE DISEASES

Ehlers–Danlos syndromes

Ehlers–Danlos syndromes consist of varying degrees of hyperelastic skin, skin haemorrhages, loose jointedness, and cutaneous pseudotumours. Ten entities have been recognized on the basis of genetics, clinical findings, and pathogenesis.

Four variants are autosomal dominant traits (types I, II, III, VIII), two are autosomal recessive (A.R.) traits (types VI, X), two are X-linked (types V, IX) and two may be A.D. or A.R. (types IV, VII). Known basic defects include (Gorlin, 1976; Byers and Holbrook, 1990):

- type IV – type 3 collagen deficiency;
- type VI – lysyl hydroxilase deficiency; and
- type VII – procollagen peptidase deficiency.

The oral mucosa is fragile and easily bruised. Gorlin (1976) noted that gingivae and periodontium are susceptible to injury and to destructive periodontal disease at an early age. Barabas (1969) reported that in the molar teeth examined, the cementum seemed disorganized and contained organic inclusions. Stewart et al. (1977) described two families, now classified as Type VIII (Byers and Holbrook, 1990), in which affected individuals had lost most of their teeth due to periodontal disease by their early 20s.

MUCOPOLYSACCHARIDOSES AND MUCOLIPIDOSES

The mucopolysaccharidoses and mucolipidoses are a heterogeneous group of approximately 20 rare, phenotypically similar but genetically distinct, inborn errors of metabolism. Most of these disorders culminate in severe disability over many years, and only seldom result in death in infancy. Specific enzyme deficiencies have been discovered for the majority of the mucopolysaccharidoses and also for a few of the mucolipidoses (Gorlin, 1976).

The mucopolysaccharidoses and mucolipidoses are good examples of genetic heterogeneity (multiple genetic causes of a similar phenotype) and leiotropism (a single gene resulting in several different diseases; the genotype can be determined directly by measuring the gene product).

The pattern of inheritance for all these disease is autosomal recessive with the exception of mucopolysaccharidosis II, which is X-linked (Goodman and Gorlin, 1977). The total incidence of the mucopolysaccharidoses has been estimated as approximately 4 in 100,000 (Legum *et al.*, 1976).

It would seem that tooth eruption is delayed in at least 50 per cent of gargoyle patients (Cawson, 1962). The gingivae are described as hyperplastic, hypertrophic, or broad and thick. Periodontal ligament changes are not reported, although a prominent feature of histology of idiopathic gingival hyperplasia is the accumulation of mucoid material among the collagen fibres (Rushton, 1957).

Delay in the appearance of teeth, especially the secondary dentition, is frequent in Hurler syndrome, and the teeth may be of an abnormal size and shape. Gingival hypertrophy leads to wide alveolar margins and encroachment of the gums onto the crowns of the teeth (Cawson, 1962). Localized bone destruction resembling dentigerous cysts is common in the mandibular molar region by the age of 3 years. Sedano *et al.* (1977) believed that these bone lesions represent hyperplastic dental follicles engorged by dermatan sulphate.

The basis of Maroteaux–Lamy disease (polydystrophic dwarfism) appears to be a deficiency of arylsulphatase B. The permanent mandibular molars are usually delayed in eruption and may be surrounded by radiolucent areas, which possibly represent accumulations of dermatan sulphate (Sedano *et al.*, 1977). The fibroblasts of mucolipidosis II (I-cell disease) contain in their cytoplasm numerous granular inclusions believed to be altered lysosomes. The gingivae are greatly enlarged and may cover the teeth or interfere with eruption. Storage material may occur around unerupted teeth, particularly the molars (Gorlin, 1976).

Connective tissue disorders are discussed further in chapter 20.

METABOLIC DISORDERS

Acatalasia

Catalase generates oxygen by rapidly decomposing hydrogen peroxide. The physiological role of catalase is not clear. It provides a pathway for breaking down hydrogen peroxide, which might otherwise accumulate within the cell. Liberated catalase usually protects surrounding tissues from hydrogen peroxide generated by polymorphonuclear leucocytes during phagocytosis. Acatalasic patients are unable to degrade exogenous or endogenous hydrogen peroxide, which accumulates in the periodontal tissues, deprives them of oxygen, and causes ulceration and necrosis of the soft and hard tissues (Delgado and Calderon, 1979). The clinical manifestations of catalase deficiency are confined to the oral tissues, specifically to the periodontium. The main oral findings in two Peruvian brothers with acatalasia examined by Delgado and Calderon (1979) were gingival necrosis and severe alveolar bone destruction; otherwise the patients were in good health.

The lesions may appear as soon as the deciduous and permanent teeth erupt. They may begin on the interdental papilla of the incisors and progress to the rest of the teeth. Ulceration and necrosis of the gingivae, vestibular fistulas, migration of teeth, and denuded root surfaces may follow.

Where teeth are absent, the alveolar mucosa is normal; after extractions, wound sockets heal normally. Antibiotic therapy and removal of dental plaque limit the progression of the gingival lesions. Gingival damage perhaps results from a lack of catalase activity in the gingivae, permitting proliferation of bacteria in dental plaque and gingival inflammation. The absence of catalase allows accumulation of hydrogen peroxide in gingival tissues. Most of the cultures obtained from necrotic gingival tissues and from dental plaque showed a predominance of catalase-negative pneumococci, which are also known to be hydrogen peroxide producers (Delgado and Calderon, 1979). *Lactobacillus acidophilus* and streptococci also generate hydrogen peroxide. Hydrogen peroxide production during the gingival inflammatory process results from phagocytosis by the polymorphonuclear leucocyte. Thus, it is postulated that the gingival lesions resulted from damage to tissue caused by hydrogen peroxide generated by organisms in gingival plaque. Some patients with acatalasia, however, do not develop gingival lesions. This could be due to their peculiar oral flora, salivary composition, immunological status, or tooth composition.

Takahara (1952) proposed that acatalasia was inherited as an autosomal recessive trait. People who are homozygous for the disorder have little or no catalase activity (Aebi and Wyss, 1978). Using spectrophotometric methods to determine the catalase activity in red blood cells, Delgado and Calderon (1979) were able to show three phenotypes – acatalasic, hypocatalasic, and normal. All carriers of acatalasia were hypocatalasic. Thirteen hypocatalasemic (carrier) individuals, including both the Peruvian parents, were found among 29 relatives of the probands examined from four generations. No other acatalasemic individuals were found. Hypocatalasic relatives of the probands did not have oral lesions, and no other abnormalities were detected. The parents of the affected children were not known to be related; however, both parents and their families came from the same small rural community. The inheritance pattern in the kindred was compatible with an autosomal recessive mode of inheritance for the disorder (Delgado and Calderon, 1979).

Hypophosphatasia

Hypophosphatasia is a disease complex in which bone fails to mineralize properly. The disease may be primary, or secondary to hypothyroidism, gross anaemia, scurvy, kwashiorkor, achondroplasia, hypothyroidism, or the incorporation of radioactive material in the bone. It is the primary disease that is considered here.

The condition is characterized usually by subnormal serum alkaline phosphatase values, the presence of phosphoethanolamine in plasma and urine, skeletal abnormalities, and premature loss of teeth. The clinical phenotype of hypophosphatasia may be attributed to defects in the formation of either bone or cementum.

At least three clinical forms of primary disease are seen (Fraser, 1957):

1. The infantile type. This is the severest form. There is severe skeletal disease present at birth and the mortality is over 50 per cent.
2. The childhood type. This is a self-limiting disease of moderate severity appearing after 6 months of age.
3. The adult type. This is characterized by the appearance of osteoporosis and bone fragility in early adult life.

A fourth clinical type may exist (Bixler *et al.*, 1974). It is characterized by low serum alkaline phosphatase activity, premature loss of deciduous incisors, and absence of bone lesions. This disorder is much milder than the foregoing types, and the serum enzyme levels, although reduced, are not so low.

The anterior teeth may be shed spontaneously or they may become mobile after relatively minor trauma. There is an absence of severe periodontal inflammation. The teeth most frequently lost are incisors. Occasionally, the dentition may appear to manifest hypereruption and to be loose in the alveolus without the evidence of either classical chronic gingivitis or periodontitis (Baer *et al.*, 1964; Kjellman *et al.*, 1973). Cementum may be completely absent as in Casson's (1969) two cases. When present, the cementum is often very thin or present only in islands.

A male hypophosphatasia patient, reported on both as a child and as an adolescent, is recorded by Watanabe *et al.* (1993). This patient was seen initially because of premature exfoliation of deciduous teeth. He was found to have low serum alkaline phosphatase, high urinary phosphoethanolamine excretion, and hypoplasia of cementum. At 15 years of age he was referred to Watanabe and co-workers with severe periodontal destruction in the permanent dentition. Oral radiographic examination showed a mirror image pattern of bone loss, which was similar to that seen in localized JP. Investigations revealed that he still had low serum alkaline phosphatase activity and high urinary excretion of phosphoethanolamine. The patient had a high antibody titre to *Porphyromonas gingivalis*, and this titre reduced during periodontal treatment. The chemotaxis of neutrophils and monocytes showed no reduction. Analysis of cell-mediated immunity revealed a slight reduction in CD2-, CD3-, and CD4-positive cells and a slight elevation in NK cell activity.

The degree of cementum aplasia in hypophosphatasia is related to the severity of the overall disease itself (Bruckner *et al.*, 1962). In affected persons, even those teeth that are not exfoliated do not have normal amounts of cementum (Beumer *et al.*, 1973). It has also been shown that the PDL fibres may lack an attachment to the cementum and may even run parallel to the root surface (Listgarten and Houpt, 1969). When cementum is absent, the PDL fibres approach, but are not attached to, the dentine.

The basic anomaly appears to lie in the matrix. Fraser and Yendt (1955) showed that the cartilage of rachitic rats would calcify in the serum of patients with hypophosphatasia. However, cartilage from the patients themselves would not calcify in serum from unaffected subjects. The cell membrane of odontoblasts and cementoblasts has been shown to have intense enzyme activity indicative of the presence of alkaline phophatase (Watanabe *et al.*, 1993). Since alkaline phophatase catalyzes matrix formation in bone and cementum, they postulated that a reduction in the production of this enzyme and its activity level is likely to result in hypoplasia and defective mineralization of alveolar bone and cementum.

It has been suggested that, because serum alkaline phosphatase activity represents a mixture of isoenzymes from bone, liver, and intestine, variation in the isoenzymes themselves may help to explain the spectrum of clinical disease (Scriver and Cameron, 1969; Aminoff *et al.*, 1971). Bixler *et al.* (1974) noted electrophoretic variation in the enzymes from one of their families, and the report by Hosenfeld and Hosenfeld (1973) also described isoenzyme electrophoretic variation in this disease complex. In cases of hypophosphatasia, non-specific tissue alkaline phosphatase is known to decrease. Whyte (1989), and Goseki *et al.* (1990) classified hypophosphatasia based on reactivity to monoclonal and polyclonal antibodies to non-specific tissue alkaline phosphatase.

A simple autosomal recessive mode of inheritance has been demonstrated for the various types of hypophosphatasia that show markedly decreased serum alkaline phosphatase activity, increased urinary excretion of phosphoethanolamine, rachitic-like bone diseases, and premature loss of deciduous incisors. Thus, the genetic patterns appear the same for the infantile, childhood, and adult types. This does not mean, however, that there is not heterogeneity within this grouping, and most workers believe there is more than a single type of hypophosphatasia. Indirect support for this comes from the observation that the heterozygous gene carriers in some families have a serum alkaline phosphatase activity that is somewhere between that of the affected and the normal (Glimcher and Krane, 1962). However, numerous other families have not shown this result. A similar problem has been observed when testing heterozygotes for phosphoethanolamine excretion (Harris and Robson, 1959). A tentative interpretation of these results has been non-penetrance, but it seems more likely that there is more than one disease entity in the entire group, all with a recessive mode of inheritance (Polan *et al.*, 1972).

There may also be a dominantly inherited form of hypophosphatasia (Bixler, 1976). Affected individuals have no bone disease, but a lowered serum alkaline phosphatase (not so severe as in the recessive form), and they show premature incisor loss. Bixler (1976) reported no example of non-penetrance, and the clinical picture was remarkably consistent. The presence of two genetic forms of hypophosphatasia, one recessive and the other dominant, makes it clear that at least two genes are involved in this disease complex, and the variability in clinical phenotype of the recessive form suggests additional genes, allelic or otherwise.

SKIN DISEASES

Hyperkeratosis palmoplantaris and periodontoclasia in childhood (Papillon–Lefèvre syndrome)

This syndrome is characterized by hyperkeratosis of the palms and soles with premature destruction of the PDL of deciduous and permanent teeth, resulting in their early loss (Gorlin *et al.*, 1964; Carvel, 1969). Following normal eruption of deciduous teeth, the gingivae become red and swollen and bleed easily. At about the same time, the palmoplantar hyperkeratosis usually begins to appear. With the full eruption of the second deciduous molars, destruction of PDL is noted. Deep periodontal pockets are formed, and these exude pus on pressure. Marked halitosis may be noted. The teeth become mobile, and radiographs show marked destruction of the supporting alveolar bone. By 4–5 years of age, the teeth are exfoliated, often in a sequence similar to that in which they erupted. The gingival inflammation resolves with the loss of the deciduous teeth. A similar process begins with the commencement of eruption of permanent teeth, although the symptoms may be more marked. By about 15 years of age, all permanent teeth except the third molars have usually been shed. When all permanent teeth are lost, the gingival tissue resumes its normal appearance (Carvel, 1969; Sedano *et al.*, 1977)

Willett *et al.* (1985) reported a patient in whom the palmoplantar keratosis appeared at the expected age but in whom the periodontal destruction was delayed and was less severe than in previously reported cases of Papillon–Lefèvre syndrome. Three further cases have been described by Brown *et al.* (1993) in which the periodontal lesions were relatively mild and in which both the palmoplantar lesions and the periodontal lesions were of late onset, occurring at approximately 20–30 years of age. Thus, there may well be a late-onset variant of the syndrome, although Brown *et al.* (1993) were unable to exclude the alternative explanation of a combination of early onset periodontitis and a form of palmoplantar keratoderma.

Other variants of Papillon–Lefèvre syndrome with mild periodontal symptoms but normal time of onset have been described by Lyberg (1982), Schroeder *et al.* (1983), and Preus and Morland (1987).

The reports on the immune status of different Papillon–Lefèvre syndrome patients have varied, with findings of both normal and deficient function in regard to neutrophil chemotactic, phagocytic, and bactericidal activity. Thus, Djawari (1978) found a marked decrease in neutrophil chemotactic, phagocytic, and bactericidal activity in an adolescent patient who had Papillon–Lefèvre syndrome with severe periodontal disease. Defective neutrophil chemotaxis in Papillon–Lefèvre syndrome, similar to that found in localized JP, was reported by Genco and Slots (1984) and by Slots and Genco (1984). However, Shams El Din *et al.* (1984) had a 15-year-old Papillon–Lefèvre syndrome patient with severe periodontal disease and normal neutrophil chemotaxis and phagocytosis but decreased bactericidal activity. The patient of Tinanoff *et al.* (1990) is interesting; they report a change of neutrophil function from defective to normal following full mouth extractions.

The relationship between immune status and severity of periodontal disease in Papillon–Lefèvre syndrome may parallel that in localized JP. A locally mediated immune impairment related to specific periodontal bacteria is suggested by Bimstein *et al.* (1990) and supported by Brown *et al.* (1993).

Gorlin *et al.* (1964) consider this condition to be an autosomal recessive trait, and they have estimated the frequency of the condition to be approximately 1 in 1,000,000. A prevalence of 1–4 per million population is suggested by Verma *et al.* (1979). The pedigrees of the three cases presented by Brown *et al.* (1993) are compatible with autosomal recessive inheritance.

There are several syndromes characterized by palmoplantar hyperkeratosis, but the Papillon–Lefèvre is the only one with precocious periodontal destruction. Histologically, the PDL is destroyed and replaced by chronic granulation tissue. There is considerable osteoclastic activity in the ligament. The cementum, along most of the root surface, is very thin except in the apical area, where some cellular cementum may be present (Martinez Lalis *et al.*, 1965). Using disc electrophoresis, Shoshan *et al.* (1970) compared collagen from clinically healthy young people with that of a 14-year-old patient with Papillon–Lefèvre syndrome. They postulated that the periodontal involvement may result from a functional imbalance of collagenolytic activity in the PDL.

REFERENCES

Aebi HE and Wyss SR (1978) Acatalasemia. In: The Metabolic Basis of Inherited Disease, 4th edition (Stanbury JB, Wyngarden IB and Frederickson DS, eds), pp 1792–1807, McGraw–Hill, New York.

Aminoff D, Austrins M and Zolfaghari SP (1971) Plasma alkaline phosphatase isozymes: isolation and characterisation of isozymes. Biochim Biophys Acta 242, 108–122.

Baer PN (1971) The case for periodontosis as a clinical entity. J Periodont 42, 516– 520.

Baer PN, Brown NC and Hamner JE (1964) Hypophosphatasia: report of two cases with dental findings. Periodontics 2, 209–215.

Baer PN and Gamble JW (1966) Autogenous dental transplants as a method of treating the osseous defect in periodontosis. Oral Surg 22, 405–410.

Baer PN and Lieberman JE (1959) Observations on some genetic characteristics of the periodontium in three strains of inbred mice. Oral Surg 12, 820–829.

Baker DL and Seymour GL (1976) The possible pathogenesis of gingival recession. J Clin Periodontol 3, 208–219.

Barabas GM (1969) The Ehlers–Danlos Syndrome. Abnormalities of the enamel, dentine, cementum and the dental pulp: an histological examination of 13 teeth from 6 patients. Br Dent J 126, 509–515.

Barros L and Witkop CJ (1963) Oral and genetic study of Chileans. 1960. III. Periodontal disease and nutritional factors. Arch Oral Biol 8, 195–206.

Beaty TH, Boughman JJ, Yang P, Astemborski JA and Suzuki JB (1987) Genetic analysis of juvenile priodontitis in families ascertained through an affected proband. Am J Hum Genet 40, 443.

Benjamin SD and Baer PN (1967) Familial patterns of advanced alveolar bone loss in adolescence (periodontosis). Periodontics 5, 82–88.

Berry AC (1978) Anthropological and family studies on minor variants of the dental crown. In: Development, Function and Evolution of Teeth (Butler PM and Josey KA, eds), pp 81–96, Academic Press, London.

Beumer J, Trowbridge HO, Silverman S and Eisenberg E (1973) Childhood hypophosphatasia and premature loss of teeth. Oral Surg 35, 631–640.

Bimstein E, Lustmann J, Sela MN, Neria ZB and Sosklne WA (1990) Periodontitis associated with Papillon–Lefèvre syndrome. J Periodontol 61, 373–377.

Bissada NF and Abdelmalek RG (1973) Incidence of cervical enamel projections and its relationship to furcation involvement in Egyptian skulls. J Periodont 44, 583–585.

Bixler D (1976) Heritable disorders affecting cementum and the periodontal structure. In: Oral Facial Genetics (Stewart RE and Prescott GE, eds), pp 262–287, Mosby, St Louis.

Bixler D (1987) Genetic aspects of dental anomalies. In: Dentistry for the Child and Adolescent (McDonald RE and Avenry DR, eds), p 108, Mosby, St Louis.

Bixler D, Poland CP, Brandt IK and Nicholas NJ (1974) Autosomal dominant hypophophatasia without skeletal disease. American Society of Human Genetics, 26th Annual Meeting, Portland, Oregan.

Borring-Møller G and Frandsen A (1978) Autolongous tooth transplantation to replace molars lost in patients with juvenile periodontitis. J Clin Periodont 5, 152–158.

Boughman JA, Beatty TH, Yang P, Goodman SB, Wooten RK and Suzuki JB (1988). Problems of genetic model testing in elary onset periodontitis. J Periodontol 59, 332–337.

Boughman JA, Halloran SL, Roulston D, *et al.* (1986) An autosomal-dominant form of juvenile periodontitis: Its localisation to chromosome 4 and linkage to dentiogenesis imperfect and Gc. J Craniofac Genet and Dev Biol 6, 341.

Boyde A and Jones SH (1972) Scanning electron microscopic studies of the formation of mineralised tissues. In: Developmental Aspects of Oral Biology (Slavkin HC and Bavetta LA, eds), pp 261–263, Academic Press, New York.

Brathall W and Björklander J (1980) Bacteria and oral fluid components: Report of the oral condition in hypogammaglobulinaemic patients. In: The Borderland between Caries and Periodontal Disease, 2nd edition, pp 159–173 (Lehner T and Cimasoni G, eds), Academic Press, London.

Brook AH and Winter GB (1970) Double teeth. A retrospective study of 'geminated' and 'fused' teeth in children. Br Dent J 129, 123–130.

Brown RH (1978) A longitudinal study of periodontal disease in Down's syndrome. NZ Dent J 74, 137–144.

Brown RS, Hays GL, Flaitz CM, O'Neill PA, Abramovitch K and White RR (1993) A possible late onset variation of Papillon–Lefèvre syndrome: report of 3 cases. J Periodontol 64, 379–386.

Bruckener RJ, Rickles NH and Porter DR (1962) Hypophosphatasia with premature shedding of teeth and aplasia of cementum. Oral Surg 15, 1351–1359.

Budtz-Jorgensen E, Ellegaard J, Ellegaard B, Jorgensen F and Kelstrup J (1978) Cell mediated immunity in juvenile periodontitis and levamisole treatment. Scand J Dent Res 86, 124–129.

Butler JH (1969) A familial pattern of juvenile periodontitis (periodontosis). J Periodontol 40, 115–118.

Byers PH and Holbrook KA (1990) Ehlers–Danlos syndrome. In: Principles and Practice of Medical Genetics, Chapter 63, pp 1065–1081 (Emery AE and Rimoin DL, eds), Churchill Livingstone, Edinburgh.

Carmichael AF (1969) The distribution of ABO blood groups in cases of periodontal disease. Dent Mag (London) 82, 225–257.

Carvel RI (1969) Palmar–plantar hyperkeratosis and premature periodontal destruction. J Oral Med 24, 73–82.

Casson M (1969) Oral manifestations of primary hypophosphatasia. Br Dent J 127, 561–566.

Cawson RA (1962) The oral changes in gargoylism. Proc R Soc Med 55, 1066–1077.

Chung CS, Runck DW, Niswander JD, Bilben S E and Kau MCW (1970) Genetic and epidemiologic studies of oral characteristics in Hawaii's school children. I. Caries and periodontal disease. J Dent Res 49, 1374–1385.

Cianciola L, Genco RJ, Patters MR, Mckenna I and van Oss CJ (1977) Defective polymorphonuclear leukocyte function in a human periodontal disease. Nature 265, 445–447.

Clark RA, Page RC and Wilde G (1977) Defective neutrophil chemotaxis in juvenile periodontitis. Infect Immun 18, 694–700.

Cogen RB, Roseman JH, Al-Goburi W, *et al.* (1986) Host factors in juvenile periodontitis. J Dent Res 65, 394–399.

Cogen RB, Wright JT and Tate AL (1992) Destructive periodontal disease in healthy children. J Periodontol 63, 761–765.

Cohen DW and Goldman HM (1960) Clinical observations on the modification of human oral tissue metabolism by local intraoral factors. Ann NY Acad Sci 85, 68–95.

Cohen MM (1960) Periodontal disturbances in the mentally subnormal child. Dent Clin N Amer, 483–489.

Cohen MM, Winer RA, Schwartz S and Shklar, G (1961) Oral aspects of Mongolism. part 1. Periodontal disease in Mongolism. Oral Surg 14, 92–107.

Cullinan MP, Sachs G, Wolf E and Seymour GJ (1980) The distribution of HLA-A and B antigens in patients and their families with periodontitis. J Periodont Res 15, 177–184.

Cutress TW, Brown RH and Guy E (1970) Occurrence of some bacterial species in dental plaque of trisomic 21 (mongoloid), other mentally retarded and normal subjects. NZ Dent J 6, 40–45.

de Grouchy G and Turleau C (1990) Autosomal disorders. In: Principles and Practice of Medical Genetics, Chapter 18, pp 252–256 (Emery AE and Rimoin WL, eds), Churchill Livingstone, Edinburgh.

Delgado WA and Calderon R (1979) Acatalasia in two Peruvian siblings. Oral Path 8, 358–368.

Di Biase DD (1971) The effects of variation in tooth morphology and position on eruption. Dent Practr 22, 95–108.

Di Biase DD (1976) Dental abnormalities affecting eruption. In: The Eruption and Occlusion of Teeth (Poole DFG and Stack MV, eds), pp 156–168, Butterworths, London.

Djawari D (1978) Deficient phagocytic function in Papillon–Lefèvre syndrome. J Clin Periodontol 156, 189–192.

Dow RS (1951) A preliminary study of periodontoclasia in Mongolian children at Polk State School. Am J Ment Defic 55, 535–538.

Duckworth R (1962) Abnormal attachment of labial mucosa in maleruption of teeth. Br Dent J 113, 312–314.

Engström GN, Engström P, Hammarstrom L and Edvard Smith CI (1992) Oral conditions in individuals with selective immunoglobulin A deficiency and common variable immunodeficiency. J Periodontol 63, 984–989.

Everett FG and Kramer GM (1972) The distolingual groove in the maxillary lateral incisor: a periodontal hazard. J Periodontol 43, 352–361.

Fourel J (1972) Periodontosis: a periodontal syndrome. J Periodontol 43, 240–255.

Frandsen A (1978) Personal communication cited by Saxén (1980).

Fraser D (1957) Hypophosphatasia. Am J Med 22, 730–746.

Fraser D and Yendt ER (1955) Metabolic abnormalities in hypophosphatasia Am J Dis Child 90, 552–554.

Friedman SA, Farber PA and Salkin LM (1976) Histopathology of juvenile periodontitis. I. Surface morphology of inflammatory cells. J Dent Res 55, B259 (abstract).

Genco RJ and Slots J (1984) Host responses in periodontal disease. J Dent Res 63, 441–451.

Genco RJ, van Dyke TE, Levine MJ, Nelson RD and Wilson ME (1986). Molecular factors influeince neutrophil defects in periodontal disease. J Dent Res 65, 1379–1391.

Gher M and Vernino A (1980) Root morphology: clinical significance in pathogenesis and treatment of periodontal disease. J Am Dent Assoc 101, 627.

Glimcher MJ and Krane SM (1962) Studies of the interactions of collagen and phosphate. I. The nature of inorganic and organophosphate binding. In: Radiosotopes and Bone (Lacroix P and Budy AM, eds), pp 393–418, Blackwell, Oxford.

Goodman RM and Gorlin, RJ (1977) Atlas of the Face in Genetic Disorders, pp 17–18. St Louis, Mosby.

Gorlin RJ (1976) Heritable mycocutaneous disorders. In: Oral Facial Genetics. (Stewart RE and Prescott GH, eds), pp 338–384, Mosby, St Louis.

Gorlin RJ, Pindborg JJ and Cohen MM (1976) Syndromes of the Head and Neck. McGraw–Hill, New York.

Gorlin RJ, Sedano H and Anderson VE (1964) The syndrome of palmar–plantar hyperkeratosis and premature periodontal destruction of the teeth J Pediatr 65, 895–908.

Gorlin RJ, Stallard RE and Shapiro BL (1967) Genetics and periodontal disease. J Periodontol 38, 5–10.

Goseki M, Oida S, Takagi Y, Okuyama T, Watanabe J and Sasaki S (1990) Immunological study on hypophosphatasia. Clin Chim Acta 190, 263–268.

Grant DA, Stern IB and Listgarten MA (1988) Periodontics, 6th edition, p460–461, Mosby, St Louis.

Gunsolley JC, Tew JG, Gooss CM, Burmeister JA and Schenkein HA (1988) Effects of race and periodontal status on antibody reactive with *Actinobacillus actinomycetemcomitans* strain Y4. J Periodont Res 23, 308–312.

Gunsolley JC, Tew JG, Conner T, Burmeister JA, Schenkein HA (1991) Relationship between race and antibody reactive with periodontitis associated bacteria. J Periodont Res 26, 59–63.

Hamner JE, Witkop CJ and Metro PS (1964) Taurodontism, report of a case. Oral Surg 18, 409–418.

Harley AF and Floyd PD (1988) Prevelance of juvenile periodontitis in school-children in Lagos, Nigeria. Commun Dent Oral Epidemiol 16, 299.

Harris H and Robson EB (1959) A genetical study of ethanolamine phosphate excretion in hypophosphatasia. Ann Hum Genet 23, 421–441.

Hart TC, Marazita ML, Gunsolley JA, Schenkein HA and Diehl SR (1991) No female preponderance in juvenile periodontitis after correction for ascertainment bias. J Periodont 62, 745.

Hart TC, Marazita ML, Schenkien HA and Diehl SR (1992) Re-interpretation of the evidence for X-linked dominant inheritance of juvenile periodontitis. J Periodont 63, 169–173.

Holt RD F(1976) The prevalence of root anomalies in children. MSc dissertation, University of London.

Holt RD and Brook AH (1979) Taurodontism: a criterion for diagnosis and its prevalence in mandibular first molars in a sample of 1,115 British school children. J Int Assoc Dent Child 10, 41–47.

Hosenfeld D and Hosenfeld A (1973) Qualitative and quantative examinations of the isoenzymes of serum alkaline phosphate in hypophosphatasia. Klin Pädiatr 185, 437–443.

Howard RD (1966) The unerupted incisor. Trans Br Soc Study Orthod 30–40.

Jacobson L, Svärdström G and Danielsson D (1978) Post juvenile periodontitis. Immunological screen of 30 patients. Swed Dent J 2, 209–212.

Johnson NP and Young MA (1963) Periodontal disease in mongols. J Periodontol 34, 41–47.

Johnson WP (1969) Treatment of palatally impacted canine teeth. Am J Orthodont 56, 589–596.

Jorgenson RJ, Levin LS, Hutcherson ST and Salinas CF (1975) Periodontosis in sibs. Oral Surg 39, 396–402.

Kaslick RS, West TL and Chasens AI (1980) Association between ABO blood groups, HL-A antigens and periodontal diseases in young adults: a follow-up study. J Periodont 51, 339–342.

Kaslick RS, West TL, Chasens AI, Terasaki PI, Lazzara R and Weinberg S (1975) Association between HL-A2 antigen and various periodontal diseases in young adults. J Dent Res 54, 424.

Keith A (1913) Problems relating to the teeth of the earlier forms of prehistoric man. Proc R Soc Med 6, 103–119.

Kerr DA (1961) The cementum: its role in periodontal health and disease. J Periodontol 32, 183–189.

Kirkham LB (1977) Periodontosis – general discussion and report of familial cases. J Wisconsin Dent Assoc 53, 347–349.

Kisling E and Krebs G (1963) Periodontal conditions in adult patients with Mongolism (Down's syndrome). Acta Odont Scand 21, 391–405.

Kjellman M, Oldfelt V, Nordenram A and Olow-Nordenram M (1973) Five cases of hypophophatasia with dental findings. Int J Oral Surg 2, 152–158.

Kogan S (1986) The prevalence, location and conformation of palato-radicular grooves in maxillary incisors. J Periodontol 57, 231.

Lavine WS, Maderazo EG, Stolman J, *et al.* (1979) Impaired neutrophil chemotaxis in patients with juvenile and rapidly progressing periodontitis. J Periodont Res 14, 10–19.

Lee KW, Lee EC and Poon KY (1968) Palatogingival grooves in maxillary incisors. Br Dent J 124, 14–18.

Legum CP, Schorr S and Berman ER (1976) The genetic mucopolysaccharidoses and mucolipidoses: review and comment. Adv Pediatr 22, 305–347.

Lehner T, Wilton JMA, Ivanyi L and Manson JD (1974) Immunological aspects of juvenile periodontitis (periodontosis). J Periodont Res 9, 261–272.

Leib AM, Berdo JK and Sabes WR (1967) Furcation involvements correlated with enamel projections from the cementoenamel junction. J Periodont 38, 330–334.

Liljenberg B and Lindhe J (1980) Juvenile periodontitis. Some microbiological, histopathological and clinical characteristics. J Clin Periodont 7, 48–61.

Listgraten MA and Houpt M (1969) Ultrastructural features of the root surface of deciduous teeth in patients with hypophophatasia. J Periodont Res 4 (suppl), 34–35.

Löe H and Brown LJ (1991) Early onset periodontitis in the United States of America. J Periodontol 62, 608–616.

Long JC, Nance WE, Waring P, Burmeister JA and Ranney RR (1987) Early onset periodontitis: A comparison and evaluation of two proposed modes of inheritance. Genet Epidemiol 4, 13.

Lyberg T (1982) Immunological and metabolic studies in two siblings with Papillon–Lefèvre syndrome. J Periodont Res 17, 563–568.

Malena DE (1972) ABO phenotypes and periodontal disease. J Dent Res 51, 1504.

Manson JD (1977) Juvenile periodontitis (periodontosis). Int Dent J 27, 114–118.

Manson JD and Lehner T (1974) Clinical features of juvenile periodontitis (periodontosis). J Periodontol 45, 636–640.

Martinez Lalis RR, Lopez Otero R and Carranza FA (1965) A case of Papillon–Lefèvre syndrome. Periodontics 3, 292–295.

Masters DH and Hoskins SW (1964) Projections of cervical enamel into molar furcations. J Periodontol 35, 48–53.

McMillan RS and Kashgarian M (1961) Relation of human abnormalities of structure and function to abnormalities of the dentition. II. Mongolism. J Am Dent Assoc 63, 368–373.

Melnick M, Shields ED and Bixler D (1976) Periodontosis: a phenotypic and genetic analysis. Oral Surg 42, 32–41.

Michalowicz BS, Aeppli D, Virag JG (1991) Periodontal findings in adult twins. J Periodontol 62, 293–299.

Mühlemann HR (1972) Karies und Parodontopathien beim Menschen in genetischen Sicht. Schweiz Monatschr Zahnheilk 82, 942–959.

Nisengard RJ, Myers D and Newman MG (1977) Human antibody titres to periodontosis – associated microbiota. J Dent Res 56, A73 (abs.).

Niswander JD (1975) Genetics of common dental disorders. Dent Clin North Am 19 197–206.

Ochsenbein C and Ross S (1973) A concept of osseous surgery and its clinical application. In: A Periodontal Point of View (Ward HL and Chas CT, eds), chapter 13, Charles C Thomas, Springfield, Illinois.

Oehlers FAC (1958) The radicular variety of dens invaginatus. Oral Surg 11, 1251–1260.

Olsson M and Lindhe J (1991) Periodontal characteristics in individuals with varying form of the upper central incisors. J Clin Periodontol 18, 78–82.

Olsson M, Lindhe J and Marinello CP (1993) On the relationship between crown form and clinical features of the gingiva in adolescents. J Clin Periodontol 20, 570–577.

Peterson RJ and Marsh CL (1979) The relationship of alpha-antitrypsin to inflammatory periodontal disease. J Periodont 50, 31–35.

Poland CP, Eversole LR, Bixler D and Christian JC (1972) Histochemical observations of hypophosphatasia. J Dent Res 51, 333–338.

Polevitzky K (1929) Blood types in pyorrhoea alvelaris. J Dent Res 9, 285 (abs.).

Potter RH (1989). Etiology of periodontitis: The heterogeneity paradigm (Guest Editorial). J Periodontol 60, 593–597.

Potter RH (1990) Genetic studies of juvenile periodontitis. J Dent Res 69, 94–95.

Pradhan AC, Chawla TN, Samuel KC and Pradhan S (1971) The relationship between periodontal disease and blood groups and secretor status. J Periodont Res 6, 294–300.

Preus HR and Morland B (1987) *In vitro* studies of monocyte function in two siblings with Papillon–Lefèvre syndrome. Scand J Dent Res 95, 59–64.

Rao SS and Tewani SV (1968) Prevalence of periodontosis among Indians. J Periodontol 39, 27–34.
Reich T, Rice J, Cloninger CR, Wette R and James J (1979) The use of multiple thresholds and segregation analysis in analysing phenotypic heterogeneity of multifactorial traits. Ann Hum Genet 42, 371–390.
Reinholdt J, Bay I and Svejgaard A (1977) Association between HLA-antigens and periodontal disease. J Dent Res 56, 1216–1263.
Reisel JH (1971) Clinical osteoporosis and periodontal disease. Ned Tijdschr Tandheelkd 78, 132–135.
Robertson PB and Cooper MD (1974) Oral manifestations of IgA deficiency. Adv Exp Med Biol 45, 497–503.
Robertson PB, Mackler BF, Wright TE and Levy BM (1980) Periodontal status of patients with abnormalities of the immune system. Observations over a 2-year period. J Periodontol 51, 70–73.
Robertson PB, Wright TE III, Mackler BF, Lenertz DM, Levy BM 1978 Periodontal status of patient with abnormalities of the immune system. J Periodont Res 13, 37–45.
Rosen FS, Wedgewood RJ, Aiuiti F, *et al.* (1983) Meeting report. Primary immunodeficiency disease. Report for the WHO by scientific group on immunodeficieny. Clin Immunol Immunopathol 28, 450–475.
Rushton MA (1957) Hereditary or idiopathic hyperplasia of the gums. Dent Practit 7, 136–146.
Sauk JJ (1980) Defects of the teeth and tooth-bearing structures. In: Textbook of Pediatric Dentistry (Braham RL and Morris ME, eds), pp 57–83, Williams and Wilkins, Baltimore.
Saxby MS (1987) Juvenile peridontitis: an epidemiological study in the West Midlands of the United Kingdom. J Clin Periodontol 14, 594.
Saxen L (1980a) Heredity of juvenile periodontitis. J Clin Periodontol 7, 276.
Saxen L (1980b) Juvenile periodontitis: a review. J Clin Periodontol 7, 1–19.
Saxen L and Nevanlinna HR (1984) Autosomal recessive inheritance of juvenile periodontitis. Test of a hypothesis. Clin Genet 25, 332–335.
Schenkein HA, Best AM, Gunsolley JC (1991) The influence of race and periodontal clinical status on neutrophil chemotactic responses. J Periodont Res 26, 272–275.
Schenkein HA, Burmeister JA, Koertge TE, *et al.* (1993) The influence of race and gender on periodontal microflora. J Periodontol 64, 292–296.
Schluger S, Yuodelis RA and Page R (1977) Periodontal Disease, 1st edition, pp 513–515, Lea and Febiger, Philadelphia.
Schroeder HE, Seger RA, Keller HU and Rateitschak-Pluss EM (1983) Behaviour of neutrophils granulcytes in a case of Papillon–Lefèvre syndrome. J Clin Periodontol 10, 618–635.
Scriver CR and Cameron D (1969) Pseudohypophosphatasia. N Engl J Med 281, 604–606.
Sedano HO, Sauk GG and Gorlin RJ (1977) Oral Manifestations of Inherited Disorders, pp 168, 191 and 194–195, Butterworths, Boston.
Seibert JS (1973) Surgical management of osseous defects. In: Periodontal Therapy, 5th edition (Goldman HM and Cohen DW, eds), pp 765–766, Mosby, St Louis.
Seibert J and Lindhe J (1989) Esthetics and periodontal therapy. In: Textbook of Clinical Periodontology, 2nd edition (Lindhe J, ed), chapter 19, pp. 477–514, Munksgaard, Copenhagen.
Shams El Dim A, Benton FR, Bottomley WK, *et al.* (1984) Hyperkeratosis, periodontosis, and chronic pyogenic infections in a 15 year old boy. Ann Allergy 53, 11–14, 55–56.
Shiloah J and Kopczyk RA (1979) Developmental variations of tooth morphology and periodontal disease. J Am Dent Assoc 99, 627–630.
Shoshan S, Finkelstein S and Rosenweig KA (1970) Disc electrophoretic pattern of gingival collagen isolated from a patient with palmar–planter hyperkeratosis. J Periodont Res 5, 255–258.
Slots J (1976) The predominant cultivable organisms in juvenile periodontitis. Scand J Dent Res 84, 1–10.
Slots J and Genco RJ (1984) Black pigmented *Bacteroides* species, *Capnocytophaga* species, and *Actinobaccillus actinomycetomcomitans* in human periodontal disease: Virulence factors in colonization, survival and tissue destruction. J Dent Res 64, 412– 421.
Smith C (1976) Statistical Resolution of Genetic Heterogeneity in Familial Disease. Ann Hum Genet 39, 281–291.
Sobel AE, Strazzulla M, Sherman BS, *et al.* (1958) Vitamin A absorption and other blood composition studies in Mongolism. Am J Ment Defic 62, 642–655.
Stewart RE, Hollister DW and Rimoin DL (1977) A new variant of the Ehlers–Danlos syndrome: an autosomal dominant disorder of fragile skin, abnormal scarring and generalised periodontitis. Birth Defects 13(3B), 85–93.
Sussman HI and Baer PN (1978) Three generations of periodontosis: Case report. Ann Dent 37, 8–11.
Swallow JN (1964) Dental disease in children with Down's syndrome. J Ment Defic Res 8, 102–118.
Sznajder N, Carraro JJ, Otero E and Carranza FA(1968) Clinical periodontal findings in trisomy 21 (Mongolism). J Periodont Res 3, 1–5.
Takahara S (1952) Progressive oral gangrene probably due to lack of catalase in the blood (acatalasemia). Report of nine cases. Lancet 2, 1101–1104.
Tinanoff N, Tanzer JM, Kornman KS and Maderazo EG (1990) Treatment of the periodontal component of Papillon–Lefèvre syndrome: A case report. J Clin Periodontol 61, 373–377.
Tollefsen T, Saltvedt E and Koppang HS (1978) The effect of immunosuppressive agents on periodontal disease in man. J Periodont Res 13, 240–250.
Tsunemitsu A, Honjo K, Kani M and Matsumura T (1964) Citric acid metabolism in periodontosis. Arch Oral Biol 9, 83–86.
van Dyke TE, Horoszeqicz HU, Cianciola LJ and Genco RJ (1980) Neutrophil chemotaxis dysfunction in human periodontitis. Infect Immun 27, 124–132.
van Dyke TE, Schweinebraten M, Cianciola LJ, Offenbacher S and Genco RJ (1985) Neutrophil chemotaxis in families with localised juvenile periodontitis. J Periodont Res 1985. 20, 503.
van Swol RL, Gross A, Setterstrom JA and D'alessandro SM (1980) Concentrations of immunoglobulins in granulation tissue from pockets of periodontosis and periodontitis patients. J Periodontol 51, 20–24.
Verma K, Chadda M and Joshi R (1979) Papillon–Lefèvre syndrome. Int J Dermatol 18, 146–149.
Watanabe H, Umeda M, Seki T and Ishikawa I (1993) Clinical and laboratory studies of severe periodontal disease in an adolescent associated with hypophosphatasia: A case report. J Periodontol 64, 174–180.
Wennstrom J, Lindhe J and Nyman S (1982) The role of keratinized gingiva in plaque-associated gingivitis in dogs. J Clin Periodontol 9, 75–85.
Wheeler RC (1961) Complete crown form and the periodontium. J Prosthet Dent 11, 722–734.
Whyte MP (1989) Alkaline phosphatase, physiological role explored in hypophosphatasia. Bone Miner Res 6, 175–218.
Willet L, Gabriel S, Kozma C and Bottomley W (1985) Papillon–Lefèvre: Rreport of a case. J Oral Med 40, 43–45.
Withers J, Brunsvold M, Killoy W and Rahe A (1981) The relationship of palato-gingival grooves to localised periodontal disease. J Periodontolol 52, 41.
Witkop CJ (1975) Hereditary defects of dentin. Dent Clin North Am 19, 25–45.
Witkop CJ, Maclean CJ and Schmidt PJ (1966) Medical and dental findings in the Brandywine isolate. Ala J Med Sci 3, 382–403.
Zimmerman BR and Baker WA (1960) Effect of geographic location and race on gingival disease in children. J Am Dent Assoc 51, 542–547.

Chapter 14

Infection and the Periodontal Ligament

HN Newman, SJ Challacombe

INTRODUCTION

To many periodontologists, the term 'periodontal disease' is synonymous with chronic inflammatory periodontal disease. Even when the inflammatory aspects attributable to infection are considered more fully, it is common to find a lack of coordination between studies of changes in periapical and lateral portions of the periodontal ligament (PDL). This chapter considers features of both lateral and periapical PDL consequent upon acute and chronic infection. Discussion of more esoteric oral infections is limited to the sparse information concerning PDL involvement by these conditions. Changes due to trauma-induced inflammation are considered in Chapter 15. Gingival changes are omitted, except where they relate to the transitional stages between gingivitis and periodontitis. As will become apparent, surprisingly few new data have surfaced in the last few years concerning the pathology of the PDL in infectious inflammatory periodontal diseases, compared with our knowledge of gingival changes in the same diseases.

LATERAL PERIODONTITIS

CHRONIC INFLAMMATORY PERIODONTAL DISEASES

The general features of these, the most widespread group of human diseases, resemble those of other long-term chronic inflammatory diseases affecting connective tissue (Page and Schroeder, 1976). The lack of research on PDL changes in chronic inflammatory periodontal diseases (CIPD) is surprising when one considers that these are responsible for much tooth loss in adult life. At the present time, it is not clear which factors determine the transition from chronic gingivitis to chronic periodontitis, or the rate of progression of periodontitis. Furthermore, mechanisms of PDL destruction have to be deduced from studies of changes in gingival connective tissue, for most of the research has concentrated on the early stages of disease.

Chronic inflammatory periodontal diseases are neither linear nor continuous in their rates of progression. Periods of quiescence, and even of acute exacerbation with abscess formation, occur (Page and Schroeder, 1976). And we remain unable to distinguish between established lesions that will remain stable and those that will advance, slowly or rapidly.

The change from chronic gingivitis to chronic periodontitis may be said to occur when the alveolar crest collagen fibres are replaced by inflammatory exudate (Goldman, 1957a,b; Heijl *et al.*, 1976). How soon after the onset of chronic gingivitis PDL changes occur in humans has not been determined. One experiment, in dogs fed a soft diet, suggested that significant loss of fibre attachment takes place after about 6 months in relation to molars, and in premolars and incisors after about 8 months (Lindhe *et al.*, 1973).

Tissue damage proceeds from the gingival connective tissue until the transseptal fibres are involved. Until recently, it was thought that the main body of the ligament showed little inflammatory change throughout the disease process (Warwick James and Counsell, 1927; Wade, 1965). Recent histological findings (Moskow and Polson, 1991) make it clear, however, that the inflammatory infiltrate can involve the ligament extensively, apical to the zone of actual ligament destruction. The principal alteration is progressive ligament destruction spreading apically from its coronal periphery. The alveolar bone seems to show more dramatic changes than the PDL (Warwick James and Counsell, 1927). The ligament fibres initially lose their attachment to bone and then to cementum (*Figs 14.1, 14.2, 14.3*). If occlusal trauma is a complication (see Chapter 15), the ligament may be involved before the bone (Macapanpan and Weinmann, 1954).

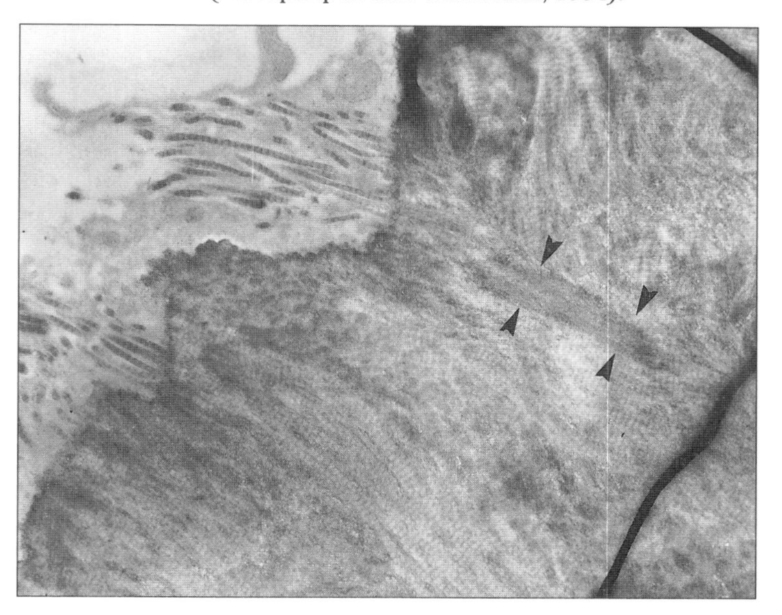

Fig. 14.1 Transmission electron micrograph showing extensive destruction of the fibre attachment to cementum. Only a few collagen fibres remain attached to the hard tissue. The matrix fibrils, which are mostly arranged in the plane of the section, exhibit the cross-banding of collagen. In one area, however, the cross-banding is absent (between the arrows). (Magnification × 14 000.) (From Selvig, 1968.)

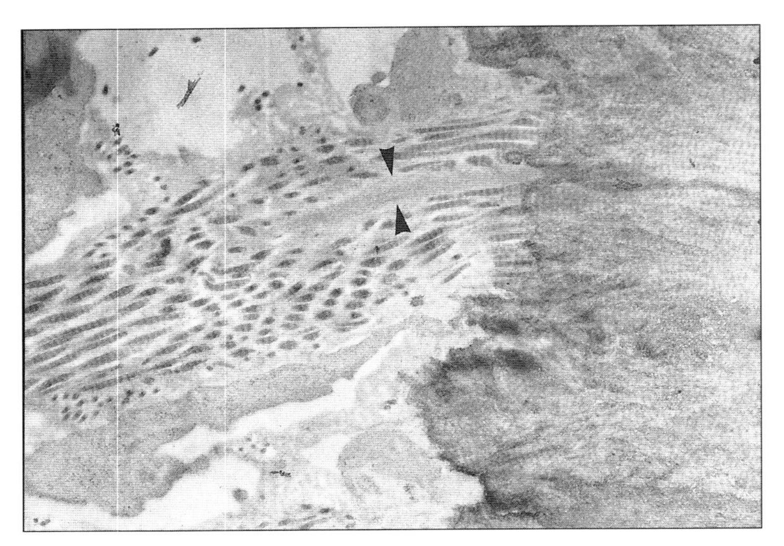

Fig. 14.2 Transmission electron micrograph of an area similar to that seen in *Fig. 14.1*. A bundle of fine, non-banded filaments is located within a collagen fibre (between the arrows). Cross-banding is present in the embedded portion of the filamentous structure. (Magnification × 14 000.) (From Selvig, 1968.)

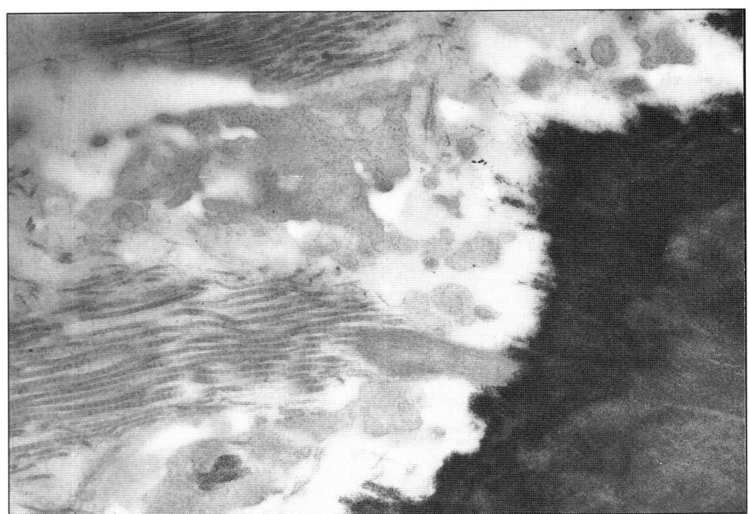

Fig. 14.3 Transmission electron micrograph showing extensive altered PDL. Only a bundle of filaments remains attached to the cementum in this area. This bundle appears to be continuous with the bundle of collagen fibrils. The periodicity of collagen is faintly visible in the embedded portion of this and other matrix fibrils. (Magnification × 14 000.) (From Selvig, 1968.)

The first part of the PDL to be involved is its interdental portion (Melcher, 1962). Resorption of interdental bone results in contact being established between contiguous ligament fibres that were previously inserted into the intervening bone. In this way, the destroyed transseptal fibres are replaced more apically, a state of affairs that persists throughout the disease process. Some of the fibres extend not simply between adjacent tooth surfaces at the same level, but from the depths of bony craters across the residual alveolar crest into the adjacent tooth cementum. This persistent transseptal fibre layer is usually densely fibrous, and it is infiltrated by small numbers of chronic inflammatory cells. It is thought to assist in walling off noxious matter from the deeper tissues (Garant, 1976). With the progression of the disease (in gnotobiotic rats), osteoclasts accumulate in the remains of the transseptal fibres, sometimes in dense groups (Irving *et al.*, 1974). Eventually this fibrous zone extends around the tooth, the bands of fibrous tissue being separated by zones of inflammatory cells (Weinmann, 1941; Fullmer, 1961; Ruben *et al.*, 1970). Fullmer (1961) observed that the initial degradation of PDL collagen occurred in regions away from the inflammatory focus.

PDL changes appear generally some distance ahead of the advancing plaque, owing to a lack of bacterial invasion and the probable diffusion of acellular toxic matter into the tissues (Newman, 1976). There is no evidence that CIPD is due to bacterial invasion. It is rare to find micro-organisms in the tissues, other than in the superficial epithelium, in disease, and all stages of tissue breakdown may be observed in the absence of whole bacterial cells (Liakoni *et al.*, 1987a,b). This applies whether dealing with moderate or advanced routine chronic adult periodontitis, or with rapidly progressive forms of CIPD, such as occur in juvenile and postjuvenile periodontitis, chronic neutropenia, or Papillon–Lefèvre syndrome (Vrahopoulos *et al.*, 1988; Joachim *et al.*, 1989, 1990; Sati *et al.*, 1991; Vaughan *et al.*, 1990). The effects of plaque on the periodontium are more likely to be due to bacterial products, particularly surface-associated materials (SAM) produced by bacteria, including those involved in periodontitis (Meghji *et al.* 1992a,b; Wilson *et al.*, 1993).

The distance from the base of the periodontal pocket to the alveolar crest seems to remain constant throughout the disease process (Stanley, 1955). This may be due to the production in the inflammatory focus of diffusible compounds that inhibit enzyme reactions in the ligament (Paunio and Mäkinen, 1969). Another characteristic that suggests that the periodontal tissues retreat in good order in spite of the more widespread inflammatory infiltrate (Moskow and Polson, 1991) is the usually almost intact epithelial lining of the periodontal pocket, which also persists throughout the disease process, and which suggests an apparent equilibrium between cell division and desquamation (Ruben *et al.*, 1970). This equilibrium may be upset by an increase in noxious stimuli of plaque or host origin, leading to ulceration at the base of the pocket. Then the adjacent epithelium shows increased mitotic activity and hyperplasia, and it penetrates the disrupted corium by extending rete pegs. The original intact transseptal fibre system seems to play a role in preventing epithelium migrating apically (Goldman, 1951).

Inflammatory and immune responses

Inflammatory and immune responses in the periodontium are virtually inseparable. Direct contact of the tissues with bacteria or their products will induce an inflammatory response and also an immune response. In this context, an inflammatory response can be considered as being non-specific, and an immune response as being specific, although the two are intimately related. Immune responses can be either protective or damaging, depending on a number of factors, including the solubility, concentration, and site of the antigen and the affinity and concentration of the response. Immune responses may amplify the inflammatory response.

Immunological mechanisms have been implicated in the pathogenesis of inflammatory periodontal diseases for many years. Studies over two decades ago suggested that advanced forms of the disease were dominated by B cells and plasma cells, while early and stable forms were dominated by T cells. These observations led to models of diseases which suggested that a T-cell macrophage immunoregulatory imbalance was important in disease pathogenesis (Seymour 1987, 1991). However, clinical studies such as that of Löe *et al.* (1986) in Sri Lanka demonstrated that gingivitis did not automatically progress to periodontitis, and suggested that patient susceptibility was of overriding importance in determining the disease outcome (Johnson, 1988). It seems that there is a sub-group of the population that is particularly susceptible to CIPD, and that this susceptibility in about 15 per cent of the population is in turn related to immune and genetic aspects.

The discovery of associations between certain diseases and the major histocompatibility complex in humans (MHC) represents one of the most important advances in clinical medicine in recent years. It also provides a firm foundation for understanding the aetiology of a range of diseases that probably includes the chronic inflammatory periodontal diseases. Associations of CIPD with the MHC have been claimed for A2 and A9 and Marggraf *et al.* (1983) and Amer *et al.* (1988) found the prevalence of HLA to be significantly elevated in CIPD, which suggests that this antigen is a marker of increased susceptibility. Other authors, however, were not able to confirm this (Reinholdt *et al.*, 1977, Kaslick *et al.*, 1980). No associations with the B, C, or D loci have yet been established (Amer *et al.*, 1988).

Table 14.1
Possible mechanisms of immune-mediated damage in chronic inflammatory periodontal disease.

Mechanisms
T-cell mediated cytotoxicity
activation of osteoclasts
immune complexes
antibody-dependent cellular cytotoxicity
inhibition of fibroblast activity
cytotoxic antibodies

Possible mechanisms of immune-mediated damage

Immune responses to antigens, or even to bacteria within the periodontium, can lead theoretically to a number of damaging immune situations. Activation of T cells within the periodontium can lead to the production of cytotoxic T cells, which can directly damage the cells within the periodontium. Alternatively, the release of cytokines may lead to osteoclast activation or to inhibition of fibroblast activity (*Table 14.1*). Since fibroblast activity can be considered to be a normal repair mechanism after inflammatory or immune-mediated damage, a continuing stimulus may lead to inhibition of fibroblasts and of this repai mechanism, and thus result in progression of the disease.

In addition to T-cell activation, humoral mechanisms may play a role via the formation of immune complexes *in situ* , with the corresponding activation of complement and neutrophil polymorphs. Complement fixing antibodies of the IgG or IgM class may be cytotoxic on their own, and this could be directed against cells within the epithelium, perhaps containing cross-reacting antigens or perhaps being innocent bystanders to an ongoing inflammatory reaction. Antibodies may also add the specific arming component to cytotoxic cells, resulting in antibody-dependent cellular cytotoxicity (see *Table 14.1*). There is evidence that each of these putative mechanisms may contribute to CIPD.

The concept that antibodies on their own may contribute to CIPD has been supported by studies that have shown antibodies to collagen both in tissue and in serum (Jonsson *et al.*, 1991, Anusaksathien *et al.*, 1992). Cell-mediated autoimmune responses to type I collagen may also contribute (Mammo *et al.*, 1982).

Cell-mediated immunity may contribute to disease activity in an autoimmune fashion (in which immunity is targeted against host antigens), or cause damage to the host as a by-product of immune responses to bacteria or their antigens (Wilde *et al.*, 1977; Ranney, 1991). Lymphocytes with natural killer cell activity do appear to be abundant within the periodontium (Kopp, 1988).

Immune complexes are a natural by-product of the binding of soluble foreign antigens with antibody. If the antibodies are of the IgG or IgM type, then the powerful complement system can be activated *in situ*. Experimental induction of CIPD with immune complexes has been demonstrated (Nisengard *et al.*, 1977).

It now seems that one of the major factors in the induction and progression of CIPD is the production of cytokines by lymphocytes within the periodontium. In this context, the resulting damage can be considered as a by-product of the immune reaction (Page, 1991). Soluble bacterial antigens diffusing into tissues activate specific lymphocytes, which secrete a number of cytokines that not only control local immune responses, but may stimulate connective tissue breakdown. Lipopolysaccharides from Gram-negative bacteria, for example, have the capacity to activate macrophages to synthesize and secrete a wide array of molecules, including interleukin 1 (IL-1), tumour necrosis factor alpha (TNF-α), prostaglandins, and hydrolytic enzymes (Meikle *et al.*, 1986).

Other microbial components can activate T lymphocytes to produce IL-2 and lymphotoxin, which have potent inflammatory activities and could play key roles in periodontal tissue breakdown. IL-2 produced by activated T-cells may then induce both fibroblasts and macrophages to produce prostaglandins, tissue inhibitors of metalloproteinases (TIMP), and collagenase (Meikle *et al.*, 1986). If collagenase is produced, then the reaction is damaging, since the enzyme will degrade extracellular matrix components, but the production of TIMP inactivates the active enzyme and blocks further degradation, and is thus protective. Activation of osteoclasts is also a by-product of such T-cell activation, leading to bone loss, and high tissue levels of bone resorptive cytokines may be found in CIPD (Stashenko *et al.*, 1991).

There are several amplification and suppression mechanisms involved, and the progression and extent of tissue degradation is likely to be determined not only by the relative concentrations and half lives of IL-1, IL-2, TNF-α and related cytokines as well as the suppressor molecules such as TGF-β and PGE_2, but also by the immunogenetic control of the production of these cytokines. IL-1 and TNF are polypeptides with multiple overlap in biological activities, and both appear to act as early mediators of inflammation and immunity (Le and Vilcek, 1987).

Inflammation, immunity, and bystander damage

The body's defence systems must cope with an enormous diversity of micro-organisms and their products, and thus neutrophils, macrophages, and lymphocytes must have the ability to destroy all of these; they must also have the potential to destroy virtually all biological host structures. It is possible that most inflammatory actions damage the host to a small degree but, whereas most tissues will regenerate to withstand small degrees of damage, chronic inflammation results in accumulative damage, and perhaps CIPD is a good example of this. The two main effector systems linking specific and non-specific immunity are neutrophils and the complement system, and both may result in extensive damage to the host (Miyasaki, 1991; Ranney, 1991). Inflammatory and immune responses to plaque bacteria and their products are summarized in *Table 14.2.*

Cytokines in the inflammatory immune response

IL-1 and TNF are two cytokines that share many properties (Le and Vilcek, 1987) and they are probably the most important mediators of chronic inflammation induced by bacteria and their products. IL-1 is a key mediator, not only in inflammation and immunity, but also in the organization of healing. Macrophages are the largest source of IL-1, but a wide variety of other cells can also produce it, and these include endothelial cells, fibroblasts, keratinocytes, and neutrophils. IL-1 and TNF have a wide variety of biological activities which are summarized in *Table 14.3.* One of the reasons for their diverse effects is that they trigger other cells to secrete further mediators and also to amplify the production of IL-1 and TNF themselves, which in turn leads to an amplification of the immune and inflammatory responses against plaque antigens. (See also Chapter 12.)

Table 14.2 Inflammation and immune responses to 'plaque bacteria' and other products.

Antigens	Effects
whole bacteria	activate complement activate neutrophils activate macrophages
bacterial capsule	polyclonal B cell activator
plaque polysaccharide matrix	polyclonal B cell activator
lipopolysaccharide	activates complement damages host cells activates neutrophils activates macrophages
enzymes	damage host cells degrade connective tissue matrix activate/degrade complement degrade antibodies
peptides/proteins	can be chemotactic for neutrophils
toxins, metabolites	damage host cells

Autoimmunity and chronic inflammatory periodontal disease

The concept of an autoimmune pathogenesis in CIPD was first suggested many years ago by Brandtzaeg and Kraus (1965). Rather than the PDL being the primary target of a misdirected immune response, it seems more likely that autoimmune mechanisms are activated as part of the inflammatory response and become directed at the components of the ligament as indirect consequences of persistent inflammation. It is now recognized, for example, that anti-idiotypic antibodies are formed in every immune response as part of the control feedback loops and it is therefore quite conceivable that, rather than clearance of antigen, the response may contribute to the damage.

Over the last decade, a number of investigators have supported the concept. The mechanism by which such autoimmunity may damage the host is essentially that of the hypersensitivity reactions described above. These may be humoral or cellular, with the common thread that the target epitopes for the responses are on host tissues. The mechanism by which such autoimmunity may arise is unclear, though recent theories of immunology have accepted that anti-idiotypes, technically autoimmune antibodies, are a normal feature of the immune response. Autoimmune reactions may be caused by:

Table 14.3 Biological effects of interleukin 1 and tumour necrosis factor

activate macrophages for bacterial killing
activate neutrophils for bacterial killing
activate B and T lymphocytes (not TNF)
cause fibroblasts to secrete collagenase
induce bone resorption by osteoclast activation
induce cells to secrete prostaglandins
induce fibroblast proliferation
induce endothelial cell proliferation
induce other cells to secrete IL-1, TNF and other cytokines

- enhanced presentation of self-antigens to increased expression or linkage with class II MHC, particularly Ia antigen;
- bacterial or viral cross-reactivity with self-antigen leading to the production of cross-reaction antibodies, as has been found in, for example, rheumatic fever;
- polyclonal activation of cells, which may produce autoantibodies;
- altered T-helper or T-suppressor cell function;
- amplification rather than suppression of anti-idiotypes; and
- genetic predisposing factors.

Autoimmunity in CIPD has recently been reviewed by Anusaksathien *et al.* (1992) and is summarized in *Table 14.4*. Evidence of autoimmunity on the humoral side includes antibody to aggregated IgG (Gargiulo *et al.*, 1982), and IgM and IgA rheumatoid factor antibody to human collagen types I and III produced by gingival mononuclear cells (Hirsch *et al.*, 1988). Antibodies to collagen types I and III, but not to type II, have been described (Ftis *et al.*, 1986; Peng, 1988). In an experimental model of gingivitis in the dog, antibodies to native DNA have been reported (Clagett and Page, 1978).

Several authors have reported cellular autoimmune function. A mechanism for damage has been demonstrated by lymphocytotoxicity for oral epithelial cells (Movius *et al.*, 1975). These cells were taken from peripheral blood, but extraction of lymphocytes from CIPD sites has demonstrated functional cytotoxic activity of extracted gingival lymphocytes (O'Neill *et al.*, 1982). As with serum antibody, cell-mediated acitivity to native and denatured collagen has also been demonstrated (Mammo *et al.*, 1982; Rupnarain *et al.*, 1990). Thus, cell-mediated reactions against whole cells and against collagen components as well as proteoglycan have been demonstrated in CIPD patients, but not controls.

Table 14.4 Evidence for autoimmunity in chronic inflammatory periodontal diseases.

Humoral
antibody to aggregated IgG in inflamed gingiva antibody to rheumatoid factor in saliva raised levels of serum antibody to human collagen type I serum IgG antibody to bovine collagen (I and II) in JP in vitro production of IgA antibody to collagen (I and II by gingival mononuclear cells)
Cellular
lymphocytoxicity for oral epithelial cells in AP toxicity to gingival fibroblasts by mononuclear cells in AP lymphocyte proliferation to native and denatured collagen in AP cellular immunity to proteoglycan detected in AP

Vascular and inflammatory cell changes

Warwick James and Counsell (1927) observed that in the initial stages of inflammation the PDL vessels were enlarged, so that the ligament appeared hyperaemic. Later, the vessels showed constriction and were surrounded by loose connective tissue. In the crestal region, infiltration by inflammatory cells was noted where small arteries traversed the coronal part of the ligament from bone to gingiva. Regarding vascular changes in the deeper ligament, there is an increase in both number and size of blood vessels in the inflamed (marmoset) ligament, most of which pass through the lamina dura (Page *et al.*, 1972) and join ligament and supracrestal vessels (Kennedy, 1974). In spontaneous 7-week periodontitis in rats fed a high sucrose diet, Garant and Cho (1979a,b) observed several features consistent with endothelial proliferation, namely, increased endothelial cell processes, penetration of the basal lamina by these processes, and increased prominence of granular endoplasmic reticulum and of Golgi complex.

Increased vascularity has been related to the accumulation of an inflammatory infiltrate (Kennedy, 1974) which seems to form in tissue planes in the transseptal fibre region between fibre bundles and in PDL lymphatics. The latter are also inflamed and contain lymphocytes and plasma cells (Bernick and Grant, 1978). Granulocytes, especially polymorphonuclear neutrophils (PMN), and macrophages account for most of the increased tissue cell content, there being an accompanying decrease in the number of fibroblasts in this location (Adams *et al.*, 1979).

Connective tissue changes

Page and Schroeder (1976) have summarized the basic features of the lesion of routine chronic adult periodontitis as comprising an acute exudative vasculitis and chronic fibrotic inflammation, the chronic cellular infiltrate consisting mainly of plasma cells, lymphocytes, and macrophages. They found clusters of plasma cells between the remains of collagen fibre bundles and around blood vessels. These findings were confirmed by Joachim *et al.* (1989, 1990), who noted that plasma cells were abundant, in various stages of integrity or degeneration, in sites of ligament breakdown, and in the absence of bacteria. While PMN also are common in such locations, and clearly produce many enzymes likely to play a role in tissue breakdown, plasma cells produce enzymes, too, apart from their well known antibody production role. Proliferation of the junctional epithelial attachment apically is followed by a mainly plasma cell infiltration of the deeper connective tissue (Orban and Weinmann, 1942; Goldman, 1957a,b). On the bony aspect of the ligament, osteoclasts are the most obvious cells. Garant (1976) also observed binucleated cells with fibroblast or osteoblast-like cytoplasm and small mononuclear cells, all rich in acid phosphatase activity like osteoclasts, next to the bone surface.

Throughout the disease process, as mentioned previously, the collagen fibre bundles remain intact, except at the cervical periphery of the PDL. Deep to this the main changes seem to be a disruption of the perivascular connective tissue (Warwick James and Counsell, 1927), which is replaced largely by ground substance, PAS-positive mucopolysaccharide (Stahl *et al.*, 1958; Toto *et al.*, 1964). Acidic glycosaminoglycans and reticulin fibres seem to be more abundant in inflamed tissue close to alveolar bone, and in areas of ground substance infiltrated by leucocytes (Stahl *et al.*, 1958; Quintarelli, 1960).

The local perivascular changes are followed by degeneration of the principal fibres of the PDL, with localized widening of the periodontal space owing to adjacent alveolar bone resorption. Capillaries proliferate with the development of loose connective tissue (Orban and Weinmann, 1942). The fibre bundles acquire an open-weave appearance, due possibly to fluid accumulation within and around them, before their disintegration (Melcher, 1962).

There seems to have been little study of non-collagenous fibres in the inflamed ligament. There are varying opinions as to the fate of oxytalan fibres. Fullmer (1962) believed they were broken down, similarly to collagen, at some distance from the inflammatory focus. Kohl and Zander (1962) observed that oxytalan resisted denaturation better than collagen.

At an ultrastructural level, the first deviation from normal ligament collagen structure appears as a relaxation of packing of fibrils within each collagen fibre. Some fibrils appear swollen, and non-banded fibrils are interposed parallel to the remaining collagen fibres (Selvig, 1966). Other fibrils have a beaded appearance, with a periodicity of beading similar to that of collagen cross-banding (Selvig, 1966; Shore *et al.*, 1989). Breakdown of the fibres is characterized by separation followed by a longitudinal splitting of component fibrils. These changes are followed by loss in orientation of the fibres and fibrils (see *Figs 14.1, 14.2, 14.3*) (Selvig, 1966, 1968). A change in collagen fibril diameters has also been recorded in the incisor PDL of 'broken mouth' sheep (Shore *et al.*, 1989). These ultrastructural findings are supported by biochemical studies which indicate that PDL from periodontitis patients is both more soluble and more unstable than that from healthy teeth (Paunio, 1965), owing apparently to deficiencies in intermolecular links rather than intramolecular links (Paunio *et al.*, 1970). As well as showing less collagen cross-linking than healthy tissue, the diseased ligament also possesses increased fibroblast activity (Paunio, 1969a,b).

There is little evidence as to changes with inflammation in the types of collagen in the ligament. There is an indication that fibroblasts from patients with chronic periodontitis synthesize a type I collagen of altered composition, $\alpha I(I)_3$, which is not synthesized by cells from normal gingiva (Page *et al.*, 1979), but produces no type III molecules.

It has been estimated that approximately 20 per cent of the diseased PDL collagen is abnormal (Narayanan and Page, 1976). The diseased ligament shows increased galactosamine–glucosamine and chondroitin sulphate–hyaluronan ratios. There is still a need for further research into changes with inflammation in this most important component of the ligament, as well as the fluid so relevant to its properties (see Chapter 4). Water-soluble proteins increase in amount but do not seem to alter in composition (Paunio, 1969a,b). One report suggests that elastic fibres occur in the ligament only in advanced disease with little overt inflammation (Popov, 1965).

Some enzyme changes have been noted in the chronically inflamed ligament, though their significance is not clear. In (hamster) periodontitis, there are reductions in fibroblast succinic dehydrogenase, and in di- and tri-phosphopyridine nucleotide diaphorase. There was a decrease in succinic dehydrogenase activity and an increase in triphosphopyridine nucleotide diaphorase activity in periodontal pocket epithelium (Carlson, 1964). This study is too isolated to permit any useful conclusions, although the fibroblast changes suggest decreased metabolic activity in diseased ligament.

The most important sequel of CIPD is the loss of teeth by exfoliation or extraction. Clearly, the loss of supporting tissue and the maintenance of unchanged occlusal load would, as in the case of deciduous root resorption, result eventually in exfoliation. It is also a common clinical finding that patients resort to softer foods when faced with the discomfort of chewing their usual diet with loose teeth. There has been little scientific study as to how CIPD affects the mobility of teeth. The effects of occlusal trauma both alone and in conjunction with infectious inflammation have attracted more attention (see Chapter 15). Picton (1962) observed no increase in mobility with the development of gingivitis over a 1 month period, but there is increased mobility in relation to teeth affected by early periodontitis, with slight horizontal bone loss (Mühlemann, 1954).

Mechanisms of periodontal ligament destruction

It seems likely that collagen breakdown in chronic periodontitis is a multifactorial process, and that mechanisms may differ at various stages of the disease (Soames and Davies, 1977). The mechanisms proposed include elements of the immune response and alterations in fibroblast activities and, from the discussion that follows, it will be seen that these may be interrelated.

Schultz-Haudt and Aas (1960) suggested that collagen loss in chronic periodontitis was primarily the result of disorganization of fibre bundles, and secondarily due to the reduced ability of ligament fibroblasts to form collagen precursors. Lymphocytes have been observed in close contact with degenerating gingival fibroblasts (Schroeder and Page, 1972). This led to the suggestion that cytotoxic activity of these lymphocytes was at least partly responsible for fibroblast lysis and for a resultant reduced rate of collagen synthesis in humans (Page and Schroeder, 1976). Damage to fibroblasts may be produced by plaque-derived substances bound to the cells, by the cytotoxic action of lymphotoxin, or by immune complex formation on the fibroblast surface with consequent complement activation (Horton *et al.*, 1972; Schluger *et al.*, 1977). There may be an important species difference regarding this phenomenon, since in rats a rapid and severe loss of periodontal tissues can occur without any apparent cytotoxic changes in the normal cells of the ligament or in those of the inflammatory infiltrate (Garant, 1976). Garant (1976) also observed close contact between lymphocytes (and small macrophages) and fibroblasts, but could find no cytoplasmic alterations within such fibroblasts.

A similar species difference may explain the contradictory finding in marmosets of increased collagen synthesis in the immediate proximity of periodontal pocket epithelium (Skougaard and Levy, 1971). It seems likely that reduced fibroblast activity occurs in the human PDL, since one of the first signs of inflammatory involvement in the human PDL is an increase in fibroblast and osteoblast glycogen content (Michel and Frank, 1970). This storage polymer also occurs between collagen fibrils, apparently owing to cell rupture (*Fig. 14.4*). Michel and Frank (1970) reasoned that glycogen accumulated because it was not being used routinely for energy. They concluded that the phenomenon indicated an upset in fibroblast metabolism induced by inflammation. A similar conclusion was reached by Rippin (1978) on the basis of similarities between rat molar and human PDL regarding structure, function and biochemistry. Unlike the extreme situation observed by Garant (1976), Rippin observed a reduced rate of collagen synthesis in the inflamed ligament, in terms of lower tritiated proline uptake. He also suggested there was no evidence of a major collagenolytic plaque or host factor and concluded that a reduced rate of collagen formation was the most likely reason for loss of ligament collagen in chronic periodontitis.

However, morphometric study suggests, at least in early gingivitis, that collagen loss is too rapid to be explained by a decrease in the rate of collagen synthesis by damaged fibroblasts (Page and Schroeder, 1976). Collagen fibrils have been observed in human fibroblasts from tissue affected by apical or juvenile periodontitis (*Figs 14.5, 14.6*) (Eley and Harrison, 1975; Garant, 1976; Garant and Cho, 1979a,b) and in beagle dog fibroblasts and

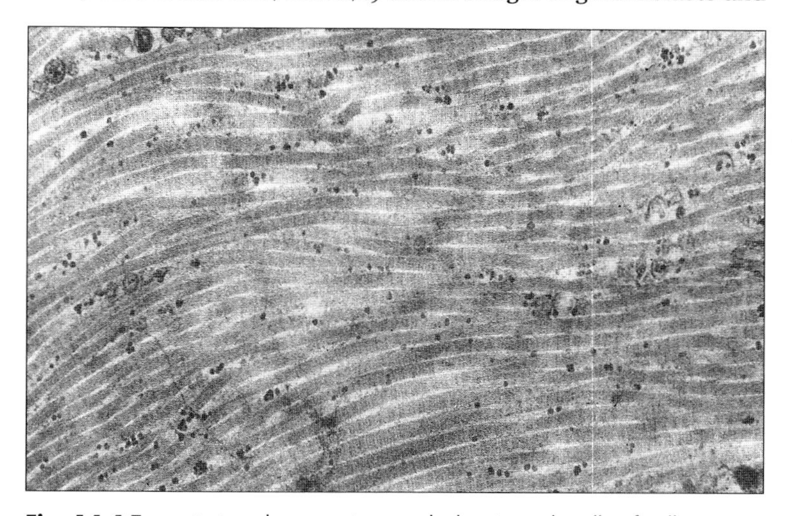

Fig. 14.4 Transmission electron micrograph showing a bundle of collagen fibres of the PDL. Between the fibrils are glycogen granules. (Magnification × 8250.) (From Michel and Frank, 1970.)

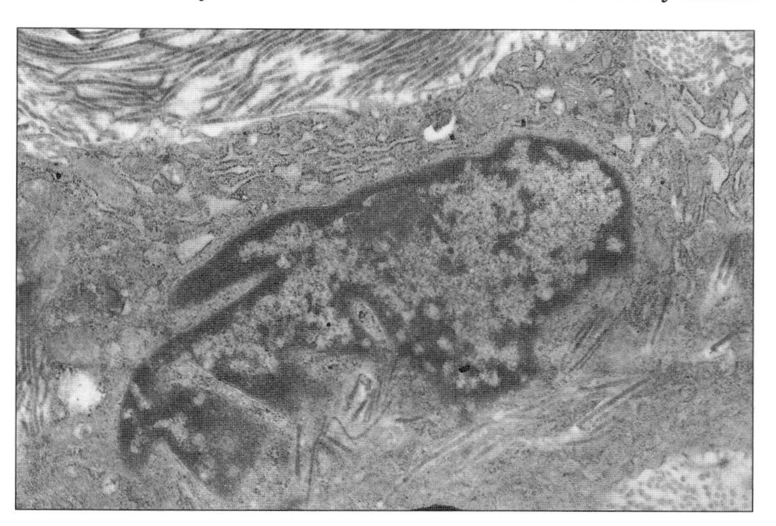

Fig. 14.5 Transmission electron micrograph showing a fibroblast containing intracellular banded collagen fibrils and rough endoplasmic reticulum, and surrounded by collagen fibrils. (Magnification × 8000.) (From Eley and Harrison, 1975.)

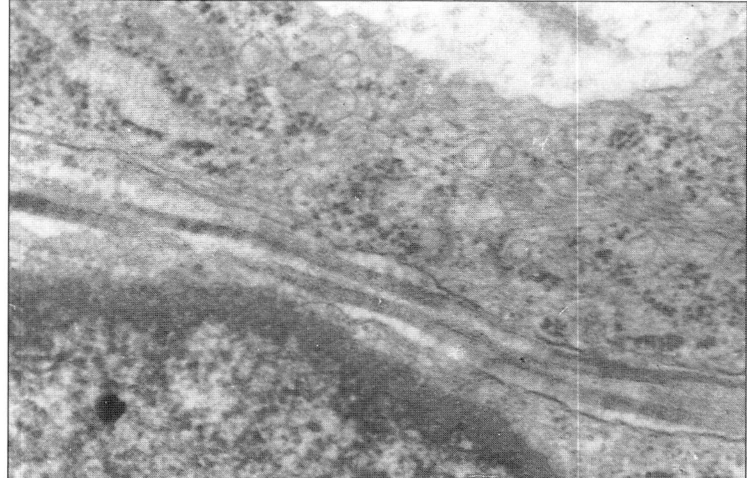

Fig. 14.6 Transmission electron micrograph showing banded collagen fibrils in an elongated membrane-bound vacuole adjacent to the nucleus, and above in a less clearly defined elongated vacuole. The plasma membrane is at the top of the micrograph. (Magnification × 38 000.) (From Eley and Harrison, 1975.)

macrophages from lesions of early chronic gingivitis (Soames and Davies, 1977). There is also evidence that both macrophages and fibroblasts can phagocytose and resorb collagen fibres (Parakkal, 1969). Soames and Davies (1977) noted that the presence of collagen within cytoplasmic vacuoles did not constitute proof of phagocytosis. However, from their observations of the frequent occurrence of intracellular fibrils, the varied orientation of fibrils within cytoplasmic vacuoles in the same cell, and the demonstration of acid hydrolase-containing bodies of similar morphology to fibril-containing vacuoles, they concluded that phagocytosis of collagen did occur, at least in early gingivitis. A similar line of reasoning and conclusion followed from Garant's (1976) work (see also Chapters 1 and 3).

On the basis of this evidence, there seems no reason why a similar situation should not exist in the inflamed PDL. There are several supporting reports for the concept of physiological phagocytosis and intracellular collagenolysis of the periodontal soft connective tissues (Ten Cate, 1972a,b; Ten Cate and Deporter, 1975). The IL-1 induced secretion of collagenase from fibroblasts in areas of inflammation is likely to be biologically important.

In a study of rapidly (7 weeks) developing gingivitis and periodontitis in rats fed a high sucrose diet, Garant and Cho (1979a) observed cytoplasmic alteration of fibroblasts limited mostly to areas adjacent to epithelium. They also noted that altered fibroblasts in this location were not usually in contact with lymphocytes, and questioned whether the deterioration of fibroblasts in gingivitis was always lymphocyte mediated. In the infiltrated dense connective tissue of advanced lesions (Garant and Cho, 1979b), they did observe a lymphocyte–fibroblast interaction, but found no changes in macrophages, endothelial cells or pericytes. They also found clusters of fibroblasts rich in intracellular collagen fibrils in the dense connective tissue of advanced lesions, and large and apparently active fibroblasts in older lesions, which they suggested represented a fibrotic or wound healing response. Although the periodontal lesions described by Garant and Cho developed rapidly, they provide further evidence for lymphocyte—fibroblast interaction and fibroblast-mediated collagenolysis as mechanisms of ligament breakdown in chronic periodontitis.

There is some evidence that extracellular collagenolysis occurs during chronic periodontitis. The ground substance seems to be affected first, since ligament hyaluronidase activity has been found to increase before that of collagenase (Paunio, 1969b). Extracellular collagenases may derive from plaque bacteria, neutrophils, macrophages, and fibroblasts. While bacterial collagenase may affect the rate of production or the activity of endogenous collagenase, the latter may be the exclusive form of the enzyme associated with the affected tissues (Fullmer *et al.*, 1969).

Lysosomal enzymes other than collagenase may have an important role in PDL destruction. This is indicated by the more rapid periodontal destruction noted in mink affected by Chediak–Higashi syndrome, in which the hereditary defect is an abundance of lysosome-like granules in leucocytes, mainly polymorphs, but also lymphocytes (Gustafson, 1969). As referred to previously, this also includes lysosomal enzymes from epithelial cell rests of Malassez (Birek *et al.*, 1980). Lysosomes from macrophages may also release enzymes that help to break down ligament connective tissue (Hamp and Folke, 1968; Paunio and Mäkinen, 1969). In one study, increases and decreases in numbers of granulocytes and macrophages in (monkey) transseptal fibres correlated respectively with initiation and slowing down of ligament destruction. This was related to the known capacity of these cells for causing cell damage, collagen degradation and bone resorption (Adams *et al.*, 1979). At the same time, these workers pointed out that the granulocytes might serve the more important function of limiting antigens to the tissue adjacent to the gingival crevice.

JUVENILE PERIODONTITIS

Juvenile periodontitis (JP) involves rapid destruction of the PDL in young people. Typically the disease is restricted initially to first molars and incisors, although, if left unchecked, it may involve the entire dentition. If diagnosed after 25 years of age, it is described as post-juvenile periodontitis (PJP). Localized and generalized forms of JP are described, without any differences other than numbers of teeth involved and rate of disease advance. There has been little study of ligament changes in other rapidly progressive forms of periodontitis (Newman *et al.*, 1993), and comparative details are considered in the section on the inflammatory–immune response (see pages 294–8).

The alveolar attachment of the PDL fibres is lost initially (Baer *et al.*, 1963). This is followed by a widening of the periodontal 'space' owing to bone resorption. The principal fibres are eventually replaced by a loose and disoriented collagen network, though they are still recognizable until the more advanced stages of the disease (Baer *et al.*, 1963). Remaining PDL fibres run parallel to the root surface (Baer *et al.*, 1963; Kaslick and Chasens, 1968a,b). The picture is one of rapid alveolar fibre destruction and apical proliferation of junctional epithelium (Bouyssou and Fourel, 1973). PDL vessels are numerous and markedly dilated, although there is minimal inflammation (Wade, 1965; Fourel, 1972). There may (Orban and Weinmann, 1942) or may not (Fourel, 1972) be proliferation of the epithelial cell rests of Malassez. There are variable numbers of plasma cells, and this will be discussed further in the section on the inflammatory–immune response (see pages 301–4).

In spite of a lack of proven aetiological factors in JP and PJP, genetic factors are suspected, although no genetic defect of collagen synthesis or metabolism has yet been demonstrated. There is no doubt that plaque is involved, its distribution being similar to that on teeth affected by routine chronic adult periodontitis, although much thinner than on the latter (Waerhaug, 1976, 1977). Several authors have suggested that immunogenetic factors might play a role but the linkage with HLA is weak. Three studies have shown an increase in HLA-A9 (Reinholt *et al.*, 1977, Cullinan *et al.*, 1980, Kaslik *et al.*, 1980) and in addition Terasaki *et al.* (1975) and Kaslik *et al.* (1980) showed a decrease in A2, a similar pattern for that found with adult periodontitis. Interestingly B15 was raised in two studies (Reinholt *et al.*, 1977, Cullinan *et al.*, 1980). However, the numbers examined in most studies have been small, and larger numbers or collaborative studies would be useful in attempting to answer the question of whether there is an immunogenetic basis for distinguishing between JP–LJP (localised juvenile periodontitis and adult periodontitis. It should be noted that other studies have failed to show any HLA linkage (Saxen and Koskimies 1984) and that if immune response genes were to be involved, then a linkage with HLA-DR rather than with HLA-A or B might be expected (see Chapter 13).

The inflammatory–immune response

The possible role of the inflammatory/immune response in CIPD has been discussed above. However, there is as yet little *in vivo* evidence that there is a direct relationship between PDL destruction and the immune–inflammatory response, and there has been little study of the possibility of genetic predisposition to rapid ligament destruction. Most, if not all, of the cellular and acellular components of the inflammatory–immune response to plaque micro-organisms and their products accumulate in the soft periodontal tissues and conceivably also in the marrow spaces of the alveolar bone. They include neutrophils, plasma cells, T lymphocytes and B lymphocytes, macrophages, immunoglobulins, complement components, and a wide range of cytokines. The severity or rate of advance of the lesion is increased by activation of the host response, perhaps by uncontrolled production of cytokines, prostaglandins, and hydrolytic enzymes. Alternatively or concomitantly, the same could result from increases in the levels of Gram-negative anaerobes in the plaque. Some research indicates a linear relationship between cell mediated immunity as assessed by peripheral blood lymphocyte transformation to plaque antigens, and the severity of periodontitis, except in rapidly progressive periodontitis (Ivanyi and Lehner, 1970, 1971; Ivanyi *et al.*, 1972; Horton *et al.*, 1972). However, there is one dissenting study (Kiger *et al.*, 1974). The greatest stimulation of peripheral blood lymphocytes seems to occur when the lesion has extended to the ligament (Patters *et al.*, 1976).

This postulated relationship between peripheral lymphocyte responses and local tissue damage is supported by work that suggests that positive lymphocyte transformation, cytotoxicity, and migration inhibition tests indicate that cell-mediated immune responses correlate with damage to periodontal tissues (Ivanyi and Lehner, 1970, 1971; Ivanyi *et al.*, 1972; Horton *et al.*, 1972). One should remember that CIPD is chronic – lasting in most patients for many years, if not for life, although it does vary greatly in severity – and that the periodontal soft tissues and alveolar bone retreat in good order ahead of the advancing front of the lesion, as described earlier. Furthermore, as in many non-specific chronic infectious inflammatory conditions, the central lesion is effectively walled off from deeper healthy tissue by zones of chronic inflammatory cells and fibrous tissue. There is additional evidence that, in most patients, the inflammatory–immune response tends to be self-limiting as the disease advances. This may also apply in CIPD, since the magnitude of lymphocyte transformation by ultrasonicates of plaque organisms is decreased significantly in cases of rapidly progressive chronic periodontitis, owing, it is postulated, to the presence of inhibitory or the absence of stimulatory factors in serum (Ivanyi *et al.*, 1972).

A further problem concerns the role of the individual components of the host response in the small amount of tissue loss that takes place. It seems that both T lymphocytes and B lymphocytes contribute to fibroblast damage through cytokine production, although there is no direct evidence for this (Mackler *et al.*, 1974) (or indeed for any other proposed mechanism!). The main inflammatory cell in the advanced lesion is the plasma cell. This may relate to the role of B lymphocytes in the production of relevant cytokines, for example IL-1. Regarding the comparative importance of T lymphocytes and B lymphocytes, there is evidence that the established human lesion is dominated by B lymphocytes (Walker, 1977), and that the T-cell role, while including other features of cell-mediated immunity, may be mainly one of helper activity (Seymour and Greenspan, 1979).

Recently, there has been a comparison of the features of the lesions in adult periodontitis, juvenile and post-juvenile periodontitis, and more severe, rapidly progressive forms of periodontitis. One of the most striking observations was the scarcity of bacteria in the affected connective tissue, regardless of disease severity or whether it was seen pre- or post-oral hygiene phase (Liakoni *et al.*, 1987a,b; Vrahopoulos *et al.*, 1988; Joachim *et al.*, 1989, 1990; Vaughan *et al.*, 1990) (*Figs 14.7, 14.8, 14.9, 14.10, 14.11, 14.12, 14.13, 14.14*). Even with rapidly progressive periodontitis in children (e.g. Kostman's syndrome, a disorder of neutrophils), there are many polymorphonuclear neutrophil leucocytes (PMN) locally at the affected site (Newman and Rule, 1983). In adult periodontitis and juvenile and post-juvenile periodontitis, and in severe rapidly progressive forms such as those due to chronic neutropenia (Vaughan *et al.*, 1990) and Papillon–Lefèvre syndrome (Vrahopoulos *et al.*, 1988), there are many PMN and plasma cells at the sites of ligament destruction, and no evident micro-organisms.

Plasma cells

The percentage density of plasma cells is significantly higher in juvenile and post-juvenile periodontitis than in adult periodontitis, as it is also in untreated lesions compared with those that had received oral hygiene. Plasma cells were more abundant in a layer deep to the neutrophils lining the basement membrane, even in areas of extensive inflammation. They were often degenerate, and were more so in juvenile and post-juvenile periodontitis, and in relatively avascular areas of connective tissue. These findings indicate an association between increase in plasma cell percentage density and increase in collagen destruction. Scarcity of Russell bodies within plasma cells suggests that immunoglobulin production and secretion are normal even in advanced or rapidly progressive lesions (Joachim *et al.*, 1989, 1990).

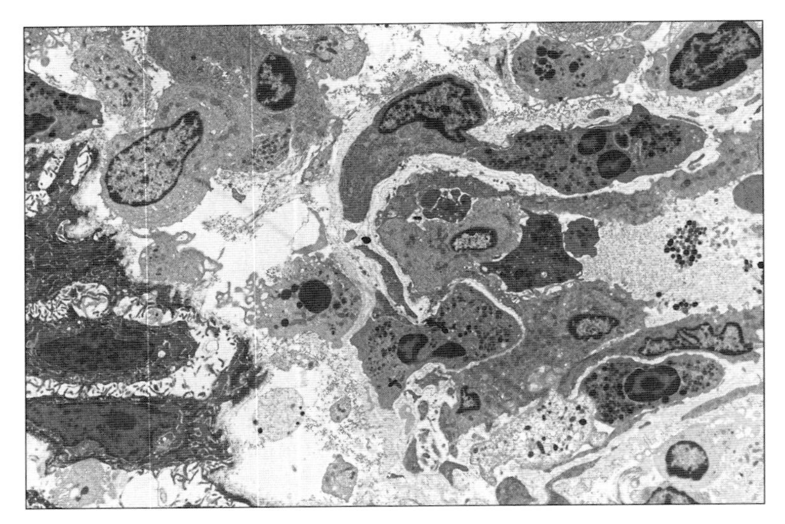

Fig. 14.7 Transmission electron micrograph showing superficial connective tissue in untreated AP. Connective tissue destruction and oedema are evident. Polymorphonuclear neutrophil leucocytes (PMN) and plasma cells are close to the epithelium. (Magnification × 1900.)

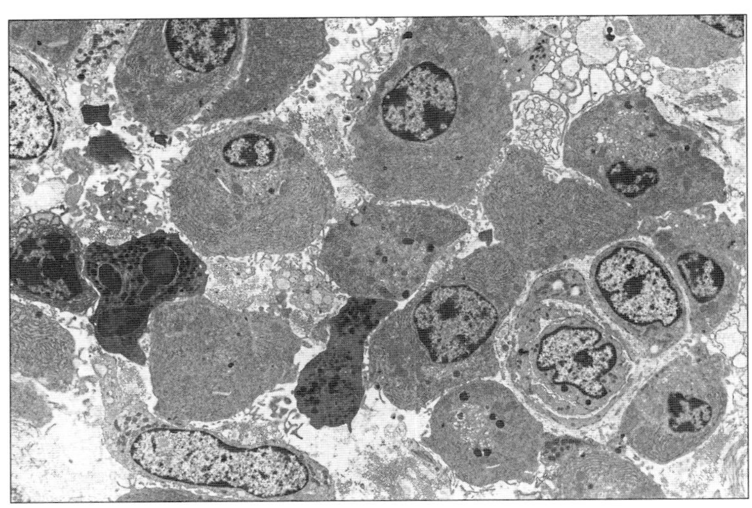

Fig. 14.8 Transmission electron micrograph showing deep connective tissue in untreated AP. At this level, also, the collagen is lysed and only leucocytes are abundant – mainly plasma cells and PMN. (Magnification × 1500.)

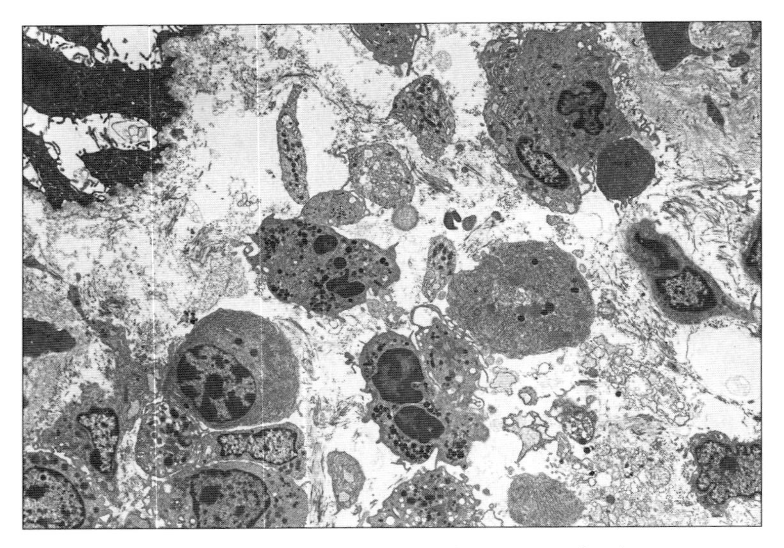

Fig. 14.9 Transmission electron micrograph showing superficial connective tissue in untreated AP. There is extensive lysis of collagen in the presence of plasma cells and degranulating PMN. (Magnfication × 1500.)

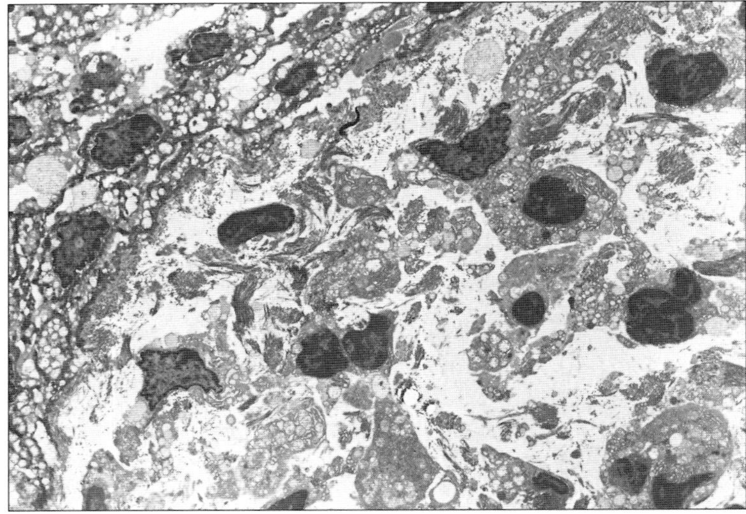

Fig. 14.10 Transmission electron micrograph showing superficial connective tissue in untreated JP. There is extensive collagen loss, but fragments are still evident, perhaps owing to a more rapid and less organized breakdown. PMN and plasma cells are present. (Magnification × 1200.)

Similarly, in a systemically related, rapidly progressive periodontitis due to chronic idiopathic neutropenia, connective tissue destruction was associated with a leucocyte accumulation that consisted mainly of plasma cells and PMN. Both cell types tended to be more degenerate than in routine chronic adult periodontitis. There was PMN lysosome loss and lymphocyte maturation within peripheral blood vessels (Vaughan *et al.*, 1990). There were similar proportions of PMN and plasma cells (the latter dominating) in the periodontitis lesions of Papillon–Lefèvre syndrome. The blood PMN count was raised (Vrahopoulos *et al.*, 1988). Owing to the reduced density of PDL fibre attachment and the thinness of the underlying cementum in Papillon–Lefèvre syndrome, a defective PDL or impaired deposition of cementum may result in an abnormal attachment more susceptible to destruction. Alternatively, the rate of disease advance may be so fast as to interfere with ligament and cementum formation (Vrahopoulos *et al.*, 1988).

While the damage does not appear to be mediated by intact bacteria, their products may certainly be involved. For example, lipopolysaccharide promotes PMN adhesion to fibroblasts, and may help to induce PMN-mediated human PDL fibroblast injury (Deguchi *et al.*, 1990). Superoxide dismutase activity is higher in

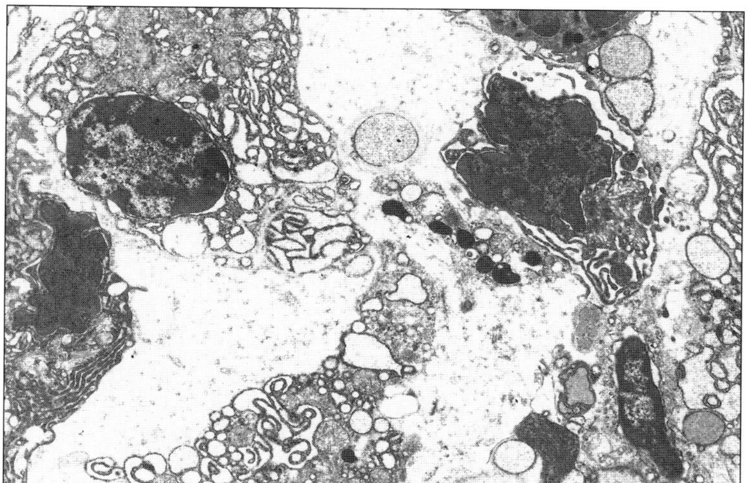

Fig. 14.11 Transmission electron micrograph showing superficial connective tissue, post-oral hygiene phase, in JP. There is still collagen loss, and degenerating plasma cells are the major cells present. (Magnification × 2500.)

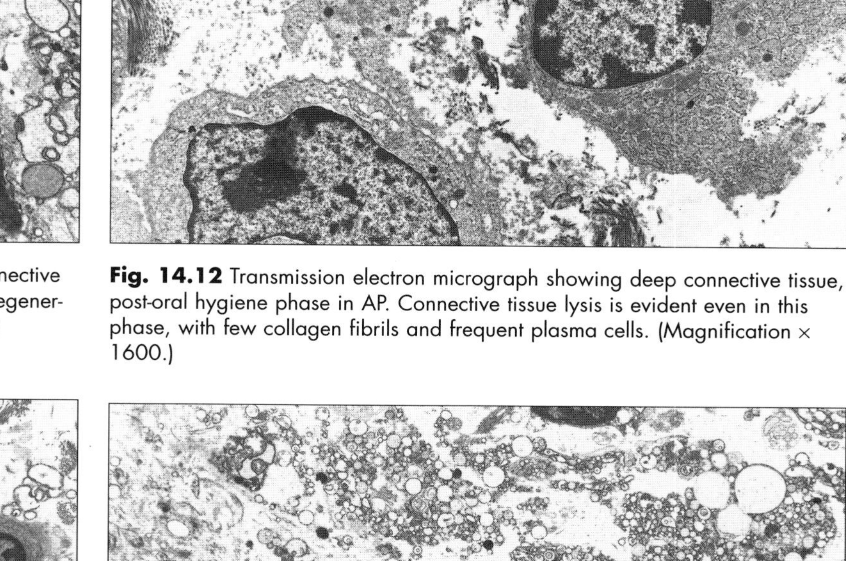

Fig. 14.12 Transmission electron micrograph showing deep connective tissue, post-oral hygiene phase in AP. Connective tissue lysis is evident even in this phase, with few collagen fibrils and frequent plasma cells. (Magnification × 1600.)

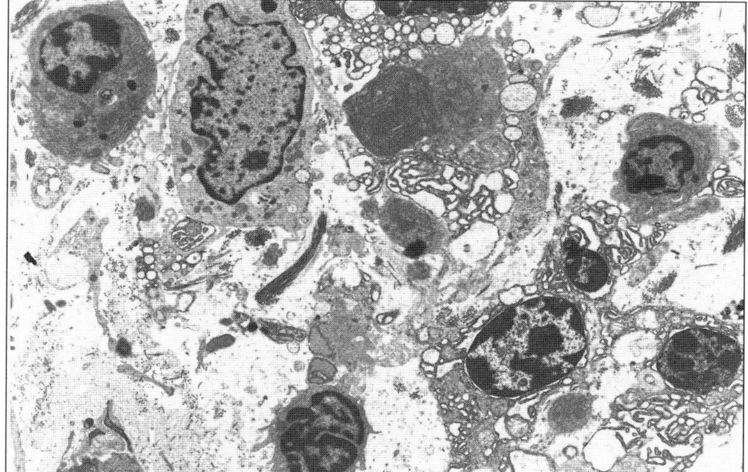

Fig. 14.13 Transmission electron micrograph showing deep connective tissue in untreated JP. Little collagen remains, and (mainly degenerate) plasma cells predominate. (Magnification × 2000.)

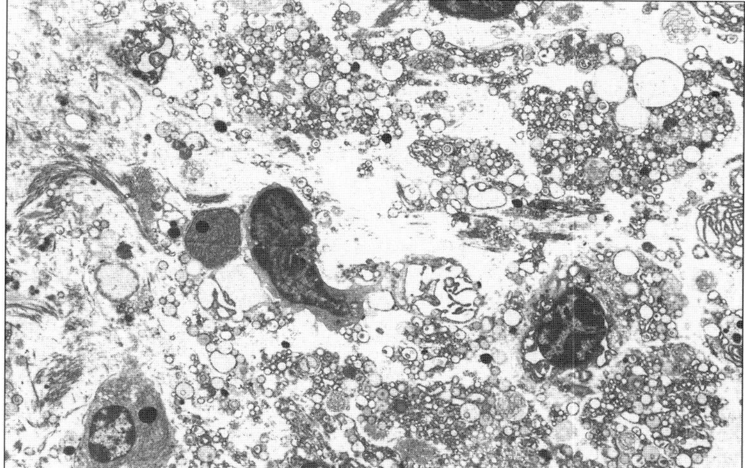

Fig. 14.14 Transmission electron micrograph showing deep connective tissue, post-oral hygiene phase in PJP. There are similar features to those seen in *Fig. 14.13*, with many degenerate plasma cells predominating. (Magnification × 1600.)

PDL than in skin, and this could reflect an increased need to protect cells and matrix components from PMN-generated reactive oxygen species (Jacoby and Davis, 1991).

One recent study indicates that the inflammatory lesion extends beyond the PDL into the alveolar bone, often before bone resorption. With advancing disease, Moskow and Polson (1991) observed deep penetration of inflammatory cells into the PDL and periapical tissues. The authors cast doubt on the perception of human periodontitis as a localized and marginal disease, in spite of the fact that the transseptal fibres reform more apically with advancing disease.

Neutrophils

Neutrophil deficiencies are currently considered the main factors in increased susceptibility to, and rapid rate of progression of, chronic periodontitis. Deficient PMN chemotaxis and phagocytosis have been demonstrated in JP patients (Cianciola *et al.*, 1977; Clark *et al.*, 1977). Polymorphs limit subgingival plaque growth (Attström and Schroeder, 1979), and there may be a defective PMN response to Gram-negative JP-related organisms (Lindhe and Socransky, 1979). It does not seem that there is any deficiency in levels of circulating PMN in JP. Indications of such deficiencies in Negroes, who are more affected by JP, are attributable almost entirely to racial differences in levels of circulating blood leucocytes. Small increases in PMN may indicate simply a response to infection (Sati *et al.*, 1991). Similarly, it used to be thought that in JP/PJP, PMN at the disease site were relatively inactive. From studies of gingival crevicular fluid PMN in JP and in healthy control patients, it is now clear that failure to phagocytose by PMN in JP is solely due to the fact that they have already ingested plaque bacteria (Newman and Addison, 1982). Furthermore, the number of PMN recovered from severely involved JP sites was about ten times the level from non-involved sites in the same patient (Murray and Patters, 1980).

As regards a possible explanation for the neutrophil defect, Daniel *et al.* (1993) have recently observed an abnormality of signal transduction in JP PMN resulting in a reduced influx of extracellular calcium, 'perhaps due to failure in plasma membrane calcium channel activation, or in an associated activation pathway'. As Daniel and co-workers mention, previously noted instances of defective chemotaxis and phagocytosis may be attributed to intracellular calcium as a mediator. Certainly, PMN in the crevice are functionally active, and their efficiency of opsonization and phagocytosis may by directly related to the degree of periodontal damage (Challacombe *et al.*, 1992).

Van Dyke *et al.* (1993) have recently reviewed the role of the host response in CIPD. They considered the biochemical basis of PMN abnormalities in localized JP (LJP). They attributed the decreased PMN chemotaxis often observed in LJP to abnormal chemotactic receptor expression, to signal transduction abnormalities, and to reduced levels of the chemotaxis-associated protein GP110. The main signal transduction abnormality was suggested to be decreased protein kinase C activity, because the activity of this enzyme is 'central to neutrophil functions such as respiratory burst and degranulation'. They hypothesized that in certain LJP cases down-regulation of PKC by increased levels of diacylglycerol renders the PMN cell surface 'incapable of responding to extracellular signals and to certain pathogenic bacteria'. Inconsistency in individual LJP cases they attributed to disease heterogeneity. They noted a further deficiency, in that LJP PMN phagosome–lysosome fusion was abnormal, but only for the disease-related species *Actinobacillus actinomycetemcomitans.*

Mast cells

Mast cells have been associated with regions of collagen breakdown, so they too could be involved in PDL destruction (Barnett, 1974). Mast cell heparin can stimulate collagenase production and activity (Sakamoto *et al.*, 1973). Mast cell neutral proteases may digest both collagen and non-collagenous ligament proteins after initial cleavage by collagenase (Page and Schroeder, 1976).

Macrophages

As mentioned earlier, macrophages, by virtue of their enzymic activity (particularly lysosomal activity and including collagenase), may have a part in tissue breakdown. In addition, activated macrophages can synthesize prostaglandins, which relate to various cytokine-mediated tissue destructive activities. Prostaglandins produce effects varying from collagen synthesis (Raisz and Koolemans-Beynen, 1974) to fibrotic ligament changes (Blumenkrantz and Söndergaard, 1972). Schluger *et al.* (1977) suggested that prostaglandins may suppress the immune response but inhibit fibroblast mitosis and the synthesis and turnover of both collagen and non-collagenous proteins. However, one experiment suggests that prostaglandins, particularly PGE_1, may increase PDL collagen resorption without affecting many fibroblasts (Rao *et al.*, 1978). Van Dyke *et al.* (1993) observed increased PGE_2 and TNF-α production in response to LPS by monocytes from patients with early-onset periodontitis.

Because of the lack of any firm experimental evidence, the precise role of the humoral response during periodontitis can only be surmised. One possibility is that immune complex formation could activate complement, resulting in C3b stimulation of hydrolytic enzyme (including collagenase) secretion by macrophages (Berglund, 1971; Schluger *et al.*, 1977). Fibroblast lysis may result from complement activation at its surface by immune complex formation between specific antibody and plaque antigens, or from the activation by immune complex of killer lymphocytes (K-cells) (Brandtzaeg, 1966). It is possible, however, for antibodies to be directly toxic to cells, to arm non-specific killer cells as well as form immune complexes. Antibodies to a wide variety of periodontal pathogens and their antigens have been demonstrated both in serum and in crevicular fluid, and although *in vivo* evidence of the cytotoxic potential is difficult to confirm, it remains very possible that antibodies contribute directly or indirectly to CIPD.

Another interesting region of histologically evident difference between healthy and periodontitis-affected sites is the basement membrane in the periodontal pocket. In disease-affected sites there were many ultrastructural changes, including breaks, absence, fragmentation, detachment, thickening, replication, and changes in electron density (Subadan *et al.*, 1990).

LATERAL PERIODONTAL ABSCESS

There has been little research into PDL changes in this condition. Its aetiology has been attributed to sudden alterations in ecology in the bacterial population of periodontal pockets, produced, for example, by scaling or probing, especially where there are deep infrabony defects or involvement of the furcations of multirooted teeth (Pritchard, 1953; McFall, 1964; Miyasoto, 1975). Acute changes are therefore superimposed generally on tissues that are already chronically inflamed. The histopathology resembles in many respects that of the periapical abscess (see the following section on suppurative apical periodontitis), with an abundance of PMN being the main feature. Chronic change results in reversion to a predominance of plasma cells and lymphocytes, with peripheral fibrosis (Stahl, 1973).

APICAL PERIODONTITIS

NON-SUPPURATIVE APICAL PERIODONTITIS

The acute form of this lesion usually follows physical trauma or chemical irritation, but it may be infective in origin. There are the typical changes associated with acute inflammation, including hyperaemia, oedema, neutrophil infiltration, and some widening of the periodontal space (Darling, 1970). The chronic variety is often a sequel to the acute form with a change to a chronic inflammatory cell infiltrate that consists mainly of plasma cells and macrophages. There is moderate vasodilatation and new capillary formation, together with fibroblast activity. This results in the formation of a granuloma, which gradually increases in volume, with associated bone resorption; a fibrous tissue layer and new bone may be found at the periphery of the lesion (Wade, 1965; Darling, 1970).

The granuloma itself consists mainly of chronic inflammatory granulation tissue composed mainly of plasma cells, lymphocytes, a few polymorphs, proliferating fibroblasts, and a varying density of collagen bundles (Gardner, 1962a) (*Figs. 14.15, 14.16, 14.17*). It varies macroscopically from a granuloma that is firm and adherent to the root apex, to a soft or haemorrhagic granuloma that is easily damaged during tooth extraction. This variation relates to differences in the density and degree of order of connective tissue fibres in the lesion (Lyons *et al.*, 1970). The fibrous tissue of the lesion is continuous at its periphery with the healthy PDL (Leuin, 1957). On a histological basis, Yanagisawa (1980) has divided periapical granulomas into four types: exudative, granulomatous, granulo-fibrous and fibrous. Cases of more than one year's duration showed much fibrosis.

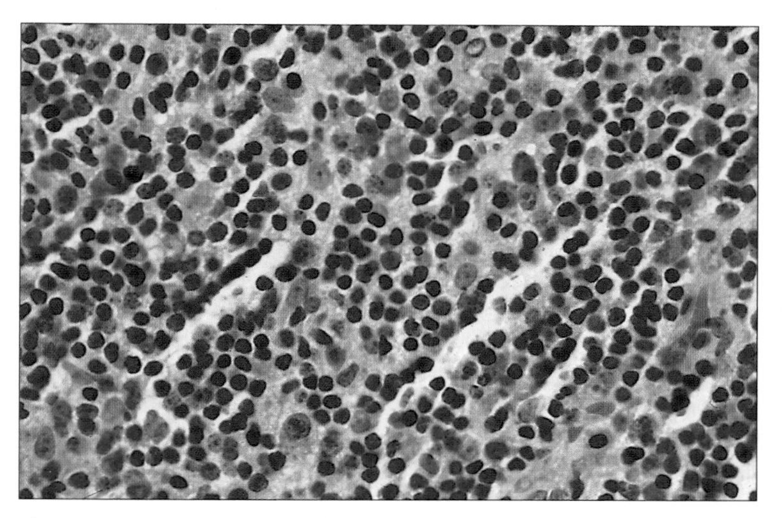

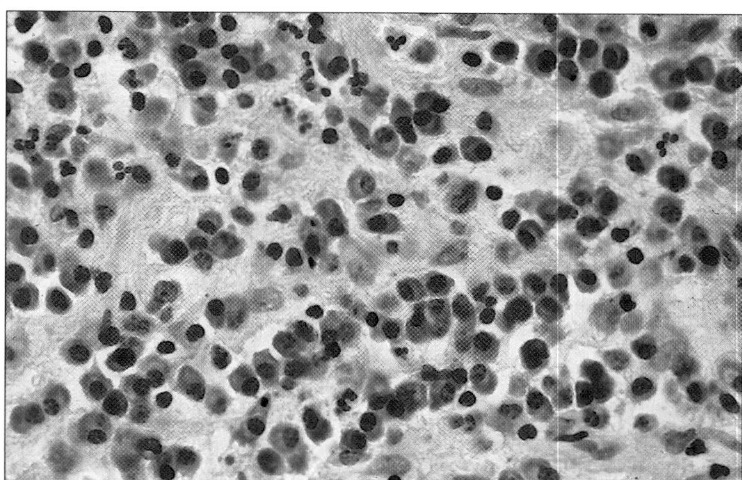

Figs 14.15, 14.16 Transmitted light micrographs showing chronically inflamed periapical tissue composed of many inflammatory cells in loose connective tissue stroma. Prominent in *Fig. 14.15* are lymphocytes and plasma cells, as well as blood vessels. In *Fig. 14.16*, many plasma cells and a few PMN are evident. (Haematoxylin and eosin; magnification × 900.) (From Morton *et al.*, 1977.)

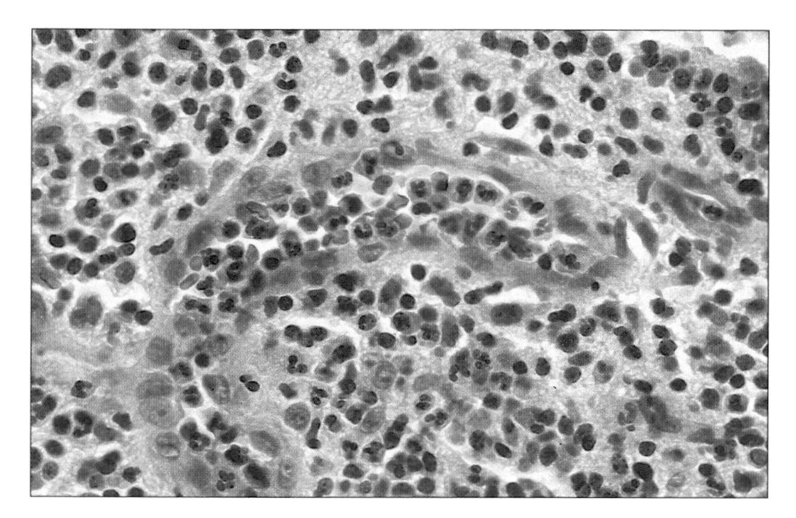

Fig. 14.17 Transmitted light micrograph showing chronically inflamed periapical tissue, including a neutrophil lesion. PMN may be prominent, and in such cases they are often seen penetrating blood vessel walls. A few macrophages are scattered through the connective tissue. (Haematoxylin and eosin; magnification × 900.) (From Morton *et al.*, 1977.)

Elimination or reduction in the severity of irritation can allow the lesion to proceed to complete repair. Ankylosis of tooth to bone can occur (Wade, 1965; Darling, 1970). There may be a widening of the PDL space, with breaks in continuity of the lamina dura, associated with granuloma formation (Narita, 1956). Root resorption, osteosclerosis, or hypercementosis can occur, but usually only in long-standing cases (Darling, 1970).

Epithelial cell rests occur in the lesion, and one (monkey) study suggests that they are larger, but not more numerous, than in normal tissues, and can eventually occupy most of a granuloma (Valderhaug, 1974). The epithelial cells in apical lesions are polygonal, adhering to each other by fewer desmosomes than in normal squamous epithelium. The cells have irregular nuclei, prominent nucleoli, and much euchromatin. There is a decrease in the nuclear–cytoplasmic ratio. Some contain lipid droplets. The cells also contain scattered polyribosomes and dilated rough endoplasmic reticulum. Their cytoplasm contains bundles of tonofilaments and keratohyalin granules, scattered mitochondria, a well-developed Golgi apparatus and occasional membrane whorls or residual myelin bodies. Micropinocytotic vesicles and large vacuoles are also present, but phagosomes are rare (Ten Cate, 1972b; Summers and Papadimitriou, 1975). It has been suggested that the stimulus causing proliferation of the epithelial cells is a local change in pH or CO_2 tension (Grupe *et al.*, 1967) (see also Chapter 1).

The epithelial (and capillary endothelial) basement membranes in these lesions are strongly PAS-positive, the intensity of staining increasing with subacute or acute inflammatory change (Diniotou *et al.*, 1975). This is indicative of connective tissue breakdown and an increase in ground substance mucopolysaccharide (Obrunik and Meduna, 1959). Diniotou *et al.* (1975) suggested that chronic inflammatory changes in apical granulomas were marked by a gradual disappearance of connective tissue mucopolysaccharides, and the replacement of reticulin by collagen. Oxytalan fibres have been found in periapical granulomas, although their significance has not been explained (Fullmer, 1960).

Lack of pain from the lesion has been associated with lack of nerve endings (Gardner, 1962a), although nerve endings are present in small numbers in at least half of chronic inflammatory periapical lesions. Following pulpectomy and root canal obturation, perapical nerves proliferate and branch within the area of chronic inflammation (Martinelli and Rulli, 1967; Lin and Langeland, 1981; Holland, 1988, 1993).

Periapical lesions contain several fat residues of tissue degeneration. These include glycerides, free and esterified cholesterol, and phospholipids (Bozzo *et al.*, 1972). Cholesterol clefts are common, the crystals themselves having been removed, of course, during routine tissue processing. The clefts are surrounded by foreign body giant cells, Russell bodies, and haemosiderin pigment (Gardner, 1962a; Leonard *et al.*, 1974). Cholesterol and other fat residues may result from fatty degeneration of cells (Gardner, 1962a). Cholesterol also forms in blood clots, which congest the many capillaries in the inflamed tissue. The disintegrating red thrombi may release their lipids to form the characteristic spindle-shaped aggregates of cholesterol crystals, which are enveloped by the endothelial walls of small vessels (Browne, 1971; Arwill and Heyden, 1973). Foam cells occur adjacent to the zone of fibrosis (Yanagisawa, 1980).

The capillaries in apical lesions are hard to discern, but may be distinguished by their high ATP-ase activity. Pericytes of the inflamed capillary endothelium show increased lysosomal function, and may form foreign body giant cells with tissue-degrading properties leading to resorption of components of the lesion (Browne, 1971; Arwill and Heyden, 1973).

Immunoglobulin-producing cells are common in periapical lesions (Morse *et al.*, 1975; Morton *et al.*, 1977). Of the plasma cells, those containing IgG are the most numerous. Some cells contain IgA, but few contain IgM (*Figs 14.18, 14.19*). In one study IgG, IgA, IgM, and IgE cells represented 70 per cent, 14 per cent, 4 per cent, and 10 per cent respectively of the immunoglobulin-containing cells that were observed (Pulver *et al.*, 1978). There is no clear evidence that immune complexes contribute to the inflammatory events or subsequent bone loss of periapical periodontitis (Morton *et al.*, 1977). Immune complexes and IgE-mediated reactions may play a role in periapical pathology (Yanagisawa, 1980). Bacteria rarely occur in inflamed periapical tissue (Block *et al.*, 1976; Langeland *et al.*, 1977).

Many lymphocytes, including T-cells (Farber, 1975), occur in the typical granuloma, and complement components, mainly C3, are also present (Kuntz *et al.*, 1977). Granulomas with marked lymphocyte infiltration are more frequent in cases that had received endodontic treatment. In contrast, an infiltrate of mainly plasma cells was more frequent in untreated cases with open pulp chambers, as was epithelial proliferation. Mast cells in exudative and granulomatous zones may release histamine, increasing vascular permeability. In the fibrous zone, mast cells may contribute to breakdown and formation of collagen and ground substance (Yanagisawa, 1980). Abundant mast cells were found in apical granulomas (Mathiesen, 1973). The ligament seems to be more resistant to the spread of periapical inflammation than the adjacent marrow spaces (Walton and Garnick, 1986).

In general, there appears to be too little information to comment usefully on the significance of these demonstrated components of the host response in periapical lesions, except to suggest that, as in lateral periodontitis, they serve to counter infection.

SUPPURATIVE APICAL PERIODONTITIS

These lesions have been reviewed by Gardner (1962a) and Darling (1970), though there is a lack of literature on the topic. The periapical suppurative lesions are composed of a focus of infection around the apical foramen which, with necrosis and the accumulation of PMN, results in pus formation. The acute central necrotic area is surrounded by a dense PMN infiltrate and some chronic inflammatory cells. This zone is encompassed by inflammatory granulation tissue and then by an area of fibrosis, the latter being more abundant in chronic lesions. External to the fibrotic zone is a region of hyperaemia, oedema, and bone resorption, producing widening of the periodontal space. The chronic lesion contains lymphocytes, plasma cells, PMN, and some bacteria and serous pus. The cavity in both acute and chronic forms centres on the root apex foramen, a lateral canal, or the furcation area of a multirooted tooth. In the chronic lesion, the central zone is surrounded by inflammatory granulation issue infiltrated with chronic inflammatory and giant cells, with a peripheral fibrous capsule between this and the alveolar bone. Pus may accumulate in the adjacent bone marrow spaces as well as the periapical PDL space (Gardner, 1962b) (*Fig. 14.20*).

RARE INFECTIONS OF THE PERIODONTAL LIGAMENT

ACTINOMYCOSIS

Periodontal lesions are usually secondary to cervicofacial actinomycosis. The rare PDL lesions often contain epithelial cell rests, which may form cysts. Chronic abscess formation is a more usual sequel. This displays a central zone of bacterial filaments surrounded by lymphocytes, PMN, endothelioid and giant cells, and a peripheral thick fibrous layer (Wade, 1965; August and Levy, 1973; Samanta *et al.*, 1975; Krolls et al., 1977). The lesion may spread to involve the jaw, or present gingivally as an enlarging painless nodule that softens, usually after several months, and breaks down, discharging yellow pus that contains typical sulphur granules (Wade, 1965). Periapical actinomycosis has also been reported with demonstrable actinomycetes in the periapical region surrounded by PMN and other inflammatory cells (August and Levy, 1973; Samanta *et al.*, 1975; Krolls *et al.*, 1977).

ACUTE NECROTIZING ULCERATIVE GINGIVITIS

Spread to involve the PDL, except in HIV infection, is uncommon, but extensive destruction of the PDL can occur (Hornstein and Gorlin, 1970). In such instances, there is loss of crestal bone, and the ligament is affected by marked vasodilatation and thrombosis, resulting in a localized ischaemic necrosis. An intense acute inflammatory infiltrate may spread to the marrow spaces, and the transseptal fibres are then usually disrupted (Cohen, 1965; Wade, 1965). Among the possible mechanisms underlying the pathogenesis may be an excessive cell-mediated immune response to one of the associated organisms, fusiform bacilli (Nisengard, 1977). Lehner (1969) found significantly depressed IgG and raised IgM concentrations within 1–4 days of onset of clinical symptoms, followed by rises in levels of IgG and IgM during the first month after onset. Complement levels appeared to be normal. Lehner suggested that these changes could be effected by a relative hypogammaglobulinaemia of the IgG class or by the (unspecified) activity of Gram-negative organisms.

Rees (1993) has reviewed HIV-related periodontitis. He describes lesions as localized or generalized. Periodontitis is aggressive, necrotizing, similar to acute necrotizing ulcerative periodontitis, and it occurs in conjunction with a rapidly destructive periodontitis suggestive of cancrum oris. It seems that CIPD may progress more rapidly in HIV infection, but in addition there are specific periodontal lesions strongly associated with HIV. These have been termed linear gingival erythema, necrotizing ulcerative gingivitis, necrotizing ulcerative periodontitis, and necrotizing stomatitis (Axell *et al.*, 1991; Williams, 1993).

TUBERCULOSIS

The oral lesion is usually a crateriform, painless ulcer with a caseated base, which may rarely extend to the PDL and cause tooth loss. If extension occurs, the lesion presents as an endosteal granuloma with a chronic sinus, which often persists after local treatment (Wade, 1965). One individual with acute disseminated miliary tuberculosis was found to have very loose teeth with numerous yellowish, pinhead-sized tubercles on the affected gingival margins. The roots of extracted teeth were covered by soft, adherent granulomatous tissue containing many tubercles (Grant and Bernick, 1972). Cases have been reported of apical granulomas containing closely packed tubercles with epithelioid and giant cells, but little caseation (Bradnum, 1961). In general, periodontal lesions are secondary to pulmonary tuberculosis (Jian, 1956).

LEPROSY

Gingival ulceration in lepromatous leprosy may spread to cause severe PDL destruction, affecting particularly the maxillary incisors (Epker and Via, 1969; Reichart *et al.*, 1976). There seem to be no reports of tuberculoid leprosy affecting the PDL. The lepromatous lesion typically causes widening of both lamina dura and PDL space. Histologically, the changes seen in the PDL are little different from those seen in non-specific chronic inflammation. Occasionally, scanty acid-fast fragmented granular bacilli, representing the degenerate forms of *Mycobacterium leprae*, occur in relation to macrophages (Reichart *et al.*, 1976).

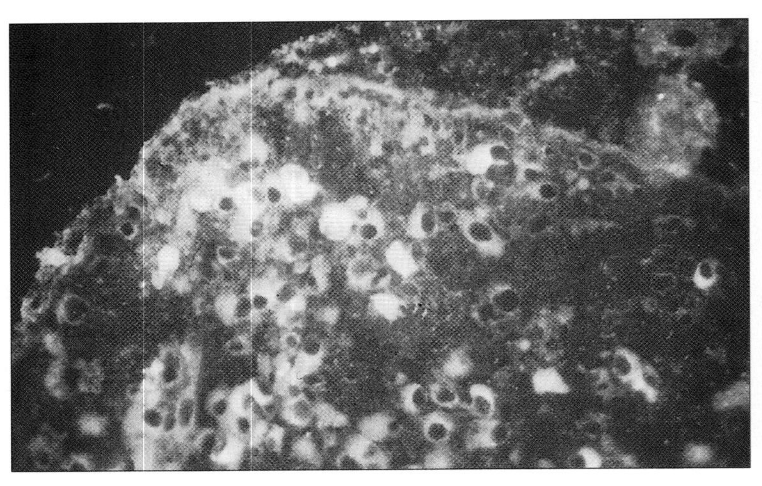

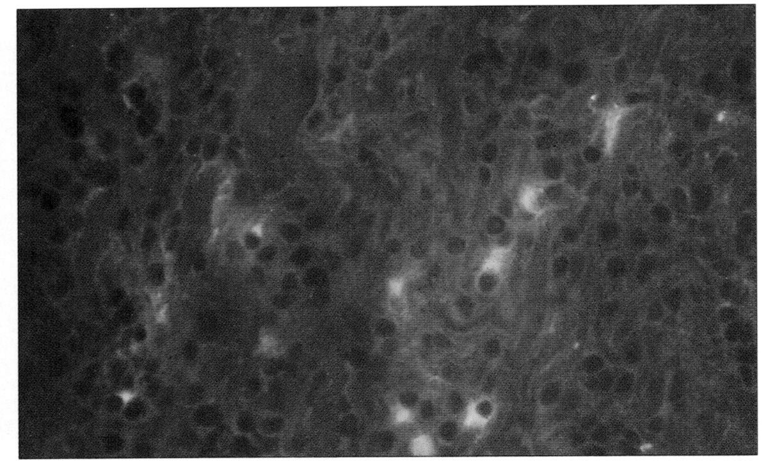

Figs 14.18, 14.19 Immunofluorescence photomicrographs of unfixed chronically inflamed periapical tissues labelled with fluoresceinated anti-human IgG and IgM respectively. Abundant IgG-containing cells are present in most instances (*Fig. 14.18*) and fewer IgM plasma cells (*Fig. 14.19*). (Magnification × 700.) (From Morton *et al.*, 1977.)

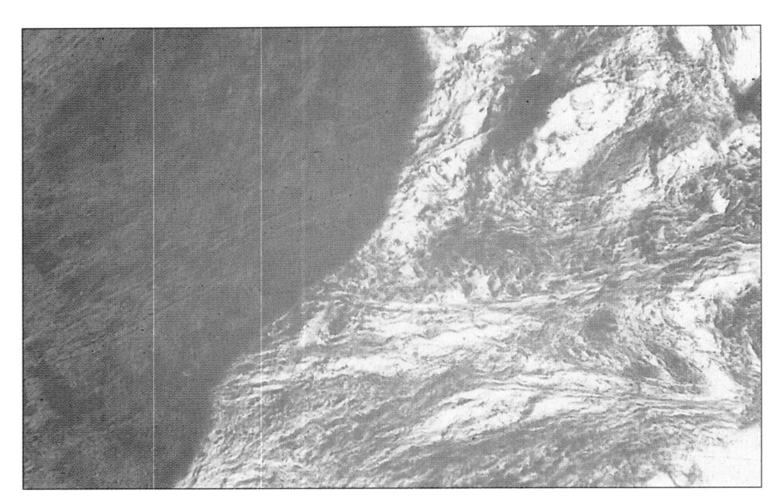

Fig. 14.20 Transmitted light micrograph, showing PDL necrosis periapically following severe inflammation. Ligament cells are not visible, and the fibres are thin and disordered. (Magnification × 25.)

ASPERGILLOSIS

A single case of aspergillosis of the nasal cavity, caused by a strain of the filamentous fungus *Aspergillus*, and arising probably from a maxillary incisor periapical abscess, has been reported in a patient debilitated by acute myelogenous leukaemia (Fields, 1977).

CYTOMEGALOVIRUS

Morgan (1993) reported a case of necrotizing periodontitis in an HIV-seropositive patient, who had cytomegalovirus-infected endothelial cells lining blood vessels in inflamed periodontal pocket wall. These cells had classical 'owl's eye' nuclei and they stained positively with a commercial polyclonal antibody to cytomegalovirus. Morgan (1993) suggested further evaluation of the possible contribution of cytomegalovirus infection to periodontal destruction in HIV-affected patients.

GLANDERS

This disease of horses is caused by the Gram-negative bacillus *Loefflerella mallei*. Human glanders, occurring usually in those working with affected animals, may on rare occasions produce destructive crateriform gingival ulcers extending in even rarer instances to alveolar bone, and leading to tooth exfoliation. The lesion develops quickly into an ulcer, which enlarges by marginal breakdown or confluence of adjacent ulcers, and discharges a yellowish, blood-streaked, oily fluid (Hornstein and Gorlin, 1970).

LEISHMANIASIS

Protozoa of the genus *Leishmania*, closely related to the trypanosomes, may cause disease in humans. On extremely rare occasions, leishmaniasis may involve the PDL, and endarteritis accelerates the process of destruction. This occurs only in the serious mucocutaneous form of the disease, in which the lesions are reported as firm, partly ulcerative, partly polypoid, severely mutilating, chronic, and progressive (Hornstein and Gorlin, 1970). Detailed PDL histopathology is lacking. In kala-azar, the most serious form of the disease, loosening of the teeth has been reported in some cases. In one report of kala-azar, there was severe periodontitis that did not respond to antiseptics or antibiotics. All teeth were loose, with extensive bone destruction and widening of the PDL space (Abbas *et al.* 1992).

HISTOPLASMOSIS

A single case of histoplasmosis as periapical pathology has been documented (Pisanty, 1979). The fungus was identified in a periapical granuloma in relation to a symptomless upper first molar, for which vitality tests had been inconclusive. There had been no periodontal pockets around the affected tooth. Histologically, large numbers of fungus-laden phagocytes were present. These contained many minute yeast-like bodies with prominent round nuclei surrounded by a clear zone and a distinct peripheral capsule, compatible with the appearance of *Histoplasma capsulatum*. Pisanty (1979) suggested that the organism had gained entry to the tissue during previous extraction of an adjoining tooth. The patient had no systemic involvement and intradermal histoplasmin skin test and chest radiography were negative. A similar case has been reported at a tooth extraction site that failed to heal (Young *et al.*, 1981).

MYIASIS

Myiasis, the term used for parasitic invasion in humans or other mammals by fly larvae (Rees, 1993), has been reported in a periodontal pocket around all the lower incisors, with advanced alveolar bone loss, and generally poor oral hygiene (Zeltser and Lustmann, 1988).

HERPES ZOSTER

Wright *et al.* (1983) reported a case of alveolar bone necrosis and tooth loss associated with herpes zoster infection of the fifth cranial nerve.

CONCLUSIONS

Surprisingly little attention has been given to changes in the PDL in the infectious inflammatory periodontal diseases, whether rare or common. Concerning the most widespread of these periodontal diseases, there is still inadequate information concerning mechanisms of ligament degradation, although there are suggestions that defective cellular host response factors, especially PMN, and a range of Gram-negative anaerobes in plaque, may accelerate the rate of tissue loss. This would point to the elaboration by live organisms or the passive release by dead or dying bacteria of factors of which some are more noxious than others to the PDL.

One of the most important features requiring clarification is the mechanism by which gingivitis spreads to involve the deeper tissues, and how this change occurs at different times and rates in different patients. There still needs to be more effort to establish the mechanisms of collagen loss, and more detail is required concerning the changes that occur in both the collagen fibre structure and the ground substance. Is collagen loss brought about directly by plaque enzymes or other factors, or by host tissue factors alone? The general details of the host response remain confusing at the present time. It is to be hoped that future research will clarify the situation *in vivo*. This should involve the subjection of periodontal tissues to a variety of putative, protective, or destructive factors in order to assess the effects of these factors (both singly and in combination), and especially to assess the effects on the rate of development and progression of chronic inflammatory periodontal disease.

ACKNOWLEDGMENT

Figures **14.7** to **14.14** inclusive are courtesy of PM Barber, F Joachim and HN Newman, Eastman Dental Institute.

REFERENCES

Abbas K, El Toum I and El Hassan AM (1992) Oral leishmaniasis associated with kala-azar. Oral Surg 73, 583–584.

Adams RA, Zander HA and Polson AM (1979) Cell population in the transseptal fibre region before, during and after experimental periodontitis in squirrel monkeys. J Periodontol 50, 7–12.

Amer A, Singh G, Darke C and Dolby AE (1988) Association between HLA antigens and periodontal disease. Tissue Antigens 31, 53–58.

Anusaksathien O, Singh G, Matthews N and Dolby AE (1992) Autoimmunity to collagen in adult periodontal disease: immunoglobulin classes in sera and tissue. J Periodont Res 27, 55–61.

Arwill T and Heyden G (1973) Histochemical studies on cholesterol-formation in odontogenic cysts and granulomas. Scand J Dent Res 81, 406–410.

Attström R and Schroeder HE (1979) Effect of experimental neutropenia on initial gingivitis in dogs. Scand J Dent Res 87, 7–23.

August OS and Levy BA (1973) Periapical actinomycosis. Oral Surg 36, 585–588.

Axell T, Baert AE, Brocheriou C *et al.* (1991) An update of the classification and diagnostic criteria of oral lesions in HIV infection. J Oral Pathol Med 20, 97–100.

Baer PN, Stanley HR, Brown K, Smith L, Gamble J and Swerdlow H (1963) Advanced periodontal disease in an adolescent (periodontosis). J Periodontol 34, 533–539.

Barnett ML (1974) The fine structure of human connective tissue mast cells in periodontal disease. J Periodont Res 9, 84–91.

Berglund SE (1971) Immunoglobulins in human gingiva with specificity for oral bacteria. J Periodontol 42, 546–551.

Bernick S and Grant DA (1978) Lymphatic vessels of healthy and inflamed gingiva. J Dent Res 57, 810–817.

Birek P, Wang HM, Brunette DM and Melcher AH (1980) Epithelial rests of Malassez *in vitro*. Phagocytosis of collagen and the possible role of their lysosomal enzymes in collagen degradation.Lab Invest 43, 61–72.

Block RM, Bushell A, Rodrigues H and Langeland K (1976) A histopathologic, histobacteriologic and radiographic study of periapical endodontic surgical specimens. Oral Surg 42, 656–678.

Blumenkrantz N and Söndergaard J (1972) Effect of prostaglandins on biosynthesis of collagen. Nature 239, 246.

Bouyssou M and Fourel J (1973) La parodontite aiguë juvénile et le syndrome de Papillon Lefèvre. Problème clinique, pathologique et étiologique. Acta Stomatol Belgica 70, 71–113.
Bozzo L, Valdrighi L and Vizioli MR (1972) Lipid components of human dental periapical lesions. Histochemical and histophysical observations. Oral Surg 34, 166–171.
Bradnum P (1961) Tuberculous sinus of face associated with an abscessed lower third molar. Dent Practit 12, 127–128.
Brandtzaeg P (1966) Local factors of resistance in the gingival area. J Periodont Res 1, 19–42.
Brandtzaeg P and Kraus FW (1965) Autoimmunity and periodontal disease. Odontol Tidskr 73, 281–393.
Browne RM (1971) The origin of cholesterol in odontogenic cysts in man. Arch Oral Biol 16, 107–114.
Carlson DR (1964) Histochemistry of oxidative enzymes in hamster periodontal disease. J Dent Res 43, 846.
Challacombe SJ, Yiel N, Stephenson PA and Wilton JMA (1992) Antibodies and opsonic activity to plaque bacteria in human gingival crevicular fluid in relation to dental caries. Microb Ecol Hlth Dis 5, 21–30.
Challacombe SJ (1993) Genetic and immune aspects of chronic inflammatory periodontal disease. In: Diseases of the Periodontium, pp 27–54 (Newman HN, Rees TD and Kinane DF, eds), Science Reviews, Northwood.
Cianciola LJ, Genco RJ, Patters MR, McKenna J and van Oss C (1977) Defective polymorphonuclear leukocyte function in a human periodontal disease. Nature 265, 445–447.
Clagett JA and Page RC (1978) Insoluble immune complexes and chronic periodontal disease in man and the dog. Arch Oral Biol 23, 153–165.
Clark RA, Page RC and Wilde G (1977) Defective neutrophil chemotaxis in juvenile periodontitis. Infect Immun 18, 694–700.
Cohen DW (1965) Pathology of periodontal diseases. In: Oral Pathology (Tiecke RW, ed), pp 131–167, McGraw Hill, New York.
Cullinan MP, Sachs J, Wolf E and Stewart GJ (1980) The distribution of HLA-A and -B antigens in patients and their families with periodontosis. J Periodont Res 15, 177–184.
Daniel MA, McDonald G, Offenbacher S and van Dyke TE (1993) Defective chemotaxis and calcium response in localized juvenile periodontitis neutrophils. J Periodontol 64, 617–621.
Darling AI (1970) Periapical inflammation of the teeth. In: Thoma's Oral Pathology, volumel 1 (Gorlin RJ and Goldman HM eds), pp 335–358, Mosby, St Louis.
Deguchi S, Hori T, Creamer H and Gabler W (1990) Neutrophil-mediated damage to human periodontal ligament-derived fibroblasts: role of lipopolysaccharide. J Periodontol Res 25, 293–299.
Diniotou M, Croisier N, Pompidou A, Mare B, Mugnier A and Schramm B (1975) Contribution à l'étude histopathologique des granulomes apexiens. Bull Groupe Eur Rech Sci Stomat Odont 18, 25–35.
EC Clearinghouse on Oral Problems Related to HIV Infection and WHO Collaborating Centre on Oral Manifestations of the Immunodeficiency Virus (1993) Classification and diagnostic criteria for oral lesions in HIV infections. J Oral Pathol Med. 22, 289–291.
Eley BM and Harrison JD (1975) Intracellular collagen fibrils in the periodontal ligament of man. J Periodont Res 10, 168–170.
Epker BN and Via WF (1969) Oral and perioral manifestations of leprosy. Report of a case. Oral Surg 28, 342–347.
Farber PA (1975) Scanning electron microscopy of cells from periapical lesions. J Endod 1, 291–294.
Fields BN (1977) Case 36–1977. Case records of the Massachusetts General Hospital. N Engl J Med 297, 546–551.
Fourel J (1972) Periodontosis: a periodontal syndrome. J Periodontol 43, 240–255.
Ftis A, Singh G and Dolby AE (1986) Antibody to collagen type I in periodontal disease. J Periodontol 57, 693–698.
Fullmer HM (1960) Observations on the development of oxytalan fibres in dental granulomas and radicular cysts. Arch Pathol 70, 59–67.
Fullmer HM (1961) A histochemical study of periodontal disease in the maxillary alveolar processes of 135 autopsies. J Periodontol 32, 206–218.
Fullmer HM (1962) A critique of normal connective tissues of the periodontium and some alterations with periodontal disease. J Dent Res 41, 223–229 and 229–234.
Fullmer HM, Baer P and Driscoll E (1969) Correlation of collagenase production to periodontal disease. J Periodont Res 4 (suppl), 30–31.
Garant PR (1976) An electron microscopic study of the periodontal tissues of germfree rats and rats mono-infected with Actinomyces naeslundii. J Periodont Res (suppl) 11, 3–79.
Garant PR and Cho MI (1979a) Histopathogenesis of spontaneous periodontal disease in conventional rats. I. Histometric and histologic study. J Periodont Res 14, 297–309.
Garant PR and Cho MI (1979b) Histopathogenesis of spontaneous periodontal disease in conventional rats. II. Ultrastructural features of the inflamed subepithelial connective tissue. J Periodont Res 14, 310–322.
Gardner AF (1962a) A survey of periapical pathology. Part I. Dent Digest 68, 162–167.
Gardner AF (1962b) A survey of periapical pathology. Part 2. Dent Digest 68, 223–227.
Gargiulo AV Jr, Robinson J, Toto PD and Gargiulo AW (1982) Identification of rheumatoid factor in periodontal disease. J Peridontol 53, 568–577.
Goldman HM (1951) The topography and role of the gingival fibres. J Dent Res 30, 331–336.
Goldman HM (1957a) The behavior of transseptal fibres in periodontal disease. J Dent Res 36, 249–259.
Goldman HM (1957b) Extension of exudate into supporting structures of teeth in marginal periodontitis. J Periodontol 28, 175–183.
Grant D and Bernick S (1972) The periodontium of ageing humans. J Periodontol 43, 660–667.
Grupe HE, Ten Cate AR and Zander HA (1967) A histochemical and radiological study of *in vitro* and *in vivo* human epithelial cell rest proliferation. Arch Oral Biol 12, 1321–1329.
Gustafson GT (1969) Increased susceptibility to periodontitis in mink affected by a lysosomal disease. J Periodont Res 4, 259–267.
Hamp SE and Folke LEA (1968) The lysosomes and their possible role in periodontal disease. Odont Tidskr 76, 353–375.
Heijl L, Rifkin BR and Zander HA (1976) Conversion of chronic gingivitis to periodontitis in squirrel monkeys. J Periodontol 47, 710–716.
Hirsch HZ, Tarkowski A, Miller EJ, Gay S, Koopman WJ and Mestecky J (1988) Autoimmunity to collagen in adult periodontal disease. J Oral Pathol 17, 456–459.
Holland GR (1988) The periapical innervation of the ferret canine and the local retrograde neural changes after pulpectomy. Anat Rec 220, 318–327.
Holland GR (1993) Neural changes in periapical lesions after systemic steroids in the ferret. J Dent Res 72, 987–992.
Hornstein OP and Gorlin RJ (1970) Infectious oral diseases. In: Thoma's Oral Pathology, volume 2 (Gorlin RJ and Goldman HM, eds), pp 708–774, Mosby, St Louis.
Horton JE, Leikin S and Oppenheim JJ (1972) Human lympho-proliferative reaction to saliva and dental plaque deposits: an in vitro correlation with periodontal disease. J Periodontol 43, 522–527.
Irving JT, Socransky SS and Heeley JD (1974) Histologic changes in experimental periodontal disease in gnotobiotic rats and conventional hamsters. J Periodont Res 9, 73–80.
Ivanyi L and Lehner T (1970) Stimulation of lymphocyte transformation by bacterial antigens in patients with periodontal disease. Arch Oral Biol 15, 1089–1096.

Ivanyi L and Lehner T (1971) Lymphocyte transformation by sonicates of dental plaque in human periodontal disease. Arch Oral Biol 16, 1117–1121.

Ivanyi L, Wilton JMA and Lehner T (1972) Cell-mediated immunity in periodontal disease: cytotoxicity, migration inhibition and lymphocyte transformation studies. Immunology 22, 141–145.

Jacoby BH and Davis WL (1991) The electron microscopic immunolocalization of a copper–zinc superoxide dismutase in association with collagen fibers of periodontal soft tissues. J Periodontol 62, 413–420.

Jian W (1956) Parodontolyses et tuberculose. Parodontol Zürich 10, 66–69.

Joachim F, Sati K, Barber P, Newman HN and Osborn J (1989) Aspects of the distribution of plasma cells at the advancing front of the lesion in chronic periodontitis: a quantitative ultrastructural study. J Parodont 8, 229–248.

Joachim F, Barber P, Newman HN and Osborn J (1990) The plasma cell at the advancing front of the lesion in chronic periodontitis. J Periodont Res 25, 49–59.

Johnson NW (1988) Detection of high-risk groups and individuals for periodontal diseases: evidence for the existence of high risk groups and approaches to their detection. J Clin Periodontol 15, 271–277.

Jonsson R, Pitts A, Lue C, Gay S and Mestecky J (1991) Immunoglobulin isotype distribution of locally produced autoantibodies to collagen type I in adult periodontitis. Relationship to periodontal treatment. J Clin Periodontol 18, 703–707.

Kaslick RS and Chasens AI (1968a) Periodontosis with periodontitis: a study involving young adult males. Part I. Review of the literature and incidence in a military population. Oral Surg 25, 305–326.

Kaslick RS and Chasens AI (1968b) Periodontosis with periodontitis: a study involving young adult males. Part II. Clinical, medical and histopathologic studies. Oral Surg 25, 327–350.

Kaslick RS, West TL and Chasens AI (1980) Association between ABO blood groups, HLA antigens and periodontal disease in young adults: a follow-up study. J Periodontol 51, 339–342.

Kennedy JE (1974) Effect of inflammation on collateral circulation of the gingiva. J Periodont Res 9, 147–152.

Kiger RD, Wright WH and Creamer HR (1974) The significance of lymphocyte transformation responses to various microbial strains. J Periodontol 45, 780–785.

Kohl J and Zander HA (1962) Fibres conjonctives 'oxytalan' dans le tissu gingival interdentaire. Paradontologie 16, 23–30.

Kopp W (1988) Density and localization of lymphocytes with natural-killer (NK) cell activity in periodontal biopsy. J Clin Periodont 15, 595–600.

Krolls SO, Westbrook SD and Hess DS (1977) Actinomycosis as periapical pathology. Case report. J Oral Med 32, 41–43.

Kuntz DS, Genco RJ, Guttuso J and Natiella JR (1977) Localization of immunoglobulins and the third component of complement in dental periapical lesions. J Endod 3, 68–73.

Langeland K, Block RM and Grossman LI (1977) A histopathologic and histobacteriologic study of 35 periapical endodontic surgical specimens. J Endod 3, 8–23.

Le J and Vilcek J (1987) Tumour necrosis factor and interleukin 1: cytokines with multiple overlapping biological activities. Lab Invest 56, 234–248.

Lehner T (1969) Immunoglobulin abnormalities in ulcerative gingivitis. Br Dent J 127, 165–169.

Leonard EP, Lunin M and Provenza DV (1974) On the occurrence and morphology of Russell bodies in the dental granuloma. An evaluation of seventy-nine specimens. Oral Surg 38, 584–590.

Leuin IS (1957) Infection and tumors arising in and from the periapical tissues. Oral Surg 10, 1291–1301.

Liakoni H, Barber PM and Newman HN (1987a) Bacterial penetration of the pocket tissues in juvenile/postjuvenile periodontitis after the presurgical oral hygiene phase. J Periodontol 58, 847–855.

Liakoni H, Barber P and Newman HN (1987b) Bacterial penetration of pocket soft tissues in chronic adult and juvenile periodontitis cases. An ultrastructural study. J Clin Periodont 14, 22–28.

Lin L and Langeland K (1981) Innervation of the inflammatory periapical lesions. Oral Surg 51, 535–543.

Lindhe J, Hamp SE and Löe H (1973) Experimental periodontitis in the beagle dog. J Periodont Res 8, 1–10.

Lindhe J and Socransky SS (1979) Chemotaxis and vascular permeability produced by human periodontopathic bacteria. J Periodont Res 14, 138–146.

Löe H, Anerud A, Boysen H and Morrison E (1986) Natural history of periodontal disease in man. Rapid, moderate and no loss of attachment in Sri Lankan laborers 14 to 46 years of age. J Clin Periodontol 13, 431–440.

Lyons DC, Yazdi I, Nonparast B and Miriohi M (1970) The histopathologic variations of the chronic dental granuloma. J Oral Med 25, 46–50.

Macapanpan LC and Weinmann JP (1954) The influence of injury to the periodontal membrane on the spread of gingival inflammation. J Dent Res 33, 263–272.

Mackler BF, Altman LC, Wahl S, Rosenstreich DL, Oppenheim JJ and Mergenhagen SE (1974) Blastogenesis and lymphokine synthesis by T and B lymphocytes from patients with periodontal disease. Infect Immun 10, 844–850.

Mammo W, Singh G and Dolby AE (1982) Enhanced cellular immune response to collagen type I in patients with periodontal disease. Int Arch Allergy Appl Immunol 67, 149–154.

Marggraf E, Keyserlingk-Eberius JJ, Komischke B and Wollert N (1983) Die Assoziation von Histocompatibilitatsantigen (HLA-Antigene) mit profunden Paradontopathien. Dtsch Zahnarzt Z 38, 585–589.

Martinelli C and Rulli MA (1967) The innervation of chronic inflammatory human periapical lesions. Arch Oral Biol 12, 593–600.

Mathiesen A (1973) Preservation and demonstration of mast cells in human apical granulomas and radicular cysts. Scand J Dent Res 81, 218–229.

McFall WT (1964) Periodontal abscess. J N Carolina Dent Soc 47, 34–36.

Meghji S, Henderson B, Nair S and Wilson M (1992a) Inhibition of bone DNA and collagen production by surface-associated material from bacteria implicated in the pathology of periodontal disease. J Periodontol 63, 736–742.

Meghji S, Wilson M, Henderson B and Kinane D (1992b) Anti proliferative and cytotoxic activity of surface-associated material from periodontopathogenic bacteria. Arch Oral Biol 37, 637–644.

Meikle MD, Heath JK and Reynolds JJ (1986) Advances in understanding cell interactions in tissue resorption: relevance to the pathogenesis of periodontal diseases and a new hypothesis. J Oral Pathol 15, 239–250.

Melcher AH (1962) Pathogenesis of chronic gingivitis. I. The spread of the inflammatory process. Dent Practit 13, 2–7.

Michel G and Frank RM (1970) Surcharge glycogénique des cellules ligamentaires et osseuses au cours des parodontolyses. Parodontologie 24, 3–9.

Miyasaki KT (1991) The neutrophil: mechanisms of controlling periodontal bacteria. J Periodontol 62, 761–774.

Miyasato MC (1975) The periodontal abscess. Periodontology 23, 53–59 (abstract).

Morgan PR (1993) Specific periodontal infections. In: Diseases of the Periodontium. (Newman HN, Rees TD and Kinane DF, eds), pp 99–107, Science Reviews, Northwood, Middlesex, UK.

Morse DR, Lasater DR and White D (1975) Presence of immunoglobulin-producing cells in periapical lesions. J Endod 1, 338–343.

Morton TH, Clagett JA and Yavorsky JD (1977) Role of immune complexes in human periapical periodontitis. J Endod 3, 261–268.

Moskow BS and Polson AM (1991) Histologic studies on the extension of the inflammatory infiltrate in human periodontitis. J Clin Periodontol 18, 534–542.

Movius D, Roger RS and Reeve CM (1975) Lymphocytotoxicity for gingival epithelial cells in periodontal disease. J Periodontol 46, 271–276.
Mühlemann HR (1954) Tooth mobility. The measuring method. Initial and secondary tooth mobility. J Periodontol 25, 22–29.
Murray PA and Patters MR (1980) Gingival crevice neutrophil function in periodontal lesions. J Periodont Res 15, 463–469.
Narayanan AS and Page RC (1976) Biochemical characterization of collagens synthesized by fibroblasts derived from normal and diseased human gingiva. J Biol Chem 251, 5464–5471.
Narita T (1956) Histopathologic study on natural healing in chronic periapical periodontitis. Bull Oral Path Tokyo 1, 163–185.
Newman HN (1976) The apical border of plaque in chronic inflammatory periodontal disease. Br Dent J 141, 105–113.
Newman HN and Addison IE (1982) Gingival crevice neutrophil function in periodontosis. J Periodontol 53, 578–586.
Newman HN, Rees TD and Kinane DF (1993) Diseases of the Periodontium. Science Reviews, Northwood, Middlesex, UK.
Newman HN and Rule DC (1983) Plaque-host imbalance in severe periodontitis. A discussion based on two cases. J Clin Periodontol 10, 137–147.
Nisengard RJ (1977) The role of immunology in periodontal disease. J Periodontol 48, 505–516.
Nisengard RJ, Beutner EH, Neugeboren NJ, Neider M and Asaro J (1977) Experimental induction of periodontal disease with Arthus-type reactions. Clin Immunol Immunopathol 8, 97–104.
Obrucnik M and Meduna J (1959) Histological and histochemical characteristics of apical granulomas. Ceskoslov Stomat 59, 317–328.
Orban B and Weinmann JP (1942) Diffuse atrophy of the alveolar bone (periodontosis). J Periodontol 13, 31–45.
O'Neill PA, Woodson DL and Mackler BF (1982) Functional characterisation of human gingival lymphocytes cytotoxic activity. J. Periodont 46, 271–276.
Page RC and Schroeder HE (1976) Pathogenesis of inflammatory periodontal disease. A summary of current work. Lab Invest 34, 235–249.
Page RC (1991) The role of inflammatory mediators in the pathogenesis of periodontal disease. J Periodont Res 26, 23–242.
Page RC, Ko SD, Hassell TM and Narayanan AS (1979) The role of fibroblast subpopulations in the connective tissue alterations of gingival and periodontal diseases. J Periodont Res 14, 266 (ahs).
Page RC, Simpson DM, Ammons WF and Shechtman LR (1972) Host tissue response in chronic periodontal disease. III. Clinical, histopathologic and ultrastructural features of advanced disease in a colony-maintained marmoset. J Periodont Res 7, 283–296.
Parakkal PF (1969) Involvement of macrophages in collagen resorption. J Cell Biol 41, 345–354.
Patters MR, Genco RJ, Reed MJ and Mashimo PA (1976) Blastogenic response of human lymphocytes to oral bacterial antigens: comparison of individuals with periodontal disease to normal and edentulous subjects. Infect Immun 14, 1213–1220.
Paunio K (1965) Studies on the connective tissue components in the periodontal membrane. Odont Tidskr 73, 613–614.
Paunio K (1969a) The age change of acid mucopolysaccharides in the periodontal membrane of man. J Periodont Res 4 (suppl), 32–33.
Paunio K (1969b) Periodontal connective tissue. Biochemical studies of disease in man. Suomen Hammas Toim 65, 249–290.
Paunio K and Mäkinen K (1969) Studies on hydrolytic enzyme activity in the connective tissue of the human periodontal ligament. Observations apart from areas of inflammation. Acta Odont Scand 27, 153–171.
Paunio KU, Mäkinen KK and Paunio IK (1970) The stability of extracted collagen molecules from human periodontal membrane. Acta Odont Scand 28, 959–966.
Peng TK (1988) Serum antibodies to native and denatured type I and III collagen in patients with periodontal disease. Proc Natl Sci Council Repub China [B] 12, 21–26.
Picton DCA (1962) A study of normal tooth mobility and the changes with periodontal disease. Dent Practit 12, 167–173.
Pisanty S (1979) Histoplasmosis as periapical pathology. J Oral Med 34, 116–118.
Popov CP (1965) Sur la présence et la signification des fibres élastiques dans le paradentium. Rev Stomatol (Paris) 66, 553–556.
Pritchard JF (1953) Management of the periodontal abscess. Oral Surg 6, 474–482.
Pulver WH, Taubman MA and Smith DJ (1978) Immune components in human dental periapical lesions. Arch Oral Biol 23, 535–543.
Quintarelli G (1960) Histochemistry of the gingiva. IV. Preliminary investigations on the mucopolysaccharides of connective tissue. Arch Oral Biol 2, 277–284.
Raisz LG and Koolemans-Beynen AR (1974) Inhibition of bone collagen synthesis by prostaglandin E_2 in organ cultures. Prostaglandins 10, 377–385.
Ranney RR (1991) Immunologic mechanisms of pathogenesis in periodontal diseases: an assessment. J Periodont Res 26, 243–254.
Rao LG, Moe HK and Heersche JNM (1978) *In vitro* culture of porcine periodontal ligament cells: response of fibroblast-like and epithelial-like cells to prostaglandin E_1, parathyroid hormone and calcitonin and separation of a pure population of fibroblast-like cells. Arch Oral Biol 23, 957–964.
Rees TD (1993) Systemic factors in periodontal disease. In: Diseases of the Periodontium (Newman HN, Rees TD and Kinane DF, eds), pp 55–93, Science Reviews, Northwood, Middlesex.
Reichart P, Ananatasan T and Reznik G (1976) Gingiva and periodontium in lepromatous leprosy. A clinical, radiological and microscopical study. J Periodontol 47, 455–460.
Reinholdt J, Bay L and Svejgaard A (1977) Association between HLA antigens and periodontal disease. J Periodontol 51, 70–73.
Rippin JW (1978) Collagen turnover in the periodontal ligament under normal and altered functional forces. II. Adult rat molars. J Periodont Res 13, 149–154.
Ruben MP, Goldman HM and Schulman SM (1970) Diseases of the periodontium. In: Thoma's Oral Pathology, volume 1 (Gorlin RJ and Goldman HM, eds), pp 394–444, Mosby, St Louis.
Rupnarain B, Singh G, Newcombe R and Dolby AE (1990) Cellular immunity to autoantigen in periodontal disease: lymphoblastic responses to differing concentrations of collagen type I. Med Sci Res 18, 141–143.
Sakamoto S, Goldhaber P and Glimcher MJ (1973) Mouse bone collagenase: the effect of heparin on the amount of enzyme released in tissue culture and on the activity of the enzyme. Calc Tissue Res 12, 247–258.
Samanta A, Malik CP and Aikat BK (1975) Periapical actinomycosis. Oral Surg 39, 458–462.
Sati K, Bulman JS and Newman HN (1991) Peripheral blood polymorphonuclear neutrophil (PMN) count in caucasian and negro patients with juvenile/post-juvenile periodontitis (JP/PJP). In: Recent Advances in Periodontology, volume 2 (Gold SI, Midda M and Mutlu S, eds), pp 225–228, Excerpta Medica, Amsterdam.
Saxén L and Koskimies S (1984) Juvenile periodontitis – no linkage with HLA-antigens. J Periodont Res 19, 441–444.
Schluger S, Yuodelis R and Page RC (1977) Pathogenic mechanisms. In: Periodontal Disease. Lea and Febiger, Philadelphia.
Schroeder HE and Page R (1972) Lymphocyte fibroblast interaction in the pathogenesis of inflammatory gingival disease. Experientia 28, 1228–1230.
Schultz-Haudt SD and Aas E (1960) Observations on the status of collagen in human gingiva. Arch Oral Biol 2, 131–142.
Selvig KA (1966) Ultrastructural changes in cementum and adjacent connective tissue in periodontal disease. Acta Odont Scand 24, 459–500.
Selvig KA (1968) Nonbanded fibrils of collagenous nature in human periodontal connective tissue. J Periodont Res 3, 169–179.

Seymour GJ (1987) Possible mechanisms involved in the immunoregulation of chronic inflammatory periodontal disease. J Dent Res 66, 2–9.

Seymour GJ (1991) Importance of the host response in the periodontium. J Clin Periodontol 18, 421–426.

Seymour GJ and Greenspan JS (1979) The phenotypic characterization of lymphocyte subpopulations in established human periodontal disease. J Periodont Res 14, 39–46.

Shore RC, Moxham BJ and Berkovitz BKB (1989) Effect of inflammatory periodontal disease ('broken mouth') on the structure of collagen fibrils in the sheep incisor periodontum. Res Vet Sci 47, 148–151.

Skougaard MR and Levy BM (1971) Collagen metabolism in periodontal membrane of the marmoset. Influence of periodontal disease. Scand J Dent Res 79, 518–572.

Soames JV and Davies RM (1977) Intracellular collagen fibrils in early gingivitis in the beagle dog. J Periodont Res 12, 378–386.

Stahl SS (1973) Marginal lesions. In: Periodontal Therapy, 5th edtion (Goldman HM and Cohen DW, eds), pp 94–142, Mosby, St. Louis.

Stahl SS, Sandler HC and Suben E (1958) Histochemical changes in inflammatory periodontal disease. J Periodontol 29, 183–191.

Stanley HR (1955) The cyclic phenomenon of periodontitis. Oral Surg 8, 598–610.

Stashenko P, Jandinski JJ, Fujiyoshi P, Rynar J and Socransky SS (1991) Tissue levels of bone resorptive cytokines in periodontal disease. J Periodontol 62, 504–509.

Subadan CJ, Barber P, Joachim F and Newman HN (1990) The basement membrane in adult and juvenile/post-juvenile periodontitis: an ultrastructural study. J Parodontol 9, 321–334.

Summers L and Papadimitriou J (1975) The nature of epithelial proliferation in apical granulomas. J Oral Pathol 4, 324–329.

Ten Cate AR (1972a) Morphological studies of fibrocytes in connective tissue undergoing rapid remodelling. J Anat 112, 401–414.

Ten Cate AR (1972b) The epithelial cell rests of Malassez and the genesis of the dental cyst. Oral Surg 34, 956–964.

Ten Cate AR and Deporter DA (1975) The degradative role of the fibroblast in the remodelling and turnover of collagen in soft connective tissue. Anat Rec 182, 1–14.

Terasaki PI, Kaslick RS, West TL and Chasens AI (1975) Low HL-A2 frequency and periodontitis. Tissue Antigens 5, 286–288.

Toto PD, Pollock RJ and Gargiulo AW (1964) Pathogenesis of periodontitis. Periodontics 2, 197–201.

Valderhaug J (1974) Epithelial rests in the periodontal membrane of teeth with and without periapical inflammation. Int J Oral Surg 3, 7–16.

Van Dyke TE, Lester MA and Shapira L (1993) The role of the host response in periodontal disease progression: implications for future treatment strategies. J Periodontol 64, 792–806.

Vaughan AG, Vrahopoulos TP, Joachim F, Sati K, Barber P and Newman HN (1990) A case report of chronic neutropenia: clinical and ultrastructural findings. J Clin Periodontol 17, 435–445.

Vrahopoulos TP, Barber P, Liakoni H and Newman HN (1988) Ultrastructure of the periodontal lesion in a case of Papillon–Lefèvre syndrome (PLS). J Clin Periodontol 15, 17–26.

Wade AB (1965) Basic Periodontology. Wright, Bristol.

Waerhaug J (1976) Subgingival plaque and loss of attachment in periodontosis as observed in autopsy material. J Periodontol 47, 636–642.

Waerhaug J (1977) Subgingival plaque and loss of attachment in periodontosis as evaluated on extracted teeth. J Periodontol 48, 125–130.

Walker DM (1977) Lymphocytes and macrophages in the gingiva. In: The Borderland Between Caries and Periodontal Disease (Lehner T, ed), pp 185–198, Academic Press, London.

Walton RE and Garnick JJ (1986) The histology of periapical inflammatory lesions in permanent molars in monkeys. J Endod 12, 49–53.

Warwick James W and Counsell A (1927) A histological investigation into so-called pyorrhoea alveolaris. Brit Dent J 48, 1237–1252.

Weinmann JP (1941) Progress of gingival inflammation into the supporting structures of the teeth. J Periodontol 12, 71–82.

Wilde G, Cooper M and Page RC (1977) Host tissue response in chronic periodontal disease. VI. The role of cell-mediated immunity. J Periodont Res 12, 179–196.

Williams DM and Clearinghouse EC (1993) On oral problems related to HIV infection. Classification and diagnostic criteria for oral lesions in HIV infection. J Oral Pathol Med 22, 289–291.

Wilson M, Meghji S, Barber P and Henderson B (1993) Biological activities of surface-associated material from *Porphyromonas gingivalis*. FEMS Immonol Med Microbiol 6, 147–156.

Wilton JMA (1988) Detection of high-risk groups and individuals for periodontal diseases. Systemic predisposition and markers of general health. J Clin Periodont 15, 339–346.

Wright WE, Davis DL, Geffen DB, Martin SE, Nelson MJ and Straus SE (1983) Alveolar bone necrosis and tooth loss: a rare complication associated with herpes zoster infection of the fifth cranial nerve. Oral Surg 56, 39–46.

Yanagisawa S (1980) Pathologic study of periapical lesions. 1. Periapical granulomas: clinical, histopathologic and immunohistopathologic studies. J Oral Pathol 9, 288–300.

Young SK, Rohrer MD and Twesme AT (1981) Spontaneous regression of oral histoplasmoss. Oral Surg 52, 267–270.

Zeltser R and Lustmann J (1988) Oral myiasis. Int J Oral Maxillofac Surg 17, 288–289.

Chapter 15

Trauma and the Periodontal Ligament

Hubert N Newman

INTRODUCTION

There have been few systematic reviews of the effects of trauma on the periodontal ligament (PDL). Periodontologists have been concerned mainly with trauma to the lateral portion of the ligament; endodontists have been interested mostly in periapical changes. There are relatively few documented instances of experimental physical and chemical injury to the PDL. Information on changes as they relate to human PDL is scarce, particularly for occlusal traumatism, even with the recent increase in interest in PDL regeneration (see Chapter 16). No one seems to have produced in experimental animals an occlusal traumatism like that which occurs in humans in the presence of dental plaque.

This review has been written with these limitations in mind. As the range of responses is limited, it again seems logical to consider the subject matter under the headings of types of traumatic factor rather than resultant damage. The first section considers the effects of occlusal trauma (including excessive orthodontic forces) and surgical trauma (including replants and transplants). The second section concerns the sequelae of endodontic injury. The final section collates information on the more abstruse forms of physical and chemical injury to which the PDL has been subjected.

Tissue damage resulting from a variety of iatrogenic procedures has not been discussed. These procedures include subgingival placement of orthodontic bands and elastics, gingival retraction cords, copper rings, impression materials, restorations with overhanging subgingival margins, and periodontal surgical procedures, since the last-named affect almost exclusively the gingival ligament. Regeneration is considered in Chapter 16.

From the studies reported, it will be shown that the PDL has a considerable potential for repair, often following comparatively severe injury. The role of occlusal trauma in chronic inflammatory periodontal disease has been less well defined. It seems that complete resolution will occur in the absence of infective matter (i.e. plaque), and that occlusal trauma is a factor in progressive PDL destruction only when combined with plaque and after the onset of periodontitis. Regarding periapical responses to injury, it seems that chemically induced damage using clinically suitable endodontic materials is often transient, and that over-instrumentation is a more significant clinical cause of periapical PDL injury.

OCCLUSAL TRAUMA

PARAFUNCTION

Early work concerning the influence of parafunction on the human PDL was summarized in the statement that functionless teeth show a poorly developed PDL, consisting merely of loose connective tissue almost devoid of fibre bundles, whereas PDL subjected to excessive abnormal function undergo hypertrophy (Kronfeld, 1931). Coolidge (1938) noted that jaws in which many teeth were missing furnished the most frequent evidence of trauma in the PDL of the remaining teeth. He listed these injuries as haemorrhage, thrombosis, and hyalinization of the PDL. In instances of severe damage, he observed tissue necrosis, likely to be increased by excessive pressure. He also noted repair following removal of trauma. Early conclusions such as these were extrapolated from jaw biopsies. Most investigators since have tried to relate PDL changes to the type of trauma. However, in none of the studies does the PDL appear to have been subjected to stresses typical of occlusal traumatism, which clinically is related to an unusually rapid rate of PDL destruction. Attempts to correlate occlusal traumatism and chronic periodontitis using human autopsy and biopsy material are inconclusive (Waerhaug, 1979).

One of the early methods of applying stress was to place a wedge (e.g. a piece of rubber dam) between two teeth (Macapanpan and Weinmann, 1954). This caused a widening of the PDL on the tension side and a narrowing on the pressure side within 3 days. After that, fibroblasts differentiated in the stretched portion of PDL near the alveolar crest. Leucocytes seemed to enter the PDL at this site. Capillary damage and small areas of haemorrhage were observed. Macapanpan and Weinmann (1954) were among many in observing that traumatism of the PDL will not by itself produce the lesion of chronic periodontitis. Further studies (Macapanpan *et al.*, 1954) revealed that the rate of mitotic activity of periodontal fibroblasts was directly proportional to the increase in width of the PDL due to tension, becoming greatest between 24 hours and 36 hours from the time of introduction of the rubber dam, and reducing to zero by 48 hours. They concluded that fibroblast proliferation is part of the process by which the damaged fibre bundles of abruptly enlarged PDL spaces are repaired.

Bhaskar and Orban (1955) produced traumatism with premature contact from high crowns placed on (monkey) premolar teeth. After 3 days there was necrosis of PDL fibres on the pressure side and widening of the PDL space and vascular thrombosis on the tension side. Both features became more pronounced after 3 weeks. Following removal of the high contacts, repair occurred within 3–6 months. Neither gingival changes nor pocket formation were observed. Similar features were noted by Glickman and Weiss (1955). In addition, they found that loss of principal fibres was most marked adjacent to bone on the pressure side, where the tissue was more vascular and cellular than normal, many of the cells being osteoclasts. The tension side contained densely packed fibre bundles and many fibroblasts and dilated blood vessels.

Wentz *et al.* (1958) fitted rhesus monkeys with high gold crowns and an appliance to produce jiggling forces. In both 3- and 6-month specimens, the PDL space was elongated apically and was three times its original lateral width. However, neither gingivitis nor periodontitis was present. Pressure (132 days) without jiggling led to depression of the tooth in its socket, altered orientation of transseptal fibres, and persistence of any necrotic areas. Such changes resolved if the pressure was removed. Glickman and Smulow (1962, 1968) suggested that excessive force was necessary to damage the PDL on the tension side. On the pressure side of their specimens, the PDL fibres underwent moderate compression, disorientation, realignment, and degeneration, and there was engorgement of blood vessels. Eventually, most fibres became aligned parallel to root and bone. The compressed PDL becomes either acellular or its cells show pyknotic nuclei (Picton, 1976; Polson *et al.*, 1976a,b). Leucocytes penetrate between the injured PDL fibres. In areas subjected to severe pressure, the PDL necroses (Glickman and Smulow, 1962, 1968). Picton (1976) suggested that this was due to prolonged ischaemia followed by autolysis.

Crumley (1964) carried out a rubber-dam-type traumatism study on rats. He observed that there was orientation of the fibre bundles on the tension side in the direction of stress between bone and cementum but poor organization in areas subjected to pressure. Using labelling with tritiated proline, he showed that most cell activity in the stressed PDL was initially osteoblastic, the PDL fibre bundles exhibiting only slight labelling. In 1 day and 3 day specimens, the Sharpey fibres in bone were relatively heavily labelled. The coronal third of the PDL adjacent to cementum showed little labelling, unlike the corresponding apical third. He found no concentration of labelling at any time in the central zone of the PDL. Silver grains were mostly over the cells (mainly fibroblasts, but including vascular endothelium) 30 minutes after ^{3}H-proline administration. Later, a small but significant number of grains was extracellular, and at 4 hours there was moderately heavy labelling of loose perivascular connective tissue. There was no dense labelling in any area of PDL exposed to pressure. At the earliest (30 minutes) and latest (72 hours) time intervals, the proportion of extracellular grains was highest in the zone of the PDL adjacent to bone. Crumley (1964) concluded that fibroblast activity was responsible for fibre production in the PDL, and that extracellular labelling in the PDL after tritiated proline administration was due to the presence of a collagen-bound derivative of the labelled proline. It should be remembered that proline labelling is not specific for collagen.

In an histological and autoradiographic study of the PDL following wedging (compressive) interdental injury in mice, Solt and Glickman (1968) observed compressive necrosis of alveolar crest and transseptal fibres after 4 days, as well as a moderate level of inflammation around the necrotic zone. Using tritiated proline, they claimed that in the injured tissue there was a decrease in collagen formation in transseptal and crestal ligaments. By 8 days, there was an increase in PDL cellularity and reorientation of transseptal and crestal fibres. New collagen formation was greatest between 4 and 8 days. By 2 weeks, there was only moderate inflammation and transseptal and alveolar crest fibres were organized into bundles. By 3 weeks, the test and control PDL were indistinguishable histologically. There was a corresponding increase in collagen formation interdentally and interradicularly in the ligaments of teeth opposing those subjected to injury, although histologically they appeared normal. Similarly, the usual pressure and tension side changes may take place in distant teeth due to trauma from occlusion (Nascimento and Sallum, 1975).

Few workers have investigated the biophysics of occlusal traumatism. Palcanis (1973) applied excessive occlusal loads for 48 hours to dog canines. He showed that the histological changes described by others resulted from microcirculatory injury due to pressure. Less severe hyperfunction, as from the placing of slightly high amalgams, leads to an increase in the gingival vascular network, but only rarely to similar changes in the PDL (Koivumaa and Lassila, 1971). Occlusal trauma caused an increase in PDL tissue fluid (Palcanis, 1973; Walker *et al.*, 1978).

There has always been difficulty in correlating histological changes with the clinical features of occlusal traumatism. Mobility of teeth may not correlate with radiographic signs such as widening of the PDL space (Posselt and Maunsbach, 1957; Mühlemann and Herzog, 1961). Glickman and Smulow (1962, 1969) attempted to correlate occlusal traumatism with the pattern of tissue destruction in chronic inflammatory periodontal disease using high gold crowns in rhesus monkeys. Their work suggested that excessive forces, particularly pressure, could determine the path of tissue damage. These and other studies using human biopsy and autopsy material have led to the conclusion that trauma from occlusion and gingival inflammation were destructive factors jointly responsible for the production of vertical patterns of PDL and alveolar bone destruction (Glickman, 1963; Glickman and Smulow, 1965, 1967). Similar studies in monkeys also showed that periodontal pockets advance more rapidly in the presence of excessive occlusal loads (Waerhaug and Hansen,

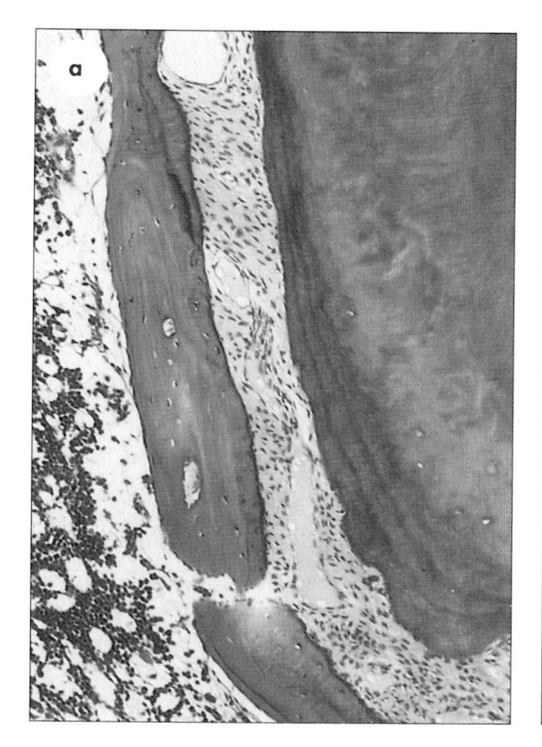

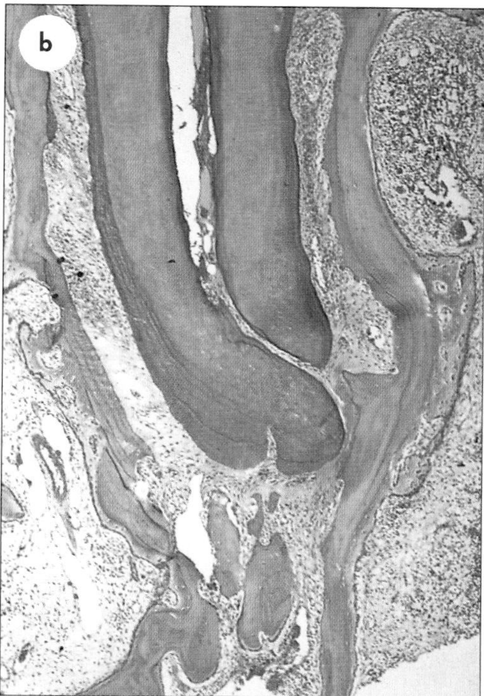

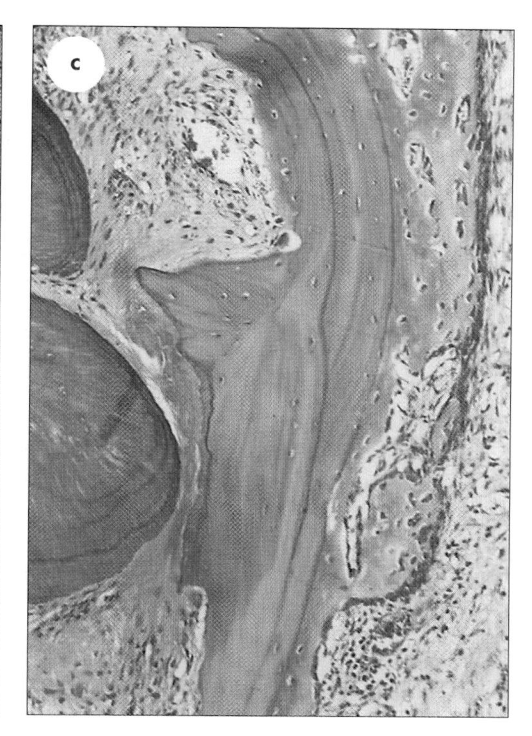

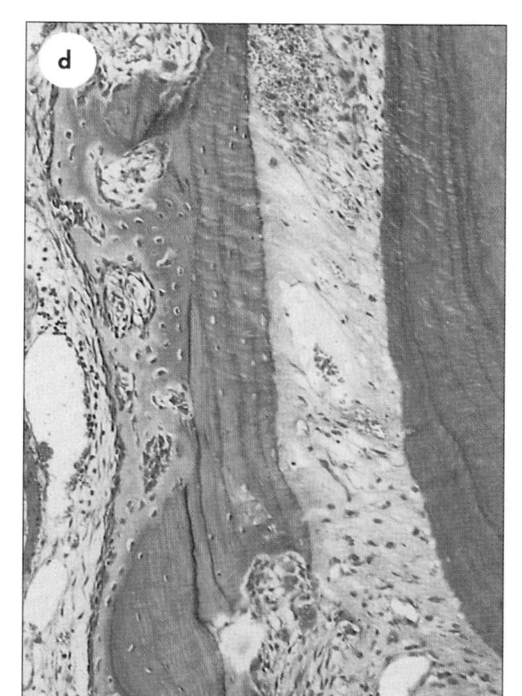

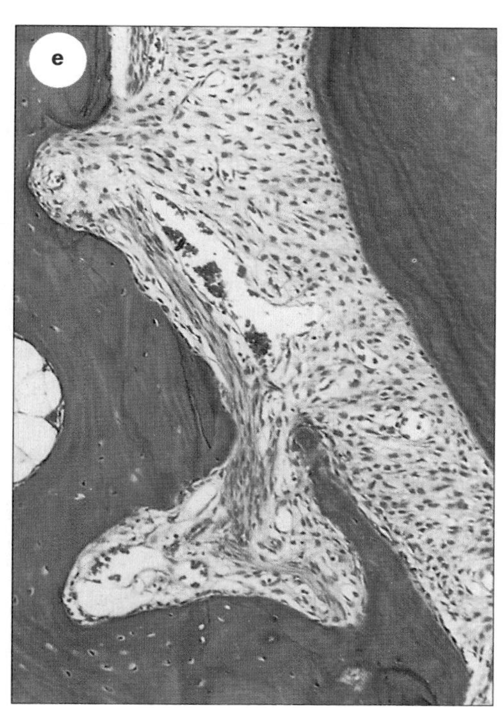

Fig. 15.1 Effects of trauma on primate (squirrel monkey) periodontal ligament. (a) Control (magnification × 35). (b) Periodontal ligament after 2 weeks of subjection to mesiodistal jiggling forces. Note increase in width of ligament on the left (tension) side (magnification × 35). (c) Same specimen as in (b). Note acellularity and narrowing of ligament in pressure area at root apex (magnfication × 140). (d) Same specimen as in (b), tension side. The ligament is wider and less cellular than normal (magnification × 150). (e) After 10 weeks of mesiodistal jiggling forces, the periodontal ligament shown in (b) has reverted to more normal appearance, but increased width of ligament is still apparent (H & E magnification × 150). (Courtesy of Dr P Dowell.)

1966) (*Fig. 15.1*). However, there is contradictory evidence, in that histological examination of human PDL subjected to occlusal hyperfunction as assessed from autopsy material showed minimal changes (Koivumaa and Lassila, 1971).

Experimental hypermobility of (dog) teeth has been achieved with a cap splint that displaced the tooth and a spring mechanism that tended to return the tooth to its original position. Over 13 days, this caused a widening of the PDL and the types of bone defect associated by earlier workers with occlusal traumatism (Svanberg and Lindhe, 1973). Similar jiggling-type forces produced prolonged hypermobility if the forces were maintained. In addition, Svanberg and Lindhe (1974) and Svanberg (1974) observed increasing width and vascularity of the alveolar crest region of the PDL on the pressure side. Trauma from occlusion neither induced gingivitis nor influenced the level or extent of established gingivitis. However, when surgically created bony pockets around the dogs' teeth were allowed to accumulate plaque, jiggling forces produced more rapid increase in pocket depth, although plaque levels and gingivitis were similar on test and control sides (Lindhe and Svanberg, 1974). Dogs with healthy periodontal tissues adapted to the altered occlusion within 6 months of the start of the experiment, whereas those animals with experimental periodontitis still showed PDL abnormalities after this time, including increased vascular leakage, leucocyte migration and osteoclastic activity.

Polson (1974), using a circumdental ligature technique to produce a progressive periodontitis in squirrel monkeys, found no evidence for occlusal trauma as a co-destructive factor in chronic inflammatory periodontal disease. Nor could others (Lindhe and Ericsson, 1976; Ericsson and Lindhe, 1977) find any evidence that jiggling-type occlusal trauma and the resulting tooth hypermobility detrimentally affect healing after periodontal surgery (in dogs), provided plaque control is maintained. Similarly, pocketing was a likely, though not invariable, sequel to conversion of a supragingival into a subgingival plaque by orthodontic means. When normal orthodontic forces were applied to plaque-free teeth, the tilting movement did not result in the formation of infrabony pockets (Ericsson *et al.*, 1977). Ericsson *et al.* (1978) showed that, in the absence of plaque, orthodontic forces moving individual teeth do not (at least in the dog) induce gingivitis. Nor were such forces, in the presence of plaque, capable of converting a gingivitis into a destructive and progressive periodontitis. In dogs with a progressive periodontitis, however, repeated jiggling mediated an enhanced rate of PDL and bone destruction (Nyman *et al.*, 1979). However, jiggling forces produced by alternate siting of wedges caused no increased bone loss unless in the presence of a pre-existing periodontitis. Jiggling trauma in the presence of periodontitis did not affect the loss of PDL attachment (Polson *et al.*, 1976a,b; Polson, 1977).

In (human) studies of occlusal hypofunction and hyperfunction, Johnson (1990) observed that hypofunction led to increased thickness of the transseptal fibre region, with decreased new bone thickness, and that hyperfunction led to a thinner transseptal fibre region and increased new bone formation (*Fig. 15.2*). In a similar (rat) experiment, hypofunction resulted in decreased PDL width after 15 days, apparently owing to bone apposition and not to any effect on cementum (Levy and Mailland, 1980). Beertsen (1987) observed that the volume density of extracellular collagen in the hypofunctional PDL decreased from 50 per cent to 30 per cent over 1 week, and that the fraction of fibrillar collagen ingested by fibroblasts increased over twofold shortly after the start of the experiment, and he related this finding to the net loss of collagen extracellularly. In rats in which surgical trauma had been applied to alveolar bone and underlying PDL and cementum, and in which occlusion had been altered by placing a high amalgam, by grinding, or by extraction, the PDL was narrower around occluding teeth, and there was a thickening of cementum at and central to the surgical site. There were, however, no significant changes at the end of the study (28 days) in relation to hypo- or hyperoccluding teeth compared to controls (El Deeb and Andreasen, 1991). Although such structural changes do occur in the PDL of teeth of non-continuous growth, this is less evident in the PDL of teeth of continuous growth (Shore *et al.*, 1982). Indeed, there is little change when the tooth has been pinned, preventing any movement (Beertsen *et al.*, 1982; Shore *et al.*, 1985).

In relation to human studies, there is still no definitive correlation between occlusal traumatism and periodontitis, other than the evidence indicating that such traumatism accelerates the rate of disease progression. Pihlstrom *et al.* (1986) observed that teeth with bi-digital mobility, functional mobility, or widened PDL space had deeper probing depth, more loss of clinical attachment, and less radiographically evident bone support than teeth without these findings. Teeth with occlusal contact in centric jaw relation that were in working, non-working, or protrusive positions, did not have more severe periodontitis than teeth without these contacts. Teeth with both functional mobility and widened PDL spaces had deeper probing depth, greater attachment loss, and less bone support than teeth without these findings. Further, given equal clinical attachment levels, teeth with functional mobility and widened PDL space had less bone support than teeth not so affected. While Ericsson and Lindhe (1984) had noted a similar rate of breakdown of PDL tissues in beagle dogs that had normal or widened PDL spaces, and that, prior to ligature placement, had normal or increased mobility respectively, the traumatic factor had not been active at the time of treatment.

In recent years, there has been little development of research into the links between parafunctional activities such as bruxism, occlusal traumatism, and periodontitis. Pierce and Gale (1988) showed that bruxing activity was decreased significantly in subjects who received nocturnal biofeedback or full coverage acrylic biteguards, but not in controls, or in those who were subjected to diurnal biofeedback.

Pihlstrom *et al.* (1986) noted increased tooth mobility, probing depth, and bone loss in relation to teeth with non-working contacts. In a longitudinal study of 82 patients and 1974 teeth, which aimed at determining whether mobility influenced treatment results, Fleszar *et al.* (1980) found that pockets of clinically mobile teeth did not respond as well as pockets of firm teeth with the same initial disease severity. Shefter and McFall (1984) observed that teeth with protrusive premature contacts had deeper pockets.

Perhaps the most significant development in this field in recent years has been the effort to establish whether or not psychological factors have a role in the relationship between occlusal dysfunction and PDL tissue behaviour. Some of this work was pioneered by Budtz-Jørgensen (1981), who produced dysfunctional

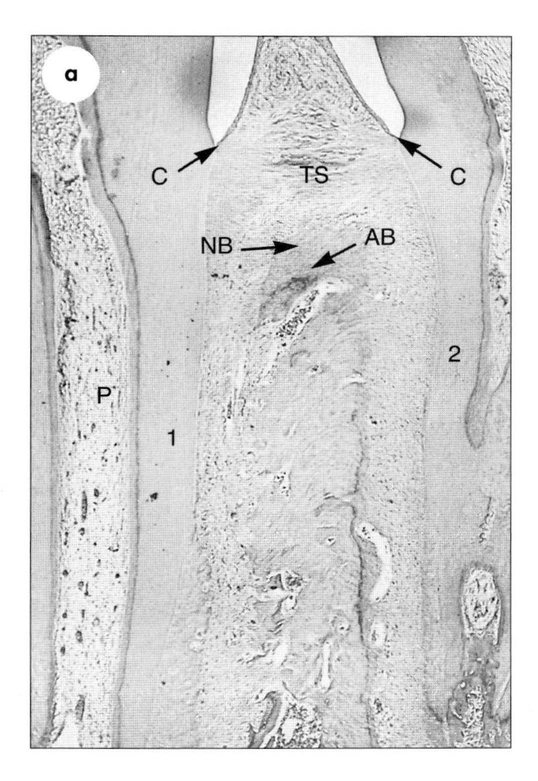

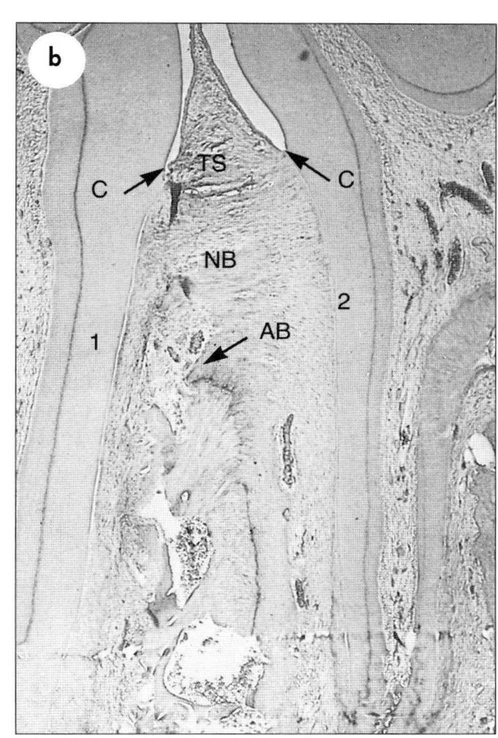

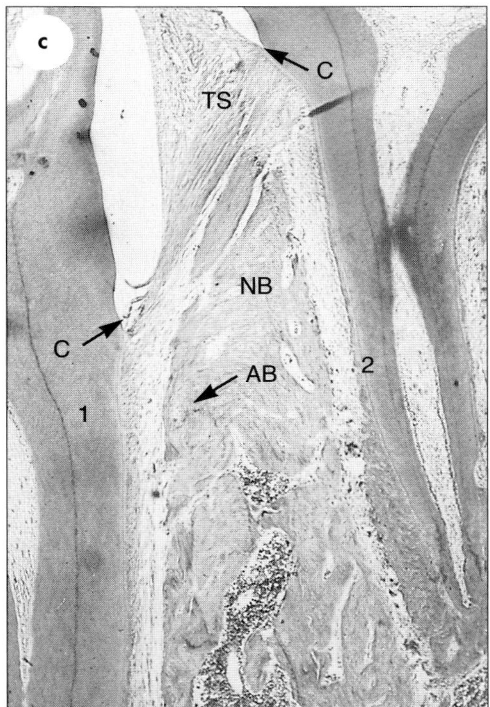

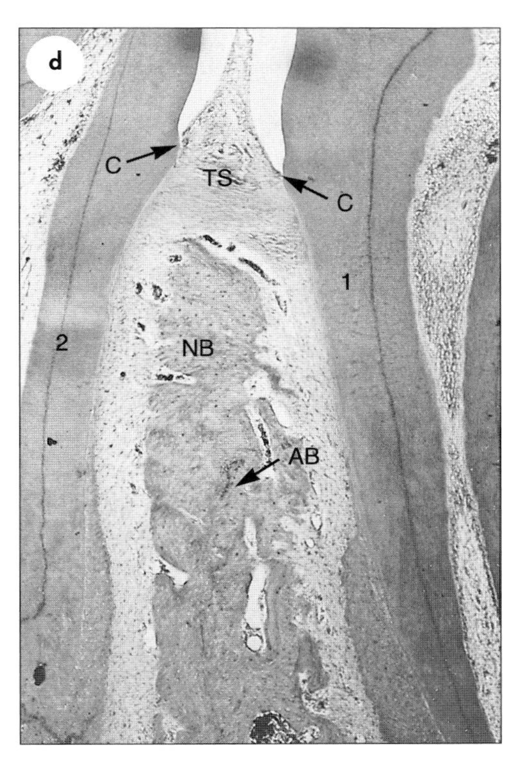

Fig. 15.2 Altered occlusal function and the periodontal ligament. (a) Interdental septum 1 week after injection of ^{3}H-proline, external control. This is a representative field for measurements as it has teeth with continuous coronal and radicular pulp chambers (P), a prominent appositional band of silver grains within interdental bone, and interdental gingiva of normal morphology (magnification × 60). (b) Interdental septum 3 weeks after injection of ^{3}H-proline, external control. There is more new bone formed at the alveolar crest than after 1 week; the transseptal ligament thickness appears to be unchanged (magnification × 60). (c) Interdental septum 5 weeks after injection of ^{3}H-proline, hypofunctional side. The second molar tooth appears to have overerupted relative to the first molar tooth. The transseptal ligament is oblique in orientation, and is thinner than in other groups (magnification × 150). (d) Interdental septum 5 weeks after injection of ^{3}H-proline, hyperfunctional side. The transseptal ligament is thicker than on the hypofunctional side (magnification × 60). (From Johnson, 1990.)

1 and 2 are adjacent molars
TS = Transseptal fibres
C = Cement–enamel junction
AB = Alveolar bone
NB = New bone
P = Pulp

occlusion in *Macaca irus* monkeys by means of occlusal splints and interferences, with resultant bruxism associated with emotional stress, and increased urinary cortisol excretion, during the experimental period.

Rugh *et al.* (1984) reviewed the evidence for a possible relation between emotional conditions and chronic inflammatory periodontal disease. De Marco (1976) had observed such a relationship between emotional stress and alveolar bone loss in military personnel on duty in Vietnam. Belting (1967) had noted a higher Russell Periodontal Index in psychiatric patients. Mellars and Herms (1947) stated that habitually excited patients had more bleeding gingivae associated with irregular alveolar bone resorption, while habitually depressed patients had little or no gingival bleeding and regular bone loss. Overall, Rugh *et al.* (1984) concluded that a correlation exists, but that there was a need for more evidence.

Perhaps the most constructive development in this field is the realization that the periodontium, like so many other organs, tissues, and systems, may be subject to the effects of emotional stress either directly or via the immune system. Psychoneuroimmunology may be expected to constitute a major area of future research into occlusal traumatism. This aspect has been reviewed by Ballieux (1991). As he points out, the role of psychosocial and personality factors, especially stress, has been established in the development of upper respiratory infections. Further, he reviewed evidence to show that antibody response was directly related to mood. He considered that immunoenhancement by psychological processes can have clinical significance in relation to inflammatory periodontal disease.

It is concluded that occlusal traumatism may be a factor in progressive destruction of the PDL, but only in the presence of active chronic periodontitis. Occlusal traumatism does not initiate attachment loss. Unfortunately, human studies are rare, and the animal experiments cited may bear little relation to human occlusal traumatism. Further research is required to establish whether interrelationships between psychological factors and the immune response are indeed related to occlusal traumatism and a related more rapidly progressive chronic periodontitis.

EXCESSIVE ORTHODONTIC FORCES

The histological response of the PDL to horizontal loads has been considered already in Chapter 11. Discussion here concerns only excessive orthodontic forces applied mainly for experimental purposes. Excessive force produced by intermaxillary elastics (in rats) (Waldo and Rothblatt, 1954) increased the width and vascularity of the PDL. As with occlusal traumatism, pressure areas showed regions of vasoconstriction by 24 hours. Tension areas showed a widened PDL space and slight vasodilation. The responses were maximal by 3 days. On the pressure side, there was haemorrhage and crushing and eventually resorption of PDL fibres. The study also confirmed that bodily movements of teeth produce most damage since they cut off the blood supply on the pressure side (Moyers, 1950). Bien (1967) posed the question: why do orthodontic forces move teeth while chewing forces, which are much greater, do not drive a tooth into the skull? He concluded that rate rather than magnitude of force was related to ligament injury. He did not make conclusions about the significance of the direction of force or of its duration.

The level of force capable of producing damage is low. Gianelly (1969) showed that forces exceeding 50 g reduced the vascular flow in the (dog) PDL, but many vessels remained patent. Forces of 150 g almost completely occluded vessels at the alveolar crest. A force of 75 g applied for 7 days did not significantly impair the structural integrity of the PDL. A 125 g force applied for 7 days resulted in many of the PDL fibres becoming aligned parallel to the long axis of the affected tooth. The 75 g and 125 g forces compressed the PDL and its blood vessels. This fits with Miura's (1973) finding that pressures of approximately 80 g/cm^2 decrease the blood flow to the PDL and at the same time compress its thickness to two-thirds of its original lateral dimension.

Orthodontic forces can delay healing of the PDL following root canal treatment and apicectomy (Baranowskyj, 1969). Singer *et al.* (1967) suggested that fewer areas of hyalinization occurred and that they were delayed and less intense in (rat) PDL subjected to orthodontic loads if the animals had previously received 100 ppm fluoride in their diet, though the mechanism was not clarified.

SURGICAL TRAUMA

In most of the numerous reports of injuries to teeth, there is little or no mention of the effects of such injuries on the PDL (Andreasen and Hjörting-Hansen, 1966). The PDL is usually mentioned as a source of repair tissue between apical and coronal portions of a fractured root (Pindborg, 1955; Arwill, 1962). Bevelander (1942) examined tissue reactions in experimental tooth fracture (in dogs). Adjacent to the fracture site, a mild inflammatory reaction was observed. In most cases the PDL formed a fibrous union between root fragments. When lateral displacement of the fragments had occurred, there was complementary alveolar resorption to allow for the maintenance of a normal width of the PDL space. Uniform width of PDL seems to be established after about 6 months. However, Blackwood (1959) still noted changes in orientation of PDL fibres, and many dilated vascular channels after about 6 months. Torn cementum appears to be repaired by bone, cementum, or an unidentified calcified tissue (Claus and Orban, 1953). Enlarged PDL spaces were observed adjacent to fracture sites (in rats) (Dreyer and Blum, 1967). The fibres were less dense and less organized. There was a downgrowth of crevicular epithelium associated with traumatic detachment of underlying PDL fibres, so that pockets of varying depths formed as far as the root apex.

In root fractures, the PDL around the apical fragment shows histological changes indicative of loss of normal function. It becomes uniformly thinner, its collagen fibres are less dense, and they are arranged mostly parallel to the root surface (Kronfeld, 1936). Its thickness ranges from 0.03–0.13 mm, which is within the limits for the PDL of embedded teeth and teeth without antagonists. By contrast, the PDL around the coronal fragment was about 0.3 mm wide, within the range typical of ligaments subjected to heavy masticatory forces, and it showed fibres that were aligned normally. Pindborg (1955) studied intra-alveolar fractures of upper central incisors and concluded that root fracture repair tissue was organized from both pulp and PDL. He also reported the proliferation in the region of the fracture line of epithelial rests of Malassez.

The response of the human PDL to surgical trauma from clinical periodontics is poorly documented, except for the extraction of teeth. The main reason is that most procedures aimed at eliminating periodontal pockets encroach minimally on healthy PDL. Therefore, correct periodontal surgery should not result in injury to any but a small portion of supracrestal PDL fibres.

Morris (1953) studied periodontal reattachment following surgical detachment around periodontally sound human anterior teeth that had been extracted for prosthetic reasons. Connective tissue healing took place against dentine or cementum. PDL fibres were aligned parallel to the root in all except the oldest (106 day) specimen, in which Sharpey fibres were present. There was apparently no attachment to the dentine of non-vital teeth (Morris, 1957).

Burkland *et al.* (1976) carried out a histological study of regeneration of the completely disrupted PDL (in the rat). The maxillary first molar was elevated and replaced immediately with the torn PDL in the original socket. After 2 days, the PDL was inflamed and necrotic and was without oriented fibres. After 5 days, some collagen fibres had united to bone and cementum. The oriented fibres were more developed cervically and less so apically. Oxytalan fibres were more abundant than in normal PDL. By 10 days, scattered areas of inflammation were still present. The transseptal and principal fibres had regained their normal orientation, and were only slightly less abundant than in normal PDL. The apical PDL now showed greater regeneration of collagen than the lateral areas. Oxytalan fibres were still more abundant than in control specimens. At 15 days, orientation of the still sparse collagen fibres appeared normal, but at 20 days oxytalan fibres were still more abundant than normal. By 30 days, some animals showed degeneration and hyalinization of part of the PDL. In others, the PDL was thinner than normal. After 50 days, the disrupted PDL was still not fully repaired, being discontinuous over areas of root resorption. It was concluded that the repair process was not maintained because of the persistence of necrotic matter leading to root resorption. Hair impaction and inflammation were absent, and bacterial contamination was only present initially. In a similar study of PDL healing adjacent to (monkey) extraction sockets, Chase and Revesz (1944) found that transseptal fibres formed and connected the teeth on either side of the socket after 5 weeks.

Hurst (1972) reasoned that oxytalan fibres may be needed in the initial healing process to hold the tooth stable until collagen fibres mature. He also noted that some mobility may be necessary for regeneration of collagen fibres after initial attachment since, of a number of splinted teeth, the only specimen that did not ankylose was that from which the splint had been dislodged accidentally after 6 weeks.

Occlusal trauma may destabilize healing. Glickman *et al.* (1966) applied a traumatic splint to the mandibular anterior teeth of dogs, which then received mucogingival surgery, consisting either of a flap reflected from the gingival margin to the fornix of the vestibule, or of an apically repositioned flap. PDL widening was observed in both groups. Collagen fibre bundles appeared well formed, and blood vessels were increased in number and appeared dilated. There were irregular areas of bone resorption covered with new bone into which new PDL fibres were inserted. Alveolar crest fibres were shorter and more nearly perpendicular to the tooth than they were in hypofunctional teeth.

Pietrokovski (1967) investigated roots fractured during extraction of (rat) teeth and left *in situ*. After 1 week, the PDL near the wound surface had lost its regular structure, and the main components of the periodontal space were blood capillaries, lymphocytes, and neutrophils. There was widening of the PDL between the apical foramen and the bony fundus. After 4 weeks, the PDL space around the root remnant was enlarged and occupied by obliquely oriented collagen fibres and many fibroblasts. Exfoliative movement of the root took place within the healing socket.

In a similar study, Johansen (1970) observed the incorporation of tritiated thymidine into the epithelial cell rests up to 6 days after attempted extraction. He suggested that the experimental injury and subsequent inflammatory response provided the stimulus for epithelial cell rest proliferation. In the case of root fracture with retention of both portions, repair seems also to depend upon the activity of the PDL, with its invagination into the fracture site, and infiltration into the same site of chronic inflammatory cells (Michanowicz *et al.*, 1971).

Melcher (1967a,b) studied the effects of mechanical injury with a saline-cooled bur on a (rat) incisor PDL. At 4 days, the disorganized PDL contained many active fibroblasts with a high cytoplasm–nucleus ratio. A well-organized cellular connective tissue formed within 1 week of injury. At 6 weeks, the PDL was wider than normal.

The same group studied the response of (mouse) molar PDL to similar bur-induced injury, which exposed but did not extirpate the PDL through a hole in alveolar bone (Gould *et al.*, 1977, 1980). The wound site was isolated by mylar film from the overlying connective tissue. It was found that most dividing progenitor cells in the wounded PDL were close to blood vessels but external to the basement lamina of the latter (Gould *et al.*, 1977). Labelling by autoradiography was apparent in some cells even 30 hours after injury, although most of the affected PDL was necrotic at this time (Gould *et al.*, 1980). Reorganization was marked by 5 days. The labelled cells were shown to be moving away from blood vessels to repopulate the reorganizing PDL. Repopulation was delayed by 88r caesium irradiation. Labelled cells taking part in repair, though mainly fibroblasts, included endothelial cells, osteoblasts, and cementoblasts. Gould and co-workers concluded that there is in (mouse) molar PDL a population of progenitor cells located very close to blood vessels, the number of these cells remaining relatively stable during the healing of a PDL wound.

No significant differences in mechanical properties or histological features were observed around subluxated teeth, whether splinted or unsplinted (Mandel and Viidik, 1989) (*Figs 15.3, 15.4*). Fourel and Mattout (1989) noted that, when human teeth were displaced, no new attachment formed except where the PDL had been preserved. They further suggested that the epithelial elements in the PDL derived from the junctional epithelium, and did not represent the rests of Malassez. Around traumatized resorbing deciduous teeth, Alexander and Swerdloff (1980) observed increased mucopolysaccharide activity and a concomitant decrease in the level of glycosaminoglycans, compared to the situation with physiologic resorption.

In relation to PDL wound healing, some PDL fibroblasts appear to be capable of differentiating into osteoblasts and cementoblasts, and these cells apparently have the phenotype of osteoblasts (Nojima *et al.*, 1990). While research into the possible effects of growth factors in PDL wound healing is still at an early stage, there is already evidence that platelet-derived growth factor and insulin-like growth factors appear to act synergistically to enhance early wound healing (in dogs) (Lynch *et al.*, 1991). Local gingival injury, whether occurring accidentally or during dental treatment, may cause osteoclastic resorption of the root surface (*Fig. 15.5*). This is likely to be prevented if PDL cells migrate coronally to form a fibrous attachment, or if epithelial cells migrate apically (Karring *et al.*, 1984). As regards electrosurgery, all that would appear relevant is that it delays PDL healing (Azzi *et al.*, 1983) (*Fig. 15.6*). There has been such extensive development in the field of periodontal tissue regeneration, that this topic forms the subject of chapter 16.

REPLANTATION AND TRANSPLANTATION

There has been much debate as to the advantages of the presence of an intact PDL on the tooth to be replanted. Perhaps the best results are obtained using unerupted teeth with only partially formed roots, as in the replacement by third molars of first molars that have been compromised by idiopathic juvenile periodontitis (Borring-Møller and Frandsen, 1978).

Following removal of PDL tissues (from dog teeth), Yoshida (1976) found that within the first few days the wound sites became filled with granulation tissue containing undifferentiated mesenchyme cells that proliferated from the PDL of adjoining teeth, periosteum and endosteum. After 7–9 days, cementoblasts were arranged on the prepared dentine surface. After 2 weeks, collagen fibre bundles were attached perpendicular to the cavity walls. After 3 weeks, new PDL had formed between the original cementum and newly formed bone. At 4 weeks, the DPL was wide, highly cellular, and vascular, but poorly organized.

For teeth with complete roots, the best results follow endodontics, washing, and avoidance of delay prior to replacement with minimal interference with residual PDL (Hammer, 1955; Andreasen, 1981; Neukam *et al.*, 1987). While root anatomy does not appear to affect the success of transplantation, more damage to the PDL was found to occur when the roots were more developed (Schliephake and Neukam, 1990).

If replantation is to have any chance of success, it is essential to maintain the viability of the PDL (Hunter, 1778; Sherman, 1968). Two important points are the avoidance of dehydration of the PDL (e.g. by short-term storage in saline – Andreasen and Schwartz, 1986), and loss of viability of its cell rests (Löe and Waerhaug, 1961). Söder *et al.* (1977) observed that after 2 hours at 20 per cent relative humidity and 25°C, no PDL cells were viable on tissue culture.

The main problem is the prevention of external resorption and ankylosis (Barbakow *et al.*, 1977). In the investigation of Simons *et al.* (1975), six human tooth roots examined 22 or 30 months after replantation all showed external resorption. There were acute and chronic inflammatory cells in the PDL. Resorbed cementum and dentine were bordered by non-inflamed fibrous connective tissue. Most roots had scattered areas of relatively normal PDL attached to unresorbed root surfaces. Similar results were obtained by Andreasen and Hjörting-Hansen (1966). Another study involved implantation of (monkey) roots in bone and in contact with replaced flaps. No new PDL formed on those portions of roots that had been exposed to plaque and then planed thoroughly prior to implantation. In areas where the PDL had been preserved, a fibrous reattachment occurred between the root and adjacent gingival tissue derived from the flaps (Nyman *et al.*, 1980).

In further studies using animals, it has been possible to follow the sequence of events more closely. Nasjleti *et al.* (1975) observed that 1 day after replantation there was only blood clot at the wound site. Granulation tissue was present at 3 days. It occupied most of the PDL space by 14 days, and at this time it was still oedematous and contained many fibroblasts, macrophages, and epithelial rests, these rests being especially conspicuous in the cervical third of the PDL space. Specimens at 3 weeks showed more cellularity and a tendency towards orientation of the new PDL collagen fibres compared to untreated specimens. Nasjelti *et al.* (1975) found that root resorption could be avoided by storage of teeth prior to replantation at +4°C for up to 1 year. Storage at –10°C resulted in moderate inflammation, followed by a failure of the PDL to organize properly; it also resulted in root resorption and ankylosis. Eventually, these teeth were exfoliated. Even those preserved at +4°C may not show resolution in the long term, PDL fibres often failing to regain or retain functional orientation, and partial or complete ankylosis may supervene (Caffesse *et al.*, 1977).

Costich *et al.* (1958) observed (in hamsters) normal fibroblast orientation around molars 3 months after replantation. Ankylosis occurred around half of the teeth; bone resorption in relation to all but one specimen. Transplantation of teeth from young to adult animals was relatively unsuccessful, most cases forming a poor attachment, although ankylosis did not occur (Hoek *et al.*, 1958).

Castelli *et al.* (1980) investigated the vascular response of (monkey) incisor PDL after replantation. Apical and cervical vessels regained patency after 4 days and the vessels of the middle third regained patency after 7 days. The difference in the time taken to regain patency is due to better blood supply to the apical and cervical regions. At 4 days, the vascular network was disordered, blood vessels intermingling with reparative cells and disrupted collagen fibres. This, the authors suggested, allowed a maximum contact area at the blood vessel–ground substance interface for nutrient supply. Areas of hyaline degeneration in the middle third of the PDL at this time were associated with a scarcity of reparative cells. By 7 days, the hyperaemic reaction was accompanied by proliferation of fibroblasts and endothelial cells. At 15 days, focal spots of increased vascular density were observed in areas undergoing reparative remodelling and in areas adjacent to cementum resorption. In areas where pre-ankylotic bony trabeculae were forming, the vasculature appeared less pronounced. Three months after replantation, the PDL vascular network had regained its normal appearance.

Andreasen *et al.* (1978) studied the effects of tissue culture on teeth scheduled for replantation. Tooth crowns were cleaned before extraction, irrigated with phosphate-buffered saline after extraction, and placed in tissue culture medium either immediately or after drying at room temperature and humidity for 1 hour. Teeth were replanted after 5, 7 or 14 days in culture medium. Normal PDL formed only in those specimens where no drying had been permitted. Some of the dried specimens showed inflammation, owing to resorption of necrotic remnants of PDL and extensive root resorption, and only a few areas of normal PDL persisted. Separation lines in the ligaments of replanted (monkey) teeth can disappear within 2 weeks of immediate replantation (Andreasen, 1980).

In another (monkey) study, the PDL was removed by scraping and the root surface decalcified before replantation (Nordenram *et al.*, 1973). The inflammatory response varied from mild to intense, the latter being seen especially periapically. About half the teeth became ankylosed. Removal of non-vital PDL resulted in slower resorption after replantation of teeth with severely damaged PDL (Lindskog *et al.*, 1983, 1985) (*Fig. 15.7*).

Rate of repair of PDL depends on the degree of preservation of existing PDL. Sharpey fibres (in dogs) have been observed at 4–6 weeks after replantation (Hammer, 1955). If the PDL has been removed, the area between cementum and bone becomes filled after 4 days with poorly formed, young connective tissue, which will form a new ligament after 2–3 months. Unfortunately, all such cases eventually undergo ankylosis (Hammer, 1955; Löe and Waerhaug, 1961). Ankylosis has been observed in such specimens as early as 30 days after replantation.

Andreasen (1981) noted that some normal PDL did form cervically around replanted teeth, despite prolonged drying or PDL removal before replantation. He ascribed this phenomenon to gingival fibroblasts. However, McCulloch and Bordin (1991) found that gingival fibroblasts grown *in vitro* failed to contribute to reformation of a PDL around replanted (dog) teeth, while PDL fibroblasts either aided or, at least, did not inhibit regeneration. They described PDL stem cells as arising from paravascular cells with small nuclei and with a high rate of proliferation. Where delay is unavoidable before transplantation, appropriate storage media are indicated. While normal saline is used commonly, when this is not available, milk has been found to be superior to saliva (Andreasen and Schwartz, 1986).

Selvig *et al.* (1990), in a study of teeth that had had non-vital soft tissues removed and been subsequently replanted after 45 minutes' delay, observed a reduced frequency of adverse healing. This was attributed to citric acid demineralization of, and prevention of, mechanical trauma to the root surface. In fact, root surfaces treated with stannous fluoride followed by tetracycline showed neither inflammatory resorption nor ankylosis. Andersson (1988) observed that the PDL of a tooth prevented from drying for 1 hour before replantation healed without resorption or ankylosis in a manner similar to that of an immediately replanted tooth. Antibiotic was recommended to be taken as soon as possible, and endontics to be carried out within 1 week of replantation.

Concerning re-establishment of the neurovascular supply to replanted teeth, Kvinnsland *et al.* (1991) demonstrated nerve regeneration in the periapical periodontium and in the pulp after replantation of (rat) molars. Concerning PDL mechanoreceptors, Loescher and Robinson (1991) noted that 1 year after replantation (of cat teeth) their characteristics were significantly different from those of control units; these differences included raised thresholds and occasional raised responses to forces applied in more than two directions. In a similar (cat) experiment, PDL reinnervation was observed by 12 weeks, and it was found that it did not differ significantly from controls unless there was apical resorption (Loescher *et al.*, 1995). Schwartz *et al.* (1987) observed allotransplanted immunogenetically matched human teeth for up to 28 years. There was no pulp survival evident in any graft. Root resorption had occurred in 92 per cent of cases, and 34 per cent had been lost in the first 2 years. They noted that despite

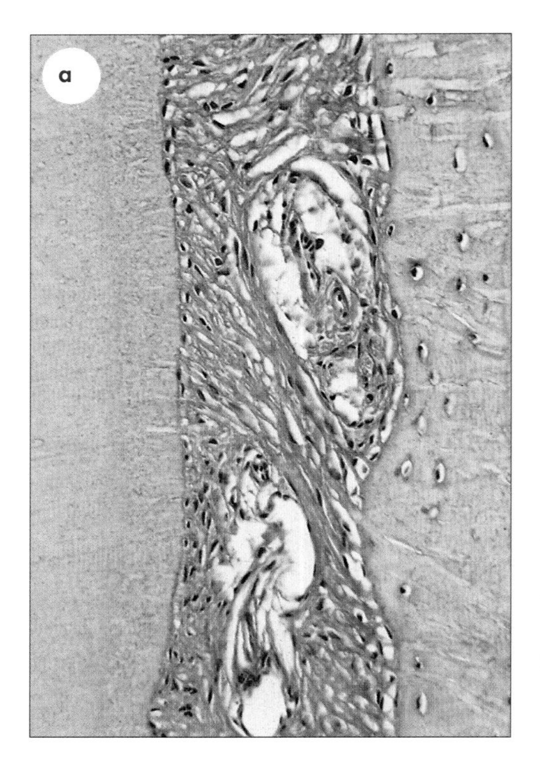

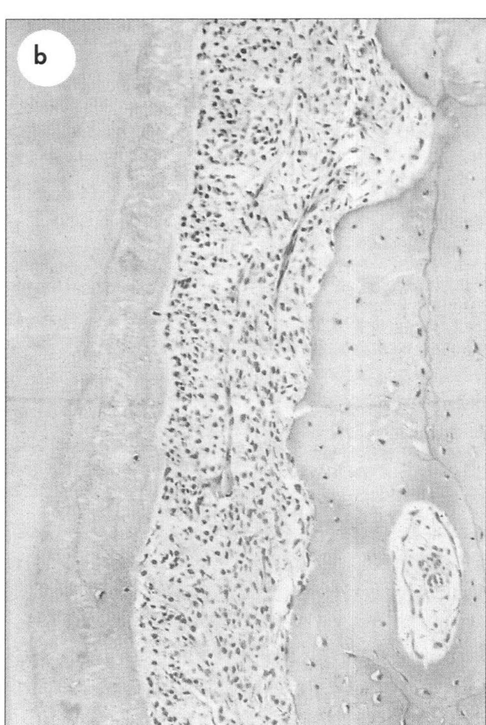

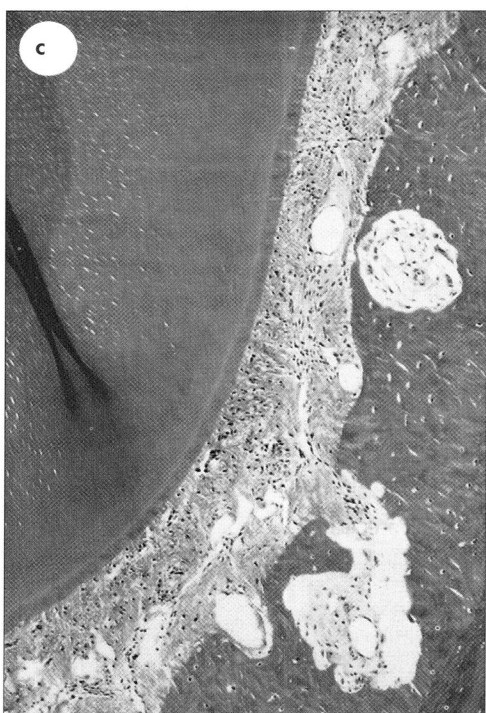

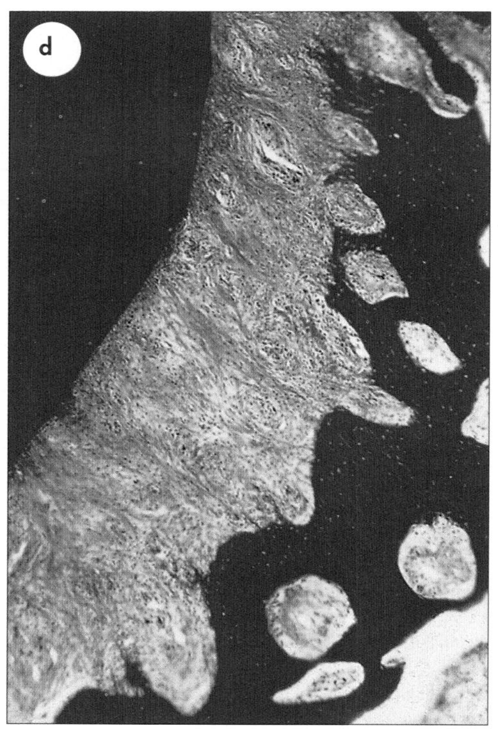

Fig. 15.3 Effect of splinting after extrusive luxation of (monkey) teeth. (a) Normal PDL with dense connective tissue bundles running at different angles. (Picrosirius and orcein staining; (magnfication × 190.) (b) PDL at 1 week after luxation. Granulation tissue filling the periodontal space completely with solid strings of endothelial cells (H & E, magnfication × 160). (c) PDL at 1 week after luxation. Granulation tissue in a narrow zone in the middle third of the ligament. (Van Gieson stain; magnfication × 125.) (d) PDL at 2 weeks after luxation. There is granulation tissue with thicker collagen fibres than are seen after 1 week. These extend into the area of bone resorption. (Van Gieson stain; magnfication × 125.) (From Mandel and Viidik, 1989.)

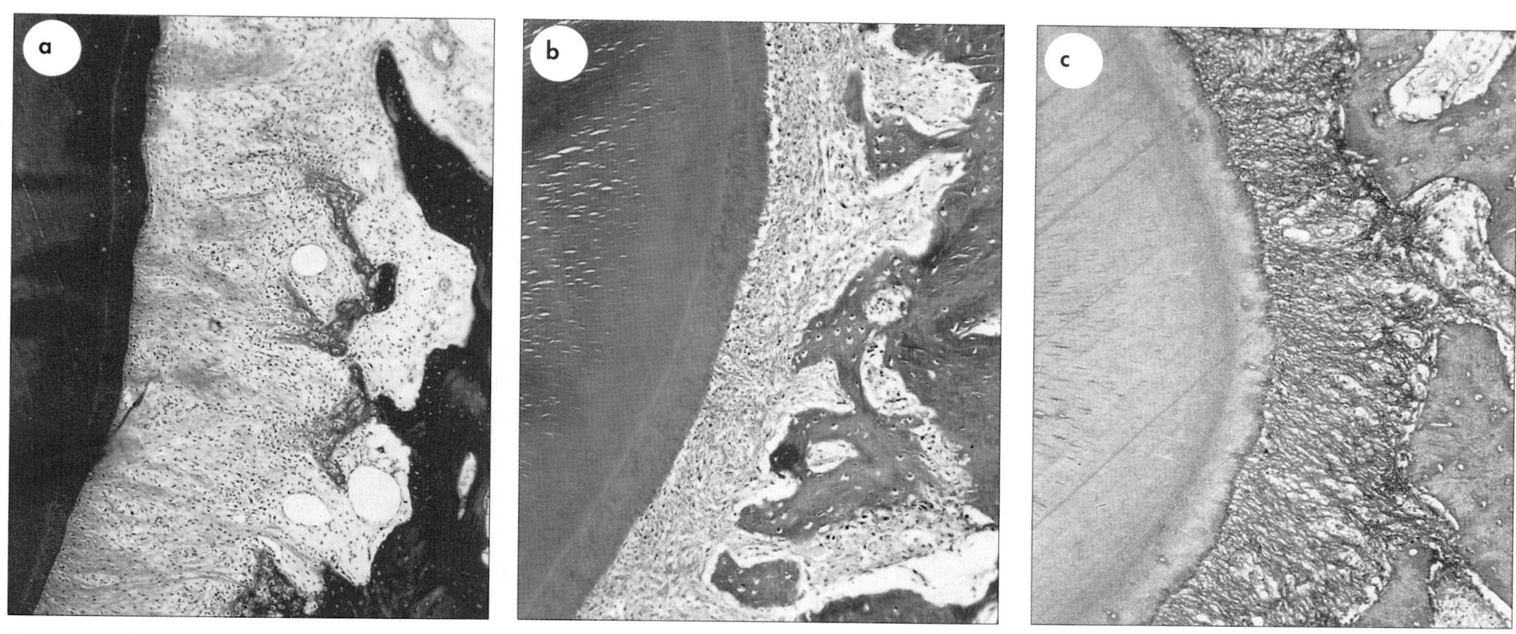

Fig. 15.4 Effects of luxation on (monkey) PDL. (a) PDL at 2 weeks after luxation. Osteoid formation parallel to the tooth at a distance equivalent to the normal ligament width can be seen. (Van Gieson stain; magnification × 125.) (b) PDL at 3 weeks after luxation. Alveolar bone has replaced the osteoid formation seen at 2 weeks. (Van Gieson stain; magnification × 125.) (c) PDL at 8 weeks after luxation. The ligament, alveolar and supporting bone did not differ from those of intact control monkey specimens. (Picrosirius and orcein stain; magnification × 125.) (Courtesy of Dr Ulla Mandel.)

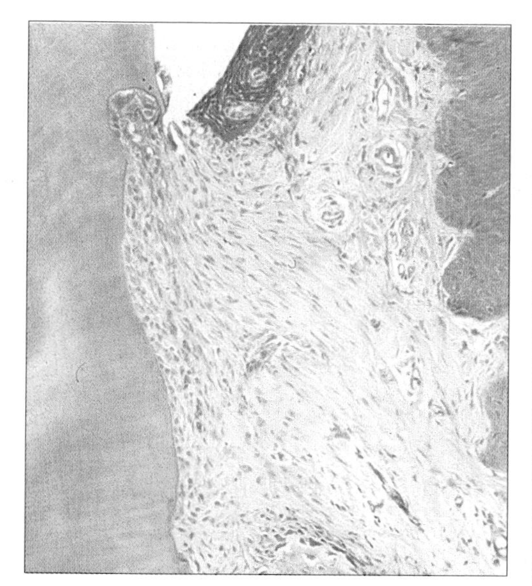

Fig. 15.5 Mechanical injury to (rat) periodontal soft tissues. Damage was produced with a flat, needle-like instrument to the cervical PDL. This specimen shows the effects at 21 days. A resorption lacuna undermines the dentine below the enamel just coronal to the cement–enamel junction. Odontoclasts are seen only in an undermining part of the lacuna (H & E magnification × 125). (Courtesy of Professor Y Kameyama.)

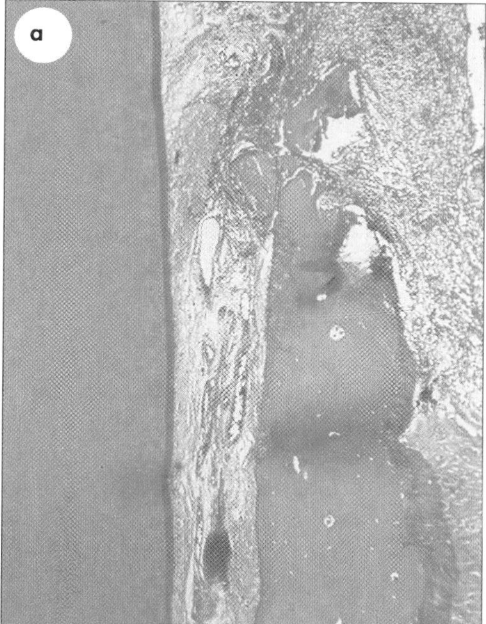

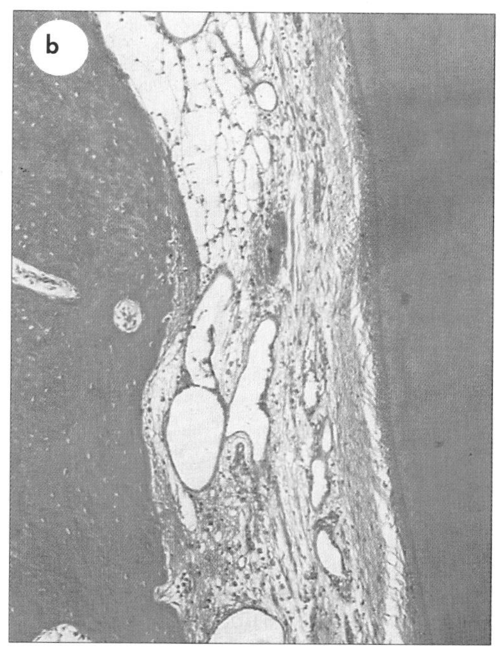

Fig. 15.6 Effect of electrosurgery on periodontal tissues. (a) Alveolar crest area 3 days after application of electrosurgery for 5 seconds. There is an acute inflammatory exudate in the line of incision across the alveolar process. The periodontal ligament space is occupied by blood vessels, cell debris, and inflammatory cells. There are areas of necrosis in the crestal bone (magnification × 25). (b) Middle third of PDL 1 week after application of electrosurgery for 1 second. Most of the PDL fibres have been destroyed and there is proliferation of blood vessels with an inflammatory exudate of polymorphonuclear leucocytes and macrophages (H & E magnification × 25). (Courtesy of Professor FA Carranza.)

progressive replacement resorption, these teeth often functioned normally for many years. Recipient age at the time of transplantation was significantly related directly to the functional time of the graft. Younger recipients had more resorption of the transplant.

Andreasen (1981) observed that replacement resorption after replantation was significantly related to the distance of the resorption site from a site with normal numbers of vital cementoblasts. He reasoned that, after replantation, minor areas of PDL damage were repaired from adjacent vital ligament, with possible surface root resorption and then repair with new cementum. If the dentine is damaged and infected, inflammatory resorption will occur. More extensive PDL damage resulted in healing, with rapid osteogenesis leading to ankylosis.

A further factor in healing after replantation is diet texture. Andersson *et al.* (1985) subjected (monkey) teeth to air drying for 1 hour, extraction, and then replantation. Those animals receiving hard diets demonstrated less ankylosis and a greater area of root surface with normal PDL than those fed soft food.

It may be concluded that the prognosis for a replanted tooth depends on the viability of its PDL, and on a minimum delay before replantation (or transplantation).

ENDODONTIC INJURY

MECHANICAL INJURY

Early studies of injury to the periapical PDL lacked experimental detail, but revealed considerable recovery properties on the part of this portion of the PDL. For example, following unspecified experimental trauma to (dog) teeth, Sippy (1928) found complete repair. Similarly, while root amputation of (cat) teeth led to ankylosis, functional stimulation resulted in renewal of normal PDL structure (Bauer, 1923). This, and similar work using dogs (Sippy, 1927), showed that loss of pulp vitality need not interfere with PDL function. Stahl (1960) observed (in rat teeth) no periapical changes 3 hours after pulp and ligament exposure. At 6 hours there was increased vascularity and cellularity of the periapical PDL, and some evidence of argyrophilic fibre formation and fuchsinophilia, indicating reticulin and ground substance formation. Between 1 day and 3 days, neutrophils became abundant, and capillaries and argyrophilic fibres proliferated. This process continued until 6 days from injury. Many disoriented fibroblasts appeared. Granulation tissue was most abundant by 10 days. After 2 weeks, it was being replaced slowly by organizing connective tissue, which appeared to wall off inflammatory cells at the apical foramen. Hyaluronic acid and collagen increased in amount. By 44 days, the periapical tissue was composed mainly of organized collagen bundles. Cysts sometimes appeared by 30 days. Epithelial cell rest proliferation was observed in five out of 20 specimens. Stahl (1960) noted that periapical tissue organized more rapidly and showed more extensive collagen formation than comparably injured gingiva, perhaps because the former was more protected from the oral environment. Similar events follow pulpectomy and root canal filling. As will be made clear, however, the chemical composition of filling materials can modify periapical healing. In general, competent endodontic treatment results in successful periapical healing, with true or pseudo-encapsulation of any filling material projecting from the apex (Kukidome, 1959; Fukunaga, 1960). Complete regeneration may take a year or more (Hiatt, 1959), and it may take the form of a relatively avascular fibrous tissue of repair rather than of a regenerated PDL (Penick, 1961).

Pulpal injury itself can lead to periapical changes. The placing of amalgam in direct contact with exposed (rat) pulps caused less periapical destruction if the restoration were not a cause of premature contact, indicating an exacerbating role for occlusal traumatism in periapical injury (Stahl *et al.*, 1958). Stahl *et al.* (1969) observed an initial reduction in labelling of (rat) periapical ligament fibroblasts by tritiated thymidine. After 24 hours, there was an increase in labelling of fibroblasts, osteoblasts, and cementoblasts, which by 4 days had spread to the adjacent PDL. The rate of proliferation had diminished by 20 days, at which time a well-circumscribed granuloma had formed. At the same time periapical vessels proliferated (Strömberg, 1971).

Seltzer and co-workers (1968, 1973) compared the effects of endodontic instrumentation short of and beyond root apices. Immediately following underinstrumentation (in rhesus monkey teeth), a slight polymorphonuclear neutrophil (PMN) infiltrate was observed periapically. In humans, 2 weeks after treatment, dilated vessels, oedema, haemorrhage, and granulation tissue were present periapically. In one case, epithelial cell rest proliferation occurred. Four to six weeks later, the response varied from mild inflammation to resolution or granuloma formation. After 90 days, apical granulomas were the commonest finding. Dilation of apical PDL blood vessels was observed at 4 days. After 11 days (Seltzer *et al.*, 1969), compression of the PDL by dentine chips was observed, with the accumulation of neutrophils and red blood cells around the latter. After about 4 weeks, chronic inflammation supervened, and it took 6–12 months for repair or further breakdown to occur. The least periapical damage resulted when root canals were underinstrumented (Seltzer *et al.*, 1969; Bhaskar and Rappoport, 1971; Davis *et al.*, 1971). Seltzer's group and others (Penick, 1961; Andreasen and Rud, 1972a) noted that the tissue of repair was usually a thickened fibrous layer which, by producing the appearance on radiographs of a widened PDL space, could give a false impression of continuing disease.

Seltzer *et al.* (1968, 1973) also noted that over-instrumentation caused profuse periapical haemorrhage and the dissemination of dentine particles beyond the apical foramina. The PDL became oedematous and an intense, mainly neutrophil inflammatory infiltrate formed. After 5–6 weeks, the PDL underwent granuloma or occasionally abscess formation. Generally, after 180 days, some epithelial rest proliferation was apparent.

Periapical abscesses need not impede completion of root formation. In a study of developing (monkey) incisors, after pulpectomy or pulpotomy, all showed complete root formation, in spite of prior abscesses (the root canals were sealed only with cotton pellets and amalgam) (Torneck and Smith, 1970). Teeth that had been 'irritated' by caries and restorations prior to endodontic treatment exhibited root canal narrowing, but no significant periapical inflammation after endodontics, provided the root canals had been underinstrumented (Seltzer *et al.*, 1968).

Root perforation appears to cause inflammation even if the defect is filled immediately. Hamamoto *et al.* (1989) noted that endodontic perforation of the pulp floor (in rats) resulted in rapid formation of cellular cementum around epithelial rests at the root apex. There were scanty collagen fibres between the rests and the cementum. After 4 weeks and 8 weeks, the epithelial islands were embedded in the cellular cementum and were undergoing degeneration. In the bifurcation area there was PDL destruction. There was some epithelial cell rest activity in the form of enlarged nucleus and cytoplasm, indicative, it was suggested, of some role in the formation of cementum. After approximal or bifurcation perforation (of dog teeth) with a machine-driven reamer followed by pulpectomy and immediate filling under aseptic conditions, the PDL at the site of injury suffered acute, and after 6 weeks, chronic inflammatory changes. These changes, again, were least when the defect was filled immediately, in this instance with chloroform-rosin and gutta-percha cones, and greatest when left open to contamination, even if restored subsequently (Lantz and Persson, 1967). Seltzer *et al.* (1970) studied the PDL effects of root perforation before and during endodontics, experimenting with varying intervals between perforation and closure. Inflammation was most severe when perforations were not closed, either immediately or at all, and the prognosis was doubtful in all cases, but better if the defect were closed immediately. A more promising prognosis for perforated roots derived from a similar (dog) study (Lantz and Persson, 1970). In this instance, however, the perforation was made after aseptic pulpectomy and root canal filling (with chloroform rosin and gutta-percha). The result was mild chronic inflammation with scattered lymphocytes and plasma cells. Inflammation was more marked when amalgam was substituted for gutta-percha, because of leakage around the amalgam. A well-organized fibrous capsule formed around gutta-percha, but only sparse collagen fibres around amalgam. If the perforations were sealed with zinc phosphate cement, there was a similar mild chronic inflammatory reaction in the periapical PDL (Lantz and Persson, 1970). Andreasen and Skougaard (1972) (in rats) showed comparable temporary inflammatory changes around perforations in vital teeth. Early ankylosis was followed after only 3 weeks by re-establishment of an intact PDL.

In a series of experiments, Paterson, Watts and co-workers noted the periapical response of pulp exposure in germ-free and gnotobiotic rats as well as in conventional animals. There were no periapical changes in the germ-free animals whereas, 7 days after pulp exposure in the conventional animals, 19 of 34 teeth showed periapical inflammation, leading to the conclusion that mechanical trauma to the pulp alone did not cause such inflammation (Paterson and Watts, 1987) (*Fig. 15.8*). In further work, the pulp was exposed to caries-related bacterial species such as *Lactobacillus casei* or *Streptococcus mutans*, in monoinfected gnotobiotic rats. *L. casei* induced pulp necrosis after direct application to the mechanically exposed pulp of previously germ-free rats. After 28 days, periapical inflammation was found in relation to about 40 per cent of teeth. Bacteria were present in these lesions (Paterson and Pountney, 1987a). The occurrence was rarer with *S. mutans* (Paterson and Pountney, 1987b) (*Fig. 15.9*). Similar responses to combinations of both species were observed by Paterson and Watts (1992). One strain of *S. mutans* was found to be more virulent than others in its periapical effects (Watts and Paterson, 1992), with about half the teeth being affected periapically. Fibrous capsule formation suggestive of an abscess was observed in some lesions, and occasionally polymorphonuclear neutrophils were found within root canals. Numerous streptococci were detected within phagocytic cells present in most of the periapical lesions. These lesions were much more extensive than in the *L. casei* study of Paterson and Pountney (1987a). In conventional rats, with pulp exposed to the oral cavity, bacterial contamination occurred, but periapical changes were rare, and bacteria were hard to find in this locus, being seen in only one specimen periapically in one of 34 sections, 14 days after pulp exposure (Watts and Paterson, 1990).

CHEMICAL INJURY

The periapical PDL response to endodontic materials seems to depend both on the texture of the filling and on its chemical composition. When the filling material is hard and compact, it tends to become encapsulated, although a loose connective tissue containing macrophages frequently forms between a 'capsule' and the filling material. When it is less compact, the filling material is resorbed more rapidly. Resorbable pastes (e.g. iodoform) produce an infiltrate that is rich in PMN, and cause necrosis of the surrounding PDL, owing to obliteration of the local blood supply (Muruzábal *et al.*, 1966). In contrast to the persistent inflammation produced by zinc oxide–eugenol, iodoform pastes rarely produce necrosis (Erausquin and Muruzábal, 1969a,b; Holland *et al.*, 1971).

Various pastes and resins have been used as root canal fillers. With Diaket (a polyvinyl resin with bismuth phosphate and an antiseptic, dihydroxydichlorophenyl-methane) and AH-26 (a compound of silver, bismuth oxide, titanium oxide, hexamethylene tetramine, and bisphenol diglycidyl ether) moderate periapical inflammatory infiltration was observed whether roots were

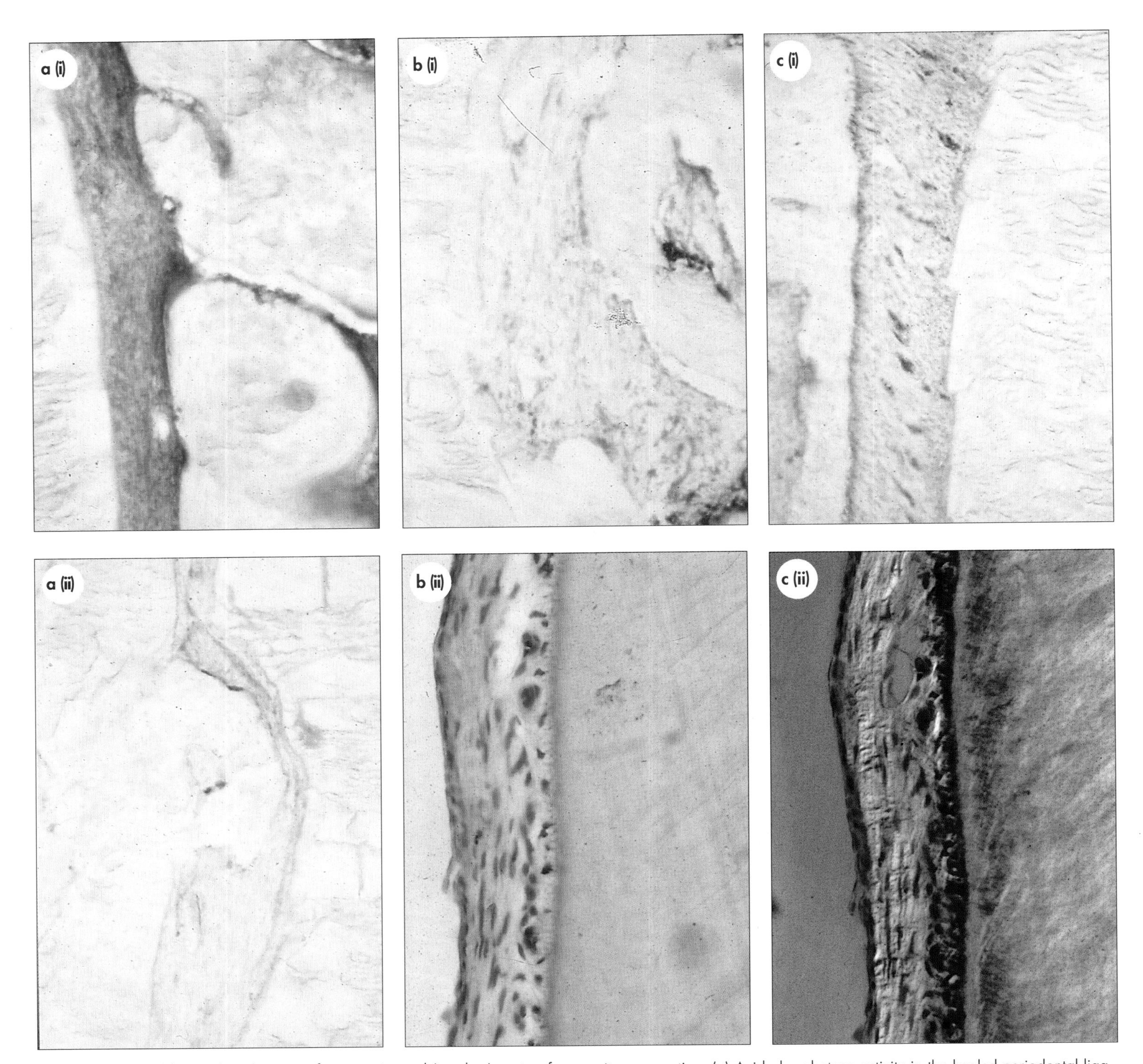

Fig. 15.7 Repair of periodontal tissues after experimental (monkey) root surface cavity preparation. (a) Acid phosphatase activity in the healed periodontal ligament (i) and in the experimental cavity (ii). The darker areas show enzyme activity, which was weaker in the PDL of the experimental cavity than in the surrounding ligament (magnfication × 25). (b) Glucose-6-phosphate dehydrogenase activity in the healed PDL (i) and in the experimental cavity (ii). Enzyme activity was higher in cells in the PDL between bone and experimental cavity dentine (magnification × 25). (c) PDL after 8 weeks in tissue culture; it contains dense connective tissue (i). By polarized light the collagen fibres may be seen to be aligned parallel to the root surface (ii) (magnification × 100). (From Lindskog *et al.*, 1983.)

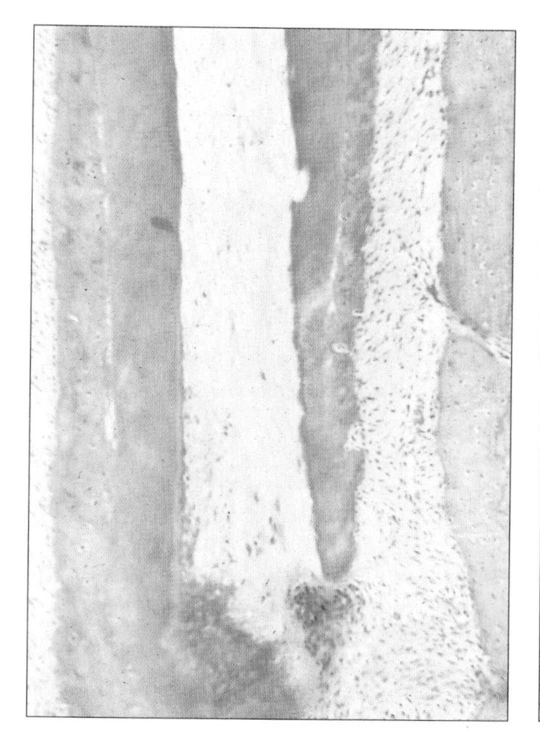

Fig. 15.8 Root apex, germ-free (rat) molar. The pulp is totally necrotic, but there is no evidence of inflammation in the periapical tissues. (H & E magnification × 75.) (From Watts and Paterson, 1992.)

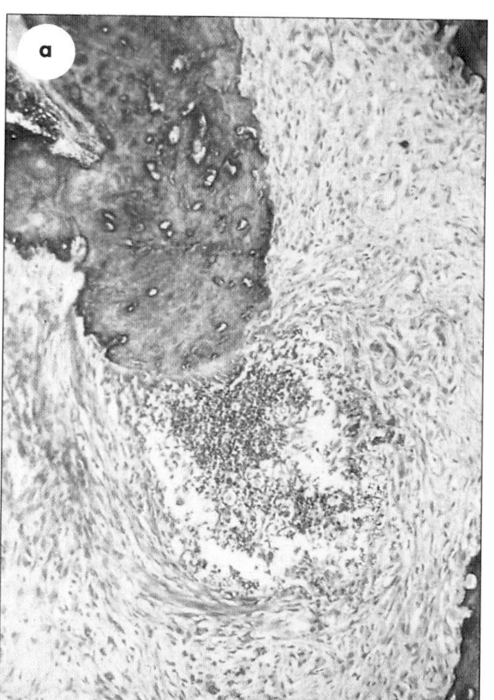

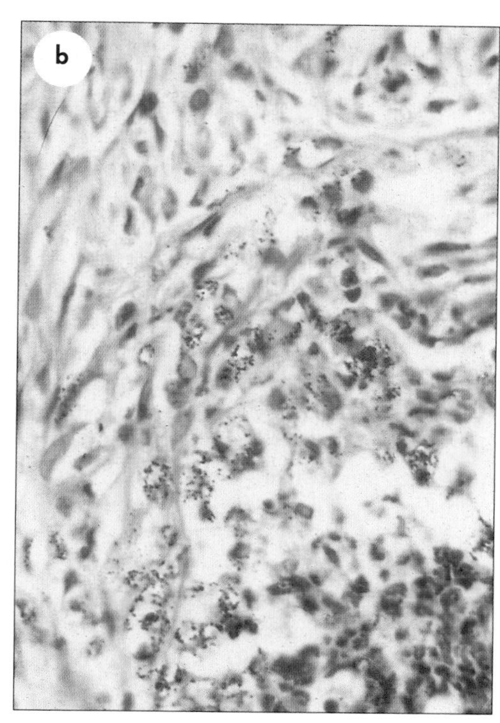

Fig. 15.9 (a) Root apex of molar from gnotobiotic rat moninfected with *Streptococcus mutans* (NCTC 10832) 28 days after mechanical pulp exposure. There is a periapical abscess with evidence of fibrous capsule formation. (Gram Weigert stain; magnification × 60.) (b) Higher magnification of periapical lesion shown in (a). A mixture of inflammatory cells is present, notably polymorphonucleocytes and macrophages containing blue-staining phagocytosed streptocooci. (Gram Weigert stain; magnification × 350.) (From Watts and Paterson, 1992.)

underfilled or overfilled. Overfilled material compressed the PDL, producing a pseudocapsule. By 15 days, the overfilled material was separated from the surrounding tissue by a fibrous layer outside a zone of macrophages, foreign-body giant cells, and stellate fibroblasts. After 30 days, only the overfilled sites showed persistent inflammation. The pseudocapsule also persisted except at the periphery of the filling material, where it had been replaced by new fibrous tissue. Diaket overfill was surrounded by a fibrous capsule with a loose structure, containing macrophages and giant cells, and the cytoplasm of these cells was loaded with particles of Diaket. AH-26 overfill disintegrated, and many phagocytes were found among the particles. The overfilled mass was often surrounded by a poorly organized fibrous capsule. By 60 days, the AH-26 overfill showed little change, and it had not been completely removed at 90 days (Muruzábal and Erausquin, 1966). This study was extended to include Riebler resin, which is basically a phenol formaldehyde resin (Erausquin and Muruzábal, 1969a). Again, the the response seemed to depend primarily on the level to which the root was filled.

Overfilling produced either necrosis of the apical PDL, or infiltration of neutrophils and macrophages, and later giant cells. This was followed by encapsulation, or occasionally by abscess or granuloma formation. This response was typical of the industrial epoxy resins and of root canal cements containing resins, the latter producing a slight but persistent neutrophil infiltrate replaced eventually by macrophages and giant cells (Erausquin *et al.*, 1966; Erausquin and Muruzábal, 1969b). Chloroform rosin and gutta-percha led to acute inflammation even when used to fill perforations immediately after the defects had been created (Lantz and Persson, 1967).

Hydron, poly-2-hydroxyethyl methacrylate, a gel that polymerizes in the presence of water, was found to produce little or no periapical reaction, although histiocytes took up the barium salt filler (Benkel *et al.*, 1976; Kronman *et al.*, 1977).

Silicone rubber used as a root canal filling produced periapical fibrotic encapsulation with slight inflammation. There was some phagocytosis by giant cells (Kasman and Goldman, 1977).

Results from root canal cements are variable. Phosphate cement has been associated with progressive periodontal destruction when used to fill root perforations (Lantz and Persson, 1967). Zinc oxide–eugenol produced a larger zone of necrosis than N2 or Kerr cements, particularly if it became mixed with tissue debris owing to instrumentation. However, all such lesions were eventually encapsulated (Erausquin and Muruzábal, 1968). Rowe (1967) used various combinations of zinc oxide, eugenol, barium sulphate, olive oil, glycyrrhetinic acid, 2 per cent cortisone acetate, paraformaldehyde, calcium hydroxide, Kri paste (iodoform paste containing a blend of parachlorphenol, camphor, and menthol), an unidentified resorbable material, Grossman's root canal sealer (zinc oxide, staybelite resin, bismuth subcarbonate, barium sulphate, eugenol, and almond oil), Ledermix cement (zinc oxide, calcium hydroxide, triamcinolone acetonide, and demethylchlortetracycline hydrochloride) and paste (water-soluble cream, triamcinolone acetonide, demethylchlortetracycline-calcium) and N2 (paraformaldehyde, an anti-inflammatory agent called hydroxydimethyl octodien, zinc oxide, barium sulphate, and oil of cloves). Results 2 weeks after pulpectomy (of cat teeth) and extension of fillings at least to apical thirds were similar, irrespective of the material used. All but one of 58 teeth showed considerable periapical inflammation with PMN and some plasma cells and lymphocytes. Using zinc oxide–eugenol, inflammation was still present after 16 weeks. The addition of barium sulphate and olive oil resulted in less inflammation. No improvement was obtained by the addition of glycyrrhetinic acid. When the latter was replaced by 2 per cent cortisone acetate, marked inflammation occurred. Paraform and glycyrrhetinic acid with zinc oxide and eugenol produced minimal inflammation. Calcium hydroxide with distilled water produced the most severe reaction, with abscess formation. None of the proprietary pastes prevented inflammation.

It should be emphasized that these reactions are usually transient, whether they occur periapically or in relation to lateral canals (Rud and Andreasen, 1972), and they do not warrant the rejection of those materials that produce only a mild inflammation for a brief period (Barker and Lockett, 1972a,b). For example, N2 (in dog teeth) showed very little periapical disturbance 3 months after placement (Barker and Lockett, 1972b).

Erausquin and Muruzábal (1968) compared the effects of filling short of, to, and beyond the root apices (of rat molars), using zinc oxide–eugenol, Grossman's, N2, and Kerr root canal cements. Overfilling produced infarction of the periapical PDL, owing to destruction, compression, or thrombosis of the apical vessels, regardless of the cement used. Necrosis was most extensive with zinc oxide–eugenol, although necrotic tissue was replaced within 4 days. Mild inflammation resulted whether the filling extended to or slightly beyond the apex. More severe inflammation occurred if the overfilled mass was not compact. Tightly packed cements resorbed very slowly.

Resorption was carried out partly by foreign body giant cells on the surface of the overfilled material. N2 tended to fragment temporarily, with the release of granules of titanium dioxide that were phagocytosed rapidly by macrophages. PMN tended to disappear 2 weeks after filling, and encapsulation of excess filling material occurred usually by 90 days. In two cases of overfill with Grossman's cement and one with zinc oxide–eugenol, bone was deposited directly on the cementum.

Similar results were obtained when acrylic polymer was added to these various root canal cements, the position of the cement in relation to the apex being of apparently greater consequence than its chemical composition (Erausquin and Muruzábal, 1968).

Erausquin (1970) tested root canal filling materials containing zinc, titanium, lead oxide, and aluminium oxides. Propylene glycol, polyethylene glycol, petrolatum–lanolin, and silicone cream were used as excipients. Zinc and lead oxides produced a moderate inflammatory infiltrate 1 week after placement, and this was still slightly evident 90 days post-operatively. Overfilled material was surrounded by fibrous tissue. Titanium dioxide produced a dense PMN infiltrate that also contained many macrophages loaded with the oxide. Granulomas and apical abscesses were frequent sequels. The reaction was more severe if petrolatum–lanolin was used as the excipient. Aluminium oxide stimulated a marked infiltrate with subsequent encapsulation. Zinc and lead oxides, which had no tendency to disperse, underwent encapsulation. Titanium and aluminium oxides tended to disperse, and this exacerbated the inflammatory response.

One of the least offensive root canal fillings seems to be calcium hydroxide, notwithstanding Rowe's (1967) early results. In studies of periapical response to root canal treatment of incompletely formed (dog) teeth, this agent was used with distilled water or as the proprietary paste Calxyl (calcium hydroxide, sodium bicarbonate, and sodium, potassium, and calcium chlorides) (Binnie and Rowe, 1973, 1974). Some canals were filled with Grossman's root canal sealer, which generally produced mild but occasionally severe inflammation not observed following the use of either calcium hydroxide preparation. Mild transient inflammation did occur soon after placement (Binnie and Rowe, 1973; Holland *et al.*, 1977).

Citrome and Hever (1979) compared a calcium hydroxide–saline paste and a collagen–calcium phosphate gel. The gel produced severe inflammation in the form of acute abscesses, followed by granulomas or cysts. Little inflammation followed the use of the calcium hydroxide–saline preparation. Calcium hydroxide used with or without iodoform produced good healing in (dog) teeth with open apices (Holland *et al.*, 1971).

Delayed calcium hydroxide treatment of (monkey) teeth subjected to experimentally induced root resorption of contaminated replanted teeth resulted in a significant shift from inflammatory resorption to ankylosis. The treatment caused an increase in ankylosis, preceded by root resorption, while ankylosis not associated with root resorption decreased. Intracanal calcium hydroxide treatment of teeth with compromised PDL may cause unnecessary resorption if left in the canal for a long time or if changed repeatedly (Lengheden *et al.*, 1990a). Immediate permanent root filling and intracanal calcium hydroxide of similar contaminated replanted teeth resulted in a shift towards ankylosis not associated with root resorption. While calcium hydroxide is suitable for teeth with healthy periapical PDL, the authors concluded that prolonged treatment of teeth that have compromised PDL should be avoided so as not to risk ankylosis (Lengheden *et al.*, 1990b).

Polycarboxylates were found to be no better than other cements, nor were there particular advantages to be gained by using them in combination with other materials, including tin hydroxide, stannous fluoride, calcium hydroxide, or calcium fluoride, which were tried in various concentrations. In most cases, the cements were forced into the periapical PDL, producing the typical overfill reaction. This invalidates this study as a test of the materials themselves (Seltzer *et al.*, 1976).

Corticosteroid-containing root canal preparations were investigated by Barker and Lockett (1972c). Prolonged contact of Ledermix paste with (dog) periapical tissues had no harmful consequences. Cortril, which contains hydrocortisone in a water-miscible base, caused severe periapical inflammation, including abscess. This was attributed to the base, although it had been shown previously (Rowe, 1967) that cortisone in a root canal cement was itself associated with marked periapical inflammation, and also with enhanced spread of bacteria from the pulp (Watts and Paterson, 1988) (*Fig. 15.10*), which prompted Watts and Paterson to advise against the endodontic use of anti-inflammatory compounds in patients at risk from bacteraemia. In their study, prednisolone and triamcinolone acetonide application to exposed (rat) pulp led to periapical inflammation.

Cortisone administered systemically is known to impair fibroblast metabolism and collagen synthesis (Dreizen *et al.*, 1971). Erausquin (1972) filled root canals with corticoid-containing materials and found only a minimal inflammatory reaction periapically if radicular pulp and dentine chips were compressed beforehand to form an apical plug between the cement and the PDL. After local application of prednisolone following pulpectomy, Strömberg (1972) observed periapical vascular proliferation in dogs that had undergone partial pulpectomy. In a similar group, which underwent total pulpectomy, a comparable increase in vascularity occurred by the third instead of the tenth day. Otherwise, no differences were noted between the groups.

The effects of amalgam were studied by Nasjleti *et al.* (1977), who found that reimplantation of rhesus monkey teeth that had been extracted and root filled and had had an amalgam restoration placed midway along the root was followed by severe inflammation. Omitting the PDL effects produced by this trauma, inflammation was more severe and prolonged in relation to the restoration.

Erausquin and Devoto (1970) investigated the potential of different root canal cements to produce ankylosis. They found this rarely followed zinc oxide–eugenol or Grossman's root canal sealer. Formaldehyde-containing derivatives caused ankylosis. Trioxymethylene powder, a constituent of N2, rarely produced ankylosis unless combined with a corticoid. If the root canal was filled with trioxymethylene-containing N2 but the vital pulp not removed, there was periapical inflammation but no ankylosis. After pulpectomy, the same N2 paste produced acute periapical inflammation followed by ankylosis or granuloma formation (Langeland, 1974). Ankylosis was less frequent and extensive when the root canal was underfilled. The addition of acrylic to the paste resulted in only slight inflammation and moderate fibrosis (Bordoni and Erausquin, 1970).

Erausquin and Devoto (1970) noted that, when healing started in the healthy PDL after periapical instrumentation, there was functional rehabilitation of the tissues; when regeneration began in the alveolar bone marrow, they observed ankylosis as a sequel. Either the newly formed fibrous tissue that had replaced necrotic PDL underwent trabecular bone formation, or the necrotic PDL calcified.

None of the root canal cements tested by Binnie and Rowe (1973) caused epithelial cell rest proliferation, and neither did various zinc and magnesium salts with water, glutaraldehyde, or eugenol. It was concluded that the presence of rests was a characteristic of the individual animal rather than a response to a particular filling material (Binnie and Rowe, 1974). Epithelial rests also proliferate following mechanical injury, e.g., attempted tooth extraction (Johansen, 1970).

Attention has been drawn above to the variability in response of the periapical PDL to a variety of endodontic procedures and filling materials, and to the short-term delay in healing in most instances. Healing showed a similar variability. The PDL may regenerate or ankylosis may occur with or without persistent mild inflammation. Fibrous scar tissue may form adjacent to healthy PDL or to an ankylosis, in the presence of varying grades of inflammation. Moderate or severe inflammation may persist in the absence of tissue repair. These conclusions were drawn from a study of 70 cases of human endodontic surgery 1–14 years after the original endodontic therapy; materials and techniques used in the original surgery were amalgam or gutta-percha, and retrograde or orthograde filling (Andreasen and Rud, 1972c). Andreasen (1973) observed that lateral PDL inflammation was

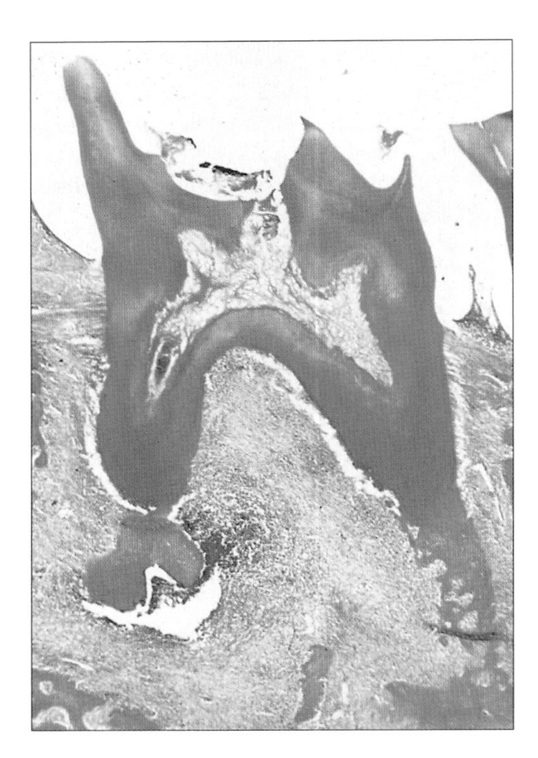

Fig. 15.10 Mechanically exposed (rat) molar pulp treated with prednisolone. The pulp is totally necrotic and there is extensive periapical inflammation. (Haematoxylin and eosin stain; magnification × 20.) (From Watts and Paterson, 1992.)

more inclined to persist after pulp necrosis in younger (rat) teeth, owing to the greater permeability of younger dentine which permitted more ready spread of necrotic pulp products.

Only isolated studies have been reported concerning the effects of drugs and poisons on the PDL. Most of them derive from endodontic studies and will be reviewed here.

The acute secondary agranulocytosis resulting from arsphenamine treatment has been associated with extensive haemorrhage and ultimately necrosis of the PDL, owing to the activity of anaerobic bacteria in periodontal pockets (Bauer, 1946). Similarly, arsenical pulp devitalizers were observed to cause acute periapical inflammation if pushed through the apex (Glasser, 1957). Arsenic supplements (20 ppm) to the diet of rats led to a slightly increased severity of chronic periodontitis (Shaw, 1973).

Attalla (1968) observed that beechwood creosote, an antiseptic used to clean root canals, caused a severe periapical reaction with abscess formation in 60 per cent of specimens (in dogs). Similar treatment with chloramine, however, produced no significant reaction.

Butyl-2-cyanoacrylate was applied in one study to exposed (rat) molar pulps. After 1 week there had been no extension of (minimal) pulpal inflammation to the PDL. Marked periapical inflammation with microabscess formation occurred in those specimens exposed to cavity liner varnish. However, widening of the apical PDL space was evident in the cyanoacrylate-treated cases after 7 weeks (Wade, 1969).

When cold cure acrylic was placed in root surface cavities in extracted (monkey) teeth, which were subsequently replanted after 4 minutes outside the mouth, inflammation and fibre disorientation were more marked and prolonged in relation to the PDL apposed to the resin, and fibres that did form remained parallel to the restoration surface (Nasjleti *et al.*, 1972).

Accidental injection of sodium hypochlorite beyond the root apex has been reported on one occasion as producing an acute periapical reaction spreading to involve the face (Becker *et al.*, 1974). Routine canal irrigation with 1 per cent NaOCl or with 1 per cent NaOCl followed by 2 per cent iodine potassium iodide produced insignificant and transient periapical inflammation (Lamers *et al.*, 1980). Watts and Paterson (1993) observed periapical PDL damage caused by hypochlorite, with collagen loss and the absence of fibrin and osteoclastic activity at the contiguous bone surface. There was an extensive, mainly polymorphonuclear infiltrate, but very few micro-organisms were present (*Fig. 15.11*).

There are few reported non-endodontic cases of chemical damage to the PDL. The local application of carbolic acid to (rat) interdental papilla resulted in loss of alveolar crest PDL fibres after 3 days. These regenerated 4 days later, but there was still diminished birefringence of the fibres after 30 days. The fibre changes were accompanied by a round-cell infiltrate (Tonna and Stahl, 1967).

Ogle and Ciancio (1971) showed that protracted exposure to anticholinergic agents was associated with a more severe periodontal response to plaque, perhaps owing to reduction in salivary flow.

PHYSICAL AGENTS

INJECTION PRESSURE

Recent years have seen the development of intraligamentary anaesthesia, in which local anaesthetic is injected under pressure directly into the PDL. Most reports describe the resultant tissue changes as localized, minor, and reversible (Galili *et al.*, 1984; Anneroth *et al.*, 1985). Granulation tissue was evident (in dogs) after 15 days. In one study there was neither bone nor cementum damage (Galili *et al.*, 1984). Tissue disruption occurs shortly after injection, and some studies (also on dogs) have shown areas of active external root resorption after 30 days (Roahen and Marshall, 1990). In a similar (monkey) study, no changes from normal were observed after 1, 3, or 30 days (Albers and Ellinger, 1988). Brännström *et al.* (1982), after 1 hour, observed fluid-filled spaces, distorted or disrupted collagen bundles, and lesions of tooth root and bone, and these had still not healed by 2 weeks.

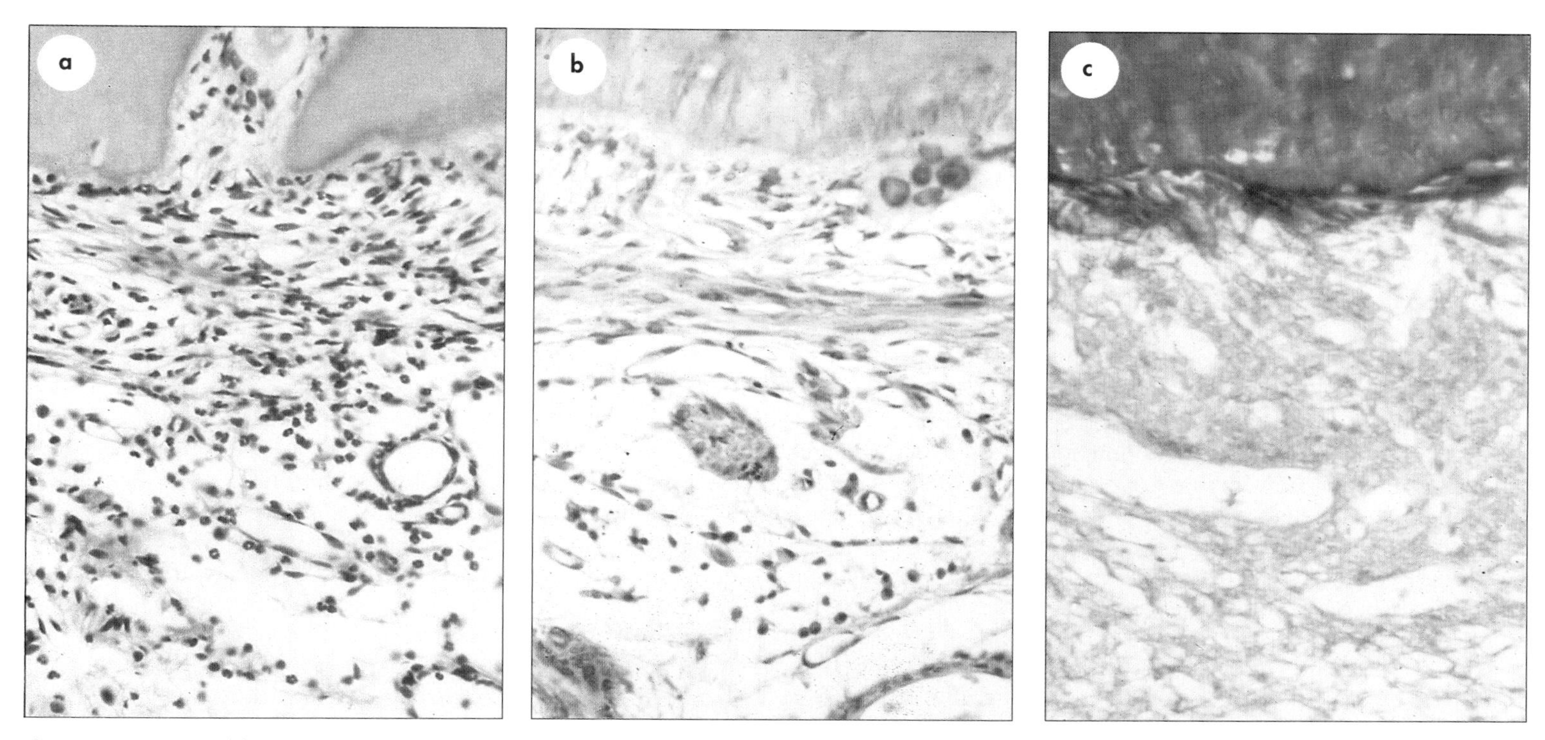

Fig. 15.11 (a) Apical foramen and adjacent periapical tissues from a (dog) upper central incisor, 2 weeks after ultrasonic instrumentation of the root canal. This is one type of response observed in these specimens, which contain mostly PMN infiltration, and it differs markedly from the changes seen in (c). (Haematoxylin and exosin stain × 75.) (b) Periapical tissues of (dog) premolar. A minimal infiltration of small round cells and macrophages is present, and the tissue structure appears unaltered. (Haematoxylin and eosin stain; magnification × 300.) (c) Periapical tissues of (dog) incisor stained to demonstrate collagen. The mesh-like tissue appears greyish, whereas normal collagen would have stained red. (Van Gieson stain; magnification × 115.) (From Watts and Paterson, 1992.)

They observed less damage with saline controls, and concluded that the effects were attributable both to physical trauma and to cytotoxic effects of the solution (prilocaine and felypressin). They advised against use of the technique for primary teeth because of a possible risk to the underlying permanent tooth germ. Tal and Stahl (1986) observed root resorption (in cats) with unmasking of dentine collagen and with some evidence of eventual interdigitation with PDL fibres.

RADIATION

Following x-radiation or radium treatment, Leist (1926) and Zerosi (1938, 1940) observed degenerative changes in (dog) PDL, with hyperaemia, exudation, and reduced principal fibres and cellularity, caused by thrombosis and vascular degeneration. By contrast, radium sulphate administered through the alveolar bone (in rabbits) led to fibrous hypertrophy and the development of cysts from epithelial cell rests (Rosenthal, 1937).

Shapiro *et al.* (1960) found that whole body irradiation of 1200 r induced (in mice) severe PDL destruction within 100 days. Two cases of radiation damage (2000 r) to child dentitions were recorded in which the PDL was widened (Fronman and Ratzkowski, 1966).

A study using kittens revealed a decrease in PDL width with loss of normal insertion of fibres following two doses of 100 r given 1 week apart. Ankylosis occurred in nearly half the animals (Winter and Kramer, 1965). Frandsen (1962) noted (in rats) extensive PDL destruction related to ulcers spreading from the overlying mucosa if the tooth and supporting tissues were irradiated. Whole-body irradiation (1000 r) resulted only in decreased cellularity of the PDL 2–58 days after irradiation. Frandsen (1963), in a further study of local roentgen irradiation (in rats), found no difference between dosages of 1725 r and 2400 r. No extensive destruction originated in the PDL, which showed only oedema or degeneration of some fibres. A dose of 1000 r to the head produced decreased PDL cellularity. A dose of 2000 r or 3000 r led to death before PDL involvement had occurred, although there had been gingival epitheliolysis. Mayo *et al.* (1962) observed that a threshold of 700 r of total-body irradiation was necessary to produce lesions (in hamsters); 1020 r from 200 kV radiation was found to produce decreased PDL vascularity, with only occasional small sclerotic blood vessels seen. There were also fewer fibroblasts, and these were smaller, rounded and more deeply staining than normal. Cementoblasts were also scarcer. A similar radiation dose from cobalt-60 produced very slight alterations, the PDL generally possessing normal vascularity and cellularity, although there was a slight decrease in collagen fibre density. Doubling the standard dose of radiation to 2040 r exacerbated the PDL changes that had been seen with half this dosage, whereas a 2040 r dose of cobalt-60 radiation made little change. Meyer *et al.* (1962) concluded that cobalt-60 radiation was much less damaging than standard high-voltage radiation. However, Zach *et al.* (1973) observed PDL inflammation when high-voltage or cobalt-60 irradiation was used. They administered fractionated doses of 333 r three times a week over 6 weeks (total 6000 r) to 34 monkeys, at a rate of 35 r per minute.

Diet texture may modify the response to radiation. While no changes were observed in mice fed a routine diet, soft food consumption resulted in disorganization of the PDL, especially along the apical third of the root, with hyalinization and fragmentation of collagen fibres and nuclear pyknosis of fibroblasts. Both groups had received 200 r whole body X-irradiation repeated once weekly until 1200 r had been given (Mayo *et al.*, 1962; Ershoff *et al.*, 1967). While the authors did not explain their findings, it is known that typical chronic inflammatory periodontal disease advances only in animals consuming diets of soft texture, owing to the the fact that these diets do not offer prevention of plaque accumulation at the site of onset (Egelberg, 1965; Newman, 1974).

Laser radiation has been found to produce PDL degeneration and inflammatory changes; these changes are attributable to the heat produced by the beam (Taylor *et al.*, 1965).

TEMPERATURE

When rats were maintained between 0°C and 2°C for up to 2 weeks, the PDL appeared more granular than fibrillar (Shklar and Glickman, 1959). Fibroblasts were reduced in number and irregular in distribution, size, and shape. Their nuclei became small, they were spherical rather than elliptical, and they stained deeply. There were fewer cementoblasts and osteoblasts. By 4 weeks, the collagen fibres looked normal, but there were still fewer fibroblasts than normal. By 4 months, no significant differences were noted between control and experimental animals. The initial changes were attributed to adrenal stress, although no clear mechanism was put forward. Heat challenge (43°C) to human PDL fibroblasts caused the production of heat stress proteins by the latter (Sauk *et al.*, 1988). Sauk *et al.* (1988) suggested that, as these proteins can increase the rate of protein translocation between intracellular membrane compartments, this could relate to a role in PDL development, repair, and regeneration. They further suggested that heat stress protein binding to steroid receptors prior to hormone binding represents a protective function (e.g. solubilizing proteins that otherwise tend to form aggregates.)

In a further study of rats exposed to the same temperature (43°C) for up to 18 months, Shklar (1966) observed decreased cellularity and separation and irregularity of collagen bundles. There were many dilated and engorged capillaries. He attributed the changes on this occasion to loss of normal function following prolonged exposure of the animals to stress. At the other extreme, mice subjected to temperatures of 42°C and 90 per cent relative humidity for 10 minutes suffered an initial depression of PDL fibroblast labelling by tritiated thymidine. Subsequent peak labelling values at 4–8 hours or 24–48 hours were double those for control tissues. Thereafter, labelling values returned to those of the control animals (McKibben and Pechersky, 1972).

A local application of high temperature to the PDL was obtained by insertion after pulpectomy of an electrosurgery tip 2.5 mm apical to the cement–enamel junction (of squirrel monkey teeth) (Atrizadeh *et al.*, 1971). Necrosis occurred 3–7 days later in the PDL near where the broach had been inserted. Fibroblasts, cementoblasts, and osteoblasts were destroyed, and there was a reduced staining of PDL fibres. At the periphery of the necrotic area, fibroblasts and blood vessels proliferated 2 weeks after injury. The vascular and cellular responses were more marked apically than coronally. Many osteoclasts were seen. Granulation tissue formation and widening of the PDL space, owing to bone resorption, proceeded. However, between 3 months and 6 months, ankylosis occurred, the PDL became less cellular than normal, and many collagen fibres were aligned parallel to the root surface. Similar findings were obtained by Line *et al.* (1974).

With the increased use of cryoprobes, there have been studies of the effects of direct freezing injury on the PDL. Tal *et al.* (1991) applied a cryoprobe at -81°C to bone 5 mm apical to the alveolar crest (in dogs). While cells were killed, extracellular matrix in the devitalized area was preserved, supporting regeneration of the cryolesion. The probe had been applied for three intervals of 10 seconds each, and sections were examined for up to 30 days after the application (*Fig. 15.12*, p. 336). At 48 hours after surgery, there were no cells in the frozen PDL, and a minimal inflammatory response. At 30 days, the PDL was repopulated so that it did not differ significantly from the untreated PDL coronal or apical to it, providing further evidence that the extracellular matrix in the devitalized tissue supported regeneration of the cryolesion. Tal and co-workers also deduced from this observation that extracellular matrix components of PDL may be important in regulating periodontal wound healing. Tal and Stahl (1986) had previously shown that cryoprobe application for 5 seconds produced loss of vitality within PDL, bone and cementum by 24 hours. Root resorption was marked.

REFERENCES

Albers DD and Ellinger RF (1988) Histologic effects of high-pressure intraligamental injections on the periodontal ligament. Quintess Int 19, 361–363.

Alexander SA and Swerdloff M (1980) Collagenolytic activity of periodontal ligament and hydroxyproline content during human deciduous root resorption. J Periodont Res 15, 434–443.

Andersson L (1988) Dentoalveolar ankylosis and associated root resorption in replanted teeth. Experimental and clinical studies in monkeys and man. Swed Dent J Suppl 56.

Andersson J, Lindskog S, Blomlöf L, Hedström KG and Hammarström L (1985) Effect of masticatory stimulation on dentoalveolar ankylosis after experimental tooth replantation. Endod Dent Traumatol 1, 13–16.

Andreasen JO (1973) Effect of pulpal necrosis upon periodontal healing after surgical injury in rats. Int J Oral Surg 2, 62–68.

Andreasen JO (1980) A time–related study of periodontal healing and root resorption activity after replantation of mature permanent incisors in monkeys. Swed Dent J 4, 101–110.

Andreasen JO (1981) Interrelation between alveolar bone and periodontal ligament repair after replantation of mature permanent incisors in monkeys. J Periodont Res 16, 228–235.

Andreasen JO and Hjörting-Hansen E (1966) Replantation of teeth. II. Histologic study of 22 replanted anterior teeth in humans. Acta Odont Scand 24, 287–300.

Andreasen JO, Reinholdt J, Rüs I, Dybdahl R, Söder PÖ and Otterskog P (1978) Periodontal and pulpal healing of monkey incisors preserved in tissue culture before replantation. Int J Oral Surg 7, 104–112.

Andreasen JO and Rud J (1972a) Correlations between histology and radiography in the assessment of healing after endodontic surgery. Int J Oral Surg 1, 161–173.

Andreasen JO and Rud J (1972b) A histobacteriologic study of dental and periapical structures after endodontic surgery. Int J Oral Surg 1, 272–281.

Andreasen JO and Rud J (1972c) Modes of healing histologically after endodontic surgery in 20 cases. Int J Oral Surg 1, 148–160.

Andreasen JO and Schwartz O (1986) The effect of saline storage before replantation upon dry damage of the periodontal ligament. Endod Dent Traumatol 2, 67–70.

Andreasen JO and Skougaard MR (1972) Reversibility of surgically induced dental ankylosis in rats. Int J Oral Surg 1, 98–102.

Anneroth G, Danielsson KH, Evers H, Hedström KG and Nordenram Å (1985) Periodontal ligament injection. An experimental study in the monkey. Int J Oral Surg 14, 538–543.

Arwill T (1962) Histopathologic studies of traumatized teeth. Odont Tidskr 70, 91–117.

Atrizadeh F, Kennedy J and Zander H (1971) Ankylosis following thermal injury. J Periodont Res 6, 159–167.

Attalla MN (1968) Effect of beechwood creosote and chloramine on periapical tissue of dogs. J Can Dent Assoc 34, 190–195.

Azzi R, Kenney EB, Tsao TF and Carranza FA (1983) The effect of electrosurgery on alveolar bone. J Periodontol 54, 96–100.

Ballieux RE (1991) Impact of mental stress on the immune response. J Clin Periodontol 18, 427–430.

Baranowskyj GRT (1969) A histologic investigation of tissueresponse to an orthodontic intrusive force on a dog maxillary incisor with endodontic treatment and root resection. Am J Orthodont 56, 623–524.

Barbakow FH, Austin JC and Cleaton-Jones PE (1977) Experimental replantation of root-canal-filled and untreated teeth in the vervet monkey. J Endod 3, 89–93.

Barker BCW and Lockett BC (1972a) Reaction of dog tissue to immediate root filling with zinc oxide cement and gutta percha. Austr Dent J 17, 1–8.

Barker BCW and Lockett BC (1972b) Periapical response to N2 and other paraformaldehyde compounds confined within or extruded beyond the apices of dog root canals. Dent Practitr 22, 370–379.

Barker BCW and Lockett BC (1972c) Reaction of dog pulp and periapical tissue to two glucocorticosteroid preparations. Oral Surg 33, 249–262.

Bauer W (1923) The histology of the periapical region after amputation. Dent Cosmos 65, 1145.

Bauer WH (1946) The supporting tissues of the tooth in acute secondary agranulocytosis (arsphenamin neutropenia). J Dent Res 25, 501–508.

Becker GL, Cohen S and Borer R (1974) The sequelae of accidentally injecting sodium hypochlorite beyond the root apices. Oral Surg 38, 633–638.

Beertsen W (1987) Collagen phagocytosis by fibroblasts in the periodontal ligament of the mouse molar during the initial phase of hypofunction. J Dent Res 66, 1708–1712.

Beertsen W, Everts V, Niehof A and Bruins H. (1982) Loss of connective tissue attachment in the marginal periodontium of the mouse following blockage of eruption. J Periodont Res 17, 640–656.

Belting CM (1967) Prevalence of periodontal disease in hospitalized populations. J Periodontol 38, 302–309.

Benkel BH, Rising DW, Goldman LB, Rosen H, Goldman M and Kronman JH (1976) Use of hydrophilic plastic as a root canal filling material. J Endod 2, 196–202.

Bevelander G (1942) Tissue reactions in experimental tooth fracture. J Dent Res 21, 481–487.

Bhaskar SN and Orban B (1955) Experimental occlusal trauma. J Periodontol 26, 270–284.

Bhaskar SN and Rappoport HM (1971) Histologic evaluation of endodontic procedures in dogs. Oral Surg 31, 526–535.

Bien SM (1967) Difficulties and failures in tooth movement – biophysical responses to mechanotherapy. Trans Eur Orthod Soc 43, 55–67.

Binnie WH and Rowe AHR (1973) A histological study of the periapical tissues of incompletely formed pulpless teeth filled with calcium hydroxide. J Dent Res 52, 1110–1116.

Binnie WH and Rowe AHR (1974) The incidence of epithelial rests, proliferations and apical periodontal cysts following root canal treatment. Br Dent J 137, 56–60.

Blackwood HJJ (1959) Tissue repair in intra-alveolar root fractures. Oral Surg 12, 360–370.

Bordoni N and Erausquin J (1970) Periapical tissue reaction to root canal filling with a paste containing 7 per cent trioxymethylene. Oral Surg 29, 907–914.

Borring-Møller G and Frandsen A (1978) Autologous tooth transplantation to replace molars lost in patients with juvenile periodontitis. J Clin Periodontol 5, 152–158.

Brannström M, Nordenvall KJ and Hedström KG (1982) Periodontal tissue changes after intraligamentary anesthesia. J Dent Child 49, 417–423.

Budtz-Jørgensen E (1981) Occlusal dysfunction and stress. An experimental study in macaque monkeys. J Oral Rehabil 8, 1–9.

Burkland GA, Heeley JD and Irving JT (1976) A histological study of regeneration of the completely disrupted periodontal ligament in the rat. Arch Oral Biol 21, 349–354.

Caffesse RG, Nasjleti CE and Castelli WA (1977) Long term results after intentional tooth reimplantation in monkeys. Oral Surg 44, 666–678.

Castelli WA, Nasjleti CE, Caffesse RG and Diaz-Perez R (1980) Vascular response of the periodontal membrane after replantation of teeth. Oral Surg 50, 390–397.

Chase SW and Revesz J (1944) Re-establishment of transseptal fibres following extraction. J Dent Res 23, 333–336.

Citrome GP and Hever MA (1979) A comparative study of tooth apexification in the dog. J Endod 5, 290–297.

Claus EC and Orban B (1953) Fractured vital teeth. Oral Surg 6, 605–613.

Coolidge ED (1938) Traumatic and functional injuries occurring in the supporting tissues of human teeth. J Am Dent Assoc 25, 343–357.

Costich ER, Hoek RB and Hayward JR (1958) Replantation of molar teeth in the Syrian hamster. J Dent Res 37, 36.

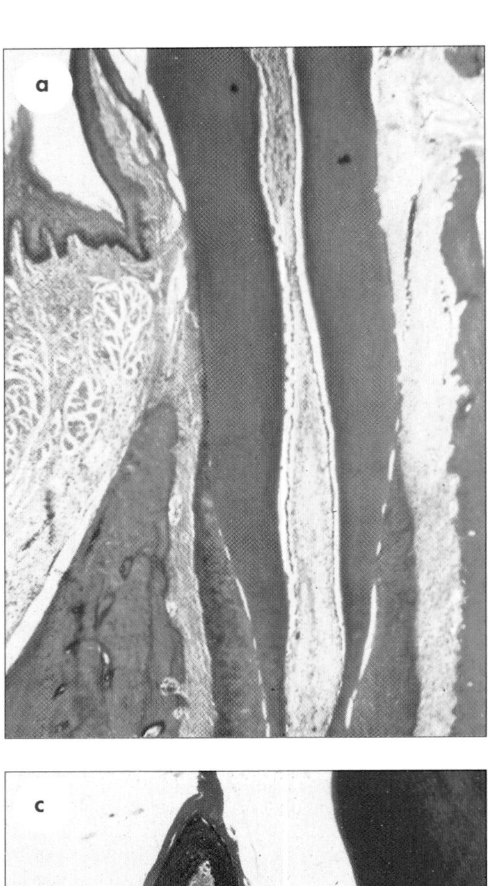

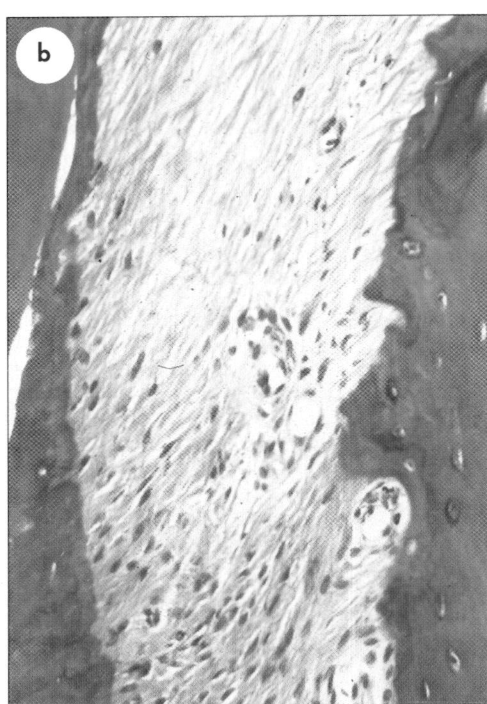

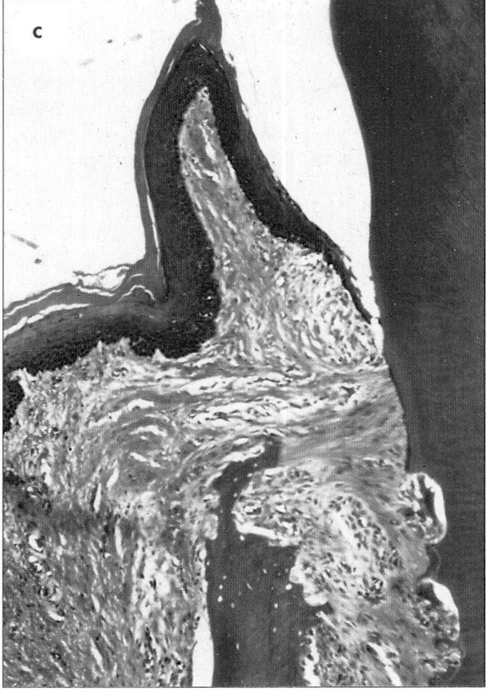

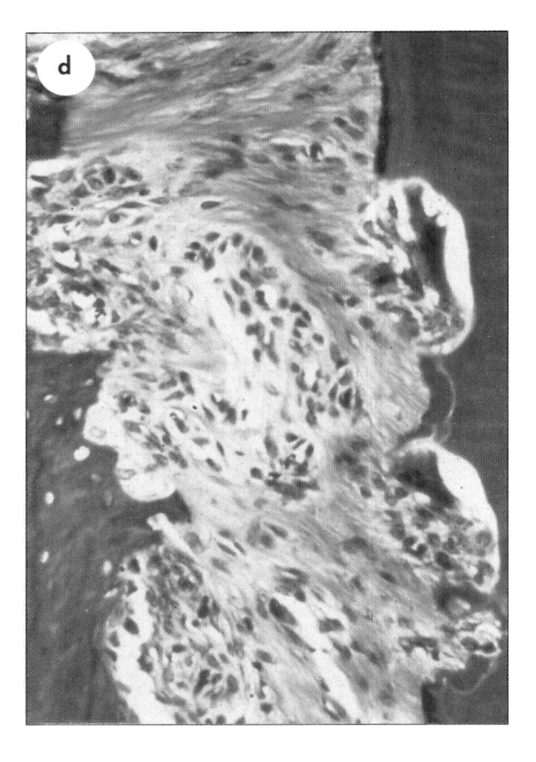

Fig. 15.12 Effect of cold on (rat) PDL. (a) 24 hours after freezing, cellularity has been lost in affected portion of the PDL (magnification × 75). (b) Same specimen as in (a), showing loss of cellularity and maintenance of functionally oriented ligament fibres (magnification × 75). (c) 14 days post-freezing, there is disorientation of the PDL and some root resorption (magnification × 25). (d) Higher magnification of area of PDL and root damage seen in (c) (H & E magnification × 75). (From Tal *et al.* 1991.)

Crumley PJ (1964) Collagen formation in the normal and stressed periodontium. Periodontics 2, 53–61.

Davis MS, Joseph SW and Buchner JF (1971) Periapical and intracanal healing following incomplete root canal fillings in dogs. Oral Surg 31, 662–675.

De Marco TJ (1976) Periodontal emotional stress syndrome. J Periodontol 47, 67–68.

Dreizen S, Levy BM and Bernick S (1971) Studies on the biology of the periodontium of marmosets. X. Cortisone induced periodontal and skeletal changes in adult cotton top marmosets. J Periodontol 42, 217–224.

Dreyer CJ and Blum L (1967) Effect of root fracture on the epithelial attachment. J Dent Assoc SA 22, 103–105.

Egelberg J (1965) Local effect of diet on plaque formation and development of gingivitis in dogs. I. Effects of hard and soft diets. Odont Rev 16, 31–41.

El Deeb ME and Andreasen JO (1991) Histometric study of the effect of occlusal alteration on periodontal tissue healing after surgical injury. Endod Dent Traumatol 7, 158–163.

Erausquin J (1970) Periapical tissue reaction to root canal fillings with zinc, titanium, lead, and aluminium oxides. Oral Surg 30, 545–554.

Erausquin J (1972) Periapical tissue response to the apical plug in root canal treatment. J Dent Res 51, 483–487.

Erausquin J and Devoto FCH (1970) Alveolodental ankylosis induced by root canal treatment in rat molars. Oral Surg 30, 105–116.

Erausquin J and Muruzábal M (1968) A tissue reaction to root canal cements in the rat molar. Oral Surg 26, 360–373.

Erausquin J and Muruzábal M (1969a) Tissue reaction to root canal fillings with absorbable pastes. Oral Surg 28, 567–578.

Erausquin J and Muruzábal M (1969b) Tissue reaction to root canal fillings with plastic cements. Oral Surg 29, 91–101.

Erausquin J, Muruzábal M, Devoto FCH and Rikles A (1966) Necrosis of the periodontal ligament in root canal overfillings. J Dent Res 45, 1084–1092.

Ericsson I and Lindhe J (1977) Lack of effect of trauma from occlusion on the recurrence of experimental periodontitis. J Clin Periodontol 4, 115–127.

Ericsson I and Lindhe J (1984) Lack of significance of increased tooth mobility on experimental periodontitis. J Periodontol 55, 447–452.

Ericsson I, Thilander B and Lindhe J (1978) Periodontal conditions after orthodontic tooth movements in the dog. Angle Orthodont 48, 210–218.

Ericsson I, Thilander B, Lindhe J and Okamoto H (1977) The effect of orthodontic tilting movements on the periodontal tissues of infected and non-infected dentitions in dogs. J Clin Periodontol 4, 278–293.

Ershoff BH, Bajwa GS, Shapiro M and Bernick S (1967) Comparative effects of a purified diet and natural food stock rations on the periodontium of mice exposed to multiple sublethal doses of total body X-irradiation. J Dent Res 46, 1051–1057.

Fleszar TJ, Knowles JW, Morrison EC, Burgett FG, Nissle RR and Ramfjord SP (1980) Tooth mobility and periodontal therapy. J Clin Periodontol 7, 495–505.

Fourel J and Mattout P (1989) Étude histologique de la cicatrisation parodontale de dents humaines déplacées chirurgicalement. J Parodontol 8, 281–288.

Frandsen AM (1962) Periodontal tissue changes induced in young rats by roentgen irradiation of the molar regions of the head. Acta Odont Scand 20, 393–410.

Frandsen AM (1963) Experimental investigations of socket healing and periodontal disease in rats. Effects of vitamin A deficiency. Acta Odont Scand 21 (suppl) 37.

Fronman S and Ratzkowski E (1966) Two cases of radiation damage to the growing dentition and their supporting structures in children. Dent Practit 16, 344–348.

Fukunaga K (1960) Healing of periapical tissues in human teeth after pulp extirpation and root canal filling. D Abs 5, 595.

Galili D, Kaufman E, Garfunkel AA and Michaeli Y (1984) Intraligamentary anesthesia – a histological study. Int J Oral Surg 13, 511–516.

Gianelly AA (1969) Force-induced changes in the vascularity of the periodontal ligament. Am J Orthodont 55, 5–11.

Glasser MM (1957) Acute periapical necrosis from arsenical pulp devitalizer. Oral Surg 10, 216–217.

Glickman I (1963) Inflammation and trauma from oclusion, codestructive factors in chronic inflammatory periodontal disease. J Periodontol 34, 5–10.

Glickman I and Smulow JB (1962) Alterations in the pathway of gingival inflammation into the underlying tissues induced by excessive occlusal forces. J Periodontol 33, 7–13.

Glickman I and Smulow JB (1965) Effect of excessive occlusal forces upon the pathway of gingival inflammation in humans. J Periodontol 36, 141–147.

Glickman I and Smulow JB (1967) Further observations on the effects of trauma from occlusion in humans. J Periodontol 38, 280–293.

Glickman I and Smulow JB (1968) Adaptive alterations in the periodontium of the rhesus monkey in chronic trauma from occlusion. J Periodontol 39, 101–105.

Glickman I and Smulow JB (1969) The combined effects of inflammation and trauma from occlusion in periodontitis. Int Dent J 19, 393–407.

Glickman I, Smulow JB, Vogel G and Passamonti G (1966) The effect of occlusal forces on healing following mucogingival surgery. J Periodontol 37, 319–325.

Glickman I and Weiss I (1955) Role of trauma from occlusion in initiation of periodontal pocket formation in experimental animals. J Periodontol 26, 14–20.

Gould TRL, Melcher AH and Brunette DM (1977) Location of progenitor cells in periodontal ligament stimulated by wounding. Anat Rec 188, 133–141.

Gould TRL, Melcher AH and Brunette DM (1980) Migration and division of progenitor cell populations in periodontal ligament after wounding. J Periodont Res 15, 20–42.

Hamamoto V, Nakajima T and Ozawa H (1989) Histological changes in periodontal tissues of rat molars following perforation of the pulp and its floor. J Oral Biol 31, 627–637.

Hammer H (1955) Replantation and implantation of teeth. Int Dent J 5, 439–457.

Hiatt WH (1959) Regeneration of the periodontium after endodontic therapy and flap operation. Oral Surg 12, 1471–1477.

Hoek RB, Costich ER and Hayward JR (1958) Homogenous transplantation of hamster second molars from young to adult animals. J Dent Res 37, 36.

Holland R, De Mello W, Nery MJ, Bernabe PFE and de Souza V (1977) Reaction of human periapical tissue to pulp extirpation and immediate root canal filling with calcium hydroxide. J Endod 3, 63–67.

Holland R, de Souza V, Tagliavini RL and Milanezi LA (1971) Healing process of teeth with open apices: histological study. Bull Tokyo Dent Coll 12, 333–338.

Hunter J (1778) The Natural History of the Human Teeth: Explaining their Structure, Use, Formation, Growth and Diseases, part I, pp 127–128, part II, pp 94–112, Johnson, London.

Hurst RVV (1972) Regeneration of periodontal and transseptal fibres after autografts in rhesus monkeys: a qualitative approach. J Dent Res 51, 1183–1192.

Johansen JR (1970) Incorporation of tritiated thymidine by the epithelial rests of Malassez after attempted extraction of rat molars. Acta Odont Scand 28, 463–470.

Johnson RB (1990) Effect of altered occlusal function on transseptal ligament and new bone thicknesses in the periodontium of the rat. Am J Anat 187, 91–97.

Karring T, Nyman S, Lindhe J and Sirirat M (1984) Potentials for root resorption during periodontal wound healing. J Clin Periodont 11, 41–52.

Kasman FG and Goldman M (1977) Tissue response to silicone rubber when used in a root canal filling. Oral Surg 43, 607–614.

Koivumaa KK and Lassila V (1971) Angiographical investigation of the influence of occlusal hyper- and hypofunction on the periodontium in rat. Suom Hammaslääk Toim 67, 102–122.

Kronfeld R (1931) Histologic study of the influence of function on the human periodontal membrane. J Am Dent Assoc 18, 1242–1274.

Kronfeld R (1936) A case of tooth fracture with special emphasis on tissue repair and adaptation following traumatic injury. J Dent Res 15, 429–446.

Kronman JH, Goldman M, Lin PS, Goldman LB and Kliment C (1977) Evaluation of intra-cytoplasmic particles in histiocytes after endodontic therapy with a hydrophilic plastic. J Dent Res 56. 795–801.

Kukidome K (1959) Histopathological study on healing of periapical tissues after infected root canal treatment of human teeth. D Abs 4, 44–45.

Kvinnsland I, Heyeraas KJ and Byers MR (1991) Regeneration of calcitonin gene-related peptide immunoreactive nerves in replanted rat molars and their supporting tissues. Arch Oral Biol 36, 815–826.

Lamers AC, van Mullem PJ and Simon M (1980) Tissue reactions to sodium hypochlorite and iodine potassium iodide under clinical conditions in monkey teeth. J Endod 6, 788–792.

Langeland K (1974) Root canal sealants and pastes. Dent Clin N Amer 18, 309–327.

Lantz B and Persson PA (1967) Periodontal tissue reactions after root perforations in dogs' teeth. A histologic study. Odont Tidskr 75, 209–220.

Lantz B and Persson PA (1970) Periodontal tissue reactions after surgical treatment of root perforations in dogs' teeth. Odont Revy 21, 51–62.

Leist M (1926) Experimentelle Untersuchungen über die Einwirkung der Röntgenstrahlen und des Radiums auf die zweite Dentition. Z Stomatol 24, 452–460.

Lengheden A, Blomlöf L and Lindskog S (1990a) Effect of immediate calcium hydroxide treatment and permanent root-filling on periodontal healing in contaminated replanted teeth. Scand J Dent Res 99, 139–146.

Lengheden A, Blomlöf L and Lindskog S (1990b) Effect of delayed calcium hydroxide treatment on periodontal healing in contaminated replanted teeth. Scand J Dent Res 99, 147–153.

Levy G and Mailland ML (1980) Étude quantitative des effets de l'hypofonction occlusale sur la largeur desmodontale et la résorption ostéoclastique alvéolaire chez le rat. J Biol Buccale 8, 17–31.

Lindhe J and Ericsson I (1976) The influence of trauma from occlusion on reduced but healthy periodontal tissues in dogs. J Clin Periodontol 3, 110–122.

Lindhe J and Svanberg G (1974) Influence of trauma from occlusion on progression of experimental periodontitis in the beagle dog. J Clin Periodontol 1, 3–14.

Lindskog S, Blomlöf L and Hammarström L (1983) Repair of periodontal tissues in vivo and in vitro. J Clin Periodontol 10, 188–205.

Lindskog S, Pierce AM, Blomlöf L and Hammarström L (1985) The role of the necrotic periodontal membrane in cementum resorption and ankylosis. Endod Dent Traumatol 1, 96–101.

Line SE, Polson AM and Zander HA (1974) Relationship between periodontal injury, selective cell repopulation and ankylosis. J Periodontol 45, 725–730.

Löe H and Waerhaug J (1961) Experimental replantation of teeth in dogs and monkeys. Arch Oral Biol 3, 176–184.

Loescher AR and Robinson PP (1991) Characteristics of periodontal mechanoreceptors supplying reimplanted canine teeth in cats. Arch Oral Biol 36, 33–40.

Loescher AR, Holland GR and Robinson PP (1993) The distribution and morphological characteristics of axons innervating the periodontal ligament of reimplanted teeth in cats. Arch Oral Biol 38, 813-822.

Lynch SE, Ruiz de Castilla G, *et al.* (1991) The effects of short-term application of a combination of platelet-derived and insulin-like growth factors on periodontal wound healing. J Periodontol 62, 458–467.

Macapanpan LC, Meyer J and Weinmann JP (1954) Mitotic activity of fibroblasts after damage to the periodontal membrane of rat molars. J Periodontol 25, 105–112.

Macapanpan LC and Weinmann JP (1954) The influence of injury to the periodontal membrane on the spread of gingival inflammation. J Dent Res 33, 263–272.

Mandel U and Viidik A (1989) Effect of splinting on the mechanical and histological properties of the healing periodontal ligament in the vervet monkey (*Cercopithecus aethiops*). Archs Oral Biol 34, 209–212.

Mayo J, Carranza FA, Epper CE and Cabrini RL (1962) The effect of total irradiation on the oral tissues of the Syrian hamster. Oral Surg 15, 739–745.

McCulloch CAG and Bordin S (1991) Role of fibroblast subpopulations in periodontal physiology and pathology. J Periodont Res 26, 144–154.

McKibben DH and Pechersky JL (1972) Effect of thermal stress on cell proliferation of the submandibular gland and periodontal ligament of CH^{3} male mice. Arch Oral Biol 17, 291–298.

Melcher AH (1967a) Wound repair in the periodontium of the rat incisor. Arch Oral Biol 12, 1645–1647.

Melcher AH (1967b) Remodelling of the periodontal ligament during eruption of the rat incisor. Arch Oral Biol 12, 1649–1651.

Mellars NW and Herms FW (1947) Investigations of neuropathologic manifestations of oral tissue. II. The psychosomatic background of certain oral manifestations. Am J Orthodont Oral Surg 33, 812–826.

Meyer I, Shklar G and Turner J (1962) A comparison of the effects of 200 kV radiation and cobalt-60 radiation on the jaws and dental structure of the white rat. A preliminary report. Oral Surg 15, 1098–1108.

Michanowicz AE, Michanowicz JP and Abou-Rass M (1971) Cementogenic repair of root fractures. J Am Dent Assoc 82, 569–579.

Miura F (1973) Effect of orthodontic force on blood circulation in periodontal membrane. Transactions of the Third International Orthodontic Congress, London, p 21.

Morris ML (1953) The reattachment of human periodontal tissues following surgical detachment: a clinical and histological study. J Periodontol 24, 270–278.

Morris ML (1957) Healing of human periodontal tissues following surgical detachment from non-vital teeth. J Periodontol 28, 222–238.

Moyers RE (1950) The periodontal membrane in orthodontics. J Am Dent Assoc 40, 22–27.

Mühlemann HR and Herzog H (1961) Tooth mobility and microscopic tissue changes produced by experimental occlusal trauma. Helv Odont Acta 5, 33–39.

Muruzábal M and Erausquin J (1966) Response of periapical tissues in the rat molar to root canal fillings with Diaket and AH-26. Oral Surg 21, 786–804.

Muruzábal M, Erausquin J and Devoto FCH (1966) A study of periapical overfilling in root canal treatment in the molar of rat. Arch Oral Biol 11, 373–383.

Nascimento A and Sallum AW (1975) Periodontal changes in distant teeth due to trauma from occlusion. J Periodont Res 10, 44–48.

Nasjleti CE, Castelli WA and Blankenship JR (1975) The storage of teeth before reimplantation in monkeys. Oral Surg 39, 20–29.

Nasjleti CE, Castelli WA and Caffesse RG (1977) Effects of amalgam restorations on the periodontal membrane in monkeys. J Dent Res 56, 1127–1131.

Nasjleti CE, Castelli WA and Keller BE (1972) Effects of acrylic restorations on the periodontium of monkeys. J Dent Res 51, 1382–1387.

Neukam FW, Reumann K and Schliephake H (1987) Experimental studies on the assessment of periodontal ligament injuries. Dtsch Zahnarzt Z 42, 186–189.

Newman HN (1974) Diet, attrition, plaque and dental disease. Br Dent J 136, 491–497.

Nojima N, Kobayashi M, Shionome M, Takahashi N, Suda T and Hasegawa K (1990) Fibroblastic cells derived from bovine PDL have the phenotypes of osteoblasts. J Periodont Res 25, 179–185.

Nordenram A, Bang G and Anneroth G (1973) A histopathologic study of replanted teeth with superficially demineralised root surfaces in Java monkeys. Scand J Dent Res 81, 294–302.

Nyman S, Karring T, Lindhe J and Plantén S (1980) Healing following implantation of periodontitis-affected roots into gingival connective tissue. J Clin Periodontol 7, 394–401.

Nyman S, Lindhe J and Ericsson I (1979) The effect of progressive tooth mobility on destructive periodontitis in the dog. J Clin Periodontol 5, 213–215.

Ogle RE and Ciancio SG (1971) The effect of anti-cholinergic agents on the periodontium. J Periodontol 42, 280–282.

Palcanis KG (1973) Effect of occlusal trauma on interstitial pressure in the periodontal ligament. J Dent Res 52, 903–910.

Paterson RC and Pountney SK (1987a) The response of the dental pulp to mechanical exposure in gnotobiotic rats mono-infected with a strain of Streptococcus mutans. Int Endod J 20, 159–168.

Paterson RC and Pountney SK (1987b) Pulp response to and cariogenicity of Lactobacillus casei in monoinfected gnotobiotic rats. Oral Surg 64, 611–624.

Paterson RC and Watts A (1987) Further studies on the exposed germ-free dental pulp. Int Endod J 20, 112–121.

Paterson RC and Watts A (1992) Pulp responses to two strains of bacteria isolated from human carious dentine *L. plantarum* (NCTC 1406) and *S. mutans* (NCTC 10919). Int Endod J 25, 134–141.

Penick EC (1961) Periapical repair by dense fibrous connective tissue following conservative endodontic therapy. Oral Surg 14, 239–242.

Picton DCA (1976) Experimental evidence on the role of abnormal contacts in the aetiology of periodontal disease. In: Mastication (Anderson DJ and B Matthews B, eds), pp 251–258, Wright, Bristol.

Pierce CJ and Gale EN (1988) A comparison of different treatments for nocturnal bruxism. J Dent Res 67, 597–601.

Pietrokovski J (1967) Extraction wound healing after tooth fracture in rats. J Dent Res 46, 233–240.

Pihlstrom BL, Anderson KA, Aeppli D and Schaffer EM (1986) Association between signs of trauma from occlusion and periodontitis. J Periodontol 57, 1–6.

Pindborg JJ (1955) Clinical, radiographic and histological aspects of intra-alveolar fractures of upper central incisors. Acta Odont Scand 13, 41–71.

Polson AM (1974) Trauma and progression of marginal periodontitis in squirrel monkeys. II. Mechanical. J Periodont Res 9, 108–113.

Polson AM (1977) Interactions between periodontal trauma and marginal periodontitis. Int Dent J 27, 107–113.

Polson AM, Meitner SW and Zander HA (1976a) Trauma and progression of marginal periodontitis in squirrel monkeys. III. Adaptation to repetitive injury. J Periodont Res 11, 279–289.

Polson AM, Meitner SW and Zander HA (1976b) Trauma and progression of marginal periodontitis in squirrel monkeys. IV. Trauma and inflammation. J Periodont Res 11, 290–298.

Posselt U and Maunsbach O (1957) Clinical and roentgenographic studies of trauma from occlusion. J Periodontol 28, 192–196.

Roahen JO and Marshall FJ (1990) The effects of periodontal ligament injection on pulpal and periodontal tissues. J Endod 16, 28–33.

Rosenthal M (1937) Experimental radium poisoning. II. Changes in teeth of rabbits produced by oral administration of radium sulphate. Am J Med Sci 193, 495–501.

Rowe AHR (1967) Effect of root filling materials on the periapical tissues. Br Dent J 122, 98–102.

Rud J and Andreasen JO (1972) Operative procedures in periapical surgery with contemporaneous root filling. Int J Oral Surg 1, 297–310.

Rugh JD, Jacobs DT, Taverna RD and Johnson RW (1984) Psychophysiological changes and oral conditions. In: Social Sciences and Dentistry. A Critical Bibliography. II (Cohen LK and Bryant PS, eds), pp 19–83, Quintessence, London.

Sauk JJ, Norris K, Foster R, Moehring J and Somerman MJ (1988) Expression of heat stress proteins by human periodontal ligament cells. J Oral Pathol 17, 496–498.

Schliephake H and Neukam FW (1990) Influence of root development and root anatomy on the occurrence of periodontal damage during removal of third molars for transplantation. A histometric study. J Oral Maxillofac Surg 48, 601–605.

Schwartz O, Frederiksen K and Klausen B (1987) Allotransplantation of human teeth. A retrospective study of 75 transplantations over a period of 28 years. Int J Oral Maxillofac Surg 16, 285–301.

Seltzer S, Green DB, de la Guardia R, Maggio J and Barnett A (1973) Vitallium endodontic implants: a scanning electron microscope, electron microprobe and histologic study. Oral Surg 35, 828–860.

Seltzer S, Maggio J, Wollard RR, Brough SO and Barnett A (1976) Tissue reactions to polycarboxylate cements. J Endod 2, 208–214.

Seltzer S, Sinai I and August D (1970) Periodontal effects of root perforations before and during endodontic procedures. J Dent Res 49, 332–339.

Seltzer S, Soltanoff W, Sinai I, Goldenberg A and Bender IB (1968) Biological aspects of endodontics. III. Periapical tissue reactions to root canal instrumentation. Oral Surg 26, 534–546.

Seltzer S, Soltanoff W, Sinai I and Smith J (1969) Biological aspects of endodontics. IV. Periapical tissue reactions to root-filled teeth whose canals had been instrumented short of their apices. Oral Surg 28, 724–738.

Selvig KA, Bjorvatn K and Claffey N (1990) Effect of stannous fluoride and tetracycline on repair after delayed replantation of root-planed teeth in dogs. Acta Odont Scand 48, 107–112.

Shapiro M, Brat V and Ershoff BH (1960) Periodontal changes following multiple sublethal doses of X-irradiation in the mouse. J Dent Res 39, 668.

Shaw JH (1973) Relation of arsenic supplements to dental caries and the periodontal syndrome in experimental rodents. J Dent Res 52, 494–497.

Shefter GJ and McFall WT (1984) Occlusal relations and periodontal status in human adults. J Periodontol 55, 368–374.

Sherman P (1968) Intentional replantation of teeth in dogs and monkeys. J Dent Res 47, 1066–1071.

Shklar G (1966) Periodontal disease in experimental animals subjected to chronic cold stress. J Periodontol 37, 377–383.

Shklar G and Glickman I (1959) The effect of cold as a stressor agent upon the periodontium of albino rats. Oral Surg 12, 1311–1320.

Shore RC, Moxham BJ and Berkovitz BKB (1982) A quantitative comparison of the ultrastructure of the PDL of impeded and unimpeded rat incisors. Arch Oral Biol 27, 423–430.

Shore RC, Berkovitz BKB and Moxham BJ (1985) The effects of preventing movement of the rat incisor on the structure of the periodontal ligament. Arch Oral Biol 30, 221–228.

Simons JHS, Jensen JL and Kimura JT (1975) Histologic observations of endodontically treated replanted roots. J Endod 1, 178–180.

Singer J, Furstman L and Bernick S (1967) A histologic study of the effect of fluoride on tooth movement in the rat. Am J Orthodont 53, 296–308.

Sippy BO (1927) Regeneration of tissues following experimentalinjury of the tooth roots. Dent Cosmos 69, 771–780.

Sippy BO (1928) Regeneration of bone, peridental membrane, and cementum, following experimental injury in dogs. J Dent Res 8, 9.

Söder PØ, Oterskog P, Andreasen JO and Modéer T (1977) effect of drying on viability of periodontal membrane. Scand J Dent Res 95, 164–168.

Solt CW and Glickman I (1968) A histologic and radiographic study of healing following wedging interdental injury in mice. J Periodontol 39, 249–254.

Stahl SS (1960) Response of the periodontium, pulp and salivary glands to gingival and tooth injury in young adult male rats. I. Periodontal tissues. II. Pulp and periapical tissues. Oral Surg 13, 613–626, 734–742.

Stahl SS, Miller SC and Goldsmith ED (1958) The influence of occlusal trauma and protein deprivation on the response of periapical tissues following pulpal exposures in rats. Oral Surg 11, 536–540.

Stahl SS, Tonna EA and Weiss R (1969) Autoradiographic evaluation of periapical responses to pulpal injury. II. Mature rats. Oral Surg 29, 270–274.

Strömberg T (1971) The apical blood vessel topography, with special reference to pulpectomy. A microangiographic and histologic study in dogs. Odont Revy 22, 163–177.

Strömberg T (1972) The effect of pulpectomy and root canal filling in the same treatment, with special reference to local prednisolone therapy. A microangiographic and histologic study in dogs. Odont Revy 23, 221–230.

Svanberg G (1974) Influence of trauma from occlusion on the periodontium of dogs with normal or inflamed gingivae. Odont Revy 25, 165–178.

Svanberg G and Lindhe J (1973) Experimental hyper-tooth-mobility in the dog. Odont Revy 24, 269–282.

Svanberg G and Lindhe J (1974) Vascular reactions in the periodontal ligament incident to trauma from occlusion. J Clin Periodontol 1, 58–67.

Tal H, Kozlovsky A and Pitaru S (1991) Healing of sites within the dog periodontal ligament after application of cold to the periodontal attachment apparatus. J Clin Periodontol 18, 543–547.

Tal H and Stahl SS (1986) Periodontal attachment responses to surgical injury in the cat. Removal of buccal bone with and without placement of foreign body at ligament periphery. J Clin Periodontol 13, 45–51.

Taylor R, Shklar G and Roeber F (1965) The effects of laser radiation on teeth, dental pulp and oral mucosa of experimental animals. Oral Surg 19, 786–795.

Tonna EA and Stahl SS (1967) A polarized light microscopic study of rat periodontal ligament following surgical and chemical gingival trauma. Helv Odont Acta 11, 90–105.

Torneck CS and Smith J (1970) Biologic effects of endodontic procedures on developing incisor teeth. I. Effect of partial and total pulp removal. Oral Surg 30, 258–266.

Wade GW (1969) Pulpal and periapical tissue response to butyl 2-cyanoacrylate. Oral Surg 28, 226–234.

Waerhaug J (1979) The angular bone defect and its relationship to trauma from occlusion and downgrowth of subgingival plaque. J Clin Periodont 6, 61–82.

Waerhaug J and Hansen ER (1966) Periodontal changes incident to prolonged occlusal overload in monkeys. Acta Odont Scand 24, 91–105.

Waldo C and Rothblatt JM (1954) Histologic response to tooth movement in the laboratory rat. J Dent Res 33, 481–486.

Walker TW, Ng GC and Burke PS (1978) Fluid pressures in the periodontal ligament of the mandibular canine tooth in dogs. Arch Oral Biol 23, 753–765.

Watts A and Paterson RC (1988) The response of the mechanically exposed pulp to prednisolone and triamcinolone acetonide. Int Endod J 21, 9–16.

Watts A and Paterson RC (1990) Detection of bacteria in histologic sections of the dental pulp. Int Endod J 23, 1–12.

Watts A and Paterson RC (1992) Pulp response to, and cariogenicity of, a further strain of Streptococcus mutans (NCTC 10832). Int Endod J 25, 142–149.

Watts A and Paterson RC (1993) Atypical apical lesions detected during a study of short-term tissue responses to three different endodontic instrumentation techniques. Endod Dent Traumatol 9, 200–210.

Wentz FM, Jarabak J and Orban B (1958) Experimental occlusaltrauma imitating cuspal interferences. J Periodontol 29, 117–127.

Winter GB and Kramer IRH (1965) Changes in periodontal membrane and bone following experimental injury in deciduous molar teeth in kittens. Arch Oral Biol 10, 279–289.

Yoshida M (1976) An experimental study on regeneration of cementum, periodontal ligament and alveolar bone in the intradentinal cavities in dogs. Shikwa Gakuho 76, 1197–1222.

Zach L, Cohen G, Scopp I and Kaplan G (1973) Experimental radioosteonecrosis in rhesus macaque jaws; therapeutic irradiation dose effect on dental extraction wound healing. Am J Phys Anthropol 38, 325–330.

Zerosi C (1938) Experimentelle Untersuchungen über die histologischen Reaktionen und Veränderungen, weiche durch Röntgen- und Radiumsbestrahlungen in dentalen und periodontalen Gewebe verursacht werden. Zahnarztl Rdsch 47, 265–272.

Zerosi C (1940) Experimentelle Forschungen über die histologischen Reaktionen und Veränderungen der dentalen und periodontalen Gewebe infolge von Roentgen- und Radiumbestrahlung. Z Stomatol 38, 278–304, 322–339.

Chapter 16
Periodontal Ligament Healing

Sven Lindskog, Leif Blomlöf

INTRODUCTION

The periodontium consists of a complex mixture of mineralized and non-mineralized tissues derived from the ectoderm and mesoderm (*Fig. 16.1*). It develops as a single phylogenetic unit (Ten Cate *et al.*, 1971; Yoshikawa and Kollar, 1981; Palmer and Lumsden, 1987; Lumsden, 1988; MacNeil and Thomas, 1993), a fact that is reflected in periodontal healing mechanisms. Although the role of vascular and nervous components in periodontal healing should not be underestimated, currently the emphasis appears to be on six other cell phenotypes: periodontal fibroblasts, gingival fibroblasts, cementoblasts, osteoblasts, junctional epithelial cells, and the epithelial cell rests of Malassez (for review, see Ben-Yehuda *et al.*, 1989; McCulloch and Bordin, 1991). The expression of any of these phenotypes yields widely different healing results, ranging from complete regeneration to formation of scar tissues (Lindskog and Blomlöf, 1992). The latter include pathological pockets (Blomlöf *et al.*, 1988a,b; Lindskog *et al.*, 1993) and long epithelial junctions (Moskow 1964; Kon *et al.*, 1969; Caton and Nyman, 1980; Caton *et al.*, 1980; Proye and Polson, 1982; Blomlöf *et al.*, 1988a,b; Lindskog *et al.*, 1993). Repair with connective tissue attachments in capsule-like arrangements (Lindskog *et al.*, 1983a, Lengheden *et al.*, 1991a,b; Lindskog *et al.*, 1993; Blomlöf and Lindskog, 1994) in combination with various mineralized tissues apposed to the root surfaces (Karring *et al.*, 1984; Bogle *et al.*, 1985; Egelberg, 1987; Lindskog and Blomlöf, 1992) appears to fall somewhere in between scar tissue formation and regeneration. At present, no clear correlations between the type of therapy and the subsequent healing reaction have been established. Additional factors, such as the patient's susceptibility to periodontal disease, degree of marginal inflammation, age, systemic illness etc, also appear to influence the outcome (for review, see Seymour and Heasman, 1992). Consequently, a wide range of prognoses can be expected, all of which are determined by the resistance of the healing tissues to the sequelae of reinfection (Lindskog *et al.*, 1993), which is the single most important factor in recurrence of periodontal pathology (Nyman *et al.*, 1977; Berg *et al.*, 1990, Ehnevid *et al.*, 1994).

This review discusses periodontal healing from the perspective of phylogenetic derivation of the healing tissues, with only limited reference to therapy-related, host-specific, and specific disease-related factors.

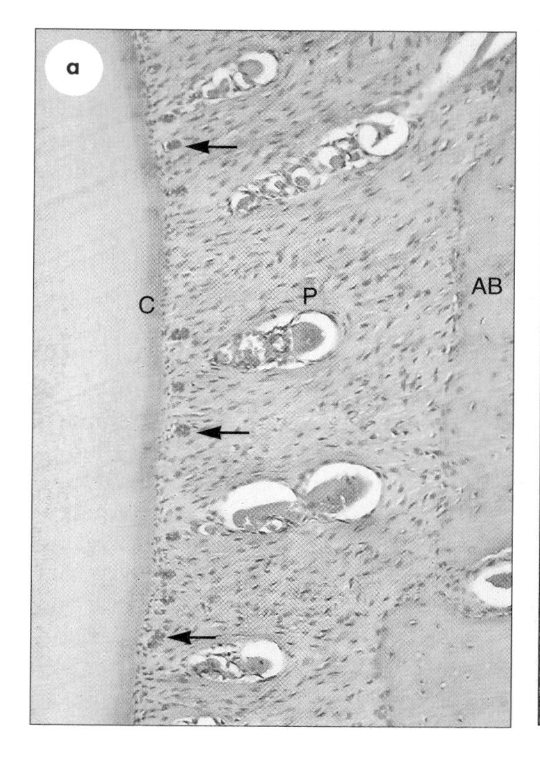

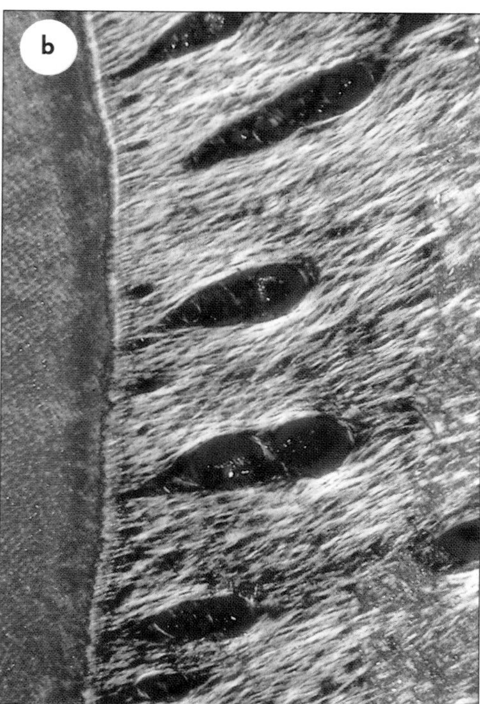

Fig. 16.1 Normal periodontium in a transversal section stained with haematoxylin and eosin from a monkey incisor (*Macaca fascicularis*) in ordinary transmitted (a) and polarized (b) light. The periodontium consists of a complex mixture of mineralized and non-mineralized tissues derived from the ectoderm (epithelial rests of Malassez – arrows) and mesoderm (cementum – C, periodontal ligament – P, alveolar bone – AB. Note the palisade-like pattern of extrinsic fibres (Sharpey fibres) in both cementum and alveolar bone and the functionally oriented periodontal fibres (a). (Magnification × 200.)

PERIODONTAL LIGAMENT HEALING

Initially, healing of wounds in the periodontal ligament (PDL) does not differ from the healing of other types of connective tissue wounds. It begins with the formation of granulation tissue subsequent to necrosis and blood clot formation, regardless of the type of periodontal challenge. Organization of the granulation tissue follows, during which a new vascular and nervous supply is re-established (Parlange and Sims, 1993). The PDL connective tissue also forms again; this includes fibroblasts and collagenous fibres (Melcher, 1970, 1976; Line *et al.*, 1974; Caton and Nyman, 1980; Caton *et al.*, 1980; Nyman *et al.*, 1982; Harrison and Jurosky, 1991; Wikesjö *et al.*, 1992). The junctional epithelium (Taylor and Cambell, 1972; Wirthlin *et al.*, 1980), and the epithelial rests of Malassez (Spouge, 1980; Brice *et al.*, 1991).

Provided that it is not infected, the marginal junctional epithelium undergoes only limited proliferation in a marginal periodontal wound (Hammarström *et al.*, 1986, Berg *et al.*, 1990). The epithelial cuff down to the cementoenamel junction is re-established within 1–2 weeks of invasive therapy (Moskow, 1964; Kon *et al.*, 1969; Taylor and Cambell, 1972; Wirthlin *et al.*, 1980; Proye and Polson, 1982), during which pocket and junctional epithelium phenotypes are re-established (Salonen *et al.*, 1989). The limited proliferation of the marginal epithelium may be explained by the presence of substances in cementum, such as sialoprotein-II and at least four other fibroblast-attachment proteins, which have been shown not to support epithelial cell attachment (Olson *et al.*, 1991). Further, a direct contact inhibition between PDL fibroblasts and marginal epithelial cells has been proposed (Pitaru *et al.*, 1991). However, if the marginal wound is infected, the accompanying inflammatory reaction appears to stimulate epithelial proliferation in a cyst-like manner, encompassing foci of necrosis and granulation tissue found in the infected areas (Berg *et al.*, 1990). In this respect, the behaviour of the epithelium is similar to that found in periapical and juxtaradicular cyst formation after pulpal infection, where the epithelial cell rests of Malassez proliferate (Jansson *et al.*, 1993a). Hence, the marginal epithelium in an infected marginal wound does *not* initially grow down along the dentine surface. It assumes this position at a later stage when the encapsulated necrotic areas have been incorporated into the periodontal pocket (Berg *et al.*, 1990).

According to current opinion, repopulation of the PDL space can be principally attributed to gingival and PDL mesenchymal phenotypes (Nyman *et al.*, 1982; McCulloch and Bordin, 1991), although an endosteal contribution from neighbouring marrow spaces should not be overlooked (Hammarström *et al.*, 1989). These different mesenchymal phenotypes have been characterized to only a limited extent *in vivo*, and most studies have been performed *in vitro* (Brunette *et al.*, 1976, 1977; Marmary *et al.*, 1976; Blomlöf and Otteskog, 1981; Piche *et al.*; 1989; Arceo *et al.*, 1991). Nevertheless, it appears that a centrally located pool of undifferentiated (ecto)mesenchymal cells in the PDL will start to proliferate when challenged (McCulloch *et al.*, 1989). Although not conclusively shown, it has been suggested that these cells are able to differentiate into PDL fibroblasts, cementoblasts, or osteoblasts (for review, see McCulloch and Bordin, 1991; McCulloch, 1993; see also Chapter 1). Healing in the PDL space may also receive contributions from the gingival connective tissue, as recently highlighted by the working principle of Guided Tissue Regeneration (Nyman *et al.*, 1982; Gottlow *et al.*, 1984). As a consequence, the resulting healing tissue varies widely, from a completely regenerated functional PDL following surface resorption (*Fig. 16.2*) incident to orthodontic tooth movement (for review, see Hammarström and Lindskog, 1992; see also Chapter 11) to the non-functional capsular arrangements seen on instrumented (mechanically denuded) root surfaces (*Figs 16.3, 16.4*) (Lindskog *et al.*, 1983a; Lindskog and Blomlöf, 1992; Blomlöf and Lindskog, 1994).

Many vital functions of the regenerating PDL cells are influenced by the substratum they settle upon (Uitto and Larjava, 1991) and, conversely, spreading of these cells on a substratum is vital in order for them to express vital healing functions (Lindskog *et al.*, 1987; Ingber and Folkman, 1989). The PDL, like other connective tissues, consists of a water-soluble matrix of proteins and polysaccharides–proteoglycans, which are predominantly collagen coated with charged glycosaminoglycans (for review, see Bartold, 1987, 1991). The glycosaminoglycans (see Chapter 4) are decisive in determining the phenotype of differentiating mesenchymal cells, as reflected in cell morphology, cell communication, and expression of surface attachment proteins (Ruoslahti, 1989). In addition, glycosaminoglycans modulate cell interaction with growth factors (for review, see Gallagher, 1989). Extrapolated to the periodontium, it has been argued that among periodontal (McCulloch and Bordin, 1991; Uitto and Larjava, 1991) and gingival–periodontal granulation tissue fibroblasts (Häkkinen and Larjava, 1992) there exist several different clones. Although this basic knowledge may yield a better understanding of PDL healing, it currently appears to be only of limited therapeutic value. Nevertheless, application to PDL wounds of bone-related growth factors (for review, see Mohran and Baylink, 1991; Finkelman, 1992) such as insulin-like growth factors (IGF-I and IGF-II), platelet-derived growth factor (PDGF), transforming growth factor-β (TGF-β) and bone morphogenetic protein (BMP) have indicated that PDL wound healing may be enhanced and even influenced towards regeneration (for review, see Caffesse and Quiñones, 1993). Of these growth factors, those that are known to promote mineralized tissue-formation (PDGF and TGF) (for review, see Mohran and Baylink, 1991) and cell division and collagen production in general (IGF-I and IGF-II) (Cook *et al.*, 1988; Tavakkol *et al.*, 1992; Kratz *et al.*, 1992; Gillery, 1992) have attracted special attention (Lynch *et al.*, 1991) (see also Chapter 12). However, the influence of the substratum (the dentine collagenous matrix and hydroxyapatite, the fibrin–fibronectin clot, etc) on the healing cells appears to be of even greater importance to PDL healing at the root surface, where it involves proliferation and differentiation not only of PDL fibroblasts but also of cementoblasts and, consequently, formation of mineralized tissue.

PDL healing and the expression of different PDL mesenchymal phenotypes is intimately associated with formation of mineralized tissues, either associated with the root surface or with the alveolar bone (Lindskog and Blomlöf, 1992). In this respect, the PDL shares not only morphological similarities with the periosteum, with which it interlaces at the alveolar crest, but also functional similarities such as a capacity to form mineralized tissue, as evidenced by its intense activity of non-specific alkaline phosphatases (NSAP) (Lilja *et al.*, 1984; Arceo *et al.*, 1991; Lindskog and Blomlöf, 1994) (*Fig. 16.5*). Interestingly, such activity is not detectable in the gingival connective tissue (see *Fig. 16.5*), despite the fact that it is virtually impossible to distinguish morphologically between PDL and gingival connective tissue.

ALVEOLAR BONE HEALING

For a long time it has been accepted that the PDL possesses an osteogenic capacity (Melcher, 1976; Nyman and Karring, 1979; Andreasen, 1980; Lilja *et al.*, 1984; Lindskog *et al.*, 1993; Lindskog and Blomlöf, 1992, 1994). Selective experimental removal of the alveolar bone will provoke regeneration of the lost bone (see *Fig. 16.6*) by the remaining root-associated PDL (Helldén, 1972; Nyman and Karring, 1979; Andreasen, 1980; Lindskog *et al.*, 1993; Lindskog and Blomlöf, 1994), which is derived from the dental follicle, the tissue that forms the alveolar bone during tooth development (see Chapter 8). In a clinical situation, regeneration of bone is, however, dependent on a number of modifying factors, such as the degree of marginal or endodontic infection and subsequent periodontal inflammation (Berg *et al.*, 1990; Blomlöf *et al.*, 1988b, 1989, 1992; Ehnevid *et al.*, 1993a, 1994; Jansson *et al.*, 1993b), as the trauma from the surgical procedure affects the quality of the remaining PDL and flap adaptation (Nyman and Karring, 1979; Wikesjö and Nilvéus, 1990). Thus, provided enough PDL tissue remains and can be encouraged to re-populate a damaged area, alveolar bone re-formation follows. Nevertheless, in clinical practice, marginal bone regeneration is not a regular finding after conventional periodontal therapy.

Under favourable conditions, PDL healing in angular osseous defects may result in clinical attachment gain and radiographic bone fill. These features, which can be evident radiographically or detected clinically during re-entry procedures (Polson and Heijl, 1978), have been taken as a sign of new attachment (for review, see Nyman *et al.*, 1989). However, experimental studies in monkeys have shown that the tissue between the newly formed alveolar bone and the root surface usually consists not only of connective tissue but also of an epithelial lining along the root surface (Caton and Nyman, 1980; Caton *et al.*, 1980). In the light of recent experimental studies, it appears likely that the connective tissue that has recolonized the root surfaces is of gingival origin (Lindskog and Blomlöf, 1994), and that the epithelium is stimulated to proliferate into the connective tissue by marginal infection (*Fig. 16.7*) (Berg *et al.*, 1990; Lindskog *et al.*, 1993). It can thus be argued that radiographically recorded bone regeneration, when it occurs following conventional periodontal therapy, is not of PDL origin but rather stems from endosteal growth from pre-existing alveolar bone.

ROOT SURFACE HEALING

New attachment (with reparative cementum, new PDL fibres, and new alveolar bone) is only occasionally found after flap surgery, and then only under certain favourable circumstances, such as in conjunction with Guided Tissue Regeneration (Nyman *et al.*, 1982; Gottlow *et al.*, 1984), implantation of freeze-dried decalcified bone (Bowers *et al.*, 1989a,b), and experimental chemical conditioning of the cementum surface (Blomlöf *et al.*, 1987, 1989; Ehnevid *et al.*, 1993b). A key factor appears to be marginal infection, as stated by Middleton and Bowers (1990): '[reparative cementum formation] will occur with equal frequency over cementum and dentine when the oral environment is excluded'. However, mineralized tissue formation on denuded root surfaces is not only a sequela to periodontal therapy, but also a near-universal finding following injuries to the dentoalveolar complex. In this context, a unified nomenclature is lacking, and all deposits of mineralized tissue on root surfaces that are not attached to alveolar bone have been regarded as reparative cementum or even regeneration of original cementum. Consequently, doubts have been expressed as to whether all newly formed mineralized tissue deposits on root surfaces should be regarded as reparative cementum and as to what criteria should be applied to define new cementum (Karring *et al.*, 1984; Bogle *et al.*, 1985; Egelberg, 1987; Lindskog and Blomlöf, 1992, 1994; Blomlöf and Lindskog, 1994).

Formation of cementum plays a key role in periodontal healing, since it serves to attach the root to the PDL, involving both PDL fibroblasts forming extrinsic collagenous fibres (Sharpey fibres) and cementoblasts forming intrinsic collagenous fibres (Schroeder, 1986). The success of PDL healing can thus be determined by the presence of (reparative or new) cementum, since it is exclusively formed by cells from the PDL (Schroeder, 1986). Consequently, accurate markers to identify dental cementum appear imperative for assessing PDL healing (MacNeil and Sommerman, 1993). This was emphasized in 1987 by Egelberg in a review article: 'Thus, different types of cementum-like deposits may form on the root surface depending upon the available conditions during healing. It is possible that only cementum formed by cementoblasts originating from the PDL can serve as a lasting attachment. Other cementum-like deposits may be subjected to subsequent resorption, exposing root dentine to resorption as well. The possibility of cementum-like deposits of various genesis needs to be investigated.' The fact that, during healing of instrumented root surfaces, reparative cementum may be seen temporarily bridging over to the alveolar bone (Andreasen

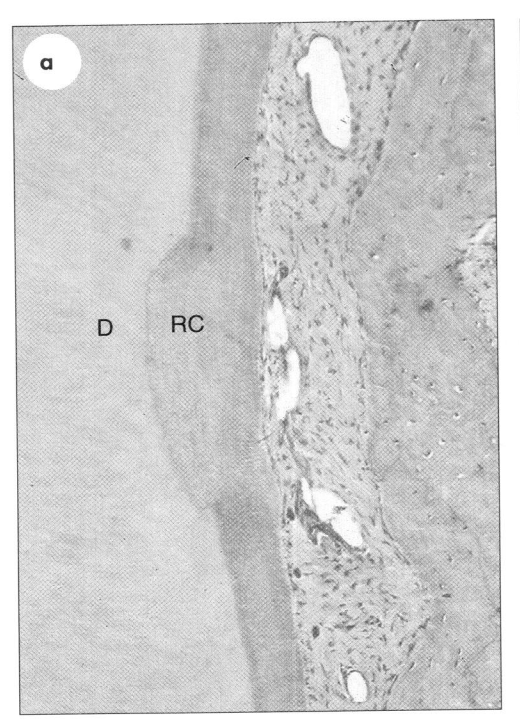

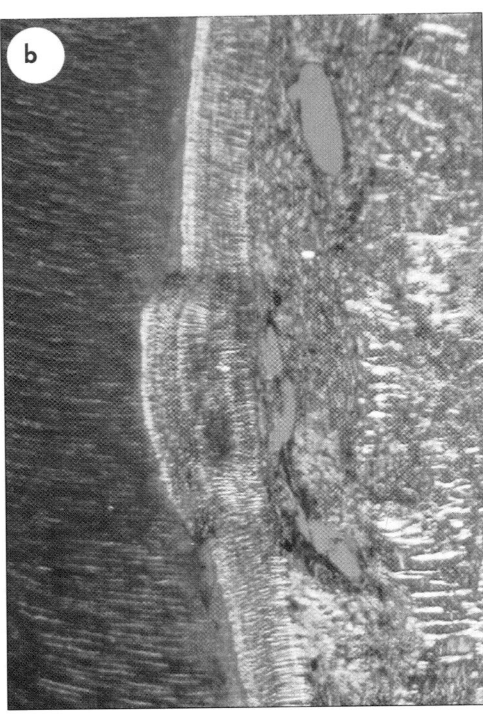

Fig. 16.2 Healed surface resorption in a transversal section stained with haematoxylin and eosin from a traumatically injured monkey incisor (*Macaca fascicularis*) in ordinary transmitted (a) and polarized (b) light. The resorbed root surface is covered by a layer of reparative cementum (RC) adheing to the dentine (D). In polarized light, the extrinsic fibres (Sharpey's fibres) of the reparative cementum display an orientation essentially perpendicular to the root surface similar to that of the surrounding original cementum (b). (H & E magnification × 250.)

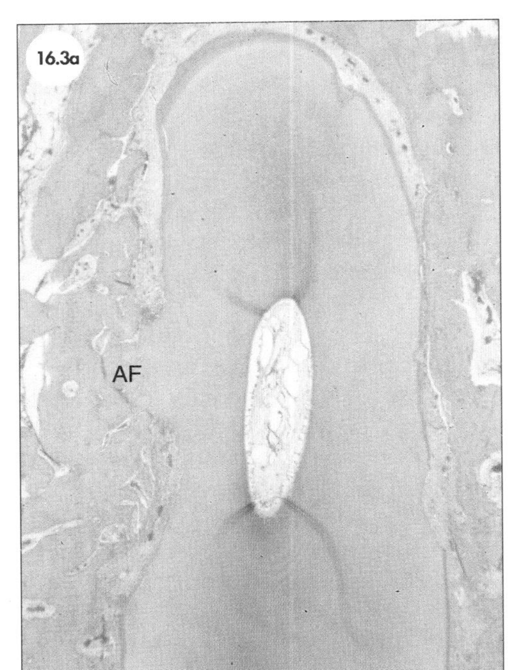

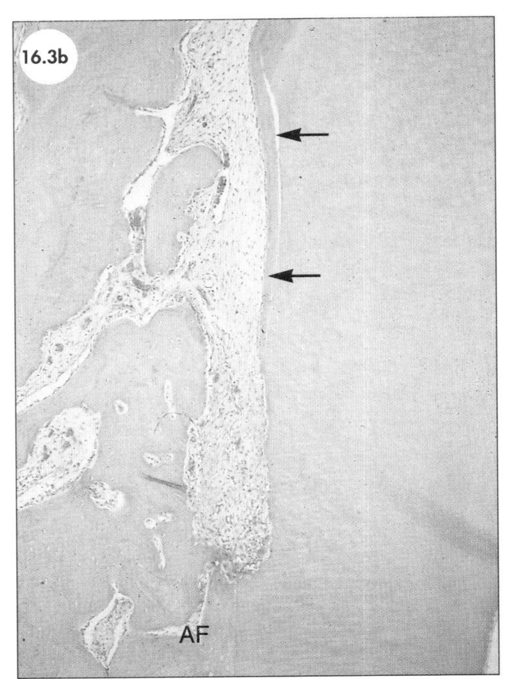

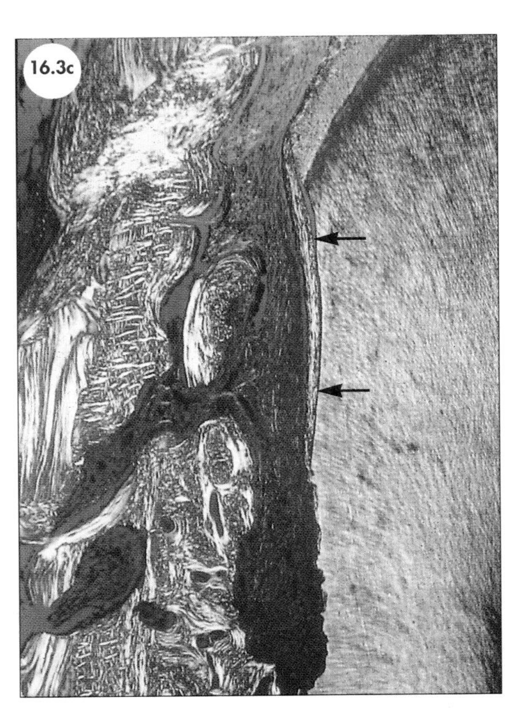

Figs 16.3, 16.4 Development of reparative cementum in longitudinal sections stained with hematoxylin and eosin from monkey incisors (*Macaca fascicularis*) in ordinary transmitted (*Figs 16.3a, 16.3b, 16.4a, 16.4b*) and polarized (*Figs 16.3c, 16.4c*) light.) (*B* and *C* are details from *A*.) Centrally, on the instrumented root surface, an ankylotic fusion (AF) undergoing resorption is seen 5 weeks after instrumentation (*Figs 16.3a, 16.3b*). At the periphery of the instrumented surface, reparative cementum is left loosely apposed to the dentine surface. Note the lamellar appearance of the reparative cementum (arrows), which resembles alveolar bone and the palisade-like structure of the original cementum in polarized light (*Fig. 16.3c*). The connective tissue fibres adjacent to the reparative cementum are not functionally oriented but rather run parallel to the root surface. The ankylotic fusion seen after 5 weeks (*Fig. 16.3)* has been completely resorbed, leaving reparative cementum loosely apposed to the dentine surface at 10 weeks after instrumentation (*Figs 16.4a, 16.4b*). The lamellar appearance of the reparative cementum (arrows) resembles alveolar bone and the palisade-like structure of the original cementum in polarized light remains (*Fig. 16.4c*). The connective tissue fibres adjacent to the reparative cementum are not functionally oriented but still run parallel to the root surface. (From Blomlöf and Lindskog, 1994.) (Magnifications: *16.3a* – × 16; *16.3b, c* – × 100; *16.4a* – × 16; *16.4b, c* – × 100.)

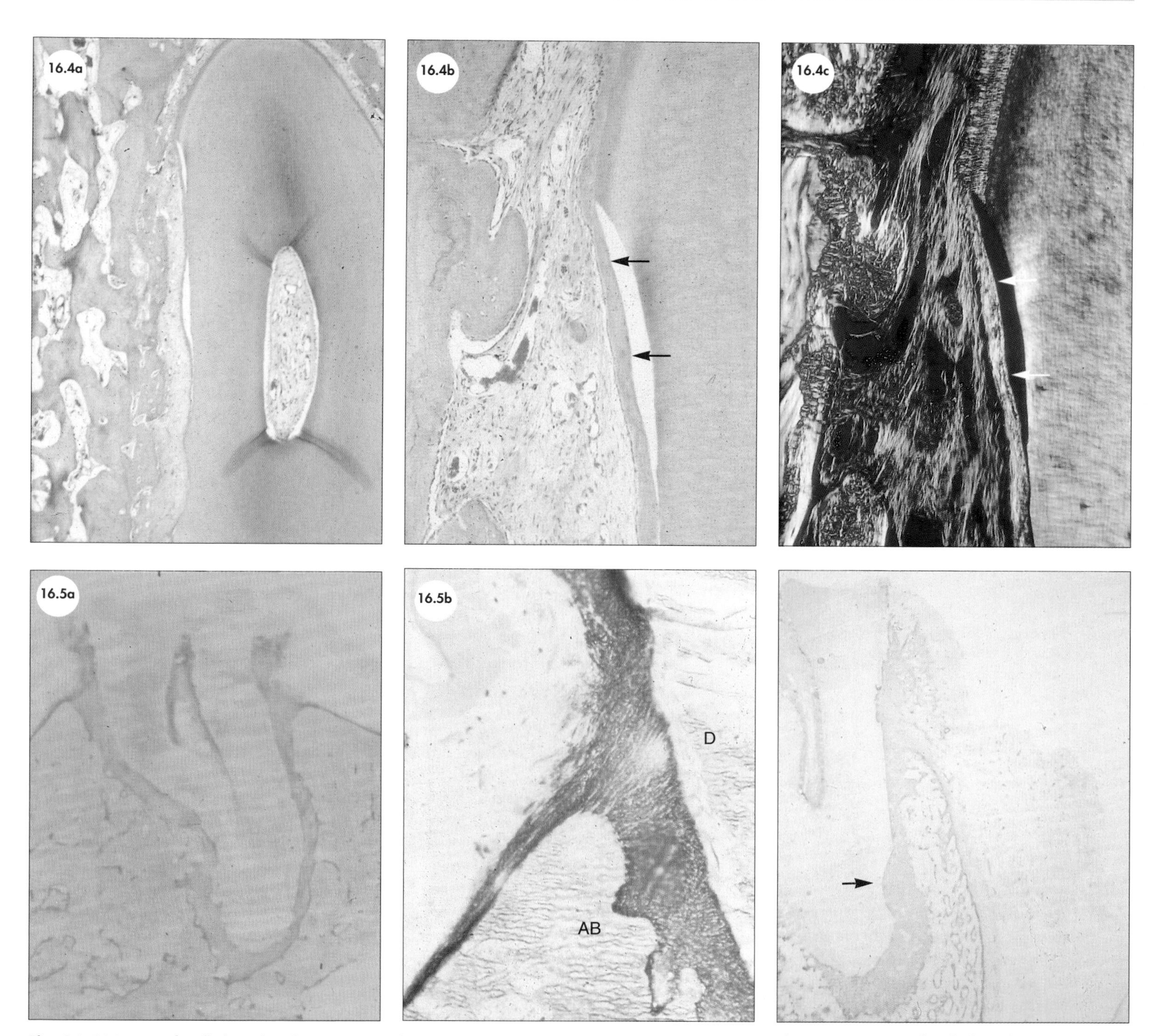

Fig. 16.5 Non-specific alkaline phosphatase activity (frozen section) in the PDL from a rat upper first molar (Sprague–Dawley) evidenced by intense blue staining (*Fig. 16.5a*). The periodontal connective tissue interlaces at the alveolar crest with the periosteum, which also shows intense enzyme activity (*Fig. 16.5b*). *Fig. 16.5b* is a detail from *Fig. 16.5a*. Note the lack of enzyme activity in the connective tissue of the gingiva except for activity in the walls of small blood vessels. Dentine (D) and alveolar bone (AB). (From Lilja *et al.*, 1984.) (Magnifications: *16.5a* – × 40; *16.5b* – × 250.)

Fig. 16.6 Non-specific alkaline phosphatase activity in a frozen undecalcified section evidenced by blue staining, 8 weeks after selective removal of the buccal bone plate in a monkey premolar (*Macaca fascicularis*). The notch in the root surface (arrow) indicates level of bone removal. Note regenerated bone coronal to this level and the intense activity of alkaline phosphatase in the PDL connective tissue extending to the enamel–cementum border. (From Lindskog and Blomlöf, 1994.) (Magnification × 16.)

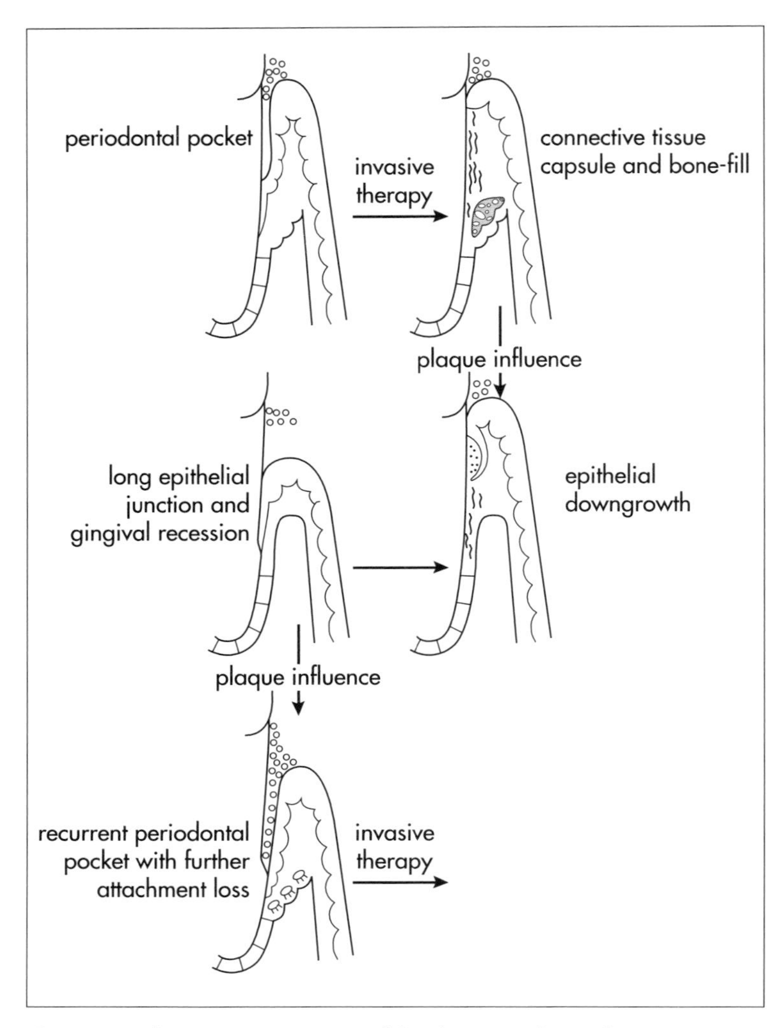

Fig. 16.7 Schematic representation of the dynamics of periodonitis.

and Skougaard, 1972; Blomlöf and Lindskog, 1994) has raised the question that perhaps bone-forming cells are responsible for the formation of reparative cementum in this situation (Bogle *et al.*, 1985; Egelberg, 1987; Lindskog and Blomlöf, 1992), as indicated by morphological findings (Lindskog and Blomlöf, 1992; Blomlöf and Lindskog, 1994), enzyme histochemical evidence (Lindskog and Blomlöf, 1994), and *in vitro* results (Melcher *et al.*, 1987).

In recent studies of the dynamics of reparative cementum formation on instrumented root surfaces, transient ankylosis was observed for up to 5 weeks (Blomlöf and Lindskog, 1994) (see *Fig. 16.3*), leaving a mineralized tissue layer loosely apposed to the dentine surface (see *Fig. 16.4*) (Lindskog and Blomlöf, 1992). The reparative cementum differed markedly from the surrounding normal cementum. Not only was it *not* attached to the dentine surface, but it also showed a lamellar appearance resembling alveolar bone. The connective tissue fibres adjacent to the reparative cementum were not functionally oriented but rather ran parallel to the root surface in a capsular arrangement (see *Figs. 16.3, 16.4*). It is interesting to note that this non-attached bone-like tissue has sometimes been observed with an intervening layer of tissue debris against the dentine surface (Lindskog and Blomlöf, 1992). This would indicate that the mineralized tissue had not formed directly on the dentine surface, but rather within the PDL space as part of a developing ankylotic fusion, only to appear associated with the root after an extended healing period. It could thus be argued that osteoblast phenotypes from the pool of undifferentiated mesenchymal cells in the PDL apical to the damaged areas (Aukhil and Iglhaut, 1988) had been attracted to the areas of resorption in the granulation–necrotic tissue (Lindskog and Blomlöf, 1992). Subsequently, stimulated by the resorptive activity, the osteoblasts started to form islands of bone-like tissue, initiating the ankylosis process (Andreasen and Skougaard, 1972; Hammarström *et al.*, 1989; Lindskog and Blomlöf, 1992, 1994). The fact that the bone-like tissue, irrespective of attachment to the dentine surface, does not routinely form a permanent ankylotic fusion with the alveolar bone is due to resorptive activity (Andreasen and Skougaard, 1972; Hammarström *et al.*, 1989; Lindskog and Blomlöf, 1992; Blomlöf and Lindskog, 1994; Lindskog and Blomlöf, 1994) followed by ingrowth of intervening PDL connective tissue and regeneration of the periodontal epithelial network (Löe and Waerhaug, 1961; Lindskog *et al.*, 1983a, 1987; Brice *et al.*, 1991; Lindskog and Blomlöf, 1992, 1994). However, when the regenerative potential of the remaining PDL connective tissue is impaired or absent, a complete ankylotic fusion will be the result (Hammarström *et al.*, 1989).

Activity of vanadate-resistant alkaline phosphatase (VRAP), an isoenzyme of non-specific alkaline phosphatase (NSAP), is intense in osteoblasts in the PDL (Hasselgren *et al.*, 1978; Lilja *et al.*, 1984). Activity of both NSAP and VRAP is detectable in the tissues around dental roots; there is a preferential localization for VRAP to periosteal and endosteal bone surfaces. Following experimental removal of the periodontium, including alveolar bone, PDL, and cementum, the subsequent spontaneous marginal healing on the exposed dentine surface has been shown to result in activity of VRAP on the healing dentine surfaces (Lindskog and Blomlöf, 1994) (*Fig. 16.8*). This adds further evidence to indicate that osteoblasts rather than cementoblasts are responsible for forming reparative cementum on instrumented root surfaces (*Fig. 16.9*) (Lindskog and Blomlöf, 1994).

Formation of reparative cementum after root resorption presents a somewhat different situation from that found when reparative cementum forms on instrumented root surfaces. In these areas of resorption, the cementum invariably shows a morphology and attachment similar to the surrounding original cementum (see *Fig. 16.2*). Limited resorption of root surfaces is inevitably followed by a repair phase involving cementoblasts derived from the cell layers closest to the cementoblasts surrounding the resorbed area (Lindskog *et al.*, 1987;

Hammarström and Lindskog, 1992). These cells start to divide (Lindskog *et al.*, 1983b) and repopulate the resorbed dentine surface from its periphery (Lindskog *et al.*, 1983b, 1987; Aukhil and Iglhaut, 1988). Although a centrally located pool of undifferentiated mesenchymal cells appears to be the largest source of regenerating cells in the PDL (McCulloch *et al.*, 1989; McCulloch, 1993), it may be argued that these root-surface-associated cell layers are the only source of cementoblast differentiation and proliferation. At present, we are unaware of the factors that stimulate repopulation of the resorbed areas. It has been suggested that the resorptive process leaves a trail ('coupling factor') which attracts reparative cells in a way similar to the mechanisms seen in bone formation following bone resorption (for review, see Parfitt, 1982). Furthermore, both the collagenous dentine matrix and the cementum contain potential stimulants of cell attachment (McAllister *et al.*, 1990), division (Miki *et al.*, 1987; Narayanan and Yonemura, 1993), and migration (Nishimura *et al.*, 1989). These stimulatory substances remain to be conclusively characterized, but some of them appear to have the -arg-gly-asp-sequence in common with many other attachment proteins (McAllister *et al.*, 1990). Limited ultrastructural evidence supports an involvement of these proteins in attaching cementoblasts to the cementoid surface layer of both reparative and original cementum (Philipsson *et al.*, 1990).

It may be concluded that there are two different types of reparative cementum resulting from repopulation of the damaged root surface areas by mesenchymal cells expressing different phenotypes (Lindskog *et al.*, 1983a, Melcher *et al.*, 1987; McCulloch and Bordin, 1991; Lindskog and Blomlöf, 1992, 1994; Tenorio *et al.*, 1993; Blomlöf and Lindskog, 1994), either a cementoblast phenotype (root resorption) or an osteoblast phenotype (instrumented root surfaces). Expression of the cementoblast phenotype may only be possible after a superficial resorption of the dentine surface. However, this can not be the only factor that promotes formation of attached reparative cementum, since resorption has also been shown to precede non-attached bone-like reparative cementum formation (Lindskog and Blomlöf, 1992; Blomlöf and Lindskog, 1994). It is likely that additional factors, such as the potency of the source of undifferentiated mesenchymal cells (most pronounced in young teeth with incomplete root closure) also determine the type of root surface healing that will occur (Blomlöf *et al.*, 1992; Lindskog and Blomlöf, 1992).

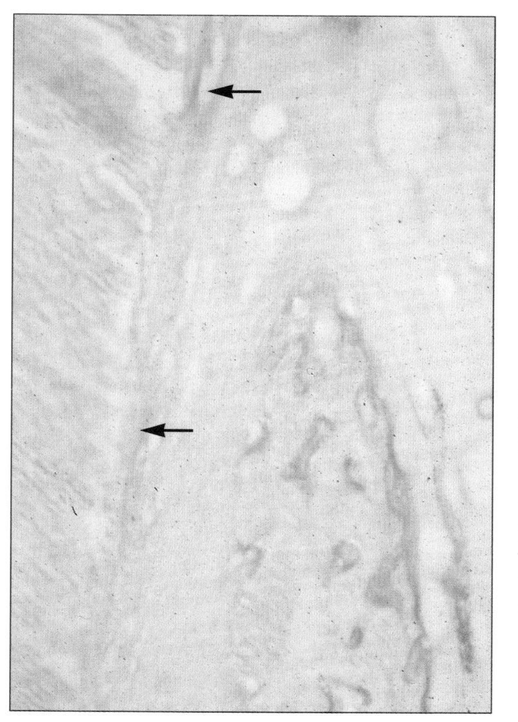

Fig. 16.8 Vanadate-resistant alkaline phosphatase activity in a frozen undecalcified section of a denuded dentine surface and on the regenerating alveolar bone 8 weeks after removal of the buccal bone plate and cementum in a monkey premolar (*Macaca fascicularis*). The enzyme activity (arrows) indicates an osteoblast origin of cells producing reparative cementum on the instrumented root surface. (Courtesy of the editor of Swedish Dental Journal, and Lindskog and Blomlöf, 1994). (Magnification × 250.)

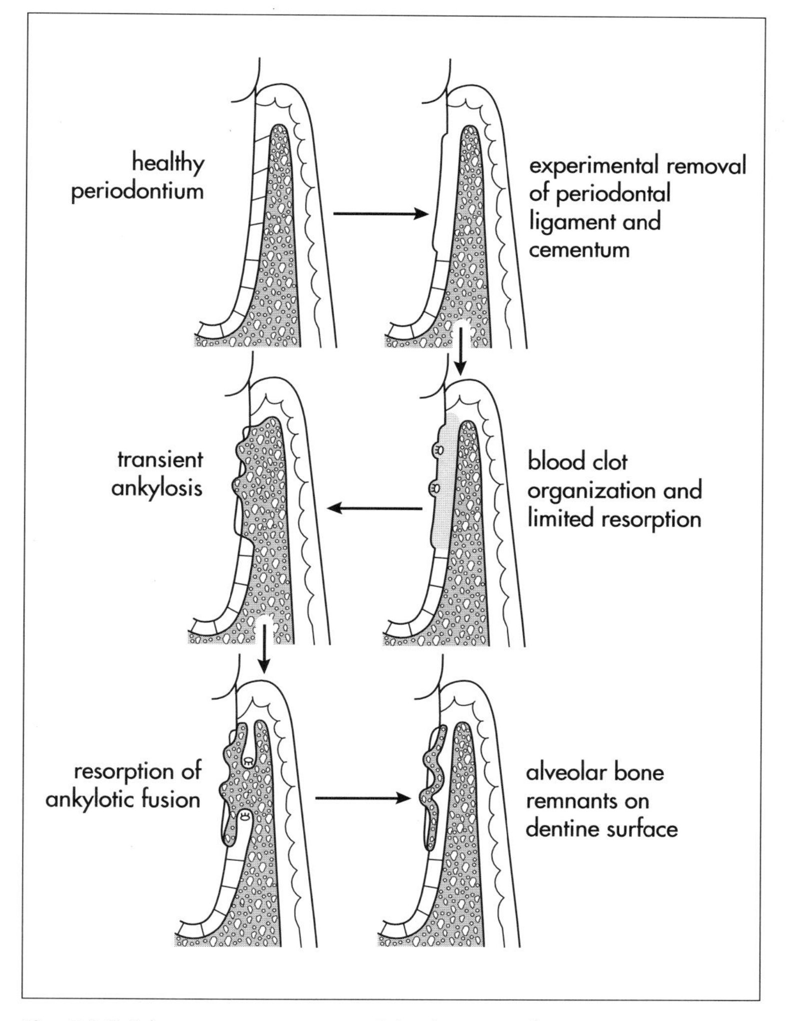

Fig. 16.9 Schematic representation of the dynamics of reparative cementum formation on an instrumented root surface.

SUMMARY AND CONCLUSIONS

Periodontal healing with new functional tooth-supporting tissues requires PDL phenotypes to repopulate the root surface and periodontal space. A mixture of gingival periodontal and endosteal–periosteal connective and epithelial tissues compete in this process. Consequently, the resulting healing tissue varies widely from a completely regenerated functional PDL, such as that seen after surface resorption incident to orthodontic tooth movement, to the non-functional capsular arrangements seen on instrumented root surfaces following periodontal scaling and root planing.

Only cells from the PDL connective tissue appear to be able to form dental cementum and bone. However, the non-attached non-functionally organized reparative cementum found on instrumented dentine surfaces in teeth with fully formed roots has several characteristics in common with bone, and it appears to be the result of a transient ankylosis produced by an osteoblastic phenotype, while the cementoblast phenotype is expressed only after a superficial resorption of the dentine surface resulting in an attached functionally organized reparative cementum.

REFERENCES

Andreasen JO (1980) Delayed replantation after submucosal storage in order to prevent root resorption after replantation. Int J Oral Surg 9, 394–403.

Andreasen JO and Skougaard MR (1972) Reversibility of surgically induced dental ankylosis in rats. Int J Oral Surg 1, 98–102.

Arceo N, Sauk JJ, Moehring J, Foster RA and Sommerman MJ (1991) Human periodontal cells initiate mineral-like nodules *in vitro*. J Periodontol 62, 499–503.

Aukhil I and Iglhaut J (1988) Periodontal ligament cell kinetics following experimental regenerative procedures. J Clin Periodontol 15, 374–382.

Bartold PM (1987) Proteoglycans of the periodontium: structure, role and function. J Periodont Res 22, 431–444.

Bartold PM (1991) Connective tissues of the periodontium. Research and clinical implications. Aust Dent J 36, 255–268.

Ben-Yehuda A, Machtei EE and Goultschein J (1989) The regeneration potential of the periodontium. J West Soc Periodontol 37, 5–11.

Berg JO, Blomlöf L and Lindskog S (1990) Periodontal and pulpal reactions following different periodontal treatments. J Clin Periodontol 17, 165–173.

Blomlöf L, Friskopp J, Appelgren R, Lindskog S and Hammarström L (1989) Influence of granulation tissue, calculus and contaminated root cementum on periodontal healing. An experimental study in monkeys. J Clin Periodontol 16, 27–32.

Blomlöf L, Lindskog S, Appelgren R, Jonsson B, Weintraub A and Hammarström L (1987) New attachment in monkeys with experimental periodontitis with and without removal of the cementum. J Clin Periodontol 14, 136–143.

Blomlöf L, Lindskog S and Hammarström L (1988a) A time-related study of healing in the marginal periodontal/root interface. Swed Dent J 14, 459–464.

Blomlöf L, Lindskog S and Hammarström L (1988b) Influence of pulpal treatments on cell and tissue reactions in the marginal periodontium. J Periodontol 59, 577–583.

Blomlöf L, Lengheden A and Lindskog S (1992) Endodontic infection and calcium hydroxide-treatment. Effects on periodontal healing in mature and immature replanted monkey teeth. J Clin Periodontol 19, 652–658.

Blomlöf L and Lindskog S (1994) Quality of periodontal healing II: Dynamics of reparative cementum formation. Swed Dent J 18, 131–138.

Blomlöf L and Otteskog P (1981) Composition of human periodontal ligament cells in tissue culture. Scand J Dent Res 89, 43–47.

Bogle G, Claffey N and Egelberg J (1985) Healing of horizontal circumferential periodontal defects following regenerative surgery in beagle dogs. J Clin Periodontol 12, 837–849.

Bowers GM, Chadroff B, Carnevale R, Mellonig J, R, Emerson J, Stevens M and Romberg E (1989a) Histologic evaluation of new attachment apparatus formation in humans (II). J Periodontol 60, 675–682.

Bowers GM, Chadroff B, Carnevale R, Mellonig J, Corio R, Emerson J, Stevens M and Romberg E (1989b) Histologic evaluation of new attachment apparatus formation in humans (III). J Periodontol 60, 683–693.

Brice GL, Sampson WJ and Sims MR (1991) An ultrastructural evaluation of the relationship between epithelial rests of Malassez and orthodontic root resorption and repair in man. Au Orthod J 12, 90–94.

Brunette DM, Melcher AH, and Moe HK (1976) Culture and origin of epithelium-like and fibroblast-like cells from porcine periodontal ligament explants and cell suspensions. Arch Oral Biol 21, 393–400.

Brunette DM, Kanoza RJ, Marmary Y, Chan J and Melcher AM (1977) Interactions between epithelial- and fibroblast-like cells in culture derived from monkey periodontal ligament. J Cell Sci 27, 127–140.

Caffesse RG and Quiñones CR (1993) Polypeptide growth factors and attachment proteins in periodontal wound healing and regeneration. Periodontology 2000 1, 60–79.

Caton J and Nyman S (1980). Histometric evaluation of periodontal surgery. I. The modified Widman flap procedure. J Clin Periodontol 7, 212–223.

Caton J, Nyman S and Zander H (1980). Histometric evaluation of periodontal surgery. II. Connective tissue attachment levels after four regenerative procedures. J Clin Periodontol 7, 224–231.

Cook JJ, Haaynes KM and Werther GA (1988) Mitogenic effects of growth hormones in cultured human fibroblasts. J Clin Invest 81, 206–212.

Egelberg J (1987) Regeneration and repair of periodontal tissues. J Periodontal Res 22, 233–242.

Ehnevid H, Lindskog S, Jansson L and Blomlöf L (1993b) Tissue formation on denuded and demineralized cementum surfaces *in vivo*. Swed Dent J 17, 1–8.

Ehnevid H, Jansson L, Lindskog S and Blomlöf L (1993a) Periodontal healing in teeth with periapical lesions – A clinical retrospective study. J Clin Periodontol 20, 254–258.

Ehnevid H, Jansson L, Lindskog S and Blomlöf L (1994) Periodontal healing in horizontal and vertical defects. J Clin Periodontol (submitted).

Finkelman RD (1992) Growth factors in bones and teeth. Calif Dent Ass J 20, 23–29.

Gallagher JT (1989) The extended family of proteoglycans: social residents of the pericellular zone. Curr Opin Cell Biol 1, 1201–1218.

Gillery P, Leperre A, Maquart FX and Borel JP (1992) Insulin-like growth factor I (IGF-I) stimulates protein synthesis and collagen gene expression in monolayer and lattice cultures of fibroblasts. J Cell Physiol 152, 389–396.

Gottlow J, Nyman S, Karring T and Lindhe J (1984) New attachment formation as the result of controlled tissue regeneration. J Clin Periodontol 11, 494–503.

Häkkinen L and Larjava H (1992) Characterization of fibroblast clones from periodontal granulation tissue *in vitro*. J Dent Res 71, 1901–1907.

Hammarström L, Blomlöf L, Feiglin B and Lindskog S (1986) Replantation of teeth and antibiotic treatment. Endod Dent Traumatol 2, 51–57.

Hammarström L, Lindskog S and Blomlöf L (1989) Dynamics of dentoalveolar ankylosis and associated root resorption. Endod Dent Traumatol 5, 163–175.

Hammarström L and Lindskog S (1992) Factors regulating and modifying dental root resorption. Proc Finn Dent Soc 88 (suppl 1), 115–123.

Harrison JW and Jurosky KA (1991) Wound healing in the tissues of the periodontium following periradicular surgery. II. The dissectional wound. J Endod 17, 544–552.

Hasselgren G, Fransén A and Hammarström L (1978) Histochemical characterization of alkaline phosphatase in developing rat teeth and bone. Scand J Dent Res 86, 325–336.

Helldén L (1972) Periodontal healing following experimental injury to root surfaces of human teeth. Scand J Dent Res 80, 197–205.

Ingber DE and Folkman J (1989) Tension and compression as basic determinants of cell form and function: Utilization of a cellular tensegrity mechanism. In: Cell shape: Determinants, regulation, and regulatory role (Stein WD and Bronner F, eds), pp3–31, Academic Press, San Diego.

Jansson L, Ehnevid L, Lindskog S and Blomlöf L (1993a) Development of periapical inflammatory lesions. Swed Dent J 17, 245–248.

Jansson L, Ehnevid L, Lindskog S and Blomlöf L (1993b) Relationship between periapical lesions and periodontal status – A clinical retrospective study. J Clin Periodontol 20, 117–123.

Karring T, Nyman S, Lindhe J, Sirirat M (1984) Potentials for root resorption during periodontal wound healing. J Clin Periodontol 11, 41–52.

Kon S, Novaes AB, Ruben MP and Golgman HM (1969) Visualization of microvascularization of the healing periodontal wound. II. Curettage. J Periodontol 40, 90–105.

Kratz G, Lake M, Ljungström K, Forsberg G, Haegerstrand A and Gidlund M (1992) Effect of recombinant IGF binding protein-1 on primary cultures of human keratinocytes and fibroblasts: selective enhancement of IGF-1 but not IGF-2r induced cell proliferation. Exp Cell Res 202, 381–385.

Lengheden A, Blomlöf L and Lindskog S (1991a) Effect of immediate cacium hydroxide treatment and permanent root-filling on periodontal healing in contaminated replanted teeth. Scand J Dent Res 99, 139–146.

Lengheden A, Blomlöf L and Lindskog S (1991b) Effect of delayed cacium hydroxide treatment on periodontal healing in contaminated replanted teeth. Scand J Dent Res 99, 147–153.

Lilja E, Lindskog S and Hammarström L (1984) Alkaline phosphatase activity and tetracycline incorporation during initial tooth movement in rats. Acta Odont Scand 42, 1–11.

Lindskog S and Blomlöf L (1992) Mineralized tissue formation in periodontal wound healing. J Clin Periodontol 19, 741–748.

Lindskog S and Blomlöf L (1994) Quality of priodontal healing IV: Enzyme histochemical evidence for an osteoblast origin of reparative cementum. Swed Dent J 18, 181–190.

Lindskog S, Blomlöf L and Hammarström L (1983a) Repair of periodontal tissues *in vivo* and *in vitro*. J Clin Periodontol 10, 188–205.

Lindskog S, Blomlöf L and Hammarström L (1983b) Mitoses and microorganisms in the periodontal membrane after storage in milk or saliva. Scand J Dent Res 91, 465–472.

Lindskog S, Blomlöf L and Hammarström L (1987) Cellular colonization on denuded root surfaces *in vivo*: cell morphology in dentin resorption and cementum repair. J Clin Periodontol 14, 390–395.

Lindskog S, Lengheden A and Blomlöf L (1993) Successive removal of periodontal tissues – Marginal periodontal healing without plaque control. J Clin Periodontol 20, 14–19.

Line SE, Polson AM and Zander MA (1974) Relationship between periodontal injury and selective cell repopulation and ankylosis. J Periodontol 45, 725–730.

Löe H and Waerhaug J (1961) Experimental replantation of teeth in dogs and monkeys. Arch Oral Biol 3, 176–183.

Lumsden AGS (1988) Spatial organization of the epithelium and the role of neural crest cells in the initial of the mammalian tooth germ. Development 103 (suppl), 155–169.

Lynch SE, de Castilla GR, Williams RC *et al.* (1991) The effect of short-term application of a combination of platelet-derived and insulin-like growth factors on periodontal healing. J Periodontol 62, 458–467.

MacNeil RL and Sommerman MJ (1993) Molecular factors regulating development and regeneration of cementum. J Periodont Res 28, 550–559.

MacNeil RL and Thomas HF (1993) Development of the murine periodontium. II. Role of the epithelial root sheath in formation of the periodontal attachment. J Periodontol 64, 285–291.

Marmary Y, Brunette DM and Meershe JNM (1976) Differences *in vitro* between cells derived from periodontal ligament and skin of *Macaca irus*. Arch Oral Biol 21, 709–716.

McAllister B, Narayanan AS, Miki Y and Page RC (1990) Isolation of a fibroblast attachment protein from cementum. J Periodont Res 25, 99–105.

McCulloch CA (1993) Basic considerations in periodontal wound healing to achieve regeneration. Periodontology 2000 1, 16–25.

McCulloch CAG, Barghava U and Melcher AH (1989) Cell death and the regulation of populations of cells in the periodontal ligament. Cell Tissue Res 255, 129–138.

McCulloch CAG and Bordin S (1991) Role of fibroblast subpopulations in periodontal physiology and pathology. J Periodont Res 26, 144–154.

Melcher AH (1970) Repair of wounds in the periodontium of the rat. Influence of periodontal ligament on osteogenesis. Arch Oral Biol 15, 1183–1204.

Melcher AH (1976) On the repair potential of periodontal tissues. J Periodontol 47, 256–260.

Melcher AH, McCulloch CAG, Cheong T, Nemeth E and Shiga A (1987) Cells from bone synthesized cementum-like and bone-like tissue *in vitro* and may migrate into periodontal ligament *in vivo*. J Periodont Res 22, 246–247.

Middleton CT and Bowers BG (1990) Histologic evaluation of cementogenesis on periodontitis-affected roots in humans. Int J Periodont Rest Dent 10, 429–435.

Miki Y, Narayanan S and Page RC (1987) Mitogenic activity of cementum components to gingival fibroblasts. J Dent Res 66, 1399–1403.

Mohran S and Baylink DJ (1991) Bone growth factors. Clin Orthop Rel Res 263, 30–48.

Moskow BS (1964) The response of the gingival sulcus to instrumentation: A histologic investigation. J Periodontol 35, 112–126.

Narayanan SA and Yonemura K (1993) Purification and characterization of a novel growth factor from cementum. J Periodont Res 28, 563–565.

Nishimura K, Hayashi M, Matsuda K, Shigeyama Y, Yamasaki A and Yamaoka A (1989) The chemoattractive potency of periodontal ligament, cementum and dentin for human gingival fibroblasts. J Periodont Res 24, 146–148.

Nyman S and Karring T (1979) Regeneration of surgically removed buccal alveolar bone in dogs. J Periodont Res 14, 86–92.

Nyman S, Gottlow J, Karring T and Lindhe J (1982) The regenerative potential of the periodontal ligament. An experimental study in the monkey. J Clin Periodontol 9, 257–265.

Nyman S, Lindhe J and Karring T (1989) Reattachment – new attachment. In: Textbook of Clinical Periodontology (Lindhe J, ed), pp450–476. Munksgaard, Copenhagen.

Nyman S, Lindhe J and Rosling B (1977) Periodontal surgery in plaque-infected dentitions. J Clin Periodontol 4, 340–249.

Olson S, Arzate H, Naraynan AS and Page RC (1991) Cell attachment activity of cementum proteins and mechanism of endotoxin inhibition. J Dent Res 70, 1272–1277.

Palmer RM and Lumsden AGS (1987) Development of periodontal ligament and alveolar bone in hemografted recombinations soft tissue enamel organs and papillary, pulpal and follicular mesenchyme in the mouse. Arch Oral Biol 32, 281–289.

Parfitt AM (1982) The coupling of bone formation to bone resorption: A critical analysis of the concept and of its relevance to the pathogenesis of osteoporosis. Metab Bone Dis Rel Res 4, 1–6.

Parlange LM and Sims MR (1993) A TEM stereological analysis of blood vessels and nerves in marmoset periodontal ligament following endodontic and magnetic extrusion. Eur J Orthod 15, 33–44.

Philipsson S, Lindskog S and Flock A (1990) Ultrastructure of cementoblast attachment. Scand J Dent Res 98, 295–300.

Piche JE, Carnes DL and Graves DT (1989) Initial characterization of cells derived from human periodontia. J Dent Res 68, 761–767.

Pitaru S, Hekmati M, Metzger Z and Savion N (1991) Epithelial-connective tissue interaction on the tooth surface: an *in vitro* model. J Periodont Res 26, 461–467.

Polson AM and Heijl LC (1978) Osseous repair in infrabony periodontal defects. J Clin Periodontol 5, 13–23.

Proye M and Polson AM (1982) Effect of root surface alterations on periodontal healing. I. Surgical denudation. J Clin Periodontol 9, 428–440.

Ruoslahti E (1989) Proteoglycans in cell regulation. J Biol Chem 264, 13369–13372.

Salonen JI, Kautsky MB and Dale BA (1989) Changes in cell phenotype during regeneration of junctional epithelium of human gingiva *in vitro*. J Periodont Res 24, 370–377.

Schroeder HE (1986) The Periodontium, pp26–33, Springer-Verlag, Berlin.

Seymour RA and Heasman, PA (1992) Drugs, Diseases, and the Periodontium, Oxford University Press, Oxford.

Spouge JD (1980) A new look at the rests of Malassez. A review of their embryological origin, anatomy, and possible role in periodontal health and disease. J Periodontol 51, 437–444.

Tavakkol A, Elder JT, Cooper KD, *et al.* (1992) Expression of growth hormone receptor, insulin-like growth factor I (IGF-I) and IGF-I receptor mRNA and proteins in human skin. J Invest Dermatol 999, 343–349.

Taylor AC and Cambell MM (1972) Reattachment of gingival epithelium to the tooth. J Periodontol 43, 281–293.

Ten Cate AR, Mills C and Solomon G (1971) The development of the periodontium: a transplantation and autoradiographic study. Anat Rec 170, 365–380.

Tenorio D, Cruchley A, Hughes FJ (1993) Immunocytochemical investigation of the rat cementoblast phenotype. J Periodont Res 28, 411–419.

Uitto VJ and Larjava H (1991) Extracellular matrix, molecules and their receptors: An overview with special emphasis on periodontal tissues. Critical Rev Oral Biol Med 2, 323–354.

Wikesjö UME and Nilvéus R (1990) Periodontal repair in dogs: effect of wound stabilization on healing. J Periodontol 61, 719–724.

Wikesjö UME, Nilvéus R and Selvig KA (1992) Significance of early healing events on periodontal repair: A review. J Periodontol 63, 158–165.

Wirthlin MR, Yaeger JE, Hancock EB and Gaugler RW (1980) The healing of gingival wounds in miniature swine. J Periodontol 51, 318–327.

Yoshikawa DK and Kollar EJ (1981) Recombination of experiments on the odontogenic roles of mouse dental papilla and dental sac tissues in ocular grafts. Arch Oral Biol 26, 303–307.

Chapter 17

Neoplastic Involvement of the Periodontal Ligament

DM Walker

INTRODUCTION

Although the nature of a number of different lesions arising in the tissues that support the teeth remains undecided, many arising in the periodontal ligament (PDL) may be reactive rather than neoplastic. By the time tumours present clinically, it is usually impossible to pinpoint the precise anatomical site of origin except in some small neoplasms in surgical specimens where the PDL remains intact. The true incidence of PDL tumours is unknown; however, a breed of mice carrying albumin-myc and albumin-ras transgenes which develop odontogenic tumours in the PDL (Gibson *et al.*, 1992) might offer a useful experimental model for future research.

Although anatomically limited in extent, the PDL has a diversity of cell types – epithelial (the rests of Malassez), or connective tissue (fibroblasts, osteoblasts, osteoclasts, cementoblasts, blood vessels, leucocytes, nerves and lymphatics) (see Chapter 1) . The possible spectrum of tumours is thus theoretically wide, even though their incidence is low. Secondary involvement of the PDL by infiltration from primary tumours arising in adjacent tissues, such as gingival carcinomas, or by blood-borne metastasis, e.g. leukaemia, may be commoner than primary neoplasia of PDL elements.

Oxytalan fibres are characteristically found in the PDL (e.g. Hamner and Fullmer, 1966; Shore *et al.*, 1984) although they are not unique to that site (see Chapter 2). In support of a PDL origin for certain tumours, oxytalan fibres have been identified in peripheral odontogenic fibromas (Wright and Jennings, 1979) and adenomatoid odontogenic tumours (Berghagen *et al.*, 1973).

Infiltration of the PDL by primary or secondary malignant tumours (especially osteosarcoma, for example) results in a widening of the PDL space in radiographs. The resulting increased mobility of the associated teeth, ('malignant loosening of teeth') is an important physical sign of neoplastic involvement of the PDL.

EPITHELIAL TUMOURS

The epithelial rests of Malassez remaining in the PDL after root development has been completed may occasionally undergo neoplastic change.

In adult life, remnants of odontogenic epithelium seem to persist routinely in the jaw bones only in the PDL of standing teeth or in the follicles of unerupted teeth. Intraosseous epithelial tumours or cysts occurring as central radiolucent swellings in the jaws in later life are likely to originate in these sites. Alternatively some neoplasms, e.g. ameloblastoma, could also arise from the lining of odontogenic cysts (Shteyer *et al.*, 1978). Extraosseous tumours of odontogenic epithelium situated exclusively in soft tissue have been documented but they are rare.

The epithelial rests of Malassez have abundant membrane receptors for epidermal growth factor (Thesleff, 1987). These are also expressed in the epithelial lining of cysts, but interestingly they could not be demonstrated by an immunohistological method in a range of odontogenic epithelial tumours (Shrestha *et al.*, 1992).

AMELOBLASTOMA

Excluding odontomes, ameloblastomas are the commonest odontogenic tumours, although their absolute incidence is low. Extraosseous peripheral ameloblastomas confined to the soft tissues of the gingiva (Buchner and Sciubba, 1987; Batsakis *et al.*, 1993; Bucci *et al.*, 1992) are even rarer.

Using *in situ* hybridization techniques for messenger RNA, it has been found that the types of intermediate filament proteins (Fuchs *et al.*, 1981; Moll *et al.*, 1982; Sun *et al.*, 1985) – such as the cytokeratins 19, 8 and 18, and vimentin – that are expressed in ameloblastomas are strongly reminiscent of those found in the epithelial layers of the enamel organs at various stages of tooth development (Heikinheimo *et al.*, 1991). The restricted range of these proteins in these tumours is contrary to the suggestion that the rare peripheral gingival ameloblastomas (Nauta *et al.*, 1992; Hernandez *et al.*, 1992) could be derived from the oral epithelium, which has a wider spectrum of cytokeratins, although this needs to be confirmed directly on a series of ameloblastomas in this location.

Antibodies for enamel proteins, specific to ameloblasts, such as amelogenin and enamelin (Saku *et al.*, 1992) have also been useful in immunohistological studies of the histogenesis of odontogenic tumours. These proteins could be demonstrated in odontogenic tumours such as adenomatoid odontogenic tumours and calcifying epithelial odontogenic tumours (Saku *et al.*, 1992). Messenger RNA specific for the amelogenin gene was expressed by ameloblastomas and developing tooth germs, confirming the odontogenic origin of the tumours (Snead *et al.*, 1992).

Ameloblastomas present at a mean age of 38.9 years and they are most prevalent in the molar or ascending ramus regions of the mandible (Small and Waldron, 1955). Maxillary tumours may be more aggressive (Bredenkamp and Zimmerman, 1989). They cause central painless slowly progressive expansion of the jaw. Radiographically there is a central monolocular radiolucency, with more complex multilocular patterns found at more advanced stages. There may be focal loss of the lamina dura and a burrowing irregular resorption of the roots of adjacent teeth. (*Figs 17.1, 17.2*). The ameloblastoma has a tendency to recur after removal. Risk factors for recurrence were found to be a follicular histological pattern (see *Fig. 17.2*), multilocular rather than monolocular radiolucency, and age above 20 years. Block resection of the tumours is followed by the lowest recurrence rate (Veno *et al.*, 1989).

CALCIFYING EPITHELIAL ODONTOGENIC TUMOUR

This neoplasm was delineated by Pindborg (1958, 1966) as a central radiolucent lesion more often encountered in the maxilla than in the mandible. It is sometimes related to an unerupted tooth. Calcification may become extensive enough to be evident in plain radiographs. Infrequently, calcifying epithelial odontogenic tumours may present as a peripheral soft tissue gingival swelling (Pindborg, 1966; Buchner and Sciubba, 1987).

The epithelial cells of the lesion are polyhedral, and they are sometimes connected by intercellular bridges. Although hyperchromatic nuclei may be encountered, mitotic activity is not a feature. Clear cell versions of the tumour have also been described (Franklin and Pindborg, 1976). One distinguishing feature is a homogeneous deposit, which may subsequently become calcified, in the stroma and the epithelium. This deposit reacts like amyloid with conventional stains. However, at the ultrastructural level, the fibrils within this material are smaller than those of true amyloid. The calcified material and tumour cells have recently been shown to contain amelogenin and enamelin (Saku *et al.*, 1992; Mori *et al.*, 1991). The tumour infiltrates locally, with a recurrence rate approaching 14 per cent.

CALCIFYING ODONTOGENIC CYST

This monolocular radiolucency is frequently diagnosed only after histological examination of a cyst enucleated from the molar region of the mandible. In the epithelial lining there are characteristic 'ghost cells', which retain outlines of nuclei and cell membranes. Calcification or even identifiable dental hard tissues in the fibrous capsule are typical (Hong *et al.*, 1991) and may be extensive enough to be evident on plain radiographs of mature lesions. Enamelin and amelogenin are also detectable in the epithelial lining (Saku *et al.*, 1992). Enucleation and curettage is the standard treatment (El-Beialy *et al.*, 1990).

Solid variants of this lesion, dentinogenic ghost cell tumours (Raubenheimer *et al.*, 1992), with a significant recurrence rate, have been described. Gingival soft tissue cases of calcifying odontogenic cyst are on record (Buchner *et al.*, 1991).

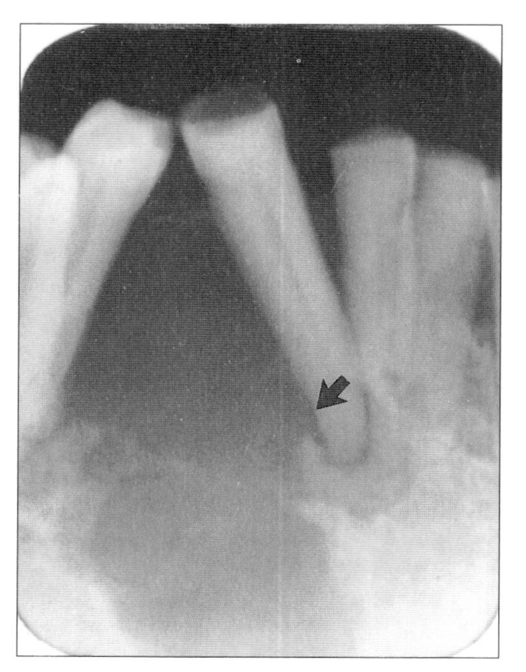

Fig. 17.1 Radiograph of an ameloblastoma of the mandible in a 61-year-old man, with displacement and loosening of teeth and involvement of periodontal ligament space of 43 (arrow).

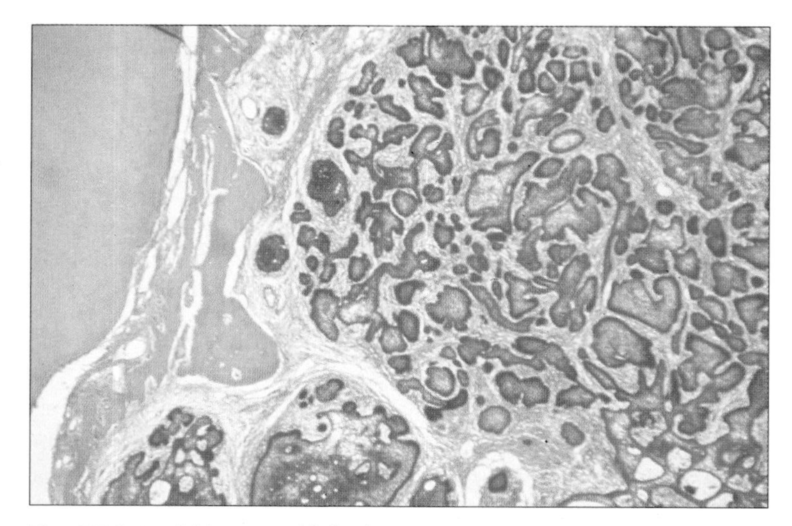

Fig. 17.2 Ameloblastoma of follicular pattern with some cystic degeneration near the root of a molar, with focal resorption of lamina dura and the root apex. The ameloblastoma appeared to involve the periodontal ligament secondarily rather than originate from the epithelial rests of Malassez within it. (Haematoxylin and eosin x 25.)

SQUAMOUS ODONTOGENIC TUMOUR

This tumour may involve the PDL as a circumscribed radiolucent lesion adjacent to the root of the associated tooth. The squamous odontogenic tumour may present as a swelling, a loosening of the tooth, or an incidental finding (Reichart and Philipsen, 1990). The neoplasms most frequently occur in the maxillary canine and mandibular molar regions. Islands of epithelium, often concentrically arranged to form laminated structures or with cystic degeneration, are encased in fibrous tissue (Pullon *et al.*, 1975; Doyle *et al.*, 1977; Hopper *et al.*, 1980).

Subsequent accounts of multiple lesions (Hopper *et al.*, 1980) and a familial tendency prompted a re-evaluation of the nature of the lesion. These findings implied that this could be a reactive hyperplasia or hamartoma of the odontogenic epithelium arising from the rests of Malassez in the PDL (Reichart and Philipsen, 1990), or from the remnants of the dental lamina in the case of gingival lesions. The fact that the lesions arise from odontogenic epithelium is also supported by the spectrum of epithelial cytokeratins (Tatemoto *et al.*, 1989).

ADENOMATOID ODONTOGENIC TUMOUR

Over half of adenomatoid odontogenic tumours present in the second decade. They occur as:

- follicular lesions, surrounding an embedded tooth, most frequently in the maxillary lateral incisor, canine, or premolar regions, mimicking a dentigerous cyst;
- extrafollicular lesions, not related to an unerupted tooth (*Fig. 17.3*);
- extra-osseous cases.

Uncommonly, the adenomatoid odontogenic tumour is contained entirely within the gingival soft tissues; in these cases it presents as an epulis.

Histologically, whorled masses of odontogenic epithelial cells form rosette-like structures (*Fig. 17.4*). Slender strands of these cells ramify in the stroma, giving a cribriform pattern. Ductal structures are a further finding of diagnostic value. Haematoxyphil globular calcified deposits or even dysplastic dentine may be prominent.

In a survey of 50 published cases, none had recurred even when incompletely removed (Philipsen *et al.*, 1991) and the lesions are generally believed to be hamartomatous proliferations of odontogenic epithelium rather than true tumours (Kramer *et al.*, 1992).

MALIGNANT EPITHELIAL TUMOUR

Local infiltration from a carcinoma of the gingiva is the usual cause of involvement of the PDL by a primary malignant epithelial tumour. Carcinomas arising as primary growths within the jaws, other than from cysts, are thought to be derived from rests of odontogenic epithelium in the PDL or in follicles surrounding unerupted teeth. These intra-alveolar carcinomas tend to have a characteristic histological alveolar pattern or a plexiform pattern with a basal columnar layer resembling pre-ameloblasts. Alternatively, they may be indistinguishable from the squamous cell carcinomas that arise from oral epithelium (Shear, 1969). Resorption of the lamina dura when infiltrating cancers involve the PDL is rapid, with consequent loosening of the teeth.

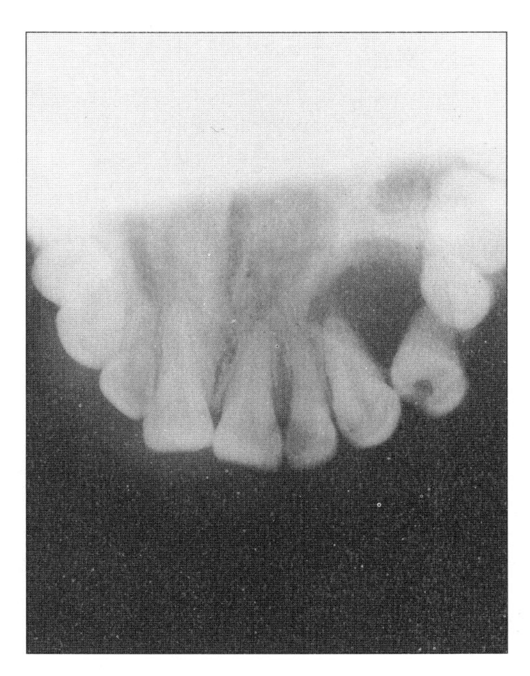

Fig. 17.3 Adenomatoid odontogenic tumour of extrafollicular type, presenting as a radiolucent painless swelling in canine region of left maxilla, in a 26-year-old woman.

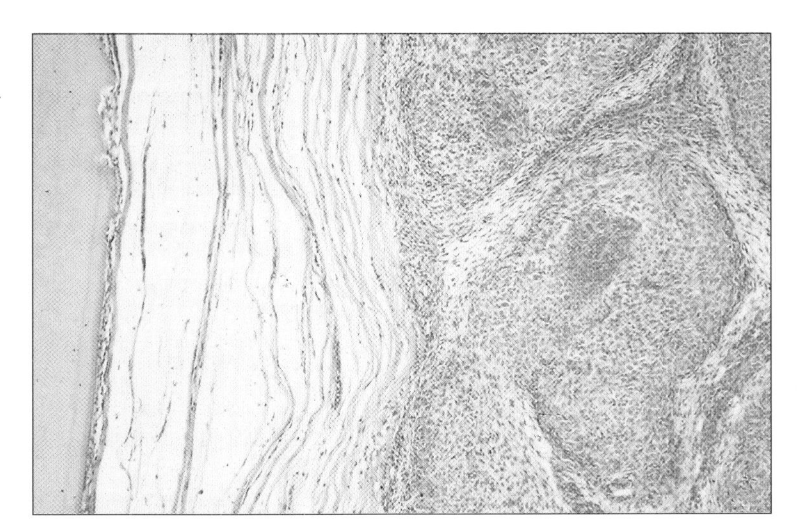

Fig. 17.4 Adenomatoid odontogenic tumour. Histology of the lesion in *Fig. 17.3*. Nodules of odontogenic epithelium near the periodontal ligament of the maxillary canine. (Haematoxylin & eosin x 60.)

Significant root resorption is unusual, histologically or radiographically. By contrast, root and lamina dura resorption in proximity to benign or locally invasive neoplasms of odontogenic epithelium, such as ameloblastomas, may be marked, possibly owing to the longer time course of these tumours before discovery.

CONNECTIVE TISSUE TUMOURS

FIBROMAS

Whereas the level of fibroblast and collagen turnover activity in the PDL is high, true fibromas originating from the fibroblast, the predominant mesenchymal cell of the PDL , are regarded as uncommon (Barker and Lucas, 1967) compared with fibrous epulides, solitary swellings of the gingiva that seem to be reactive hyperplasias triggered by dental plaque. Microscopically, a moderately cellular collagenous fibrous tissue predominates, with a diffuse inflammatory infiltrate and occasionally metaplastic woven bone. True fibromas are, by contrast, well demarcated (Barker and Lucas, 1967).

ODONTOGENIC FIBROMA

These present as an expanding central radiolucency (*Figs 17.5, 17.6*) of the jaws (Gardner, 1980). They probably originate in the PDL or from the dental follicle of unerupted teeth (Gardner, 1980). They often contain strands of odontogenic epithelium, dysplastic dentine, cementum-like material, or acellular calcific deposits (*Fig. 17.7*). Peripheral extraosseous variants limited to the soft tissue of the gingiva may occur (Slabbert and Altini, 1991), and diffuse rather than localized forms of these lesions associated with ocular and skin lesions have now been described (Weber *et al.*, 1992). The status of peripheral odontogenic fibroma as a hamartoma or an odontogenic neoplasm is in dispute (Slabbert and Altini, 1991).

The histogenesis of radiolucent fibrous tumours of the jaws lacking any odontogenic epithelium or dental hard tissues is open to question, although they have been classified as odontogenic because of their location in the tooth-bearing segment of the jaws.

ODONTOGENIC MYXOMA

These are radiolucent tumours of the jaw, usually involving the mandible (*Fig. 17.8*), but occasionally involving or even confined to soft tissues of the gingiva (*Fig. 17.9*). Their characteristic histological feature (*Fig. 17.10*) is of fibroblasts and myofibroblasts widely dispersed in abundant deposits of glycosaminoglycans in the stroma. Those tumours with a significant content of collagen have been called myxofibromas. Odontogenic myxomas have a reputation for being locally aggressive. It has been proposed that jaw myxomas are derived from pulpal ectomesenchyme of developing teeth. However, myxomas express only vimentin whereas the mesenchymal cells of tooth germs contain both S-100 and vimentin (Lombardi *et al.*, 1992).

FIBROMATOSES AND FIBROUS HISTIOCYTOMA

This group of fibrous tissue proliferations occurs particularly in children and young people (Stout, 1953, 1954). One characteristic is their tendency to occur at specific sites, such as desmoids in the rectus abdominis, retroperitoneal fibrosis, Dupuytren's contracture of the palmar fascia, and fibromatosis colli in the neck. They have been subdivided into benign reactive fibrous lesions, such as fibrous histiocytoma, fibrous proliferations of childhood, desmoid tumours, and fibrosarcoma (Enzinger and Weiss, 1983).

FIBROUS HISTIOCYTOMA

Some of the fibrous histiocytomas presenting as a central radiolucent swelling in the jaws may arise from the PDL . The collagen bundles are typically arranged in a storiform (matted) pattern, and histiocytes and giant cells may also be present. Malignant fibrous histiocytomas are distinguished by their rapid growth and tendency to local recurrence, and they may metastasize via the bloodstream (i.e. behaving like a sarcoma) (O'Brien and Stout, 1964; Van Hale *et al.*, 1981; Amornman *et al.*, 1991). The tumours are derived from a fibroblast or primitive mesenchymal stem cell. Some cells may subsequently express some features of histiocytes (Fletcher, 1987).

Tumours of the jaws with abundant collagen and cytologically uniform fibroblasts with normal mitoses are identical to the desmoplastic fibromas (desmoid tumours of bone) that are found in other parts of the skeleton. They have a reputation for local infiltration and recurrence unless adequately resected (Vally and Altini, 1990; Kwon *et al.*, 1989). They must be distinguished from well-differentiated fibrosarcomas, which have metastatic potential (Dahlin, 1967; de Vito *et al.*, 1989).

FIBROSARCOMA

With the recognition as distinct entities of such conditions as fibrous histiocytoma, fasciitis, and fibromatosis, fibrosarcomas are now much less frequently diagnosed (Eversole *et al.*, 1973). They may arise within the jaw bone, particularly in the mandible (Eversole *et al.*, 1973), generally as a slowly growing swelling, which initially is often painless. Later the teeth become mobile and the mucosa is ulcerated. Some of these tumours may arise in the PDL . Fibrosarcomas of the gingiva may be purely soft tissue lesions presenting as an epulis without resorption of the alveolar bone (O'Day *et al.*, 1964; Fletcher and Crabb, 1961; Mellor and Wood, 1982). Compared with those at other sites, fibrosarcomas of the jaws seldom metastasize, but when they do it is usually to the lungs, and at a late stage (Reade and Radden, 1966; MacFarlane, 1972).

NERVE SHEATH TUMOURS

Although the PDL is richly innervated (see Chapter 7), true neuromas do not seem to have been reported. Nerve sheath tumours such as the neurilemmoma and neurofibroma occur in the gingivae, however, and they sometimes involve the PDL, though often only secondarily.

Neurilemmoma (Schwannoma)

These are usually solitary, except occasionally in neurofibromatosis when multiple neurilemmomas may occur. Periodontal tumours are usually located in the gingiva, rather than in the PDL. Typically they are circumscribed neoplasms with a defined fibrous capsule, and they exhibit a histological spectrum varying between Antoni A type, in which the nuclei of the Schwann cells are aligned in parallel rows, to Antoni B where there is a more pleomorphic population of randomly distributed cells (Hatziotis and Asprides, 1967). The Schwann cells are immunoreactive for S-100 protein.

Neurofibroma

These present either as benign solitary lesions or as multiple tumours as part of an inheritable neurofibromatosis. The neurofibromatoses are a family of generalized proliferations of nerve sheath elements, and the genes responsible have been identified (Riccardi, 1990). The commonest, type 1 (von Recklinghausen's disease of nerves), is due to an autosomal dominant gene with varied expressivity, and has an incidence of between 1 in 2000 and 1 in 4000. The mouth is affected in approximately 4–7 per cent of cases (Preston *et al.*, 1952). A mutation involving a 285 base-pair Alu sequence has been detected on chromosome 17 (Wallace *et al.*, 1991).

Solitary neurofibromas may form an epulis (Walker, 1993) or, in neurofibromatosis, they may present as small gingival tumours. They are sometimes noted as a chance radiographic finding of widening of the inferior dental canal or its mental branch or as a radiolucency around the crowns of buried teeth (Langford and Rippin, 1990).

GIANT CELL GRANULOMAS

These occur more commonly as peripheral giant cell granulomas within soft tissue as an epulis. The giant cell epulis is a reddish-purple solitary swelling of the gingiva, often with superimposed ulceration or bleeding when traumatized. The incidence is highest in the fourth decade and there is an excess of female patients (Cooke, 1952).

Central giant cell granulomas are less frequently found than giant cell epulides, and they present as an intra-osseous radiolucent expansion of the jaw (*Fig. 17.11*).

Giant cell granulomas are vascular proliferations with focal aggregations of multinucleated cells, stromal cells and collagen fibres (*Fig. 17.12*). Haemorrhage and haemosiderin deposits are frequent. In more mature lesions osteoid or woven bone are deposited by osteoblasts (Flanagan *et al.*, 1988) that contain alkaline phosphatase.

The aetiology and significance of giant cell granulomas remain controversial. The haemosiderin deposits or erythrocytes, found in the stroma and sometimes also observed intracellularly in the multinucleated giant cells, suggested a traumatic origin to some earlier authors (Cooke, 1952; Bernier and Cahn, 1954; Bhaskar *et al.*, 1971; Thompson *et al.*, 1983). It was alternatively hypothesized that the lesions were reactive, stimulated by plaque and calculus. The giant cells might be formed by the fusion of histiocytes (Cooke, 1952; Pepler, 1958), endothelial cells (Sapp, 1972), fibroblasts (Bartel and Piatowska, 1977), pericytes (Andersen *et al.*, 1973) or myofibroblasts.

Giant cells cultured in explants have the functional properties of osteoclasts in that they can excavate bone *in vitro*. Consistent with this, they have the appropriate phenotypic membrane calcitonin receptors (Flanagan *et al.*, 1988), which the stromal cells lack. Flanagan *et al.* (1988) also suggested that the osteoblast cells containing alkaline phosphatase, forming woven bone in the granulomas, could provide a signal, inducing giant cell infiltration of the lesions.

At the usual stage of presentation, however, it is usually impossible to determine exactly where central giant cell granulomas begin, and the proportion of these jaw lesions that is derived from the PDL remains undetermined. Earlier theories suggested ingeniously that the giant cells might be derived from periodontal osteoclasts that have remained after physiological resorption of primary teeth, but osteoclasts, like any other cell, have a finite life and the notion seems improbable. Curettage or local excision of the central giant granulomas is recommended and is also the recommended treatment for any recurrences. Wide resection is unnecessary.

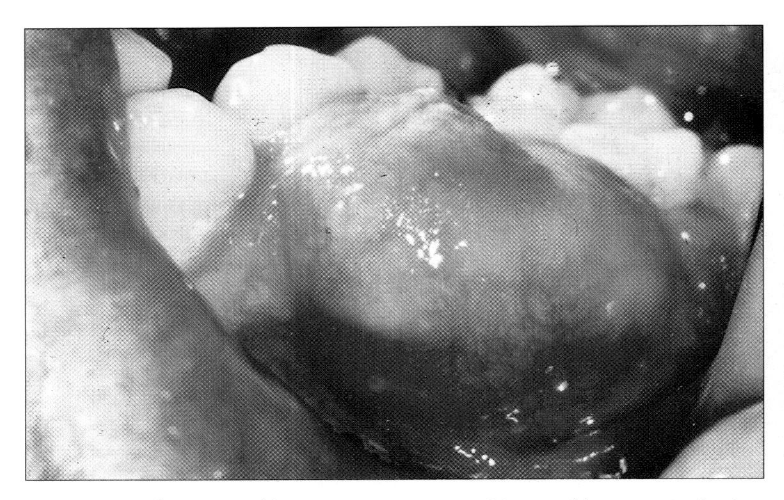

Fig. 17.5 Odontogenic fibroma presenting in a 28-year-old man as a slowly-expanding lesion of the left side of the mandible and buccal gingiva. There is superficial surface ulceration due to trauma from the opposing maxillary teeth.

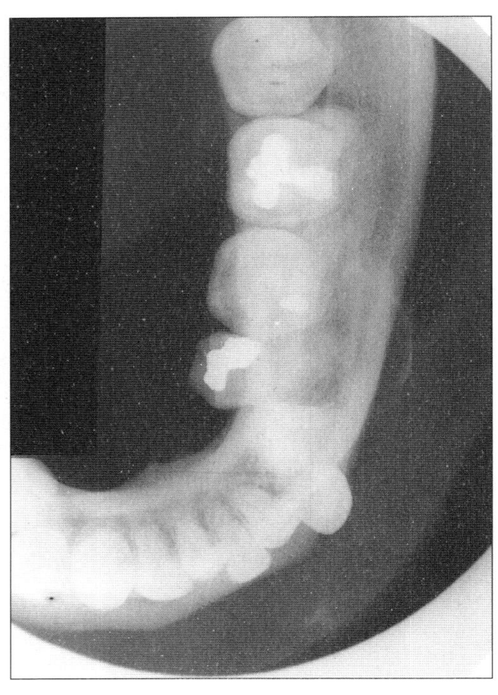

Fig. 17.6 Radiograph of same patient as in *Fig. 17.5*, showing buccal expansion of the mandible by the radiolucent odontogenic fibroma.

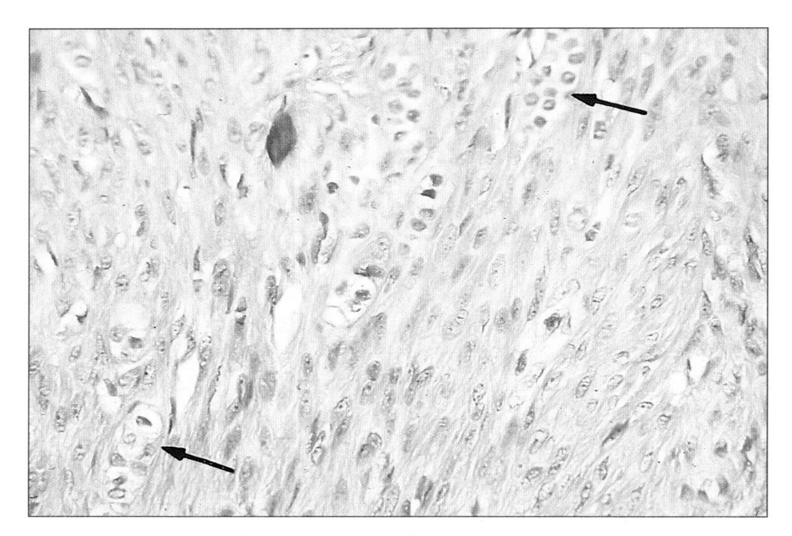

Fig. 17.7 Histology of the odontogenic fibroma in *Figs 17.5 and 17.6*. Moderately cellular bundles of collagen have been deposited, containing a cellular haematoxyphil calcific deposit and clusters of odontogenic epithelium (arrows). (Haematoxylin and eosin x 250.)

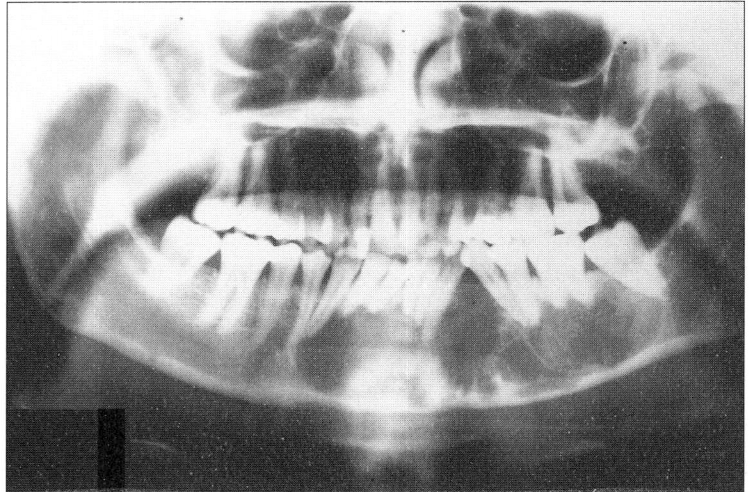

Fig. 17.8 Odontogenic myxoma of the mandible, presenting as a central radiolucency with displacement of teeth, characteristically subdivided by coarse bone trabeculae resulting in a multilocular appearance.

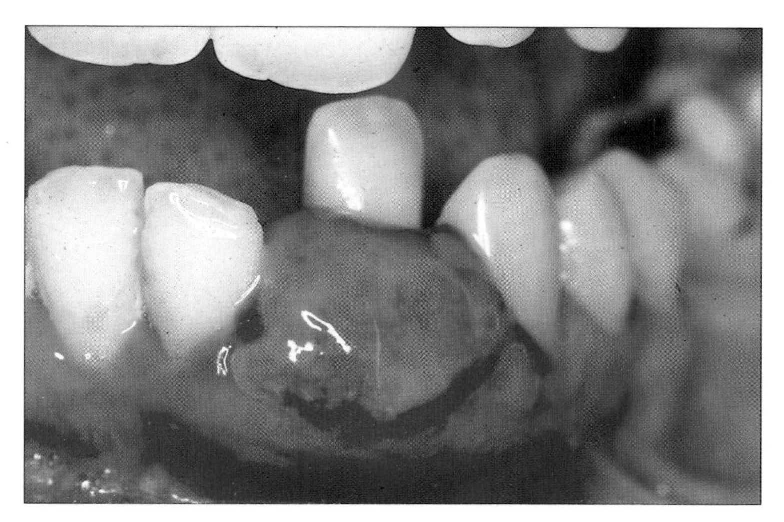

Fig. 17.9 An odontogenic myxoma with involvement of the gingiva.

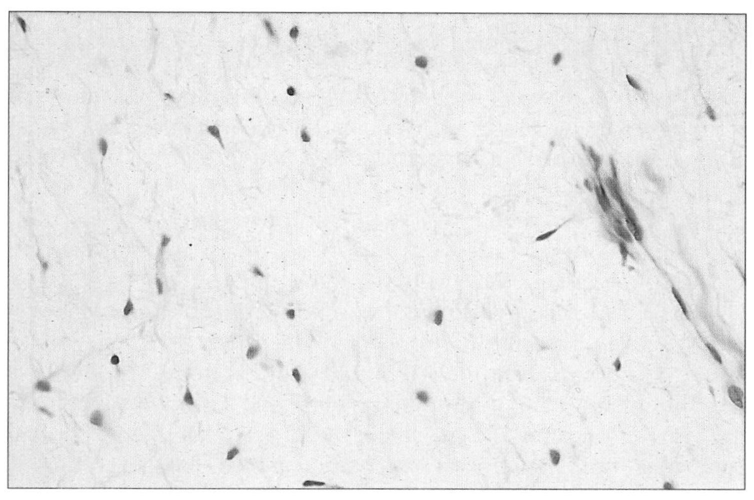

Fig. 17.10 Histological appearances in an odontogenic myxoma. The spindle-shaped cells are widely separated in a myxomatous matrix. (Haematoxylin and eosin x 250.)

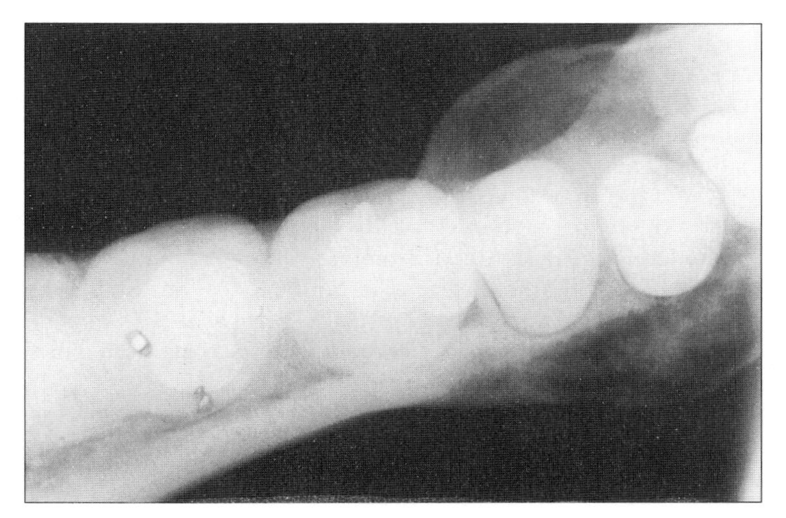

Fig. 17.11 A central giant cell granuloma presenting as a radiolucent mandibular swelling, causing buccal and lingual enlargement.

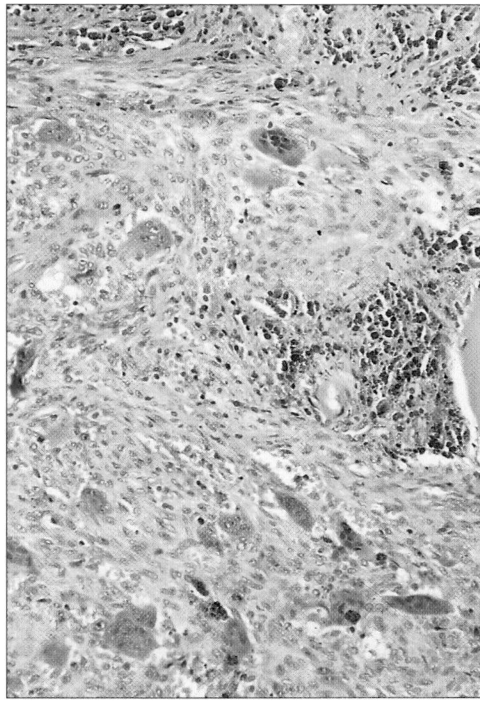

Fig. 17.12 Microscopic findings in a central giant cell granuloma. There are multinuclear giant cells, round or polygonal stromal cells, haemosiderin deposits and residual trabeculae of lamellar bone. (Haematoxylin and eosin x 125.)

CONGENITAL EPULIS

The congenital epulis (congenital gingival granular cell tumour) of the newborn occurs as a pedunculated swelling of the gum pads that is noted at birth or shortly after (Henefer *et al.*, 1979). It is usually situated in the midline or incisor regions of the maxilla, although similar swellings have been reported in the lower jaw. Multiple lesions are also on record. Females are more often affected than males. The swelling seems painless.

Microscopically, the congenital epulis has much in common with the granular cell tumour, the so-called myoblastoma, which usually occurs in adult life (Herschfus and Wolter, 1970; Bernier and Thompson, 1946). Although the overlying stratified squamous gingival epithelium is unremarkable and lacks the epithelial hyperplasia of the mucosa overlying the granular cell tumour, both lesions feature solid masses of large rounded, or polyhedral cells with abundant eosinophilic granules in their cytoplasm. Interstitial spindle-shaped or polygonal cells may also be found. Mitotic activity is uncommon. Patients who have had both lesions are on record (Dixter *et al.*, 1975). Although it might seem reasonable to suppose that the congenital epulis and the granular cell tumour are analogous (Bernier and Thompson, 1946) even though they occur at different sites, the different age spectrum has yet to be explained.

The histogenesis of these rare lesions is still being researched. It was initially thought that the congenital epulis was derived from pulpal mesenchymal cells or odontogenic epithelium. Immunocytochemistry of the granular cells detected neurone-specific enolase and vimentin but they reacted negatively for S-100. From this evidence and from ultrastructural evidence, it was postulated that they may be nerve-related mesenchymal cells (Tucker *et al.*, 1990). The interstitial cells had neuroendocrine characteristics in that they were positive for S-100 protein, cytokeratin, vimentin, and neurone-specific enolase (Takahashi *et al.*, 1990).

The behaviour of the congenital epulis mirrors that of granular cell tumours elsewhere in the mouth in that it does not recur after excision and may regress spontaneously (Jenkins and Hill, 1989).

TUMOURS OF CEMENTUM AND ALLIED LESIONS

Except when applied to the roots of teeth, cementum is difficult to distinguish from bone and indeed may be regarded as a specialized layer of thin bone applied to dentine. Although the pattern of collagen fibre arrangement in normal bone and cementum may differ, especially when viewed in polarized light, this difference may not be apparent in pathological states. This difficulty in differentiating cementum from bone particularly applies in hard-tissue lesions in the tooth-bearing segment of the jaws – the problem is implicit in the use of terms such as cemento-ossifying fibroma (Kramer *et al.*, 1992). More recently, cells have been cultured from explants of tumours of human cementum, which proved capable of synthesizing cementum-like attachment proteins (Arzate *et al.*, 1992). A more reliable classification of this group of tumours may result from this approach.

The second challenge is in distinguishing cemental neoplasms, such as benign cementoblastomas and cemento-ossifying fibromas, from cemental dysplasias, such as periapical cemental dysplasia and florid cemento-osseous dysplasia.

TUMOURS OF CEMENTUM

Benign cementoblastoma

More than half of these tumours of PDL elements occur in the first two decades of life. They are commoner in males than females. Typically the cementoblastoma forms a knob-like swelling fused to the roots of a mandibular premolar or permanent first molar (Eversole *et al.*, 1973; Abrams *et al.*, 1974; Corio *et al.*, 1976; Schneider and Bise, 1990). Early lesions may be detected as an asymptomatic radiolucency as an incidental x-ray finding (*Fig. 17.13*). Eventually a swelling of the jaw is noticed, characteristically accompanied by pain (Forsslund *et al.*, 1988). The tooth root is partly replaced by a mass of calcified cementum containing cementocytes, often with prominent reversal lines (*Fig. 17.14*). The periphery has radially aligned columns of the mineralized tissue, an incompletely mineralized outer layer ('cementoid') and a cellular peripheral rim of fibrous tissue containing cementoblasts. There are similarities between this lesion and an osteoid osteoma or an osteoblastoma (Slootweg, 1992), but the situation of the cementoblastoma attached to the roots of the teeth – and often partly replacing them – and a fine fibrillar birefringent pattern of cementum viewed under polarized light is sufficiently distinctive (Giansanti, 1970). Antibodies to cementum-derived attachment proteins (Arzate *et al.*, 1992) might be also useful in distinguishing the cementoblastoma from allied bone tumours.

The progressive growth of many benign cementoblastomas is consistent with their classification as odontogenic tumours, although documented recurrences after attempts at excision are uncommon.

Cemento-ossifying fibroma

The difficulty in differentiating between cementum or bone is acknowledged in the current WHO nomenclature of odontogenic tumours (Kramer *et al.*, 1992). It is suggested that primitive cells in the PDL have the potential of differentiating into pre-osteoblasts, pre-fibroblasts, and pre-cementoblasts (Sciubba and Younai, 1989). Cemento-ossifying fibromas occur as solitary lesions with a central radio-opacity and a radiolucent periphery. They are usually found in the molar or premolar region of the jaws, more often the mandible than the maxilla, usually in middle age, as an expanding swelling. Histologically, roughly spherical, calcified deposits of cementum are seen in fibrous tissue; these deposits fuse to form coarser masses in the centre of the tumour. Dentine has also recently been identified in essentially similar lesions (Burkhardt, 1989).

Management by excision usually gives a satisfactory outcome.

CEMENTO-OSSEOUS DYSPLASIAS

Periapical cemental dysplasia

This is generally agreed to be a non-progressive, non-neoplastic change occurring as multiple periapical radiolucencies that subsequently mineralize. The condition is generally associated with mandibular incisor teeth in middle-aged women (Stafne, 1934; Vegh, 1976).

Florid cemento-osseous dysplasia (gigantiform cementoma)

Initially termed gigantiform cementomas, these have been redesignated florid cemento-osseous dysplasia, following the account of florid osseous dysplasia, a similar or identical condition, by Melrose and co-workers (Melrose *et al.*, 1976). They present as multiple swellings of the jaws, with a bilateral distribution, in upper or lower jaw (Punnia-Moorthy, 1980). The condition is most often found in middle-aged black females in the USA. In plain radiographs, the irregular opaque masses are not surrounded by a radiolucent rim, a point of difference from the cemento-ossifying fibroma. Histologically, there are cellular masses of cementum in a sparse fibrous stroma (Thompson and Altini, 1989). Although the lesions may gradually become more extensive, their multifocal and symmetrical distribution are more in keeping with a generalized dysplasia of cementum or bone than a neoplastic change. Some cases are familial.

TUMOURS OF BONE

OSTEOMA

Most osteomas of the jaws are subperiosteal, forming a slowly enlarging hard protruberance covered by normal mucosa. Those that originate from the osteoblasts of the PDL as central osteomas seem rare. They must be distinguished from non-neoplastic masses of bone, including idiopathic bone sclerosis, fibrous dysplasia, chronic sclerosing osteomyelitis, and cemental tumours.

The multiple osteomas in the jaws in Gardner's syndrome (Gardner, 1962) may be central or peripheral. Osteomas or cementomas continuous with the roots of molar teeth may be a feature. The gene responsible for this spectrum of manifestations – familial adenomatous polyposis syndrome involving premalignant polyps of the large bowel, skin tumours, osteomas, and epidermal cysts – has been localized to chromosome 5 (Bodmer *et al.*, 1987).

OSTEOSARCOMA

Malignant primary tumours of bone are infrequent compared with secondary metastases to the skeleton. A radiological appearance of a symmetrical widening of the PDL space, displacement and loosening of the associated teeth, rapid swelling of the jaw, and eventual ulceration of the overlying mucosa is typical of an osteosarcoma involving the PDL (Gardner and Mills, 1976) (*Figs 17.15, 17.16, 17.17*).

Formation of osteoid by malignant osteoblasts is the key histopathological finding. Osteosarcomas are less common in the jaws than in other bones, and they present approximately 10 years later than extragnathic tumours (Garrington *et al.*, 1967). Metastases to the lungs and other sites are less frequent than from osteosarcomas arising in other sites in the skeleton, and they occur later in the natural history of the malignancy.

SECONDARY TUMOURS

About 1 per cent of oral malignancies are metastatic deposits (Goveia and Bahn, 1978; Fantasia and Chen, 1979; El-Dibany *et al.*, 1984; Dahl *et al.*, 1981; Zachariades, 1989) and the primary tumour is usually situated below the level of the clavicles (Hartman *et al.*, 1973; de-Padua-Bertelli *et al.*, 1970; Mace, 1978; Adler, 1973; Cherry and Glass, 1977; Hatziotis *et al.*, 1973; Angelopoulos *et al.*, 1972; Schofield, 1974; Levy and Smith, 1974; Mosby *et al.*, 1973), most frequently in the lungs, breast, kidney, adrenal glands, prostate, thyroid, gut, and uterus (Zachariades, 1989).

Metastatic tumours are the commonest malignancies of the skeleton (de-Padua-Bertelli *et al.*, 1970) and they are most commonly responsible for central malignant tumours of the jaws (Hartman *et al.*, 1973; Mace, 1978). They occur more often in the mandible, especially the angle and ascending ramus region, than in the maxilla. The preferential localization of metastases in the orofacial region to the region of the angle and ascending ramus of the mandible has been attributed to the persistence of red marrow at this site.

In comparison, the frequency of secondary tumours presenting in the oral and perioral soft tissues is low (Hatziotis *et al.*, 1973). The gingivae were involved in 15 per cent of reported cases of metastases to the mouth (Zachariades, 1989), slightly more frequently in the maxillary gingivae than in the mandibular gingivae.

To become established, however, a metastatic cell has to adhere to the vascular endothelium, penetrate the vessel wall, and then proliferate in its new milieu. It seems that a complex interaction between the metastatic cell and the local host tissues

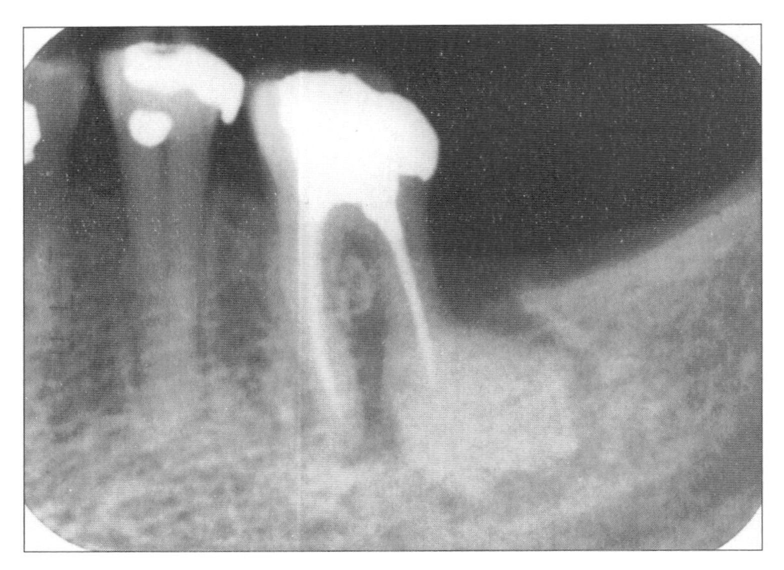

Fig. 17.13 Radiograph of benign cementoblastoma, appearing as a radiopaque mass fused to the root of a right mandibular molar. Endodontic treatment has been attempted. Secondary bacterial infection has supervened. The differential diagnosis included a focal sclerosing osteitis.

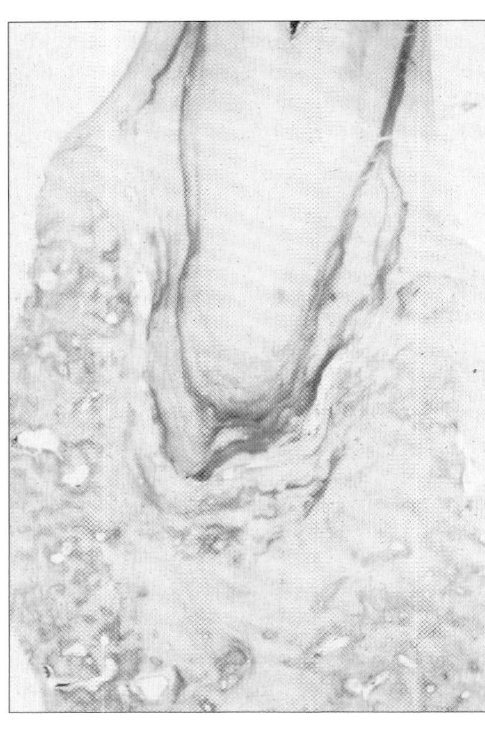

Fig. 17.14 Histological appearances of the same benign cementoblastoma as in *Fig. 17.13*. Sheets of cementum have been laid down, with reversal lines. There is evidence of bacterial infection. (Picrothionin x 30.)

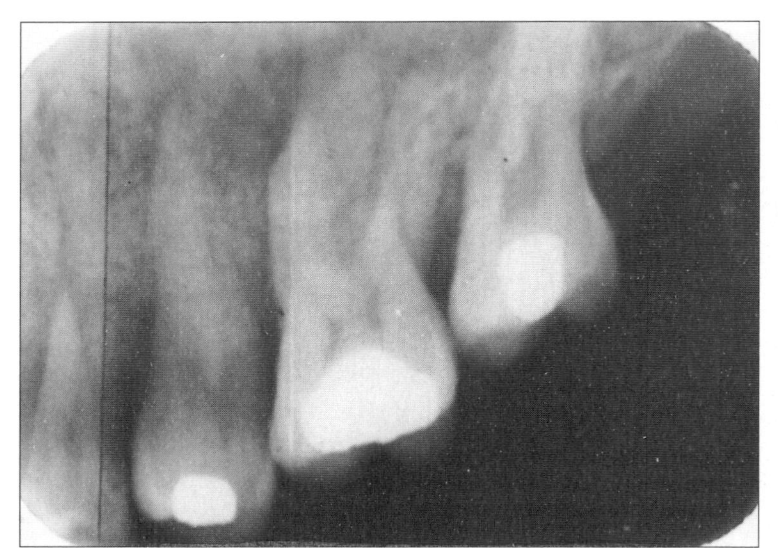

Fig. 17.15 Osteosarcoma of left maxilla in a 28-year-old man. Radiograph showing diffuse rarefaction of the alveolar bone, with widening of the molar periodontal ligament space.

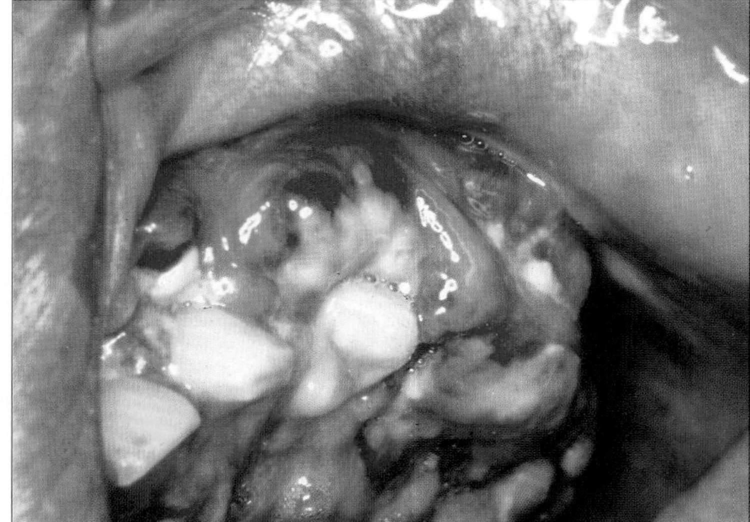

Fig. 17.16 Osteosarcoma of left maxilla. Same case as in *Fig. 17.15* following extraction of the molar teeth. The tumour has formed an ulcerated growth fungating from the sockets.

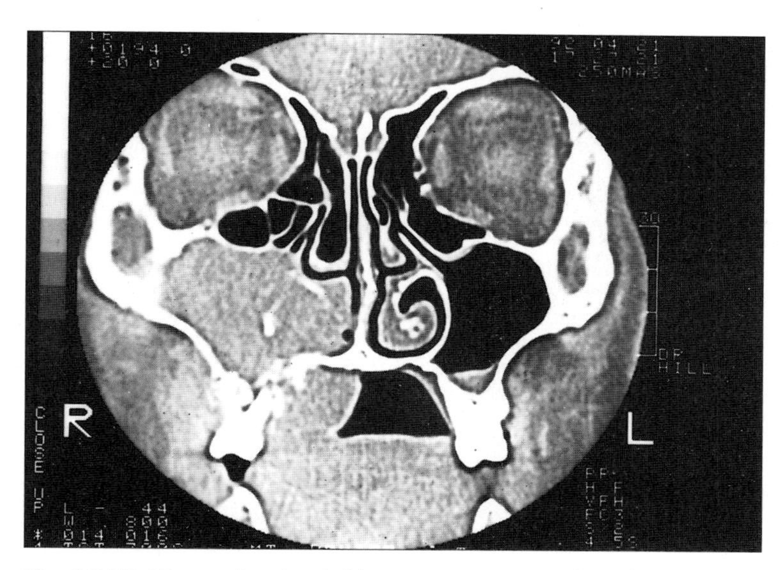

Fig. 17.17 CT scan of a chondroblastic osteosarcoma in the right maxilla in a 31-year-old male, presenting as a palatal swelling. The infiltrative tumour has eroded the floor, medial and lateral wall of the right antrum and the alveolar bone supporting the right maxillary molar.

(Evans, 1991) determines whether the tumour cell will lodge and then proliferate in the PDL .

Involvement of the PDL by secondary deposits has been observed from miscellaneous primary tumours (Zachariades, 1989; Ellis *et al.*, 1977) including carcinoma of the pancreas (Schofield, 1974) and lung (Cherry and Glass, 1977), adenocarcinoma of the colon (Levy and Smith, 1974), malignant melanoma (Mosby *et al.*, 1973; Adatia, 1982), choriocarcinoma (Bakeen *et al.*, 1976), retinoblastoma (Zegarelli, 1976), hepatocellular carcinoma (Yacabucci *et al.*, 1972), and multiple myeloma (Ozaki and Yamanaka, 1988).

Malignant lymphoma of either Hodgkin's type (Forman and Wesson, 1969) or non-Hodgkin's type (Adatia, 1982; Mittelman and Kaban, 1976) involving the jaws may occur. However, Burkitt's lymphoma is unusual in its predilection for the jaws, and Adatia (1982) has described loosening of the teeth in African children, with loss of the lamina–dura radiographic appearance. The PDL is infiltrated by the lymphoma spreading between the collagen fibres. Although teeth may be displaced, the PDL attachment to cementum, bone or gingivae may be retained until a late stage. Teeth may regain their usual position, and tooth development may continue after successful cytotoxic drug therapy for the lymphoma.

In acute leukaemia, infiltration of the gingivae and PDL accompanied by enlargement, redness, or pain of the gums is relatively common (Stafford *et al.*, 1980).

KAPOSI'S SARCOMA

Until recently in the Western world, Kaposi's sarcoma was seen usually in elderly patients as an indolent benign purple skin eruption of the distal extremities. More recently, it has been reported associated with AIDS in a younger age group – particularly male homosexuals, infrequently in intravenous drug abusers and in affected women. Widespread disease with involvement of intra-abdominal viscera tends to follow.

Kaposi's sarcoma was reported as being present in as many as 36 per cent of male homosexuals with AIDS and, in 50 per cent or more of these patients, the lesions were oral or perioral (Marcusen and Sooy, 1985).

In the mouth, the palate, gingiva and tongue are most often affected (Pindborg *et al.*, 1988). Kaposi's sarcoma of the gingiva and PDL usually appears as an epulis, with displacement of teeth with radiological evidence of a widened PDL space and local bone destruction. More recent research suggests that Kaposi's sarcoma may be a reactive multifocal blood vessel proliferation in response to some angiogenic growth factor rather than a true malignancy (Bayley *et al.*, 1990).

REFERENCES

Abrams AM, Kirby JW and Melrose RJ (1974) Cementoblastoma. A clinical-pathologic study of seven new cases. Oral Surg 38, 394–403.

Adatia AK (1982) Neoplastic involvement of the periodontal ligament. In: The Periodontal Ligament in Health and Disease, Chapter 16, 1st Edition, pp. 359–371 (Berkovitz BK, Moxham BJ, Newman HN, eds). Pergamon Press, Oxford, New York.

Adler CI, Sotereanos GG, Valdiviesco JG (19730 Metastatic bronchogenic carcinoma to the maxilla: report of case. J Oral Surg 31, 543–546.

Amornman R, Prempree T and Perez RA (1991) Malignant fibrous histiocytoma of the gingiva. A clinicopathological study. J Fla Med Assoc 78, 149–152.

Andersen L, Arwill T, Feterskov O, Heyden G and Philipsen HP (1973) Oral giant cell granulomas: an enzyme histochemical and ultrastructural study. Acta Pathol Microbiol Scand (Section A) 81, 617–629.

Angelopoulos AP, Tilsn HB and Stewart FW (1972) Metastatic neuroblastoma of the mandible: review of the literature and report of case. J Oral Surg 30, 93–106.

Arzate H, Olson SW, Page RC and Narayanan AS (1992) Isolation of human tumor cells that produce cementum proteins in culture. Bone Miner 18, 15–30.

Bakeen G, Hiyarat AM and Al-Ubaidy SS (1976) Chorio-epithelioma presenting as a bleeding gingival mass. Oral Surg 41, 467–471.

Barker DS and Lucas RB (1967) Localised fibrous overgrowths of the oral mucosa. Brit J Oral Surg 5, 86–92.

Bartel H and Piatowska D (1977) Electron microscopic study of peripheral giant-cell reparative granuloma. Oral Surg 43, 82–96.

Batsakis JG, Hicks MJ, Flaitz CM (1993) Peripheral epithelial tumors. Ann Otol Rhinol Laryngol 102, 322–324.

Bayley AC and Lucas SB (1990) Kaposi's sarcoma or Kaposi's disease? A personal reappraisal. In: The Pathobiology of Tumours, Chapter 7 (Fletcher CDM and McKee PH, eds). Churchill Livingstone, Edinburgh.

Berghagen N, Bergstrom J and Valerius–Olsson H (1973) Adenomatoid odontogenic tumour. Periodontal aspects of diagnosis and treatment. Sven Tandlak Tidskr 66, 467–474.

Bernier JL and Thompson HC (1946) Myoblastoma. J Dent Res 25, 253–260.

Bernier JL and Cahn, LR (1954) The peripheral giant cell reparative granuloma. J Amer Dent Ass 49, 141–148.

Bhaskar SN, Cutright DE, Beasley JD and Perez B (1971) Giant cell reparative granuloma (peripheral): Report of 50 cases. J Oral Surg 29, 110–115.

Bodmer WF, Bailey CJ, Bodmer J, Bussy HJ, Ellis A, Gorman P, Lucibello FC, Murday VA, Rider SH, Scambler P, Sheer D, Solomon E and Spurr NK (1987) Localization of the gene for familial adenomatous polyposis on chromosome 5. Nature 328, 614–616.

Bredenkamp JK and Zimmerman MC (1989) Maxillary ameloblastoma. Arch Otolaryngol Head Neck Surg 115, 99–104.

Bucci E, Lo-Muzio L, Mignogna MD and de-Rosa G (1992) Peripheral ameloblastoma: case report. Acta Stomatol Belg 89, 267–269.

Buchner A, Merrell PW, Hansen LS and Leider AS (1991) Peripheral (extraosseous) calcifying odontogenic cyst: A review of forty-five cases. Oral Surg 72, 65–70.

Buchner A and Sciubba JJ (1987) Peripheral epithelial odontogenic tumours: a review. Oral Surg 63, 688–697.

Burkhardt A (1989) Dentin formation in so-called 'fibro-osteo-cemental' lesions of the jaw: histologic, electron microscopic & immuno-histochemical investigations. Oral Surg 68, 729–738.

Cherry CQ and Glass RT (1977) Large-cell carcinoma metastatic to the jaw. Oral Surg 44, 358–361.

Cooke BED (1952) The giant cell epulis: Histogenesis and natural history. Br Dent J 93, 13–16.

Corio RL, Crawford BE and Schaberg SJ (1976) Benign cementoblastoma. Oral Surg 41, 524–530.

Dahl EC, Synhorst JB and Lilly GE (1981) Gingival metastasis from a tracheal adenoid cystic carcinoma. J Oral Surg 39, 446–448.

Dahlin DC (1967) Bone tumors, 2nd Edition, pp.212–221. Charles C. Thomas, Springfield, Ill.

de Vito MA, Tom LWC, Boran TV and Quinn PD (1989) Desmoplastic fibroma of the mandible. Ear Nose Throat J 68, 553–556.

de-Padua-Bertelli AP, Queiroz-Costa F and Miziara JE (1970) Metastatic tumors of the mandible. Oral Surg 30, 21–28.

Dixter CT, Konstat MS, Giunta JL, Schreier E and White GE (1975) Congenital granular-cell tumor of alveolar ridge and tongue. Report of two cases. Oral Surg 40, 270–277.

Doyle JL, Grodjesk JE, Dolinsky HB and Rafel SS. Squamous odontogenic tumour: report of three cases. J Oral Surg 35, 994–996.

El-Beialy RR, El-Mofty S and Refai K (1990) Calcifying odontogenic cyst: case report and review of literature. J Oral Maxillofac Surg 48, 637–640.

El-Dibany MH, Azab AS and Kutty AS (1984) Breast carcinoma metastatic to the maxillary gingiva. J Oral Max-fac Surg 42, 459–461.

Ellis GL, Jensen JL, Reingold IM and Barr RJ (1977) Malignant neoplasms metastatic to gingivae. Oral Surg 44, 238–245.

Enzinger FM and Weiss SW (1983) Soft Tissue Tumors, pp15–70. CV Mosby, St Louis.

Evans CW (1991) The Metastatic Cell: Behaviour and Biochemistry, pp178–205. Chapman and Hall, London/New York.

Eversole LR, Sabes WR and Dauchess VG (1973) Benign cementoblastoma. Oral Surg 36, 824–830.

Eversole LR, Schwartz WD and Sabes WR (1973) Central and peripheral fibrogenic and neurogenic sarcoma of the oral region. Oral Surg 36, 49–62.

Fantasia JE and Chen L–C (1979) A testicular tumor with gingival metastasis. Oral Surg 48, 64–68.

Flanagan AM, Tinkler SM, Horton MA, Williams DM and Chambers TJ (1988) The multinucleate cells in giant cell granulomas of the jaw are osteoclasts. Cancer 62, 1139–1145.

Fletcher CDM (1987) Malignant fibrous histiocytoma. Histopathology 11, 433–437.

Fletcher JP and Crabb HSM (1961) Fibrosarcomatous epulis. Oral Surg 14, 1091–1098.

Forman GH and Wesson CM (1969) Hodgkin's disease of the mandible. Br J Oral Surg 7, 146–152.

Forsslund HG, Bodin I and Julin P (1988) Undiagnosed benign cementoblastoma in a patient with a 6-year pain condition. Oral Surg 66, 243–248.

Franklin CD and Pindborg JJ (1976) The calcifying epithelial odontogenic tumor. A review and analysis of 113 cases. Oral Surg 42, 753–765.

Fuchs EV, Coppock SM, Green H and Cleveland D (1981) Two distinct classes of keratin genes and their evolutionary significance. Cell 27, 75–84.

Gardner DG (1980) The central odontogenic fibroma: An attempt at clarification. Oral Surg 50, 425–432.

Gardner DG and Mills DM (1976) The widened periodontal ligament of osteosarcoma of the jaws. Oral Surg 41, 652–656.

Gardner EJ (1962) Follow-up study of a family group exhibiting dominant inheritance for a syndrome including intestinal polyps, osteomas, fibromas and epidermal cysts. Am J Hum Genet 14, 376–390.

Garrington GE, Scofield HH, Cornyn J and Hooker SP (1967) Osteosarcoma of the jaws. Analysis of 56 cases. Cancer 20, 377–391.

Giansanti JS (1970) The pattern and width of the collagen bundles in bone and cementum. Oral Surg 30, 508–514.

Gibson CW, Lally E, Herold RC, Decker S, Brinster RL and Sandgren EP (1992) Odontogenic tumors in mice carrying albumin-myc and albumin-ras transgenes. Calcif Tissue Int 51, 162–167.

Goveia G and Bahn S (1978) Asymptomatic hepato-cellular carcinoma metastatic to the mandible. Oral Surg 45, 424–430.

Hamner JE and Fullmer HM (1966) Oxytalan fibres in benign fibro-osseous jaw lesions. Arch Path 82, 35–39.

Hartman GL, Robertson GR, Sugg WE and Hiatt WR (1973) Metastatic carcinoma of the mandibular condyle: report of case. J Oral Surg 31, 716–717.

Hatziotiz JC and Asprides H (1967) Neurilemmoma (Schwannoma) of the oral cavity. Oral Surg 24, 510–526.

Hatziotis JC, Constantinidou H and Papanayotou PH (1973) Metastatic tumors of the oral soft tissues. Oral Surg 36, 544–550.

Heikinheimo K, Sandberg M, Happonen R–P, Virtanen I and Bosch FX (1991) Cytoskeletal gene expression in normal and neoplastic human odontogenic epithelia. Lab Invest 65, 688–701.

Henefer EP, Abaza NA and Anderson SP (1979) Congenital granular-cell epulis. Report of a case. Oral Surg 47, 515–518.

Hernandez G, Sanchez C, Caballero T and Moskow B (1992) A rare case of a multicentric peripheral ameloblastoma of the gingiva. A light and electron microscopic study. J Clin Periodontol 19, 281–287.

Herschfus L and Wolter JG (1970) Granular-cell myoblastoma of the oral cavity. Oral Surg 29, 341–352.

Hong SP, Ellis GL and Hartman KS (1991) Calcifying odontogenic cyst: a review of ninety-two cases with re-evaluation of their nature as cysts or neoplasms, the nature of ghost cells and subclassification. Oral Surg 72, 56–64.

Hopper TL, Sadeghi EM and Pricco, DF. Squamous odontogenic tumor: Report of a case with multiple lesions. Oral Surg 50, 404–410.

Jenkins HR and Hill CM (1989) Spontaneous regression of congenital epulis of the newborn. Arch Dis Child 64, 145–147.

Kramer IRH, Pindborg JJ and Shear M (1992) International Histological Classification of Tumours No. 5. Histological Typing of Odontogenic Tumours, Jaw Cysts and Allied Lesions. World Health Organization. Springer-Verlag, Berlin.

Kwon PHJ, Horswell BB and Gatto DJ (1989) Desmoplastic fibroma of the jaws: Surgical management and review of the literature. Head Neck 11, 67–75.

Langford RJ and Rippin JW (1990) Bilateral intra-osseous neurofibroma of the mandible. Br J Oral Max-Fac Surg 28, 344–346.

Levy B and Smith WK (1974) A jaw metastasis from the colon. Oral Surg 38, 769–772.

Lombardi T, Samson J, Bernard JP, Di-Felice R, Fiore-Donna G, Mulhausser J, Maggiano N (1992) Comparative immunohistochemical analysis between jaw myxoma and mesenchymal cells of tooth germ. Pathol Res Pract 188, 141–144.

Mace MC (1978) Condylar metastasis from mammary adenocarcinoma. Brit J Oral Surg 15, 227–230.

MacFarlane WI (1972) Fibrosarcoma of the mandible with pulmonary metastases. Br J Oral Surg 10, 168–174.

Marcusen DC and Sooy CD (1985) Otolaryngolic and head and neck manifestations of acquired immunodeficiency syndrome. Laryngoscope 95(4), 401–5.

Mellor TK and Wood GD (1982) Fibrosarcoma presenting as an epulis. Br Dent J 153, 67–69.

Melrose RJ, Abrams AM and Mills BG (1976) Florid osseous dysplasia. A clinical-pathologic study of 34 cases. Oral Surg 41, 62–82.

Mittelman D and Kaban LB (1976) Recurrent non-Hodgkin's lymphoma presenting with gingival enlargement. Report of a case. Oral Surg 42, 792–800.

Moll R, Franke WW, Schiller DL, Geiger B and Krepler R (1982) The catalog of human cytokeratins: patterns of expression in normal epithelia, tumors and cultured cells. Cell 31, 11–24.

Mori M, Yamada K, Kasai T, Yamada T, Shimokawa H and Sasaki S (1991) Immunohistochemical expression of amelogenins in odontogenic epithelial tumours and cysts. Virchow's Archiv. A. Path Anat Histopathol 418, 319–325.

Mosby EL, Sugg WE and Hiatt WR (1973) Gingival and pharyngeal metastasis from a malignant melanoma. Report of a case. Oral Surg 36, 6–10.

Nauta JM, Panders AK, Schoots CJ, Vermey A, Roodenburg JL (1992) Peripheral ameloblastoma. A case report and review of the literature. Int J Oral Maxillofacial Surg 21, 40–44.

O'Brien JE and Stout AP (1964) Malignant fibrous xanthoma. Cancer 17, 1445–1455.

O'Day RA, Soule EK and Gores RJ (1964) Soft tissue sarcomas of the oral cavity. Mayo Clin Proc 39, 1069–1081.

Ozaki M and Yamanaka H (1988) A case of IgD myeloma with extraosseous spread to the gingiva. Oral Surg 65, 726–730.

Pepler WJ (1958) The histochemistry of giant cell tumours, osteoclastoma and giant cell epulides. J Path Bact 76, 505–510.

Philipsen HP, Reichart PA, Zhang KH, Nikai H and Yu QX (1991) Adenomatoid odontogenic tumour: Biologic profile based on 499 cases. J Oral Pathol Med 20,149–158.

Pindborg JJ (1955) Calcifying epithelial odontogenic tumours. Acta Path Microbiol Scand Suppl. 111, 71(Abs).

Pindborg JJ (1958) A calcifying epithelial odontogenic tumour. Cancer 11, 838–843.

Pindborg, JJ. The calcifying epithelial odontogenic tumor. Review of the literature and report of an extra-osseous case. Acta Odont Scand 1966;24:419–430.

Pindborg, JJ, Schiodt, M & Holmstrup, P. Oral lesions in patients with HIV infection. World Health Organisation Collaborative Centre for Oral Manifestations of the Human Immunodeficiency Virus, 1988.

Preston FW, Walsh WS and Clarke TH (1952) Cutaneous neurofibromatosis (von Recklinghausen's disease): Clinical manifestations and incidence of sarcoma in 61 male patients. Arch Surg 64, 813–827.

Pullon PA, Shafer WG, Elzay RP, Kerr DA and Corio RL (1975) Squamous odontogenic tumor: Report of six cases of a previously undescribed lesion. Oral Surg 40, 616–630.

Punnia-Moorthy A (1980) Gigantiform cementoma: review of the literature and a case report. Br J Oral Surg 18, 221–229.

Raubenheimer EJ, van-Heerden WF, Sitzmann F and Heymer B (1992) Peripheral dentinogenic ghost cell tumor. J Oral Pathol Med 21, 93–95.

Reade PC and Radden BG (1966) Oral fibrosarcoma. Oral Surg 22, 217–225.

Reichart PA and Philipsen HP (1990) Squamous odontogenic tumor. J Oral Pathol Med 19, 226–228.

Riccardi VM (1990) Neurofibromatosis. In Konnard, C (Ed) Recent Advances in Clinical Neurology, pp.187–208. Churchill Livingstone, London.

Saku T, Okabe H, Shimokawa H (1992) Immunohistochemical demonstration of enamel proteins in odontogenic tumors. J Oral Pathol Med 21, 113–119.

Sapp JP (1972) The ultrastructure and histogenesis of peripheral giant cell reparative granuloma of the jaws. Cancer 30, 1119–1129.

Schneider MS and Bise RN (1990) Cementoma: presentation predicates approach. J Cranio Fac Surg 1, 143–146.

Schofield JJ (1974) Oral metastatic deposit from carcinoma of the head of the pancreas. Br Dent J 137, 553–356.

Sciubba JJ and Younai F (1989) Ossifying fibroma of the mandible. J Oral Pathol Med 18, 315–321.

Shear M (1969) Primary intra-alveolar epidermoid carcinoma of the jaw. J Pathol 97, 645–651.

Shore RC, Moxham BJ and Berkovitz BKB (1984) Oxytalan fibres in the periodontal ligament. INSERM 125, 565–572.

Shrestha P, Yamada K, Higashiyama H, Takagi H and Mori M (1992) Epidermal growth factor receptor in odontogenic cysts and tumors. J Oral Pathol Med 21, 314–317.

Shteyer A, Lustmann NJ and Lewin-Epstein J (1978) The mural ameloblastoma: a review of the literature. J Oral Surg 36, 866–872.

Slabbert H de V, Altini M (1991) Peripheral odontogenic fibroma: A clinicopathologic study. Oral Surg 72, 86–90.

Slootweg PJ (1992) Cementoblastoma and osteoblastoma: a comparison of histologic features. J Oral Pathol Med 21, 385–389.

Small IA and Waldron CA (1955) Ameloblastomas of the jaws. Oral Surg 8, 281–297.

Snead ML, Luo W, Hsu DD-J, Melrose RJ, Lau EC and Syenman G (1992) Human ameloblastoma tumors express the amelogenin gene. Oral Surg 74, 64–72.

Stafford R, Sonis S, Lockhart P and Sonis A (1980) Oral pathoses as diagnostic indicators in leukemia. Oral Surg 50, 134–139.

Stafne, EC. Periapical osteofibrosis with formation of cementomas. J Amer Dent Ass 1934;21:1822–1829.

Stout AP (1953) Tumours of the Soft Tissues. Atlas of Tumour Pathology Section 2 Fascicle 5. Armed Forces Institute of Pathology, Washington, DC.

Stout AP (1954) Juvenile fibromatoses. Cancer 7, 953–978.

Sun, T-T, Tseng SCG, Huang A, Cooper D, Schermer A, Lynch MH, Weiss R, Eichner R (1985) Monoclonal antibody studies of mammalian epithelial keratins: a review. Ann NY Acad Sci 455, 307–329.

Takahashi H, Fujita S, Satoh H and Okabe H (1990) Immunohistochemical study of congenital gingival granular cell tumor (congenital epulis). J Oral Pathol Med 19, 492–496.

Tatemoto Y, Okada Y and Mori M (1989) Squamous odontogenic tumor: Immunohistochemical identification of keratins. Oral Surg 67, 63–67.

Thesleff I (1987) Epithelial cell rests of Malassez bind epidermal growth factor intensely. J Periodont Res 22, 419–421.

Thompson SH, Bischoff P and Bender S (1983) Central giant cell granuloma of the mandible. J Oral Maxillo-Fac Surg 41, 743–746.

Thompson SH and Altini M (1989) Gigantiform cementoma of the jaws. Head Neck 11, 538–544.

Tucker MC, Rusnock EJ, Azumi N, Hoy GR and Lack EE (1990) Gingival granular cell tumors of the newborn: an ultrastructural and immunohistochemical study. Arch Pathol Lab Med 114, 895–898.

Vally IM and Altini HM (1990) Fibromatoses of the oral & paraoral soft tissues and jaws. Oral Surg 69, 191–198.

Van Hale HMcM, Handlers JP, Abrams AM and Strams G (1981) Malignant fibrous histiocytoma, myxoid variant metastatic to the oral cavity. Report of a case and review of the literature. Oral Surg 51, 165–163.

Vegh T (1976) Multiple cementomas (periapical cemental dysplasia). Report of a case. Oral Surg 42, 404–406.

Veno S, Mushimoto K and Shirasu R (1989) Prognostic evaluation of ameloblastoma based on histological & radiographic typing. J Oral Maxillofacial Surg 47, 11–15.

Walker DM (1993) Periodontal neoplasia. In: Diseases of the Periodontium, Chapter 4, pp 135–169. Science Reviews Ire, in press (Newman HN, ReesTD and KinaneDF,eds).

Wallace MR, Andersen LB, Saulino AM, Gregory PE, Glover TW and Collins FS (1991) A *de novo Alu* insertion results in neurofibromatosis type 1. Nature 353, 864–866.

Weber A, van Heerden WF, Ligthelm AJ, Raubenheimer EJ (1992) Diffuse peripheral odontogenic fibroma: report of 3 cases. J Oral Pathol Med 21, 82–84.

Wright BA and Jennings EH (1979) Oxytalan fibres in peripheral odontogenic fibromas. A histochemical study of eighteen cases. Oral Surg 48, 451–453.

Yacabucci E, Mainous EG and Kramer HS (1972) Hepatocellular carcinoma, diagnosed following metastasis to the mandible. Oral Surg 33, 888–893.

Zachariades N (1989) Neoplasms metastatic to the mouth, jaws and surrounding tissues. J Cranio Max-Fac Surg 17, 283–290.

Zegarelli DJ (1976) Primary and metastatic intraoral carcinoma. NY State Dent J 42, 478–481.

Chapter 18

Periodontal Ligament Features in Blood and Lymphoreticular Disorders

DF Kinane, RM Browne

INTRODUCTION

The periodontal ligament (PDL) is a vascular tissue with a significant proportion of its volume made up of blood and lymph vessels and their contents. The circulation of large numbers of red and white blood cells within the PDL is a significant feature, as disorders of these cells will lead to a disruption of the PDL and so normal periodontal function will be lost. In many instances such effects are functional rather than morphological, and thus no overt changes are demonstrable. In a number of disorders, however, the PDL may exhibit clinical or microscopical changes, and it is likely that most of these changes would occur secondarily to two other events.

Firstly, epidemiological studies have established that gingivitis is almost universally present in children and additionally that by the age of 15 years many have lost some bone around one or more teeth. The prevalence and severity of periodontitis increases steadily throughout life and is a prominent cause of tooth loss after 30 years of age. During simple gingival inflammation and in the more advanced lesions of chronic periodontitis, one of the most prominent histopathological changes is the dense leucocyte infiltration in gingival tissues and in close proximity to the coronal portion of the PDL. These cells include the omnipresent polymorphonuclear leucocytes and the lymphocytes, macrophages, and plasma cells, the latter being characteristic of chronic inflammation (*Fig. 18.1*). These leucocytes are crucial to the tissues' ability to respond to the variety of challenges made on them from the microbes of the subgingival plaque. These toxic, antigenic, and chemical insults affect both the immune and inflammatory systems, which are intricately linked and interdependent on each other. These are crucial systems and thus back-up systems exist such that many otherwise serious defects are not fatal, but these defects can nevertheless predispose to diseases such as chronic periodontitis.

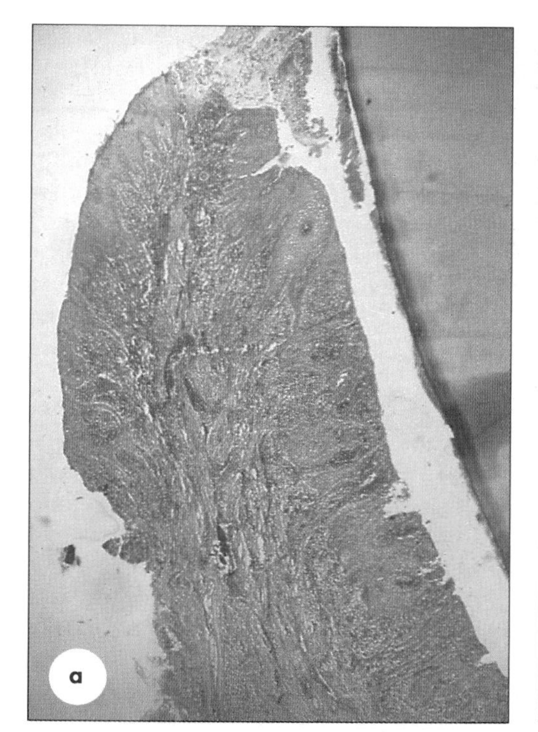

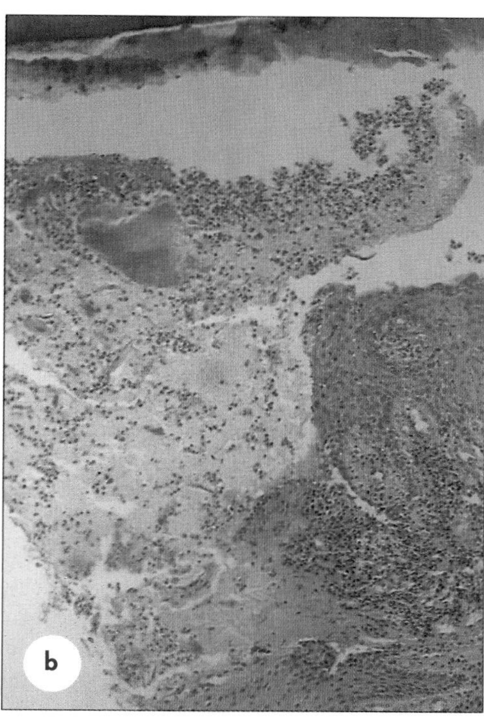

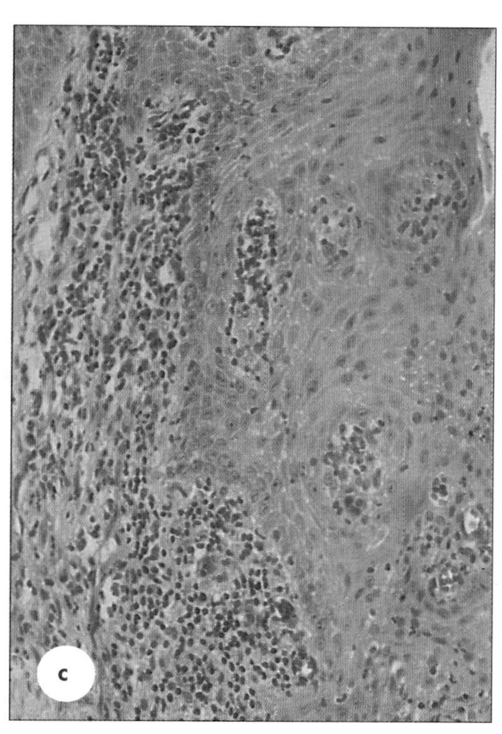

Fig. 18.1 (a) Section of gingival pocket lining of a chronic inflammatory periodontal site, showing the marked and variable leucocyte infiltrate (H & E, magnification × 20). (b) Higher power view of the coronal portion of the periodontal pocket shown in (a) (H & E, magnificatin × 90). The marked polymorphonuclear infiltrate can be seen within the gingival epithelium and connective tissue and in the crevicular plaque and fluid. (c) Higher power view of the base of the pocket shown in (a) (H & E, magnification × 100). The leucocyte infiltrate is made up of a variety of cell types, including lymphocytes, plasma cells, macrophages, and polymorphonuclear leucocytes.

Other non-defence-related cells, such as the red blood cells, have crucial roles in maintaining gas exchange and nutrient supply to the PDL. The platelets are another non-defence-related haematological element; platelets are needed for efficient haemostasis of this well-perfused tissue, which, when inflamed, is commonly hyperaemic and haemorrhagic. Thus the pivotal role of the blood cells in the maintenance of a stable PDL means that systemic haematological disorders can have a profound effect on the periodontium. In addition, specific periodontal diseases, such as the early-onset forms of periodontitis, are increasingly being linked with functional leucocyte abnormalities, which could feasibly manifest their effects through damage to the PDL.

Secondly, the PDL of the teeth are surrounded by alveolar bone and its marrow spaces. The marrow spaces of the jaws contain scattered lymphocytes and histiocytes and, in certain parts (especially in children), erythropoietic tissue. The PDL may thus be affected by abnormalities of its own cells, of the cells of the marrow spaces of the alveolar bone, and of leucocytes that become lodged in these areas, such as occurs in lymphomas and secondaries of other tumours, and in deposition of proteins and other molecules, e.g. amyloidosis and granulomas.

This chapter will thus concentrate on blood and lymphoreticular disorders that affect the PDL through reduction in the tissue's host resistance, and on those disorders that result in invasion by blood or lymphoid cells or deposition of substances that disrupt or replace the PDL. The leukaemias are one example of a condition that fits both categories, but they will be discussed in the section covering the host response defects, although the invasion of these leucocytes into the PDL and other periodontal tissues is also covered.

As might be expected, the commonest changes in the PDL are related to haematological disorders that reduce the host response of the periodontium to microbial plaque.

BLOOD DYSCRASIAS AFFECTING THE IMMUNE AND INFLAMMATORY RESPONSES OF THE PERIODONTAL LIGAMENT

Haematological disorders can be broadly grouped into haemostatic disorders, red blood cell disorders, and the white blood cell disorders. Although the white blood cell (or leucocyte) disorders make up most of the haematological disorders affecting the periodontium, the haemostatic and red blood cell disorders can also crucially affect the integrity of the periodontium.

DISORDERS OF HAEMOSTASIS

The platelets or thrombocytes are essential in haemostasis, both in repair of blood vessel wear and tear by replacing endothelial cells, and in arresting haemorrhage. Defective haemostasis can arise in three basic ways:

- from abnormalities of the coagulation factors involved in the clotting mechanism;
- from defective platelet function; and
- from impaired support of the blood vessels.

Defective platelet function may be a consequence of reduced numbers (thrombocytopenia), increased numbers (thrombocytosis), or of abnormalities in their metabolism (thrombocytosthenia). Thrombocytosthenic disorders and impaired support of blood vessels that occur in avitaminosis C, are discussed on page 367.

Haemophilia

Defective haemostasis arising as a consequence of abnormalities of coagulation factors, haemophilia, is due to deficiencies of factors VIII, IX, and XI; 80 per cent of cases are due to deficiencies of factor VIII (antihaemophilic globulin), 15 per cent due to deficiencies of factor IX (Christmas factor, plasma thromboplastic component). and 1–2 per cent are due to deficiencies of factor XI (plasma thromboplastin antecedent) – these disorders are called haemophilia A, B, and C respectively (Green, 1974; Grossman, 1975). In addition, in von Willebrand's disease there is a deficiency of factor VIII (Nilsson *et al.*, 1957) as well as defective platelet function (Hellem, 1960).

Haemorrhaging after scaling in these patients is predictable and supplementing haemostatic mechanisms via alterations in anticoagulant therapy, platelet transfusions, or clotting factor supplements should be considered, particularly before surgery. The extent of the deficiency varies very much from patient to patient and from time to time in the same patient, and hence the clinical manifestations are variable. In classical haemophilia, haemophilia A, levels of antihaemophilic globulin at 25 per cent or less of normal are likely to lead to prolonged haemorrhage after dental extractions; levels at 5 per cent or less may lead to spontaneous haemorrhage (Green, 1974), including gingival haemorrhage. Spontaneous gingival haemorrhage has also been reported in factor X (Stuart–Prower factor) deficiency (Bhoweer *et al.*, 1977) as well as in deficiencies of factors VIII, IX and XI.

Thrombocytopenia

A reduction in the numbers of circulating platelets – thrombocytopenia – results in a prolongation of the bleeding time together with defective clot retraction. The outstanding clinical sign is the presence of numerous petechial haemorrhages and a purpuric rash on the skin, but this rash can also involve the oral mucosa. Most commonly thrombocytopenic purpura is secondary to drug toxicity, and can occur at any age; less commonly it arises as idiopathic thrombocytopenic purpura, which usually occurs in young adults. This form of the disease is believed to be an autoimmune condition and is accompanied by the presence of antiplatelet antibodies in the plasma, which leads to their agglutination (Harrington *et al.*, 1956) and subsequent lysis in the spleen (McKelvy *et al.*, 1976). The platelet–antiplatelet complexes can also lead to complement activation in the tissues (Yeager,

1975) and thus to destruction of the peripheral blood vessels. Such changes can occur in the gingiva, where the capillaries may exhibit extensive serofibrinous perivascular exudation (McKelvy *et al.*, 1976). As a consequence, there may be gingival haemorrhage (Laskin, 1974; Yeager, 1975), and/or swelling (McKelvy *et al.*, 1976).

There is a third, rare form of thrombocytopenia, thrombotic thrombocytopenic purpura, which is accompanied by thrombosis of the terminal arterioles and capillaries (Moschcowitz, 1925). It most commonly affects adolescents and young adults and runs a rapidly fatal course (Amorosi and Ultmann, 1966; Hill and Cooper, 1968). Although there are no significant oral features clinically, it has been demonstrated that the gingival vessels exhibit the same changes as elsewhere, and they provide an invaluable site for biopsy for confirmation of the diagnosis (Schwartz *et al.*, 1972; Goldenfarb and Finch, 1973; Fox *et al.*, 1977). The arterioles and capillaries contain hyaline thrombi, which occlude their lumens, and there is endothelial proliferation. The aetiology of this form of the disease is unknown, but drug sensitivity and autoimmunity may both be factors (Fox *et al.*, 1977).

Defective platelet function (thrombocytosthenia), such as occurs in uraemia (Merril and Peterson, 1970) and in Glanzmann's thrombasthenia, may also lead to gingival bleeding (Nixon *et al.*, 1975). In Glanzmann's thrombasthenia, there are normal numbers of platelets, but they fail to aggregate normally in response to adenosine diphosphate and collagen, thus leading to defective clot retraction. Adensonine diphosphate activation of platelet thromboplastic factor is also inhibited in uraemia.

In general, although no PDL changes have been reported related to haemostasis problems, periodontal home care can be problematic e.g. cases of thrombocytopenic purpura have been reported in which severe gingival haemorrhage occurred after scaling (Peltier and Olivier, 1961) and thus by limiting treatment options and patient home care, these disorders could indirectly be detrimental to the periodontium in a susceptible host.

RED BLOOD CELL DISORDERS

Four types of red blood cell disorders are worthy of comment: anaemia; sickle cell disease; acatalasia; and polycythaemia.

Anaemia

Anaemia is the state in which there is an inadequate quantity of circulating haemoglobin. The anaemias fall into two major groups, those consequent upon a deficiency of some factor essential for the development or maturation of the erythrocytes and those consequent upon the excessive loss or breakdown of the erythrocytes once they have been formed. In both groups the oral mucosa may exhibit pallor, owing to the lowered concentration of circulating haemoglobin. In addition, there are other striking features, particularly in the lingual mucosa, which may be present in the deficiency anaemias (Ferguson, 1975). For example, iron, cyanocobalamin, and folic acid, in addition to being essential for the formation of erythrocytes, are important constituents of enzymes and co-enzymes involved in general cellular metabolism. Thus, other cell systems that exhibit marked cell turnover, such as the oral epithelium, are also directly affected (Jones, 1973).

On the other hand, there is no evidence that the anaemia of iron deficiency has any direct effect upon the PDL. In a study of 752 patients with periodontal disease, no correlation was obtained between the haematocrit, haemoglobin concentration, or erythrocyte count and the level of disease (Lainson *et al.*, 1968). A similar lack of correlation has also been observed in rats (Deutsch *et al.*, 1969). However, there does not appear to have been any attempt to correlate serum iron levels with periodontal disease, although it is known that the lymphocytes from sideropenic patients exhibit deficient immune responses (Joynson *et al.*, 1972). In humans, there is no clear evidence that the megaloblastic anaemias of vitamin B_{12} or folic acid deficiency have any direct effect upon the periodontal tissues, although there are reports that gingivitis and periodontitis are features of folate deficiency in humans (Day *et al.*, 1938) and other primates (Dreizen *et al.*, 1970; Siddons, 1974).

Mild anaemia is a variable feature of ascorbic acid, riboflavin, and pyridoxine deficiency in humans (Ferguson, 1975). Swollen haemorrhagic gums together with accelerated progression of established periodontal disease leading to destruction of the PDL and loosening of the teeth are also common features of ascorbic acid deficiency (scurvy) (Dreizen, 1971; Hodges *et al.*, 1971; Schluger *et al.*, 1977). However, there is no evidence that the anaemia is of significance in these changes. It is more likely that it is the defective hydroxylation and cross-linking of secreted tropocollagen molecules which are dependent upon the presence of ascorbic acid, that leads to them. Such defective collagen metabolism results in weakening of the walls of capillaries (Priest, 1970) and other small vessels, and in the inadequate maintenance of the fibres of the PDL (Dreizen *et al.*, 1969). However, there is evidence that plaque must be present for the periodontal changes to occur, so that avitaminosis C may lead also to an altered host response to local irritation (Wolbach and Bessy, 1942; Glickman, 1948, 1964; El-Ashiry *et al.*, 1964; O'Leary *et al.*, 1969; Schluger *et al.*, 1977).

Since it is primarily the direct effect of the deficient factor upon the oral tissues rather than the anaemia itself that causes the important changes in the deficiency anaemias, it would be anticipated that none would occur in anaemias that arise from an excessive rate of destruction of the erythrocytes, i.e. the haemolytic anaemias and haemoglobinopathies. There is indeed no association between this group of anaemias and lesions of the PDL. However, there are characteristic changes in the alveolar bone in some of the haemoglobinopathies, notably the sickle cell disease and to a lesser extent thalassaemia.

Aplastic anaemia, a bone marrow disorder characterized by markedly reduced haemopoietic tissue, has been associated with severe periodontal destruction. There is, however, a concomitant generalized pancytopenia associated with this condition, which will greatly reduce white blood cell numbers and, if the defensive leucocytes are thus depleted, will predispose to periodontal destruction.

Sickling disorders

Sickle cell disease is characterized by the presence of haemoglobin S in the erythrocytes. In haemoglobin S, valine is substituted for glutamic acid in the β-chain of the molecule, and this leads to a rigidity and distortion of the shape of the erythrocyte, which then takes on the characteristic sickle appearance (Catena, 1975). The disorder is transmitted as a non-sex-linked dominant and is of variable expressivity according to whether the subject is heterozygous or homozygous and to the penetrance of the gene. The heterozygous form, or sickle cell trait, is the commoner, and it affects 8–11 per cent of US Negroes (Catena, 1975). Anaemia, which affects particularly the homozygotes, results from haemolytic episodes brought on by such factors as hypoxia and infection. As a result of the anaemia there is erythroplasia of bone marrow, which results in generalized osteoporosis, including osteoporosis of the alveolar bone. Indeed, osteoporosis can be detected here before in other bones (Robinson and Sarnat, 1952), probably owing to the greater definition obtained on intraoral radiographs rather than to any predilection of this site.

In the jaws, there is a generalized osteoporosis with fewer, but sharply defined, trabeculae, which show a characteristic 'step-ladder' pattern in the alveolar bone, the trabeculae arising from a distinct lamina dura, which remains intact (Robinson and Sarnat, 1952; Morris and Stahl, 1954; Prowler and Smith, 1965; Catena, 1975). All reports stress that the PDL space remains normal. In addition, irregular osteosclerotic areas may be present (Prowler and Smith, 1965; Catena, 1975), probably indicative of past focal infarcts that have repaired by bone sclerosis. The changes are more obvious and more prevalent in homozygotes than in those with sickle-cell trait (Prowler and Smith, 1965). In addition to the bone changes, abnormalities of tooth structure may also occur (Soni, 1966).

Sickling disorders result in red blood cells changing shape (sickling) during hypoxic states. Crawford (1988) examined patients with sickling disorders and reported no differences in age-matched controls for periodontal destruction or gingival inflammation. This is despite the report by Onwubalili (1983), which claimed these patients had an increased general susceptibility to infection, owing to local vascular occlusion.

Similar bone changes to those seen in sickle cell disease have also been reported in homozygous haemoglobin C disease (Halstead, 1970). In haemoglobin C, lysine is substituted for glutamic acid in the β-chain of the molecule. This disorder is much less common than the heterozygous form of haemoglobin C disease, which affects only approximately 2 per cent of US Negroes (Smith and Conley, 1953).

In thalassaemia (Cooley's anaemia), osteoporosis may also affect the alveolar bone although it is not an outstanding feature (Catena, 1975). In thalassaemia, which affects predominantly the races living around the Mediterranean Sea, the defect lies in the rate of globin synthesis in the β-chain of the haemoglobin molecule. It is transmitted as an autosomal recessive.

Acatalasia

This is a rare, inherited disorder caused by the lack of catalase in cells, especially red blood cells and white blood cells. Catalase is used by these cells to convert the reactive hydrogen peroxide to oxygen and water. This catalase neutralization is thought to protect these cells from harmful oxidizing agents which could denature haemoglobin and produce local hypoxia and necrosis of the gingiva. A report by Delgado and Calderon (1979) indicated that severe periodontal destruction and gingival necrosis is likely in these patients; this is possibly linked to colonization by bacteria that reduce hydrogen peroxide and to the lack of neutralizing catalase activity in the gingiva. The condition is so rare that this is the only available report, and confirmatory evidence is needed for this indication of catalase's crucial role in preserving periodontal integrity in cases of poor oral hygiene.

Polycythaemia

This condition is characterized by an increase in red blood cells (RBC) caused by overproduction by the bone marrow, and also in platelets and white blood cells (polycythaemia rubra vera). Patients have a florid complexion and may be deeply cyanosed. Significant bleeding on brushing and during clinical scaling is common, although this can be markedly reduced by good plaque control. Sluggish blood flow and thrombosis may also occur and this increases the possibility of strokes. Occasionally patients with polycythaemia have gingival bleeding, which is probably a consequence of thrombocytosis (Ferguson, 1975). Thrombocytosis, an increase in the number of circulating platelets, may accompany polycythaemia and leukaemia, and results in defective thromboplastic generation.

LEUCOCYTE DISORDERS

The majority of haematological disorders affecting the periodontium are related to white cell function or numbers. White blood cell defects can be considered under two main headings: disorders of white cell number (quantitative disorders) and disorders in white cell function (qualitative disorders).

DISORDERS OF WHITE CELL NUMBER

Leucopenia is regarded as being present when the white cell count drops below 3000 per mm^3; agranulocytosis is a virtual absence of granulocytes from the blood. Disorders in which there are excessive numbers of leucocytes are termed leukaemias. The main disorders of white cell number that have detrimental effects on the PDL are depletion or absence of circulating polymorphonuclear leucocytes (PMNs) – neutropenia – and the leukaemias.

Neutropenia

The neutropenias are a heterogeneous group characterized by a decrease or an absence of circulating PMNs. In general, quantitative PMN deficiencies are accompanied by generalized PDL destruction whereas functional defects (see below) are often associated with localized destruction affecting only the PDL of certain teeth (Wilton *et al.*, 1988). There are several types and descriptions of neutropenias; these include: agranulocytosis, familial neutropenia, and chronic idiopathic neutropenia.

Agranulocytosis

Agranulocytosis, by strict definition, means a depletion of all granulocytes (neutrophils, eosinophils, monocytes, and basophils) in the blood, but it is generally used to describe an extremely severe neutropenia, which is often due to adverse drug reactions. The majority of cases of agranulocytosis that are a consequence of drug toxicity (Mishkin *et al.*, 1976) are acute and rapidly fatal, owing to overwhelming infection, most commonly by Gram-negative organisms. In addition to the cytotoxic and immunosuppressive agents given for the treatment of malignant disease and immune disorders, the drugs most commonly associated with agranulocytosis are the aminopyrines, phenothiazines, barbiturates, arsenicals, sulphonamides, thiouracils, gold, and anti-malarials (Pretty *et al.*, 1965; Cohen, 1977). Although ulceration of the oral mucosa, including the gingiva, is a frequent occurrence, the PDL is rarely involved, probably because of the short clinical course of the disorder. For example, it has been demonstrated in dogs that severe leucopenia induced either with nitrogen mustard (Attström and Egelberg, 1971a) or anti-neutrophil serum (Attström and Egelberg, 1971b) over periods of 4 days results in no change in the gingival index (Rylander *et al.*, 1975; Attström and Schroeder, 1979).

Agranulocytosis may also occur as part of the complete cessation of haematopoiesis that occurs in aplastic anaemia. Again, although mucosal ulceration is a usual feature, involvement of the PDL as part of the overall necrotizing stomatitis is rare (Stamps, 1974; Lerman and Grodin, 1977).

Sometimes a more chronic course may ensue, in which case there may be extensive gingival ulceration resembling the lesions of acute ulcerative gingivitis, together with exposure of necrotic alveolar bone, destruction of the PDL, and increased mobility of the affected teeth (Swenson *et al.*, 1965).

This ulceration and necrosis of the marginal gingiva and involvement of the PDL can be seen in relatively severe neutropenia, which is often drug-induced. This is associated with bleeding, and occasional involvement of the attached gingiva (Awbrey and Hibbard, 1973). Histologically, the ulcerated marginal gingiva and PDL regions exhibit little or no PMN infiltration.

Involvement of the PDL is a more important feature of the rare conditions of congenital neutropenia and cyclical neutropenia. In these conditions, which affect the polymorphonuclear leucocytes and not the other forms of granulocyte, there is a persistent or cyclical absence or reduction of the cells to very low levels in the circulation. In more protracted forms of the disease, such as cyclic, chronic, and familial benign neutropenia, the lesions are frequently severe. The gingivae may be oedematous, hyperaemic, and hyperplastic, with areas of partial desquamation (Kyle and Linman, 1970; Baer and Benjamin, 1974). These features are often accompanied by severe destruction of the PDL, deep periodontal pockets, and extensive, generalized bone loss involving the permanent dentition (Levine, 1959; Smith 1964; Baehni *et al.*, 1983). Occasionally, the PDL destruction and bone resorption may be seen in the deciduous dentition of these patients with this condition (Lampert and Fesseler, 1975).

In congenital neutropenia, there is persistent neutropenia with a differential count usually below 5 per cent and often a relative lymphocytosis, monocytosis, and eosinophilia. Approximately 70 per cent of these patients die in the first 3 years of life (Mishkin *et al.*, 1976), but some survive into adolescence. In these, severe periodontitis is a characteristic feature, with extensive destruction of the alveolar bone and PDL, and rapid loosening and premature loss of both the deciduous and permanent dentition (Levine, 1959; Cutting and Lang, 1964; Andrews *et al.*, 1965; Davey and Konchak, 1969; Gates, 1969; Kyle and Linman, 1970; Miller *et al.*, 1971; Awbrey and Hibbard, 1973; Lampert and Fesseler, 1975; Vann and Oldenburg, 1976; Mishkin *et al.*, 1976; Reichart and Dornow, 1978). This rapid periodontal destruction occurs despite rigorous oral hygiene and is presumably a consequence of uninhibited irritation of the tissues by the plaque micro-organisms, caused by deficient phagocytosis. In support of this is the observation that, despite the neutropenia, extraction sockets heal normally (Andrews *et al.*, 1965; Mishkin *et al.*, 1976). Furthermore, necrotizing periodontitis has been demonstrated in rats in which granulocytopenia was induced for 30–60 days with either methyl folic acid (Franklin *et al.*, 1947; Pindborg, 1949) or neoarsphenamine (Bauer, 1946).

Familial neutropenia occurs in several forms – some of these forms are transmitted as an autosomal recessive (Kostman, 1956; Andrews *et al.*, 1965; MacGillwray *et al.*, 1964; Matsaniotis *et al.*, 1966); others forms of the disease are transmitted as a dominant (Cutting and Lang, 1964); most cases, however, have no familial pattern. In some cases, it has been demonstrated that there is a failure of the normal granulocyte maturation in the bone marrow, such that cells in this line do not progress beyond the myelocyte or metamyelocyte stage (Cutting and Lang, 1964; Gates, 1969;

Mishkin *et al.*, 1976); in other cases, there are normal numbers of mature neutrophils in the marrow but these do not enter the circulation (i.e. they are not released properly from the marrow – Mintz and Sachs, 1973); and in yet other cases the neutrophils do not respond well to chemical or inflammatory stimuli in the other tissues (Miller *et al.*, 1971). In this last type of case, the neutrophils exhibit normal phagocytosis but respond weakly to chemotactic stimuli. A slight monocytosis can occur, and in some forms of the disease monocyte activity is enhanced. Presumably these features compensate for the lack of neutrophils (Biggar *et al.*, 1974; Kay *et al.*, 1976). The periodontal manifestations include fiery red oedematous gingivitis, which is often hyperplastic (*Fig. 18.2*) and accompanied by periodontal bone loss (Deasy *et al.*, 1980).

Cyclic neutropenia

This is a rare condition, characterized by cyclical depletion of PMN numbers, typically in cycles of 3 weeks (Reimann and Debaradinis, 1949), although it can be between 2 weeks and 5 weeks. The episode of neutropenia is usually short with the cell count increasing again after 5–8 days, but the patient's PMN count never returns to normal and the differential blood cell count for PMNs is at least 40 per cent less than normal. The cyclical depression of PMN numbers is thought to be due to a disorder of haematopoietic control (Zucker-Franklin *et al.*, 1977) – i.e. there is a complete suppression of neutrophil leucopoiesis or a maturation arrest at the promyelocyte stage in the bone marrow. Despite the periods of neutropenia, these patients usually remain in good health, although they are subject to recurrent infections.

The most common oral symptom is recurrent oral ulceration, crops of ulcers coinciding with the periods of neutropenia (Cohen and Morris, 1961). Periodontal manifestations include inflamed gingiva (*Fig. 18.3*), gingival ulceration (*Fig. 18.4*), periodontal attachment and bone loss (Gorlin and Chaudhry, 1960; Cohen and Morris 1961; Rylander and Ericsson, 1981; Scully *et al.*, 1982; Prichard, 1984; Spencer and Fleming 1985; Long *et al.*, 1983). In some patients there are reports of advanced periodontal disease with bifurcation and trifurcation involvement and marked increase in tooth mobility (Page and Good, 1957; Gorlin and Chaudhry, 1960; Cohen and Morris, 1961; Telsey *et al.*, 1962; Wade and Stafford, 1963; Cohen, 1965; Binon and Dykema, 1974). Since such cases are usually diagnosed in the first decade, rapidly progressing periodontal disease may be an early diagnostic feature of the condition. In general, neither the extent of the periodontitis nor the number of patients exhibiting this feature is as great as in congenital neutropenia, presumably because the neutropenia occurs for only short periods.

Despite the obvious decrease in host defences caused by neutrophil depletion in familial benign chronic neutropenia, periodontitis is not always inevitable (Deasy *et al.*, 1976). Deasy *et al.* (1976) described a family that exhibited familial benign chronic neutropenia and showed that, although several individuals within this family were neutropenic, not all were affected either by recurrent infections or by inflammatory periodontal disease. One neutropenic sibling who was free from periodontal disease had good oral hygiene, whereas her neutropenic brother, with poor oral hygiene, had fiery-red oedematous gingiva and early generalized periodontitis. These findings might be explained by the variable expressivity of the disorder between the siblings, or by the interaction of the environment (e.g. the oral hygiene) on this disorder.

Chronic idiopathic neutropenia

This condition is characterized by a persistent neutropenia from birth, which is not cyclical and does not appear to be inherited. The periodontal manifestation is a severe persistent gingivitis, which is oedematous and hyperplastic (Kyle and Linman, 1970; Kalkwarf and Gutz, 1981). However, these authors gave no indication of detrimental effects on the PDL or of periodontal bone loss.

Leukaemia

Leukaemia is a serious malignant disease characterized by the neoplastic proliferation of the leucocyte precursor cells within the haemopoetic tissues such that there is usually a marked increase in circulating white blood cells and infiltration of these cells into tissues, particularly the lymph nodes. All leucocyte types may be involved – granulocytes (myeloid), monocytes, and lymphocytes.

The disease may be acute or chronic. In acute leukaemias, the cell type is commonly a stem cell precursor or blast cell, and patients are usually under 20 years of age or over 55 years of age. Chronic leukaemias occur mainly in people aged over 40 years, and the component cell type is well differentiated. The acute leukaemias are broadly classified into acute lymphocytic and acute myelogenous leukaemia (non-lymphocytic). The chronic leukaemias are chronic myeloid (granulocytic) leukaemia and chronic lymphocytic leukaemia, which is the commonest leukaemia (and is twice as common as chronic myeloid leukaemia). In all leukaemias, the normal marrow function will be impaired, and thus anaemia, infections, and thrombocytopenia are common.

Several factors are implicated in the aetiology of leukaemia – namely, radiation, chemical injury, genetic factors, immune deficiency, and viral infections. Periodontal lesions are common in patients with leukaemia, particularly the acute forms of the disease. Gingival enlargement, which is usually generalized and variable in its severity, was apparent in 36 per cent of the individuals with acute forms of leukaemia (*Fig. 18.5*) and in 10 per cent of those with chronic forms (*Fig. 18.6*) (Lynch and Ship, 1967a,b). Gingival swelling due to actual infiltration by leukaemic cells is relatively uncommon, and when present it is usually a feature of acute monocytic leukaemia, although it has been reported in other forms, including chronic lymphocytic leukaemia (Presant, Safdar and Cherrick, 1973; Sydney and Serio, 1981). This swelling is considered to be a consequence of plaque-induced chronic inflammation, since a marked improvement is brought about by systemic management of the disease and the institution of an effective oral hygiene programme (Barrett, 1984). Gingival tissues are considered more susceptible to leukaemic cell infiltration because of their microanatomy and because of the constitutive expression of endothelial adhesion molecules, which enhance leucocyte infiltration and the steady state of mild gingival inflammation that is present even in clinically healthy gingiva (Moughal *et al.*, 1992). Gingival bleeding is also a common sign in both acute and chronic leukaemia (see *Fig. 18.6*) (Stafford *et al.*, 1980). This probably relates to the associated thrombocytopenia and the fact that the gingival epithelium may be thin and atrophic. In some cases there is rapid loss of alveolar bone (Curtis, 1971) but this is usually due to an exacerbation of a pre-existing periodontitis or a result of chemotherapy or radiotherapy treatment regimes.

Evidence for involvement of the PDL is, on the other hand, largely circumstantial and not well documented. There are a number of clinical reports in which reference is made to the presence of generalized bone loss (Keene *et al.*, 1972; Presant *et al.*, 1973; Segelman and Doku, 1977), increased mobility of teeth (McCarthy and Karcher, 1946; Stern and Cole, 1973; Michaud *et al.*, 1977; Pogrel, 1978) and protrusion of teeth (Mallett *et al.*, 1947; Taliano and Wakefield, 1966; Smillie and Cowman, 1969). Since most of these occurred in adults, the extent to which the periodontal changes were a consequence of a pre-existing chronic periodontitis and not due to leukaemia infiltration is not clear. However, more definitive evidence is derived from radiological studies, particularly in children, in whom bone changes as a consequence of chronic periodontitis are unlikely. Curtis (1971) studied the oral radiographs of 214 children with leukaemia and observed bone changes in 87 of them (41 per cent). There was a significant difference between children with active disease (62 per cent) and those in remission (5 per cent), and between patients with acute lymphocytic leukaemia (65 per cent) and acute myelogenous leukaemia (47 per cent). The most characteristic changes were a loss of the lamina dura around erupted teeth, with widening of the PDL space, and loss of the crypt outline around unerupted teeth. Similar changes have been mentioned in other case reports (Bender, 1944; Sinrod, 1957; Taliano and Wakefield, 1966; Stern and Cole, 1973; Michaud *et al.*, 1977).

In children, the changes are most commonly observed around the last developing molar tooth (Curtis, 1971) and involve the periapical part of the periodontium rather than the crestal part. The involvement of the periapical part of the PDL before the crestal part in leukaemia is confirmed from histological studies in both AKR (Carranza and Cabrini, 1966) and CFW mice (Flanagan *et al.*, 1970). In both these studies, no infiltration of the gingiva was present. It has therefore been suggested (Curtis, 1971) that the primary event is infiltration of the marrow spaces by the leukaemic cells, which spread to involve the lamina dura and PDL of the involved teeth. Since haemopoietic bone marrow persists longest in the posterior and molar regions of the jaws in children, this might account for the more frequent involvement of the molar teeth (Curtis, 1971; Jones, 1975) in the early stages of leukaemia. Infiltration of the pulp has also been reported both in humans (Sinrod, 1957; Duffy and Driscoll, 1958; Smillie and Cowman, 1969) and in mice (Carranza and Cabrini, 1966; Flanagan *et al.*, 1970). As far as can be determined, such infiltration usually occurs only in the pulps of incompletely formed or continuously forming teeth, both of which have open apices.

The pathogenesis of the destructive changes in the periodontal tissues in leukaemia is unclear. The relative frequency of gingival changes, including hyperplasia, haemorrhage, and ulcerative necrosis, are considered a consequence of the high incidence of pre-existing chronic gingivitis. Several authors have emphasized that the gingival changes are less marked or even suppressed if excellent oral hygiene measures are maintained (Sinrod, 1957; McGowan *et al.*, 1970; Segelman and Doku, 1977; Pogrel, 1978; Carranza, 1979). Gingival biopsy reveals a dense infiltrate of the gingiva with leukaemic cells, the infiltrate characteristically being separated from the gingival epithelium by a narrow band of normal connective tissue (*Fig. 18.7*) (Sinrod, 1957; Lucas, 1976a). Leukaemic cells have been variously reported as exhibiting defective immune responses (Dupuy *et al.*, 1971), and also impaired phagocytosis (Lehrer *et al.*, 1972). Thus in sites where, prior to the disease, inflammation already existed, such as in the gingiva in chronic gingivitis, greater numbers of cells would be attracted.

There is no information on the mechanisms of tissue destruction once the leukaemic cells have arrived in the tissues. However, several authors have observed blood vessels occluded by dense aggregates of leukaemic cells (Burkett, 1940; Sinrod, 1957; Bodey, 1971; Segelman and Doku, 1977) and noted that this may lead to necrosis of the gingiva and PDL. Intravascular leucocyte thrombi and aggregates are a particular feature of myelogenous leukaemia (McKee and Collins, 1974) and occur in sites other than the PDL with increasing frequency proportional to the circulating leucocyte count. Although no such study has been made of the PDL, the incidence of leukaemic cell infiltration of non-ulcerated labial mucosa in acute myelogenous leukaemia shows a similar relationship to the circulating leucocyte count (Basu and Pollock, unpublished).

However, the circulating level of leucocytes is probably only one of many factors, since radiological changes in alveolar bone have been reported in preleukaemia when the circulating leucocytes are still within normal limits (Deasy *et al.*, 1976). Whether bone resorption is a consequence of a direct effect of the release of lysosomal enzymes from the leukaemic cells or of stimulation of osteoclasts is uncertain. In studies of leukaemia in mice, particular note was made of the paucity of osteoclasts in histological examination of the alveolar bone, despite the marked destruction of the lamina dura and adjacent bone (Carranza and Cabrini, 1966). On the other hand, marked odontoclastic activity can occur in the PDL in acute leukaemia.

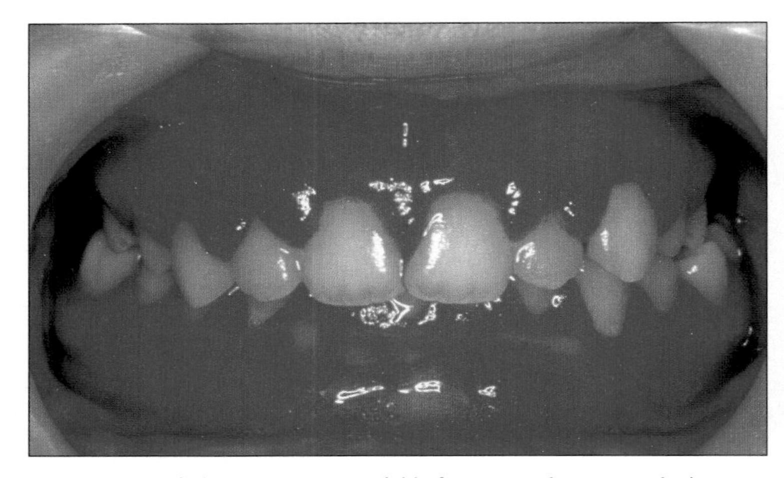

Fig. 18.2 Familial neutropenia in a child of 13 years showing marked gingival inflammation with fiery red oedematous gingiva.

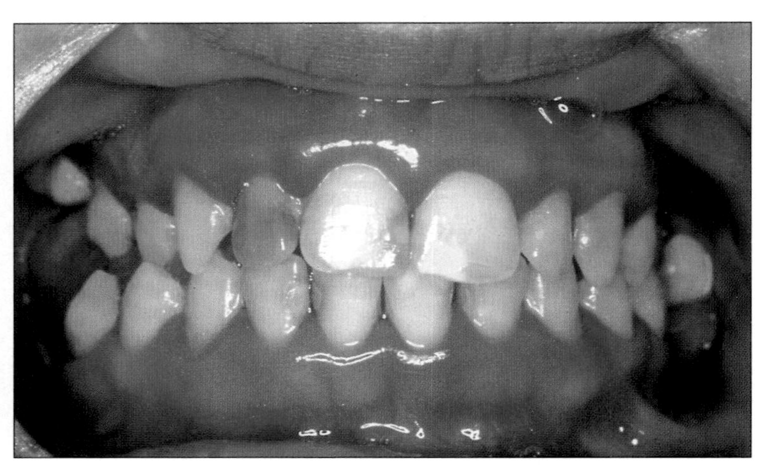

Fig. 18.3 The periodontal manifestations of cyclic neutropenia include inflamed gingiva with marked periodontal pocketing and bone loss.

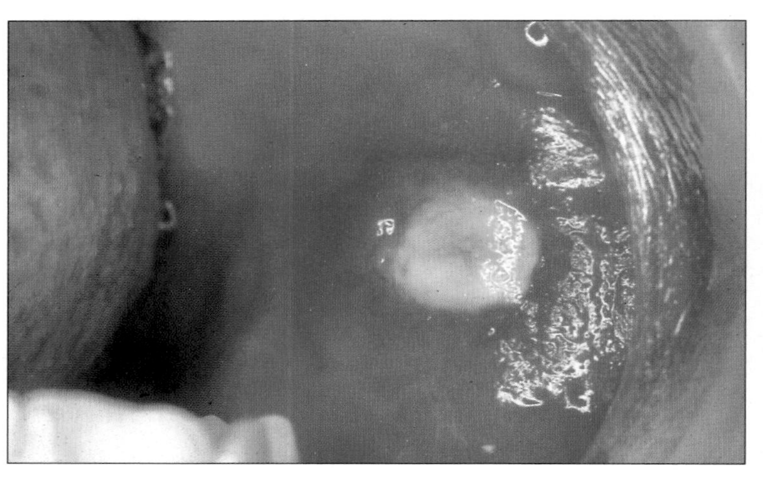

Fig. 18.4 Neutropenic ulceration is a common oral manifestation of cyclic neutropenia.

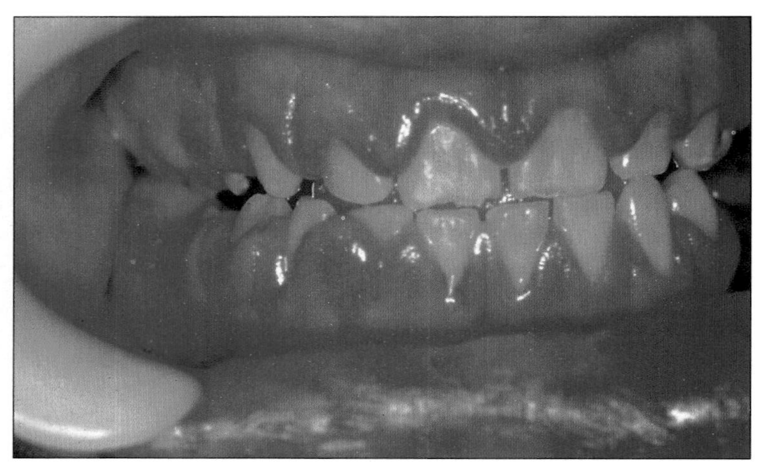

Fig. 18.5 Generalized and variable gingival enlargement seen in a 12-year-old male with acute myeloblastic leukaemia.

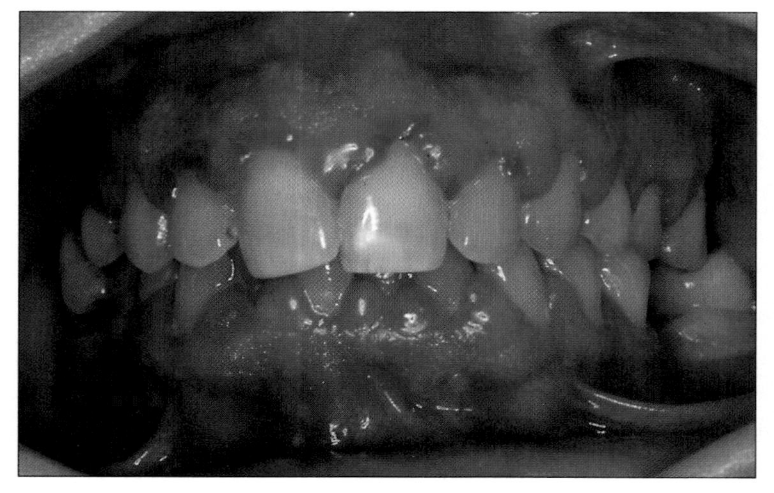

Fig. 18.6 Gingival enlargement in a patient with chronic lymphocytic leukaemia.

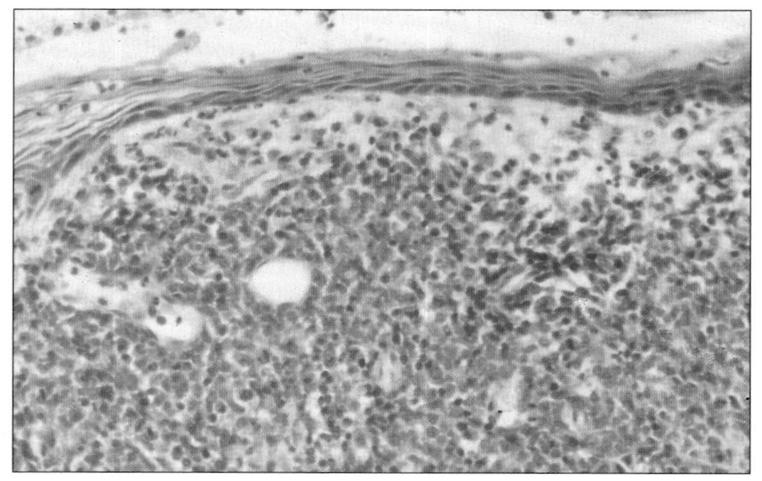

Fig. 18.7 Acute monocytic leukaemia. The gingiva is densely infiltrated by abnormal monocytic cells, but a small band of fibrous tissue persists between the infiltrate and the surface epithelium. (Haematoxylin and eosin × 330.)

Another factor of possible significance is the change in the oral flora in leukaemic patients. Leukaemic patients are particularly susceptible to infections (Hersh *et al.*, 1965), partly as a consequence of their defective immune responses, and partly because of the myelosuppression, immunosuppression, and cytotoxicity that are side effects of the chemotherapeutic treatment of the disease (Dreizen *et al.*, 1974). In the course of the disease, particularly during periods of remission in acute myelogenous leukaemia, patients are granulocytopenic for approximately 50 per cent of the time (Bodey *et al.*, 1966), and it is during such periods that they are particularly prone to infection. The infections are caused predominantly by opportunist organisms, in particular the Gram-negative bacilli and *Candida* species (Dreizen *et al.*, 1974). In the oral cavity, *Escherichia coli*, *Klebsiella* and *Pseudomonas* are commonly cultured from patients with leukaemia (Bodey, 1971; Brown *et al.*, 1973), whereas they are rare in the mouths of healthy patients. The reason for this change in the oral flora is unclear, although it should be noted that there is a reduction in the level of parotid secretory IgA in patients with acute myelogenous leukaemia (Brown *et al.*, 1973; Basu *et al.*, 1978) and acute lymphoblastic leukaemia (Schiliro *et al.*, 1977).

In addition to the above micro-organisms, infections of the oral mucosa associated with *Candida albicans* (Bodey, 1971; McGowan *et al.*, 1970; Segelman and Doku, 1977; Michaud *et al.*, 1977) are not uncommon. In one study, *Candida* were recovered from the mouths of 93 per cent of patients (Segelman and Doku, 1977). Less commonly, acute ulcerative gingivitis has been reported (Michaud *et al.*, 1977; Segelman and Doku, 1977).

Preleukaemia

Preleukaemia, as the name implies, is a syndrome of haematological abnormalities that often proceeds to leukaemia (30 per cent of patients with preleukaemia become leukaemic). Anaemia, neutropenia, and platelet deficiency are all possible, and this preleukaemic condition may last for 6–24 months before leukaemia develops. A 13-year-old preleukaemic syndrome child with severe periodontal destruction was reported by Deasy *et al.* (1976). The gingivae were hyperplastic, oedematous, and haemorrhagic. There was pocketing of 10 mm, extensive bone loss, and the teeth were very mobile. The authors suggested that neutropenia and an impairment of phagocytic activity and immune mechanisms might be responsible for the tissue destruction.

The frequency of involvement of the PDL is, therefore, uncertain. However, changes occur in children, probably as a result of secondary invasion from the marrow spaces, and in adults as a consequence of spread of tumour cells attracted into periodontal tissues that have previously altered by chronic periodontal disease. Whether this difference between children and adults is a consequence of the different incidence of the various forms of leukaemia in the two groups or of the different prevalence of pre-existing inflammatory changes, or of other factors, is unclear.

DISORDERS OF WHITE CELL FUNCTION

Disorders of leucocyte function, primarily of neutrophil function, are commonly associated with severe PDL destruction.

Chediak–Higashi syndrome

Chediak–Higashi syndrome (Chediak, 1952; Higashi, 1954) is a genetically transmitted disease that is characterized by partial oculocutaneous albinism, photophobia, nystagmus, recurrent pyogenic infections, and abnormally large granules in all the granulocytic cells of the body (Kritzler *et al.*, 1964; Blume and Wolff, 1972). It is transmitted as an autosomal recessive, and has not been reported in Negroes. In humans, death usually occurs before the age of 20, either from recurrent infections or from an accelerated, lymphoma-like stage of the disease in which there is widespread lymphohistiocytic infiltration, pancytopenia, thrombocytopenia, lymphadenopathy, and hepatosplenomegaly (Kritzler *et al.*, 1964). It is not clear whether this stage of the disease is reactive (Padgett *et al.*, 1967; Blume and Wolff, 1972) or neoplastic (Dent *et al.*, 1966).

Abnormal, large granules are present within the polymorphonuclear leucocytes, eosinophils, basophils and their precursors, and under the electron microscope these cells have been demonstrated to be lysosomally derived (White, 1966). These abnormalities in the cytoplasmic granules result in impaired killing of certain micro-organisms. The primary defect may be in the regulation of membrane activation. PMNs ingest micro-organisms into phagosomes but the cytoplasmic granules coalesce into large secondary granules, with much reduced enzymatic potential; fusion of phagosome and lysosome to form the bactericidal phagolysosome is impaired. There is also a report of defective chemotactic attraction (Clark and Kimball, 1971). In addition, there is granulocytopenia, possibly as a result of intramedullary breakdown of the abnormal cells (Blume *et al.*, 1968).

Those affected are thus very susceptible to bacterial infections, owing to the reduced functional capacity of the PMN. Humans (Hamilton and Giansanti, 1974) and other animals (Lavine *et al.*, 1976) with Chediak–Higashi syndrome exhibit generalized, severe gingivitis, extensive loss of alveolar bone, and premature loss of teeth (Temple *et al.*, 1972). At all stages of the disease in animals the tissues are densely infiltrated by PMNs, but plasma cells and lymphocytes are relatively scarce (Lavine *et al.*, 1976). While the observed tissue destruction could result theoretically from the release of PMN lysosomal enzymes and neutral proteases, a more likely explanation is that it reflects a failure of the PMNs to protect the host tissue because of functional defects. The chemotactic response of PMNs in Chediak–Higashi syndrome was found to be impaired in one study (Clark and Kimball, 1971) and in another was reported to be only 40 per cent of normal (Edland *et al.*, 1968). As would be expected, a reduction in the intracellular killing of bacteria by PMNs of patients with this syndrome has also been observed (Clark *et al.*, 1972), and following phagocytosis the cells remained intact for long periods with ineffective delivery of peroxidase to the phagosome (Renshaw *et al.*, 1974).

Associated with the decreased numbers of circulating granulocytes, which are abnormal, patients exhibit severe gingivitis and advanced periodontitis, leading to marked mobility and loss of teeth even before the end of the first decade (Weary and Bender, 1967; Gillig and Caldwell, 1970; Blume and Wolff, 1972; Tempel *et al.*, 1972; Hamilton and Giansanti, 1974). It is generally believed that this accelerated tissue destruction is a consequence of defective protection by the abnormal leucocytes, allowing unhindered periodontal breakdown by the plaque micro-organisms (Lavine *et al.*, 1976) rather than increased tissue destruction by the abnormal cells. It has been demonstrated that leucocytes from patients with Chediak–Higashi syndrome exhibit no cytotoxic effect upon HeLa cells in tissue culture (Taubman *et al.*, 1974).

The periodontal tissues are infiltrated densely by lymphocytes and plasma cells, which are, in some areas, closely packed into 'abscesses' (Gustaffson, 1969). Relatively few polymorphonuclear leucocytes inflitrate the PDL. Radiographically, there is extensive bone loss around the affected teeth, often with a 'moth-eaten' appearance (Lavine *et al.*, 1976). In addition to periodontitis there may be gingival haemorrhage (Blume and Wolff, 1972), mucosal ulceration, and glossitis (Gillig and Caldwell, 1970).

Chronic granulomatous disease

This is a rare disease, with at least two genetic forms, autosomal recessive and X-linked recessive. The defect in this disease is in the ability of phagocytic cells, both PMN and monocytes, to perform killing by the oxidative pathway after ingestion. As a consequence, multiple purulent granulomas develop in the lymph nodes, spleen, liver, skin, and lungs, and the child seldom survives to adolescence (Berendes *et al.*, 1957; Johnston and Baehner, 1971). Hydrogen peroxide cannot be produced as there is a defect in the activation of the enzyme NADPH oxidase. As a consequence, superoxide and hydrogen peroxide generation are defective in the phagocyte, and intracellular killing is inefficient. Bacteria that produce catalase – *staphylococci* and *pseudomonas* in particular – are not eliminated and these organisms flourish and cause infections. It is thought that catalase-negative organisms cannot break down their endogenous hydrogen peroxide, which builds up in phagosomes and results in death of the organisms. Granulomas and microabscesses are commonly present. The definitive test for this condition is the nitroblue tetrazolium reduction test, which, when applied to PMNs from these patients, indicates an inability to reduce this substrate, owing to ineffective oxidative metabolism.

Photosensitivity dermatoses are also common in patients who are heterozygous for chronic granulomatous disease (i.e. carriers). Males who have the X-linked recessive form of the disease have PMNs that lack nitroblue tetrazolium-reducing ability – i.e. the PMNs have no oxidative killing capacity – and death soon after birth is the norm. Their female siblings may carry the same defective gene on an X chromosome and by a process of Lyonization may have a very much reduced proportion of nitroblue tetrazolium-reducing PMNs after stimulation with phorbyl myristate acetate. These siblings usually exhibit photosensitivity dermatoses, and occasional oral mucosal erythema (Wolf and Ebel, 1978; Allan and Straton, 1983) but they do not seem to be in any way more predisposed to chronic gingivitis or periodontitis than normal. The use of the drug Septrin (trimethoprim with sulphamethoxazole) appears to be effective in heterozygous carriers, but long-term use may also mask any periodontal susceptibility in these individuals.

Kinane (1993) describes a family with the X-linked recessive form of chronic granulomatous disease. Female carriers suffered from photosensitivity dermatoses and had very much reduced nitroblue tetrazolium-reducing ability within their phagocytes. The family were initially uncovered because of the death of a male child whose mother had only 10 per cent nitroblue tetrazolium function in her peripheral blood PMNs (compared to 100 per cent function in controls). The child's polymorphonuclear leucocytes were checked for their nitroblue tetrazolium activity, which showed a totally negative nitroblue tetrazolium response, and the child died within a few days of birth. The reduced nitroblue tetrazolium levels are a consequence of the Lyonization process whereby one X chromosome is masked such that the other X chromosome (with or without the defective gene) controls the phenotype of the phagocyte. All of the female carriers in this series were examined for oral and periodontal lesions, and although erythema of the gingiva and oral mucosa with occasional ulceration were seen, there were no periodontal manifestations attributable to this condition. For practical purposes, these patients should be treated as normal but with the recognition that erythema of the mucosa and ulceration are likely and may be episodic – these episodes tend to occur with skin rashes related to their photosensitivity dermatoses.

Infectious mononucleosis

Infectious mononucleosis (glandular fever) is a systemic lymphoproliferative disease that is characterized by the presence of large numbers of atypical mononuclear cells in the peripheral blood. It is commonest in spring and autumn. It occurs almost exclusively in adolescents and young adults (Hoagland, 1960; Dunnet, 1963), among whom it is believed that kissing is an important mode of transmission (Cassingham, 1971). Most commonly there is a febrile illness with ulceromembranous pharyngitis and generalized lymphadenopathy involving variable numbers of lymph nodes, but almost invariably those in the posterior triangle of the neck (Banks, 1967).

The most striking oral feature is a palatal enanthematous eruption (Shiver *et al.*, 1956; Caird and Holt, 1958; Courant and Sobkov, 1969). Less commonly there may be an ulcero-membranous gingivitis, which resembles acute ulcerative gingivitis (Contratto, 1944; Fraser-Moodie, 1959; Banks, 1967; Valentine, 1971). This is sometimes associated with partially erupted lower third molars, where it resembles pericoronitis (Fraser-Moodie, 1959; Banks, 1967). It is not clear whether the PDL is involved under these circumstances.

The striking finding in infectious mononucleosis is the presence of heterophil antibodies in the serum, which cause the lysis of sheep red blood cells (Paul and Bunnell, 1932). The association between the presence of these antibodies and infection with Epstein–Barr virus was first demonstrated in 1968 (Henle *et al.*, 1968; Niederman *et al.*, 1968), and it is now widely accepted that this is the most frequent causative virus (Evans, 1974). The incubation period is uncertain, estimates varying from a few days to several weeks (Hoagland, 1964; Valentine, 1971). However, there are some patients with all the clinical features of infectious mononucleosis who do not have heterophil antibodies in their serum, and there is evidence that, whereas some of these may also be a consequence of infection with Epstein–Barr virus (Evans *et al.*, 1968; Klemola *et al.*, 1970), approximately half are associated with cytomegalovirus infection (Klemola and Kaariainen, 1965; Klemola *et al.*, 1970; Jordan *et al.*, 1973) or, occasionally, with other unknown agents (Evans, 1972; Jordan, 1975).

Leucocyte adhesion deficiency syndrome

Two studies have described severe inflammatory periodontal disease in young patients with leucocyte adhesion deficiency syndrome (Page *et al.*, 1985; Waldrop *et al.*, 1987), a rare autosomal recessive disease. Children with deficiencies in expression of the LFA family of adhesins have been reported as suffering from severe periodontal infections (Springer *et al.*, 1984). LFA-1 has a crucial role in the presentation of antigen by cells termed 'antigen presenting cells', to lymphocytes which then mount an immune response. The binding of LFA-1 to the intercellular adhesion molecule-1 (ICAM-1) is crucial in antigen presentation and in the binding of leucocytes to vascular endothelium and other surfaces; these processes permit leucocytes to leave the blood vessels at postcapillary venule sites and then accumulate at sites of inflammation. Leucocyte adhesion deficiency disease may have other forms apart from the LFA-1 deficient form (LAD-1), such as LAD-2, which is associated with an inability to sialize selectin molecules, which results in impairment of adhesion. Clinically, both forms exhibit periodontitis. Variations in density of LFA-type receptors or lack of specific LFA receptors may be involved in the aetiology of various forms of periodontal disease. So far Genco *et al.* (1986) have found no evidence of adhesion abnormalities in localized juvenile periodontitis patients. Demonstration of an abnormality in the CD11 family of leucocyte adhesion receptors on neutrophils is reported to be diagnostic for prepubertal periodontitis (Altman *et al.*, 1985). Abnormalities in a cell surface molecule that is designated GP110 and the suppression of *in vitro* neutrophil chemotaxis (related presumably to a reduced number of cell surface receptors) are considered indicative of localized juvenile periodontitis (van Dyke *et al.*, 1990). These tests of chemotaxis and receptor expression cannot be considered diagnostic, as many patients do not exhibit chemotactic defects, and the diagnosis can more easily be made by clinical and radiographic examination (Page, 1992).

LEUCOCYTE-RELATED CONDITIONS THAT AFFECT THE PDL THROUGH INVASION OR DEPOSITION

MALIGNANT LYMPHOMAS

Malignant lymphomas are neoplastic lesions of the cells of the lymphoreticular system. They occur predominantly in the lymph nodes. The cervicofacial lymph nodes are commonly involved, although, since the spread of tumour cells to involve other groups of lymph nodes is often rapid, other groups of nodes are usually also affected. In approximately 10 per cent of cases (Rosenberg *et al.*, 1961), the tumour is first noted in the head and neck region.

Malignant lymphomas are subdivided into two main groups, the non-Hodgkin's lymphomas and Hodgkin's disease, which, respectively, account for 60 per cent and 40 per cent of all lymphomas. The majority of lymphoid neoplasms arise in lymph nodes or other recognized lymphoid tissue, including the pharyngeal tonsils. However, a few occur in other extranodal sites, most commonly the gastrointestinal tract, but less frequently the salivary gland, oral mucosa, and bone. Such extranodal lymphomas account for up to 40 per cent of non-Hodgkin's lymphomas, but only occasional lesions of Hodgkin's disease arise extranodally. There is a form of lymphoma, Burkitt's lymphoma, in which involvement of the jaw is a particular characteristic (Burkitt, 1958) (see Chapter 16).

Non-Hodgkin's lymphomas

The classification of non-Hodgkin's lymphomas was originally based on the histological features of the tumours (Rappaport, 1966, 1977). With the advent of immunocytochemistry and the identification of numerous phenotypic cell markers, the classification has become complex and no single classification is generally accepted. The updated Keil classification is widely used in Europe (Stansfield *et al.*, 1988) and broadly divides lymphomas into low-grade and high-grade tumours according to their histological characteristics. The extranodal lymphomas that might affect the periodontium are derived predominantly from the mucosa-associated lymphoid tissue (MALT) (Isaacson, 1990) and share, in common with lymphomas arising from this tissue in other sites, a low grade of clinical behaviour. They tend to remain localized for relatively long periods before spreading, often to other mucosal tissues. Lymphomas arising in the bone marrow, on the other hand, tend to be more aggressive. Both types of tumour are predominantly of B cell origin, probably mostly being derived from 'centrocyte-like' cells that normally surround the B-cell follicles (Howell *et al.*, 1987; Takahashi *et al.*, 1989). They are usually diffuse rather than nodular in structure. Occasional T-cell lymphomas, some of them associated with human T_0cell lymphocytic virus, have been reported, particularly in Japan (Kurihara *et al.*, 1990). The PDL may become secondarily involved.

In the head and neck region, Waldeyer's ring is the commonest site of origin (Wong *et al.*, 1975), the gingivae, floor of mouth, vestibular sulcus, and cheek accounting for approximately 8 per cent. Males are affected twice as commonly as females and the tumours become increasingly common with age. Most patients are over 50, and the peak incidence is in the seventh decade. In the maxilla, the tumour may arise in the antrum, which is the commonest site of origin of lymphomas involving this bone (Steg *et al.*, 1959). In patients who are positive for human immune deficiency virus, the tumour may contain Epstein–Barr virus genome (Green and Eversole, 1989; Kaugars and Burns, 1989).

The most common complaint is of a painful swelling (Steg *et al.*, 1959), which may involve the bone of the maxilla and mandible or be restricted to the gingivae (Silverman, 1955; Orsos, 1958; Harvey and Thomson, 1966; Calderwood, 1967; Mittelman and Kaban, 1976). In dentate jaws, mobility of the teeth is an outstanding feature (Seldin *et al.*, 1954; Gerry and Williams, 1955; Kennedy, 1957; Cook, 1961; Chaudhry and Vickers, 1962; Tillman, 1965; Keusch *et al.*, 1966; Binnie *et al.*, 1971; Mittelman and Kaban, 1976), owing to the destruction of the PDL and alveolar bone. Thus the radiographic features associated with such lesions are predominantly those of poorly defined areas of osteolysis (Seldin *et al.*, 1954; Gerry and Williams, 1955; Steg *et al.*, 1959; Cook, 1961; Blake and Beck, 1963; Gould and Main, 1969; Binnie *et al.*, 1971), although in one report there is specific reference to the loss of the lamina dura and to the appearance of floating teeth (Blake and Beck, 1963).

The occurrence of primary intraosseous lymphomas in bone was first established by Parker and Jackson (1949), and, in the jaws, it is likely that involvement of the PDL is secondary to that of the bone marrow spaces. When the PDL is involved, it is infiltrated by dense sheets of lymphocytic cells, which results in destruction of the fibre bundles and the adjacent alveolar bone (*Fig. 18.8*). Depending on the stage of differentiation of the neoplastic cells, they will vary in appearance from small lymphocytes with darkly staining nuclei to larger, less well-differentiated cells of the centrocytic–centroblastic type, with vesicular nuclei and poorly defined cytoplasm (*Fig. 18.9*). Resorption of the roots of the teeth has been reported (Blake and Beck, 1963; Keusch *et al.*, 1966). Immunoperoxidase techniques indicate that the tumour cells exhibit a monoclonality with regard to both immunoglobulins and κ-short chains and the λ-short chains, similar to that exhibited by non-Hodgkin's lymphomas in lymph nodes.

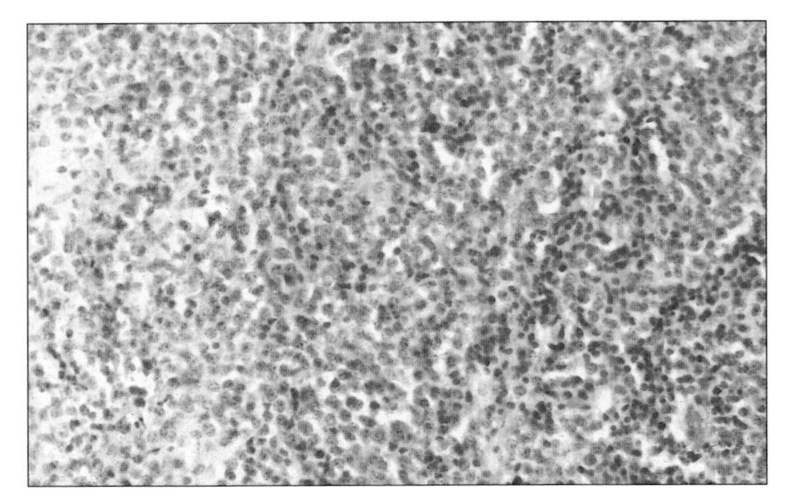

Fig. 18.8 Non-Hodgkin's, low-grade B-cell lymphoma. The tissue is occupied by well-differentiated small and large lymphoid cells, and all normal structure is destroyed. (Haematoxylin and eosin × 330.)

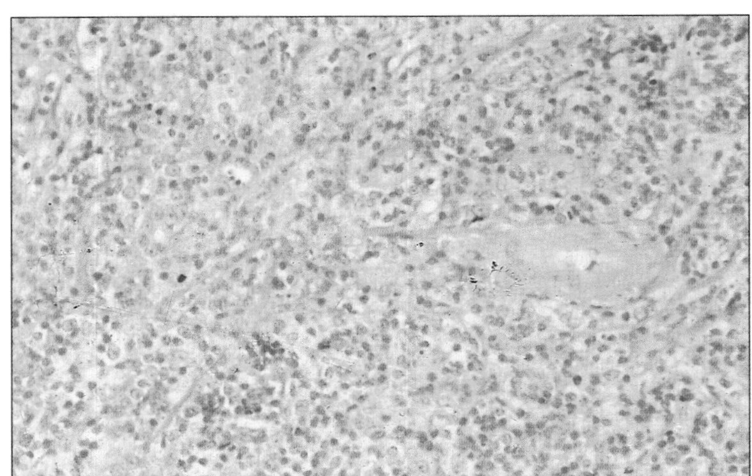

Fig. 18.9 Non-Hodgkin's, high-grade B-cell lymphoma. The tissue is infiltrated by lymphoid cells with clear vesicular nucleii and poorly defined cytoplasm. A residual blood vessel survives. (Haematoxylin and eosin × 330.)

Burkitt's lymphoma

In this form of malignant lymphoma, extranodal lesions are frequent and commonly affect the jaws in children living in the central part of Africa and in New Guinea (Burkitt, 1958). In the endemic regions of the world, Burkitt's tumour affects the jaws in 50–60 per cent of cases; other bones are only rarely involved (Burkitt, 1958, 1964; Burkitt and Davies, 1961; Edington *et al.*, 1964; Davies, 1964; Adatia, 1968a,b; Wright, 1971).

The cytological appearance of Burkitt's lymphoma is distinctive, being composed of sheets of undifferentiated lymphoblastic cells of remarkably uniform appearance, each with a round to oval nucleus containing coarsely shaped chromatin and one to four prominent nucleoli. Their cytoplasm is vacuolated and strongly pyroninophilic (WHO Bulletin, 1969), owing to the large numbers of ribosomes. Scattered among these malignant cells are varying numbers of large macrophages, which are reactive rather than neoplastic in type and whose cytoplasm frequently contains substantial quantities of nuclear debris. Their scattered distribution among the tumour cells forms a characteristic 'starry-sky' pattern. The tumour cells have the characteristics of B lymphocytes and are probably derived from germinal follicles (Schnitzer and Weaver, 1979).

In regions where it is endemic (Africa, the Middle East, New Guinea) the tumour is rare in children under 2 years and over 15 years (Burkitt, 1958; Anaissie *et al.*, 1985; Anavi *et al.*, 1990), and the peak involvement of the jaws is at the age of 3 years (Kramer, 1965; Adatia, 1968b). Involvement of the jaws becomes decreasingly common as the age of the patient increases. This association probably explains the less frequent involvement of the jaws in Burkitt's lymphoma occurring in non-endemic areas, where only 15–18 per cent have jaw involvement (Adatia, 1968b; Sariban *et al.*, 1984), since the average age of these patients is rather greater (Schnitzer and Weaver, 1979). In any event, involvement of the jaws is uncommon after the age of 15.

The maxilla is involved approximately twice as commonly as the mandible (Burkitt, 1964; Adatia, 1968b; Patton *et al.*, 1990) and the tumour usually first affects the molar regions. More than one quadrant is commonly affected, simultaneous involvement of all four being the most frequent form of multiple presentation (Adatia, 1968b). Radiological studies suggest that more than one jaw is involved in 83 per cent of patients. Loosening of the primary molars is the earliest sign and usually precedes the onset of swelling. There is rapid dissemination of the tumour cells through the posterior parts of the jaws so that varied radiological changes may be seen, including scattered foci of radiolucency, which may coalesce to form larger areas (Adatia, 1968b), loss of the lamina dura (Adatia, 1966, 1968b; Hesseling *et al.*, 1989), focal enlargement of the PDL space (Adatia, 1970), and enlargement of the crypts around unerupted teeth (Adatia, 1966; Hesseling *et al.*, 1989). There is rapidly progressive infiltration of the tumour cells among the fibres of the PDL and dental follicle, resulting in their displacement and destruction. Active osteoclastic resorption accounts for the breakdown of the alveolar bone. Subsequently, the entire attachment between the tooth and bone is disrupted and the tooth may be displaced out of the remains of its socket, thus forming a radiological image of floating teeth.

The pulp is also frequently infiltrated by tumour cells penetrating through the incompletely closed apex of developing teeth. Outward displacement of the epithelial diaphragm may occur, leading to the formation of hook-like deformities in the roots of those teeth where dentinogenesis continues (Adatia, 1968b, 1973).

The genome for Epstein–Barr virus is present in the tumour cells of 97 per cent of African patients (Ziegler, 1977), although this close association is not a feature of cases reported in non-endemic areas (Pagano *et al.*, 1973; Judson *et al.*, 1977). The significance of this association in the pathogenesis of Burkitt's lymphoma remains uncertain, although there is some evidence of overexpression of c-mcg oncogene (Syrjanen *et al.*, 1992). The presence of Epstein–Barr virus genome has also been found in Burkitt-like lymphomas occurring in patients with AIDS (Green and Eversole, 1989; Vallejo *et al.*, 1989). The aetiology of the other forms of non-Hodgkin's lymphoma affecting the jaws is unknown, although it has been demonstrated that implantation of a known carcinogen, dimethylbenzanthrocene, into extraction sockets in hamsters results in lymphoma formation (Mesrobian and Shklar, 1971).

Hodgkin's disease

Hodgkin's disease is the commonest form of malignant lymphoma. It is a multicentric condition that affects the lymph nodes and many other tissues, in particular the spleen and liver. The cervical lymph nodes are commonly involved, and this is the presenting symptom in approximately half of cases (Forman and Wesson, 1970). As in the non-Hodgkin's lymphomas, males are affected approximately twice as often as females. Hodgkin's disease occurs particularly in adolescents and young adults and after the age of 50. There is accumulating evidence for the presence of Epstein–Barr virus in affected tissues (Weiss *et al.*, 1987).

Bone involvement is not commonly reported, being observed radiologically in 8–15% of cases (Steiner, 1943; Tiwari, 1973). However, much greater involvement has been reported in histological studies of autopsy material, and Steiner (1943) found tumour foci in 78.6 per cent of cases. The areas most commonly affected were the vertebrae, pelvis, sternum, and ribs. Tumour deposits in the jaws are rare and are found in only 0–0.86 per cent of cases (Steiner, 1943; Jackson and Parker, 1945; Fuscilla and Hannam, 1961; Tiwari, 1973). It is not surprising, therefore, that there are few clinical reports of lesions involving the mouth and jaws. In three of the four cases with involvement of the PDL (Ames, 1958; Meyer *et al.*, 1959; Forman and Wesson, 1970; Tiwari, 1973), the lesion arose in the mandibular molar region in patients who were under treatment for the disease. In the fourth case the maxilla was primarily involved. The typical radiological changes were the presence of a diffuse irregular radiolucency in relation to the roots of the involved teeth, together with loss of the lamina dura. Clinically, tenderness and looseness of the teeth were a feature.

Histologically, the nodal lesions of Hodgkin's disease are characterized by the presence of Reed–Sternberg cells. Reed–Sternberg cells have large vesicular nuclei with prominent acidophilic nucleoli. Classically, they are binucleate and the two nuclei are arranged in a mirror-image pattern, although mononuclear and multinuclear forms occur. In addition, there are varying numbers of lymphocytes, plasma cells, eosinophils, and polymorphonuclear leucocytes. The lesions are classified into four distinct types, namely lymphocyte dependent, nodular sclerosing, mixed cellularity, and lymphocyte depleted, according to the proportions of the constituent cells (Lukes and Butler, 1966). Such a classification is of clinical importance, since the prognosis is substantially better in the first two types than in the last two. The paucity of data on the extranodal lesions involving the jaws does not allow any conclusion as to whether a similar classification can be applied to these lesions.

Herpes zoster is common in patients with Hodgkin's disease – it occurs in approximately 15 per cent of patients (Wilson *et al.*, 1972; Goffinet *et al.*, 1972). It is generally considered that Hodgkin's disease is a neoplasm of T lymphocytes and is accompanied by defects of cell-mediated immunity. It is likely that these defects contribute to the increased incidence of herpes zoster infections. However, the precise relationship between the two is unclear, since the changes in immune responsiveness occur early in the disease and herpes zoster infections are usually late complications (Cassazza *et al.*, 1966; Goffinet *et al.*, 1972). As a rare complication of herpes zoster infections of the trigeminal nerve in Hodgkin's disease, necrosis of the alveolar process and PDL may occur, leading to loosening and exfoliation of the teeth (Delaire *et al.*, 1964; Chenitz, 1976; Vickery and Midda, 1976).

MALIGNANT GRANULOMA AND WEGENER'S GRANULOMATOSIS

Malignant granuloma classically arises within the nose, usually in the midline, but the oral tissues may become secondarily affected. It is a destructive, granulomatous lesion which causes progressive necrosis of the midline of the face, usually culminating in rapid death (Batsakis, 1979). Very occasionally, the oral lesion may be the first sign (Garrett and Ludman, 1965; Hamilton *et al.*, 1965; Butler and Thompson, 1972), in which case pain associated with the maxillary teeth is the commonest symptom. Irregular bone loss related to the teeth, with loss of the lamina dura, may be present radiographically.

The lesion is characterized by a diffuse granulomatous infiltrate of lymphocytes and histiocytes accompanied by varying amounts of necrosis and fibrosis (*Fig. 18.10*). The cellular infiltrate is usually well differentiated and is often angiocentric in its distribution. Vasculitis may be present.

A more disseminated type of the disease is recognized (Friedman, 1964) although such variants may represent a form of Wegener's granulomatosis (Wegener, 1936). This condition is characterized by a triad of features: necrotizing granulomatous lesions of the upper and lower respiratory passages; generalized focal necrotizing vasculitis of arteries and veins, usually affecting the lungs; and glomerulitis with necrosis and thrombosis of the capillary loops, often accompanied by capsular adhesion (Godman and Churg, 1954). As with the malignant granuloma, the oral tissues may be involved, oral ulceration being the commonest feature (Walton, 1958; Reed *et al.*, 1963; Scott and Finch, 1972a). Gingivitis may also occur, and some cases exhibit an unusual form of granulomatous gingivitis in the early stages, which may be pathognomonic (Morgan and O'Neil, 1956; Reed *et al.*, 1963; Cawson, 1965; Kakehashi *et al.*, 1965; Brooke, 1969; Scott and Finch, 1972a; Edwards and Buckerfield, 1978). The gingiva is erythematous and granular, the changes spreading beyond the mucogingival junction; they may be localized in the early stages, but they usually become segmental or panoral in distribution. The term 'strawberry gums' has been applied to this condition (Israelson *et al.*, 1981; Cohen and Meltzer, 1981; Raustia *et al.*, 1985; Cohen *et al.*, 1990; Parson *et al.*, 1992). Areas of irregular bone loss, with destruction of the lamina dura and PDL of the affected teeth, are often present. In Wegener's granulomatosis there is a polymorphic infiltrate of inflammatory cells with numerous polymorphonuclear leucocytes, lymphocytes, and macrophages. Some of these cells are multinucleated, and both the foreign body and Langerhan's type are seen (*Fig. 18.11*). Tissue eosinophilia is frequently a prominent feature. Vasculitis with fibrinoid necrosis is not a significant finding in the periodontal lesions. Neutrophil anticytoplasmic autoantibodies are often present in the serum (van der Worde *et al.*, 1985; Nolle *et al.*, 1989).

The aetiology and pathogenesis of both disorders are poorly understood, although hypersensitivity (Edwards and Buckerfield, 1978) and selective immunodeficiency (Shillitoe *et al.*, 1974) may be factors. It is clear that some forms of malignant granuloma are due to peripheral T-cell lymphoma (Lippman *et al.*, 1987; Gaulard *et al.*, 1988; Chott *et al.*, 1988; Platt *et al.*, 1989; Harabuchi *et al.*, 1992) and they may arise in HIV-positive patients (Gold *et al.*, 1990). Epstein–Barr virus genome has been identified in some lesions (Harabuchi *et al.*, 1992), and this may play a role.

PLASMACYTOMA AND MULTIPLE MYELOMA

Plasma cell tumours rarely affect the jaws, and when they do it is usually as a manifestation of multiple myelomatosis. Deposits of myeloma in the jaws most frequently arise in patients with established disease (Sherman, 1951), although occasionally the jaw lesions may be the first manifestations (Wolff and Nolan, 1944;

Meloy *et al.*, 1945; Calman, 1952; Ewing and Foote, 1952; Silverman and Shklar, 1962; Lewin and Cataldo, 1967). This is probably explicable from the observation that the tumour has a predilection for bones containing active haematopoietic marrow, and since multiple myelomatosis is uncommon before the sixth decade it is not surprising that the jaws are only infrequently involved, and that the mandible is involved more often than the maxilla (Bruce and Quentin-Royer, 1953). However, it has been pointed out that deposits of myeloma can often be demonstrated histologically in bones in the absence of radiological changes (Linarzi, 1951), and it is likely that the jaws are involved more frequently than is generally reported (Bruce and Quentin-Royer, 1953; Cataldo and Meyer, 1966; Willis, 1967). It is suggested that myelomatosis is a multifocal disease rather than a single neoplasm that metastasizes (Christopherson and Miller, 1950) and therefore it also sometimes occurs as a solitary tumour or a plasmacytoma (Stout and Kenney, 1949; Christopherson and Miller, 1950; Ewing and Foote, 1952). However, it is possible that if most solitary lesions are followed up long enough, disseminated lesions will eventually appear (Lucas, 1976b).

Solitary tumours may arise within the bones of the jaws, most commonly in the mandible (Spitzer and Price, 1948; Christopherson and Miller, 1950; Ewing and Foote, 1952; Lane, 1952; Hinds *et al.*, 1956; Whitlock and Hughes, 1960) or in the overlying soft tissue (Stout and Kenney, 1949; Ewing and Foot, 1952). In the soft tissue sites, particularly when there is involvement of the gingiva, it may be difficult to distinguish between a solitary plasma cell neoplasm and dense infiltrations of plasma cells, which are believed to be reactive. Plasma cell infiltration is a feature of chronic periodontal disease, particularly in progressive chronic periodontitis and chronic hyperplastic gingivitis, although some authorities consider that when such infiltrates are prominent, they represent a specific disease process that has variably been called plasmacytosis (Poswillo, 1967; Ginwalla *et al.*, 1977) or plasma cell granuloma of the gingiva (Bhaskar *et al.*, 1968; Warson and Preis, 1969; Acevedo and Buhler, 1977). It is still not clear if they are distinct diseases or merely extreme variants of the chronic inflammatory process.

Whether the tumours are multiple or solitary, infiltration of the PDL may occur by spread of tumour cells from the medullary spaces of the mandible and maxilla or from the overlying soft tissues. Pain is the commonest complaint, but looseness of the teeth may be an early feature (Meloy *et al.*, 1945; Calman, 1952; Bruce and Quentin-Royer, 1953; Whitlock and Hughes, 1960; Orleans and Blewitt, 1965; Nally, 1968; Wood, 1975). When there is infiltration of the PDL, there is usually radiographic evidence of irregular destruction of the lamina dura around the involved teeth (Calman, 1952; Bruce and Quentin-Royer, 1953; Whitlock and Hughes, 1960; Orlean and Blewitt, 1965; Nally, 1968; Wood, 1975), together with solitary or multiple 'punched-out' areas of radiolucency of variable size, which may become confluent. Occasionally there may be single or multiple gingival swellings (Stout and Kenney, 1949; Bruce and Quentin-Royer, 1953; Smith, 1957; Orlean and Blewitt, 1965). In multiple myelomatosis there is often widespread replacement of the normal haematopoietic marrow tissue by tumour cells, which may result in thrombocytopenia, and as a result postextraction haemorrhage (Ramon *et al.*, 1965) or delayed healing (Meloy *et al.*, 1945; Spitzer and Price, 1948; Hinds *et al.*, 1956) may occur.

When the PDL is involved in plasma cell tumours, its structure is progressively destroyed by the dense infiltrate of plasma cells (*Fig. 18.12*). They may exhibit some pleomorphism, and binucleate and occasionally multinucleate forms may be present. The tumour has a scant stroma of reticulin fibres, within which deposition of amyloid sometimes occurs. Occasionally, there is active resorption of the tooth root.

In patients with multiple tumours, abnormal monoclonal immunoglobulin paraproteins can be demonstrated in the serum, and Bence–Jones protein is found in the urine – these abnormal proteins are not usually present in solitary tumours. In addition, amyloidosis arises as a complication of multiple myelomatosis in 7–15 per cent of cases (Gold, 1961), and deposits of amyloid may occur in the oral mucosa, particularly in the tongue (Cahn, 1957; Tillman, 1957; Raubenheimer *et al.*, 1988). Such deposits have also been demonstrated in the gingiva (Calkins and Cohen, 1960). Multiple myelomatous masses can form within the PDL and surrounding tissues; these masses cause gingival bleeding (particularly in the retromolar areas), destruction of alveolar bone and ligament, and expansion of the buccal cortical plates (Petit and Ripamonti, 1990).

Deposition of amyloid in the gingiva in primary and secondary amyloidosis (Symmers, 1956) is probably more common than in myelomatosis, although the frequency has varied greatly in different reports (from 0–78 per cent) (Selikoff and Robizeb, 1947; Gorlin and Gottsegen, 1949; Symmers, 1956; Cooke, 1958; Calkins and Cohen, 1960; Trieger *et al.*, 1960; Lovett *et al.*, 1965; Pettersson and Wegelius, 1972; van der Waal *et al.*, 1973). In the early stages, the deposits occur only in the walls of the small blood vessels and sinusoids and at the basement membrane of the gingival epithelium, and they do not, therefore, cause any clinical signs. There are no reports of deposits in the walls of the blood vessels of the PDL in humans, although they have been demonstrated experimentally in mice 22 weeks after the subcutaneous injection of casein (Miller and Clark, 1968). Furthermore, there is a report of a primary form of the disease in two siblings, aged 7 and 12, in whom, in addition to gingival hyperplasia, there was loosening of some of the teeth, although there was no histological examination of the PDL (Hornova and Dluhosova, 1968).

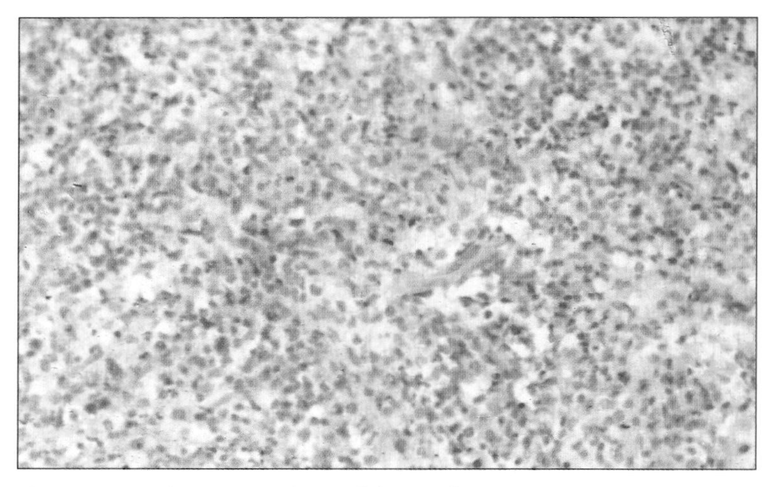

Fig. 18.10 Malignant granuloma of the maxilla. There is mixed lymphohistiocytic infiltrate, together with scattered polymorphonuclear leucocytes. (Haematoxylin and eosin × 330.)

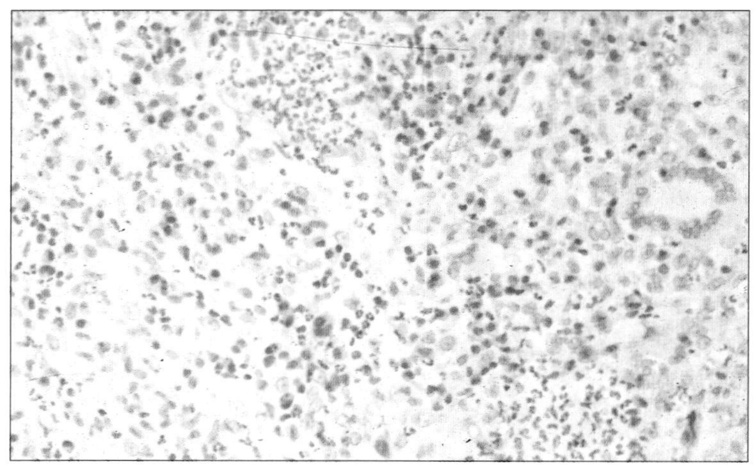

Fig. 18.11 Wegener's granulomatosis. A gingival biopsy containing a polymorphic infiltrate of polymorphonuclear leucocytes, lymphocytes, eosinophils and macrophages, some of them multinucleate. (Haematoxylin and eosin × 330.)

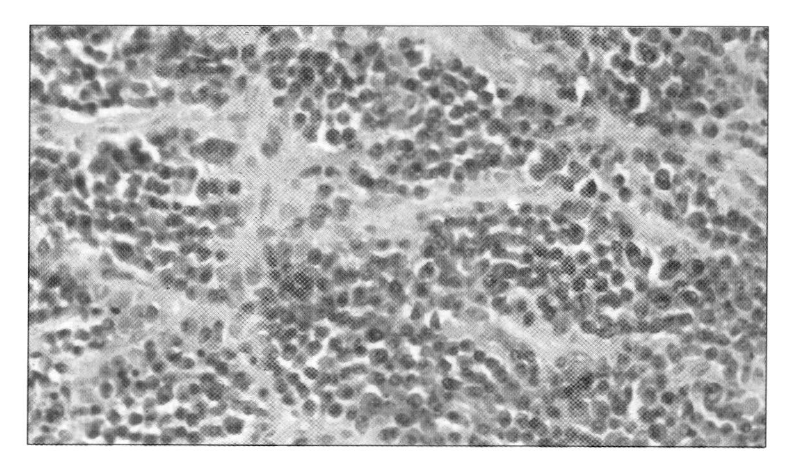

Fig. 18.12 Myelomatosis. The tissue is infiltrated by groups of pleomorphic plasma cells. (Haematoxylin and eosin × 330.)

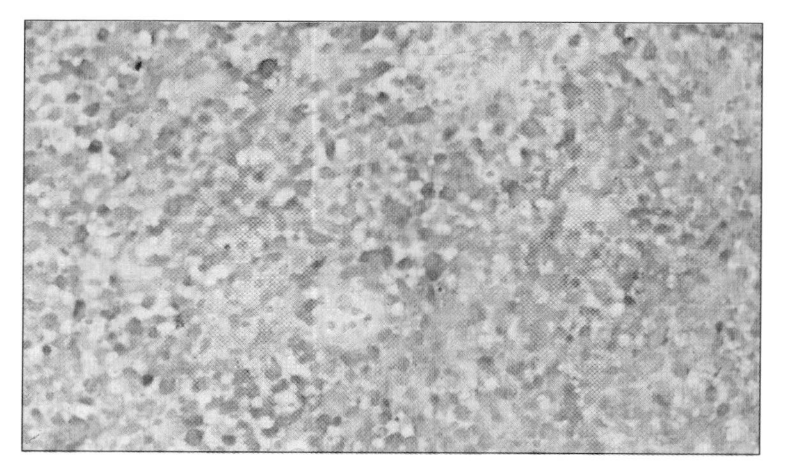

Fig. 18.13 Langerhan's cell histiocytosis. Many of the cells are positive for S-100 protein. (Immunoperoxidase × 330.).

LANGERHANS CELL HISTIOCYTOSIS (HISTIOCYTOSIS X)

Histiocytosis X was originally believed to be a disorder of histiocytes, of unknown aetiology, characterized by infiltration of the affected tissues by non-lipid-containing histiocytes. It is now known that these cells are Langerhan's cells containing Birbeck granules evident by electron microscopy and reacting positively with S-100 and HLA-DR antigens (*Fig. 18.13*) (Stewart *et al.*, 1986). The group of conditions is therefore now referred to as Langerhan's cell histiocytosis.

Three forms of the Langerhan's cell histiocytosis have been identified – Letterer–Siwe disease, Hand–Schüller–Christian disease, and eosinophilic granuloma.

Letterer–Siwe disease is the acute disseminated form in which almost any tissue of the body may be affected. This eponym was first proposed by Abt and Denenholz (1936) after the original descriptions of the disease (Letterer, 1924; Siwe, 1933). If not present at birth, it is usually manifest during the first 6 months of life and is rapidly fatal.

Hand–Schüller–Christian disease, named eponymously after the original descriptions (Hand, 1893; Schüller, 1915; Christian, 1919), is the chronic disseminated form of the disease and affects particularly the skeleton and certain viscera, notably the lungs, liver and spleen. The original descriptions drew attention to a triad of features – exophthalmos, diabetes insipidus, and multiple skeletal lesions, although this triad is probably present in only 10 per cent of cases. The disease is usually diagnosed in the first decade of life and is fatal in 30–70 per cent of cases.

Eosinophilic granuloma (Lichtenstein and Jaffe, 1940) is the localized form of the disease. It usually affects only one bone, but it can be multifocal. It is usually diagnosed in adolescents and adults before the age of 30, and is only rarely fatal. It is widely believed that these three disorders are variants of the same disease process and as such there are many examples which do not fit clearly into one category.

Oral lesions are common in Langerhan's cell histiocytosis, and have been variably reported in 10–77 per cent of cases (Sleeper, 1951; Blevins *et al.*, 1959; Sedano *et al.*, 1969; Lucaya, 1971; Sigala *et al.*, 1972; Hartman, 1980). Of greater importance is the fact that the oral lesions are the presenting symptoms in 10–28% of cases (Blevins *et al.*, 1959; Sedano *et al.*, 1969; Lucaya, 1971; Sigala *et al.*, 1972). In Letterer–Siwe disease and Hand–Schüller–Christian disease, the commonest change is the presence of ulcerative necrotic enlargement of the gingiva, together with looseness of the teeth (Blevins *et al.*, 1959; Johnson and Mohnac, 1967; Sedano *et al.*, 1969; Sigala *et al.*, 1972; Scott and Finch, 1972b; Dinardo and Wetmore, 1989). These changes most commonly occur in the mandible and usually first affect the molar teeth and subsequently spread to involve the anterior teeth. The ulcerative necrotic lesions lead to marked halitosis. The bone loss may progress rapidly and lead to premature loss of the primary and permanent teeth (Hartman, 1980).

Radiographically there is advanced bone loss around the affected teeth, with loss of the lamina dura (Winther *et al.*, 1972) and often marked areas of radiolucency. The destruction of alveolar bone may be so complete that the teeth, particularly in the molar regions, have the appearance of floating in the alveolar bone (Keusch *et al.*, 1966; Fasulo and Vangaasbeek, 1966; Boggs and McMahon, 1968; Schofield and Gardner, 1971; Betts and McNeish, 1972; Uthman, 1974). Several authors have emphasized that Langerhan's cell histiocytosis is an important cause of advanced periodontal disease in children (Kaufman, 1951; Holst *et al.*, 1953; Blevins *et al.*, 1959; Meranus *et al.*, 1968; Schofield and Gardner, 1971; Hartman, 1980; Shaw and Glenwright, 1988; Dinardo and Wetmore, 1989). In addition, cyst-like osteolytic lesions may be present.

In eosinophilic granuloma, osteolytic lesions of the jaws are the more common presentation. These are often associated with the apical regions of the teeth. They therefore simulate (both clinically and radiologically) a periapical granuloma, abscess, or cyst, and they may, at first, be treated as such (Whitehead, 1972; Carraro *et al.*, 1972; Pringle *et al.*, 1992; Dagenais *et al.*, 1992). However, the lesions recur and spread to involve adjacent teeth or other parts of the jaw. They can be extensive and predispose to pathological fracture (MacMillan *et al.*, 1991).

In all forms of Langerhan's cell histiocytosis, the PDL of the involved teeth is extensively infiltrated and destroyed by the dense histiocytic infiltrate. In Letterer–Siwe disease and Hand–Schüller–Christian disease, the infiltrate consists of large numbers of histiocytes (*Fig. 18.14*); these histiocytes contain varying numbers of fat droplets (Georgiewa *et al.*, 1965; Ritter, 1966; Markert, 1967), which sometimes assume such large proportions as to give the cells the appearance of foam cells, particularly in Hand–Schüller–Christian disease. Varying numbers of eosinophils are present. As the lesion progresses, there may be some fibrosis. Occasionally resorption of the cementum of the tooth root occurs (Carraro *et al.*, 1967; Dagenais *et al.*, 1992).

In eosinophilic granuloma, the cellular infiltrate is more mixed and contains variable proportions of histiocytes, lymphocytes, and eosinophils, although the latter usually predominate (*Fig. 18.15*).

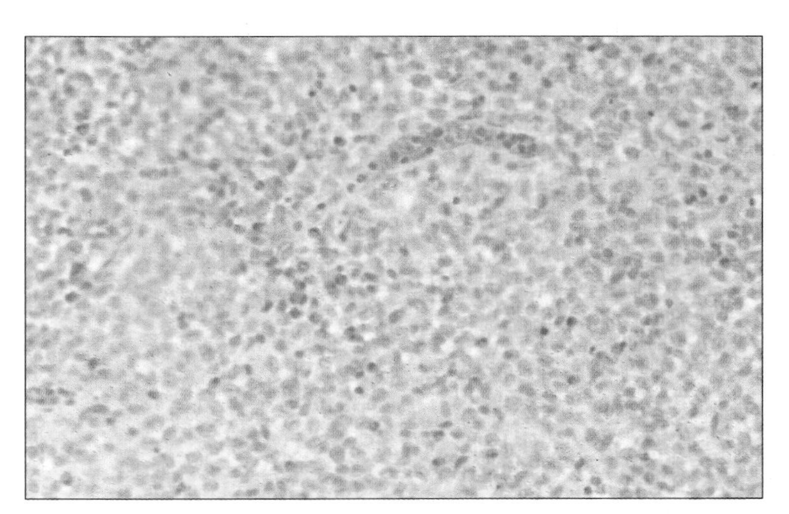

Fig. 18.14 Langerhan's cell histiocytosis (Hand–Schüller–Christian disease). The tissue is infiltrated by large numbers of histiocyte-like cells and only occasional eosinophils. (Haematoxylin and eosin × 330.)

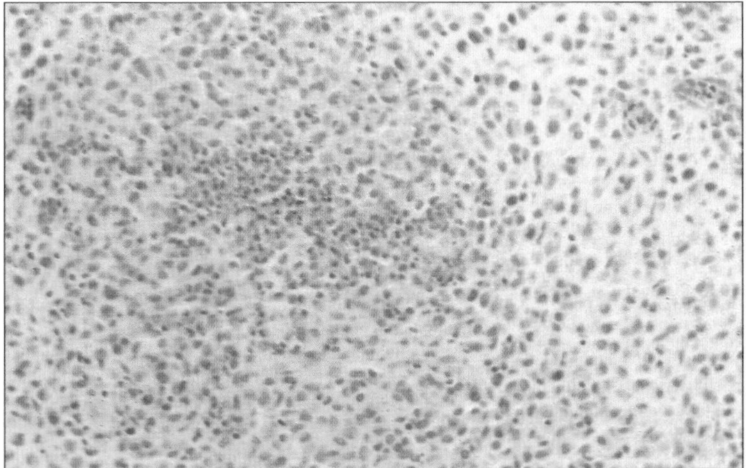

Fig. 18.15 Langerhan's cell histiocytosis (eosinophilic granuloma). Eosinophilic microabscesses, often with central necrosis, are a prominent feature among the histiocyte infiltrate. (Haematoxylin and eosin × 330.)

The eosinophils are typically formed into focal groups, the centres of which are often necrotic. The focal areas of necrosis may become confluent and form a predominant feature of the lesion. As the lesion progresses, there is increasing fibrosis and the characteristic cellular infiltrate may become decreasingly conspicuous.

The aetiology of Langerhan's cell histiocytosis is unknown, and although it is generally believed that the acute disseminated form (Letterer–Siwe disease) is neoplastic and that the chronic multifocal form (Hand–Schüller–Christian disease) and eosinophilic granuloma are reactive, the evidence for this is slight.

CONCLUSION

Microbial dental plaque is undoubtedly the main aetiological agent in chronic inflammatory periodontal disease that leads to destruction of the PDL, but the actual form of disease progression depends on the host defences to this challenge. Systemic disorders or other systemic factors may modify the normal defences and predispose individuals to specific forms and patterns of periodontal disease.

The blood cells have a vital role in supplying oxygen, haemostasis, and protection to the tissues of the periodontium. Absence, depletion, or dysfunction of these cells has effects throughout the body but particularly in the finely balanced host–parasite relationship within the gingival crevice and periodontal pocket. In this region, the leucocytes are crucial in supplying the inflammatory and immune responses to microbial insult. The red blood cells are needed for gas exchange, and the platelets are needed for control of bleeding. Systemic haematological disorders can, therefore, have profound effects on the periodontium by denying any of these functions necessary for its integrity.

The polymorphonuclear neutrophil leucocyte is undoubtedly crucial to the defence of the periodontium. To exert this protective function several activities of PMNs must be integrated – chemotaxis, phagocytosis, and killing or neutralization of the ingested organism or substance. Patients with either quantitative (neutropenia) or qualitative (chemotactic or phagocytic) PMN deficiencies exhibit severe destruction of the periodontal tissues, which is strong evidence that PMNs are an important component of the host's protective response to dental plaque. Quantitative deficiencies are generally accompanied by destruction of the periodontium of all teeth, whereas qualitative defects are often associated with localized destruction affecting only the periodontium of certain teeth (Wilton *et al.*, 1988).

Leukaemias, which give excessive numbers of leucocytes in the blood and tissues, also cause a greatly depleted bone marrow function. It is arguably the results of this depletion of the haemopoietic tissues, with the concomitant anaemia, thrombocytopenia, neutropenia, and reduced range of specific immune cells, which gives the characteristic periodontal features – anaemic gingival pallor, gingival bleeding, neutropenic ulceration, and decreased inflammatory and immune response to periodontal infection. Leukaemic features are further complicated by the potential for the proliferating leucocytes to infiltrate the gingiva and result in gingival enlargement.

Although relatively uncommon, invasion, replacement, and deposition into the tissues of the PDL by such conditions as leukaemias, lymphomas, granulomatous lesions, and myelomas can result in widespread damage to the PDL such that tooth mobility and tooth loss are evident.

In broad terms, leukaemias result in gingival problems, whereas destruction of the PDL follows neutrophil deficiencies or functional defects such as deficiency of leucocyte adhesion receptors. It is difficult to determine precisely the role any blood or lymphoreticular disorder may play in the disruption of the PDL. Apart from the multiple effects these disorders may produce, treatment of these disorders and the patient's own oral hygiene levels greatly influence the survival of the PDL. In addition, the rarity of the cases and the necessity of cross-sectional observations with few subjects necessitates care in inference. These disorders do, however, permit us to determine the relative importance of particular processes and cells in the maintenance of the PDL. Although the roles of many of these mechanisms have not been fully elucidated, further research on these and other haematological factors may help our understanding of the susceptibility of the PDL to disruption.

REFERENCES

Abt A and Denenholz EJ (1936) Letterer–Siwe's disease. Am J Dis Child 51, 499–522.

Acevedo A and Buhler JE (1977) Plasma cell granuloma of the gingiva. Oral Surg 43, 196–200.

Adatia AK (1966) Burkitt's tumour in the jaws. Br Dent J 120, 315–326.

Adatia AK (1970) Dental aspects. In: Burkitt's Lymphoma, p 36 (Burkitt DP and Wright DH, eds). Churchill Livingstone, Edinburgh.

Adatia AK (1968b) Dental tissues and Burkitt's tumour. Oral Surg 25, 221–234.

Adatia AK (1968a) Response of the dental elements to chemotherapy of Burkitt's tumour. Int Dent J 18, 646–654.

Adatia AK (1973) Dental changes in Burkitt's lymphoma. Pathol Microbiol 39, 196–203.

Allan D and Straton AG (1983). Chronic granulomatous disease with associated oral lesions. Br Dent J 154, 110–112.

Altman LC, Page RC, Vandesteen GE, Dixon LI and Bradford C (1985). Abnormalities of leukocyte chemotaxis in patients with various forms of periodontitis. J Periodont Res 20, 553–563.

Ames MI (1958) Oral manifestations of Hodgkin's disease. Oral Surg 11, 155–157.

Amorosi EL and Ultmann JE (1966) Thrombotic thrombocytopenic purpura: report of 26 cases and review of the literature. Medicine 45, 139–159.

Anaissie E, Geha S, Allam C, Jabbour J, Khalyl M and Salem P (1985) Burkitt's lymphoma in the Middle East. A study of 34 cases. Cancer 56, 2539–2543.

Anavi Y, Kaplinsky C, Calderon S and Azizov R (1990) Head, neck and maxillofacial childhood Burkitt's lymphoma. A retrospective analysis of 31 patients. J Oral Maxillofac Surg 48, 708–713.
Andrews RG, Benjamin S, Shore N and Canter S (1965) Chronic benign neutropenia of childhood with associated oral manifestations. Oral Surg 20, 719–725.
Artzi A, Gorsky M and Raviv M (1989) Periodontal manifestations of adult onset of histiocytosis X. J Periodontol 60, 57–66.
Attström R and Egelberg J (1971a) Effect of experimental leucopenia on chronic gingival inflammation in dogs. I Induction of leucopenia by nitrogen mustard. J Periodont Res 6, 194–199.
Attström R and Schroeder HE (1979) Effect of experimental neutropenia on initial gingivitis in dogs. Scand J Dent Res 87, 7–23.
Attström R and Egelberg J (1971b) Effect of experimental leucopenia on chronic gingival inflammation in dogs. II. Induction of leucopenia by heterologous anti-neutrophil serum. J Periodont Res 6, 200–210.
Awbrey JJ and Hibbard ED (1973) Congenital agranulocytosis. Oral Surg 35, 526–530.
Baehni PC, Payot P, Tsai C and Cimasoni G (1983) Periodontal status associated with chronic neutropenia. J Clin Periodontol 10, 222–230.
Baer PN and Benjamin SD (1974). Oral manifestations of systemic diseases associated with resorptive lesions of the alveolar bone. In: Periodontal Disease in Children and Adolescents, pp 183–194 and pp 206–209, Lippincott, Philadelphia.
Banks P (1967) Infectious mononucleosis: a problem of differential diagnosis to the oral surgeon. Br J Oral Surg 4, 227–234.
Barrett PA (1984). Gingival lesions in leukaemia: a classification. J Periodontol 55, 585–588.
Basu MK, Pollock A and Gordon PA (1978) Serum and salivary immunoglobulin in acute myelogenous leukaemia. Proceedings of the 17th Congress of the International Society of Haematology, p 792, Paris.
Batsakis JG (1979) Tumours of the Head and Neck. Clinical and Pathological Considerations, 2nd edition, pp 492–500, Williams and Wilkins, Baltimore.
Bauer W (1946) The supporting tissues of the tooth in acute secondary agranulocytosis (arsphenamin neutropenia). J Dent Res 25, 501–508.
Bender IB (1944) Bone changes in leukaemia. Am J Orthod 30, 556–563.
Berendes H, Bridges RA and Good RA (1957) A fatal granulomatosis of childhood: the clinical study of a new syndrome. Minn Med 40, 309–312.
Betts PR and McNeish AS (1972) Oral manifestations of Letterer–Siwe disease. Arch Dis Child 47, 463–464.
Bhaskar SN, Levin MP and Frisch J (1968) Plasma cell granuloma of periodontal tissues: report of 45 cases. Periodontics 6, 272–276.
Bhoweer AL, Shirwatkar LG and Desai AJ (1977) Possible congenital deficiency of factor X (Stuart–Prower): a case report, Ann Dent 36, 1–7.
Biggar WD, Holmes B, Page AR, Deinard AS, L'Esperance P and Good R A (1974) Metabolic and functional studies of monocytes in congenital neutropenia. Br J Haematol.28, 233–243.
Binnie WH, Bret Day RC and Lynn AH (1971) Lymphosarcoma presenting with oral symptoms. Br Dent J 130, 235–238.
Binon PP and Dykema RW (1974) Rehabilitative management of cyclic neutropenia. J Prosthet Dent 31, 52–60.
Blake MN and Beck L (1963) Reticulum cell sarcoma: report of a case. J Oral Surg 21, 165–168.
Blevins C, Dahlin DC, Lovestedt SA and Kennedy RLJ (1959) Oral and dental manifestations of histiocytosis X. Oral Surg 12, 473–483.
Blume RS, Bennett JM, Yankee RA and Wolff SM (1968) Defective granulocyte regulation in the Chediak–Higashi syndrome. N Engl J Med 279, 1009–1015.
Blume RS and Wolff SM (1972) The Chediak–Higashi syndrome: Studies in four patients and a review of the literature. Medicine 51, 245–280.
Bodey, GP (1971) Oral complications of the myeloproliferative diseases. Postgrad Med 49, 115–121.
Bodey GP, Buckley M, Sathe YS and Freireich EJ (1966) Quantitative relationships between circulating leukocytes and infection in patients with acute leukaemia. Ann Intern Med 64, 328–340.
Boggs DC and McMahon LJ (1968) Hand–Schüller–Christian disease presenting as gingivitis. Oral Surg 26, 261–264.
Brooke RI (1969) Wegener's granulomatosis involving the gingivae. Br Dent J 127, 34–36.
Brown LR, Dreizen S and Bodey GP (1973) Effect of immuno-suppression on the human oral flora. Comparative immunology of the oral cavity. DHEW Publication No (NIH) 73–428, 204–220.
Bruce KW and Quentin-Royer R (1953) Multiple myeloma occurring in the jaws. Oral Surg 6, 729–744.
Burkett LW (1940) Histopathologic explanation for oral lesions in acute leukaemia. Am J Orthod 30, 516–523.
Burkitt D (1964) A lymphoma syndrome dependent upon the environment. Part I. Clinical aspects. In: Symposium on Lymphomatous Tumours in Africa, (Roulet FC, ed), p 80, Karger, Basel.
Burkitt D and Davies JNP (1961) Lymphoma syndrome in Uganda and tropical Africa. Med Press 245, 367–369.
Burkitt D (1958) A sarcoma involving jaws in African children. Br J Surg 46, 218–224.
Butler DJ and Thompson H (1972) Malignant granuloma. Br J Oral Surg 9, 208–221.
Cahn L (1957) Oral amyloid as a complication of myelomatosis. Oral Surg 10, 735–742.
Caird FI and Holt PR (1958) The enanthema of glandular fever. Br Med J 1, 85–87.
Calderwood RG (1967) Primary reticulum cell sarcoma of gingiva. Oral Surg 24, 71–77.
Calkins E and Cohen AS (1960) Diagnosis of amyloidosis. Bull Haematol Dis 10, 215–218.
Calman HI (1952) Multiple myeloma. Report of a case first observed in the maxilla. Oral Surg 5, 1302–1311.
Carranza FA (1979) Glickman's Clinical Periodontology (5th edition), pp 529–530, Saunders, Philadelphia.
Carranza RL and Cabrini FA (1966) Histochemistry of periodontal tissues. A review of the literature. Int Dent J 16, 466–479.
Carraro JJ, Sznajder N, Barros R and Lalis RM (1972) Periodontal involvement in eosinophilic granuloma. J Periodontol 43, 427–432.
Carraro JJ, De Sereday M and Sznajder N (1967) Oral manifestations of histocytosis X. J Periodontol 38, 521–525.
Cassazza AR, Duvall CP and Carbone PP (1966) Infection in lymphoma. Histology, treatment and duration in relation to incidence and survival. J Am Med Assoc 197, 710–716.
Cassingham RJ (1971) Infectious mononucleosis. A review of the literature, including recent findings on etiology. Oral Surg 31, 610–623.
Cataldo E and Meyer I (1966) Solitary and multiple plasma cell tumours of the jaws and oral cavity. Oral Surg 22, 628–639.
Catena DL (1975) Oral manifestations of the haemoglobinopathies. Dent Clin North Am 19, 777–785.
Cawson RA (1965) Gingival changes in Wegener's granulomatosis. Br Dent J 118, 30–32.
Chaudhry AP and Vickers RA (1962) Primary reticulum cell sarcoma of the mouth. Report of a case. J Oral Surg 20, 159–162.
Chediak MM (1952) Nouvelle anomalie leucocytaire de caractère constitutionel et familial. Rev Hematol 7, 362–367.
Chenitz JE (1976) Herpes zoster in Hodgkin's disease: unusual oral sequelae. J Dent Child 43, 184–186.
Chott A, Rappersberger K, Schlossarek W and Radaszkiewicz T (1988) Peripheral T-cell lymphoma presenting primarily as lethal midline granuloma. Hum Pathol 19, 1093–1101.
Christian HA (1919) Defects in membranous bones, exophthalmos and diabetes insipidus, an unusual syndrome of dyspituitarism. Med Clin North Am 3, 849–871.

Christopherson WM and Miller AJ (1950) A re-evaluation of solitary plasma-cell myeloma of bone. Cancer 3, 240–252.

Clark RA and Kimball HR (1971) Defective granulocyte chemotaxis in the Chediak–Higashi syndrome. J Clin Invest 50, 2645–2652.

Clark RA, Kimball AS and Balestra DJ (1972). Abnormal bactericidal, metabolic and lysosomal functions of Chediak–Higashi syndrome leukocytes. J Clin Invest 51, 649–665.

Cohen DW and Morris AL (1961) Periodontal manifestations of cyclic neutropenia. J Periodontol 32, 159–168.

Cohen MM (1977) Stomatologic alterations in childhood, Part III. J Dent Child 44, 396–400.

Cohen L (1965) Recurrent oral ulceration and cutaneous infections associated with cyclical neutropenia. Dent Practitr 16, 97–98.

Contratto AW (1944) Infectious mononucleosis. A study of one hundred and ninety-six cases. Arch Intern Med 73, 449–459.

Cohen PS and Meltzer JA (1981) Strawberry gums – a sign of Wegener's granulomatosis – a distinct gingival lesion. J Am Med Assoc 246, 2610–2611.

Cohen RE, Cardoza TT, Drinnan AJ, Aquire A and Neiders ME (1990) Gingival manifestations of Wegener's granulomatosis. J Periodontol 61, 705–709.

Cook HP (1961) Oral lymphomas. Oral Surg 14, 690–704.

Cooke BED (1958) Biopsy procedures. Oral Surg 11, 750–761.

Courant P and Sobkov T (1969) Oral manifestations of infectious mononucleosis. J Periodontol 40, 279–283.

Crawford J (1988) Periodontal disease in sickle cell disease subjects. J Periodontol 59, 164–169.

Curtis AB (1971) Childhood leukaemias: osseous changes in jaws on panoramic dental radiographs. J Am Dent Assoc 83, 844–847.

Cutting HD and Lang JE (1964) Familial benign chronic neutropenia. Ann Intern Med 61, 876–887.

Dagenais M, Pharoah MJ and Sikorski MA (1992) The radiographic characteristics of histiocytosis X. A study of 29 cases that involve the jaws. Oral Surg Oral Med Oral Pathol 74, 230–236.

Davey KW and Konchak PA (1969) Agranulocytosis. Dental case report. Oral Surg 28, 166–171.

Davies JNP (1964) Lymphomas and leukemias in Uganda Africans. In: Symposium on Lymphomatous Tumours in Africa, Paris, 1963 (Roulet FC, ed), p 67, Karger, Basel.

Day PL, Langston WC and Darby WJ (1938) Failure of nicotinic acid to prevent nutritional cytopenia in the monkey. Proc Soc Exp Biol Med 38, 860–863.

Deasy MJ, Vogel R, Macedo-Sobrinho B, Gertzman G and Simon B (1980) Familial benign chronic neutropenia associated with periodontal disease. J Periodontol 51, 206–210.

Deasy MJ, Vogel RI, Annes IK and Simon BI (1976) Periodontal disease associated with preleukaemic syndrome. J Periodontol 47, 41–45.

Delaire J, Gallard A, Billet J and Renaud Y (1964) Le zona et ses manifestations faciales. Acta Odontostomatol 65, 7–22.

Delgado W and Calderon R (1979). Acatalasia in two Peruvian siblings. J Oral Path 8, 358–368.

Dent PB, Fish LA, White JG and Good RA (1966) Chediak–Higashi syndrome. Observations on the nature of the associated malignancy. Lab Invest 15, 1634–1642.

Deutsch CM, Dreizen S and Stahl SS (1969) The effects of chronic iron deficiency anaemia on the periodontium of the adult rat. J Periodontol 40, 736–739.

Dinardo LJ and Wetmore RF (1989) Head and neck manifestations of histiocytosis X in children. Laryngoscope 99, 721–724.

Dreizen A (1971) Oral indications of the deficiency states. Postgrad Med 49, 97–102.

Dreizen S, Bodey GP and Brown LR (1974) Opportunist Gram-negative bacillary infections in leukaemia. Oral manifestations during immunosuppression. Postgrad Med 55, 133–139.

Dreizen S, Levy BM and Bernick S (1969) Studies on the biology of the periodontium of marmosets. VII. The effect of vitamin C deficiency on the marmoset periodontium. J Periodont Res 4, 274–280.

Dreizen S, Levy BM and Bernick S (1970) Studies on the biology of the periodontium of marmosets. VII. The effect of folic acid deficiency on the marmoset oral mucosa. J Dent Res 49, 616–620.

Duffy JH and Driscoll EJ (1958) Oral manifestations of leukaemia. Oral Surg 11, 484–490.

Dunnet WN (1963) Infectious mononucleosis. Br Med J 1, 1187–1191.

Dupuy JM, Kourilsky FM, Fradelizzi D, *et al.* (1971) Depression of immunologic reactivity of patients with acute leukaemia. Cancer 27, 323–331.

Edington GM, Maclean CHU and Okubadejo OA (1965) 101 necropsies on tumours of the reticulo-endothelial system in Ibadan, Nigeria, with special reference to childhood lymphoma. In: Symposium on Lymphomatous Tumours in Africa, Paris, 1963 (Roulet FC, ed), p 236, Karger, Basel.

Edland CM, Hadlow WJ, Kennedy RC, Bayte, CC and Jackson TA (1968) Alentian disease of mink: properties of the aetiological agent and the host responses. J Infect Dis 118, 510–526.

Edwards MB and Buckerfield JP (1978) Wegener's granulomatosis: a case with primary mucocutaneous lesions. Oral Surg 46, 53–63.

El-Ashiry GM, Ringsdorf WMJ and Cheraskin E (1964) Local and systemic influences in periodontal disease. II. Effect of prophylaxis and natural versus synthetic vitamin C upon gingivitis. J Periodontol 35, 250–259.

Evans AS (1974) The history of infectious mononucleosis. Am J Med Sci 267, 189–195.

Evans AS (1972) Infectious mononucleosis and other monolike syndromes. N Engl J Med 286, 836–838.

Evans AS, Niederman JC and McCollum RW (1968) Seroepidemiologic studies of infectious mononucleosis with EB virus. N Engl J Med 279, 1121–1127.

Ewing MR and Foote FW (1952) Plasma-cell tumours of the mouth and upper air passages. Cancer 5, 499–513.

Fasulo CP and Vangaasbeek JB (1966) Hand–Schüller–Christian disease. Medical and surgical problems involved. Oral Surg 22, 555–563.

Ferguson, MM (1975) Oral mucous membrane markers of internal disease. Part II: disorders of the endocrine system, haematopoietic system and nutrition. In: Oral Mucosa in Health and Disease (Dolby AE, ed), pp 232–299, Blackwell, Oxford.

Flanagan V, Brown LR, Roth GD, Hoover DR, Nielsen AH and Werder AA (1970) Histopathologic changes in the oral tissue of leukaemic and non-leukaemic mice. J Periodontol 41, 526–531.

Forman GH and Wesson CM (1970) Hodgkin's disease of the mandible. Br J Oral Surg 7, 146–152.

Fox PC, Gordon RE and Williams AC (1977) Thrombotic thrombocytopenic purpura: report of a case. J Oral Surg Anaesth Hosp Dent Serv 35, 921–923.

Franklin, AL, Stokstad, ELR, Belt, M and Jukes, TH (1947) Biochemical experiments with a synthetic preparation having an action antagonistic to that of pteroylglutamic acid. J Biol Chem 169, 427–435.

Fraser-Moodie, W (1959) Oral lesions in infectious mononucleosis. Oral Surg 12, 685–691.

Friedman, I (1964) Midline granuloma. Proc. R Soc Med 57, 289–297.

Fuscilla IS and Hannam A (1961) Hodgkin's disease in bone. Radiology 77, 53–60.

Garrett JR and Ludman H (1965) Delayed healing of an extraction socket caused by a malignant granulomatous condition. Br J Oral Surg 3, 92–96.

Gates GF (1969) Chronic neutropenia presenting with oral lesions. Oral Surg 27, 563–567.

Gaulard P, Henni T, Maralleau JP, *et al.* (1988) Lethal midline granuloma (polymorphic reticulosis) and lymphomatoid granulomatosis. Evidence for a monoclonal T-cell lymphoproliferative disorder. Cancer 62, 705–710.

Genco RJ, van Dyke TE, Levine MJ, Nelson RD and Wilson ME (1986) Molecular factors influencing neutrophil defects in periodontal disease. J Dent Res.65, 1370–1391.

Georgiewa S, Georgiev G, Hadjiolov AI, and Zanruschanov I (1965) Histiochemie der Lipide in den Reticulohistiocyten bei einem Fail von Letterer–Siwescher Krankheit. Arch Klin Exp Dermatol 221, 348–357.
Gerry RG and Williams SF (1955) Primary reticulum cell sarcoma of the mandible. Oral Surg 8, 568–581.
Gillig JL and Caldwell CH (1970) The Chediak–Higashi Syndrome: case report. J Dent Child 37, 527–529.
Ginwalla TMS, Bhoweer AL and D'Silva IR (1977) Plasmacytosis of the gingiva. J Oral Med 32, 75–78.
Glickman I (1964) Nutrition in the prevention and treatment of gingival and periodontal diseases. J Dent Med 19, 179–183.
Glickman I (1948) Acute vitamin C deficiency and periodontal disease. II. The effect of acute vitamin C deficiency upon the response of the periodontal tissues of the guinea pig to artificially induced inflammation. J Dent Res 27, 201–210.
Godman GC and Churg J (1954) Wegener's granulomatosis. Pathology and review of the literature. Arch Pathol 58, 533–553.
Goffinet DR, Glatstein EJ and Merigan TC (1972) Herpes zoster varicella infections and lymphoma. Ann Intern Med 76, 235–240.
Gold JE, Ghali V, Gold S, Brown JC and Zalusky R (1990) Angiocentric immunoproliferative lesion/T-cell non-Hodgkin's lymphoma and the acquired immune deficiency syndrome: a case report and review of the literature. Cancer 66, 2407–2413.
Gold BG (1961) Amyloidosis. J Oral Surg 19, 136–139.
Goldenfarb PB and Finch SC (1973) Thrombotic thrombocytopenic purpura: a ten year survey. J Am Med Assoc 644–647.
Gorlin RJ and Chaudhry AP (1960) The oral manifestations of cyclic (periodic) neutropenia. Arch Dermatol 82, 344–347.
Gorlin RJ and Gottsegen R (1949) The role of the gingival biopsy in secondary amyloid disease. Oral Surg 2, 864–866.
Gould JF and Main JHP (1969) Primary lymphosarcoma of the maxillary alveolar process. Oral Surg 28, 106–108.
Green D (1974) Haemophilia. Postgrad Med 55, 129–133.
Green TL and Eversole LR (1989) Oral lymphomas in HIV-infected patients: association with Epstein–Barr virus DNA. Oral Surg Oral Med Oral Pathol 67, 437–442.
Grossman RC (1975) Orthodontics and dentistry for the haemophilic patients. Am J Orthod 68, 391–403.
Gustaffson GT (1969) Increased susceptibility to periodontitis in mink affected by a lysosomal disease. J Periodont Res 4, 259–267.
Halstead HL (1970) Oral manifestations of haemoglobinopathies. A case of homozygous haemoglobin C disease diagnosed as a result of dental radiographic changes. Oral Surg 30, 615–623.
Hamilton MK, Sherrer EL and Schwartz DS (1965) Lethal midline granuloma: report of a case. J Oral Surg 23, 514–520.
Hamilton RE and Giansanti JS (1974) The Chediak–Higashi Syndrome. Oral Surg 37, 754–761.
Hand A Jr (1893) Polyuria and tuberculosis. Arch Pediatr 10, 673.
Harabuchi Y, Kataura, A, Kobayashi, K, *et al.* (1992) Lethal midline granuloma (peripheral T-cell lymphoma) after lymphomatoid papulosis. Cancer 70, 835–839.
Harabuchi Y, Yamanaka N, Kataura A, *et al.* (1990) Epstein–Barr virus in nasal T-cell lymphomas in patients with lethal midline granuloma. Lancet i, 128–130.
Harrington WJ, Minnich V and Arimura G (1956) The autoimmune thrombocytopenias. Prog Hematol 1, 166–192.
Hartman KS (1980) Histiocytosis X: A review of 114 cases with oral involvement. Oral Surg 49, 38–54.
Harvey W and Thomson AD (1966) A case of reticulum cell sarcoma of gums and skin. Br J Oral Surg 3, 152–157.
Hellem AJ (1960) The adhesiveness of human blood platelets in vitro. Scand J Clin Lab Invest 12 (suppl 51).
Henle G, Henle W and Diehl V (1968) Relation of Burkitt's tumour-associated herpes type virus to infectious mononucleosis. Proc Natl Acad Sci USA 59, 74–101.
Hersh EM, Bodey GP, Nies BA and Freireich EJ (1965) The causes of death in acute leukaemia. A study of 414 patients from 1954–1963. J Am Med Assoc 193, 105–109.
Hesseling P, Wood RE, Nortje CJ and Mouton S (1989) African Burkitt's lymphoma in Cape province of South Africa and in Namibia. Oral Surg 68, 162–166.
Higashi O (1954) Congenital giantism of peroxidase granules. Tohuku J Exp Med 59, 315–332.
Hill JB and Cooper WM (1968) Thrombotic thrombocytopenic purpura. Treatment with corticosteroids and splenectomy. Arch Intern Med 122, 353–358.
Hinds EC, Pleasants JE and Bell WE (1956) Solitary plasma cell myeloma of the mandible. Oral Surg 9, 193–202.
Hoagland RJ (1964) The incubation period of infectious mononucleosis. Am J Public Health 54, 1699–1705.
Hoagland RJ (1960) The clinical manifestations of infectious mononucleosis. Am J Med Sci 240, 55–63.
Hodges RE, Hood J, Canham JE, Sauberlich HE and Baker EM (1971) Clinical manifestations of ascorbic acid deficiency in man. Am J Clin Nutr 24, 432–443.
Holst G, Husted E and Pindborg JJ (1953) On the eosinophilic bone granuloma with regard to localisation in the jaws and relation to general histiocytosis. Acta Odont Scand 10, 148–179.
Hornova J and Dluhosova A (1968) Primary amyloidosis of gingiva and conjunctiva and mental disorder in a brother and sister. Oral Surg 25, 457–464.
Howell RE, Handlers JP, Abrams AM and Melrose RJ (1987) Extranodal oral lymphoma. Part II. Relationships between clinical features and the Lukes–Collins classification of 34 cases. Oral Surg 64, 597–602.
Isaacson PG (1990) Lymphomas of mucosa-associated lymphoid tissue (MALT). Histopathol 16, 617–619.
Israelson H, Binnie WH and Hurt WC (1981) The hyperplastic gingivitis of Wegener's granulomatosis. J Periodontol 52, 81–87.
Jackson H and Parker F (1945) Hodgkin's disease. IV. Involvement of certain organs. N Engl J Med 232, 547–559.
Johnson RP and Mohnac AH (1967) Histocytosis X: report of 7 cases. J Oral Surg 25, 7–21.
Johnston RB Jr and Baehner RL (1971) Chronic granulomatous disease: correlation between pathogenesis and clinical findings. Pediatrics 48, 730–739.
Jones JH (1973) The oral mucous membrane marker of internal disease. Br Dent J 134, 81–87.
Jones JH (1975) Healthy and diseased gingiva. Practitioner 214, 356–364.
Jordan MC (1975) Nomenclature for mononucleosis syndromes. J Am Med Assoc 234, 45–46.
Jordan MC, Rousseau WE, Stewart JA, Noble GR and Chin TDY (1973) Spontaneous cytomegalovirus mononucleosis. Clinical and laboratory observations in nine cases. Ann Intern Med 79, 153–160.
Joynson DMH, Jacobs A, Walker DM and Dolby AE (1972) Defect of cell mediated immunity in patients with iron-deficiency anaemia. Lancet ii, 1058–1059.
Judson SC, Henle W and Henle G (1977) A cluster of Epstein–Barr virus associated American Burkitt's lymphoma. N Engl J Med 297, 464–468.
Kakehashi S, Hamner JE, Baer PN and McIntyre JA (1965) Wegener's granulomatosis. Report of a case involving the gingiva. Oral Surg 19, 120–127.
Kalkwarf KL and Gutz DP (1981). Periodontal changes associated with chronic idiopathic neutropenia. Pediatr Dent 3, 189–195.
Kaufman M (1951) Eosinophilic granuloma of bone. J Oral Surg 9, 273–281.
Kaugars GE and Burns JC (1989) Non-Hodgkin's lymphoma of the oral cavity associated with AIDS. Oral Surg Oral Med Oral Pathol 67, 433–436.

Kay AB, White AG, Barclay GR, *et al.* (1976) Leukocyte function in a case of chronic benign neutropenia of infancy associated with circulating leucoagglutinins. Br J Haemat 32, 451–457.

Keene JJ, Hussman L and Bruner G (1972) Terminal oral manifestations of acute lymphoblastic leukaemia. J Oral Med 27, 117–119.

Kennedy DJ (1957) Reticulum cell sarcoma of the maxilla. Oral Surg 10, 819–823.

Keusch KD, Poole CA and King DR (1966) The significance of 'floating teeth' in children. Radiology 86, 215–219.

Kinane DF (1993) Haematological disorders and the periodontium. In: Diseases of the Periodontium (Newman HN, Rees TD and Kinane D, eds), pp 175–202, Science Reviews, Northwood, Middlesex.

Klemola E, von Essen R, Henle G and Henle, W (1970) Infectious mononucleosis-like disease with negative heterophil agglutination test: clinical features in relation to Epstein–Barr virus and cytomegalovirus antibodies. J Infect Dis 121, 608–614.

Klemola E and Kaariainen L (1965) Cytomegalovirus as a possible cause of a disease resembling infectious mononucleosis. Br Med J 2, 1099–1102.

Kostman R (1956) Infantile genetic agranulocytosis (agranulocytosis infantilis hereditaria), new recessive lethal disease in man. Acta Paediat Stockh Suppl 105, 1–78.

Kramer IRH (1965) Malignant lymphoma of children in Africa. Int Dent J 15, 200–208.

Kritzler RA, Terner JY, Lindenbaum J, *et al.* (1964) Chediak–Higashi syndrome. Cytologic and serum lipid observations in a case and family. Am J Med. 36, 583–594.

Kurihara K, Kohno H, Miyamoto N, Chikamosi Y and Kondo T (1990) Pathologic characteristics of human T-cell lymphotropic virus (HTLV)–related extranodal orofacial lymphomas. Oral Surg Oral Med Oral Pathol 70, 199–205.

Kyle RA and Linman JW (1970) Gingivitis and chronic idiopathic neutropenia: report of two cases. Proc Staff Meeting Mayo Clin 45, 494–504.

Lainson PA, Brady PP and Fraleigh CM (1968) Anaemia, a systemic cause of periodontal disease. J Periodontol 39, 35–38.

Lampert F and Fesseler A (1975) Periodontal changes during chronic benign granulocytopenia in childhood. J Clin Periodontol 2, 105–110.

Lane SL (1952) Plasmacytoma of the mandible. Oral Surg 5, 434–442.

Laskin JL (1974) Oral haemorrhage after the use of quinidine. J Am Dent Assoc 88, 137–139.

Lavine WS, Page RC and Padgett GA (1976) Host response in chronic periodontal disease. V. The dental and periodontal status of mink and mice affected by Chediak–Higashi syndrome. J Periodontol 47, 621–635.

Leader RW, Padgett GA and Gorham JR (1963) Studies of abnormal leucocyte bodies in the mink. Blood 22, 477–484.

Lehrer RI, Goldberg LS, Apple MA and Rosenthal NP (1972) Refractory megaloblastic anaemia with myeloperoxidase-deficient neutrophils. Ann Intern Med 76, 447–453.

Lerman RL and Grodin MA (1977) Necrotising stomatitis in a pediatric burn victim. J Dent Child 44, 36–38.

Letterer E (1924) Aleukamische Retikulose. Frankf Z Pathol 30, 377–394.

Levine S (1959) Chronic familial neutropenia with marked periodontal lesions. Oral Surg 12, 310–314.

Lewin RW and Cataldo E (1967) Multiple myeloma discovered from oral manifestations: report of a case. J Oral Surg 25, 68–72.

Lichtenstein L and Jaffe HL (1940) Eosinophilic granuloma of bone, with report of a case. Am J Pathol 16, 595–604.

Lichtenstein L (1964) Histiocytosis X (eosinophilic granuloma of bone, Letterer–Siwe disease, Hand–Schüller–Christian disease): further observations of pathological and clinical importance. J Bone Joint Surg 46, 76–90.

Lichtenstein L (1953) Histocytosis X: Integration of eosinophilic granuloma of bone 'Letterer–Siwe disease', and 'Schüller–Christian disease' as related manifestations of a single nosologic entity. Arch Pathol 56, 84–102.

Linarzi LR (1951) Diagnostic and therapeutic aspects of multiple myeloma. Med Clin North Am 35, 189–226.

Lippman SM, Grogan TM, Spier CM, *et al.* (1987) Lethal midline granuloma with a novel T-cell phenotype as found in peripheral T-cell lympoma. Cancer 59, 936–939.

Long LM, Jacoway JR and Bawden JW (1983). Cyclic neutropenia: case report of two siblings. Pediatr Dent 5, 142–144.

Lovett DW, Cross KR and van Allen M (1965) The prevalence of amyloids in gingival tissues. Oral Surg 20, 444–448.

Lucas, RB (1976a) Pathology of Tumours of the Oral Tissues (3rd edtion), p 250, Churchill Livingstone, Edinburgh.

Lucas RB (1976b) Pathology of Tumours of the Oral Tissues (3rd edition), p 254, Churchill Livingstone, Edinburgh.

Lucaya J (1971) Histocytosis X. Am J Dis Child 121, 289–295.

Lukes R and Butler JJ (1966) The pathology and nomenclature of Hodgkin's disease. Cancer Res 26, 1063–1081.

Lynch MA and Ship II (1967a) Initial oral manifestations of leukaemia. J Am Dent Assoc 75, 932–940.

Lynch MA and Ship II (1967b) Oral manifestations of leukaemia: a postdiagnostic study. J Am Dent Assoc 75, 1139–1144.

MacGillwray JB, Pacie JV, Henry JRK, Sacker LS and Tigard JPM (1964) Congenital neutropenia: a report of five cases. Acta Paediatr Stockh 53, 188–203.

Macmillan AR, Oliver AJ, Radden BG and Lay MF (1991) Langerhan's cell disease associated with pathological fracture of the mandible. Aust Dent J 36, 451–455.

Mallett SP, Golan HP, England LC and Kutch JH (1947) Acute myelogenous leukemia with primary oral manifestations. J Oral Surg 5, 209–214.

Markert J (1967) Zur Ultrastruktur des eosinophilen Granulom des Knochens. Frankf Z Pathol 76, 157–163.

Matsaniotis N, Kossoglau K, Karpouzas J and Anastasea-Vlachou K (1966) Chromosomes in Kostmann's disease. Lancet ii, 104.

Matthews JB and Basu MK (1983) Primary extra-nodal lymphoma of the oral cavity: an immunohistochemical study. Br J Oral Surg 21, 159–170.

McCarthy FP and Karcher DH (1946) The oral lesions of monocytic leukaemia. N Engl J Med 234, 787–790.

McGowan DA, Gorman JM and Otridge DW (1970) Intensive dental care in adult acute leukaemia. Dent Practit 20, 239–243.

McKee LC and Collins RD (1974) Intravascular leukocyte thrombi and aggregates as a cause of morbidity and mortality in leukaemia. Medicine 53, 463–478.

McKelvy B, Satinover F and Sanders B (1976) Idiopathic thrombocytopenic purpura manifesting as gingival hypertrophy: case report. J Periodontol 47, 661–663.

Meloy TM, Gunter JH and Sampson DA (1945) Mandibular lesion as first evidence of multiple myeloma. Am J Orthod 31, 685–689.

Meranus H, Carlin R, Surprenant P and Seldin R (1968) Histiocytosis X: problems in diagnosis. Oral Surg 26, 759–768.

Merril A and Peterson LJ (1970) Gingival haemorrhage secondary to uraemia. Review and report of a case. Oral Surg 29, 530–535.

Mesrobian AZ and Shklar G (1971) Experimental oral malignant lymphoma using alveolar socket carcinogen implantation. J Periodontol 42, 105–108.

Meyer G, Roswit B and Unger SM (1959) Hodgkin's disease of the oral cavity. Am J Roentg 81, 430–432.

Michaud M, Baehmer RL, Bixler D and Kafrany AH (1977) Oral manifestations of acute leukaemia in children. J Am Dent Assoc 95, 1145–1150.

Miller AS and Clark PG (1968) Experimental amyloidosis: deposition in the general and oral tissues of mice. J Oral Surg 26, 175–179.

Miller ME, Oski FA and Harris MB (1971) Lazy-leucocyte syndrome. A new disorder of leucocyte formation. Lancet i, 665–668.

Mintz U and Sachs L (1973) Normal granulocyte colony forming cells in the bone marrow of Yemenite Jews with genetic neutropenia. Blood 41, 745–751.

Mishkin DJ, Akers JO and Darby CP (1976) Congenital neutropenia. Report of a case and a biorationale for dental management. Oral Surg 42, 738–745.
Mittelman D and Kaban LB (1976) Recurrent non-Hodgkin's lymphoma presenting with gingival enlargement. Oral Surg 42, 792–800.
Morgan AD and O'Neil R (1956) The oral complications of polyarteritis and giant cell granulomatosis (Wegener's granulomatosis). Oral Surg 9, 845–857.
Morris AL and Stahl SS (1954) Intra-oral roentgenographic changes in sickle cell anaemia. A case report. Oral Surg 7, 787–791.
Moschcowitz E (1925) An acute febrile pleiochromic anemia with hyaline thrombosis of the terminal arterioles and capillaries. An undescribed disease. Arch Intern Med 36, 89–93.
Moughal NA, Adonogianaki E, Thornhill MH and Kinane DF (1992) Endothelial cell leukocyte adhesion molecule-1 (ELAM-1) and intercellular adhesion molecule-1 (ICAM-1) expression in gingival tissue during health and experimentally induced gingivitis. J Periodont Res 27, 623–630.
Nally FE (1968) Myeloma-like plasma cell lesion of the maxilla. Ir J Med Sci 7, 227–236.
Niederman JC McCollum RW, Henle G and Henle W (1968) Infectious mononucleosis: clinical manifestations in relation to EB virus antibodies. J Am Med Assoc 203, 205–209.
Nilsson IM, Blomback M, Jorres E, Blomback B and Johansson SA (1957) On an inherited autosomal haemorrhagic diathesis with antihemophilic globulin (AHG) deficiency and prolonged bleeding time. Acta Med Scand 159, 179–188.
Nixon KC, Keys DW and Brown G (1975) Oral management of Glanzmann's thrombasthenia. A case report. J Periodontol 46, 364–367.
Nolle B, Specks U, Ludermann J, Rohsbeck MS, Deremee RA and Gross WL (1989) Anticytoplasmic autoantibodies: their immunodiagnostic value in Wegener's granulomatosis. Ann Intern Med 111, 28–40.
O'Leary TJ, Rudd KD, Crump PP and Krause RE (1969) The effect of ascorbic acid supplementation on tooth mobility. J Periodontol 40, 284–286.
Onwubalili K (1983). Sickle cell disease and infection. Infect Immun 7, 2–9.
Orlean SL and Blewitt G (1965) Multiple myeloma with manifestation of a bony lesion in the maxilla. Oral Surg 19, 817–824.
Orsos S (1958) Primary lymphosarcoma of the gingivae. Oral Surg 11, 426–430.
Padgett GA, Leader RW, Gorham JR and O'Mary CC (1964) The familial occurrence of the Chediak–Higashi syndrome in mink and cattle. Genetics, Princeton 49, 505–512.
Padgett GA, Reiquam CW, Gorham JR, Henson JB and O'Mary CC (1967) Comparative studies of the Chediak–Higashi syndrome. Am J Path 51, 553–571.
Pagano JS, Huang CH and Levine P (1973) Absence of Epstein–Barr viral DNA in American Burkitt's lymphoma. N Engl J Med 289, 1395–1399.
Page AR and Good RA (1957) Studies on cyclic neutropenia: a clinical and experimental investigation. Am J Dis Child 94, 623–661.
Page RC (1992) Host response tests for diagnosing periodontal diseases. J Periodontol 63, 356–366.
Page RC, Sims TJ, Geissler F, Altman LC and Baab DA (1985) Defective neutrophil and monocyte mobility in patients with early onset periodontitis. Infect Immun 47, 169–175.
Parker F Jr and Jackson H Jr (1949) Primary reticulum cell sarcoma of bone. Surgery 68, 45–53.
Parson E, Seymour RA, Macleod RI, Nand N and Ward MK (1992) Wegener's granulomatosis – a distinct gingival lesion. J Clin Periodontol 19, 64–66.
Patton LL, McMillan CW and Webster WP (1990) Americal Burkitt's lymphoma: a 10-year review and case study. Oral Surg 69, 307–316.
Paul JR and Bunell WW (1932) The presence of heterophile antibodies in infectious mononucleosis.
Peltier JR and Olivier RM (1961) Oral manifestations of idiopathic thrombocytopenic purpura. J Oral Surg 19, 130–135.
Petit JC and Ripamonti U (1990) Multiple myeloma of the periodontium. A case report. J Periodontol 61, 132–137.
Petterson T and Wegelius D (1972) Biopsy diagnosis of amyloidosis in rheumatoid arthritis. Malabsorption caused by intestinal amyloid deposits. Gastroenterology 62, 22–27.
Pindborg JJ (1949) The effect of methyl folic acid on the periodontal tissues in rat molars (experimental granulocytopenia). Oral Surg 2, 1485–1496.
Platt JC, Tomich CE and Campbell S (1989) Malignant lymphoma presenting as a midline lethal granuloma. J Oral Maxillofac Surg. 47, 511–513.
Pogrel MA (1978) Acute leukaemia. An atypical case presenting with gingival manifestations. Int J Oral Surg 7, 119–122.
Poswillo D (1967) Plasmacytosis of the gingiva. Br J Oral Surg 5, 194–202.
Presant CA, Safdar SH and Cherrick H (1973) Gingival leukaemic infiltration in chronic lymphocytic leukaemia. Oral Surg 36, 672–674.
Pretty HM, Gosselin G, Colpron G and Long LA (1965) Agranulocytosis: a report of 30 cases. Can Med Assoc J 93, 1058–1064.
Prichard JF, Ferguson DM, Windmiller J and Hart WC (1984) Prepubertal periodontitis affecting the deciduous dentition and the permanent dentition in a patient with cyclic neutropenia: a case report and discussion. J Periodontol 55, 114–122.
Priest RE (1970) Formation of epithelial basement membrane is restricted by scurvy in vitro and is stimulated by vitamin C. Nature 225, 744–745.
Pringle GA, Daley TD, Veinot LA and Wysocki GP (1992) Langerhan's cell histiocytosis in association with periapical granulomas and cysts. Oral Surg 74, 186–192.
Prowler JR and Smith EW (1965) Dental bone changes occurring in sickle cell diseases and abnormal haemoglobin traits. Radiol 65, 762–769.
Ramon Y, Marberg K, Samra H and Kaufman A (1965) Severe post-extraction bleeding as a presenting feature in a case of multiple myeloma. Oral Surg 19, 720–722.
Rappaport H (1966) Tumours of haematopoietic system. In: Armed Forces Institute of Pathology, Atlas of Tumor Pathology, Section II, Fascicle 8, Washington DC.
Rappaport H (1977) In: Berard CW, Discussion II: round table discussion of histopathological classification. Cancer Treat Rep 61, 1037–1048.
Raubenheimer EJ, Danth J and Pretorius J (1988) Multiple myeloma and amyloidosis of the tongue. J Oral Pathol 17, 554–559.
Raustia AM, Autio-Harmainen HI, Knuuttila MLE and Raustia JM (1985) Ultrastructural findings and clinical follow-up of 'strawberry gums' in Wegener's granulomatosis. J Oral Pathol 14, 581–587.
Reed WB, Jensen AK, Konwaler BE and Hunter D (1963) The cutaneous manifestations in Wegener's granulomatosis. Acta Derm Venereol (Stockh) 43, 250–264.
Reichart PA and Dornow H (1978) Gingivo-periodontal manifestations in chronic benign neutropenia J Clin Periodontol 5, 74–80.
Reimann HA and Debaradinis CT (1949) Periodic (cyclic) neutropenia, an entity: collection of sixteen cases. Blood 4, 1109–1116.
Renshaw HW, Davis WC, Fudenberg HH and Padgett GA (1974) Leukocyte dysfunction in the bovine homologue of the Chediak–Higashi syndrome in humans. Infect Immun 10, 928–937.
Ritter RA (1966) Histiocytosis X: a case report with electron microscopic observations. Cancer 19, 1155–1169.
Robinson IB and Sarnat BG (1952) Roentgen studies of the maxillae and mandible in sickle cell anaemia. Radiology 58, 517–523.
Rosenberg SA, Diamond HD, Jaslowitz B and Craver LF (1961) Lymphosarcoma: a review of 1269 cases. Medicine 49, 31–84.
Rylander H, Attström R and Lindhe J (1975) Influence of experimental neutropenia in dogs with chronic gingivitis. J Periodont Res 10, 315–323.

Rylander H and Ericsson I (1981). Manifestations and treatment of periodontal disease in a patient suffering from cyclic neutropenia. J Clin Periodontol 8, 77–80.
Sariban E, Donhu A and McGrath IT (1984) Jaw involvement in American Burkitt's lymphoma. Cancer 53, 1777–1782.
Schiliro G, Pizzarelli G, Russo A and Sciacca A (1977) Dental care in leukaemia. N Engl J Med 296, 109.
Schluger S, Yuodelis RA and Page RC (1977) Periodontal Disease, p 98, Lea and Febiger, Philadelphia.
Schnitzer B and Weaver DK (1979) Lymphoreticular disorders. In: Tumours of the Head and Neck, 2nd edition, pp 448–491 (Batsakis JG, ed). Williams and Wilkins, Baltimore.
Schofield IDF and Gardner DG (1971) Histiocytosis X: a case diagnosed from the oral findings. J Can Dent Assoc 37, 343–346.
Schuller A (1915) Über eigenartige Schadeldefekte im Jugendalter. Fortschr Geb Rontgenstr 23, 12–18.
Schwartz J, Rosenberg A and Cooperberg AA (1972) Thrombotic thrombocytopenic purpura: a successful treatment of two cases. Can Med Assoc J 106, 1200–1205.
Scott J and Finch LD (1972a) Wegener's granulomatosis presenting as gingivitis. Oral Surg 34, 920–933.
Scott J and Finch LD (1972b) Histiocytosis X with oral lesions. J Oral Surg 30, 748–753.
Scully C, Macfadyen E and Campbell A (1982) Oral manifestations in cyclic neutropenia. Br J Oral Surg 20, 96–101.
Sedano HO, Cernea P, Hoske G and Gorlin RJ (1969) Histiocytosis X: clinical, radiologic and histologic findings with special attention to oral manifestations. Oral Surg 27, 760–771.
Segelman AE and Doku HC (1977) Treatment of the oral complications of leukaemia. J Oral Surg 35, 469–477.
Seldin HM, Seldin SD and Rakower W (1954) Oral lymphosarcoma. J Oral Surg 12, 3–15.
Selikoff IJ and Robizek EH (1947) Gingival biopsy for the diagnosis of generalised amyloidosis. Am J Pathol 23, 1099–1111.
Shaw L and Glenwright HD (1988) Histiocytosis X: an oral diagnostic problem. J Clin Periodontol 15, 321–315.
Sherman RA (1951) Resumé of the roentgen diagnosis of tumours of the jaw bones. Oral Surg, 4, 1427–1443.
Shillitoe EJ, Lehner T, Lessof MH and Harrison DFN (1974) Immunological features of Wegener's granulomatosis. Lancet i, 281–284.
Shiver CB, Berg P and Frenkel EP (1956) Palatine petechiae, an early sign in infectious mononucleosis. J Am Med Assoc 161, 592–594.
Siddons RC (1974) Experimental nutritional folate deficiency in the baboon (*Papio cynocephalus*). Br J Nutr 32, 579–587.
Sigala JL, Silverman S, Brody HA and Kushner JH (1972) Dental involvement in histiocytosis. Oral Surg 33, 42–48.
Silverman LM (1955) Lymphosarcoma of gingivae. Oral Surg 8, 1108–1114.
Silverman LM and Shklar G (1962) Multiple myeloma: report of a case. Oral Surg 15, 301–309.
Sinrod HS (1957) Leukaemia as a dental problem. J Am Dent Assoc 55, 809–818.
Siwe S (1933) Die Reticuloendotheliose – ein neues Krankheitsbild unter den Hepatosplenomegalien. Z Kinderheilk 52, 212–217.
Sleeper EL (1951) Eosinophilic granuloma of bone. Its relationship to Hand–Schüller–Christian and Letterer–Siwe diseases, with emphasis upon oral symptoms and findings. Oral Surg 4, 896–918.
Smillie AC and Cowman SC (1969) Pulp and periapical involvement in leukaemia. NZ Dent J 65, 32–34.
Smith DB (1957) Multiple myeloma involving the jaws. Oral Surg 10, 910–919.
Smith EW and Conley CL (1953) Filter paper electrophoresis of human haemoglobins with special reference to the incidence and clinical significance of Hemoglobin C. Bull Johns Hopkins Hosp 93, 94–106.
Smith JF (1964) Cyclic neutropenia. Oral Surg 18, 312–320.
Soni NN (1966) Microradiographic study of dental tissues in sickle cell anaemia. Arch Oral Biol 11, 561–564.
Spencer P and Fleming JE (1985). Cyclic neutropenia: a literature and report of a case. J Dent Child 52, 108–113.
Spitzer R and Price LW (1948) Solitary myeloma of the mandible. Br Med J 1, 1027–1028.
Springer TA, Thompson WS and Miller (1984) Inherited deficiency of the MAC-1, LFA-1, P150,95 glycoprotein family and its molecular basis. J Exp Med 160, 1901–1918.
Stafford R, Sonis S, Lockhart P and Sonis A (1980). Oral pathoses as diagnostic indicators in leukaemia. Oral Surg 50, 134–138.
Stamps JT (1974) The role of oral hygiene in a patient with idiopathic aplastic anaemia. J Am Dent Assoc 88, 1025–1027.
Stansfield AG, Diebold J and Noel H (1988) Updates Kiel classification for lymphomas. Lancet i, 292–293.
Steg RF, Dahlin DC and Gores RJ (1959) Malignant lymphoma of the mandible and maxillary region. Oral Surg 12, 128–141.
Steiner PE (1943) Hodgkin's disease. The incidence, distribution, nature and possible significance of lymphogranulomatous lesions in the bone marrow. A review of the original data. Arch Pathol 36, 627–637.
Stern MH and Cole WL (1973) Radiographic changes in the mandible associated with leukaemic cell infiltration in a case of acute myelogenous leukaemia. Oral Surg 36, 343–348.
Stewart JCB, Regezi JA, Lloyd RV and McClatchey RD (1986) Immunohistochemical study of idiopathic histiocytosis of the mandible and maxilla. Oral Surg 61, 48–53.
Stout AP and Kenney FR (1949) Primary plasma-cell tumours of the upper air passages and oral cavity. Cancer 2, 261–277.
Swenson HM, Redish CH and Manne M (1965) Agranulocytosis: two case reports. J Periodontol 36, 466–470.
Sydney SB and Serio F (1981). Acute monocytic leukaemia diagnosed in a patient referred because of gingival pain. J Am Dent Assoc 103, 886–887.
Symmers WStC (1956) Primary amyloidosis: a review. J Clin Pathol 9, 187–211.
Syrjanen S, Kallio P, Sainio P, Chang F and Syrjanen K (1992) Epstein–Barr virus – EBV genomes and c-myc oncogene in Burkitt's lymphomas. Scand J Dent Res 100, 176–179.
Takahashi H, Tsuda N, Teguka F and Okabe H (1989) Primary extranodal non-Hodgkin's lymphoma of the oral region. J Oral Pathol Med 18, 84–91.
Taliano AD and Wakefield BG (1966) Atypical oral symptoms in acute myeloblastic leukaemia: report of a case. J Oral Surg 24, 440–444.
Taubman SB, Cogen RB and Lepow AH (1974) Granule enzymes from human leukocytes. Their effects on HeLa cells. Proc Soc Exp Biol Med 145, 952–957.
Telsey B, Beube FE, Zegarelli EV and Kutscher AH (1962) Oral manifestations of cyclical neutropenia associated with hypergamma-globulinaemia. Oral Surg 15, 540–543.
Temple TR, Kimball HR, Kakehashi S and Amen CR (1972) Host factors in periodontal disease: periodontal manifestations of Chediak–Higashi syndrome. J Periodont Res Suppl 10, 26–27.
Tillman HM (1965) Malignant lymphomas involving the oral cavity and surrounding structures. Oral Surg 19, 60–72.
Tillman HM (1957) Oral manifestations of generalised systemic amyloid disease. Oral Surg 10, 743–748.
Tiwar RM (1973) Hodgkin's disease of maxilla. J Laryngol Otol 87, 85–88.
Trieger N, Cohen AS and Calkins E (1960) Gingival biopsy as a diagnostic aid in amyloid disease. Arch Oral Biol 1, 187–192.
Uthman AA (1974) Hand–Schüller–Christian disease. J Oral Med 29, 22–24.
Valentine WN (1971) Infectious mononucleosis. In: Cecil-Loeb Textbook of Medicine (Beeson PB and McDermott, eds), pp 1565–1566, Saunders, Philadephia.
Vallejo GH, Garcia MD, Lopez A, Mendieta C and Moskow BS (1989) Unusual periodontal findings in an AIDS patient with Burkitt's lymphoma. J Periodontol 60, 723–727.

van der Waal I, Fehmers MCO and Kraal ER (1973) Amyloidosis: its significance in oral surgery. Oral Surg 36, 469–481.

van der Worde FJ, Rasmussen N and Lobatto S (1985) Autoantibodies against neutrophils and monocytes: tool for diagnosis and marker of disease activity in Wegener's granulomatosis. Lancet i, 425–429.

van Dyke TE, Offenbacher S, Kalmar J, Arnold RR and Soskolne WA (1990) Reactor paper: risk factors involving host defense mechanisms. In: Risk Assessment in Dentistry (Baker JD, ed), pp 105–108, University of North Carolina Press, Chapel Hill.

Vann WF and Oldenburg TR (1976) Atypical hereditary neutropenia: case reports of two siblings. J Dent Child 43, 265–269.

Vickery I and Midda M (1976) Dental complications of cytotoxic therapy in Hodgkin's disease – a case report. Br J Oral Surg 13, 282–288.

Wade AB and Stafford JL (1963) Cyclical neutropenia. Oral Surg 16, 1443–1448.

Waldrop TC, Anderson DC, Hallmon WW, Schmalsteig FC and Jacobs RL (1987) Periodontal manifestations of the heritable Mac-1, LFA-1 deficiency syndrome. Clinical, histopathologic, and molecular characteristics. J Periodontol 58, 401–416.

Walton EW (1958) Giant cell granuloma of the respiratory tract (Wegener's granulomatosis). Br Med J 2, 265–270.

Warson R and Preis F (1969) A nonexophytic plasma-cell granuloma of the mandible. Oral Surg 28, 791–796.

Weary PE and Bender AS (1967) Chediak–Higashi syndrome with severe cutaneous involvement. Occurrence in two brothers 14 and 15 years of age. Arch Intern Med 119, 381–386.

Wegener F (1936) Über generalisierte, septische Gafasserkrankungen. Verh Dtsch Ges Pathol 29, 202–209.

Weiss LM, Strickler JG, Warnke RA, Purtilo DT and Sklar J (1987) Epstein–Barr viral DNA in tissue of Hodgkin's tissue. Am J Pathol 129, 86–91.

White JG (1966) The Chediak–Higashi syndrome: a possible lysosomal disease. Blood 28, 143–156.

Whitehead FIH (1972) Histiocytosis X. Br J Oral Surg 10, 199–204.

Whitlock RIH and Highes NC (1960) Solitary myeloma of mandible. Oral Surg 13, 23–32.

WHO Bulletin (1969) Histopathological definition of Burkitt's tumor. Memorandum Rev Bull WHO 40, 601.

Willis RA (1967) Pathology of Tumours, 4th edition, pp 795–802, Butterworths, London.

Wilson JF, Marsa GW and Johnson RE (1972) Herpes zoster in Hodgkin's disease. Clinical, histologic and immunologic correlations. Cancer 29, 461–465.

Wilton JMA, Griffiths GS, Curtis MA, *et al.* (1988) Detection of high-risk groups and individuals for periodontal diseases. J Clin Periodontol 6, 339–346.

Winther JE, Fejerskov O and Philipsen HP (1972) Oral manifestations of histiocytosis X. Arch Derm Stockh. 52, 75–79.

Wolbach SB and Bessy OA (1942) Tissue changes in vitamin deficiencies. Physiol Rev 22, 233–289.

Wolf JE and Ebel LK (1978) Chronic granulomatous disease: report of a case and review of the literature. J Am Dent Assoc 96, 292–295.

Wolff E and Nolan LE (1944) Multiple myeloma first discovered in the mandible. Radiol 42, 76–78.

Wong DS, Fullmer LM, Butler JJ and Shullenberger CC (1975) Extranodal non-Hodgkin's lymphoma of the head and neck. Am J Roentg 123, 471–481.

Wood GD (1975) Myelomatosis: a case report. Br Dent J 139, 472–474.

Wright DH (1971) Burkitt's lymphoma: a review of the pathology, immunology, and possible etiologic factors. Pathol Ann 6, 337–363.

Yeager DA (1975) Idiopathic thrombocytopenic purpura: report of a case. J Am Dent Assoc 30, 640–643.

Ziegler JL (1977) Treatment results of 54 American patients with Burkitt's lymphoma are similar to the African experience. N Engl J Med 297, 75–80.

Zucker-Franklin D, L'Esperance P and Good RA (1977) Congenital neutropenia: an intrinsic cell defect demonstrated by electron microscopy of soft agar colonies. Blood 49, 425–436.

Chapter 19
Periodontal cysts

KW Lee

INTRODUCTION

The periodontal ligament (PDL) is occasionally involved by non-neoplastic cysts. These pathological lesions are soft tissue sacs containing fluid, semi-fluid or gas, and they may contain pus when secondarily infected. They are frequently, but not always, lined by epithelium. The epithelium that lines these cysts originates in the majority of cases from the odontogenic apparatus; in a few areas of the jaws, it is possible that the epithelium may be non-odontogenic in origin.

Oral cysts that do not involve the PDL are not discussed in the present chapter. Readers are referred to Shear (1992) for a recent account of these entities.

ODONTOGENIC CYSTS

INFLAMMATORY PERIODONTAL CYSTS

Radicular (dental, periapical) cyst

The radicular cyst is the commonest non-neoplastic cyst involving the PDL. It usually arises as a result of chronic inflammatory changes at the periapical region of a non-vital tooth, commonly the end result of caries. Less commonly it may arise as a result of trauma, or the presence of a developmental defect, e.g. an invagination or evagination allowing direct bacterial ingress. Chronic inflammatory changes consequent to the spread of infection to the periapical tissues lead to the formation of a periapical granuloma. This is a mass of granulation tissue with fibroblasts, capillaries and a diffuse infiltrate of lymphocytes, plasma cells, macrophages and polymorphonuclear leucocytes. Within this mass, proliferated epithelium is seen. This is presumed to originate from epithelial cell rests of Malassez in the PDL (*Fig. 19.1*). Further proliferation of epithelium leads to tissue breakdown and the formation of a cavity lined with stratified squamous epithelium. If the causative tooth is removed, leaving behind the cyst, this is referred to as a residual cyst.

The exact mechanism of cystic change is still unknown, but there are three main hypotheses (Stones, 1951; Soames and Southam, 1993):

1. As the mass of epithelium proliferates, stimulated by the inflammation, the cells in the central part of the mass become removed from their blood supply and undergo degeneration. This breakdown leads to cavity formation, and the rest of the epithelium forms a lining around this cavity.
2. The mass of proliferating epithelium encircles connective tissue islands forming loops around them. As a result of enzymatic action, this core of connective tissue may break down and liquefy, undergoing cavity formation.
3. The periapical granuloma frequently undergoes abscess formation. When an abscess cavity is formed, the epithelium within the granuloma proliferates to line the abscess cavity and converts it into a cyst. A modification to this hypothesis suggests the oral epithelium as a possible alternative source of epithelium for the lining. The oral epithelium is deemed to have proliferated through the opening of a sinus through which the pus has tracked (Warwick James and Counsell, 1932).

Summers (1974) examined frozen sections of human periapical granulomas histochemically for aminopeptidase activity and proteolytic activity. He found that aminopeptidase activity was located in the mesodermal polymorphonuclear leucocytes and macrophages, and that maximal activity appeared within connective tissue not as yet surrounded by epithelium, although there was some activity in the epithelium from migrated polymorphonuclear leucocytes. The finding of aminopeptidase activity in the mesoderm within the proliferating loops of epithelium suggested to him that cavitation in granulomas was due to enzymic proteolytic activity occurring in the mesoderm.

Shear (1992) believed that both intraepithelial and connective tissue breakdown were feasible and that they might operate independently of one another. There was morphological evidence in support of the intraepithelial breakdown hypothesis, as the proliferating epithelial masses showed considerable intercellular oedema. The intercellular accumulations of fluid coalesced to form microcysts containing epithelial and inflammatory cells. As Summers (1974) also found weak proteolytic activity within the proliferating epithelium, this suggested that the cells were undergoing autolysis. The microcysts might increase in size by coalescing with adjacent microcysts.

Enlargement of the cyst

Regardless of the mode of pathogenesis of the cyst, once a cavity is formed, the cyst gradually expands within the marrow spaces and the surrounding bone is resorbed. The mechanism of cyst expansion is also imperfectly understood. The classical explanation is that the cyst fluid exerts a higher osmotic pressure than the surrounding tissues, and this results in attraction of fluid into the

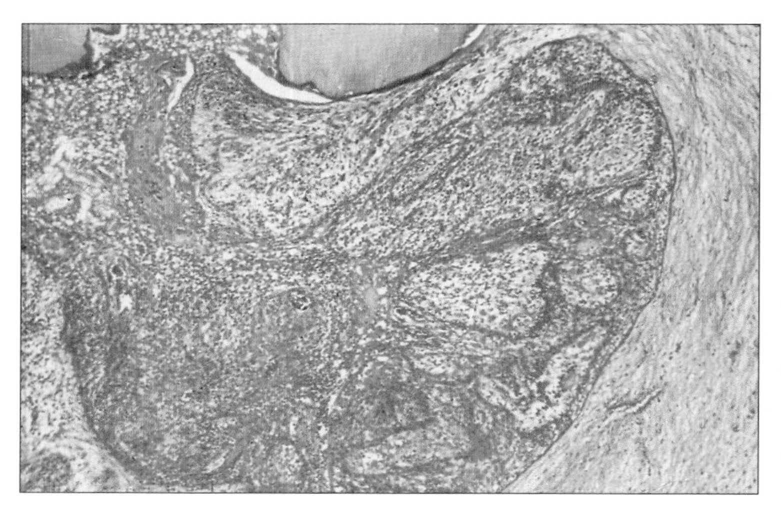

Fig. 19.1 Strands of proliferating epithelium within a periapical granuloma. (Haematoxylin and eosin × 65.)

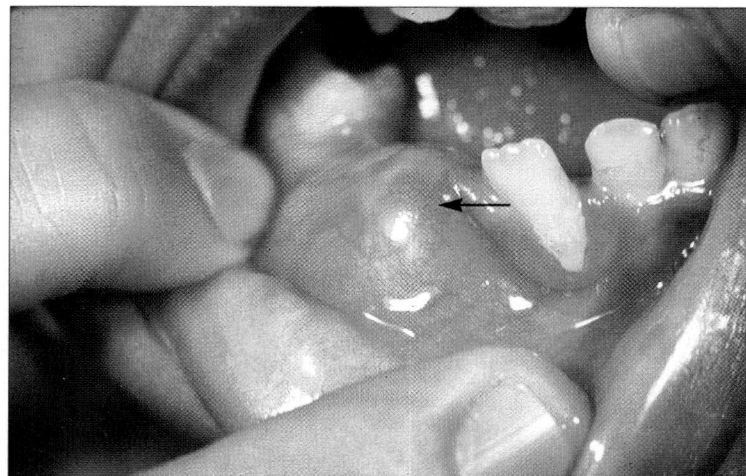

Fig. 19.2 Radicular cyst presenting as a translucent bluish fluctuant swelling (arrow).

cyst cavity, which in turn exerts a pressure effect on the surrounding bone, leading to osteoclastic resorption. Toller (1970) has shown that the mean osmolality of the fluid from twenty-one radicular cysts was 290±14.93 milliosmoles compared to a mean serum osmolality of 279±4.68 milliosmoles. The increased osmotic pressure of the cyst fluid probably arises as a result of lytic products of the epithelial and inflammatory cells in the cyst cavity. Skaug (1976a) measured the intracystic fluid pressure of apical cysts by means of a pressure transducer after cannulation of the cyst cavity, and he found that the average radicular cyst exerted a pressure of +47 mm Hg. Smith (1991) has recently reviewed the evidence, and he considers oversimplistic Toller's view that cyst fluid is just a dialysate of blood which passes through a semipermeable cyst lining into the lumen. The presence of higher molecular weight proteins and glycosaminoglycans in cyst fluids and the presence of immunoglobulin-producing plasma cells in the cyst capsule indicate that inflammation and local tissue metabolism contribute to the content of cyst fluids and also that molecules of high molecular weight can enter the cyst lumen through intercellular channels and discontinuities of the epithelial lining.

Using a tissue culture technique, Harris (1978) showed that odontogenic cyst linings may liberate significant quantities of bone-resorbing prostaglandins. Chromatography on silica gel-impregnated paper further revealed that the prostaglandins were principally PGE-2, PGE-3 and PGF-3a. Matejka *et al.* (1985) also found that PGE-2 was the predominant prostaglandin synthesized but they also found evidence of PGI-2. They believed that the surrounding granulation tissue with its associated inflammatory cells was the likely site of this synthesis. They suggested that the synthesis of leucotrienes was the mediator, at least in part, of this increase of PGI-2. Further studies by Meghji *et al.* (1989) have demonstrated a macromolecular factor with the characteristics of interleukin-1 (IL-1) in radicular and dentigerous cyst walls. They believe that the released IL-1 could lead to osteoclastic resorptions, and the connective tissue cells to produce prostaglandins and collagenases which will be responsible for further osteoclast activation and destruction of the bone matrix. Several of the cytokines with known inflammatory and osteolytic activity (IL-1, tumour necrosis factor, IL-6, IL-8) and cellular adhesion receptors ICAM-1 and ELAM-1 have been immunocytochemically localized in radicular cysts by Bando *et al.* (1993).

On the outer aspect of the bone, osteoblastic activity attempts to compensate by laying down new bone. However, resorption outstrips repair, and the covering bone is gradually thinned and eventually produces the eggshell crackling on pressure. When the bone is thinned sufficiently, a translucent bluish fluctuant swelling is seen clinically (*Fig. 19.2*). In the maxilla, the enlargement may be buccal or palatal, while in the mandible the enlargement is usually on the buccal aspect. On aspiration, a straw coloured fluid rich in cholesterol crystals is obtained. These crystals appear in a smear preparation as rhomboid plates with one corner cut off.

Fate of radicular cysts

Seward (1992) states that there is good circumstantial evidence that some small radicular cysts will regress if the necrotic pulp remnants and bacteria are removed from the root canal of the causative tooth and the canal effectively filled. This echoes views expressed by Oehlers (1970) and Bhaskar (1972). As previously indicated, the removal of the causative tooth results in a residual cyst. The fate of these cysts may depend on symptomatology; High and Hirschmann (1988) reported that asymptomatic cysts tend to decrease in size with increasing age but do not completely resolve. The case for non-surgical treatment of radicular cysts has yet to be established (Shear, 1992).

Radiological features

Radiographically, a typical radicular cyst appears as a well-circumscribed radiolucent area with a radiopaque margin (*Fig.*

19.3). When the cyst is secondarily infected, the radiopaque margin is replaced by an irregular radiolucent zone. It is generally accepted that, in the early stages, it is not possible to tell if a periapical radiolucency is a granuloma, a cyst or an abscess.

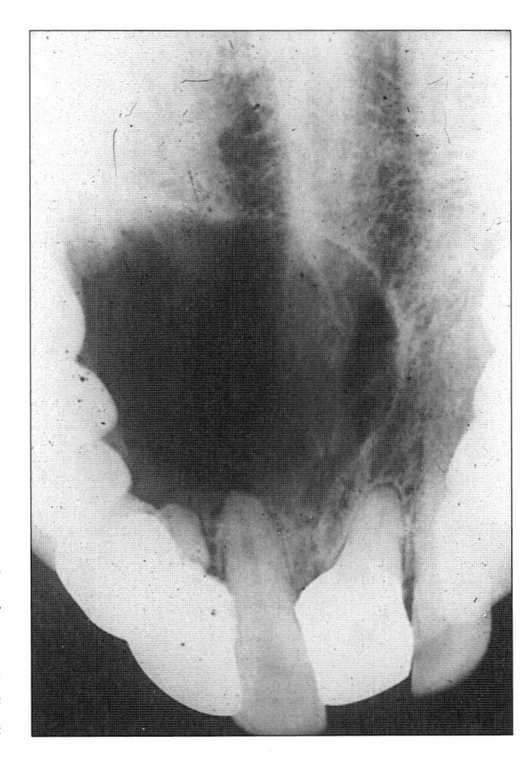

Fig. 19.3 Radiograph of a radicular cyst. Note the well-circumscribed radiolucent area with a radiopaque margin.

Histology

The soft tissue sac that makes up the cyst is lined with a non-keratinized stratified squamous epithelium of varying thickness. Near the causative tooth, the epithelium may proliferate in the form of arcades or rings around islands of connective tissue (*Fig. 19.4*). Sometimes the lining is incomplete or discontinuous, owing either to secondary infection that has caused destruction of the epithelium, or to an inherent incompleteness *de novo*. Goblet and ciliated cell metaplasia of the superficial cells may be seen (*Fig. 19.5*). Nodules of cholesterol are often seen attached to the cyst sac in areas of epithelial discontinuity.

The source of the cholesterol in the cyst is a subject of considerable debate. Browne (1971a) found a statistically significant correlation ($p<0.01$) between the presence of cholesterol and haemosiderin. He postulated that disintegrating red blood cells provided the main source of cholesterol, in a form that crystallized readily in the tissues. Shear (1992) thought that the β-lipoproteins in the plasma might also serve as a source. As the

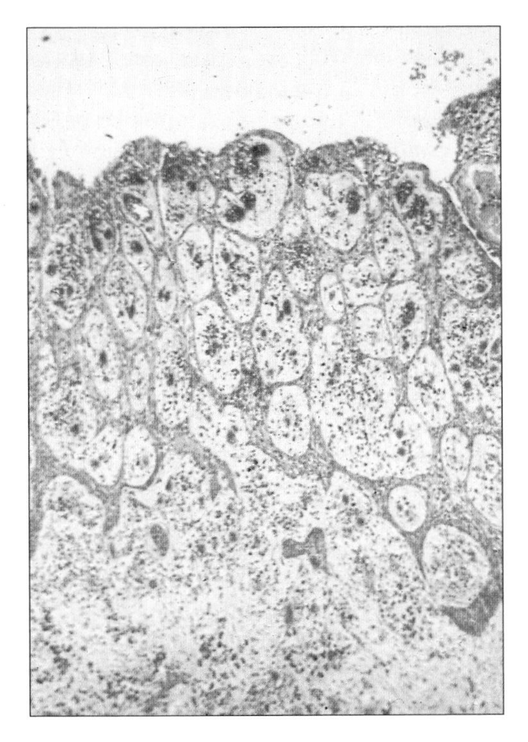

Fig. 19.4 Proliferating epithelium making arcades or rings around islands of connective tissue in the superficial part of the cyst lining. (Haematoxylin and eosin × 25.)

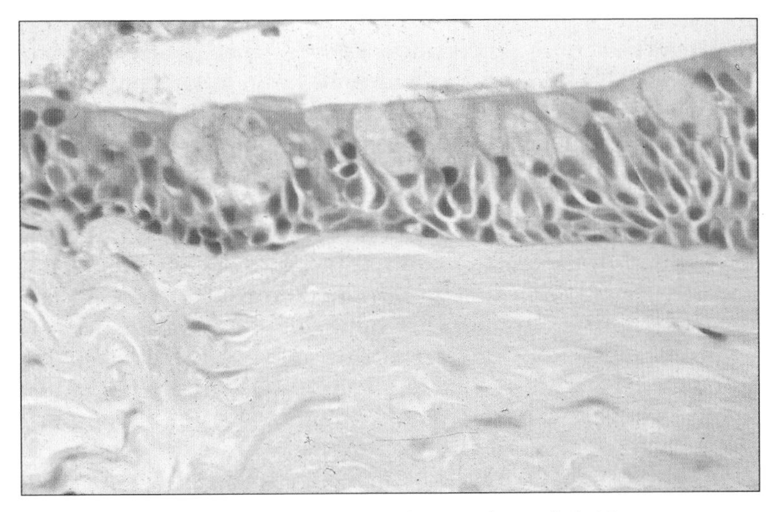

Fig. 19.5 Goblet and ciliated cell metaplasia in the epithelial lining. (Haematoxylin and eosin × 250.)

β-lipoproteins passed through the fragile, thin-walled blood vessels in the inflamed portions of the cyst wall, they split into cholesterol and its esters, which were retained, and other lipid components, such as phospholipids, which were absorbed by the lymphatics. Once the cholesterol crystals were deposited in the fibrous wall of the cyst, they were extruded by a foreign-body giant-cell reaction through the epithelial lining into the cyst lumen. Skaug (1976b) examined the lipoprotein content of cyst fluids by cellulose acetate membrane (CAM) electrophoresis and immunoelectrophoresis. By CAM electrophoresis, cyst fluids showed α-1-lipoprotein and β-lipoprotein bands but no pre-β-lipoprotein band. The relative amount of α-1-lipoprotein was higher in cyst fluid than in serum. Single radial immunodiffusion showed that the content of β-lipoprotein was low. Skaug hypothesized that the cholesterol in cysts was derived, in part at least, from the β-lipoprotein originating from the plasma. Garrett and Winstone (1991) have carried out histochemical and ultrastructural studies, and they suggest that the deposition of cholesterol appears to be the consequence of a complex set of events which leads to a failure of foamy macrophages to remove the excess lipid and its subsequent deposition.

Hyaline bodies of Rushton are occasionally seen within the epithelium lining the cyst (*Fig. 19.6*). They are straight, curved, or of hair-pin shape, and sometimes laminated. There is considerable uncertainty about the nature and origin of these hyaline bodies. Early investigations (Rushton, 1955; Shear, 1961) suggested that they may be keratinous in nature. Bouyssou and Guilheim (1965), Hodson (1966, 1967) and Sedano and Gorlin (1968) suggested a haèmatogenous origin. Morgan and Johnson (1974) concluded from histochemical and ultrastructural studies that they were a secretory product of odontogenic epithelium deposited on the surface of particulate matter, such as cell debris or cholesterol crystals, in a manner analogous to the formation of dental cuticle on the unerupted portions of enamel surfaces. Allison (1977) studied these bodies by electron microprobe analysis and revealed that they contained sulphur, chlorine, calcium, and, in some instances, iron. His microradiographic studies showed that the density increased progressively towards the core and he concluded that his observations conformed with the hypothesis that hyaline bodies originated as epithelial secretions.

In an electron-microscopic investigation, El-Labban (1979) observed that the lamellar type of hyaline body was composed of alternating electron-dense and electron-lucent layers, the outermost layer always being electron-dense. The granular type of hyaline body was composed of amorphous material in which fragments of red blood cells were seen. She concluded that the granular type formed from degenerating red blood cells and that the lamellar type might have resulted from segregation of components within the mass.

Browne and Matthews (1985) investigated hyaline bodies with an immunoperoxidase technique for keratin, factor VIII-related antigen, haemoglobin and fibrinogen. They found only fibrinogen in the cases of some circular and polycyclic forms and their results were negative for the others. Immunohistochemical and scanning electron microscopic studies and x-ray microanalysis have been carried out recently by Rühl *et al.* (1989) and Philippou *et al.* (1990) and they support the view that these bodies are a product of the epithelium. Matthews (1991) has reviewed all the published data to date and concurs with this view.

The connective tissue wall of the cyst is usually divisible into two zones:

- a subepithelial, vascular, granulation tissue zone that is diffusely infiltrated with chronic inflammatory cells, including lymphocytes, plasma cells and macrophages, which may be laden with lipids (foam cells) or haemosiderin; and
- a more collagenous zone of fibrous tissue that lies outside the granulation tissue zone forming a capsule.

The myofibroblast, a cell type with the features of both smooth muscle and fibroblasts, was first recognized in granulation tissue by Gabbiani *et al.* (1971). These cells show the presence of parallel bundles of microfilaments that have many electron-opaque areas (dense bodies), and they have a well-developed rough endoplasmic reticulum and multiple nuclear indentations (Skalli and Gabbiani, 1988). Their presence in the granulation tissue zone of radicular cysts was detected by Lee and El-Labban (1976, 1980). Harris (1978) suggested that they may contribute to the elasticity of the fibrous wall. Myofibroblasts are considered in connection with the eruptive mechanism in Chapter 9.

Buchner and David (1978) demonstrated that some of the pigmented cells showed sudanophilia, acid-fastness, PAS-positivity, a silver reduction capacity and yellow autofluorescence in ultraviolet light. They concluded that these cells may be macrophages containing lipopigments in the form of ceroids. They suggested that the ceroids were formed from locally liberated lipids with haemosiderin acting as an oxidation catalyst.

Immunological studies suggest that both humoral and cell-mediated reactions have been implicated in the pathogenesis of radicular cysts. IgG is the predominant class of immunoglobulin demonstrated in the immunoglobulin-containing cells. T lymphocytes predominate in the lymphocyte population and T helper cells (CD4) were found to be more numerous than suppressor–cytotoxic (CD8) cells (Nilsen *et al.*, 1984), although others have found that the reverse is the case. Gao *et al.* (1988) demonstrated HLA-DR-positive cells and lysosymes and α-1-antitrypsin-positive cells were always near the epithelium of granulomas and cysts. They speculated that activated T cells in periapical granulomas produced lymphokines that may act on the rests of Malassez to cause proliferation and altered differentiation leading to cyst formation. Matthews and Browne (1987) suggested that these HLA-DR-positive cells may be antigen-presenting cells responding to the antigens in the cyst fluid.

There is considerable doubt if a cyst within the PDL forms as a result of an inflammatory process in a periodontal pocket. Main (1970) refers to it as an inflammatory collateral cyst. Shear records

13 cysts under this heading over a period of 33 years and considers that the explanation for this may be that drainage occurs more readily from the gingival crevice than from the apical periodontium and that the conditions may not be conducive to cyst formation. The author remains unconvinced of its existence.

Paradental cyst

Craig (1976) described a cyst related to partly erupted mandibular third molars which had been involved by pericoronitis (*Fig. 19.7*). He found that the available teeth always possessed an enamel projection extending from the amelocemental junction into the buccal bifurcation. The cyst was lined with a non-keratinized stratified squamous epithelium and was histologically indistinguishable from a radicular cyst. He concluded that these enamel projections might have a role in the pathogenesis of paradental cysts that appeared to originate from the reduced enamel epithelium (*Fig. 19.8*). Further series of reported cases have appeared in recent years (Ackermann *et al.*, 1987; Fowler and Brannon, 1989; Vedtofte and Praetorius, 1989). A similar lesion affecting principally the permanent first mandibular molar in children has been referred to as a mandibular infected buccal cyst. The association with enamel spurs has not been confirmed in all cases.

DEVELOPMENTAL CYSTS

Dentigerous (follicular) cyst

A dentigerous cyst is one that encloses the crown of an unerupted tooth. Dentigerous cysts are less common than radicular cysts. The pathogenesis is uncertain, but it is not thought to be of inflammatory origin. Following completion of crown development, the dental organ shrinks to a few layers of cells to become the reduced enamel epithelium. Accumulation of fluid between either the enamel surface and the reduced enamel epithelium, or, more commonly, between the layers of the reduced enamel epithelium itself, results in the formation of a cyst that envelops the crown of the unerupted tooth. Main (1970) suggested that the accumulation of fluid is the result of obstruction of venous outflow due to pressure exerted by the tooth on an impacted follicle. This is thought to induce a transudation of fluid across the capillary walls. Experimental production of dentigerous cysts has been performed by Atkinson (1972, 1976, 1977), Rivière and Sabet (1973) and Al-Talabani and Smith (1980), among others.

Clinical features

Dentigerous cysts present as painless fluctuant swellings in the maxilla or mandible, associated with a missing tooth. The mandibular third molar, maxillary canine, supernumerary mesioden, and mandibular premolar are the teeth most frequently involved. Pain is not usually a feature unless the cyst is secondarily infected.

Radiological features

Radiographs show a well-circumscribed radiolucent area related to the crown of the associated tooth (*Fig. 19.9*). In central dentigerous cysts, the radiolucency envelops the crown, while in lateral dentigerous cysts, the radiolucent area lies on one side of the crown. It is important to remember that not all radiographs showing these features will turn out to be dentigerous cysts at operation, as a number of these will be superimposed images, and the cyst and tooth may not be in dentigerous relationship with each other.

Histology

The epithelium lining the cyst is usually a non-keratinized stratified squamous epithelium (*Fig. 19.10*) attached to the tooth at the level of the amelocemental junction (*Fig. 19.11*). Goblet and ciliated cell metaplasia are common, and hyaline bodies are seen occasionally. The connective tissue capsule is uniform unless the cyst becomes inflamed or infected, and islands of odontogenic epithelium are seen in the fibrous wall (Kramer *et al.*, 1992). The enamel of the associated tooth is usually normal, although Crabb (1963) examined ground sections of these teeth by polarized light and observed that there were areas of lower mineralization in the sub-surface enamel corresponding to zones of natural enamel caries. He thought that these areas might be related to faults in mineralization or to an attack on the enamel surface by cyst fluid. The experimental production of dentigerous cysts by Al-Talabani and Smith (1980 – see above) showed that some cysts were associated with enamel hypoplasia. They suggested that their cysts formed at an early stage of tooth development with a consequent effect on enamel development.

Odontogenic keratocyst (primordial cyst)

Much confusion surrounds the use of the terms odontogenic keratocyst and primordial cyst. The terms are used here synonymously, as recommended by the World Health Organization (WHO, 1978). The term 'primordial cyst' was originally used by Robinson to designate a cyst that developed in place of a tooth (Robinson, 1975). Hence, to be diagnosed as having a primordial cyst, patients had to show an incomplete dentition with no history of tooth loss. Where a full dentition existed, supernumerary tooth germs were postulated. Philipsen (1956) coined the term 'odontogenic keratocyst' to describe cysts of odontogenic origin which possessed linings of keratinized stratified squamous epithelium. These were thought to be radicular or dentigerous cysts where inflammation had subsided. Shear (1960) detailed several criteria whereby primordial cysts could be diagnosed histologically, and Pindborg and Hansen (1963) correlated these criteria with many of their odontogenic keratocysts. They further focused attention on the clinical behaviour of this cyst and showed that they had a high recurrence rate (62 per cent in their series), a finding endorsed by Toller (1967), who found a recurrence rate of 51 per cent. The detailed clinical and histological features of the

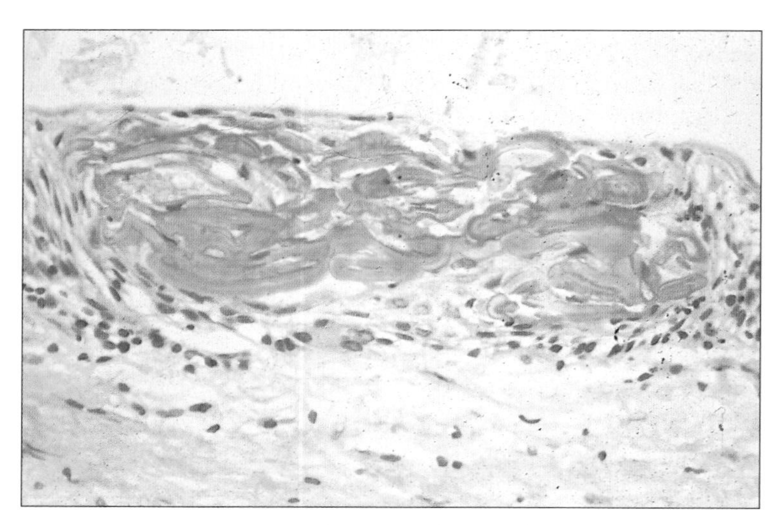

Fig. 19.6 Hyaline bodes of Rushton within the epithelial lining. (Haematoxylin and eosin × 100.)

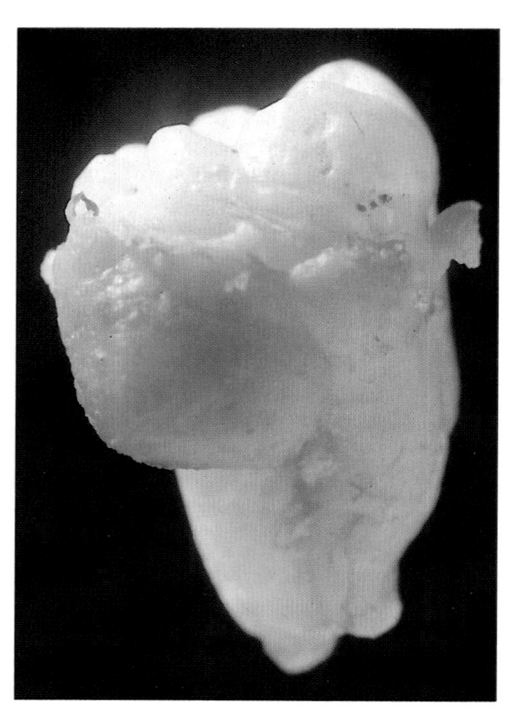

Fig. 19.7 Paradental cyst associated with an impacted mandibular third molar.

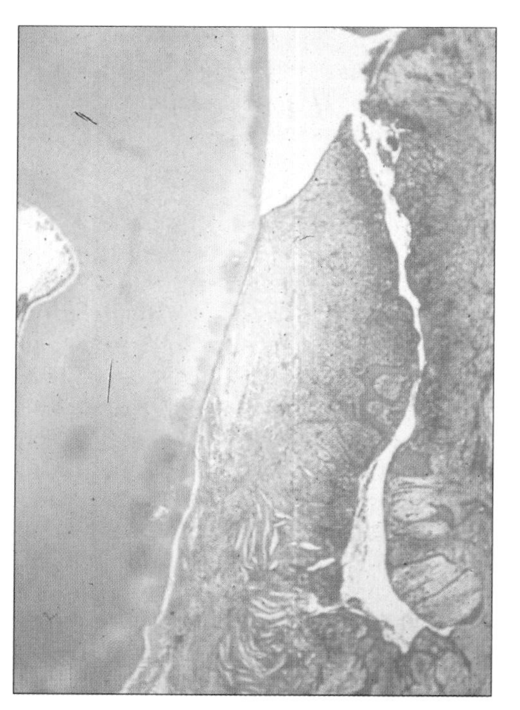

Fig. 19.8 Paradental cyst apparently arising from reduced enamel epithelium adjacent to the root of an impacted mandibular third molar. (Haematoxylin and eosin × 10.)

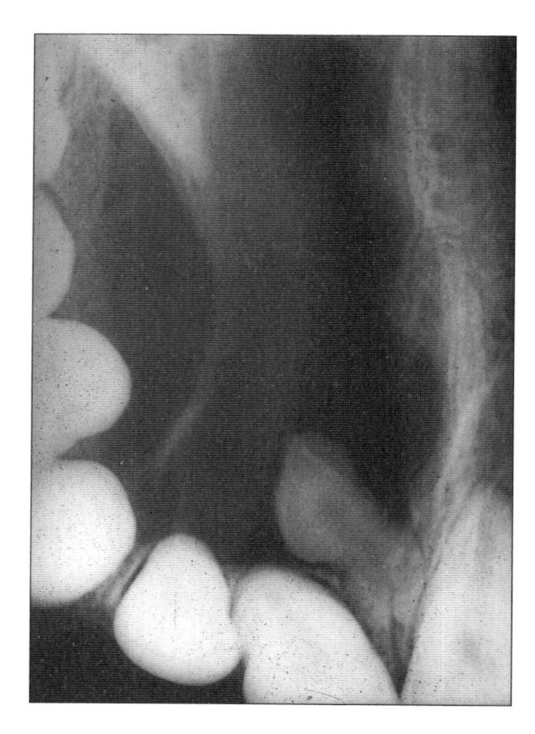

Fig. 19.9 Radiograph of a dentigerous cyst. The radiolucent area is associated with the conical supernumerary tooth.

condition have been reviewed by Browne (1970, 1971b) and Brannon (1976, 1977).

It is thought (Kramer, 1974) that it is no longer necessary to postulate tooth germs that failed to develop into teeth as the source of epithelium for the development of a keratocyst, and there is general acceptance that it is an odontogenic cyst of developmental origin that has formed from primordial odontogenic epithelium. Stoelinga and Peters (1973) suggested, however, that these cysts originate from the oral mucosa, as they were able to observe epithelial islands only within the oral mucosa superficial to the operated keratocysts and the developing dental lamina in human foetuses. Gustafson *et al.* (1989) have illustrated their paper with material from the author's (KWL) department, a keratocyst apparently having its origin in the mucosal basal epithelium (*Fig. 19.12*).

The lesion commonly develops in the region of the angle of the mandible and presents radiographically as a multilocular cyst (*Fig. 19.13*). Clinical swelling is often not marked, even when radiographic examination reveals extensive involvement of the mandible. In addition, the cyst may develop in the tooth-bearing part of the jaws, presenting clinically and radiographically as a lateral periodontal cyst, a globulomaxillary cyst, a median

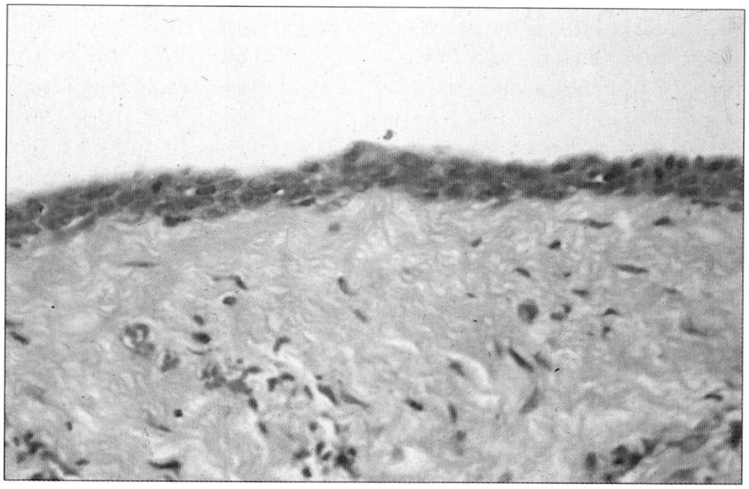

Fig. 19.10 Typical lining of a dentigerous cyst, consisting of a thin non-keratinized stratified squamous epithelium, overlying uninflamed fibrous tissue. (Haematoxylin and eosin × 100.)

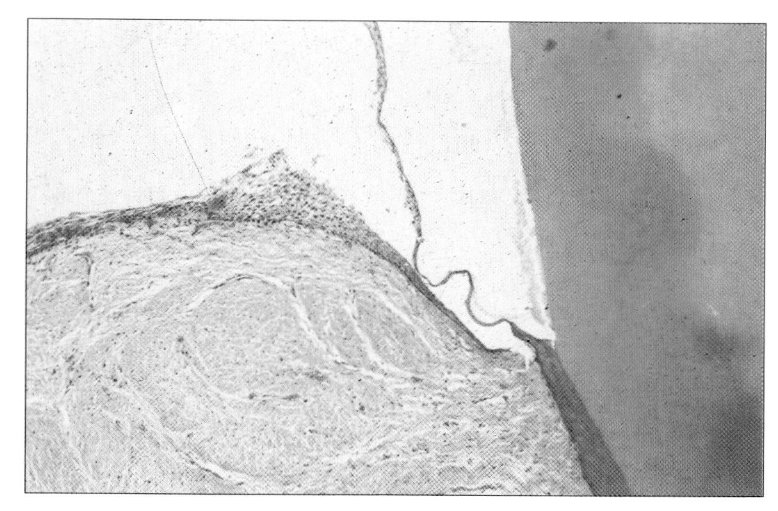

Fig. 19.11 Attachment of the cyst to the tooth at the level of the amelocemental junction. Note the relationship of the cyst lining to reduced enamel epithelium. (Haematoxylin and eosin × 60.)

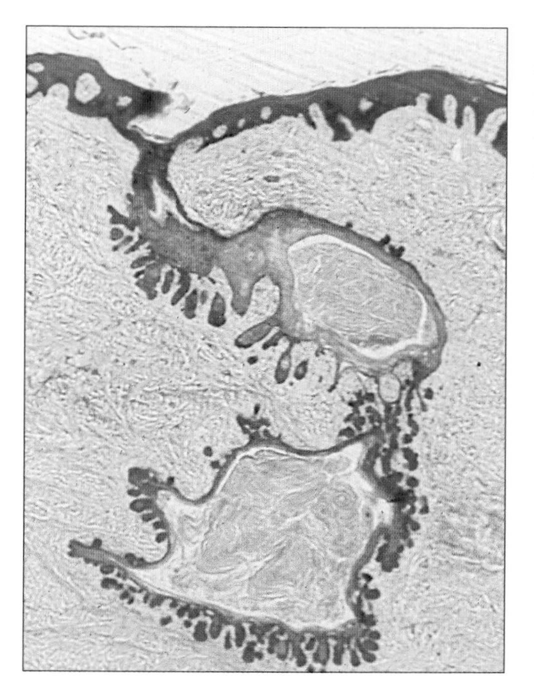

Fig. 19.12 A 'daughter' keratocyst apparently originating from mucosal epithelium. (Haematoxylin and eosin × 100.)

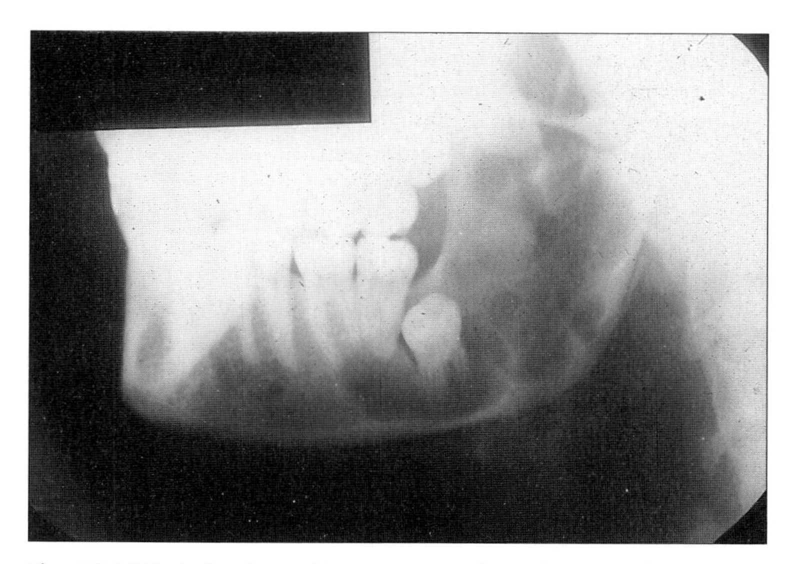

Fig. 19.13 Typical radiographic appearance of an odontogenic keratocyst. Note the multilocular appearance of the radiolucent area affecting the angle and ascending ramus of the mandible.

mandibular or a median alveolar cyst; this contributes to the confusion that surrounds several of the so-called 'fissural' cysts. Less commonly, the cyst exists in true dentigerous relationship with a tooth, but it is assumed that this is a secondary dentigerous cyst. In edentulous mouths they may also be misdiagnosed as residual radicular cysts.

On aspiration, a material resembling inspissated pus without the characteristic smell is often obtained. Smears prepared from the aspirate reveal the presence of squames, and the soluble protein content of the aspirate has been shown to be frequently less than 4 g per 100 ml. These two findings have been used by Kramer and Toller (1973) to complement the accuracy of preoperative diagnoses.

Histology

The criteria listed for the diagnosis of primordial cysts by Shear (1960) were as follows:

1. The epithelium is keratinized or parakeratinized and is about five to eight cells thick.
2. The basal layer is cuboidal or columnar and the nuclei are intensely basophilic.
3. The epithelium is devoid of rete processes and the underlying connective tissue is free from inflammatory cell infiltration (*Fig. 19.14*).

These histological criteria remain the most important for the identification of the odontogenic keratocyst. Subsequently, additional features have been observed. These include the increased mitotic activity of the linings when compared to those of cysts with non-keratinized epithelial linings; the frequent separation of epithelium from connective tissue; the presence of islands of odontogenic epithelium and daughter cysts in the fibrous wall (*Fig. 19.15*), and the change from a keratinized to a non-keratinized lining when inflammation supervenes, with features becoming indistinguishable from those of radicular and dentigerous cysts. Parakeratinized linings are the predominant form of keratinization; orthokeratinized linings are less frequently seen. El-Labban and Aghabeigi (1990) investigated the blood vessels in keratocysts stereologically and ultrastructurally. They noted that fenestrated capillaries were found only in keratocysts and not in non-keratinized cysts, and they suggested that this may indicate a rapid transfer of fluid to meet the demand of active proliferating epithelium.

Enlargement of the cyst

Kramer (1974) has suggested that keratocysts enlarge by accumulation of keratin within the cyst cavity. If one part of the epithelial lining is producing keratin at a greater rate, this locally increased production of a rather firm material might account for the uneven pushing out of the cyst wall. Harris and Toller (1975) suggest as an alternative explanation the fact that keratocysts are poor bone resorbers and extend preferentially along the cancellous bone with little resorption and expansion to the dense cortex.

Clinical behaviour

The high recurrence rate of the odontogenic keratocyst is probably attributable to several factors:

- the cyst lining is friable and thus small fragments of cyst may be left behind during removal, resulting in recurrence;
- the higher mitotic activity is an indicator of a more active epithelium – Toller (1967) suggested that the epithelial linings of keratocysts have intrinsic growth, and Ahlfors *et al.* (1984) also proposed that they should be regarded as benign cystic neoplasms; and
- the presence of islands of odontogenic epithelium and daughter cysts in the fibrous wall.

Many series of cases have been studied since the 1960s, with recurrence rates varying from 3–59 per cent (see Shear, 1992). The type of operative procedure employed, the histology and the variability in the follow-up period probably contribute to the vast difference in results. For instance, Niemeyer *et al.* (1985) found that the highest frequency of recurrences occurred in those patients treated by cystostomy. Wright (1981) suggested that orthokeratinized keratocysts may be less aggressive than the parakeratinized type. Vuhahula *et al.* (1993) have recently suggested that jaw cysts with orthokeratinization may represent cysts other than keratocysts. This view, however, has been well documented in earlier literature (Browne, 1991).

Histochemistry, immunology, and molecular biological studies

Donoff *et al.* (1972) demonstrated that explants of keratocysts exhibit collagenase activity, which might be related to the expansile growth of keratocysts within bone. Magnusson (1978) studied the activity of NADH2 and NADPH2-diaphorase, glucose-6-phosphate dehydrogenase, glutamate dehydrogenase, acid phosphatase, leucine aminopeptidase, and ATPase in keratocysts. He found that the oxidative enzymes showed strong activity in keratocyst epithelium, which contrasted with weak activity in other cysts. Acid phosphatase activity was similarly strong in keratocysts, while the fibrous walls of keratocysts showed a high activity of leucine aminopeptidase.

There are 19 types of keratin now known to exist. In addition to keratins 13, 14, and 19, which are found in simple and non-keratinized stratified squamous epithelium, keratins 10 and 11, which are typical of keratinizing epithelia, have been demonstrated in keratocyst linings (Morgan *et al.*, 1987; Matthews *et al.*, 1988). Hormia *et al.* (1987) were able to demonstrate only cytokeratins 7, 17, and 19; they failed to find cytokeratins 1, 9, 10, and 11. Gao *et al.* (1989) likewise found that there was very weak expression of keratin 10 and suggested that this may be a reflection of the parakeratinization process or that it may be related to developmental differences. They further found that keratin 16, which is associated with high proliferative activity, was strongly positive in suprabasal cells, and they suggested that this may further reflect the high intrinsic growth potential of the keratocyst. Smith and Matthews (1991) have reviewed the most recent published data.

Ogden *et al.* (1992) have detected the presence of p53 protein, the gene product of a tumour suppressor gene, within the lining of five of 12 keratocysts. The protein was absent in dentigerous and radicular cysts. They used an immunoperoxidase technique with the polyclonal antibody CM-1, but as the antibody recognizes both wild and mutant forms of p53, identification does not imply association with malignant disease.

Multiple keratocysts (multiple naevoid basal cell carcinoma syndrome)

Odontogenic keratocysts occur as part of the multiple naevoid basal cell carcinoma syndrome. In this syndrome, which involves autosomal dominant inheritance with complete penetrance and extremely variable expressivity, the patients exhibit frontal and temporoparietal bossing, giving the skull a somewhat pagetoid appearance. Multiple cysts occur in the jaws, and lesions microscopically indistinguishable from basal cell carcinomas occur on the skin of the face and neck, back and thorax, abdomen and upper extremities. In addition, there are skeletal anomalies and intracranial calcifications. The skin lesions usually appear between puberty and 35 years of age as papules varying from flesh-coloured to pale brown. The jaw cysts are typical keratocysts with epithelial islands and microcysts in the connective tissue of the fibrous wall, which may account for the high recurrence rate of cysts seen in patients with naevoid basal cell carcinoma syndrome. Donatsky *et al.* (1976) showed that 85 per cent of the patients experienced recurrence within 2 years of cyst removal. Skeletal anomalies are present in 60 per cent of patients; the commonest anomaly is a splayed or bifid rib. Other costal anomalies include synostosis, partial agenesis, pseudoarthrosis, and cervical rudimentary ribs. Intracranial calcifications occur chiefly in the form of lamellar calcifications of the falx cerebri. Congenital communicating hydrocephaly and medulloblastomas have also been described in these patients. It has been shown that malignant transformation of cells *in vitro* with acetylaminofluorene occurs at a faster rate in cells from patients with the syndrome than in cells from normal individuals, and that fibroblasts from these patients were defective in their repair of potentially lethal damage (Gorlin *et al.*, 1990).

Woolgar *et al.* (1987a,b,c) compared the clinical presentation and histological features of single keratocysts to those occurring in the syndrome. They found that syndrome cysts occurred more commonly in females and that they tended to occur at a younger age. Histologically syndrome cysts had significantly higher numbers of satellite cysts, solid islands of epithelial proliferation, odontogenic rests, and numbers of mitotic figures.

Lateral periodontal cyst

The term 'lateral periodontal cyst' has been applied to at least three different entities, none of which truly represents the entity under discussion. Radicular cysts which form on the lateral aspect of the root as a result of inflammatory changes related to lateral canals have been called lateral periodontal cysts. Odontogenic keratocysts that fulfil the definition anatomically have likewise been referred to as lateral periodontal cysts. Still other cysts in this location have been shown to take origin from the reduced enamel epithelium and probably represent residual dentigerous cysts. This is one of the modes of origin of the lateral periodontal cyst suggested by Shear and Pindborg (1975). Lateral periodontal cysts should, however, be diagnosed only after these entities have been excluded.

Defined in this way, the lateral periodontal cyst is a developmental cyst of the PDL, with cystic change taking place within epithelial cell rests in this location. Altini and Shear (1992) have considered the relative merits of the reduced enamel epithelium, remnants of dental lamina and the cell rests of Malassez, as the source of the epithelium from which the cyst is derived, and they continue to favour reduced enamel epithelium as the source. Support for this view has come from immunocytochemical studies, in which cytokeratin 18 has been found in a lateral periodontal cyst (botryoid variety) and in some dentigerous cysts.

Clinically, lateral periodontal cysts are found chiefly distal to the mandibular third molar or in the canine–premolar region (*Fig. 19.16*). They are usually discovered on incidental radiographic examination and seldom grow to large size. Multilocular variants are recognized by some authorities, but these may represent botryoid, glandular, or sialo-odontogenic cysts (see below).

Histology

The lining is composed of a thin non-keratinized stratified squamous epithelium backed by fibrous tissue. Shear and Pindborg (1975) state that plaque formation is an important characteristic of the epithelium. These plaques are localized thickenings of the epithelial lining (*Fig. 19.17*). While some of these are small others are larger and extend into the cyst cavity. Some cysts contain a number of plaques. The cells of the plaque are sometimes fusiform, with their long axes parallel to the basement membrane. Frequently they are large and clear, showing the features of intracellular oedema, and contain small pyknotic nuclei.

Botryoid, glandular and sialo-odontogenic cysts

A multilocular cystic lesion that was distinctive in macroscopic appearance in that it resembled a cluster of grapes was reported by Weathers and Waldron (1973). Further cases similar in appearance have been described in national and international meetings of pathological societies in recent years and the names of glandular and sialo-odontogenic cysts have been proposed (Padayachee and van Wyk, 1987; Gardner *et al.*, 1988). Whether these cysts represent variants of a single entity or are different entities remains to be established. The smaller lesions, which could be enucleated in entirety, probably account for the macroscopic appearance; these cysts tend not to recur. The larger lesions, which are usually removed piecemeal and therefore do not demonstrate the macroscopic descriptive feature, show a more aggressive behaviour with multiple recurrences, raising the speculation as to whether, like the odontogenic keratocyst, they should be regarded

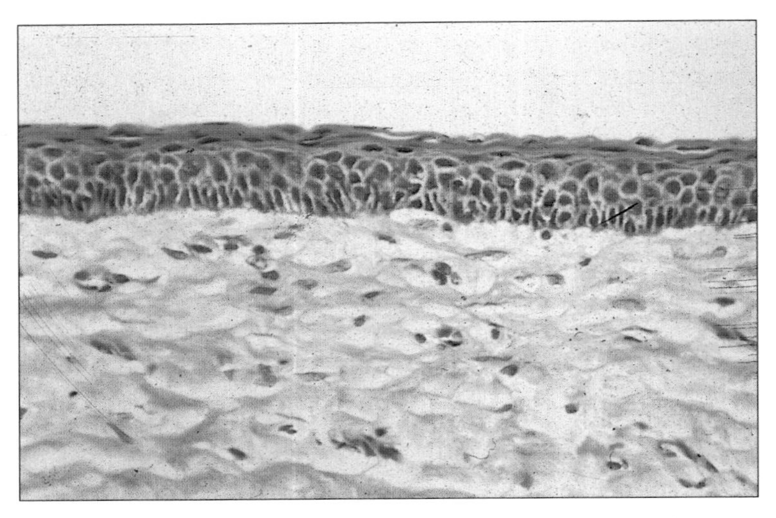

Fig. 19.14 Histological appearance of the lining of an odontogenic keratocyst. The thin parakerationized stratified squamous epithelium is devoid of rete processes, the basal layer is cuboidal or columnar, and the underlying fibrous connective tissue is uninflamed. (Haematoxylin and eosin × 250.)

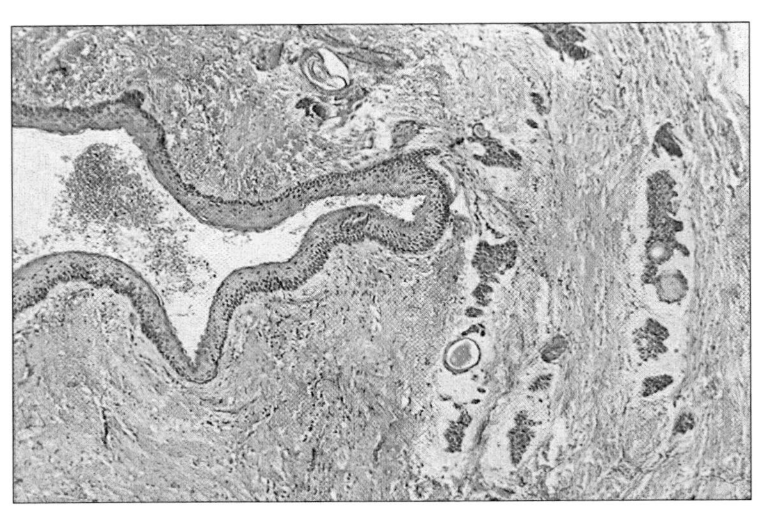

Fig. 19.15 Islands of odontogenic epithelium in the fibrous wall of an odontogenic keratocyst. (Haematoxylin and eosin × 250.)

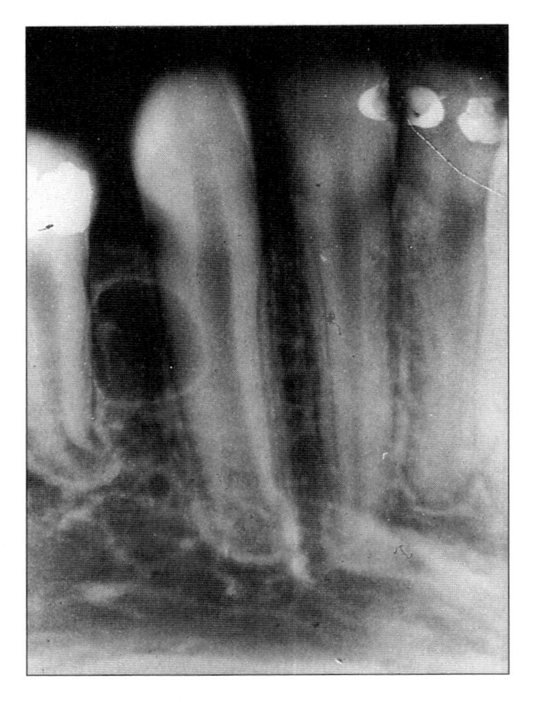

Fig. 19.16 Radiograph of a lateral periodontal cyst in the canine-premolar region.

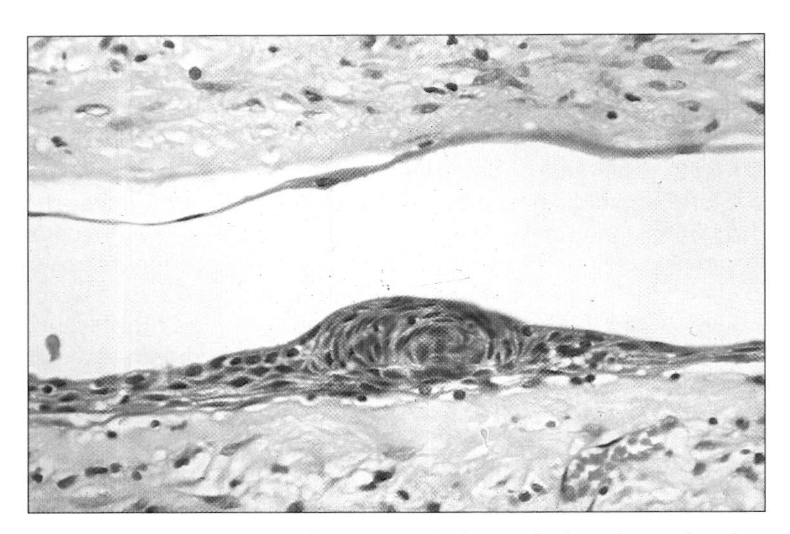

Fig. 19.17 Epithelial plaque formation in the lining of a lateral periodontal cyst. (Haematoxylin and eosin × 250.)

as a benign cystic neoplasm. They occur in the tooth-bearing parts of the jaws and thus may involve the PDL (*Fig. 19.18*). The mandible is more often involved than the maxilla. The histology is distinctive in the glandular or sialo variant, with a thin non-keratinized squamous epithelium containing areas with columnar and cuboidal cells on the surface, forming a brush-border or even cilia. Small ductal lumina containing eosinophilic secretions are also prominent (*Fig. 19.19*). Numerous goblet cells may be present, mainly within the superficial layers of the epithelium. Daughter cysts are prominent. In the botryoid cyst, the cyst lining may be indistinguishable from a lateral periodontal cyst with multiple areas of plaque formation or clear cells (Kaugars, 1986).

Calcifying odontogenic cyst

The calcifying odontogenic cyst was delineated as an entity by Gorlin *et al.* in 1962. Before then, it was probably regarded as an atypical ameloblastoma. The clinical and radiographical presentation is as for any cyst involving the PDL. However, radiopaque foci may be associated with the lesion, for it may occur in association with a complex odontome and its calcifications may become large enough to be visible radiographically. Confusion has arisen, however, because the WHO classification of odontogenic tumours lists it as an odontogenic tumour, as it has many of the features of a neoplasm. However, most people regard the simplest form as a non-neoplastic cyst and agree with Praetorius *et al.* (1981) that it probably comprises two entities: a cyst and a neoplasm. The present discussion will confine itself to the non-neoplastic cyst (see Praetorius *et al.*, 1981, and Hong *et al.*, 1991, for a consideration of the neoplasm).

Histology

The lesion has a spectrum of appearances (Kramer *et al.*, 1992). In its simplest form, the cyst is lined with an epithelium of tall columnar basal cells, the nuclei being polarized away from the basal end of the cell. Faintly eosinophilic cells (ghost cells) are prominent within the remainder of the epithelium (*Fig. 19.20*). These may undergo calcification and become visible on the radiograph. In addition to these features, the cyst may show areas of dysplastic dentine adjacent to the epithelium. As islands of odontogenic epithelium mimicking that of ameloblastoma are often seen within the fibrous wall, these foci of dysplastic dentine may distinguish the cyst from an ameloblastoma. Areas of complex odontome sometimes form within the cyst wall, and the calcified masses of ghost cells may extrude into the fibrous wall, producing a foreign body giant-cell reaction.

The ultrastructure of the cyst has been studied by Chen and Miller (1975). They identified four types of cells. These were the basal cell, the stellate reticulum type cell, the ghost cell, and the hornified cell. The first two contained various amounts of tonofilaments and organelles. The ghost cell contained coarse bundles of tonofilaments intermingled with dilated membranous organelles. The hornified cell contained densely packed tono-

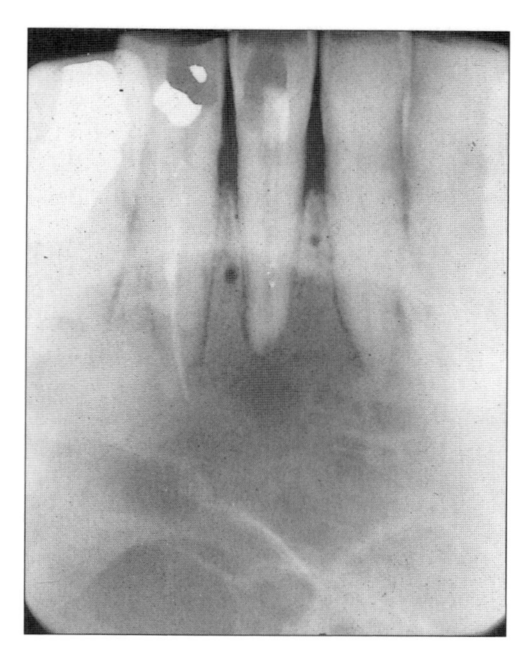

Fig. 19.18 Radiograph of a sialo-odontogenic cyst in the symphyseal region. Before its characterization, it would probably have been regarded as a median mandibular cyst.

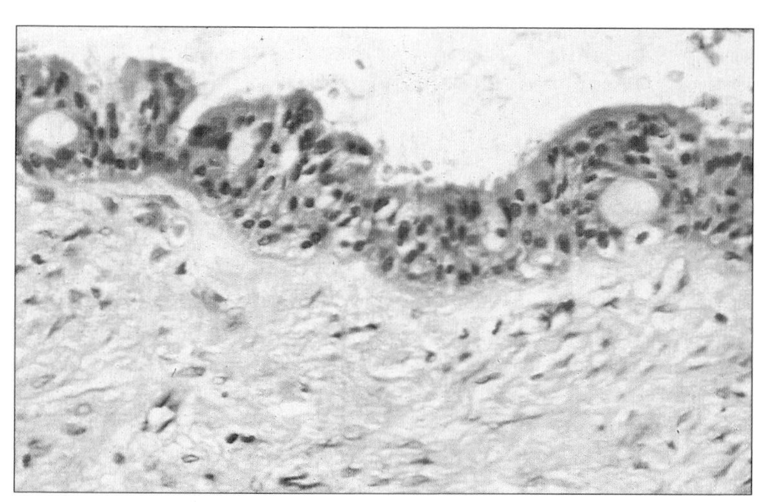

Fig. 19.19 Lining of a glandular or sialo-odontogenic cyst. Small ductal lumina are seen within the non-keratinized squamous cell epithelium, with cuboidal cells on the surface. (Haematoxylin and eosin × 250.)

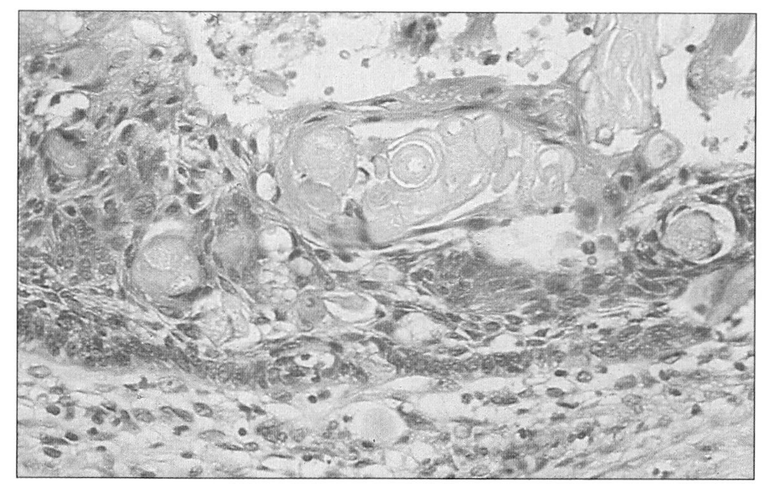

Fig. 19.20 Lining of a calcifying odontogenic cyst. The basal layer is columnar and ghost cells are prominent within the superficial layers of the epithelium. (Haematoxylin and eosin × 250.)

filaments. The authors considered that the hornified cells may have derived from either the stellate reticulum type of cell or the ghost cells. Both the hornified cells and the ghost cells were considered as non-vital cell residues, and the mineralization of these cells was regarded as dystrophic calcification.

The fluid contents of odontogenic cysts

Browne (1976) determined the proportion of soluble protein and total protein content of fluids from various odontogenic cysts. He found that radicular cysts contained an average of 51.19 per cent albumin, 17.25 per cent β-globulin, 22.04 per cent γ-globulin, and 6.30 g per 100 ml protein. Dentigerous cysts contained an average of 61.35 per cent albumin, 12.60 per cent globulin and 4.86 g per 100 ml protein. He also determined the immunoglobulin content by single radial immunodiffusion and found that radicular cysts contained an average of 488.9 mg per 100 ml IgA, 2535.4 mg per 100 ml IgG, and 135.6 mg per 100 ml IgM. Dentigerous cysts contained an average of 308.4 mg per 100 ml IgA, 1618.2 mg per 100 ml IgG, and 155.6 mg per 100 ml IgM. Odontogenic keratocysts contained mean levels of 135.6 mg per 100 ml IgA, 491.9 mg per 100 ml IgG, and 54.1 mg per 100 ml IgM. Compared to serum, the fluid of radicular cysts contained higher quantities of soluble protein, made up of proportionally less albumin and more α-globulins and γ-globulins. The protein was likely to be derived from an inflammatory exudate modified by some activity of the cyst wall. Dentigerous cysts contained similar quantities of soluble protein, but it was thought that the fluid was less modified by cellular activity of the cyst wall.

Skaug (1977) also determined the soluble proteins in fluids from non-keratinizing jaw cysts. He too found that the fluids from non-keratinizing cysts contained the main proteins found in plasma and exhibited the characteristics of an inflammatory exudate. He found that the non-immunoglobulin proteins occurred in concentrations lower than those of autologous serum, and that there was an inverse relationship between the concentrations in cyst fluids of non-immunoglobulin proteins and their molecular weights. These low relative concentrations of macromolecular non-immunoglobulin proteins showed that there was no free passage of plasma proteins into the cyst fluid. Presumably, selective protein passage was due to restricted vascular permeability and a molecular sieve effect exerted by the cyst capsule. With respect to immunoglobulins, he found that cyst fluid contained on average IgG, IgA, and IgM concentrations that were respectively 1.2, 1.7, and 0.9 times those of autologous serum. He considered that the immunoglobulins of cyst fluid were partly produced locally and partly derived from plasma.

A distinctive antigen, named the keratocyst antigen (KCA), has been reported by Kuusela *et al.* (1982, 1987) as being present in keratocyst fluids. It is a soluble component of 60–68 KDa molecular weight, present in most keratocyst fluids but absent from the fluids of non-keratinizing cysts. Southgate *et al.* (1986) have shown that the major protein fraction in keratocyst fluid appears to be a novel antigenic marker of squamous epithelium. The fraction has mobility anodal to albumin on electrophoresis and was shown to be a non-serum protein. Using an antiserum to keratocyst fluid absorbed with human serum, non-serum components were localized in squamous keratinizing epithelium, principally in the upper layers. No localization was seen in non-squamous epithelium or in non-keratinized squamous epithelial cysts. Douglas and Craig (1986, 1987) demonstrated a keratocyst-specific antigen X and subsequently characterized it as being antigenically identical with lactoferrin. Quantitation of lactoferrin in keratinizing and non-keratinizing cyst fluids by Smith *et al.* (1988a) and Douglas and Craig (1989), however, revealed detectable levels in the fluids of all types of cyst, although keratocyst fluids had the highest levels of lactoferrin. The source of lactoferrin was suggested to be neutrophils.

Smith *et al.* (1984, 1986, 1988b,c) studied the role of glycosaminoglycans in odontogenic cysts by examining cyst fluids, cyst connective tissue, and tissue extracts. They found that hyaluronic acid showed the highest incidence. Heparin sulphate was higher in keratocysts compared to other cyst types, and appreciable amounts of chondroitin-4-sulphate were also observed. The investigative aspects of cyst fluids have recently been reviewed comprehensively (Smith, 1991).

NON-ODONTOGENIC CYSTS

Nasopalatine cyst

The nasopalatine cyst occurs in the maxillary incisor region, characteristically as a heart-shaped area of radiolucency between the two maxillary central incisors (*Fig. 19.21*). Clinically it appears as a fluctuant swelling palatal to the maxillary incisors. Occasionally, it may present as a swelling on the labial aspect of the alveolus or both. Very large cysts extend posteriorly and these probably account for most of the median palatal cysts that have been reported.

Histology

Nasopalatine cysts are thought to originate from epithelial remnants of the nasopalatine duct. The cyst is lined with either pseudostratified ciliated columnar epithelium (*Fig. 19.22*) or non-keratinized stratified squamous epithelium or both. Dendritic melanocytes have been found in the basal layers of the epithelium (El-Bardaie *et al.*, 1989). Those lined with squamous epithelium are thought to have arisen from the oral end of the duct, while those originating from the nasal end are lined with respiratory epithelium. Those originating in an intermediate position are lined by both. Shear (1992) feels that this should not be regarded as a rule, but that variability of the linings is suggestive of their origin from pluripotential epithelium or as the result of metaplasia. In the fibrous wall are found thick-walled blood vessels, nerves (*Fig.*

19.23), and occasionally mucous glands, cartilage, and adipose tissue. This is thought to be due to the inclusion of the long nasopalatine nerves and vessels, which traverse the incisive canal.

Globulomaxillary cyst

Situated between the maxillary lateral incisor and the maxillary canine, the globulomaxillary cyst was at one time thought to have arisen as a result of enclavement of epithelium between the globular and maxillary processes. However, the modern embryological view is that there is no meeting of facial processes in this region and that there is continuity of the ectoderm in the earliest stages, with the 'facial processes' being due to growth of the underlying mesenchyme (Arey, 1965). It is therefore unlikely that the cyst develops from enclaved epithelium in early embryological development of the anterior maxilla.

Most cysts in this region are either radicular cysts, related to the maxillary lateral incisor or canine, or odontogenic keratocysts. It is also necessary to exclude a cyst arising from a palatal invagination in the maxillary lateral incisor. Shear (1992) points out that a number of them fulfil the criteria for the diagnosis of a lateral periodontal cyst, being lined with a thin non-keratinized stratified squamous epithelium with areas of localized plaque formation. Most authorities no longer regard it as an entity.

Median cysts

These are two rare cyst entities that may involve the PDL in the median region of the jaws. The median mandibular cyst is in the symphyseal region, and the median alveolar cyst lies between the maxillary teeth in front of the incisive foramen. The existence of these cysts as entities has also been seriously questioned, and most will be shown to be radicular cysts, lateral periodontal cysts, or odontogenic keratocysts (Kramer *et al.*, 1992).

Solitary bone cyst

The solitary bone cyst is alternatively known as a traumatic or haemorrhagic bone cyst. Although it chiefly involves the basal bone, the PDL may become involved as a result of extension to the alveolar bone. Radiographically this may be seen as a scalloping outline around the roots of the teeth (*Fig. 19.24*).

The cyst occurs in young people and is usually detected by routine radiographic examination, as it causes little or no expansion of bone. The cyst cavity is either empty or contains a small amount of serosanguinous fluid. Seward (1963) stated that, upon careful aspiration, these lesions yield a golden-yellow fluid that contains a high concentration of bilirubin. The tenuous fibrous lining lacks an epithelium and the surrounding bone exhibits osteoclastic resorption (*Fig. 19.25*).

The pathogenesis of the cyst is obscure. Howe (1965) reviewed the literature and proposed the following hypothesis. Disruption of a thin-walled sinusoid in the red bone marrow leads to the formation of an intramedullary haematoma. This haemorrhage may result from trauma. Resorption of the affected bone marrow and trabeculae occurs, this process being triggered partly by a rise in intramedullary pressure and partly by the action of breakdown products of haemolysis and a resultant rise in hydrogen ion concentration. The bone cavity so formed enlarges by means of osteoclastic action aided by transudation into the lesion from the breakdown of the blood proteins. Finally, the pressure falls, bone resorption ceases, and the resultant serous fluid is absorbed by cellular action, leaving an empty cavity within the bone. Hosseini (1978–1979) has suggested that solitary bone cysts might result from the failure of differentiation of osteogenic cells and that they might originate as multiple bursa-like synovial cavities, which later coalesce to form a larger connective-tissue lined defect.

NEOPLASTIC CHANGE IN PERIODONTAL CYSTS

Rarely, neoplastic change may take place in periodontal cysts. Examples of radicular, dentigerous and odontogenic keratocysts undergoing carcinomatous change have been reported in the literature (Gardner, 1975; Van der Wall *et al.*, 1985; High *et al.*, 1987; Macleod and Soames, 1988). There is a clinical suspicion that odontogenic keratocysts are more likely to undergo a neoplastic change than other cysts, but there are no statistical data to support such a contention.

As these are relatively rare events, there is no justification to regard cysts as precancerous lesions. The DNA content of cells from a keratocyst that had undergone malignant transformation was examined by High *et al.* (1987) using flow cytometry. As malignant transformation progressed, they found a large additional peak to the right of the diploid G_0–G_1 peak, and this represented a DNA aneuploid G_0–G_1 component with a DNA index of 2.0. Control material showed a single large peak on the left-hand side of the channel number scale, representing cells in G_0–G_1 phase that are diploid.

There is also a long-standing view that the dentigerous cyst is a potential ameloblastoma (Cahn, 1933). This view arose from a study of lesions which appeared clinically and radiologically to be dentigerous cysts but proved in fact to be ameloblastomas, and Cahn advanced the view that all dentigerous cysts should be considered as potential ameloblastomas. Shear (1992) feels that the confusion may have arisen for three reasons. Firstly, an unerupted tooth may be involved by an ameloblastoma, and this may be interpreted incorrectly as a dentigerous cyst on radiographs. Secondly, when a biopsy of an ameloblastoma is taken, the tissue biopsied may be an expanded locule lined apparently by a thin layer of epithelium similar to a non-neoplastic cyst. Thirdly, non-neoplastic islands of odontogenic epithelium in the wall of non-neoplastic cysts may be interpreted as ameloblastoma. Lucas (1984) and Shear (1992) concluded that, while such a change is theoretically possible, it must be an extremely rare occurrence.

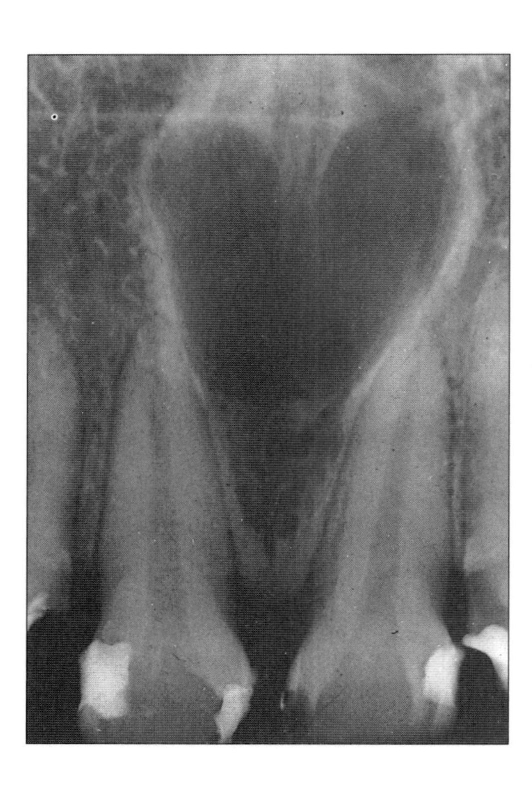

Fig. 19.21 Nasopalatine cyst presenting as a heart-shaped area of radiolucency between the two maxillary central incisor teeth.

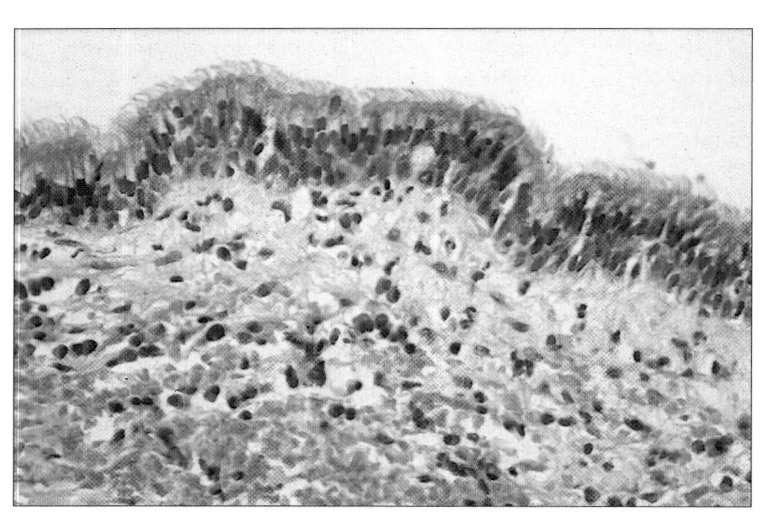

Fig. 19.22 Pseudostratified ciliated columnar epithelium lines this nasopalatine cyst. (Haematoxylin and eosin × 250.)

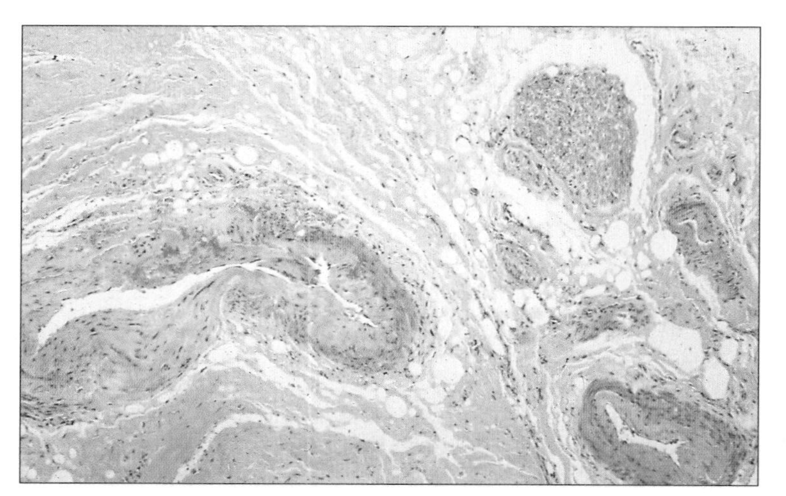

Fig. 19.23 Thick-walled blood vessels and nerve bundles in the fibrous wall of a nasopalatine cyst. (Haematoxylin and eosin × 60.)

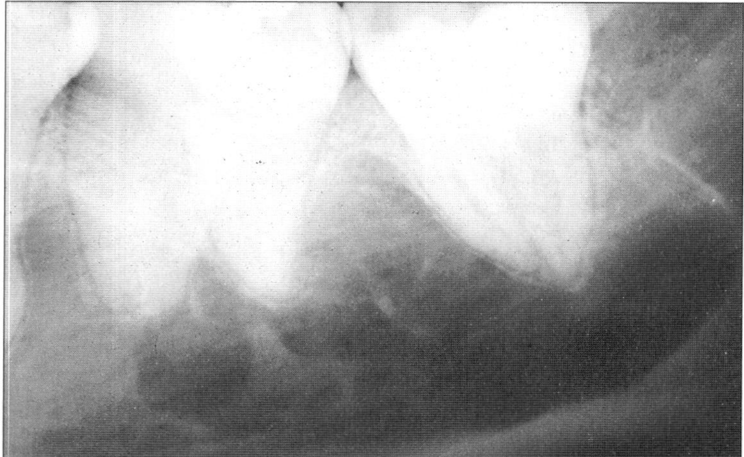

Fig. 19.24 Radiograph of a solitary bone cyst with scalloping outline around the roots of the teeth.

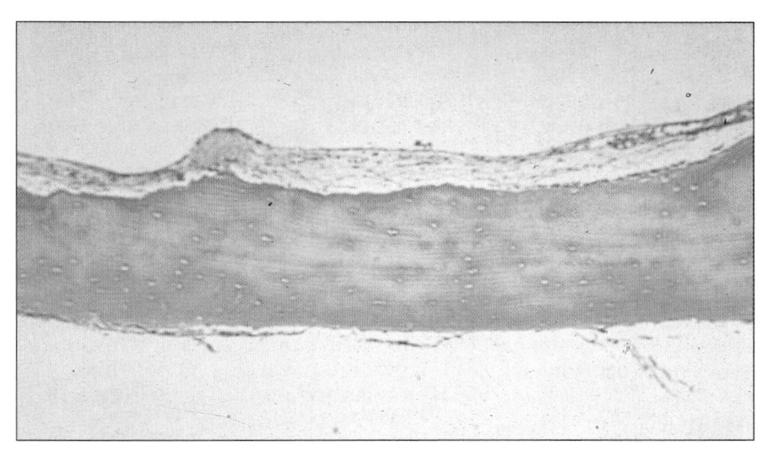

Fig. 19.25 Lining of a solitary bone cyst, consisting of a tenuous fibrous tissue without epithelium and outer bony wall. (Haematoxylin and eosin × 60.)

REFERENCES

Ackermann G, Cohen M and Altini M (1987) The paradental cyst: a clinico-pathological study of 50 cases. Oral Surg 64, 308–312.

Ahlfors E, Larsson A and Sjögren S (1984) The odontogenic keratocyst: a benign cystic tumour? J Oral Maxillofac Surg 42, 10–19.

Al-Talabani NG and Smith CJ (1980) Experimental dentigerous cyst and enamel hypoplasia: their possible significance in explaining the pathogenesis of human dentigerous cysts. J Oral Pathol 9, 82–91.

Allison RT (1977) Microprobe and microradiographic studies of hyaline bodies in odontogenic cysts. J Oral Pathol 6, 44–50.

Altini M and Shear M (1992) The lateral periodontal cyst. An update. J Oral Pathol Med 21, 245–250.

Arey LB (1965) Developmental anatomy (7th edition), p 205, Saunders, Philadelphia, London.

Atkinson ME (1972) A histological study of tooth grafts in an inbred strain of mice. J Oral Pathol 1, 115–124.

Atkinson ME (1976) A histological study of odontogenic cysts formed following mouse molar tooth transplantation. J Oral Pathol 5, 347–357.

Atkinson ME (1977) An autoradiographic study of experimental odontogenic cyst formation in the mouse. J Oral Pathol 6, 382–386.

Bando Y, Henderson B, Meghji S, Poole S and Harris M (1993) Immunocytochemical localization of inflammatory cytokines and vascular adhesion receptors in radicular cysts. J Oral Pathol Med 22, 221–227.

Bhaskar SN (1972) Non-surgical resolution of radicular cysts. Oral Surg Oral 34, 458–468.

Bouyssou M and Guilheim A (1965) Recherches morphologiques et histochimiques sur les corps hyalins intrakystiques de Rushton. Bull Group Int Rech Sci Stomat 8, 81–104.

Brannon RB (1976, 1977) The odontogenic keratocyst. A clinico-pathological study of 312 cases. Part I. Oral Surg 42, 54–72. Part II Ibid 43, 233–255.

Browne RM (1970) The odontogenic keratocyst – clinical aspects. Br Dent J 128, 225–231.

Browne RM (1971a) The origin of cholesterol in odontogenic cysts in man. Arch Oral Biol 16, 107–113.

Browne RM (1971b) The odontogenic keratocyst – histological features and their correlation with clinical behaviour. Br Dent J 131, 249–259.

Browne RM (1976) Some observations on the fluids of odontogenic cysts. J Oral Pathol 5, 74–87.

Browne RM (1991) The structure of odontogenic cysts. In: Investigative Pathology of the Odontogenic Cyst (Browne RM, ed), pp 22–51, CRC Press, Boca Raton, Florida.

Browne RM and Matthews JB (1985) Intra-epithelial hyaline bodies in odontogenic cysts; an immunoperoxidase study. J Oral Pathol 14, 422–428.

Buchner A and David R (1978) Lipopigment in odontogenic cysts. J Oral Pathol 7, 311–317.

Cahn LR (1933) The dentigerous cyst is a potential ameloblastoma. Dent Cosmos 75, 889–893.

Chen SY and Miller AS (1975) Ultrastructure of the keratinizing and calcifying odontogenic cyst. Oral Surg 39, 769–780.

Crabb HSM (1963) Areas simulating carious lesions in the enamel of teeth from dentigerous cysts. Br Dent J 114, 499–511.

Craig GT (1976) The paradental cyst. A specific inflammatory odontogenic cyst. Br Dent J 141, 9–14.

Donatsky O, Hjørting-Hansen E, Philipsen HP and Fejerskov O (1976) Clinical, radiologic, and histopathological aspects of 13 cases of naevoid basal cell carcinoma syndrome. Int J Oral Surg 5, 19–28.

Donoff RB, Harper E and Guralnick WC (1972) Collagenolytic activity in keratocysts. J Oral Surg 30, 879–884.

Douglas CW and Craig GT (1986) Recognition of protein apparently specific to odontogenic keratocyst fluids. J Clin Pathol 39, 1108–1115.

Douglas CW and Craig GT (1987) Evidence for the presence of lactoferrin in odontogenic keratocyst fluids. J Clin Pathol 40, 914–921.

Douglas CW and Craig GT (1989) Quantitation of lactoferrin in odontogenic cyst fluids. J Clin Pathol 42, 180–183.

El-Bardaie A, Nikai H and Takata T (1989) Pigmented nasopalatine duct cyst: report of two cases. Int J Oral Maxillofac Surg 18, 138–139.

El-Labban NG (1979) Electron microscopic investigation of hyaline bodies in odontogenic cysts. J Oral Pathol 8, 81–93.

El-Labban NG and Aghabeigi B (1990) A comparative stereologic and ultrastructural study of blood vessels in odontogenic keratocysts and dentigerous cysts. J Oral Pathol Med 19, 442–446.

Fowler CB and Brannon RB (1989) The paradental cyst: a clinico-pathological study of 6 new cases and review of literature. J Oral Maxillofac Surg 47, 243–248.

Gabbiani G, Ryan GB and Majno G (1971) Presence of modified fibroblasts in granulation tissue and their possible role in wound contraction. Experientia 27, 549–550.

Gao Z, Mackenzie IC, Rittman BR, Korzun AK, Williams DM and Cruchley AT (1988) Immunocytochemical examination of immune cells in periapical granulomas and odontogenic cysts. J Oral Pathol 17, 84–90.

Gao Z, Mackenzie IC, Cruchley AT, Williams DM, Leigh I and Lane EB (1989) Cytokeratin expression of the odontogenic epithelium in dental follicles and developmental cysts. J Oral Pathol Med 18, 63–67.

Gardner AF (1975) A survey of odontogenic cysts and their relationship to squamous cell carcinoma. J Can Dent Assoc 41, 161–167.

Gardner DG, Kessler HP, Morency R and Schaffner DL (1988) The glandular odontogenic cyst: an apparent entity. J Oral Pathol 17, 359–366.

Garrett JR and Winstone KMS (1991) Cholesterol in the walls of odontogenic cysts – a histochemical and ultrastructural study. In: Investigative Pathology of the Odontogenic Cyst (Browne RM, ed), pp 175–190, CRC Press, Boca Raton, Florida.

Gorlin RJ, Cohen MM and Lewin S (1990) Syndromes of the Head and Neck. (3rd edition), pp 372–378, Oxford University Press, Oxford.

Gorlin RJ, Pindborg JJ, Clausen FP and Vickers RA (1962) The calcifying odontogenic cyst – a possible analogue of the cutaneous calcifying epithelioma of Malherbe. Oral Surg 15, 1235– 1245.

Gustafson G, Lindahl B, Dahl E and Svensson A (1989) The naevoid basal cell carcinoma syndrome – Gorlin's syndrome. Multiple jaw cysts and skin cancer. Swed Dent J 13, 131–139.

Harris M (1978) Odontogenic cyst growth and prostaglandin-induced bone resorption. Ann R Coll Surg Engl 60, 86–91.
Harris M and Toller PA (1975) Pathogenesis of dental cysts. Br Med Bull 31, 159–163.
High AS and Hirschmann N (1988) Symptomatic residual radicular cysts. J Oral Pathol 17, 70–72.
High AS, Quirke P and Hume PJ (1987) DNA ploidy studies in a keratocyst undergoing subsequent malignant transformation. J Oral Pathol 16, 135–138.
Hodson JJ (1966) Origin and nature of the cuticula dentis. Nature 209, 990–993.
Hodson JJ (1967) The distribution, structure, origin and nature of the dental cuticle of Gottlieb. Periodontics 5, 237–256, 295–302.
Hong SS, Ellis GL and Hartman KS (1991) Calcifying odontogenic cyst. A review of ninety-two cases with revaluation of their nature as cysts or neoplasms, the nature of ghost cells and subclassification. Oral Surg 72, 56–64.
Hormia M, Ylipaavalniemi P, Nagle RB and Virtanen I (1987) Expression of cytokeratins in odontogenic jaw cysts. Monoclonal antibodies reveal distinct variations between different cyst types. J Oral Pathol 16, 338–346.
Hosseini M (1978–79) Two atypical solitary bone cysts. Br J Oral Surg 16, 262–269.
Howe GL (1965) 'Haemorrhagic cysts' of the mandible. Br J Oral Surg 3, Part I, 55–76, Part II, 77–91.
Kaugars GE (1986) Botryoid odontogenic cyst. Oral Surg 62, 555–559.
Kramer IRH (1974) Changing views on oral disease. Proc R Soc Med 67, 271–276.
Kramer IRH, Pindborg JJ and Shear M (1992) Histological Typing of Odontogenic Tumours, 2nd edition. Springer-Verlag, Berlin, Heidelberg.
Kramer IRH and Toller PA (1973) The use of exfoliative cytology and protein estimations in preoperative diagnosis of odontogenic keratocysts. Int J Oral Surg 2, 143–151.
Kuusela P, Hormia M, Tuompo H and Ylipaavalniemi P (1982) Demonstration and partial characterization of a novel soluble antigen present in keratocysts. Oncodevel Biol Med 3, 283–290.
Kuusela P, Ylipaavalniemi P and Thesleff I (1987) The relationship between keratocyst antigen and keratin. J Oral Pathol 15, 287–291.
Lee KW and El-Labban NG (1976) Presence of cells with morphological features of smooth muscle in the fibrous walls of radicular cysts. J Dent Res 55 (special issue) D110.
Lee KW and El-Labban NG (1980) A light and electron-microscopic study of smooth muscle-like cells in the walls of radicular (dental) cysts in man. Arch Oral Biol 25, 403–408.
Lucas RB (1984) Pathology of Tumours of the Oral Tissues, 4th edition, pp 49–51. Churchill Livingstone, Edinburgh.
MacLeod RI and Soames JV (1988) Squamous cell carcinoma arising in an odontogenic keratocyst. Br J Oral Maxillofac Surg 26, 52–57.
Magnusson BC (1978) Odontogenic keratocyst. A clinical and histological study with special reference to enzyme histochemistry. J Oral Pathol 7, 8–18.
Main DMG (1970) The enlargement of epithelial jaw cysts. Odont Revy 21, 29–49.
Matejka M, Porteder H, Ulrich W, Watzek G and Sinzinger H (1985) Prostaglandin synthesis in dental cysts. Br J Oral Maxillofac Surg 23, 190–194.
Matthews JB (1991) Hyaline and foreign bodies in cyst walls. In: Investigative Pathology of the Odontogenic Cyst (Browne RM, ed), pp 191–209, CRC Press, Boca Raton, Florida.
Matthews JB and Browne RM (1987) An immunocytochemical study of inflammatory cell infiltrates and epithelial expression of HLA-DR in odontogenic cysts. J Oral Pathol 16, 112–117.
Matthews JB, Mason GI and Browne RM (1988) Epithelial cell markers and proliferating cells in odontogenic jaw cysts. J Pathol 156, 283–290.
Meghji S, Harvey W and Harris M (1989) Interleukin I-like activity in cystic lesions of the jaws. Br J Oral Maxillofac Surg 27, 1–11.
Morgan PR and Johnson NW (1974) Histological, histochemical and ultrastructural studies on the nature of hyaline bodies in odontogenic cysts. J Oral Pathol 3, 127–147.
Morgan PR, Shirlaw PJ, Johnson NW, Leigh IM and Lane EB (1987) Potential applications of anti-keratin antibodies in oral diagnosis. J Oral Pathol 16, 212–222.
Niemeyer K, Schlien HP, Habel G and Mentler C (1985) Behandlungsergebnisse und Langzeitbeobachtungen bei 62 Patienten mit keratocysten. Dtsch Zahnarztl Z 40, 632–640.
Nilsen R, Johannessen AC, Skaug N and Matre R (1984) In–situ characterization of mononuclear cells in human dental periapical inflammatory lesions using mononuclear antibodies. Oral Surg 58, 160–165.
Oehlers FAC (1970) Periapical lesions and residual dental cysts. Br J Oral Surg 8, 103–113.
Ogden GR, Chisholm DM, Kiddie RA and Lane DP (1992) p53 protein in odontogenic cysts. J Clin Pathol 45, 1007–1010.
Padayachee A and van Wyk CW (1987) Two cystic lesions with features of both the botryoid odontogenic cyst and central mucoepidermoid tumour; sialo–odontogenic cyst? J Oral Pathol 16, 499–504.
Philippou S, Rühl GH and Mandelartz E (1990) Scanning electron microscopic studies and x-ray microanalysis of hyaline bodies in odontogenic cysts. J Oral Pathol Med 19, 447–452.
Philipsen HP (1956) Om keratocyster (kolesteatom) i kaeberne. Tandlaegebladet 60, 963–981.
Pindborg JJ and Hansen J (1963) Studies of odontogenic cyst epithelium. 2. Clinical and roentgenologic aspects of odontogenic keratocysts. Acta Pathol Microbiol Scand [A] 58, 283–294.
Praetorius F, Hjørting-Hansen E, Gorlin RJ and Vickers RA (1981) Calcifying odontogenic cyst. Range, variations and neoplastic potential. Acta Odontol Scand 39, 227–240.
Rhül GH, Philippou S and Mandelartz E (1989) Zur Histogenese von Hyalinen Bodies in Odontogenen Zysten. Dtsch Z Mund Kiefer Gerichts Chir 13, 145–154.
Rivière GR and Sabet TY (1973) Experimental follicular cyst in mice – a histological study. Oral Surg 36, 205–213.
Robinson HBG (1975) Primodial cyst vs keratocyst. Oral Surg 40, 362–364.
Rushton MA (1955) Hyaline bodies in the epithelium of dental cysts. Proc R Soc Med 48, 407–409.
Sedano JO and Gorlin RJ (1968) Hyaline bodies of Rushton. Some histochemical considerations concerning their aetiology. Oral Surg 26, 198–201.
Seward GR (1963) Radiology in general dental practice. Br Dent J 115, 231.
Seward GR (1992) Treatment of cysts. In: Cysts of the Oral Regions (Shear M, ed), pp 227–256. Butterworth–Heinmann, Oxford.
Shear M (1960) Primordial cysts. J Dent Assoc S Afr 15, 211–217.
Shear M (1961) The hyaline and granular bodies in dental cysts. Br Dent J 110, 301–307.
Shear M (1992) Cysts of the Oral Regions, 3rd edition. Butterworth–Heinemann, Oxford.
Shear M and Pindborg JJ (1975) Microscopic features of the lateral periodontal cyst. Scand J Dent Res 83, 103–110.
Skalli O and Gabbiani G (1988) The biology of the myofibroblast relationship to wound contraction and fibro-contractive diseases. In: The Molecular and Cellular Biology of Wound Repair (Clark RAF and Henson PM, eds), pp 373–402, Plenum Publications, New York.
Skaug N (1976a) Intracystic fluid pressure in non-keratinizing jaw cysts. Int J Oral Surg 5, 59–65.
Skaug N (1976b) Lipoproteins in fluids from non-keratinizing jaw cysts. Scand J Dent Res 84, 98–105.
Skaug N (1977) Soluble proteins in fluids from non-keratinizing jaw cysts in man. Int J Oral Surg 6, 107–121.

Smith AJ (1991) Odontogenic cyst fluids. In: Investigative Pathology of the Odontogenic Cyst (Browne RM, ed), pp 123–128, CRC Press, Boca Raton, Florida.

Smith AJ and Matthews JB (1991) Odontogenic epithelium and its residues. In: Investigative Pathology of the Odontogenic Cyst (Browne RM, ed), pp 53–85. CRC Press, Boca Raton, Florida.

Smith G, Smith AJ and Browne RM (1984) Glycosaminoglycans in fluid aspirates from odontogenic cysts. J Oral Pathol 13, 614–621.

Smith G, Smith AJ, and Browne RM (1986) Analysis of odontogenic cyst fluid aspirates. IRCS Med Sci 14, 304.

Smith AJ, Matthews JB, Mason GI and Browne RM (1988a) Lactoferrin in aspirates of odontogenic cyst fluids. J Clin Pathol 41, 1117–1119.

Smith G, Smith AJ and Browne RM (1988b) Histochemical studies on glycosaminoglycans of odontogenic cysts. J Oral Pathol 17, 55–59.

Smith G, Smith AJ and Browne RM (1988c) Quantification and analysis of glycosaminoglycans in human odontogenic cyst linings. Arch Oral Biol 33, 623–626.

Soames JV and Southam JC (1993) Oral Pathology, p72, Oxford University Press, Oxford.

Southgate J, Whicher JT, Davies JD, O'Reillay DStJ and Matthews RW (1986) A protein of squamous keratinizing epithelium from odontogenic keratocyst fluid. Virchows Arch [A] 409, 705–713.

Stoelinga PJW and Peters JH (1973) A note on the origin of keratocysts of the jaws. Int J Oral Surg 2, 37–44.

Stones HH (1951) Oral and Dental Diseases (2nd edition), pp805–809, Livingstone, Edinburgh.

Summers L (1974) The incidence of epithelium in periapical granulomas and the mechanism of cavitation in apical dental cysts in man. Arch Oral Biol 19, 1177–1180.

Toller PA (1967) Origin and growth of cysts of the jaws. Ann R Coll Surg Engl 40, 306–336.

Toller PA (1970) The osmolality of fluids from cysts of the jaws. Br Dent J 129, 275–278.

van der Wall I, Rauhamaa R, van der Kwast WAM and Snow GB (1985) Squamous cell carcinoma arising in the lining of odontogenic cysts. Int J Oral Surg 14, 146–152.

Vedtofte P and Praetorius F (1989) The inflammatory paradental cyst. Oral Surg 68, 182–188.

Vuhahula E, Nikai H, Ijuhin N, *et al.* (1993) Jaw cysts with orthokeratinization analysis of 12 cases. J Oral Pathol Med 22, 35–40.

Warwick James W and Counsell A (1932) A histological study of the epithelium associated with chronic apical infection of the teeth. Br Dent J 53, 463–483.

Weathers DR and Waldron CA (1973) Unusual multilocular cysts of the jaw (Botryoid odontogenic cyst) Oral Surg 36, 235–241.

Woolgar JA, Rippin JW and Browne RM (1987a) A comparative histological study of odontogenic keratocysts in basal cell nevus syndrome and control patients. J Oral Pathol 16, 75–80.

Woolgar JA, Rippin JW and Browne RM (1987b) The odontogenic keratocyst and its occurrence in nevoid basal cell carcinoma syndrome. Oral Surg 64, 727–730.

Woolgar JA, Rippin JW and Browne RM (1987c) A comparative study of the clinical and histological features of recurrent and non-recurrent odontogenic keratocysts. J Oral Pathol 16, 124–128.

World Health Organization (1978) Application of the International Classification of Diseases to Dentistry and Stomatology, Geneva.

Wright JM (1981) The odontogenic keratocyst. Orthokeratinized variant. Oral Surg 51, 609–618.

Chapter 20

Soft Connective Tissue Disorders and the Periodontal Ligament

DM Chisholm, AD Gilbert

INTRODUCTION

The connective tissue disorders comprise a group of diseases affecting connective tissues; at present they can only be classified together on the basis of the similarity of the tissue changes (Bunim and Black, 1957). The strongest link that binds together the various connective tissue diseases is a common histopathological pattern – an increase in interfibrillary ground substance, proliferation of fibroblasts, mononuclear cell infiltration and fibrinoid necrosis. Although the aetiology of these disorders is unknown, strong evidence suggests that they have an autoimmune basis. They are all associated with the production of autoantibodies that bind to predominantly intracellular antigens (Vyse and Walport, 1993). Despite unresolved problems concerning aetiology and pathogenesis, in all probability the diseases are multifactorial, with genetic, infective, immunological, and environmental components playing varying parts.

Because of their multiorgan involvement, the connective tissue disorders can alter the oral environment by impeding oral hygiene, so that periodontal disease occurs as a secondary consequence of the primary disease state. Involvement of the periodontal ligament (PDL) as a direct result of a connective tissue disorder appears to obtain with certainty for progressive systemic sclerosis (scleroderma), but only speculatively for some of the other 'collagen diseases'.

Apart from these autoimmune diseases, an understanding of heritable disorders of connective tissue is also important. Study has developed around, for example, Marfan's syndrome, osteogenesis imperfecta, and pseudoxanthoma elasticum. The concept that such disorders may represent generalized single-gene-determined defects of one or other elements of connective tissue is a fundamental one. Thus, a common pathway defined at the molecular level may be predicted. Inclusion of the mucopolysaccharides among heritable disorders of connective tissue arises from the fact that storage material is mucopolysaccharide, not lipid (Brante, 1952). The search for the basic defects in heritable disorders includes cell culture methods and biochemical methods for the characterization of the severe forms of collagen and other connective tissue problems. Methods for studying the genes themselves by recombinant DNA technology make it easier to study the gene or the messenger RNA than the protein gene product.

This chapter is concerned mainly with progressive systemic sclerosis, and only brief mention is made of other disorders. In addition, although not belonging to the classic group of connective tissue disorders, information will also be given about the effects of lathyrogens on the PDL, the heritable disorders, and atrophy of the tissue caused by reduced function.

PROGRESSIVE SYSTEMIC SCLEROSIS

CLINICAL FINDINGS

Progressive systemic sclerosis (PSS) or scleroderma is a chronic disease characterized by diffuse sclerosis of the skin, gastrointestinal tract, cardiac muscle, lung, and kidney (Winkelman, 1971). There are at least three distinct clinical variants together with a range of scleroderma-like syndromes, which have been reviewed by Rocco and Hurd (1986).

All forms of the disease are commoner among females, with a 3:1 female-to-male ratio. Most cases are detected in adults, with an average age of 40 years. The onset is usually insidious, and among the clinical changes in skin are induration, hyperpigmentation, and telangiectasia. Raynaud's phenomenon (digital arterial insufficiency provoked by cold) is a common feature, while calcification of subcutaneous tissue (calcinosis universalis) tends to be a late manifestation. Accordingly, the clinical symptoms vary depending upon the extent of involvement and which organs are involved. Diffuse scleroderma may manifest the so-called CREST phenomenon, which includes calcinosis; Raynaud's disease; oesophagitis; sclerodactyly, and telangiectasia. Thus, cardiac, pulmonary, renal, and gastrointestinal symptoms are predictably present. Morphoea or localized scleroderma is a localized benign, self-limiting form of the disease affecting the skin (Fleischmajer *et al.*, 1966).

The clinical association of PSS with other connective tissue diseases (including systemic lupus erythematosus, rheumatoid arthritis, Sjögren's syndrome, and mixed connective tissue disease) suggests an immunological cause or causes. Although some evidence of cell-mediated cytotoxicity against embryonic fibroblasts is available, inflammatory cell infiltration is slight and humoral changes are not directly suggestive of a pathogenic mechanism. Hypergammaglobulinaemia and circulating serum autoantibodies are often present. The hypergammaglobulinaemia is usually polyclonal, and rheumatoid factors are often found. The fluorescent antinuclear antibody test shows a speckled or nucleolar pattern in 70 per cent of cases. Those patients with mixed connective tissue disease have high levels of anti-ribonuclease-sensitive extractable nuclear antigen (Rothfield and Rodman, 1968; Sharp *et al.*, 1972).

Weisman and Calcaterra (1978) found that 80 per cent of PSS patients show head and neck manifestations, while 30 per cent have head and neck features as the presenting symptoms. These features included dysphagia, tight facial skin and telangiectasia, decreased mouth opening (*Fig. 20.1*), microstomia, and dryness of the mouth. PSS may also present as the connective tissue manifestation of Sjögren's syndrome. Involvement of the lips and cheeks restricts mastication and temporomandibular joint movement. Indeed, the joint may become fixed. Induration and immobility of the tongue interfere with mastication, swallowing, and speech. Exposure of the teeth following lip retraction (*Fig. 20.2*) may result in increased caries and inflammatory periodontal disease, while immobile mucous membranes are particularly susceptible to trauma from mastication or dentures.

RADIOGRAPHIC FINDINGS

Radiographically, there is often widening of the periodontal space (*Fig. 20.3*). This feature is found in 30–100 per cent of cases (Stafne and Austin, 1944; Rowell and Hopper, 1977; White *et al.*, 1977). Rowell and Hopper (1977) found no direct relationship between widening of the PDL and other systemic changes. Generalized radiographical widening of the PDL is detected in fewer than 30 per cent of patients with PSS, though a higher prevalence is observed in the diffuse as opposed to focal forms of the disease (Wood and Lee, 1988). A significant difference in the mean PDL width between scleroderma patients and controls (0.15 mm versus 0.08 mm) has been reported (Marmary *et al.*, 1981). Thickening of the PDL is associated with an insidious gingival recession. A meticulous approach to periodontal therapy is required and, if tooth extraction should become necessary, a surgical technique is advisable. In spite of the wider PDL, however, the teeth in scleroderma are not hypermobile (Fullmer and Witte, 1962; Jayson, 1976). Posterior teeth seem to be affected more than anterior teeth.

HISTOLOGY AND HISTOCHEMISTRY

Investigations of PDL affected by scleroderma have revealed that it is up to 3 mm thick, with collagen fibres in apical and middle thirds of the PDL running almost parallel to the root, and an absence of cellular cementum (Stafne and Austin, 1944; Gores, 1957). Continuity of the fibres seems to be lost a short distance from the cementum. Scattered through the fibrous tissue are many spicules of bone. The walls of blood vessels are thickened and their lumina narrowed (Stafne and Austin, 1944; Gores, 1957) as in other tissues affected by the disease (Krogh, 1950). Bailey (1976) observed that sites of PSS contain many thin, apparently newly formed fibres reminiscent of embryonic collagen.

In a detailed histological and histochemical study, Fullmer and Witte (1962) showed that the PSS-affected PDL contained collagen, oxytalan, and elastin fibres. The collagen was denser, more mature, and more hyalinized than normal, especially adjacent to the teeth. The number of oxytalan fibres increased proportionately with the collagen. The fibres were aligned normally in the transseptal region. Elsewhere they were aligned almost parallel to the root, with occasional sites of indiscriminate orientation. Some sites contained many mast cells. These workers found no alteration in cementum, either in amount or in type. They concluded that the thickening of the PDL was due to bone resorption and a proportionate increase in collagen and oxytalan fibre content, including areas of degenerating fibres. Sclerosis and hyalinization of collagen and development of elastic fibres were most marked adjacent to the cementum.

Regarding possible chemical factors underlying the PDL changes in PSS, it has been shown that there is a considerable increase in the proportion of reducible aldimine bond cross-links in connective tissue affected by scleroderma. These intermolecular cross-links (which are responsible for the high tensile strength of collagen fibres) are replaced by more stable non-reducible cross-links during maturation (Herbert *et al.*, 1974; Jayson, 1976). The older tissue from the centre of lesions in morphoea (the localized form of PSS) also contains lower levels of detectable cross-links than younger tissue from the edge of the lesion, where collagen is being synthesized (Herbert *et al.*, 1974). Jayson (1976) was unable to find a serum factor that might cause the increased production of collagen (as shown by ^{3}H-proline uptake in skin cultures) that occurs in sites of active PSS (Herbert *et al.*, 1974). Cross-links are discussed in Chapter 3.

PATHOLOGICAL MECHANISMS

Recent research into the mechanisms of disease in PSS has focused on microvascular pathosis, immunological abnormalities, and changes in fibroblast gene product regulation. Ultrastructural studies have shown a reduction in vessel basement membrane replication, gaps between endothelial cells, plasma protein leakage, and endothelial cell degeneration. Immunocytochemical markers show mononuclear infiltrate to be HLA-DR-expressing T lymphocytes and macrophages. A reduction in epidermal Langerhan's cells has been noted (Andrews *et al.*, 1986). The endothelial damage may be due to immune complex deposition. Immunofluorescence studies show IgM and complement factors in renal vessels but not in skin. Fluorescent antibody markers reveal deposition of type I procollagen, type III collagen, and fibronectin. A unique antibody to centromere protein (anti-CENP) is encountered in some forms of PSS and also in Raynaud's phenomenon (Earnshaw *et al.*, 1986). Cell mediated immunological alterations include decreased levels of circulating T lymphocytes with normal B cell numbers and an increase in OKT4–OKT8 ratio. Fibroblast regulatory mediators synthesized by activated mononuclear cells have a role in PSS. Fibroblast proliferation with accentuated fibrillogenesis is thus promoted. Defective fibroblast function is reflected morphologically in the fact that collagen fibril periodicity is normal while fibre diameter is decreased.

Thus, morphological findings, cell phenotype cell markers, humoral and cellular immune abnormalities, and fibroblast deregulation support immunological mechanisms in the pathogenesis of PSS.

Fibroblasts within the skin of PSS patients constitute a phenotypically heterogeneous population with regard to expression of collagen, cytokines, and cytokine receptors. By *in situ* hybridization techniques, PSS skin is shown to contain a sub-population of fibroblasts that are stimulated for expression of type VI collagen. This sub-population is larger than that found in normal skin. The heterogeneity in collagen production among PSS fibroblasts can also be demonstrated *in vitro* following sorting by flow cytometric analysis. An isoform of a cytokine known to be a potent modulator of collagen expression, transforming growth factor-β_2 (TGF-β_2), is overexpressed in and around inflammatory infiltrates in biopsies of skin from scleroderma patients. PSS fibroblasts grown in tissue culture express slightly elevated levels of transcripts for TGF-β_1, as demonstrated by Northem analysis. Osteonectin mRNA, widely distributed in developing tissues (Young *et al.*, 1986), is elevated in fibroblasts cultured from the affected skin of PSS patients. The affinity of epidermal growth factor receptors on fibroblasts derived from skin of PSS patients is decreased compared with that of receptors on normal fibroblasts. Receptors for platelet-derived growth factor-β (PDGF-β) are detectable by immunohistochemical staining in dermal vessels and fibroblasts in PSS but not in normal skin (Unemori and Amento, 1991).

TREATMENT

The drug D-penicillamine is used in the treatment of PSS, because it binds to the aldehyde cross-link precursor, thus inhibiting cross-linking, and producing a more fragile fibre. The drug has no effect on mature sclerodermatous collagen (Herbert *et al.*, 1974).

As mentioned above, with the exception of PSS there is little evidence of direct PDL involvement in these collagen disorders, although periodontitis may result indirectly from difficulties in maintaining satisfactory oral hygiene. However, a fortuitous case of juvenile periodontitis has been diagnosed in a patient with disseminated dermatomyositis (Newman and Dunn, unpublished finding). Bailey (1976) has reviewed the sparse information available concerning possible PDL effects in some other connective tissue disorders. (Developmental disorders are considered in more detail in Chapter 13).

LATHYRISM

Lathyrism is the name given to the condition caused by administering drugs that specifically inhibit cross-link formation in both collagen and elastin, acting on the enzyme lysyl oxidase (Siegel and Martin, 1970). This results in fragile collagen fibres in the connective tissues, at least in those in which collagen is turning over, such as the PDL. The drugs include aminoacetonitrile, β-aminopropionitrile (β-APN), and cysteamine. Inhibition of lysyl oxidase occurs by β-APN release *in vivo* by an amidase or protease from the precursor, β-(γ-glutamyl) aminopropionitrile, which is present in legumes (Kagan, 1986).

These drugs have been of particular use in studying eruptive mechanisms (see Chapter 9). Since collagen contraction has been implicated in generating the eruptive force, the effects on eruption rates following the administration of lathyrogens have been studied. By inhibiting cross-linking, these drugs should significantly reduce any contraction occurring during collagen maturation and thus retard eruption. However, though lathyritic drugs retard impeded eruption in continuously growing rodent incisors (e.g. Sarnat and Sciaky, 1965; Thomas, 1965; Berkovitz *et al.*, 1972; Michaeli *et al.*, 1975), there is little effect on unimpeded eruption rates (e.g. Berkovitz *et al.*, 1972; Tsuruta *et al.*, 1974).

Following administration of lathyritic agents to rodents, loss of tooth support owing to damage of PDL fibres is indicated by looseness of the teeth and the subsequent ease with which they can be extracted (Dasler, 1954; Sciaky and Ungar, 1961; Berkovitz *et al.*, 1972). Interference with the tooth-support mechanisms is also indicated by the occurrence of dilaceration of the root, particularly the continuously growing maxillary incisors.

The most significant change occurring in the PDL of the rat dentition is a gradual hyalinization of its structure (Gardner *et al.*, 1958; Sciaky and Ungar, 1961; Krikos *et al.*, 1965; Sarnat and Sciaky, 1965; Thomas, 1965). The collagen fibres lose their coarse, fibrous appearance and characteristic orientation. Instead, they appear as fine fibrils embedded in increased amounts of amorphous, eosinophilic material, which is surrounded by palisading fibroblasts. The fibrils lack any preferential orientation. The palisading cells bordering the cell-free, hyalinized zone are more cuboidal than normal fibroblasts (see *Fig. 20.3*). The general histological appearance seems to be related to the mechanical stresses placed on the tooth, since, if the opposing teeth are extracted, the PDL appears normal (Krikos *et al.*, 1965). For a more detailed description of the lathyritic PDL, the reader is referred to the ultrastructural studies of Cho and Garant (1984a,b) and Shore *et al.* (1984).

Since copper is a co-factor of lysyl oxidase, its deficiency results in effects that resemble lathyrism. D-penicillamine too, acts preferentially on collagen that cross-links in soft tissues. Thus, lathyrogens have been important in revealing that the functional ability of collagen and elastin depends on a system of covalent cross-links between the polypeptide chains of the proteins.

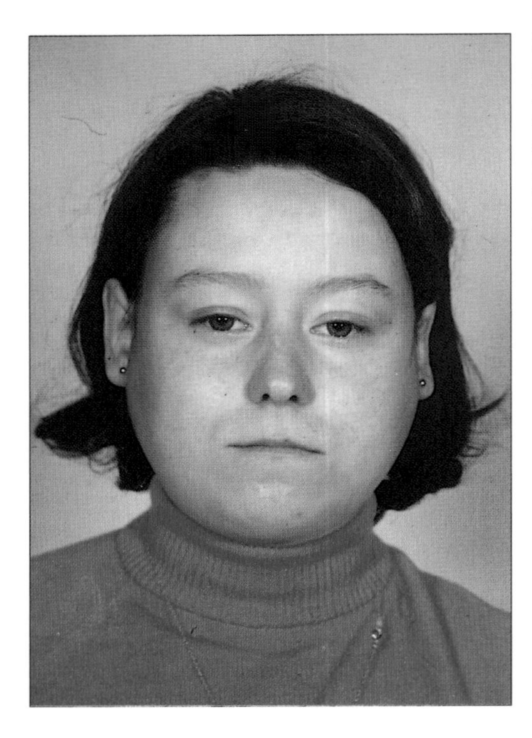

Fig. 20.1 Progressive systemic sclerosis. Female patient with expressionless, mask-like appearance. Rigidity of lips in this case resulted in difficulty in mastication.

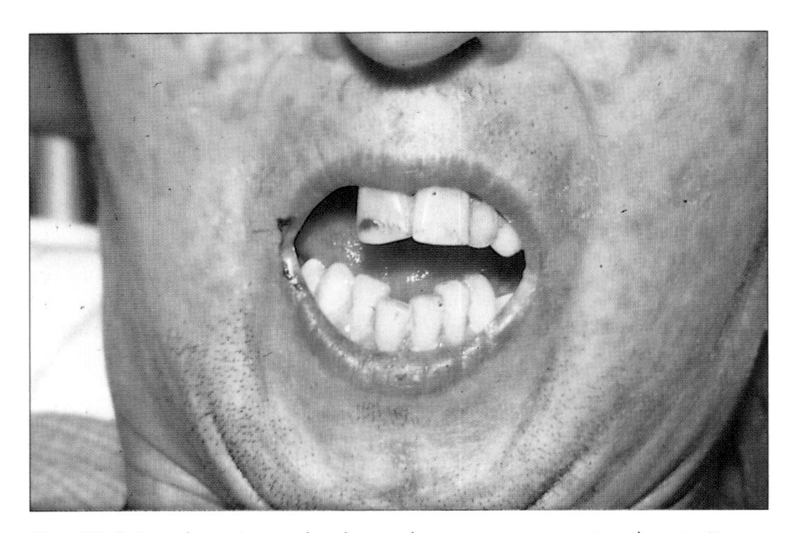

Fig. 20.2 Female patient with advanced progressive systemic sclerosis. Lip retraction together with acquired microstomia results in exaggerated prominence of upper anterior dentition.

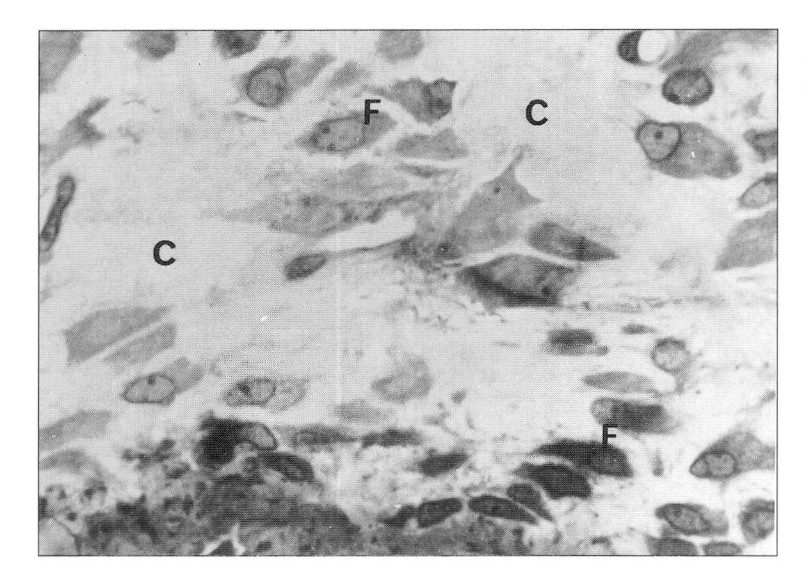

Fig. 20.3 Semi-thin section section of lathyrtic periodontal ligament showing cell-free hyalinized regions (C) between palisading cuboidal fibroblasts. Magnification × 1000. (Shore et al., 1984.)

MUCOPOLYSACCHARIDOSES AND MUCOLIPIDOSES

Current classifications of the heritable disorders of connective tissue seek to use the data derived from amino acid and cDNA sequencing, and from such information it is possible to identify three groups of molecules on the basis of the respective size of their collagenous triple helices (Miller, 1985). Grouping of collagenous molecules, based on size and physicochemical properties, is not completely satisfactory since it ignores the biological role of the individual collagens. An alternative is to classify according to structure and function, and further classifications based on gene structure seem likely to emerge. Collagens are now known to constitute a family of at least 13 proteins, which can be divided into two categories: fibrillar collagens, which form discrete fibrils with characteristic cross-striations; and non-fibrillar collagens. The structure of the genes for collagen contribute to this division in two categories. A better understanding of connective tissue matrix components, including their structure and variability, has been gained in recent years. Matrix glycoproteins with adhesive properties are, for example, fibronectin and collagen together with the more recently identified laminin (see Chapters 3 and 4).

The family of collagens represents a series of highly vulnerable gene–protein systems. This can be explained by the fact that the folding of the pro-α chains and the assembly of collagen monomers into fibrils both depend highly on the principle of nucleated growth, in which every sub-unit of the system must have the correct structure. DNA analysis has shown, for example, that most patients with the potentially lethal type IV variant of Ehlers–Danlos syndrome have mutations in the gene for type III procollagen (Vandenberg, 1993).

The degradation of connective tissue matrix is a normal event in physiological remodelling, associated with morphogenesis and growth, as well as angiogenesis, cell migration, and wound healing. The resorption is brought about both by resident connective tissue and by infiltrating cells, and is regenerated by cell–cell and cell–matrix interactions. It seems that the accelerated breakdown of connective tissue occurring in chronic inflammatory periodontal disease is mainly due to a failure of the normal regeneration of degradative processes. Although much of the connective tissue degradation taking place in periodontal tissue is mediated by proteolytic enzymes, much attention has been focused on the action of proteinases released by invading neutrophils, macrophages, and bacterial enzymes. Local tissue responses to bacterial products may be of greater significance in the pathogenesis of the disease, and the induction of matrix metalloproteinases (MMPs) may be an important process (Meikle *et al.*, 1986). The interaction of bacterial antigens with inflammatory cells resulting in the production if interleukin-1 (IL-1) may be crucial, and this may, in turn, induce MMPSs (Heath *et al.*, 1987). These cytokines may induce destruction of periodontal connective tissue through MMP stimulation (Meikle *et al.*, 1989). Collagenase activity in crevicular fluid is greater in patients with chronic periodontitis than controls. This collagenase appears to be tissue derived (Villela *et al.*, 1987) rather than from neutrophils.

MODES OF INHERITANCE

The mucopolysaccharidoses (MPS) are conditions in which there are inherited defects of ground substance metabolism, characterized by intralysosomal storage of glycosaminoglycans (GAGs). In each of the entities (such as Hurler's syndrome, Hunter's syndrome, and Morquio's disease) this is due to the deficiency of a single specific lysosomal enzyme normally involved in the hydrolytic breakdown of GAGs. All the disorders have a slow course and they all reduce life expectancy. Except for Hunter's disease, with its X-linked recessive mode of inheritance, all types of MPS are autosomal recessive disorders (Leroy and Wiesmann, 1993).

The oligosaccharidoses are inherited as autosomal recessive traits with the implication of a 1 in 4 recurrence risk for the sibs of probands. In sialidosis, an oligosaccharidosis, the clinical condition is due to the isolated deficiency of the glycoprotein sialidase. In childhood dysmorphic sialidosis (Spranger syndrome), gingival hypertrophy is mild to moderate, teeth are spaced, and the tongue is enlarged. Gingival hypertrophy is also seen in syndromes due to deficiency of β-D-galactosidase.

PERIODONTAL EFFECTS

The conditions have received little attention, however, as to their possible periodontal effects. The only histological finding seems to be the presence, in some cases around some teeth affected by delayed eruption, of hyperplastic dental follicles containing excess dermatan sulphate (Gorlin *et al.*, 1976). Gorlin *et al.* (1976) also noted that gingival and alveolar enlargement can occur. Teeth may be widely spaced. Dental abscesses have been noted in the final stages of MPS III. Eruption of permanent molars is retarded in MPS VI, and some of the affected teeth may be deeply buried and angulated in the mandible. The teeth may also be surmounted by radiolucent bony defects, which represent the accumulation of dermatan sulphate in hyperplastic follicles (Gorlin *et al.*, 1976). Dorst (1972, cited in Gorlin *et al.*, 1976) has reported on the accumulation of storage material about unerupted first permanent molars in some cases of gangliosidosis. Tooth spacing has been found in mucolipidoses. In mucolipidosis II, the teeth may be buried in hypertrophied alveolus and gingiva, and they may not erupt at all. There is accumulation of storage material about the crowns of unerupted first molars (as in gangliosidosis). Widely spaced teeth also occur in mannosidosis and aspartylglucosaminuria (Gorlin *et al.*, 1976).

Heritable disorders of connective tissue that manifest premature ageing include progenia, an example of generalized premature ageing, and pseudoxanthoma elasticum and cutis laxia, which represent the premature appearance of cutaneous ageing. Ageing is defined as progressive, time-dependent deterioration in the ability of an organism to respond adaptively to environmental change (Balin and Allen, 1986). This process of biological attrition must affect component parts of the PDL.

EHLERS–DANLOS SYNDROME

The Ehlers–Danlos syndrome (EDS) (see also Chapter 13) is a heterogeneous group of heritable disorders of connective tissue affecting skin, ligaments, joints, blood vessels, and internal organs. At least 10 types have been described. EDS IV is due to deficiency of collagen III, and EDS VIII is a rare, dominantly inherited disorder of unknown cause. Oral aspects of EDS include gingival mucosal fragility, which leads to bleeding (Barabas and Barabas, 1967). In turn, chronic inflammatory periodontal disease with early tooth loss and alveolar bone resorption is not uncommon (Gorlin *et al.*, 1990). This is a hallmark of EDS VIII but is also quite typical of EDS IV. Dental and joint problems of the temporomandibular region are common. Gingival fibrinoid deposits have been described (Slootweg and Beemer, 1987).

The gene for an autosomal dominant form of juvenile periodontitis is located on chromosome 4 and linked to the trait for dentinogenesis imperfecta type III (Broughman *et al.*, 1986). Early loss of teeth also occurs in Papillon–Lefèvre syndrome and in hypophosphatasia.

GENOKERATOSES

The benign disorders of keratinization are heritable and known as the genokeratoses. These disorders, which affect the oral mucous membranes (including the gingiva as white patch lesions), include white sponge naevus, hereditary benign intraepithelial dyskeratosis, keratosis follicularis, pachyonychia congenita, and dyskeratosis congenita. A skin or oral mucosal biopsy contains the macromolecules present in most connective tissues – collagens, elastin, glycoproteins, and proteoglycans. The matrix components are interactive and interdependent, and modifications of one of them by extrinsic (environmental) or intrinsic (systemic, genetic, age-related) factors may have consequences for the tissue as a whole.

Light and electronmicroscopic studies of skin from patients with inherited connective tissue disorders suggest that there is a limited change in the repertoire of collagen fibrils, and a greater range of abnormal structure in dermal elastic fibrils than in collagen fibrils; these studies also suggest that the morphology of fibroblasts gives a clue to defects in matrix components. Similar structural abnormalities result from different molecular defects, and a molecular defect in one connective tissue molecule has consequences for the structural properties of another connective tissue component. Characteristic patterns of structural change in the matrix may be able to be used to confirm diagnosis (Holbrook and Byers, 1989).

WHITE SPONGE NAEVUS

White sponge naevus is inherited as an autosomal dominant trait with equal expressivity in males and females. The white folded mucosal lesions are usually bilateral and may affect all parts of the oral cavity. Most lesions are asymptomatic and are not premalignant. The characteristic histopathological features include parakeratosis, acanthosis, and oedema. Fine structural studies indicate a keratization maturation defect, in as much as spinous cells differentiate early with an increase in tonofilaments, while desquamation of superficial keratinocytes is impaired. Keratin genes appear to be expressed early during the cell maturation cycle.

KERATOSIS FOLLICULARIS

Keratosis follicularis (Darier–White disease) is an autosomal dominant disorder with a typical clinical and histopathological presentation. The skin lesions, which are seborrhoeic, tend to coalesce to form verrucoid plaques. Oral lesions are white and papular, and intraepithelial change includes acantholysis of prickle cells. An immunological disorder may co-exist with the keratinocyte maturation or attachment defect, and cell-mediated abnormalities in keratosis follicularis have been reported (Soppi *et al.*, 1982). An immunohistochemical study of keratins has shown differences in various layers of the epidermis (Burge *et al.*, 1988). It should be noted that isolated lesions indistinguishable from Darier–White disease do occur and are referred to as warty dyskeratosis.

DYSKERATOSIS CONGENITA

Dyskeratosis congenita is characterized by oral, skin, and nail lesions. The condition is inherited as an X-linked disorder, and it is associated with pancytopenia. The oral lesions may progress to squamous cell carcinoma. Ultrastructural studies suggest defects in cell maturation (McKay *et al.*, 1991).

VERRUCIFORM XANTHOMA

Verruciform xanthoma is a rare cause of white oral lesions and may be mistaken clinically for a simple papilloma, although the histopathological features are characteristic. Parakeratinized cells extend deeply into the underlying spinous layer and stain an unusual orange colour with routine stains. Large, foamy cells with diastase-resistant, PAS-positive granules are noted in the papillary corium. The lesions appear to have no relationship with systemic diseases such as hyperlipidaemias. A review by Nowparast *et al.* (1981) indicated that some 16 per cent of cases reported in the literature affected the gingiva.

FOCAL MUCINOSIS

A rare condition, oral focal mucinosis, has been described (Tomich, 1974). Histological and histochemical features of the condition, which may affect the gingiva, are similar to cutaneous focal mucinosis. The cause is unknown, but the fibroblastic overproduction of hyaluronic acid may play a part.

The key to at least some of the disorders of the epidermis lies in understanding the mechanism of regeneration of keratinization, the molecular biology of intermediate filament genes, and epithelial-connective tissue interactions.

DISUSE ATROPHY

The subject of connective-tissue disorders affecting the PDL, on a practical basis, may include atrophy due to reduced function. The main features are narrowing of the PDL and reduction in the number of principal fibres (Henry and Weinmann, 1951). The remaining collagen fibres are oriented more or less parallel to the long axis of the root, and the PDL shows reduced rate of collagen turnover (Henry and Weinmann, 1951; Ruben *et al.*, 1970). In spite of the term 'atrophy', some PDL function appears to persist even if only from contact of teeth with surrounding oral soft tissues. The atrophic PDL is thought to adapt poorly to sudden stress (Ruben *et al.*, 1970). In mouse molars, loss of function without any apparent infection caused progressive PDL atrophy. This led to almost total disappearance of the PDL within 900 days (the approximate life span of the animal). At this time, only traces of PDL remained (Cohn, 1965). PDL around rat molars 3 days after extraction of the opponent teeth showed increased remodelling of collagen, as measured by ^{3}H-proline uptake (Kanoza *et al.*, 1980). This, the authors suggested, was related to reactivated eruption, although it seems unrelated to the long-term atrophic changes described previously.

REFERENCES

Andrews BD, Friou GJ, Barr RJ, *et al* (1986) Loss of epidermal Langerhan's cells and endothelial cell HLA-DR antigens in the skin in progressive systemic sclerosis. J Rheum 13, 341.

Barabas GM and Barabas AP (1967) The Ehlers–Danlos syndrome. A report of the oral and haematological findings in nine cases. Br Dent J 123, 473.

Bailey AJ (1976) In: The Eruption and Occlusion of Teeth (Poole DFG and Stack MV, eds), pp 277–278, Butterworths, London.

Balin AK and Allen RG (1986) Mechanisms of biologic ageing. Dermatol Clin 4, 347–358.

Berkovitz BKB, Migdalski A and Solomon M (1972) The effect of the lathyritic agent aminoacetonitrile on the unimpeded eruption rate in normal and root-resected rat lower incisors. Arch Oral Biol 17, 1755–1763.

Brante G (1952) Gargoylism: A mucopolysaccharidosis. Scand J Clin Lab Invest 4, 43–46.

Broughman JA, Halloran SL, Roulston D, *et al.* (1986) An autosomal-dominant form of juvenile periodontitis: Its localization to chromosome 4 and linkage to dentiniogenesis imperfecta and 6c. J Craniofac Genet Dev Biol 6, 341–350.

Bunim JJ and Black RL (1957) Connective tissue (collagen) diseases. Annu Rev Med 8, 389–406.

Burge SM, Fenton DA, Dawler RP and Leigh IM (1988) Darier's disease: an immunohistochemical study using monoclonal antibodies to human cytokeratins. Br J Dermatol 118, 629–640.

Cho MI and Garant PR (1984a) The effect of beta aminoproprionitrile on the periodontal ligament: I. Ultrastructure of fibroblasts and matrix. J Periodont Res 19, 247–260.

Cho MI and Garant PR (1984b) The effect of beta aminoproprionitrile on the periodontal ligament: II. Radioautographic study of collagen secretion by fibroblasts. Anat Rec 209, 41–52.

Cohn SA (1965) Disuse atrophy of the periodontium in mice. Arch Oral Biol 10, 909–919.

Dasler W (1954) Incisor ash versus femur ash in sweet pea lathyrism (odoratism). J Nutr 54, 397–402.

Earnshaw W, Bordwell BL, Marino C and Rothfield N (1986). Three human chromosomal autoantigens are recognised by sera from patients with anti-centromere antibodies. J Clin Invest 77, 426–436.

Fleischmajer R, Lara JV and Krol S (1966) Localized scleroderma: A histochemical and chemical study. Arch Dermatol 94, 531–535.

Fullmer HM and Witte WE (1962) Periodontal membrane affected by scleroderma. Arch Pathol 73, 184–189.

Gardner AF, Dasler W and Weinmann JP (1958) Masticatory apparatus of albino rats in experimental lathyrism. J Dent Res 37, 492–515.

Gores RJ (1957) Dental characteristics associated with acrosclerosis and diffuse scleroderma. J Am Dent Assoc 54, 755–759.

Gorlin RJ, Pindborg JJ and Cohen MM (1976). Syndromes of the Head and Neck (2nd edition), pp 476–509, McGraw–Hill, New York.

Gorlin RJ, Cohen MM and Levin LS (1990) Ehlers–Danlos syndromes. In Syndromes of the Head and Neck (3rd edition), pp 429–441, Oxford University Press, New York.

Heath JK, Atkinson SJ, Hembry RM, Reynolds JJ and Meikle MC (1987) Bacterial antigens induce collagenase and prostaglandin E_2 synthesis in human gingival fibroblasts through a primary effect on circulating mononuclear cells. Infect Immun 55, 2148–2154.

Henry JL and Weinmann JP (1951) The pattern of resorption and repair of human cementum. J Am Dent Assoc 42, 270–290.

Herbert CM, Lindberg KA, Jayson MIV and Bailey AJ (1974) Biosynthesis and maturation of skin collagen in scleroderma, and effect of D-penicillamine. Lancet i, 187–192.

Holbrook KA and Byers PH (1989) Skin is a window on heritable disorders of connective tissue. Am J Med Genet 34, 105–121.

Jayson MIV (1976) Collagen studies in connective tissue diseases. In: The Eruption and Occlusion of Teeth (Poole DFG and Stack MV, eds), pp 267–270, 277, Butterworths, London.

Kagan HM (1986) Characterization and regulation of lysyl oxidase. In: Regulation of Matrix Accumulation (Mecham RP, ed), pp 321–398, Academic Press, Orlando, Florida.

Kanoza RJJ, Kelleher L, Sodek J and Melcher AH (1980) A biochemical analysis of the effect of hypofunction on collagen metabolism in the rat molar periodontal ligament. Arch Oral Biol 25, 663–668.

Krikos GA, Beltran R and Cohen A (1965) Significance of mechanical stress on the development of periodontal lesions in lathyritis rats. J Dent Res 44, 600–607.

Krogh HW (1950) Dental manifestations of scleroderma. Report of case. J Oral Surg 8, 242–244.

Leroy JG and Wiesmann U (1993) Disorders of lysosomal enzymes. In: Connective Tissue and its Heritable Disorders, pp 613–639, Wiley–Liss, New York.

McKay GS, Ogden GR and Chisholm DM (1991) Lingual hyperkeratosis in dyskeratosis congenita – preliminary ultrastructural report. J Oral Pathol 20, 196–199.

Marmary Y, Glaiss R and Pisanty S (1981) Scleroderma: oral manifestations. Oral Surg 52, 32–37.

Meikle MC, Heath JK and Reynolds JJ (1986) Advances in understanding cell interactions in tissue resorption: Relevance to the pathogenesis of periodontal diseases and a new hypothesis. J Oral Path 15, 239–250.

Meikle MC, Atkinson SJ, Ward RV, Murphy G and Reynolds JJ (1989) Gingival fibroblasts degrade type 1 collagen fibres when stimulated with tumour necrosis factor and interleukin-1: Evidence that breakdown is mediated by metalloproteinases. J Periodont Res 24, 207–213.

Michaeli Y, Pitura S, Zajicek G and Weinreb MM (1975) Role of attrition and occlusal contact in the physiology of the rat incisor. IX. Impeded and unimpeded eruption in lathyritis rats. J Dent Res 54, 891–896.

Miller EJ (1985). The structure of fibril-forming collagens. Ann NY Acad Sci 460, 1–13.

Nowparast B, Howell FV and Rick GM (1981) Verruciform xanthoma: A clinicopathologic review and report of fifty-four cases. Oral Surg. 51, 619–625.

Rocco VK and Hurd ER (1986) Scleroderma and scleroderma-like disorders. Seminars in Arthritis and Rheumatism 16, 22–42.

Rothfield NF and Rodman GP (1968) Serum antinuclear antibodies in progressive systemic sclerosis. Arthritis Rheum 11, 607–616.

Rowell NR and Hopper FE (1977) The periodontal membrane in systemic sclerosis. Brit J Dermatol 96, 15–20.

Ruben MP, Goldman HM and Schulman SM (1970) Diseases of the periodontium. In: Thoma's Oral Pathology, volume 1 (Gorlin RJ and Goldman HM, eds), pp 394–444, Mosby, St Louis.

Sarnat H and Sciaky I (1965) Experimental lathyrism in rats; effects of removing incisal stress. Periodontics 3, 128–134.

Sciaky I and Ungar H (1961) Effects of experimental lathyrism on the suspensory apparatus of incisors and molars in rats. Ann Dent 20, 90–99.

Sharp GC, Irwin WS and Tan EM (1972) Mixed connective tissue disease. Am J Med 52, 148–159.

Shore RC, Berkovitz BKB and Moxham BJ (1984) Histological study, including ultrastructural quantification, of the periodontal ligament in the lathyritic rat mandibular dentition. Arch Oral Biol 29, 263–273.

Siegel RC and Martin GR (1970) Collagen cross-linking. Enzymatic synthesis of lysine-derived aldehydes and the production of cross-linked components. J Biol Chem 245, 1653–1658.

Slootweg PJ and Beemer FA (1987) Gingival fibrinoid deposits in Ehlers–Danlos syndrome. J Oral Pathol 16, 150–152.

Soppi AM, Soppi E and Jansen CT (1982) Cell-mediated immunity in Darier's disease: effect of systemic retinoid therapy. Br J Dermatol 118, 629–640.

Stafne EC and Austin LT (1944) A characteristic dental finding in acrosclerosis and diffuse scleroderma. J Oral Surg 30, 25–29.

Thomas NR (1965) The Process and Mechanisms of Tooth Eruption. PhD thesis, University of Bristol.

Tomich CE and Burkes EJ (1971) Warty dyskeratoma (isolated dyskeratosis follicularis) of the oral mucosa. Oral Surg 31, 798–807.

Tomich CE (1974) Oral focal mucinosis. Oral Surg 38, 714–724.

Tsuruta M, Eto K and Chiba M (1974) Effect of daily or 4-hourly administrations of lathyrogens on the eruption rates of impeded and unimpeded mandibular incisors of rats. Arch Oral Biol 19, 1221–1226.

Unemori EN and Amento EP (1991) Connective tissue metabolism including cytokines in scleroderma. Curr Opin Rheumatol 3, 953–959.

Vandenberg P (1993) Molecular basis of heritable connective tissue disease. Biochem Med Metab Biol 49, 1–12.

Villela B, Cogen RB, Barlolucci AA and Birkedal-Hansen H (1987) Collagenolytic activity in crevicular fluid from patients with chronic adult periodontitis, localized juvenile periodontitis and gingivitis, and from healthy control subjects. J Periodont Res 22, 381–389.

Vyse TJ and Walport MJ (1993) Connective tissue diseases: advances in diagnosis and management. Br J Hosp Med 50, 121–132.

Weisman RA and Calcaterra TC (1978) Head and neck manifestations of scleroderma. Ann Otol Rhinol Laryngol 87, 332–339.

White SC, Frey NW, Blaschkne DD, *et al.* (1977) Oral radiographic changes in patients with progressive systemic sclerosis (scleroderma). J Am Dent Assoc 94, 1178–1182.

Winkelmann RK (1971) Classification and pathogenesis of scleroderma. Mayo Clin Proc 46, 83–91.

Wood RE and Lee P (1988) Analysis of the oral manifestations of systemic sclerosis (scleroderma). Oral Surg 65, 172–176.

Young MF, Bolander ME, Day AA, *et al.* (1986) Osteonectin mRNA: distribution in normal and transformed cells. Nucleic Acids Res 14, 4483–4497.

Chapter 21
The Effects of Hormones and Nutritional Factors on the Periodontal Ligament

Martin M Ferguson, Justin G Wall

INTRODUCTION

While there is limited data on the influence of the hormonal or nutritional status on the condition of the periodontal ligament (PDL), knowledge about this is important for appreciating how changes outside the normal range of metabolism induce a pathological disturbance. It also allows for understanding the normal structure and function of the tissue. Clinical observations indicate that there is an association between endocrine or nutritional factors, but research on the precise mechanisms remains scanty.

The condition of connective tissue in any site is governed by its anabolism and catabolism, which in turn are influenced by local biochemical factors, the availability of essential dietary substances, and controlling factors, both neurogenic and hormonal. It is appropriate, therefore, to propose that a first step towards improving the understanding of the mechanisms that control the metabolism of the PDL involves a detailed appreciation of the manner of synthesis and degradation of its various components. Information concerning the formation of PDL fibres, ground substance, and cells are described in Chapters 3, 4, and 1 respectively. As these reviews indicate, much still needs to be elucidated, and consequently the understanding of hormonal and nutritional influences is handicapped. A further complication is the compartmentalization of PDL research. It is apparent that many of the problems related to this tissue can be solved only by an approach that is more integrated than has been attempted hitherto. An additional difficulty arises because some of the changes seen in connective tissues are common to several kinds of nutritional or hormonal imbalances and are, therefore, nonspecific. Further, in humans, nutritional deficiencies are often multiple rather than being a simple factor.

The functional state of the PDL also appears to have a bearing on these matters: it seems likely that the age of the tissue plays a role in its sensitivity to a given substrate deficiency. Also, it has been suggested that the higher the rate of turnover of a connective tissue, the more easily its metabolism is influenced (Neuberger *et al.*, 1951; Neuberger and Slack, 1953; Neuberger, 1955). On this basis, the rapid turnover of the PDL (see Chapter 3) suggests that it is vulnerable to hormonal and nutritional disturbances.

Nutritional status and endocrine functions are often interrelated, and hence a nutritional deficiency can affect the functional state of endocrine glands. In spite of this integration, for the present purposes, the effects of hormones and diet will be discussed separately.

Finally, three general points concerning this topic must be borne in mind. Firstly, what little is known is based on studies of relatively gross deficiencies or excesses of dietary factors or hormones. Secondly, much of the information is based on animal experiments, and extrapolation to humans may not always be appropriate. Finally, much work has been done on the dietary factors and hormones and their effects on fibroblast and collagen synthesis. Hence consideration of this in respect to the PDL can be done, albeit with reservation.

HORMONES AND THE PERIODONTAL LIGAMENT

Metabolic control leading to body homoeostasis is regulated by the secretions of the endocrine system. The actions of most hormones are widespread and involve many tissues, and influences that act on, in particular, fibroblasts and osteoblasts at any site in the body may be anticipated to act on these cells in the same way in the PDL. In addition, the immune system is also influenced by endocrine and nutritional factors, which is of particular relevance in the periodontium.

The variation in the molecular configuration of hormones is considerable, and target cell receptor mechanisms differ. Whereas steroids attach to cytoplasmic receptors and subsequently to nuclear receptors, it is thought that other hormones bind to surface receptor mechanisms on the plasma membrane and exert their effect mainly by altering intracellular secondary messengers.

The production rates of different hormones are frequently interrelated and, in any experimental procedure that is designed to alter a particular hormonal status, other compensatory fluctuations should be recognized. Furthermore, the nervous system has a significant influence upon the endocrine system. For example, the anterior pituitary gland is regulated by the activity of the hypothalamus and higher centres. Consequently, experimental procedures affecting one system can lead to compensatory changes in the other.

PITUITARY GLAND

The pituitary gland secretes a series of peptide hormones from both the anterior and posterior lobes.

Hypophysectomy in rats has been seen to result in reduced vascularity of the PDL of incisors and molars (Schour and van Dyke, 1932a,b; Schour, 1934; Shapiro and Shklar, 1962). Degeneration of the ligament with cystic degeneration and calcification of many of the epithelial rests has also been reported. Further, the junctional epithelium is often atrophic or absent. Whether such changes are the direct result of the hypophysectomy or are attributable to the reduction in blood supply or to changes in other endocrine glands has not been established.

Since the PDL appears to be the site of the eruptive mechanism (see Chapter 9), a hormonal effect on eruption may be regarded as evidence in favour of the view that the hormone has produced PDL changes. Following hypophysectomy, decreased eruption has been reported in the rat incisor (Schour and van Dyke, 1931, 1932a,b, 1934; Baume *et al.*, 1954a; Bryer, 1957; Garren and Greep, 1960; Kusner *et al.*, 1973). Hypopituitarism was associated with delayed eruption and hyperpituitarism with accelerated eruption (Schour and Massler, 1943). Studies (Baume *et al.*, 1954b; Bryer, 1957) confirm that the pituitary effects on eruption are not due to changes in blood levels of growth hormone but most probably act through the thyroid gland (Baume *et al.*, 1954c; Domm and Wellband, 1961) or the adrenal cortex (Domm and Wellband, 1961). Growth hormone and thyroxine produce the same eruption rate as thyroxine alone (Baume *et al.*, 1954c).

With respect to the anterior pituitary, only growth hormone LGH, by regulating plasma IGF (Blom *et al.*, 1992), is known to influence the oral tissues: this may be either from the direct action or secondarily by the stimulation of somatedin, a sulphation factor from the liver and kidneys. In children, an excessive secretion of growth hormone leads to gigantism and, depending upon the age of onset, the rate of tooth eruption may be increased. Conversely, in hypopituitarism there is a decrease in the secretion of growth hormone and dental eruption is retarded. These effects are also seen in the eruption of the rat incisor (e.g. Schour and van Dyke, 1932a,b). In the acromegalic adult there is enlargement of the entire facial skeleton and this is particularly striking in the mandible. The expansion of the dental arches results in the teeth being spaced apart. Stahl and Joly (1958) observed that the injection of growth hormone resulted in increased cellularity of the PDL. Administration of cortisone to young adult male rats was associated with reduced cellularity of the PDL. The effect was reversed by somatotropic hormone (Stahl and Gerstner, 1960).

Negligible information is available about the effects of the hormones of the posterior pituitary. However, Litvin and De Marco (1973) claim that twice-daily injections of antidiuretic vasopressin to rabbits increased the unimpeded rate of eruption of their incisors.

THYROID GLAND

The action of thyroxine and triiodothyronine is to increase generally the basic metabolic rate. Calcitonin, a peptide from the C-cells of the thyroid, suppresses osteoclastic activity and also causes a reduction in the plasma calcium and phosphorus concentrations. The effect of calcitonin on the periodontium is considered along with other aspects of calcium metabolism.

When the thyroid is excised from rats, the enamel organ undergoes partial atrophy (Baume and Becks, 1952). Thyroidectomy in the new-born rat has been reported to produce a reduction in cellularity of the incisor PDL (Baume *et al.*, 1954c). This effect was reversed with the administration of thyroxine or growth hormone. In rabbits, surgically induced hypothyroidism causes degeneration and fragmentation of PDL collagen fibres (Rosenberg *et al.*, 1961).

The experimental excision of the thyroid gland must include the C-cells of the thyroid itself and, possibly, the parathyroid glands. An alternative procedure has been to dose animals with propylthiouracil, with the intention of selectively blocking thyroxine and triiodothyronine synthesis, although other peroxidases may be influenced. In rats treated in this manner, there is both a delay in the organization of the collagen fibres and a decrease in the amount of fibres in the PDL: myxoid tissue becomes apparent relatively early and is particularly prominent adjacent to the alveolar bone surface (Paynter, 1954; Pinto, 1974). Likewise in rabbits there is a decreased cellularity, hydropic degeneration, and interstitial oedema (Rosenberg *et al.*, 1961). In thiouracil-induced hypothyroidism in the rat, Glickman and Pruzansky (1947) have reported retardation of alveolar bone apposition. Hypothyroidism is also associated with delayed eruption of human teeth (Schour and Massler, 1943, Garn *et al.*, 1965).

Thyroidectomy has resulted in decreased dental eruption in the rat (Baume *et al.*, 1954a; Bryer, 1957; Domm and Wellband, 1961), while a similar effect occurs after administration of propylthiouracil (Garren and Greep, 1955; Bryer, 1957). Baume *et al.* (1954c) found that growth hormone did not restore the eruption rate after thyroidectomy.

Early eruption occurs in hyperthyroidism in humans. An increase in the eruption rate of rats has followed the administration of thyroxine (Herzberg and Schour, 1941; Bryer, 1957; Schumer and Wells, 1958; Moxham and Berkovitz, 1980), thyroid gland powder (Garren and Greep, 1955; Bryer, 1957) and triiodothyroacetic acid (Schumer and Wells, 1958). Thyroid powder (Garren and Greep, 1955) and thyroxine (Baume *et al.*, 1954c) have been found to substitute for lost thyroid tissue.

Goldman (1943) has reported that hyperthyroidism in guinea pigs, produced by the administration of very large doses of thyroxine, results in an increased periodontal vascularity. Also, a widened PDL space was seen. In rats fed thyroid extract for up to 16 weeks, an increase in the PDL width and vascularity was also reported (Baume and Becks, 1952).

Hypothyroidism in rabbits has been observed to lead to the degeneration, fragmentation, and moderate disorganization of the PDL fibres. There was also diminished cellularity and areas of hydropic degeneration. Hyperthyroidism produced a highly cellular, well-organized, slightly thickened PDL (Baume *et al.*, 1954c; Rosenberg *et al.*, 1961). The combination of growth hormone with thyroxine produces a more vascular and cellular PDL than normal (Baume *et al.*, 1954c). The interaction of thyroid and hydrocortisone and their effects on eruption is discussed in Chapter 9.

PARATHYROID GLANDS

Parathormone is a polypeptide secreted by the parathyroid glands in response to low concentrations of plasma calcium and magnesium. The action of parathormone is to increase intestinal absorption of calcium, increase bone resorption, and inhibit phosphorus reabsorption in the renal tubules. In bone, parathormone appears to cause calcium resorption by affecting both the osteocytes and the osteoclasts. Collagen formation may also be inhibited. Dewhirst *et al.* (1987) suggested that an interaction between interleukin-1 (IL-1) and parathyroid hormone in stimulating bone resorption may be an aetiological factor in periodontal disease.

The influence of parathormone on the PDL is discussed in the section on calcium metabolism.

ADRENAL GLANDS

The adrenal cortex is a source of glucocorticosteroids, mineralocorticosteroids, and some sex hormones: the adrenal medulla secretes adrenaline. Shklar (1965) has studied the effects of adrenalectomy on the periodontal tissues. He reported that although there was a marked reduction in osteoblastic activity in the interdental septum in rats, no changes in PDL collagen fibres were seen. Glickman *et al.* (1953) observed a loss of tooth-supporting bone in adrenalectomized mice. Shklar (1965) reported that osteogenesis in alveolar bone, which was reduced in adrenalectomized rats, was restored by cortisone replacement. With respect to the hormones of the adrenal cortex, no changes in the gingivae or PDL are described in hypoadrenocorticism (Addison's disease). A reduced rate of eruption of rat incisors was reported by Garren and Greep (1960) and Domm and Wellband (1960, 1961) following adrenalectomy.

Administration of high doses of cortisone to mice leads to a reduction in cellularity and loss of definition of fibre bundles of the PDL and to osteoporosis of the alveolar bone (Glickman *et al.*, 1953; Applebaum and Seeling, 1955; Glickman and Shklar, 1955; Stahl and Gerstner, 1960; Labelle and Schaffer, 1966). Glickman *et al.* (1953) reported that cortisone injections in mice result in vascular disturbances within the PDL and degenerative changes within the collagen fibres. In addition, osteoporosis occurred in the alveolar bone. The simultaneous administration of oestrogen caused an increase in the number of fibroblasts with larger than normal nuclei. It also increased the number of PDL fibres, although these lacked the normal arrangement (Glickman and Shklar, 1954). Hydrocortisone also caused a loss of ligament fibres in rats. The effect was almost completely prevented by fluoride (Zipkin *et al.*, 1965; Lipari *et al.*, 1974). Mucopolysaccharide synthesis is also affected with diminished production of hyaluronic acid, chondroitin-6-sulphate and heparin (Kofoed and Bozzini, 1970). The changes in alveolar bone can be inhibited by the administration of relatively high doses of fluoride (Zipkin *et al.*, 1965; Lipari *et al.*, 1974).

Some of the above effects of glucocorticoid administration may be due to suppression of the immune response. In marmosets, to which cortisone was given, there was a substantial reduction in the number of acute and chronic inflammatory cells within the gingivae and this seemed to facilitate invasion of the papillae by numerous micro-organisms (Dreizen *et al.*, 1971). In addition, there was reduced fibroblast activity, with a decrease in the size and number of fibroblasts and impaired collagen synthesis; collagen bundles became thinned and fibrillar degeneration occurred, with oedema of the PDL. These findings have also been noted with dexamethasone administration, where the alveolar bone of the marmosets became osteoporotic and the PDL fibres reduced in quantity, owing to a reduction in collagen synthesis (Sallum *et al.*, 1976). Safkan and Knuuttila (1984), in a case-controlled study of multiple sclerosis sufferers on long-term steroid therapy, found no difference in the incidence of periodontal disease between cases and controls.

Regarding tooth eruption, Domm and Wellband (1960) found that daily doses of cortisone resulted in a significant increase in the eruption of rat incisors. Ball (1977) noted that maintaining mature rats in a hyperglucocorticoid state, with weekly subcutaneous injections of methylprednisolone acetate, produced a significant increase in the eruption rates of the mandibular incisors. In all of these studies the eruption rates were impeded. It has been shown, however, that hydrocortisone also increases unimpeded rates in normal (Moxham and Berkovitz, 1980) and root-resected (Berkovitz, 1971) teeth. Parmer *et al.* (1951) and Domm and Marzano (1954) noted that cortisone hastened tooth eruption in new-born rats.

No information is available on the effects of adrenaline on the PDL. However, there have been studies on the effects of noradrenaline on tooth support and the eruptive mechanism. Slatter and Picton (1972) and Wills *et al.* (1976) have recorded changes in mobility of macaque monkey teeth with intrusive loading following the submucosal injection of noradrenaline. Similar influences were reported by Körber (1961) for horizontal tooth mobility. Moxham (1979) and Myhre *et al.* (1979) have observed intrusive movements of previously erupting rabbit incisors after noradrenaline administration. Tooth mobility is considered in detail in Chapter 10.

PANCREATIC ISLETS

Insulin is secreted from the β-cells in the islets of Langerhans, and it has widespread effects on carbohydrate, protein, and lipid metabolism. In diabetes mellitus there is a lack of available insulin; this has a number of possible causes, including lack of insulin secretion, altered plasma membrane surface receptors for insulin, and antibodies directed against insulin. The severity of diabetes mellitus is variable but is generally more marked in the juvenile-onset, insulin-dependent form.

In uncontrolled diabetes mellitus there is hyperglycaemia and ketosis. Vascular changes develop, with thickening of blood vessel walls and basement membrane due to deposition of mucoprotein and collagen. Anoxia of the arterial intima is thought to lead to the development of atherosclerosis.

Chronic inflammatory periodontal disease is more severe in diabetics, whether adequately or inadequately controlled (Williams, 1928; Rutledge, 1940; Lovestedt and Austin, 1943; Mackenzie and Millard, 1963; Belting *et al.*, 1964; Cheraskin and Ringsdorf, 1965; Chinn *et al.*, 1966; Glavind *et al.*, 1968; Cohen *et al.*, 1969, 1970, 1971; Hove and Stallard, 1970; Bernick *et al.*, 1975; Ringelberg *et al.*, 1977), though not all studies show a correlation in controlled diabetes (Benveniste *et al.*, 1967; El Geneidy *et al.*, 1974). Opinions still differ regarding the exact relationship between diabetes and oral disease. Some claim that when the two conditions coexist, it is coincidental, there being no cause-and-effect relationship (e.g. Badanes, 1933; Bonheim, 1943; O'Leary *et al.*, 1962; Reeve and Winkelmann, 1962; Ulrich, 1962; Mackenzie and Millard, 1963). It is often presumed that diabetes alters the response of the periodontal tissue to local irritants. Shklar *et al.* (1962), Cohen *et al.* (1963), and Cohen *et al.* (1969) have shown an increase in chronic inflammatory periodontal disease in laboratory animals.

The histopathological changes in the PDL in diabetics have received limited attention. Vascular changes comparable to those found elsewhere in the body, with thickening of the walls, have been noted in some small blood vessels of the PDL (Russell, 1966, 1967; Keene, 1969a,b, 1972). Necrotic foci in the PDL collagen have also been reported (Benveniste *et al.*, 1967). There is more basement membrane material (Keene, 1969a,b; Listgarten *et al.*, 1974). The thickening of the vessels is due to increased collagen production and the thickening of the capillary basement lamina is due to periendothelial deposition of basement-membrane-like material. These changes may impede the diffusion of oxygen and the elimination of waste products, and this may explain the poor tissue response to plaque in diabetes (Frantzis *et al.*, 1971). Following the induction of diabetes in rats by the drug alloxan, Bissada *et al.* (1966) observed infrequent fragmentation of the bundles of PDL collagen fibres and widening of the ligament, caused by alveolar bone resorption. The fibres became disorganized and the collagen appeared more granular than fibrillar. The PDL was more vascular than normal and the blood capillaries were engorged, many being thrombosed. If local irritants were present, there was degeneration and oedema of the PDL, especially in the furcation regions. Unlike human diabetes, no histological changes in the vessels were apparent. In other animal studies, osteoporosis and reduction in height of alveolar bone have been reported without much change in the PDL. Sheenan and Cohen (1970) saw no PDL changes in animals with autosomal recessive diabetes. The combination of excessive occlusal forces with alloxan-induced diabetes results in greater periodontal tissue destruction, possibly since repair mechanisms are inhibited (Glickman *et al.*, 1966). Post-surgical periodontal healing is also delayed in these animals, although local irritants were a more significant delaying factor than the diabetes (Glickman *et al.*, 1966).

Another animal model for studying the effects of diabetes on the periodontium has been a strain of hamster with hereditary diabetes. In these, the PDL shows a reduction in the numbers of fibroblasts and collagen fibres. The remaining fibroblasts are smaller than normal with small deeply staining pyknotic nuclei. The osteoblast layer on bone is absent. Chronic periodontitis is more severe than in control animals (Shklar *et al.*, 1962).

SEX HORMONES

The principal sources of steroid sex hormones are the testes, which secrete androgens, and the ovaries, which secrete oestrogens and progestogens. The action of female sex hormones upon the periodontium has attracted substantial attention, owing to the increased severity of chronic inflammatory periodontal disease. However, most information available concerns the gingivae and not the PDL.

An increased incidence of gingivitis in females has been reported both at puberty (Massler *et al.*, 1950; Parfitt, 1957; Sutcliffe, 1972) and during pregnancy (Ziskin and Nesse, 1946; Maier and Orban, 1949; Hilming, 1952; Löe and Silness, 1963; Löe, 1965; Cohen *et al.*, 1969; Hugoson, 1971; Adams *et al.*, 1974). Löe and Silness (1963) concluded from their study that there was no permanent periodontal damage from pregnancy gingivitis. Oral contraceptives most frequently include a synthetic oestrogen and progestogen. Several workers have considered that ingestion of oral contraceptives increases the prevalence of gingivitis, although this finding is not unanimous (Lindhe and Bjorn, 1967; Lynn, 1967; Lindhe *et al.*, 1968; Kaufman, 1969; Sperber, 1969; El Ashiry *et al.*, 1970; Klinger and Klinger, 1970; Knight and Wade, 1974; Pearlman, 1974). Knight and Wade (1974) reported that oral contraceptives had no effect on plaque accumulation or gingivitis, but that they were associated with more severe periodontitis, which they attributed to an altered host response. Current opinion indicates that it is progesterone that is most probably responsible for the major gingival inflammatory changes (Lindhe and Brånemark, 1967a,b,c). The reason for this requires elucidation: one possibility is that progesterone has a direct action upon capillary permeability (Mohammed *et al.*, 1974). More recently it has been shown that progesterone in physiological concentrations stimulates the cell-mediated immune response to a standard antigenic challenge in vitro. A progestogen-binding protein has been identified in leucocytes (Ferguson *et al.*, 1981). Certain parameters of the immune system are stimulated by progesterone and this includes production of prostaglandins by macrophages (Smith *et al.*, 1986).

Although oestrogen receptors have not been identified in leucocytes, oestradiol accumulates in phagocytosing human polymorphoneutrophils (Ferguson *et al.*, 1984) and NK lymphocyte cytosis is decreased (Ferguson and MacDonald, 1985). This non-receptor mode of action may be related to the interaction of oestrogens in the peroxidative pathway, possibly including prostaglandin synthesis (Conn *et al.*, 1988).

In terms of histopathology, most attention has focused on the gingival inflammatory response, which is attributed to fluctuations in sex steroid levels. Again, there is negligible information on possible changes in the PDL.

Wojcicki *et al.* (1987) studied the relationship of bacteria, puberty, and periodontal disease, and concluded that the changes in the periodontal microbiota are related to changes within the PDL space that occur at the time of puberty. At present, there is no clear consensus as to whether the gingivitis potentiated by these hormones is beneficial or detrimental in the long term.

Oestrogen receptors were not detected in the rabbit gingiva (Rubright *et al.*, 1973) and histological studies failed to show any response to systemic oestradiol administration (Rubright *et al.*, 1971). In mice, injections of oestradiol have been reported to produce sclerosis of the alveolar bone (Stahl *et al.*, 1950). On the other hand, Aufdemorte and Sheridan (1981), using tritiated testosterone and oestrogen in baboons, found pronounced oestrogen uptake in the lamina propria and periosteal fibroblasts of male baboons but a reduced level of uptake in females.

That sex hormones have an effect on the PDL is indicated by the observation of there being a progressive increase in horizontal tooth mobility during pregnancy (Mühlemann, 1951; Mühlemann *et al.*, 1965; Rateitschak, 1967). It was reported that this increased mobility returned to previous levels at full term. Friedman (1972) claims that horizontal tooth mobility does not change during the menstrual cycle. Sex hormones may also have effects on tooth eruption. It is documented that the development and eruption of teeth is earlier in girls than boys (e.g. Cattell, 1928; Garn *et al.*, 1958; van Wagenen and Hurme, 1950), although the role of sex hormones is uncertain. Van Wagenen and Hurme (1950) accelerated canine eruption by injecting male monkeys with testosterone. Gonadectomy in squirrels resulted in a slight retardation in eruption (Schour, 1936).

Increased secretion of gonadotrophin has been found to result in early eruption and formation of the teeth in humans (Rushton, 1941). Hypergonadism is associated with more advanced deciduous eruption; hypogonadism has no marked effect on eruption but cases have occurred in which eruption has been slightly accelerated (Schour and Massler, 1943). Methyltestosterone has anacalciphylactic effects and has been found to reduce the periodontal damage caused by dihydrotachysterol intoxication (Ratcliff and Krajewski, 1966).

Histologically, when oestrogen was administered to 6-week-old mice for a period of 5 weeks, an increase in the cellularity of the PDL was observed (Shklar and Glickman, 1956). However, when the drug was given for 10 weeks, a reduction in both cellularity and collagen bundles was reported. These findings could be interpreted as the result of a possible decrease in the amount of FSH. Subsequently, Piroshaw and Glickman (1957) assessed the effects of oöphorectomy in young adult mice. They observed a reduction in fibre density and cellularity in the PDL which reduced over one year, indicating a reduced susceptibility to the hormone with increasing age. Differentiation of mesenchyme cells to form osteoblasts and cementoblasts was impaired. There was no evidence of adrenal compensation (Glickman and Quintarelli, 1960). Schneider (1967) has noted fibrosis of the periodontal vasculature in oöphorectomized rats. Shklar *et al.* (1967) reported an increased cellularity of the PDL in hypophysectomized rats receiving testosterone.

UROGASTRONE – EPIDERMAL GROWTH FACTOR

Epidermal growth factor (EGF) is a substance that has been isolated from mouse submandibular salivary glands. It accelerates incisor tooth eruption and eyelid opening (Cohen, 1962; Carpenter, 1978). An almost identical 53-residue polypeptide, called urogastrone, has been found in human urine; it is thought to originate both in the submandibular glands and in Brunner's glands of the duodenum (Gregory, Holmes and Willshire, 1979; Gregory, Walsh and Hopkins, 1979). It is secreted in submandibular and parotid saliva, where its concentration is similar to its concentration in plasma. While a range of individual cell receptors have been recorded, there is no clear effect of this hormone upon the PDL.

NUTRITION AND THE PERIODONTAL LIGAMENT

One of the major contributions to the marked prolongation of the mean length of life in developed areas has been a sufficient availability of food of good quality. However, it is only in this century that the concept of diseases caused by nutritional deficiency has evolved. A balanced diet is one containing proportional amounts of protein, minerals, fatty acids, and vitamins. Carbohydrate is basically utilized for the production of energy. It is unusual for a single constituent to be deficient in the diet of humans and the clinical descriptions of nutritional deficiency may be due to a group of essential nutrients. However, it is possible to regulate the dietary intake in experimental animals, although it must still be appreciated that metabolism of the many nutrients is interrelated (e.g. folic acid and vitamin B_{12}), and a change in one nutrient will inevitably involve others.

Surprisingly few studies have been undertaken on the influence of nutritional factors on the connective tissues of the PDL per se, although work has been done on nutritional factors, fibroblasts, and collagen synthesis. Two general points arise. Firstly, although animal experiments have shown that deficiency or excess of nutrients in the diet can markedly affect the health of the periodontal tissues, the evidence for similar periodontal changes in humans is less convincing. Secondly, it is possible that some nutritional disturbances by themselves do not initiate lesions but perhaps modify the response to local irritants.

FOOD TEXTURE

The texture of the diet is often not considered when assessing nutritional influences on health. Attention has been directed to the importance of dietary fibre (Robertson, 1972; Burkitt, 1973; Cleave *et al.*, 1973; Eastwood, 1973; Heaton, 1973; Southgate, 1973; Trowell, 1973). There has been little correlation between the advent of soft, fibre-deficient diet and dental health. This is remarkable considering that probably the most significant factor in chronic inflammatory periodontal disease is the loss of natural masticatory function, leading to the accumulation of dental plaque at sites prone to this condition (Newman, 1974). One of the means of inducing chronic periodontitis in experimental animals is to feed them soft diets (Egelberg, 1965; Carlsson and Egelberg, 1965a,b).

Diet consistency can affect the PDL not only indirectly in relation to the formation of local irritants (Ainamo, 1972; Newman, 1974), but also directly by influencing the pattern of mastication, and hence the mode of support offered by the PDL. The previous loading history has a bearing upon the reactions of a tooth to the application of a force (see Chapter 10). In mammalian dentitions where food having a 'natural' texture is masticated, there is some evidence that the extraction of teeth is usually more difficult, that the muscles of mastication are stronger, and that biting pressures are heavier than where the diet has a soft consistency (Baaregaard, 1949; Davies and Pedersen, 1955). The effects of soft diet regarding more severe periodontitis apply both to domesticated animals (Keyes and Litkins, 1946; Klingsberg and Butcher, 1959, Hatt *et al.*, 1968; Ferguson, 1969) and humans (Sim Wallace, 1904; Colyer, 1931; Waugh, 1937; Waugh, 1940; Begg, 1954; Beyron, 1964; Klatsky and Klatell, 1943; Taylor, 1962, 1963; Rugg-Gunn, 1968; Lavelle, 1973). There is evidence, for the continuously growing incisors of rodents, that eruption (a property of the PDL, see Chapter 10) is influenced by biting behaviour and the degree of attrition (e.g. Ness, 1964). Further, Shore *et al.* (1982) have shown that the periodontal tissues of these teeth show changes in resistance to loading when removed from the bite. Even in teeth of limited growth, attrition may be accompanied by compensatory eruption (Philippas, 1952; Begg, 1954; Picton, 1957; Saråns, 1957; Brothwell and Carr, 1962; Murphy, 1959, 1964; Tait, 1965; Newman and Levers, 1979). Thompson and Kendrick (1964) and Ainamo and Talari (1976) claim that eruption in humans is independent of attrition, since it has been shown to occur in the absence of attrition. Vigorous masticatory function is associated with a widening of the PDL (Coollidge, 1937). Aukes *et al.* (1987) suggest that chewing pattern depends on the texture of the masticated food, hard and tough food requiring more vertical movements and soft food requiring less vertical movements.

For information concerning the effects on the PDL of disuse of a tooth, see Chapter 3.

CARBOHYDRATES

Carbohydrates are a group of hydrated carbon compounds derived most abundantly from plant origin. Humans have a limited storage capacity for glucose – a well-fed 70 kg individual would have 500 g of glucose available as circulating glucose or in the storage form, glycogen. Glucose can be synthesized de novo in the body from protein or lipid and it is the major source of energy in the tricarboxylic acid cycle of oxidative phosphorylation. Certain tissues require glucose exclusively as an energy source; these tissues include red blood cells and the adrenal medulla.

Some findings exist suggesting that refined carbohydrates in the diet influence the severity of chronic inflammatory periodontal disease in humans (Holloway *et al.*, 1963) and in laboratory animals (Frandsen *et al.*, 1953; Auskaps *et al.*, 1957; Stahl, 1962, 1963a,b). However, others report no correlation (Shannon and Gibson, 1964). Further, there is no evidence showing a direct effect of carbohydrates per se on the PDL, though in some circumstances there could be an influence as a result of modifying the diet consistency.

PROTEINS

Since the PDL shows a high turnover rate for many of its constituents, particularly collagen (e.g. Sodek, 1978; see also Chapter 3), a deficiency of dietary protein might be expected to produce changes within it.

In rats fed protein-deficient diets, there is a reduction in PDL collagen fibres, particularly the transseptal component (Stein and Ziskin, 1949; Chawla and Glickman, 1951; Frandsen *et al.*, 1953; Stahl *et al.*, 1958; Ten Cate *et al.*, 1976). Similar changes have been reported in monkeys (Goldman, 1954) and pigs (Platt and Stewart, 1962), where the PDL is less cellular, with oedema and disorganization of fibre bundles. There is a reduction in the number of cementoblasts as well as fibroblasts, and occlusal trauma exacerbates these effects (Chawla and Glickman, 1951; Stahl *et al.*,

1955; Stahl *et al.*, 1957; Miller *et al.*, 1957). Periodontal healing is delayed in rats fed a protein-deficient diet (Stahl, 1962, 1963a,b).

The only report of the effects of an amino acid deficiency on the PDL appears to be that of Bavetta and Bernick (1956), who described severe alveolar destruction with loss of attachment of the PDL in tryptophan-deficient rats.

Bryer (1957) assessed the effect of a deficiency of proteins on eruption of the rat incisor, reporting that acute protein deficiency, (accompanied by weight loss of 25–45 per cent) had little effect.

FATTY ACIDS

Only two fatty acids (the unsaturated fatty acids linoleic acid and linolenic acid) are essential dietary components for humans, as the body can synthesize the other fatty acids. It is probable that essential fatty acid deficiency is manifested by an inability to synthesize prostaglandins (El-Attar *et al.*, 1978) and leukotrienes. If essential fatty acid deficiency leads to a reduction in the production of prostaglandin and leukotrienes, it is possible that periodontal changes may result. These changes would be due, in part, to an altered inflammatory reaction (El-Attar, 1978). El-Attar (1990) demonstrated inhibition of prostaglandin-E2 and prostaglandin-F2 with polyunsaturated fatty acid (n-3 and n-6) supplementation in human gingival fibroblasts. Much work has been done on disorders of lipid metabolism and fibroblasts, and it is suggested by Emami *et al.* (1992) that an inability to utilize particular fatty acids affects fibroblast function in the metabolism of particular prostaglandins. It is conceivable that a deficiency in fatty acid metabolism similarly affects fibroblast function. Changes have been observed within the periodontal tissues of rats fed on fatty-acid-deficient diets. Rao *et al.* (1965) reported an increase in cellularity of the PDL with resorption of adjacent cementum and alveolar bone. Prout and Tring (1971, 1973) fed young rats a fat-free diet and noted that the collagen fibre bundles of the molar PDL became more vascular, irregular, and disorientated.

VITAMINS

Vitamins are essential organic factors that cannot be synthesized within the body and are required in only small amounts. They are classified into fat-soluble vitamins (vitamins A, D, E, and K) and water-soluble vitamins (vitamin B complex and vitamin C).

Vitamin A

Vitamin A is concerned with the control of epithelial differentiation and bone formation. In dogs, vitamin A deficiency has been reported to be associated with periodontal inflammation (Mellanby M, 1929; Mellanby H, 1941; Frandsen, 1963). Rats deficient in vitamin A have been observed to have a widened (molar) PDL (Boyle and Bessey, 1941) and areas of hyaline necrosis where the roots impact against bone (Boyle, 1947). The experiments of Wolbach and Howe (1933), Schour *et al.* (1941) and Bryer (1957) suggest that eruption is retarded in rats deficient in vitamin A. Bryer (1957) reported that there was a marked decrease in vascularity of the PDL and claimed that new osteoid tissue also resulted in a decrease in width of the PDL. Whereas Glickman and Stoller (1948) found deeper periodontal pockets in rats deficient in vitamin A, Miglani (1959) found no direct effects on the PDL. It is possible that any such changes are secondary to salivary gland dysfunction (Salley *et al.*, 1959; Hayes *et al.*, 1970).

In rats, excessive intake of vitamin A may be associated with alveolar bone resorption (Wolbach and Bessey, 1942; Ferguson, 1969). One case of periodontal inflammation in humans has been described by De-Menezes *et al.* (1984).

Vitamin D

The principal action of vitamin D is to elevate plasma calcium and phosphate concentration by stimulating their intestinal absorption and by resorption of bone. Dietary cholecalciferol is absorbed from the alimentary tract and converted into 25-hydroxy-cholecalciferol in the liver. This passes into the circulation and is subsequently transformed into 1,25-dihydroxy-cholecalciferol in the kidney; this is the active form of vitamin D. Synthesis of 1,25-dihydroxycholecalciferol is regulated by plasma levels of calcium, phosphate, and parathyroid hormone, and possibly by plasma levels of calcitonin. Deficiency of vitamin D results in rickets in children and osteomalacia in adults. Both conditions are characterized by defective mineralization of the organic matrix. Hinek and Poole (1988), in rat experiments, have demonstrated variabilty in the effect of vitamin D deficiency depending on the tissue type examined. Overall they found both 1,25-dihydroxycholecalciferol and 24,25-dihydroxycholecalciferol were required for maximum stimulation of calcification and maximum increases in C-propeptide content in vitamin D depleted animals. The effects of vitamin D on the PDL are considered under the section concerned with mineralization factors (p.424).

Vitamin E

This group of tocopherols act as antioxidants, protecting unsaturated fatty acids, vitamin A, and vitamin C. In the continuously growing incisors of rats, deficiency of this vitamin is associated with atrophic changes in the enamel organ (Irving, 1942; Pindborg, 1952) and in the PDL (Schneider and Pose, 1969).

Cohen and Meyer (1993) found vitamin E supplementation decreased the extent and severity of bone loss in preconditioned rat teeth that were subjected to orthodontic rotation. They concluded that, in the rat, vitamin E may have a protective effect, particularly in the presence of pre-existing periodontal inflammation. Igarashi *et al.* (1989) suggest that vitamin E deficiency promotes the peroxidation of lipids and accelerates the cross-linking of collagen in skin.

Cerna *et al.* (1990), in a study of 39 healthy pregnant women, found a negative association between vitamins A and E and periodontal health, which peaked in the eighth month of pregnancy. Immediately preterm, the 'vitamineamia' resolved, as did the periodontitis, but it is dificult to attribute this to vitamin status or hormonal changes preterm.

Vitamin K

Vitamins K_1 and K_2 are necessary for the hepatic synthesis of clotting factors. Deficiency does not lead to any direct periodontal changes. However, there may be increased gingival bleeding, owing to failure of the clotting mechanism. Zubarev and Sharaev (1992) found a positive association with vitamin K dosing and collagen, hexosamine-containing polymers in reimplanted dog teeth.

Vitamin B complex

This group of water-soluble vitamins are essential co-enzymes for the metabolism of carbohydrates, proteins, and fats. The vitamin B complex includes thiamine (vitamin B_1), riboflavin (vitamin B_2), nicotinic acid (niacin) or nicotinic acid amide (niacinamide), pantothenic acid, pyridoxine (vitamin B_6) biotin, para-aminobenzoic acid, inositol, choline, folic acid, and vitamin B_{12} (cyanocobalamin).

Severe periodontal destruction has been reported in rats and primates that are deficient in riboflavin (Tomlinson, 1939; Topping and Fraser, 1939; Chapman and Harris, 1941), nicotinic acid and pantothenic acid (Tomlinson, 1939; Becks *et al.*, 1943; Ziskin *et al.*,1947). Mice fed a pantothenic-acid-deficient diet for 2 weeks were reported to have a wider PDL in which epithelial rest proliferation had occurred, together with an increase in the size of blood vessels on the bone side of the PDL (Levy, 1949). In a study of deficiencies of niacin, riboflavin, pyridoxine, pantothenic acid and folic acid in adult dogs (Afonsky, 1955), PDL involvement with alveolar crest fibre destruction was seen only with folic acid deficiency. Masse *et al.* (1990) have shown that chicks deficient in vitamin B_6 had significantly thickened collagen fibres in the articular fibrocartilage of the tibial metatarsal joint. They concluded that vitamin-B_6-deficient cross-linking may be responsible for the alteration in cartilage histology. Myers *et al.* (1986), however, found a 50 per cent reduction in L-proline incorporation into lung collagen in rats. There is also some evidence of a relationship between folic acid deficiency and partial necrosis of the PDL (Pindborg, 1949; Shaw, 1962).

Kretsch *et al.* (1991) found no change in periodontal status in eight healthy, non-pregnant women fed a controlled diet that was deficient in vitamin B_6 over 12 days.

Vitamin C

Vitamin C is involved in oxidation-reduction reactions and is concerned particularly with proline hydroxylation in the synthesis of collagen. Its other actions are less well understood, but it is also involved in the formation of epithelial basement membranes (Priest, 1970). Franceschi (1992) proposes that the collagen matrix produced by cells treated with ascorbic acid provides a permissive environment for tissue-specific gene expression, supporting the claim that vitamin C is required for the differentiation of mesenchyme-derived connective tissue, such as muscle, bone and cartilage. Deficiency of vitamin C leads to scurvy, with widespread disorders in bones and connective tissue as a result of defective collagen synthesis (e.g. Wolbach, 1953).

In the guinea pig, vitamin C deficiency leads to a failure in collagen formation and destruction of existing fibres in the PDL (Wolbach and Howe, 1926; Boyle *et al.*, 1937; Glickman and Stoller, 1948; Hunt and Paynter, 1959). Healing of gingival wounds is delayed and collagen formation is disordered (Turesky and Glickman, 1954). Peterkofsky (1991) found in guinea pigs, however, that this disorganization may occur as a result of overall calorific deficiency rather than as a result of vitamin C deficiency with a eucalorific diet.

Waerhaug (1960) reported that, in monkeys, a diet deficient in vitamin C results in breakdown of collagen fibres, although those in the epithelial cuff appeared to be more resistant. Widening of the PDL can occur, which may be attributed to resorption of the adjoining alveolar bone (Dreizen *et al.*, 1969). Østergaard (1975) claims that the hydroxyproline content of the PDL is decreased by 66 per cent in monkeys that are deficient in ascorbic acid, thus explaining the reduction in PDL collagen in these animals. Touyz (1984) suggests that, although certain infections and systemic diseases cause gingival bleeding, avitaminosis C does not cause commonly encountered periodontal disease, though it does aggravate established periodontitis. Melnick *et al.* (1988), in a case-control study of 60 subjects and matched controls, showed patients with a history of acute necrotizing ulcerative gingivitis ingested significantly less vitamin C than controls.

Deficiency of vitamin C is associated with a decreased rate of eruption of both impeded and unimpeded guinea pig incisors (Dalldorf and Zall, 1930; Berkovitz, 1974).

MINERALIZATION FACTORS

This section is concerned with the hormonal and nutritional factors that are involved in calcification and seem to affect PDL development and function.

Decreased availability of calcium may result from a dietary deficiency of the mineral or from a deficiency of vitamin D. A similar effect may be induced by renal disease or by excision or dysfunction of the parathyroid glands. Calcium metabolism is regulated by a series of interactions and an alteration of any one of these must inevitably result in a sequence of compensatory changes. It can be difficult, therefore, to separate primary from secondary actions. Hence, for any *in vivo* experimental procedure, cognizance should be taken of these potential effects if they have not been recorded.

One way of overcoming this difficulty is to examine the effect of individual factors in organ or tissue culture. In one such investigation (Rao *et al.*, 1978), the influence on periodontal fibroblasts of calcitonin, parathormone, and prostaglandin-E^1 was examined. This showed that, while calcitonin or parathormone had no effect on cyclic-AMP production, prostaglandin-E^1 caused a very significant elevation. A study using hamster periodontal tissue also showed no effect of calcitonin (El Kafrawy and Mitchell, 1976). Tissue culture of fibroblasts is considered further in Chapter 1.

Another approach involves feeding animals with diets in which only one factor is changed, the other factors being maintained at 'normal' levels. Weinmann and Schour (1945a,b) fed young dogs a diet that was deficient in vitamin D but had normal levels of calcium and phosphorus; they reported that this resulted in narrowing of the PDL, probably as a result of failure of the normal resorptive processes associated with the alveolar bone. There was also evidence of hyaline degeneration and partial obliteration of the PDL. Similar changes have been described by Bryer (1957) for the rat incisor and partial ligament necrosis has also been observed in monkeys deficient in vitamin D (Tomlinson, 1939). In contrast, however, Oliver (1969) found the PDL of young rats to be unaltered by such a diet. Where there was a deficiency of both vitamin D and calcium, with phosphorus levels remaining normal, Becks and Weber (1931) reported the presence of destructive changes within the PDL. They observed a widened PDL, with blood-containing, cyst-like structures in some sites.

Rats placed on a calcium-deficient diet show osteoporotic changes in alveolar bone (Ferguson and Hartles, 1963, 1966) and a reduction in the number and diameter of PDL fibres (Oliver, 1969). Parathormone administration, which is analogous to calcium deficiency, has been shown to stimulate osteoclastic activity in the rat periodontium (Roberts, 1975). Studying cell kinetics in the rat maxillary first molar following the injection of parathyroid extract, Roberts (1975) found an increased cellularity of the PDL that could be accounted for only partly by local cell proliferation. He concluded that there must have been an influx of migrating cells into the PDL. Uhrbom *et al.* (1984), in response to a suggestion by Henrikson (1968) that periodontal disease in humans was caused by calcium deficiency, found no statistically significant relationship between calcium deficiency and supplementation and periodontal disease in 66 people with periodontal disease monitored for 180 days.

There seem to be no reports of changes in the PDL associated with a deficiency of phosphorus, though osteoporotic changes in alveolar bone have been described (Ferguson and Hartles, 1966). That there might be changes in the periodontium is indicated by reports that tooth eruption may be retarded in experimental animals fed a phosphorus-deficient diet (Burrill, 1943), although Bryer (1957) reported no change in eruption rates for rat incisors.

When high doses of vitamin D (in the form of dihydrotachysterol) are given to rats to induce local calcification, there is widespread degeneration, loss in fibre orientation, and oedema of the PDL. Capillaries become enlarged, some haemorrhage is present, calcification of the transseptal fibres may occur, and multiple foci of calcification appear throughout the PDL (Ratcliff and Itokazu, 1964; Moskow, Baden and Zengo, 1966; Bernick *et al.*, 1971). The effects are reduced by ferric dextran (Ratcliff and Itokazu, 1964) and methyltestosterone (Ratcliff and Krajewski, 1966). Pitaru *et al.* (1982) found in rats that a group found to be 1,25-dihydroxycholecalciferol toxaemic had disturbances in the dental and periodontal fibroblasts. In particular, there was hypercementosis and bone-like tissue formation in the PDL, which in the incisors was considerably enlarged; furthermore, some molars were ankylosed. Alveolar changes and PDL disruption have been reported in rabbits that are overfed with vitamin D (Cai,1992). Hypervitaminosis D in the hamster is said to result in narrowing of the PDL, with calcification of the principal fibres (particularly for the molars) (Fahmy *et al.*, 1961).

As regards the effects of mineralization factors on tooth eruption, the eruption rate in rats was found to fall with vitamin D deficiency and excess (Bryer, 1957). There seems to be no effect on eruption of phosphorus deficiency. Removal of the parathyroids does not appear to affect tooth eruption of the rat incisor (Schour *et al.*, 1937; Bryer, 1957). Ziskin *et al.* (1940) reported that replacement therapy of parathormone extract had no effect on eruption. The eruption of human teeth in subjects suffering from hypoparathyroidism and hyperparathyroidism is not affected (Schour and Massler, 1943).

INORGANIC ELEMENTS

The effects of calcium and phosphorus are considered in the preceding section.

Widening of the PDL has been observed with magnesium deficiency (Klein *et al.*, 1935; Becks and Furuta, 1943). Furthermore, the eruption rate of rat incisors has been reported to decrease in animals fed magnesium-deficient diets (Klein *et al.*, 1935; Becks and Furuta, 1939, 1941; Gagnon *et al.*, 1942; Bernick and Hungerford, 1965; Kusner *et al.*, 1973). These effects may be related to the role of Mg^{++} ions in several enzyme systems. Only one study suggested a relationship between magnesium deficiency and the severity of periodontitis (Klein *et al.*, 1935).

Fluoride appears to reduce the destructive effects of excessive orthodontic tooth movement, at least in rats (Singer *et al.*, 1967). In this study, female rats were given 100 ppm fluoride in distilled water and orthodontic elastics were inserted between molar teeth. It was observed that there were fewer areas of PDL hyalinization in fluoride-treated animals than in controls. Hellsing and Hammarström (1991) found a significant reduction in pressure-side osteoclast numbers in orthodontically moved teeth in rats treated with sodium fluoride. Although it has been suggested that fluoride reduces the rate of eruption of the rat molar (Smith, 1934; Ness, 1964), Berkovitz (1974) has reported that rats given 25–100 ppm fluoride exhibited no changes in incisor eruption rates.

Severe iron deficiency has been related to periodontal destruction in dogs (Hall and Robinson, 1937). In humans, however, there does not seem to be a clear correlation between iron-deficiency anaemia and chronic inflammatory periodontal disease. From clinical observations, Lainson *et al.* (1968) gained the impression that patients with moderate to severe periodontitis sometimes had subnormal levels of iron. Animal experiments have not yet revealed any effects of iron deficiency on PDL (Deutsch *et al.*, 1969).

Although cobalt is said to retard the eruption of the rat incisor (Bryer, 1957), no reports concerning the influence of this inorganic element on the structure of the PDL have been published. Even with Bryer's work, doubts may be expressed about his conclusions since the eruption rates were only marginally reduced (from 1.83–1.70 mm per 48 hours).

REFERENCES

Adams D, Carney JS and Dicks DA (1974) Pregnancy gingivitis: a survey of 100 antenatal patients. J Dent 2, 106–111.

Afonsky D (1955) Oral lesions in niacin, riboflavin, pyridoxine, folic acid and pantothenic acid deficiencies in adult dogs. Oral Surg 8, 867–876.

Ainamo J (1972) Relationship between occlusal wear of the teeth and periodontal health. Scand J Dent Res 80, 505–509.

Ainamo J and Talari A (1976) Eruptive movements of teeth in human adults. In: The Eruption and Occlusion of Teeth (Poole DFG and Stack MV, eds), pp 97–107, London, Butterworths.

Applebaum E and Seeling A (1955) Histological changes in jaws and teeth of rats following nephritis, adrenalectomy and cortisone treatment. Oral Surg 8, 888–891.

Aufdemorte TB and Sheridan PJ (1981) Nuclear uptake of sex steroids in gingiva of the baboon. J Periodontol 52, 430–434.

Aukes JN, Felling FA and Kayser AF (1989) Interaction between food texture and dental health. Ned Tijdschr Tandheelkd 96, 406–408.

Auskaps AM, Gupta OP and Shaw JH (1957) Periodontal disease in the rice rat. III. Survey of dietary influences. J Nutr 63, 325–343.

Baaregaard A (1949) Dental conditions and nutrition among natives in Greenland. Oral Surg 2, 995–1007.

Badanes, BB (1933) Diabetes, acidosis and the significance of acid mouth. Dent Cosmos 75, 476–484.

Ball PC (1977) The effect of adrenal glucocorticoid administration on eruption rates and tissue dimensions in rat mandibular incisors. J Anat 124, 157–163.

Barrett MT (1935) The effects of thymus extract (Hanson) on the early eruption and growth of the teeth of white rats. Dent Cosmos 77, 1088–1093.

Baume LJ and Becks H (1952) The effect of thyroid hormone in dental and paradental structures. Paradentologie 6, 89–109.

Baume LJ, Becks H and Evans HM (1954b) Hormonal control of tooth eruption. III. The response of the incisors of hypophysectomized rats to growth hormone, thyroxin or the combination of both. J Dent Res 33, 104–114.

Baume LJ, Becks H and Evans HM (1954c) Hormonal control of tooth eruption. I. The effect of thyroidectomy on the upper rat incisor and the response to growth hormone, thyroxin or the combination of both. J Dent Res 33, 80–90.

Baume LJ, Becks H, Ray JC and Evans HM (1954a) Hormonal control of tooth eruption. II. The effects of hypophysectomy on the upper rat incisor following progressively longer intervals. J Dent Res 33, 91–103.

Bavetta LA and Bernick S (1956) Effect of tryptophan deficiency on bones and teeth of rats. II. Effect of prolongation. Oral Surg 9, 308–315.

Becks H and Furuta WJ (1939) Effect of magnesium deficient diets on oral and dental tissues. I. Changes in the enamel epithelium. J Am Dent Assoc 26, 883–891.

Becks H and Furuta WJ (1941) Effect of magnesium deficient diets on oral and dental tissues. II. Changes in the dental structures. J Am Dent Assoc 28, 1083–1088.

Becks H and Furuta WJ (1943) Effects of magnesium deficient diets on oral and dental structures. IV. Changes in paradental bone structure. J Dent Res 22, 215–217.

Becks H, Wainwright WW and Morgan AF (1943) Comparative study of oral changes in dogs due to deficiencies of pantothenic acid, nicotinic acid and unknowns of the B-vitamin complex. Am J Orthodont 29, 1813–2207.

Becks H and Weber M (1931) The influence of diet on the bone system with special reference to the alveolar process and the labyrinthine capsule. J Am Dent Assoc 18, 197–264.

Begg PR (1954) Stone Age Man's dentition – with reference to anatomically correct occlusion, the aetiology of malocclusion, and a technique for its treatment. Am J Orthodont 40, 292–312 and 373–383.

Belting CM, Hiniker JJ and Dummett CO (1964) Influence of diabetes mellitus on the severity of periodontal disease. J Periodontol 35, 476–480.

Benveniste R, Bixler D and Conneally PM (1967) Periodontal disease in diabetics. J Periodontol 38, 271–279.

Berkovitz BKB (1971) Effects of surgical interference and drug administration on eruption in the rat mandibular incisor. J Dent Res 50, 654 (abstract).

Berkovitz BKB (1974) Effect of fluoride on eruption rates of rat incisors. J Dent Res 53, 334–337.

Bernick S, Cohen DW, Baker L and Laster L (1975) Dental disease in children with diabetes mellitus. J Periodontol 46, 241–245.

Bernick S, Ershoff BH and Lal JB (1971) Effects of hypervitaminosis D on bones and teeth of rats. Int J Vitam Nutr Res 41, 480–489.

Bernick S and Hungerford GF (1965) Effect of dietary magnesium deficiency on the bones and teeth of rats. J Dent Res 44, 1317–1324.

Beyron H (1964) Occlusal relations and mastication in Australian aborigines. Acta Odont Scand 22, 597–678.

Bissada NF, Schaffer EM and Lazarow A (1966) Effect of alloxan diabetes and local irritating factors on the periodontal structures of the rat. Periodontics 4, 233–240.

Blockley CH and Baenzigen PE (1942) An investigation into the connection between the vitamin C content of the blood and periodontal disturbances. Br Dent J 73, 57–61.

Blom S, Holmstrup P and Dabelsteen E (1992) The effect of insulin-like growth factor-I and human growth hormone on periodontal ligament fibroblast morphology, growth pattern, DNA synthesis, and receptor binding. J Periodontol 63, 960–968.

Bonheim F (1943) The endocrine system in periodontal disease. In: Textbook of periodontia (2nd edition) (Miller SC, ed), pp 520–553, Blakiston, Philadelphia.

Boyle PE (1947) Effects of vitamin A deficiency on the periodontal tissues. Am J Orthodont 33, 744–748.

Boyle PE and Bessey OA (1941) The effect of acute vitamin A deficiency on the molar teeth and paradontal tissues with a comment on deformed incisor teeth in this deficiency. J Dent Res 20, 236–237 (abstract).

Boyle PE, Bessey DA and Wolbach SD (1937) Experimental alveolar bone atrophy produced by ascorbic acid deficiency and its relation to pyorrhoea alveolaris. Proc Soc Exp Biol Med 36, 733–735.

Brothwell DR and Carr HG (1962) The dental health of the Etruscans. Br Dent J 113, 207–210.

Bryer LW (1957) An experimental evaluation of the physiology of tooth eruption Int Dent J 7, 432–478.

Burkitt DP (1973) Some diseases characteristic of modern Western civilisation. Br Med J 1, 274–278.

Burrill DY (1943) The effect of low phosphorus intake on the growth of the jaws in dogs. J Am Dent Assoc 30, 513–523.

Cai JJ (1992) Effect of vitamin D over-dosage on the tooth and bone development of rabbits. Chung Hua Kou Chiang Hsueh Tsa Chih 27, 296–299.

Carlsson J and Egelberg J (1965a) Effect of diet on early plaque formation in man. Odont Revy 16, 112–125.

Carlsson J and Egelberg J (1965b) Local effect of diet on plaque formation and development of gingivitis in dogs. II. Effect of high carbohydrate versus high protein–fat diets. Odont Revy 16, 42–49.

Carneiro J and Fava de Moraes F (1965) Radio-autographic visualisation of collagen metabolism in the periodontal tissue of the mouse. Arch Oral Biol 10, 833–848.

Carpenter G (1978) The regulation of cell proliferation: advances in the biology and mechanisms of action of epidermal growth factor. J Invest Dermatol 71, 283–287.

Cattell P (1928) The eruption and growth of the permanent teeth. J Dent Res 8, 279–287.

Cerna H, Vesely J, Nastoupilova E, Lechner J, Fingerova H and Pohanka J (1990). Periodontium and vitamin E and A in pregnancy. Acta Univ Palacki Olomuc Fac Med 125, 173–179.

Chapman OD and Harris AE (1941) Oral lesions associated with dietary deficiencies in monkeys. J Infect Dis 69, 7–17.

Chawla TN and Glickman I (1951) Protein deprivation and the periodontal structures of the albino rat. Oral Surg 4, 578–602.

Cheraskin E and Ringsdorf WM (1965) Gingival state and carbohydrate. J Dent Res 44, 480–486.

Chinn H, Brody H, Silverman S and di Raimondo V (1966) Glucose tolerance in patients with oral symptoms. J Oral Ther Pharmacol 2, 261–269.

Cleave TL, Campbell GD and Painter NS (1973) Diabetes Coronary Thrombosis and the Saccharine Disease (2nd edition), Wright, Bristol.

Cohen DW, Friedman L, Shapiro J and Kyle GC (1969) Studies on periodontal patterns in diabetes mellitus. J Periodont Res 4 (suppl), 35–36.

Cohen DW, Friedman LA, Shapiro J, Kyle GC and Franklin S (1970) Diabetes mellitus and periodontal disease: two year longitudinal observations. J Periodontol 41, 709–712.

Cohen DW, Shapiro J, Friedman L, Kyle GC and Franklin S (1971) Diabetes mellitus and periodontal disease. II. 3 year longitudinal study. J Dent Res 50, 206 (abstract).

Cohen ME and Meyer DM (1993). Effect of dietary vitamin E supplementation and rotational stress on alveolar bone loss in rice rats. Arch Oral Biol 38, 601–606.

Cohen MM, Shklar G and Yerganian G (1963) Pulpal and periodontal disease in Chinese hamsters with hereditary diabetes mellitus. Oral Surg 16, 104–112.

Cohen S (1962) Isolation of a mouse submaxillary gland protein accelerating incisor eruption and eyelid opening in the newborn animal. J Biol Chem 237, 1555–1562.

Colyer F (1931) Abnormal Conditions of the Teeth of Animals in their Relationship to Similar Conditions in Man, pp 39–63, 81–1908, The Dental Board of the United Kingdom, London.

Coolidge ED (1937) The thickness of the human periodontal membrane. J Am Dent Assoc Dent Cosmos 24, 1260–1270.

Conn IG , Skellern GG, Sweeney D and Steer ST (1988) Co-oeidation of arachadonic acid and methimazole by prostaglandin endoperoxidase synthetase. Pharmacology 36, 45.

Dalldorf and Zall C (1930) Tooth growth in experimental scurvy. J Exp Med 52, 57–63.

Davies TGH and Pedersen PO (1955) The degree of attrition of the deciduous teeth and first permanent molars of primitive and urbanised Greenland natives. Br Dent J 99, 35–43.

De-Menezes AC, Costa IM and El GM (1984) Clinical manifestations of hypervitaminosis A in human gingiva. A case report. J Periodontol 55, 474–476.

Deutsch CM, Dreizen S and Stahl SS (1969) The effects of chronic iron deficiency anaemia on the periodontium of the adult rat. J Periodontol 40, 736–739.

Dewhirst FE, Ago JM, Peros WJ and Stashenko P (1987). Synergism between parathyroid hormone and interleukin 1 in stimulating bone resorption in organ culture. J Bone Miner Res 2, 127–134.

Domm LV and Marzano R (1954) Observations on the effect of certain hormones on the growth rate of the incisors of the albino rat. Anat Rec 118, 383–384.

Domm LV and Wellband WA (1960) Effect of adrenalectomy and cortisone on eruption rate of incisors of young female albino rats. Proc Soc Exp Biol 104, 582–584.

Domm LV and Wellband WA (1961) Effect of adrenalectomy, thyroidectomy, thyro-adrenalectomy and cortisone on eruption rate of incisors in adult female rats. Proc Soc Exp Biol 107, 268–272.

Dreizen S, Levy BM and Bernick S (1969) Studies on the biology of the periodontium of marmosets. VII. The effect of vitamin C deficiency on the marmoset periodontium. J Periodont Res 4, 274–280.

Dreizen S, Levy BM and Bernick S (1971) Studies on the biology of the periodontium of marmosets. Cortisone induced periodontal and skeletal changes in adult cotton top marmosets. J Periodontol 42, 217–224.

Eastwood M (1973) Vegetable dietary fibre food – fad or farrago. In: Getting the Most out of Food, Chapter 8, pp 39–59. van der Berghs and Jurgens, London

Egelberg J (1965) Local effect of diet on plaque formation and development of gingivitis in dogs. I. Effect of hard and soft diets. Odont Revy 16, 31–41.

El-Ashiiry GM, El Kafrawy AH, Nasr MF and Younis H (1970) Comparative study of the influence of pregnancy and oral contraceptives on the gingiva. Oral Surg 30, 472–475.

El-Ashiry GM, Ringsdorf WM and Cheraskin E (1964) Local and sytemic influences in periodontal disease. II. Effect of prophylaxis and natural versus synthetic vitamin C upon gingivitis. J Periodontol 35, 250–259.

El-Attar TMA (1978) Prostaglandins: Physiology, biochemistry, pharmacology and clinical applications. J Oral Pathol 7, 175–208, 239–282.

El-Attar TM, Lin HS and Platt RD (1990) Comparison of the inhibitory effect of polyunsaturated fatty acids on prostaglandin synthesis. II. Fibroblasts. Prostaglandins Leukot Essent Fatty Acids 39, 135–139.

El Geneidy AK, Stallard RE, Fillios LC and Goldman HM (1974) Periodontal and vascular alteration: their relationship to the changes in tissue glucose and glycogen in diabetic mice. J Periodontol 45, 394–401.

El Kafrawy AH and Mitchell DF (1976) Dental and periodontal effects of calcitonin in hamsters. J Dent Res 55, 554.

Emami S, Rizzo WB, Hanley KP, Taylor JM, Goldyne ME and Williams ML (1992) Peroxisomal abnormality in fibroblasts from involved skin of CHILD syndrome. Case study and review of peroxisomal disorders in relation to skin disease. Arch Dermatol 128, 1213–1222.

Fahmy H, Rodgers WE, Mitchell DF and Bremer HE (1961) Effects of hypervitaminosis D on the periodontium of the hamster. J Dent Res 40, 870–877.

Ferguson HW (1969) Effect of nutrition on the periodontium. In: Biology of the Periodontium (Melcher AH and Bowen WH, eds), pp 421–451, Academic Press, London.

Ferguson HW and Hartles RL (1963) Effect of vitamin D on the bones of young rats receiving diets low in calcium or phosphorus. Arch Oral Biol 8, 407–418.

Ferguson HW and Hartles RL (1966) The effect of diets deficient in calcium or phosphorus in the presence and absence of supplement of vitamin D on the incisor teeth and bone of adult rats. Arch Oral Biol 11, 1345–1364.

Ferguson MM (1983) Stimulation of the immune response by progesterone. In: Immunological Factors in Human Contraception (Schulman DF, ed), pp 124–127, Field Education Italia.

Ferguson MM, Alexander WD, Connell JMC, Lappin AG *et al.* (1984) Peroxidase activity in relation to iodide, 17β-oestradiol and thioureylene drug uptake in human polymorphoneutrophils. Biochem Pharmacol 33, 757–762.

Ferguson MM, Cowan S, Leake R (1981) Progestogen binding entity in human leukocytes. J Dent Res 60, 1160.

Ferguson MM, MacDonald FG (1985). Oestrogen as an inhibitor of human NK cell cytolysis. FEBS Lett 191, 145.

Franceschi RT (1992) The role of ascorbic acid in mesenchymal differentiation. Nutr Rev 50, 65–70.

Frandsen AM (1963) Periodontal tissue changes in vitamin A deficient young rats. Acta Odont Scand 21, 19–34.

Frandsen AM, Becks H, Nelson MM and Evans HM (1953) Effects of various levels of dietary protein on he periodontal tissues of young rats. J Periodontol 24, 135–142.

Frantzis TG, Reeve CM and Brown AL (1971) The ultrastructure of capillary basement membranes in the attached gingiva of diabetic and non-diabetic patients with periodontal disease. J Periodontol 42, 406–411.

Friedman LA (1972) Horizontal tooth mobility and the menstrual cycle. J Periodont Res 7, 125–130.

Gagnon T, Schour I and Patras MC (1942) Effect of magnesium deficiency on dentine apposition and eruption in the incisor of rat. Proc Soc Exp Biol 49, 662–666.

Garn SM Lewis AB and Blizzard, RM (1965) Endocrine factors in dental development. J Dent Res 44 (suppl) 243–258.

Garn SM, Lewis AB, Koski K and Polachek DL (1958) The sex difference in tooth calcification. J Dent Res 37, 561–567.

Garren L and Greep RO (1955) Effects of thyroid hormone and propylthiouracil on eruption rate of upper incisor teeth in rats. Proc Soc Exp Biol 90, 652–655.

Garren L and Greep RO (1960) Effect of adrenal cortical hormones on eruption rate of incisor teeth in the rat. Endocrinology 66, 625–628.

Glavind L, Lund B and Löe H (1968) The relationship between periodontal state and diabetes duration, insulin dosage and retinal changes. J Periodontol 39, 341–343.

Glickman I and Dines MM (1963) Effect of increased ascorbic acid blood levels on the ascorbic acid level in treated and non-treated gingiva. J Dent Res 42, 1152–1158.

Glickman I and Pruzansky S (1947) Propyl-thiouracil-hypothyroidism in the albino rat – its effect on the jaws. J Dent Res 26, 471 (abstract).

Glickman I and Quintarelli J (1960) Low oestrogen levels due to oöphorectomy in rats. J Periodontol 31, 31–37.

Glickman I and Shklar G (1954) Modification of the effect of cortisone upon alveolar bone by the systemic administration of estrogen. J Periodontol 25, 231–239.

Glickman I and Shklar G (1955) The steroid hormones and tissues of the periodontium. A series of related experiments in white mice. Oral Surg 8, 1179–1191.

Glickman I, Smulow JB and Moreau J (1966) Effect of alloxan diabetes upon the periodontal response to excessive occlusal forces. J Periodontol 37, 146–155.

Glickman I and Stoller M (1948) The periodontal tissues of the albino rat in vitamin A deficiency. J Dent Res 27, 758 (abs).

Glickman I, Stone IC and Chawla TN (1953) The effect of the systemic administration of cortisone upon the periodontium of white mice. J Periodontol 25, 87–96.

Goldman HM (1943) Experimental hyperthyroidism in guinea pigs. Am J Orthod Oral Surg 29, 665–681.

Goldman HM (1954) The effects of dietary protein deprivation and of age on the periodontal tissues of the rat and spider monkey. J Periodontol 25, 87–96.

Gregory H, Holmes JE and Willshire IR (1979) Urogastrone–epidermal growth factor. In: Methods in Hormone Radioimmunoassay (Jaffe BM and Behrman HR, eds), pp 927–941, Academic Press, London.

Gregory H, Walsh S and Hopkins CR (1979) The identification of urogastrone in serum, saliva and gastric juice. Gastroenterology 77, 313–318.

Hall JF and Robinson HBG (1937) Alveolar atrophy in anemic dogs. J Dent Res 16, 345–346 (abstract).

Hatt SD, Lyle-Stewart W and Cresswell E (1968) Periodontal disease in sheep. Dent Practitr 19, 123–127.

Hayes KC, McCombs HC and Faherty TP (1970) The fine structure of vitamin A deficiency. I. Parotid duct metaplasia. Lab Invest 22, 81–89.

Heaton KW (1973) Are we getting too much out of food? Nutrition 27, 170–183.

Hellsing E and Hammarström L (1991) The effects of pregnancy and fluoride on orthodontic tooth movements in rats. Eur J Orthod, 13, 223–230.

Henrikson PA (1968) Periodontal disease and calcium deficiency, an experimental study in the dog. Acta Odont Scand 26 (suppl 50), 1–132.

Herzberg F and Schour I (1941) Effects of thyroxine on rate of eruption and dentine apposition. J Dent Res 20, 276 (abstract).

Hilming F (1952) Gingivitis gravidarum. Oral Surg 5, 734–751.

Hinek A and Poole AR (1988) The influence of vitamin D metabolites on the calcification of cartilage matrix and the C-propeptide of type II collagen (chondrocalcin). J Bone Miner Res 3, 421–429.

Holloway PJ, James PMC and Slack GL (1963) Dental disease in Tristan da Cunha. Br Dent J 115, 19–25.

Hove KA and Stallard RE (1970) Diabetes and the periodontal patient. J Periodontol 41, 713–758.

Hugoson A (1971) Gingivitis in pregnant women. A longitudinal clinical study. Odont Revy 22, 65–84.

Hunt AM and Paynter KJ (1959) The effects of ascorbic acid deficiency on the teeth and periodontal tissues of guinea pigs. J Dent Res 38, 232–243.

Irving JT (1942) Enamel organ of the rat's incisor tooth in vitamin E deficiency. Nature 150, 122–123.

Igarashi A, Uzuka M and Nakajima K (1989) The effects of vitamin E deficiency on rat skin. Br J Dermatol 121, 43–9.

Kaufman AY (1969) An oral contraceptive as an etiologic factor in producing hyperplastic gingivitis and a neoplasm of the pregnancy tumour type. Oral Surg 28, 666–670.

Keene JJ (1969a) Observations of small blood vessels in human nondiabetic gingiva. J Dent Res 48, 967.

Keene JJ (1969b) A histochemical evaluation for small vessel calcification in human nondiabetic and diabetic gingival biopsy specimens. J Dent Res 48, 968.

Keene JJ (1972) An alteration in human diabetic arterioles. J Dent Res 51, 569–572.

Keyes PH and Litkins RC (1946) Plaque formation, periodontal disease, and dental caries in Syrian hamsters. J Dent Res 25, 166 (abstract).

Klatsky M and Klatell JS (1943) Anthropological studies in dental caries. J Dent Res 22, 267–274.

Klein H, Orent ER and McCallum EV (1935) The effect of magnesium deficiency on the teeth and their supporting structures in rats. Am J Physiol 112, 256–262.

Klinger G and Klinger G (1970) Untersuchungen über den Einfluss oraler Kontraseptiva auf die Mund- und Vaginalschleimhaut. Dtsch Stomatol 20, 664–669.

Klingsberg J and Butcher EO (1959) Aging, diet, and periodontal lesions in the hamster. J Dent Res 38, 421.

Knight GM and Wade AB (1974) The effects of hormonal contraceptives on the human periodontium. J Periodont Res 9, 18–22.

Körber KH (1961) Elektronisches Messen der Zahnbeweglichkeit. Dtsch Zahnärztebl 16, 605–613.

Kofoed JA and Bozzini CE (1970) The effect of hydrocortisone on the concentration and synthesis of acid mucopolysaccharides in the rat gingiva. J Periodont Res 5, 259–262.

Kretsch MJ, Sauberlich HE and Newbrun E (1991) Electroencephalographic changes and periodontal status during short-term vitamin B-6 depletion of young, nonpregnant women. Am J Clin Nutr 53, 1266–1274.

Kusner W, Michaeli Y and Weinreb MM (1973) Role of attrition and occlusal contact in the physiology of the rat incisor. VI. Impeded and unimpeded eruption in hypophysectomized and magnesium-deficient rats. J Dent Res 52, 65–73.

Labelle RE and Schaffer EM (1966) The effects of cortisone and induced local factors on the periodontium of the albino rat. J Periodont 37, 483–490.

Lainson PA, Brady PP and Fraleight CM (1968) Anaemia, a systemic cause of periodontal disease? J Periodontol 39, 35–38.

Lavelle CLB (1973) Alveolar bone loss and tooth attrition in skulls from different population samples. J Periodont Res 8, 395–399.

Levy BM (1949) Effects of pantothenic acid deficiency on the mandibular joints and periodontal structures of mice. J Am Dent Assoc 38, 215–223.

Lindhe J, Birch J and Brånemark PI (1968) Vascular proliferation in pseudopregnant rabbits. J Periodont Res 3, 12–20.

Lindhe J and Bjorn AL (1967) Influence of hormonal contraceptives on the gingiva of women. J Periodont Res 2, 1–6.

Lindhe J and Brånemark PI (1967a) The effect of sex hormones on vascularisation of a granulation tissue. J Periodont Res 3, 6–11.

Lindhe J and Brånemark PI (1967b) Changes in microcirculation after local application of sex hormones. J Periodont Res 2, 185–1913.

Lindhe J and Brånemark PI (1967c) Changes in vascular permeability after local application of sex hormones. J Periodont Res 2, 259–265.

Lindhe J, Brånemark PI and Birch J (1968) Microvascular events in cheek pouch wounds of oöphorectomised hamsters following intramuscular injections of female sex hormones. J Periodont Res 3, 21–23.

Lipari WA, Blake LC and Zipkin I (1974) Preferential response of the periodontal apparatus and the epiphyseal plate to hydrocortisone and fluoride in the rat. J Periodontol 45, 879–890.

Listgarten MA, Ricker FH, Laster L, Shapiro J and Cohen DW (1974) Vascular basement lamina thickness in the normal and inflamed gingiva of diabetics and non-diabetics. J Periodontol 45, 676–684.

Litvin PE and De Marco TJ (1973) The effect of a diuretic and antidiuretic on tooth eruption. Oral Surg 35, 294–298.

Löe H (1965) Periodontal changes in pregnancy. J Periodontol 36, 209–217.

Löe H and Silness J (1963) Periodontal disease in pregnancy. Acta Odont Scand 21, 533–551.

Lovestedt SA and Austin LT (1943) Periodontoclasia in diabetes mellitus. J Am Dent Assoc 30, 273–275.

Lynn BP (1967) 'The Pill' as an etiological agent in hypertrophic gingivitis. Oral Surg 24, 333–334.

Mackenzie RA and Millard HD (1963) Interrelated effects of diabetes, arteriosclerosis and calculus on alveolar bone loss. J Am Dent Assoc 66, 191–198.

Maier AW and Orban B (1949) Gingivitis in pregnancy. Oral Surg 2, 334–373.

Masse PG, Colombo VE, Gerber F, Howell DS and Weiser H (1990) Morphological abnormalities in vitamin B6 deficient tarsometatarsal chick cartilage. Scanning Microsc 4, 667–73.

Massler M, Schour I and Chopra B (1950) Occurrence of gingivitis in suburban Chicago school children. J Periodontol 21, 146–164.

Mellanby H (1941) The effect of maternal dietary deficiency of vitamin A on dental tissues in rats. J Dent Res 20, 489–509.

Mellanby M (1929) Diet and the teeth. Part 1. Dental structure in dogs. Spec Rep Ser Med Res Coun Lond No. 140.

Melnick SL, Alvarez JO, Navia JM, Cogen RB and Roseman JM (1988) A case-control study of plasma ascorbate and acute necrotizing ulcerative gingivitis. J Dent Res 67, 855–860.

Miglani DC (1959) The effect of vitamin A deficiency on the periodontal structures of rat molars with emphasis on cementum resorption. Oral Surg 12, 1372–1386.

Miller SC, Stahl SS and Goldsmith ED (1957) The effects of vertical occlusal trauma on the periodontium of protein-deprived young adult rats. J Periodontol 28, 87–97.

Mohammed AH, Waterhouse JP and Friederici HHR (1974) The microvasculature of the rabbit gingiva as affected by progesterone: an ultrastructural study. J Periodontol 45, 50–60.

Moskow BS, Baden E and Zengo A (1966) The effects of dihydrotachysterol and ferric dextran upon the periodontium in the rat. Arch Oral Biol 11, 1017–1026.

Moxham BJ (1979) The effects of some vaso-active drugs on the eruption of the rabbit mandibular incisor. Arch Oral Biol 24, 759–763.

Moxham BJ and Berkovitz BKB (1980) A quantative assessment of the effects of axially directed extrusive loads on displacement of the impeded and unimpeded rabbit mandibular incisor. Arch Oral Biol 26, 208–215.

Mühlemann HR (1951) Periodontometry. A method for measuring tooth mobility. Oral Surg 4, 1220–1233.

Mühlemann HR, Savdis S and Rateitschak KH (1965) Tooth mobility – its causes and significance. J Periodontol 36, 148–153.

Murphy TR (1959) Compensatory mechanisms in facial height adjustment to functional tooth attrition. Aust Dent J 4, 312–323.

Murphy TR (1964) Reduction of the dental arch by approximal attrition. Br Dent J 116, 483–488.

Myers BA, Dubick MA, Gerriets JE, Reiser KM, Last JA and Rucker RB (1986) Lung collagen and elastin after ozone exposure in vitamin B-6-deficient rats. Toxicol Lett 30, 55–61.

Myhre L, Preus HR and Aars H (1979) Influences of axial load and blood pressure on the position of the rabbit's incisor tooth. Acta Odont Scand 37, 153–159.

Ness AR (1964) Movement and forces in tooth eruption. In: Advances in Oral Biology (Staple PH, ed), pp 33–75, Academic Press, London.

Neuberger A (1955) Stoffwechsel von Kollagen unter normal Bedingungen. Symp Soc Exp Biol 9, 72–84.

Neuberger A, Perrone JC and Slack HG (1951) The relative metabolic inertia of tendon collagen in the rat. Biochem J 49, 199–204.

Neuberger A and Slack HGB (1953) The metabolism of collagen from liver, bone, skin and tendon in the normal rat. Biochem J 53, 47–52.

Newman HN (1974) Diet, attrition, plaque and dental disease. Br Dent J 136, 491–497.

Newman HN and Levers BGH (1979) Tooth eruption and function in an early Anglo-Saxon population. J R Soc Med 72, 341–350.

O'Leary TM, Shannon IL and Prigmore JR (1962) Clinical and systemic findings in periodontal disease. J Periodontol 33, 243–251.

Oliver WM (1969) The effect of deficiencies of calcium, vitamin D or calcium and vitamin D and or variations in the source of dietary protein on the supporting tissues of the rat molar. J Periodont Res 4, 56–60.

Østergaard E (1975) The collagen content of skin and gingival tissues in ascorbic acid-deficient monkeys. J Periodont Res 10, 103–114.

Parfitt GJ (1957) A five year longitudinal study of the gingival condition of a group of children in England. J Periodontol 28, 26–32.

Parmer LG, Katonah E and Argrist AA (1951) Comparative effects of ACTH, cortisone, corticosterone, deoxycorticosterone, pregnenolone, on growth and development in infant rats. Proc Soc Exp Biol 77, 215–218.

Paynter KJ (1954) The effect of propylthiouracil on the development of molar teeth in rats. J Dent Res 33, 364–376.

Pearlman BA (1974) An oral contraceptive drug and gingival enlargement; the relationship between local and systemic factors. J Clin Periodontol 1, 47–51.
Perlitsch M, Nielsen AG and Stanmeyer WR (1961) Ascorbic acids levels and gingival health in personnel wintering over in Antarctica. J Dent Res 40, 789–799.
Peterkofsky B (1991) Ascorbate requirement for hydroxylation and secretion of procollagen: relationship to inhibition of collagen synthesis in scurvy. Am J Clin Nutr 54, 11355–11405.
Philippas GG (1952) Evidence of function on healthy teeth; the evidence of ancient Athenian remains. J Am Dent Assoc 45, 443–453.
Picton DCA (1957) Calculus, wear and alveolar bone loss in the jaws of sixth-century Jutes. Dent Practit 7, 301–303.
Pindborg JJ (1949) The effect of methyl folic acid on the periodontal tissues in rat molars (experimental granulocytopenia). Oral Surg 2, 1485–1496.
Pindborg JJ (1952) Effect of vitamin E deficiency on the rat incisor. J Dent Res 31, 805–811.
Pinto ACG (1974) Effect of hypothyroidism obtained experimentally in the periodontium of rat. J Periodontol 45, 217–221.
Piroshaw NA and Glickman I (1957) The effect of ovariectomy upon the tissues of the periodontium and skeletal bones. Oral Surg 10, 133–147.
Pitaru S, Blaushild N, Noff D and Edelstein S (1982) The effect of toxic doses of 1,25-dihydroxycholecalciferol on dental tissues in the rat. Arch Oral Biol 27, 915–923.
Platt BS and Stewart RJC (1962) Transverse trabecula and osteoporosis in bones in experimental protein–calorie deficiency. Br J Nutr 16, 483–495.
Priest RE (1970) Formation of epithelial basement membrane is restricted by scurvy in vitro and is stimulated by vitamin C. Nature 225, 744–745.
Prout RES and Tring FC (1971) Effect of fat-free diet on ameloblast and enamel formation in incisors of rats. J Dent Res 50, 1559–1561.
Prout RES. and Tring FC (1973) Dentinogenesis in incisors of rats deficient in essential fatty acids. J Dent Res 52, 462–467.
Rao LG, Moe HK and Heersche JNM (1978) *In vitro* culture of porcine periodontal ligament cells: response of fibroblast-like and epithelial-like cells to prostaglandin E1 parathyroid hormone and calcitonin and separation of a pure population of fibroblast-like cells. Arch Oral Biol 23, 957–964.
Rao SS, Shourie KL and Sharkwaller GB (1965) Effect of dietary fat variations on the periodontium. Periodontics 3, 66–76.
Ratcliff PA and Itokazu H (1964) The effect of dihydrotachysterol and ferric dextran on the teeth and periodontium of the rat. J Oral Therapy Pharmacol 1, 7–22.
Ratcliff PA and Krajewski J (1966) The influence of methyl testosterone on dihydrotachysterol intoxication as it affects the periodontium. J Oral Therapy Pharmacol 2, 353–361.
Rateitschak KH (1967) Tooth mobility changes in pregnancy. J Periodont Res 2, 199–206.
Reeve CM and Winkelmann RK (1962) Glycogen storage in gingival epithelium of diabetic and non-diabetic patients. J Dent Res 40, 31 (abstract).
Restarski JS and Pijoun M (1944) Gingivitis and vitamin C. J Am Dent Assoc 31, 13–23.
Ringelberg ML, Dixon DO, Francis AD and Plummer RW (1977) Comparison of gingival health and gingival crevicular fluid flow in children with and without diabetes. J Dent Res 56, 108–111.
Roberts WE (1975) Cell kinetic nature and diurnal periodicity of the rat periodontal ligament. Arch Oral Biol 20, 465–471.
Robertson J (1972) Changes in the fibre of the British diet. Nature 238, 290–292.
Rosenberg MM, Goldman HM and Garber E (1961) Effects of experimental thyrotoxicosis and myxoedema on the periodontium of rabbits. J Dent Res 40, 708–709 (abstract).
Rubright WC, Higa LH and Yannone ME (1971) Histological quantification of the biological effects of estradiol benzoate on the gingiva and genital mucosa of castrated rabbits. J Periodont Res 6, 55–64.
Rubright WC, Termon SA and Yannone ME (1973) A comparative study of an *in vitro* ^{3}H-17β-estradiol binding in gingiva skeletal muscle and uterus of ovariectomised rabbits. J Periodont Res 8, 304–313.
Rugg-Gunn AJ (1968) Caries resistance in the Kuria Muria Islands. Report of a dental health survey. Br Dent J 124, 75–77.
Rushton MA (1941) Cases of accelerated and retarded dentition. Br Dent J 71, 277–279.
Russell BG (1966) Gingival changes in diabetes mellitus. Acta Pathol Microbiol Scand 68, 161–168.
Russell BG (1967) The dental pulp in diabetes mellitus. Acta Pathol Microbiol Scand 70, 319–320.
Rutledge CE (1940) Oral and roentgenographic aspects of teeth and jaws of juvenile diabetics. J Am Dent Assoc 27, 1740–1750.
Safkan B and Knuuttila M (1984). Corticosteroid therapy and periodontal disease. J Clin Periodontol 11, 515–522.
Salley JJ, Bryson WF and Eshleman J (1959) The effect of chronic vitamin A deficiency on dental caries in the Syrian hamster. J Dent Res 38, 1038–1043.
Sallum AW, Do Nascimento A, Bozzo L and De Toledo S (1976) The effect of dexamethasone in traumatic changes of the periodontium of marmosets (Callithrix jacchus). J Periodontol 47, 63–66.
Sarnås KV (1957) Growth changes in skulls of ancient man in North America. An x-ray cephalometric investigation of some cranial and facial changes during growth in the Indian knoll skeletons. Acta Odont Scand 15, 213–271.
Schneider HG (1967) Veränderungen am Parodont der Ratte nach Overektomie. Der Einfluss der Kastration auf das Epithel der Gingiva propria. Parodontologie Acad Rev 1, 106–114.
Schneider HG and Pose G (1969) Influence of tocopherol on the periodontium of molars in rats fed a diet lacking in vitamin E. Arch Oral Biol 14, 431–433.
Schour I (1934) The effects of hypophysectomy on the periodontal tissues. J Periodontol 5, 15–24.
Schour I (1936) Changes in the incisor of the 13-lined ground squirrel (Citellus tridecemlineatus) following bilateral gonadectomy. Anat Rec 65, 177–199.
Schour I, Chandler SB and Tweedy WR (1937) Changes in teeth following parathyroidectomy. Am J Pathol 13, 945–970.
Schour I, Hoffman MM and Smith MC (1941) Changes in incisor teeth of albino rats with vitamin A deficiency and effects of replacement therapy. Am J Pathol 17, 529–533.
Schour I and Massler M (1943) Endocrines and dentistry. J Am Dent Assoc 30, 595–603, 763–773, 943–950.
Schour I and van Dyke HB (1931) Histologic changes in the rat incisor following hypophysectomy. J Dent Res 11, 873–875.
Schour I and van Dyke HB (1932a) Changes in the teeth following hypophysectomy. I. Changes in the incisor of the white rat. Am J Anat 50, 397–433.
Schour I and van Dyke HB (1932b) Effect of replacement therapy on eruption of the incisor of the hypophysectomized rat. Proc Soc Exp Biol Med 29, 378–382.
Schour I and van Dyke HB (1934) Changes in teeth following hypophysectomy. II. Changes in the molar of the white rat. J Dent Res 14, 69–91.
Schumer S and Wells H (1958) Effect of thyroxine and triiodothyroacetic acid on incisor eruption rate. J Dent Res 37, 980 (abstract).
Shannon IL and Gibson WA (1964) Oral glucose tolerance responses in healthy young adult males classified as to caries experience and periodontal status. Periodontics 2, 292–297.
Shapiro S and Shklar G (1962) The effect of hypophysectomy on the periodontium of the albino rat. J Periodontol 33, 364–371.
Shaw JH (1962) The relation of nutrition to periodontal disease. J Dent Res 41, 264–274.

Sheenan R and Cohen M (1970) The periodontium of diabetic mice. J Dent Res 49, 111 (abstract).

Shklar G (1965) The effect of adrenalectomy and cortisone replacement on the periodontium of the rat. Periodontics 3, 239–242.

Shklar G, Chauncey HH and Shapiro S (1967) The effect of testosterone on the periodontium of normal and hypophysectomized rats. J Periodontol 38, 203–210.

Shklar G, Cohen MM and Yerganian G (1962) A histopathologic study of periodontal disease in the Chinese hamster with hereditary diabetes. J Periodontol 33, 14–21.

Shklar G and Glickman I (1956) The effect of oestrogenic hormone on the periodontium of white mice. J Periodontol 27, 16–23.

Shore RL, Moxham BJ and Berkowitz BKB (1982) A quantitative comparison of the ultrastructure of the periodontal ligament of impeded and unimpeded rat inscisors. Arch Oral Biol 27, 423–430.

Sim Wallace J (1904) Physical deterioration in relation to the teeth. Br Dent J 25, 861–867.

Singer J, Furstman L, Bernick S (1967) A histologic study of the effect of fluoride on tooth movement in the rat. Am J Orthodont 53, 296–308.

Slatter JM and Picton DCA (1972) The effect on intrusive tooth mobility of noradrenaline injected locally in monkeys (Macaca irus). J Periodont Res 7, 144–150.

Smith MA, Ferguson MM, Lucie NP, Mairs RJ and Smith JG (1986). Progesterone inhibits proliferation of human marrow colony forming cells (CFU–GM) through increased prostaglandin production by marrow macrophages. Br J Haematol 63, 649–658.

Smith MC (1934) Effects of fluoride upon rate of eruption of rat incisors and its correlation with bone development and body growth. J Dent Res 14, 139–144.

Sodek, J (1978) A comparison of collagen and non-collagenous protein metabolism in rat molar and incisor periodontal ligament. Arch oral Biol 23, 977–982.

Southgate DAT (1973) Dietary fibre. Plant Foods for Man 1, 45–47.

Sperber GH (1969) Oral contraceptive hypertrophic gingivitis. J Dent Assoc SAfr 24, 37–40.

Stahl SS (1962) The effect of a protein free diet on the healing of gingival wounds in rats. Arch Oral Biol 7, 551–556.

Stahl SS (1963a) Healing of gingival wounds in female rats fed on low-protein diet, J Dent Res 42, 1511–1516.

Stahl SS (1963b) Soft tissue healing following experimental gingival wounding in female rats of various ages. Periodontics 1, 142–146.

Stahl SS and Gerstner R (1960) The response of the oral mucosa and periodontium to simultaneous administration of cortisone and somatotrophic hormone in young adult male rats. Arch Oral Biol 1, 321–324.

Stahl SS and Joly O (1958) Response of periodontal tissues to intraoral injections of somatotropic hormone in young adult male rats. Oral Surg 11, 475–483.

Stahl SS, Miller SC and Goldsmith ED (1957) The effects of vertical occlusal trauma on the periodontium of protein-deprived young adult rats. J Periodontol 28, 87–97.

Stahl SS, Miller SC and Goldsmith ED (1958) Effects of protein deprivation on the periodontium of young adult male hamsters. J Dent Res 37, 984 (abstract).

Stahl SS, Sandler HC and Cahn L (1955) The effects of protein deprivation upon the oral tissues of the rat and particularly upon periodontal structures under irritation. Oral Surg 8, 760–768.

Stahl SS, Weinmann JP, Schour I and Brady AM (1950) The effect of estrogen on the alveolar bone and teeth of mice and rats. Anat Rec 107, 21–41.

Stein G and Ziskin DE (1949) The effect of a protein free diet on the teeth and periodontium of the albino rat. J Dent Res 28, 529 (abstract).

Stuhl F (1943) Vitamin C subnutrition in gingivo-stomatitis. Lancet i, 640–642.

Sutcliffe P (1972) A longitudinal study of gingivitis and puberty. J Periodont Res 7, 52–58.

Tait RV (1965) Tooth grinding in preventive dentistry. Dental Magazine and Oral Topics 82, 119–121.

Taylor RMS (1962) Non-metrical studies of the human palate and dentition in Moriori and Maori skulls. J Polynes Soc 71, 167–187.

Taylor, RMS (1963) Cause and effect of wear of teeth. Further non-metrical studies of the teeth and palate in Moriori and Maori skulls. Acta Anat 53, 97–157.

Ten Cate AR, Deporter DA and Freeman E (1976) The role of fibroblasts in the remodelling of periodontal ligament during physiologic tooth movement. Am J Orthod 69, 155–168.

Thompson JL and Kendrick GS (1964) Changes in the vertical dimensions of the human male skull during the third and fourth decades of life. Anat Rec 150, 209–213.

Tomlinson TH (1939) Oral pathology in monkeys in various experimental dietary deficiencies. U S Publ Health Rep 54, 1, 431–439.

Topping NH and Fraser HF (1939) Mouth lesions associated with dietary deficiencies in monkeys. U S Publ Health Rep 54, 416–431.

Touyz LZ (1984) Vitamin C, oral scurvy and periodontal disease. S Afr Med J, 65, 838–42.

Trowell H (1973) Dietary fibre, coronary heart disease and diabetes mellitus. I. Historical aspects of fibre in the food of western man. Plant Foods for Man 1, 11–16.

Turesky S and Glickman I (1954) Histochemical evaluation of gingival healing in experimental animals on adequate and vitamin C deficient rats. J Dent Res 33, 273–280.

Ulrich K (1962) Über Vorkommen und Ursachen von Parodontopathien bei jugendlichen Diabets mellitus. Dtsch Zahnarztl Z 17, 221–225.

Uhrbom E and Jacobson L (1984) Calcium and periodontitis: clinical effect of calcium medication. J Clin Periodontol, 11, 230–41.

van Wagenen G and Hurme VC (1950) Effects of testosterone propionate on permanent canine tooth eruption in the monkey. (Macaca mulatta). Proc Soc Exp Biol 73, 296–301.

Waerhaug J (1960) The role of ascorbic acid in periodontal tissue. J Dent Res 39, 1089 (abstract).

Waugh LM (1937) Dental observations among Eskimo. V11: Survey of mouth conditions, nutritional study, and gnathodynamometer data in most primitive and populous native village in Alaska. J Dent Res 16, 355–356 (abstract).

Waugh LM (1940) On the biting strength of Alaskan Eskimos. J Dent Res 19, 324–325 (abstract).

Weinmann JP and Schour I (1945a) Experimental studies in calcification. I. The effect of a rachitogenic diet on the dental tissues of the white rat. Am J Pathol 21, 821–831.

Weinmann JP and Schour I (1945b) Experimental studies in calcification. II. The effect of a rachitogenic diet on the alveolar bone of the white rat. Am J Pathol 21, 833–855.

Williams JB (1928) Diabetic periodontoclasia. J Am Dent Assoc 15, 523–529.

Wills DJ, Picton DCA and Davies WIR (1976) A study of the fluid systems of the periodontium in macaque monkeys. Arch Oral Biol 21, 175–185.

Wojcicki CJ, Harper DS and Robinson PJ (1987) Differences in periodontal disease-associated microorganisms of subgingival plaque in prepubertal, pubertal and postpubertal children. J Periodontol, 58, 219–223.

Wolbach SB (1953) Experimental scurvy: its employment for the study of intercellular substances. Proc Nutr Soc 12, 247–255.

Wolbach SB and Bessey OA (1942) Tissue changes in vitamin deficiencies. Physiol Rev 22, 233–2849.

Wolbach SB and Howe PR (1933) The incisor teeth of albino rats and guinea pigs in vitamin A deficiency and repair. Am J Pathol 9, 275–279.

Wolbach SB and Howe PR (1926) Intracellular substance in experimental scorbutus. Arch Pathol 1, 1–24.

Zipkin I, Bernick S and Menczel J (1965) A morphological study of the effect of fluoride on the periodontium of the hydrocortisone-treated rat. Periodontics 3, 111–114.

Ziskin DE and Nesse GJ (1946) Pregnancy gingivitis. Am J Orthodont Oral Surg 32, 390–432.

Ziskin DE, Salmon TN and Applebuam R (1940) The effect of thyroparathyroidectomy at birth and at 7 days on dental and skeletal development of rats. J Dent Res 19, 93–102.

Ziskin DE, Stein G, Gross P and Runne E (1947) Oral, gingival and periodontal pathology induced in rats on a low pantothenic acid diet by toxic doses of zinc carbonate. Am J Orthodont Oral Surg 33, 407–446.

Zubarev ON and Sharaev PN (1992) The effect of vicasol and pelentan on the biopolymers of the periodontium. Eksp Klin Farmakol 55, 60–61.

INDEX

Note: periodontal ligament is referred to as `PDL' throughout; page numbers in *italics* refer to figures and tables.